Campbell-Walsh UROLOGY

EDITORS

Louis R. Kavoussi, MD

Chairman
The Arthur Smith Institute for Urology
North Shore-Long Island Jewish Health System
Manhasset, New York
Professor of Urology
New York University School of Medicine
New York, New York

Andrew C. Novick, MD

Chairman
Glickman Urological Institute
Cleveland Clinic Foundation
Professor of Surgery
Cleveland Clinic Lerner College of Medicine of
Case Western Reserve University
Cleveland, Ohio

Alan W. Partin, MD, PhD

David Hall McConnell Professor and Director
James Buchanan Brady Urological Institute
Johns Hopkins Medical Institutions
Baltimore, Maryland

Craig A. Peters, MD

John E. Cole Professor of Urology
University of Virginia
Charlottesville, Virginia

Campbell-Walsh
UROLOGY

NINTH EDITION

EDITOR-IN-CHIEF

Alan J. Wein, MD, PhD(Hon)

Professor and Chair
Division of Urology
University of Pennsylvania School of Medicine
Chief of Urology
University of Pennsylvania Medical Center
Philadelphia, Pennsylvania

Volume 4

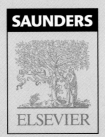

SAUNDERS

ELSEVIER

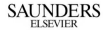

1600 John F. Kennedy Blvd.
Ste 1800
Philadelphia, PA 19103-2899

CAMPBELL-WALSH UROLOGY

ISBN 13: 978-0-7216-0798-6
ISBN 10: 0-7216-0798-5
E-dition ISBN 13: 978-1-4160-2966-3
ISBN 10: 1-4160-2966-4
International Edition ISBN 13: 978-0-8089-2353-4
ISBN 10: 0-8089-2353-6

Notice

Knowledge and best practice in this field are constantly changing. As new research and experience broaden
our knowledge, changes in practice, treatment, and drug therapy may become necessary or appropriate.
Readers are advised to check the most current information provided (i) on procedures featured or (ii) by
the manufacturer of each product to be administered, to verify the recommended dose or formula, the
method and duration of administration, and contraindications. It is the responsibility of the practitioner,
relying on his or her own experience and knowledge of the patient, to make diagnoses, to determine
dosages and the best treatment for each individual patient, and to take all appropriate safety precautions. To
the fullest extent of the law, neither the publisher nor the editors assume any liability for any injury and/or
damage to persons or property arising out of or related to any use of the material contained in this book.

Note that the term ESWL has been trademarked by Dornier MedTech in the United States. The generic
term for extracorporial shock wave lithotripsy is SWL. As the use of ESWL has become part of the
vernacular of urology, some of the authors have elected to use this term in their chapters.

The Publisher

Library of Congress Cataloging-in-Publication Data
Campbell-Walsh urology.—9th ed. / editor-in-chief, Alan J. Wein; editors, Louis R. Kavoussi . . . [et al.].
    p. ; cm.
    Rev. ed. of: Campbell's urology / editor-in-chief, Patrick C. Walsh; editors, Alan B. Retik . . . [et al.]. 8th
ed. ©2002.
    Includes bibliographical references and index.
    ISBN 0-7216-0798-5 (set)
        1. Urology.   I. Campbell, Meredith F. (Meredith Fairfax).   II. Wein, Alan J.   III. Kavoussi,
Louis R.   IV. Campbell's urology.   V. Title: Urology.
    [DNLM: 1. Urogenital Diseases.   2. Urology—methods. WJ 100 c192 2007]
    RC871.C33 2007
    616.6—dc22

                                                                          2006041807

Acquisitions Editor: Rebecca Schmidt Gaertner
Developmental Editor: Anne Snyder
Publishing Services Manager: Tina Rebane
Project Manager: Norm Stellander
Design Direction: Ellen Zanolle

Printed in China
Last digit is the print number: 9 8 7 6 5 4 3 2 1

To our families, our teachers, and our residents, all of whom have suffered our behavior in various ways and are responsible for our ability to do what we do.

CONTRIBUTORS

Paul Abrams, MD, FRCS
Professor of Urology,
Bristol Urological Institute,
Southmead Hospital,
Bristol, United Kingdom
Overactive Bladder

Mark C. Adams, MD
Professor, Division of Pediatric Urology,
Vanderbilt Children's Hospital,
Vanderbilt University Medical Center,
Nashville, Tennessee
Urinary Tract Reconstruction in Children

Mohamad E. Allaf, MD
Assistant Professor,
James Buchanan Brady Urological Institute,
Johns Hopkins Medical Institutions,
Baltimore, Maryland
Diagnosis and Staging of Prostate Cancer

J. Kyle Anderson, MD
Assistant Professor,
Department of Urologic Surgery,
Veterans Affairs Medical Center,
University of Minnesota Medical School,
Minneapolis, Minnesota
*Surgical Anatomy of the Retroperitoneum, Adrenals,
Kidneys, and Ureters*

Karl-Erik Andersson, MD, PhD
Professor, Lund University;
Head Physician, Clinical Chemistry and Pharmacology,
Lund University Hospital,
Lund, Sweden
*Pharmacologic Management of Storage and
Emptying Failure*

Kenneth W. Angermeier, MD
Associate Professor,
Prosthetic Surgery and Genitourethral Reconstruction,
Glickman Urological Institute,
Cleveland Clinic Foundation,
Cleveland, Ohio
Surgery of Penile and Urethral Carcinoma

Rodney A. Appell, MD
Professor, Scott Department of Urology,
Baylor College of Medicine;
F. Bantley Scott Chair in Urology,
St. Luke's Episcopal Hospital,
Houston, Texas
Injection Therapy for Urinary Incontinence

Dean G. Assimos, MD
Professor,
Division of Surgical Sciences,
Head, Section of Endourology and Nephrolithasis,
Department of Urology,
Wake Forest University School of Medicine,
Winston-Salem, North Carolina
Pathophysiology of Urinary Tract Obstruction

Anthony Atala, MD
W. Boyce Professor and Chair,
Department of Urology,
Wake Forest University School of Medicine;
Director, Wake Forest Institute for Regenerative Medicine,
Winston-Salem, North Carolina
*Tissue Engineering and Cell Therapy:
Perspectives for Urology*

Darius J. Bägli, MDCM, FRCSC, FAAP, FACS
Associate Professor of Surgery,
Institute of Medical Science,
University of Toronto;
Director of Urology Research,
Research Institute,
The Hospital for Sick Children,
Toronto, Ontario, Canada
Reflux and Megaureter

John M. Barry, MD
Professor of Surgery,
Head, Division of Urology and Renal Transplantation,
The Oregon Health & Science University School
    of Medicine;
Staff Surgeon, Doernbecher Children's Hospital,
Portland, Oregon
Renal Transplantation

Georg Bartsch, MD
Professor and Chairman,
Department of Urology,
Medical University of Innsbruck,
Innsbruck, Austria
Surgery of Testicular Tumors

Stuart B. Bauer, MD
Professor of Surgery (Urology),
Harvard Medical School;
Senior Associate in Urology,
Children's Hospital,
Boston, Massachusetts
*Anomalies of the Upper Urinary Tract
Voiding Dysfunction in Children: Non-Neurogenic and
Neurogenic*

Clair J. Beard, MD
Assistant Professor, Harvard Medical School;
Vice-Chair, Division of Radiation Oncology,
Dana-Farber Cancer Institute,
Brigham and Women's Hospital,
Boston, Massachusetts
Radiation Therapy for Prostate Cancer

Arie S. Belldegrun, MD, FACS
Professor of Urology,
Chief, Division of Urologic Oncology,
Roy and Carol Doumani Chair in Urologic Oncology,
David Geffen School of Medicine,
University of California, Los Angeles,
Los Angeles, California
Cryotherapy for Prostate Cancer

Mark F. Bellinger, MD
Professor of Urology,
Children's Hospital of Pittsburgh,
University of Pittsburgh Medical Center,
Pittsburgh, Pennsylvania
*Abnormalities of the Testes and Scrotum and
Their Surgical Management*

Mitchell C. Benson, MD
George F. Cahill Professor and Chairman,
J. Bently Squier Urological Clinic,
Columbia University Medical Center,
New York, New York
Cutaneous Continent Urinary Diversion

Sam B. Bhayani, MD
Assistant Professor of Surgery,
Department of Urology,
Washington University School of Medicine,
St. Louis, Missouri
Urinary Tract Imaging: Basic Principles

Jay T. Bishoff, MD
Associate Clinical Professor of Surgery,
University of Texas Health Science Center,
San Antonio, Texas;
Director,
Endourology Section,
Wilford Hall Medical Center,
Lackland AFB, Texas
Laparoscopic Surgery of the Kidney

Jerry G. Blaivas, MD
Clinical Professor of Urology,
Weill Medical College of Cornell University;
Attending,
New York-Presbyterian Hospital,
Lenox Hill Hospital,
New York, New York
*Urinary Incontinence: Epidemiology, Pathophysiology,
Evaluation, and Management Overview*

Jon D. Blumenfeld, MD
Associate Professor of Medicine,
Weill Medical College of Cornell University;
Director of Hypertension,
Director of The Susan R. Knafel Polycystic Kidney
    Disease Center,
The Rogosin Institute;
Associate Attending Physician,
New York-Presbyterian Hospital,
New York, New York
*Pathophysiology, Evaluation, and Medical Management
of Adrenal Disorders*

Michael L. Blute, MD
Professor of Urology,
Mayo Medical School;
Chairman, Department of Urology,
Mayo Clinic,
Rochester, Minnesota
Surgery of the Adrenal Glands

Joseph G. Borer, MD
Assistant Professor of Surgery,
Department of Urology,
Harvard Medical School;
Assistant in Urology,
Children's Hospital Boston,
Boston, Massachusetts
Hypospadias

George J. Bosl, MD
Chairman, Department of Medicine,
Patrick M. Byrne Chair in Clinical Oncology,
Memorial Sloan-Kettering Cancer Center,
New York, New York
Surgery of Testicular Tumors

Charles B. Brendler, MD
Professor and Chief, Section of Urology,
University of Chicago School of Medicine,
Chicago, Illinois
*Evaluation of the Urologic Patient: History, Physical
Examination, and Urinalysis*

Gregory A. Broderick, MD
Professor of Urology,
Mayo Medical School,
Mayo Clinic,
Jacksonville, Florida
*Evaluation and Nonsurgical Management of Erectile
Dysfunction and Premature Ejaculation*

James D. Brooks, MD
Associate Professor,
Department of Urology,
Stanford University Medical Center,
Stanford, California
Anatomy of the Lower Urinary Tract and Male Genitalia

Ronald M. Bukowski, MD
Professor of Medicine,
Cleveland Clinic Lerner College of Medicine of
    Case Western Reserve University;
Director, Experimental Therapeutics,
Cleveland Clinic Foundation,
Cleveland, Ohio
    Renal Tumors

Arthur L. Burnett, MD
Professor of Urology, Cellular and Molecular Biology,
Johns Hopkins University School of Medicine;
Staff Urologist, The Johns Hopkins Hospital,
Baltimore, Maryland
    Priapism

Jeffrey A. Cadeddu, MD
Associate Professor,
Clinical Center for Minimally Invasive Urologic
    Cancer Treatment;
Department of Urology,
University of Texas Southwestern Medical Center,
Dallas, Texas
    *Surgical Anatomy of the Retroperitoneum, Adrenals,
    Kidneys, and Ureters*

Anthony A. Caldamone, MD, MMS, FAAP, FACS
Professor of Surgery and Pediatrics,
Department of Urology,
Brown University School of Medicine;
Head of Pediatric Urology,
Hasbro Children's Hospital,
Providence, Rhode Island
    Prune Belly Syndrome

Steven C. Campbell, MD, PhD
Professor of Surgery,
Cleveland Clinic Lerner College of Medicine of
    Case Western Reserve University;
Section of Urological Oncology,
Glickman Urological Institute,
Cleveland Clinic Foundation,
Cleveland, Ohio
    Renal Tumors
    Non–Muscle-Invasive Bladder Cancer (Ta, T1, and CIS)

Douglas A. Canning, MD
Professor of Urology,
University of Pennsylvania School of Medicine;
Director, Division of Urology,
Children's Hospital of Philadelphia,
Philadelphia, Pennsylvania
    Evaluation of the Pediatric Urology Patient

Michael Carducci, MD
Associate Professor of Oncology and Urology,
Johns Hopkins University School of Medicine;
Staff Physician, The Sidney Kimmel Comprehensive Cancer
    Center at Johns Hopkins,
Baltimore, Maryland
    Treatment of Hormone-Refractory Prostate Cancer

Michael C. Carr, MD, PhD
Associate Professor of Surgery in Urology,
University of Pennsylvania School of Medicine;
Attending Surgeon, Pediatric Urology,
Children's Hospital of Philadelphia,
Philadelphia, Pennsylvania
    *Anomalies and Surgery of the Ureteropelvic Junction in
    Children*

Peter R. Carroll, MD
Professor and Chair,
Department of Urology,
University of California, San Francisco, School of Medicine;
Surgeon in Chief, Comprehensive Cancer Center,
University of California, San Francisco, Cancer Center,
San Francisco, California
    Treatment of Locally Advanced Prostate Cancer

H. Ballentine Carter, MD
Professor of Urology and Oncology,
James Buchanan Brady Urological Institute,
Johns Hopkins Medical Institutions,
Baltimore, Maryland
    Basic Instrumentation and Cystoscopy
    Diagnosis and Staging of Prostate Cancer

Anthony J. Casale, MD
Professor and Chairman,
Department of Urology,
University of Louisville;
Chief of Urology,
Kosair Children's Hospital,
Louisville, Kentucky
    Posterior Urethral Valves and Other Urethral Anomalies

William J. Catalona, MD
Professor of Urology,
Feinberg School of Medicine,
Northwestern University;
Director, Clinical Prostate Cancer Program,
Robert H. Lurie Comprehensive Cancer Center,
Northwestern Memorial Hospital,
Chicago, Illinois
    *Definitive Therapy for Localized Prostate Cancer—
    An Overview*

David Y. Chan, MD
Assistant Professor of Urology and Pathology,
Director of Outpatient Urology,
James Buchanan Brady Urological Institute,
Johns Hopkins Medical Institutions,
Baltimore, Maryland
    Basic Instrumentation and Cystoscopy

Michael B. Chancellor, MD
Professor of Urology,
McGowan Institute of Regenerative Medicine,
University of Pittsburgh School of Medicine,
Pittsburgh, Pennsylvania
    Physiology and Pharmacology of the Bladder and Urethra

C. R. Chapple, BSc, MD, FRCS (Urol)
Professor of Urology (Hon),
Sheffield Hallam University;
Consultant Urological Surgeon,
Royal Hallamshire Hospital,
Sheffield, United Kingdom
  *Retropubic Suspension Surgery for Incontinence
  in Women*

Robert L. Chevalier, MD
Benjamin Armistead Shepherd Professor and Chair,
Department of Pediatrics,
University of Virginia;
Pediatrician-In-Chief,
University of Virginia Medical School,
Charlottesville, Virginia
  *Renal Function in the Fetus, Neonate, and Child
  Congenital Urinary Obstruction: Pathophysiology*

Ben H. Chew, MD, MSc, FRCSC
Assistant Professor of Urology,
University of British Columbia,
Vancouver, British Columbia, Canada
  Ureteroscopy and Retrograde Ureteral Access

George K. Chow, MD
Assistant Professor,
Department of Urology,
The Mayo Clinic,
Rochester, Minnesota
  Surgery of the Adrenal Glands

Ralph V. Clayman, MD
Professor of Urology,
University of California, Irvine, Medical Center;
Chair of the Department of Urology,
University of California, Irvine, School of Medicine,
Orange, California
  Basics of Laparoscopic Urologic Surgery

Craig V. Comiter, MD
Associate Professor of Surgery/Urology,
Instructor of Obstetrics and Gynecology,
University of Arizona;
Chief, Section of Urology,
Director, Urology Residency,
University of Arizona Health Sciences Center,
Tucson, Arizona
  *Surgical Treatment of Male Sphincteric Urinary
  Incontinence: The Male Perineal Sling and Artificial
  Urinary Sphincter*

Michael J. Conlin, MD
Associate Professor of Surgery,
Director, Minimally Invasive Urologic Surgery,
Division of Urology and Renal Transplantation,
The Oregon Health & Science University School
  of Medicine,
Portland, Oregon
  Renal Transplantation

Juanita Crook, MD
Associate Professor of Radiation Oncology,
University of Toronto;
Radiation Oncologist,
University Health Network,
Princess Margaret Hospital,
Toronto, Ontario, Canada
  Radiation Therapy for Prostate Cancer

Douglas M. Dahl, MD
Assistant Professor of Surgery,
Department of Urology,
Harvard Medical School;
Assistant in Urology,
Massachusetts General Hospital,
Boston, Massachusetts
  Use of Intestinal Segments in Urinary Diversion

Anthony V. D'Amico, MD, PhD
Professor of Radiation Oncology,
Harvard Medical School;
Professor and Chief of Genitourinary Radiation Oncology,
Dana-Farber Cancer Institute,
Brigham and Women's Hospital,
Boston, Massachusetts
  Radiation Therapy for Prostate Cancer

John W. Davis, MD
Assistant Professor of Urology,
University of Texas MD Anderson Cancer Center,
Houston, Texas
  Tumors of the Penis

John D. Denstedt, MD, FRCSC
Professor of Urology,
Chairman, Department of Surgery,
Schulich School of Medicine and Dentistry,
The University of Western Ontario,
London, Ontario, Canada
  Ureteroscopy and Retrograde Ureteral Access

Theodore L. DeWeese, MD, PhD
Professor of Oncology,
Johns Hopkins University School of Medicine;
Radiation Oncologist-in-Chief,
Department of Radiation Oncology and Molecular
  Radiation Science,
Johns Hopkins Medical Institutions,
Baltimore, Maryland
  Radiation Therapy for Prostate Cancer

David A. Diamond, MD
Associate Professor of Surgery,
Department of Urology,
Harvard Medical School;
Associate in Urology,
Children's Hospital,
Boston, Massachusetts
  Sexual Differentiation: Normal and Abnormal

Roger R. Dmochowski, MD, FACS
Professor,
Department of Urologic Surgery,
Vanderbilt University Medical Center,
Nashville, Tennessee
Tension-Free Vaginal Tape Procedures

Steven G. Docimo, MD
Professor of Urology,
Vice Chairman of Urology,
University of Pittsburgh School of Medicine;
Director of Urology,
Division of Pediatric Urology,
Children's Hospital of Pittsburgh,
Pittsburgh, Pennsylvania
Pediatric Endourology and Laparoscopy

Marcus Drake, DM, MA
Consultant Urological Surgeon,
Bristol Urological Institute,
Southmead Hospital,
Bristol, United Kingdom
Overactive Bladder

James A. Eastham, MD
Associate Professor,
Department of Urology,
Memorial Sloan-Kettering Cancer Center,
New York, New York
Expectant Management of Prostate Cancer

Louis Eichel, MD
Clinical Associate Professor of Urology,
University of Rochester School of
    Medicine and Dentistry;
Director of Minimally Invasive Surgery,
Center for Urology,
Rochester, New York
Basics of Laparoscopic Urologic Surgery

Mario A. Eisenberger, MD
R. Dale Hughes Professor of Oncology and Urology,
The Sidney Kimmel Comprehensive Cancer Center at
    Johns Hopkins,
Johns Hopkins University School of Medicine,
Baltimore, Maryland
Treatment of Hormone-Refractory Prostate Cancer

Alaa El-Ghoneimi, MD, PhD
Professor of Pediatric Surgery,
University of Paris;
Senior Surgeon,
Hospital Robert Debré,
Paris, France
*Anomalies and Surgery of the Ureteropelvic Junction
in Children*

Jack S. Elder, MD
Professor and Vice Chairman,
Department of Urology,
Case Western Reserve University School of Medicine;
Division of Pediatric Urology,
Children's Hospital,
Cleveland, Ohio
*Abnormalities of the Genitalia in Boys and
Their Surgical Management*

Jonathan I. Epstein, MD
Professor of Pathology, Urology, and Oncology,
The Reinhard Professor of Urologic Pathology,
Johns Hopkins University School of Medicine;
Director of Surgical Pathology,
Johns Hopkins Medical Institutions,
Baltimore, Maryland
Pathology of Prostatic Neoplasia

Andrew P. Evan, PhD
Chancellor's Professor,
Department of Anatomy and Cell Biology,
Indiana University School of Medicine,
Indianapolis, Indiana
Surgical Management of Upper Urinary Tract Calculi

Robert L. Fairchild, PhD
Professor of Pathology,
Case Western Reserve University School of Medicine;
Staff, Department of Immunology,
Cleveland Clinic Foundation,
Cleveland, Ohio
Basic Principles of Immunology

Amr Fergany, MD, MB, BCh
Staff, Section of Urologic Oncology,
Section of Laparoscopic Surgery and Robotics,
Glickman Urological Institute,
Cleveland Clinic Foundation,
Cleveland, Ohio
Renovascular Hypertension and Ischemic Nephropathy

James H. Finke, PhD
Professor of Molecular Medicine,
Cleveland Clinic Lerner College of Medicine of
    Case Western Reserve University;
Staff, Department of Immunology,
Cleveland Clinic Foundation,
Cleveland, Ohio
Basic Principles of Immunology

John M. Fitzpatrick, MCh, FRCSI, FRCS(Glas), FRCS
Professor and Chairman,
Department of Surgery,
University College, Dublin;
Professor of Surgery and Consultant Urologist,
Mater Misericordiae University Hospital,
Dublin, Ireland
*Minimally Invasive and Endoscopic Management
of Benign Prostatic Hyperplasia*

Robert C. Flanigan, MD
Albert J. Jr. and Claire R. Speh Professor and Chair,
Department of Urology,
Stritch School of Medicine,
Loyola University;
Chair of the Department of Urology,
Loyola University Medical Center,
Maywood, Illinois
Urothelial Tumors of the Upper Urinary Tract

Stuart M. Flechner, MD
Professor of Urology,
Cleveland Clinic Lerner College of Medicine of
    Case Western Reserve University;
Director of Clinical Research,
Section of Renal Transplantation,
Glickman Urological Institute,
Cleveland Clinic Foundation,
Cleveland, Ohio
Basic Principles of Immunology

Tara Frenkl, MD, MPH
Assistant Professor of Urology,
Director, Female Urology and Reconstructive Surgery,
Robert Wood Johnson Medical School,
The University of Medicine and Dentistry of New Jersey,
New Brunswick, New Jersey
Sexually Transmitted Diseases

Dominic Frimberger, MD
Assistant Professor of Urology,
University of Oklahoma Health Sciences Center;
Pediatric Urologist,
Children's Hospital of Oklahoma,
Oklahoma City, Oklahoma
Bladder Anomalies in Children

John P. Gearhart, MD
Professor of Pediatric Urology,
Johns Hopkins University School of Medicine;
Chief of Pediatric Urology,
The Johns Hopkins Hospital,
Baltimore, Maryland
Exstrophy-Epispadias Complex

Glenn S. Gerber, MD
Associate Professor,
Department of Surgery (Urology),
University of Chicago School of Medicine,
Chicago, Illinois
*Evaluation of the Urologic Patient: History, Physical
Examination, and Urinalysis*

Inderbir S. Gill, MD, MCh
Professor of Surgery,
Head, Section of Laparoscopic and Robotic Urology,
Glickman Urological Institute,
Cleveland Clinic Foundation,
Cleveland, Ohio
Laparoscopic Surgery of the Urinary Bladder

Kenneth I. Glassberg, MD
Professor of Urology,
Columbia University College of Physicians and Surgeons;
Director, Division of Pediatric Urology,
Morgan Stanley Children's Hospital of
    New York-Presbyterian,
New York, New York
Renal Dysgenesis and Cystic Disease of the Kidney

David A. Goldfarb, MD
Head, Section of Renal Transplantation,
Glickman Urological Institute,
Cleveland Clinic Foundation,
Cleveland, Ohio
Etiology, Pathogenesis, and Management of Renal Failure

Irwin Goldstein, MD
Editor-In-Chief,
The Journal of Sexual Medicine,
Milton, Massachusetts
*Urologic Management of Women With
Sexual Health Concerns*

Marc Goldstein, MD, FACS
Professor of Urology and Reproductive Medicine,
Surgeon-In-Chief, Male Reproductive Medicine and Surgery,
Executive Director, Men's Service Center,
Cornell Institute for Reproductive Medicine,
Weill Medical College of Cornell University;
Senior Scientist, Center for Biomedical Research,
The Population Council,
New York, New York
*Male Reproductive Physiology
Surgery of the Scrotum and Seminal Vesicles*

Leonard G. Gomella, MD
Professor and Chairman,
Department of Urology,
Jefferson Medical College;
Director,
Jefferson Prostate Diagnostic Center,
Kimmel Cancer Center,
Thomas Jefferson University Hospital,
Philadelphia, Pennsylvania
Ultrasonography and Biopsy of the Prostate

Mark L. Gonzalgo, MD, PhD
Associate Professor of Urology and Oncology,
Johns Hopkins Medical Center,
Baltimore, Maryland
Management of Invasive and Metastatic Bladder Cancer

Richard W. Grady, MD
Associate Professor of Urology,
The University of Washington School of Medicine;
Director, Clinical Research,
Children's Hospital & Regional Medical Center,
Seattle, Washington
*Surgical Techniques for One-Stage Reconstruction of
the Exstrophy-Epispadias Complex*

Matthew B. Gretzer, MD
Assistant Professor of Clinical Surgery,
Department of Surgery/Urology,
University of Arizona Health Science Center,
Tucson, Arizona
  Prostate Cancer Tumor Markers

Mantu Gupta, MD
Associate Professor,
Columbia University College of Physicians and Surgeons;
Director of Endourology, and Director of
  Kidney Stone Center,
Columbia University Medical Center New York-
  Presbyterian Hospital,
New York, New York
  Percutaneous Management of the Upper Urinary Tract

Ethan J. Halpern, MD
Professor of Radiology and Urology,
Jefferson Prostate Diagnostic Center,
Thomas Jefferson University,
Philadelphia, Pennsylvania
  Ultrasonography and Biopsy of the Prostate

Misop Han, MD, MS
Assistant Professor,
Department of Urology,
James Buchanan Brady Urological Institute,
Johns Hopkins Medical Institutions,
Baltimore, Maryland
  *Retropubic and Suprapubic Open Prostatectomy
  Definitive Therapy for Localized Prostate Cancer—
  An Overview*

Philip M. Hanno, MD, MPH
Professor of Urology,
University of Pennsylvania School of Medicine;
Medical Director, Department of Clinical Effectiveness
  and Quality Improvement,
University of Pennsylvania Health System,
Philadelphia, Pennsylvania
  *Painful Bladder Syndrome/Interstitial Cystitis and
  Related Disorders*

Matthew P. Hardy, PhD
Professor, Department of Urology,
Weill Medical College of Cornell University;
Member, Population Council,
The Rockefeller University,
New York, New York
  Male Reproductive Physiology

David M. Hartke, MD
Resident Physician,
Department of Urology,
University Hospitals of Cleveland;
Case Western Reserve University School of Medicine,
Cleveland, Ohio
  Radical Perineal Prostatectomy

Jeremy P. W. Heaton, MD, FRCSC, FACS
Professor of Urology,
Assistant Professor Pharmacology and Toxicology,
Queen's University,
Kingston, Ontario, Canada
  Androgen Deficiency in the Aging Male

Sender Herschorn, BSc, MDCM, FRCSC
Professor and Chairman, Division of Urology,
Martin Barkin Chair in Urological Research,
University of Toronto;
Attending Urologist,
Director, Urodynamics Unit,
Sunnybrook Health Sciences Centre,
Toronto, Ontario, Canada
  *Vaginal Reconstructive Surgery for Sphincteric
  Incontinence and Prolapse*

Khai-Linh V. Ho, MD
Endourology Fellow,
Mayo Clinic,
Rochester, Minnesota
  Lower Urinary Tract Calculi

Thomas H. S. Hsu, MD
Assistant Professor of Urology,
Director of Laparoscopic and Minimally
  Invasive Surgery,
Department of Urology, Stanford University
  School of Medicine;
Director of Laparoscopic, Robotic, and Minimally
  Invasive Urologic Surgery,
Stanford University Medical Center,
Stanford, California
  Management of Upper Urinary Tract Obstruction

Mark Hurwitz, MD
Assistant Professor,
Harvard Medical School;
Director, Regional Program Development,
Department of Radiation Oncology,
Dana-Farber/Brigham and Women's Cancer Center,
Boston, Massachusetts
  Radiation Therapy for Prostate Cancer

Douglas Husmann, MD
Professor of Urology,
Vice Chairman,
Department of Urology,
Mayo Clinic,
Rochester, Minnesota
  Pediatric Genitourinary Trauma

Jonathan P. Jarow, MD
Professor of Urology,
James Buchanan Brady Urological Institute,
Johns Hopkins Medical Institutions,
Baltimore, Maryland
  Male Infertility

Thomas W. Jarrett, MD
Professor of Urology,
Chairman, Department of Urology,
George Washington University,
Washington, DC
  Management of Urothelial Tumors of the Renal Pelvis

Christopher W. Johnson, MD
Clinical Instructor of Urology,
Weill Medical College of Cornell University,
New York, New York;
Assistant Attending,
North Shore-Long Island Jewish Health System,
Manhasset, and St. Francis Hospital, Roslyn, New York
  *Tuberculosis and Parasitic and Fungal Infections of
  the Genitourinary System*

Warren D. Johnson, Jr., MD
B. H. Kean Professor of Tropical Medicine,
Chief, Division of Internal Medicine and Infectious Diseases,
Weill Medical College of Cornell University;
Attending Physician,
New York-Presbyterian Hospital, Cornell Campus,
New York, New York
  *Tuberculosis and Parasitic and Fungal Infections of
  the Genitourinary System*

Deborah P. Jones, MD
Associate Professor of Pediatrics,
University of Tennessee Health Science Center;
Attending, Le Bonheur Children's Medical Center,
Children's Foundation Research Center,
Memphis, Tennessee
  Renal Disease in Childhood

J. Stephen Jones, MD, FACS
Associate Professor of Surgery (Urology),
Vice Chairman, Glickman Urological Institute,
Cleveland Clinic Lerner College of Medicine of
  Case Western Reserve University,
Cleveland Clinic Foundation,
Cleveland, Ohio
  Non–Muscle-Invasive Bladder Cancer (Ta, T1, and CIS)

Gerald H. Jordan, MD, FACS, FAAP
Professor of Urology,
Eastern Virginia Medical School,
Norfolk, Virgina
  Peyronie's Disease
  Surgery of the Penis and Urethra

Mark L. Jordan, MD
Harris L. Willits Professor and Chief,
Division of Urology,
University of Medicine and Dentistry of New Jersey,
New Jersey Medical School;
Chief of Urology, University Hospital,
Newark, New Jersey
  Renal Transplantation

David B. Joseph, MD
Professor of Surgery,
University of Alabama at Birmingham;
Chief of Pediatric Urology,
The Children's Hospital of Alabama,
Birmingham, Alabama
  Urinary Tract Reconstruction in Children

John N. Kabalin, MD
Adjunct Assistant Professor of Surgery,
Section of Urologic Surgery,
University of Nebraska College of Medicine,
Omaha, Nebraska;
Regional West Medical Center,
Scottsbluff, Nebraska
  *Surgical Anatomy of the Retroperitoneum, Adrenals,
  Kidneys, and Ureters*

Martin Kaefer, MD
Associate Professor, Indiana University,
Riley Hospital for Children,
Indianapolis, Indiana
  *Surgical Management of Intersexuality, Cloacal
  Malformation, and Other Abnormalities of the
  Genitalia in Girls*

Irving Kaplan, MD
Assistant Professor of Radiation Oncology,
Harvard Medical School;
Radiation Oncologist,
Beth Israel Deaconess Medical Center,
Boston, Massachusetts
  Radiation Therapy for Prostate Cancer

Louis R. Kavoussi, MD
Chairman, The Arthur Smith Institute for Urology,
North Shore-Long Island Jewish Health System,
Manhasset, New York;
Professor of Urology,
New York University School of Medicine,
New York, New York
  Laparoscopic Surgery of the Kidney

Mohit Khera, MD, MBA, MPH
Fellow, Division of Male Reproductive Medicine
  and Surgery,
Scott Department of Urology,
Baylor College of Medicine,
Houston, Texas
  Surgical Management of Male Infertility

Antoine Khoury, MD, FRCSC, FAAP
Chief of Urology,
Senior Associate Scientist,
The Hospital for Sick Children;
Professor of Surgery,
The University of Toronto,
Toronto, Ontario, Canada
  Reflux and Megaureter

Adam S. Kibel, MD
Associate Professor, Division of Urologic Surgery,
Washington University School of Medicine,
St. Louis, Missouri
Molecular Genetics and Cancer Biology

Roger Kirby, MD, FRCS
Professor and Director, The Prostate Centre;
Visiting Professor, St. George's Hospital,
Institute of Urology,
London, United Kingdom
*Evaluation and Nonsurgical Management of Benign
Prostatic Hyperplasia*

Eric A. Klein, MD
Professor of Surgery,
Cleveland Clinic Lerner College of Medicine of
    Case Western Reserve University;
Head, Section of Urologic Oncology,
Glickman Urological Institute,
Cleveland Clinic Foundation,
Cleveland, Ohio
Epidemiology, Etiology, and Prevention of Prostate Cancer

John N. Krieger, MD
Professor of Urology,
University of Washington School of Medicine;
Chief of Surgical Urology,
VA Puget Sound Health Care System,
Seattle, Washington
Urological Implications of AIDS and HIV Infection

Bradley P. Kropp, MD
Professor of Urology,
University of Oklahoma Health Science Center;
Chief, Pediatric Urology,
Children's Hospital of Oklahoma,
Oklahoma City, Oklahoma
Bladder Anomalies in Children

John S. Lam, MD
Clinical Instructor in Urology,
David Geffen School of Medicine,
University of California, Los Angeles;
Attending Urologist,
University of California, Los Angeles, Medical Center,
Los Angeles, California
Cryotherapy for Prostate Cancer

Herbert Lepor, MD
Professor and Martin Spatz Chair,
Department of Urology,
New York University School of Medicine;
Chief of Urology,
New York University Medical Center,
New York, New York
*Evaluation and Nonsurgical Management of Benign
Prostatic Hyperplasia*

Ronald W. Lewis, MD
Witherington Chair in Urology,
Professor of Surgery (Urology) and Physiology,
    and Chief of Urology,
Medical College of Georgia,
Augusta, Georgia
Vascular Surgery for Erectile Dysfunction

James E. Lingeman, MD
Director of Research,
Methodist Hospital Institute for Kidney Stone Disease;
Volunteer Clinical Professor,
Department of Urology,
Indiana University School of Medicine,
Indianapolis, Indiana
Surgical Management of Upper Urinary Tract Calculi

Richard E. Link, MD, PhD
Associate Professor of Urology,
Director, Division of Endourology and Minimally
    Invasive Surgery,
Scott Department of Urology,
Baylor College of Medicine,
Houston, Texas
Cutaneous Diseases of the External Genitalia

Larry I. Lipshultz, MD
Professor of Urology,
Scott Department of Urology,
Lester and Sue Smith Chair in Reproductive Medicine,
Chief, Division of Male Reproductive Medicine
    and Surgery,
Baylor College of Medicine,
Houston, Texas
Surgical Management of Male Infertility

Mark S. Litwin, MD, MPH
Professor of Urology and Health Services,
David Geffen School of Medicine,
University of California, Los Angeles;
University of California, Los Angeles, School of
    Public Health,
Los Angeles, California
Outcomes Research

Yair Lotan, MD
Assistant Professor,
Department of Urology,
University of Texas Southwestern Medical Center;
Attending,
Parkland Health and Hospital Systems,
Zale Lipshy University Medical Center,
Veterans Affairs Medical Center,
Dallas, Texas
*Urinary Lithiasis: Etiology, Epidemiology,
and Pathogenesis*

Tom F. Lue, MD
Professor and Vice Chair,
Emil Tanagho Endowed Chair,
Department of Urology,
University of California School of Medicine, San Francisco,
San Francisco, California
*Physiology of Penile Erection and Pathophysiology of
Erectile Dysfunction*
*Evaluation and Nonsurgical Management of
Erectile Dysfunction and Premature Ejaculation*

Donald F. Lynch, Jr., MD
Professor and Chairman,
Department of Urology,
Professor of Obstetrics and Gynecology,
Eastern Virginia School of Medicine;
Urologic Oncologist,
Sentara Hospitals;
Consultant Urologist,
Jones Institute for Reproductive Medicine,
Norfolk, Virginia
Tumors of the Penis

Michael Marberger, MD, FRCS(Ed)
Professor and Chairman,
Department of Urology,
Medical University of Vienna,
Vienna, Austria
Ablative Therapy of Renal Tumors

Fray F. Marshall, MD
Professor and Chairman,
Department of Urology,
Emory University School of Medicine,
Atlanta, Georgia
Surgery of Bladder Cancer

Brian R. Matlaga, MD, MPH
Assistant Professor of Urology,
Johns Hopkins University School of Medicine;
Director of Stone Disease,
Johns Hopkins Bayview Medical Center,
Baltimore, Maryland
Surgical Management of Upper Urinary Tract Calculi

Ranjiv Mathews, MD
Associate Professor of Pediatric Urology,
James Buchanan Brady Urological Institute,
Johns Hopkins Medical Institutions,
Baltimore, Maryland
Exstrophy-Epispadias Complex

Julian Mauermann, MD
Senior Resident,
Department of Urology,
Medical University of Vienna,
Vienna, Austria
Ablative Therapy of Renal Tumors

Sarah J. McAleer, MD
Chief Resident, Department of Urology,
Brigham and Women's Hospital,
Boston, Massachusetts
*Tuberculosis and Parasitic and Fungal Infections of the
Genitourinary System*

Jack W. McAninch, MD
Professor of Urological Surgery,
Department of Urology,
University of California, San Francisco, School of Medicine;
Chief of Urology, San Francisco General Hospital,
San Francisco, California
Renal and Ureteral Trauma

John D. McConnell, MD
Professor of Urology, Department of Urology,
Executive Vice-President for Health Systems Affairs,
University of Texas Southwestern Medical Center,
Dallas, Texas
*Benign Prostatic Hyperplasia: Etiology, Pathophysiology,
Epidemiology, and Natural History*

W. Scott McDougal, AB, MD, MA(Hon)
Walter S. Kerr, Jr. Professor of Urology,
Harvard Medical School;
Chief of Urology, Massachusetts General Hospital,
Boston, Massachusetts
Use of Intestinal Segments in Urinary Diversion

Elspeth M. McDougall, MD, FRCSC
Professor of Urology,
Irvine Medical Center,
University of California, Irvine,
Irvine, California
Basics of Laparoscopic Urologic Surgery
Percutaneous Management of the Upper Urinary Tract

Edward J. McGuire, MD
Professor, Department of Urology,
University of Michigan,
Ann Arbor, Michigan
Pubovaginal Sling

James M. McKiernan, MD
Assistant Professor, Department of Urology,
Herbert Irving Comprehensive Cancer Center,
Columbia University;
Assistant Attending Urologist,
New York-Presbyterian Hospital,
New York, New York
Cutaneous Continent Urinary Diversion

Alan W. McMahon, MD
Associate Professor, Department of Medicine,
Division of Nephrology and Transplant Immunology,
University of Alberta,
Edmonton, Alberta, Canada
Renal Physiology and Pathophysiology

Maxwell V. Meng, MD
Assistant Professor,
Department of Urology,
University of California, San Francisco,
San Francisco, California
   Treatment of Locally Advanced Prostate Cancer

Edward M. Messing, MD
W. W. Scott Professor,
Chairman, Department of Urology,
Professor of Pathology and Oncology,
University of Rochester School of Medicine and Dentistry,
Rochester, New York
   Urothelial Tumors of the Bladder

Michael E. Mitchell, MD
Professor and Chief of Pediatric Urology,
University of Washington School of Medicine,
Children's Hospital & Regional Medical Center,
Seattle, Washington
   *Surgical Techniques for One-Stage Reconstruction of the
   Exstrophy-Epispadias Complex*

Drogo K. Montague, MD
Professor of Surgery,
Cleveland Clinic Lerner College of Medicine of
   Case Western Reserve University;
Head, Section of Prosthetic Surgery and
   Genitourethral Reconstruction,
Glickman Urological Institute,
Cleveland Clinic Foundation,
Cleveland, Ohio
   Prosthetic Surgery for Erectile Dysfunction

Alvaro Morales, MD, FRCSC, FACS
Emeritus Professor,
Queen's University;
Director, Center for Advanced Urological Research,
Kingston General Hospital,
Kingston, Ontario, Canada
   Androgen Deficiency in the Aging Male

Allen F. Morey, MD
Clinical Associate Professor of Urology,
University of Texas Health Science Center;
Chief, Urology Service,
Brooke Army Medical Center,
San Antonio, Texas
   Genital and Lower Urinary Tract Trauma

John Morley, MB, BCh
Dammert Professor of Gerontology,
   and Director of Geriatrics, St. Louis University Medical
   Center;
Director of GRECC, St. Louis Veterans Affairs Hospital,
   St. Louis, Missouri
   Androgen Deficiency in the Aging Male

Michael J. Morris, MD
Assistant Member,
Memorial Sloan-Kettering Cancer Center;
Instructor in Medicine,
Weill Medical College of Cornell University;
Assistant Attending Physician,
Memorial Hospital for Cancer and Allied Diseases,
New York, New York
   *The Clinical State of the Rising PSA Level after Definitive
   Local Therapy: A Practical Approach*

M. Louis Moy, MD
Assistant Professor,
Division of Urology,
University of Pennsylvania Medical School;
University of Pennsylvania Health System,
Philadelphia, Pennsylvania
   Additional Therapies for Storage and Emptying Failure

Ricardo Munarriz, MD
Assistant Professor of Urology,
Boston University School of Medicine,
Boston, Massachusetts
   Vascular Surgery for Erectile Dysfunction

Stephen Y. Nakada, MD
Professor of Surgery,
University of Wisconsin School of Medicine and
   Public Health;
Chairman of Urology,
University of Wisconsin Hospital and Clinics,
Madison, Wisconsin
   Management of Upper Urinary Tract Obstruction

Joseph V. Nally, Jr., MD
Staff, Department of Nephrology and Hypertension,
Cleveland Clinic Foundation,
Cleveland, Ohio
   Etiology, Pathogenesis, and Management of Renal Failure

Joel B. Nelson, MD
Frederic N. Schwentker Professor,
Chair, Department of Urology,
University of Pittsburgh School of Medicine;
Chairman of Urology,
University of Pittsburgh Medical Center;
Co-Chair, Prostate and Urological Diseases Program,
University of Pittsburgh Cancer Institute,
Pittsburgh, Pennsylvania
   Hormone Therapy for Prostate Cancer

Michael T. Nguyen, MD
Fellow, Pediatric Urology,
The Children's Hospital of Philadelphia,
Philadelphia, Pennsylvania
   Evaluation of the Pediatric Urology Patient

J. Curtis Nickel, MD
Professor of Urology, Queen's University;
Staff Urologist, Department of Urology,
Kingston General Hospital,
Kingston, Ontario, Canada
  *Inflammatory Conditions of the Male Genitourinary
  Tract: Prostatitis and Related Conditions, Orchitis,
  and Epididymitis*

Peter T. Nieh, MD
Assistant Professor, Department of Urology,
Emory University School of Medicine,
Atlanta, Georgia
  Surgery of Bladder Cancer

Victor W. Nitti, MD
Associate Professor and Vice-Chairman,
Department of Urology,
New York University School of Medicine;
Attending Physician,
New York University Hospitals Center,
New York, New York
  *Urinary Incontinence: Epidemiology, Pathophysiology,
  Evaluation, and Management Overview*

H. Norman Noe, MD
Professor of Urology,
Chief, Pediatric Urology,
University of Tennessee,
Saint Jude's Children's Research Hospital,
Memphis, Tennessee
  Renal Disease in Childhood

Andrew C. Novick, MD
Chairman, Glickman Urological Institute,
Cleveland Clinic Foundation;
Professor of Surgery,
Cleveland Clinic Lerner College of Medicine of
  Case Western Reserve University,
Cleveland, Ohio
  *Renovascular Hypertension and Ischemic Nephropathy
  Renal Tumors
  Open Surgery of the Kidney*

Seung-June Oh, MD, PhD
Associate Professor, Department of Urology,
Seoul National University Hospital,
Seoul National University College of Medicine,
Seoul, Korea
  Pubovaginal Sling

Carl A. Olsson, MD
John K. Lattimer Professor and Chairman Emeritus,
Columbia University College of Physicians and Surgeons;
Attending, New York-Presbyterian Hospital,
New York, New York
  Cutaneous Continent Urinary Diversion

Michael C. Ost, MD
Fellow, Endourology and Laparoscopy,
Institute of Urology,
North Shore-Long Island Jewish Medical Center,
New Hyde Park, New York
  Percutaneous Management of the Upper Urinary Tract

Vernon M. Pais Jr., MD
Assistant Professor,
Department of Surgery,
Division of Urology,
University of Kentucky School of Medicine;
University of Kentucky Medical Center,
Lexington, Kentucky
  Pathophysiology of Urinary Tract Obstruction

John M. Park, MD
Associate Professor of Urology,
University of Michigan Medical School;
Chief of Pediatric Urology,
University of Michigan Health System,
Ann Arbor, Michigan
  Normal Development of the Urogenital System

Alan W. Partin, MD, PhD
David Hall McConnell Professor and Director,
James Buchanan Brady Urological Institute,
Johns Hopkins Medical Institutions,
Baltimore, Maryland
  *Retropubic and Suprapubic Open Prostatectomy
  Prostate Cancer Tumor Markers
  Diagnosis and Staging of Prostate Cancer
  Anatomic Radical Retropubic Prostatectomy*

Christopher K. Payne, MD
Associate Professor of Urology,
Director,
Female Urology and Neurourology,
Stanford University Medical School,
Stanford, California
  *Conservative Managment of Urinary Incontinence:
  Behavioral and Pelvic Floor Therapy, Urethral and
  Pelvic Devices*

Margaret S. Pearle, MD, PhD
Professor of Urology and Internal Medicine,
University of Texas Southwestern Medical Center,
Dallas, Texas
  Urinary Lithiasis: Etiology, Epidemiology, and Pathogenesis

Craig A. Peters, MD
John E. Cole Professor of Urology,
University of Virginia,
Charlottesville, Virgina
  *Congenital Urinary Obstruction: Pathophysiology
  Perinatal Urology
  Pediatric Endourology and Laparoscopy*

Andrew C. Peterson, MD, FACS
Assistant Professor of Surgery,
Uniformed Services University of the Health Sciences,
Bethesda, Maryland;
Program Director,
Urology Residency,
Madigan Army Medical Center,
Tacoma, Washington
  Urodynamic and Videourodynamic Evaluation of Voiding Dysfunction

Curtis A. Pettaway, MD
Associate Professor of Urology, and
  Associate Professor of Cancer Biology,
Department of Urology,
University of Texas MD Anderson Cancer Center,
Houston, Texas
  Tumors of the Penis

Paul K. Pietrow, MD
Director of Minimally Invasive Surgery,
Hudson Valley Urology,
Poughkeepsie, New York
  Evaluation and Medical Management of Urinary Lithiasis

Louis L. Pisters, MD
Associate Professor of Urology,
Department of Urology,
University of Texas MD Anderson Cancer Center,
Houston, Texas
  Cryotherapy for Prostate Cancer

Elizabeth A. Platz, ScD, MPH
Associate Professor,
Department of Epidemiology,
Johns Hopkins Bloomberg School of Public Health,
Johns Hopkins Medical Institutions,
Baltimore, Maryland
  Epidemiology, Etiology, and Prevention of Prostate Cancer

Jeannette Potts, MD
Senior Clinical Instructor,
Department of Family Medicine,
Cleveland Clinic Lerner College of Medicine of
  Case Western Reserve University;
Staff Physician,
Glickman Urological Institute,
Cleveland Clinic Foundation,
Cleveland, Ohio
  Sexually Transmitted Diseases

Glenn M. Preminger, MD
Professor of Urologic Surgery,
Duke University Medical Center,
Durham, North Carolina
  Evaluation and Medical Management of Urinary Lithiasis

Raymond R. Rackley, MD
Professor of Surgery (Urology),
Cleveland Clinic Lerner College of Medicine of
  Case Western Reserve University,
Co-Head, Section of Female Urology and Voiding
  Dysfunction,
The Glickman Urological Institute,
Cleveland Clinic Foundation,
Cleveland, Ohio
  Electrical Stimulation for Storage and Emptying Disorders

John R. Ramey, MD
Jefferson Prostate Diagnostic Center,
Departments of Urology and Radiology,
Kimmel Cancer Center,
Thomas Jefferson University,
Philadelphia, Pennsylvania
  Ultrasonography and Biopsy of the Prostate

Robert E. Reiter, MD
Professor of Urology,
Member, Molecular Biology Institute,
Associate Director,
Prostate Cancer Program,
Geffen School of Medicine,
University of California, Los Angeles,
Los Angeles, California
  Molecular Genetics and Cancer Biology

Neil M. Resnick, MD
Professor of Medicine,
Chief, Division of Gerontology and Geriatric Medicine,
Director, University of Pittsburgh Institute on Aging,
University of Pittsburgh and University of Pittsburgh
  Medical Center,
Pittsburgh, Pennsylvania
  Geriatric Incontinence and Voiding Dysfunction

Martin I. Resnick, MD
Lester Persky Professor and Chair,
Department of Urology,
Cleveland Clinic Lerner College of Medicine of
  Case Western Reserve University,
Cleveland Clinic Foundation,
Cleveland, Ohio
  Radical Perineal Prostatectomy

Alan B. Retik, MD
Professor of Surgery (Urology),
Harvard Medical School;
Chief, Department of Urology,
Children's Hospital,
Boston, Massachusetts
  *Ectopic Ureter, Ureterocele, and Other Anomalies of
  the Ureter
  Hypospadias*

Jerome P. Richie, MD
Elliot C. Cutler Professor of Urologic Surgery,
Chairman, Harvard Program in Urology,
Harvard Medical School,
Brigham and Women's Hospital,
Boston, Massachusetts
Neoplasms of the Testis

Richard Rink, MD
Professor, Indiana University,
Riley Hospital for Children,
Indianapolis, Indiana
*Surgical Management of Intersexuality, Cloacal
Malformation, and Other Abnormalities of the
Genitalia in Girls*

Michael L. Ritchey, MD
Professor of Urology,
Mayo Clinic College of Medicine,
Phoenix, Arizona
Pediatric Urologic Oncology

Ronald Rodriguez, MD, PhD
Associate Professor of Urology, Medical Oncology, Radiation
  Oncology, Cellular and Molecular Medicine,
Johns Hopkins University School of Medicine,
Baltimore, Maryland
*Molecular Biology, Endocrinology, and Physiology of the
Prostate and Seminal Vesicles*

Claus G. Roehrborn, MD
Professor and Chairman, Department of Urology,
University of Texas Southwestern Medical Center,
Dallas, Texas
*Benign Prostatic Hyperplasia: Etiology, Pathophysiology,
Epidemiology, and Natural History*

Jonathan A. Roth, MD
Assistant Professor of Urology and Pediatrics,
Temple University Children's Hospital,
Temple University,
Philadelphia, Pennsylvania
Renal Function in the Fetus, Neonate, and Child

Eric S. Rovner, MD
Associate Professor of Urology,
Department of Urology,
Medical University of South Carolina,
Charleston, South Carolina
Urinary Tract Fistula
Bladder and Urethral Diverticula

Thomas A. Rozanski, MD
Professor, Department of Urology,
The University of Texas Health Science Center;
Chief, Medical Operations,
University Hospital,
San Antonio, Texas
Genital and Lower Urinary Tract Trauma

Arthur I. Sagalowsky, MD
Professor of Urology and Surgery,
Chief of Urologic Oncology,
Dr. Paul Peters Chair in Urology in Memory of Rumsey
  and Louis Strickland,
The University of Texas Health Science Center,
Dallas, Texas
*Management of Urothelial Tumors of the Renal Pelvis
and Ureter*

Jay I. Sandlow, MD
Associate Professor and Vice-Chair,
Department of Urology,
Medical College of Wisconsin;
Director of Andrology and Male Infertility,
Froedtert Memorial Lutheran Hospital,
Milwaukee, Wisconsin
Surgery of the Scrotum and Seminal Vesicles

Richard A. Santucci, MD
Associate Professor and Chief of Urology,
Wayne State University School of Medicine,
Detroit, Michigan
Renal and Ureteral Trauma

Peter T. Scardino, MD
Chair, Department of Surgery,
Head, Prostate Cancer Program,
Memorial Sloan-Kettering Cancer Center,
New York, New York
Expectant Management of Prostate Cancer

Harriette Scarpero, MD
Assistant Professor,
Department of Urologic Surgery,
Vanderbilt University Medical Center,
Nashville, Tennessee
Tension-Free Vaginal Tape Procedures

Anthony J. Schaeffer, MD
Herman L. Kretschmer Professor and Chair,
Department of Urology,
Northwestern University Feinberg School of Medicine;
Chief of Urology,
Northwestern Memorial Hospital,
Chicago, Illinois
Infections of the Urinary Tract

Edward M. Schaeffer, MD, PhD
Department of Urology,
James Buchanan Brady Urological Institute,
Johns Hopkins Medical Institutions,
Baltimore, Maryland
Infections of the Urinary Tract

Howard I. Scher, MD
Professor of Medicine,
Weill Medical College of Cornell University;
Member, Department of Medicine,
Memorial Sloan-Kettering Cancer Center;
Attending Physician,
Memorial Hospital for Cancer and Allied Diseases,
New York, New York
The Clinical State of the Rising PSA Level after Definitive Local Therapy: A Practical Approach

Peter N. Schlegel, MD
Professor and Chairman,
Department of Urology,
Professor of Reproductive Medicine,
Weill Medical College of Cornell University;
Staff Scientist, The Population Council;
Urologist-in-Chief, New York-Presbyterian Hospital;
Associate Physician, Rockefeller University Hospital,
New York, New York
Male Reproductive Physiology

Steven M. Schlossberg, MD
Professor, Eastern Virginia Medical School,
Norfolk, Virginia
Surgery of the Penis and Urethra

Richard N. Schlussel, MD
Assistant Professor, Department of Urology,
Columbia University;
Assistant Professor, Division of Pediatric Urology,
Morgan Stanley Children's Hospital of New York-
    Presbyterian,
Columbia University Medical Center,
New York, New York
Ectopic Ureter, Ureterocele, and Other Anomalies of the Ureter

Francis X. Schneck, MD
Associate Professor of Urology,
Children's Hospital of Pittsburgh,
University of Pittsburgh Medical Center,
Pittsburgh, Pennsylvania
Abnormalities of the Testes and Scrotum and Their Surgical Management

Mark P. Schoenberg, MD
Professor of Urology and Oncology,
Director of Urologic Oncology,
James Buchanan Brady Urological Institute,
Johns Hopkins Medical Institutions,
Baltimore, Maryland
Management of Invasive and Metastatic Bladder Cancer

Martin J. Schreiber, Jr., MD
Chairman,
Department of Nephrology and Hypertension,
Cleveland Clinic Foundation,
Cleveland, Ohio
Etiology, Pathogenesis, and Management of Renal Failure

Joseph W. Segura, MD
Consultant in Urology,
Carl Rosen Professor of Urology,
Department of Urology,
The Mayo Clinic,
Rochester, Minnesota
Lower Urinary Tract Calculi

Jay B. Shah, MD
Chief Resident,
Columbia College of Physicians and Surgeons;
Department of Urology,
Columbia University Medical Center,
New York, New York
Percutaneous Management of the Upper Urinary Tract

Robert C. Shamberger, MD
Robert E. Gross Professor of Surgery,
Harvard Medical School;
Chief of Surgery, Children's Hospital,
Boston, Massachusetts
Pediatric Urologic Oncology

David S. Sharp, MD
Fellow, Department of Urology,
Memorial Sloan-Kettering Cancer Center,
New York, New York
Surgery of Penile and Urethral Carcinoma

Joel Sheinfeld, MD
Vice-Chairman, Department of Urology,
Memorial Sloan-Kettering Cancer Center,
New York, New York
Surgery of Testicular Tumors

Linda M. Dairiki Shortliffe, MD
Professor and Chair, Department of Urology,
Stanford University School of Medicine;
Chief of Pediatric Urology,
Stanford Hospital and Clinics,
Lucile Salter Packard Children's Hospital,
Stanford, California
Infection and Inflammation of the Pediatric Genitourinary Tract

Daniel A. Shoskes, MD, FRCSC
Professor of Surgery, Cleveland Clinic Lerner College of
    Medicine of Case Western Reserve University;
Urologist, Glickman Urological Institute,
Cleveland Clinic Foundation,
Cleveland, Ohio
Renal Physiology and Pathophysiology

Cary L. Siegel, MD
Associate Professor of Radiology,
Division of Diagnostic Radiology,
Mallinckrodt Institute of Radiology,
Washington University School of Medicine,
St. Louis, Missouri
Urinary Tract Imaging: Basic Principles

Mark Sigman, MD
Associate Professor of Surgery (Urology),
Brown University,
Providence, Rhode Island
   Male Infertility

**Jennifer D.Y. Sihoe, MD, BMBS(Nottm),
   FRCSEd(Paed), FHKAM(Surg)**
Specialist in Pediatric Surgery,
Division of Pediatric Surgery and Pediatric Urology,
The Chinese University of Hong Kong,
Prince of Wales Hospital,
Hong Kong, China
   *Voiding Dysfunction in Children: Non-Neurogenic and
   Neurogenic*

Donald G. Skinner, MD
Professor and Chair,
Department of Urology,
Keck School of Medicine of the University of Southern
   California, Norris Cancer Center,
Los Angeles, California
   Orthotopic Urinary Diversion

Arthur D. Smith, MD
Professor, Department of Urology,
Albert Einstein School of Medicine,
New York, New York;
Chairman Emeritus, Department of Urology,
North Shore-Long Island Jewish Medical Center,
New Hyde Park, New York
   Percutaneous Management of the Upper Urinary Tract

Joseph A. Smith, Jr., MD
Professor,
Department of Urologic Surgery,
Vanderbilt University School of Medicine,
Vanderbilt University Medical Center,
Nashville, Tennessee
   *Laparoscopic and Robotic-Assisted Laparoscopic Radical
   Prostatectomy and Pelvic Lymphadenectomy*

Jonathan Starkman, MD
Clinical Instructor,
Department of Urologic Surgery,
Vanderbilt University Medical Center,
Nashville, Tennessee
   Tension-Free Vaginal Tape Procedures

David R. Staskin, MD
Director, Section of Voiding Dysfunction,
Female Urology and Urodynamics,
New York Hospital-Cornell;
Associate Professor, Urology and Obstetrics and Gynecology,
Weill Medical College of Cornell University,
New York, New York
   *Surgical Treatment of Male Sphincteric Urinary
   Incontinence: The Male Perineal Sling and Artificial
   Urinary Sphincter*

Graeme S. Steele, MD
Assistant Professor of Surgery,
Harvard Medical School;
Urologist, Brigham and Women's Hospital,
Boston, Massachusetts
   Neoplasms of the Testis

John P. Stein, MD
Associate Professor in Urology,
Keck School of Medicine of the University of Southern
   California, Norris Cancer Center,
Los Angeles, California
   Orthotopic Urinary Diversion

John T. Stoffel, MD
Assistant Professor of Urology,
Tufts University School of Medicine,
Boston, Massachusetts;
Senior Staff Urologist, Department of Urology,
Lahey Clinic Medical Center,
Burlington, Massachusetts
   Pubovaginal Sling

Jack W. Strandhoy, PhD
Professor, Department of Physiology and Pharmacology,
Wake Forest University School of Medicine,
Winston-Salem, North Carolina
   Pathophysiology of Urinary Tract Obstruction

Stevan B. Streem, MD (*deceased*)
Head, Section of Stone Disease and Endourology,
Glickman Urological Institute,
Cleveland Clinic Foundation,
Cleveland, Ohio
   Management of Upper Urinary Tract Obstruction

Li-Ming Su, MD
Associate Professor of Urology,
Director of Laparoscopic and Robotic Urologic Surgery,
James Buchanan Brady Urological Institute,
Johns Hopkins Medical Institutions,
Baltimore, Maryland
   *Laparoscopic and Robotic-Assisted Laparoscopic Radical
   Prostatectomy and Pelvic Lymphadenectomy*

Anthony J. Thomas, Jr., MD
Head, Section of Male Infertility,
Glickman Urological Institute,
Cleveland Clinic Foundation,
Cleveland, Ohio
   Surgical Management of Male Infertility

Ian M. Thompson, MD
Glenda and Gary Woods Distinguished Chair in
   Genitourinary Oncology,
Henry B. and Edna Smith Dielman Memorial Chair in
   Urologic Science,
The University of Texas Health Science Center,
San Antonio, Texas
   Epidemiology, Etiology, and Prevention of Prostate Cancer

Sandip P. Vasavada, MD
Associate Professor of Surgery (Urology),
Cleveland Clinic Lerner College of Medicine of
    Case Western Reserve University;
Co-Head, Section of Female Urology and
    Voiding Dysfunction,
Glickman Urological Institute,
Cleveland Clinic Foundation,
Cleveland, Ohio
    Electrical Stimulation for Storage and Emptying Disorders

E. Darracott Vaughan, Jr., MD
James J. Colt Professor and Chairman Emeritus of Urology,
Weill Medical College of Cornell University,
New York-Presbyterian Hospital,
New York, New York
    *Pathophysiology, Evaluation, and Medical Management of
    Adrenal Disorders*

Robert W. Veltri, PhD
Associate Professor,
Department of Urology
Johns Hopkins University School of Medicine,
Baltimore, Maryland
    *Molecular Biology, Endocrinology, and Physiology of the
    Prostate and Seminal Vesicles*

Patrick C. Walsh, MD
University Distinguished Service Professor of Urology,
James Buchanan Brady Urological Institute,
Johns Hopkins Medical Institutions,
Baltimore, Maryland
    Anatomic Radical Retropubic Prostatectomy

George D. Webster, MD
Professor of Urologic Surgery,
Department of Urology,
Duke University Medical Center,
Durham, North Carolina
    *Urodynamic and Videourodynamic Evaluation of
    Voiding Dysfunction*

Alan J. Wein, MD, PhD(Hon)
Professor and Chair,
Division of Urology,
University of Pennsylvania School of Medicine;
Chief of Urology,
University of Pennsylvania Medical Center,
Philadelphia, Pennsylvania
    Pathophysiology and Classification of Voiding Dysfunction
    *Lower Urinary Tract Dysfunction in Neurologic Injury
    and Disease*
    *Pharmacologic Management of Storage and
    Emptying Failure*
    Additional Therapies for Storage and Emptying Failure

Robert M. Weiss, MD
Donald Guthrie Professor and Chief,
Section of Urology,
Yale University School of Medicine,
New Haven, Connecticut
    Physiology and Pharmacology of the Renal Pelvis and Ureter

Howard N. Winfield, MD, FRCS
Professor, Department of Urology,
Director, Laparoscopy and Minimally Invasive Surgery,
The University of Iowa Hospitals and Clinics,
University of Iowa,
Iowa City, Iowa
Surgery of the Scrotum and Seminal Vesicles

J. Christian Winters, MD
Clinical Associate Professor,
Louisiana State University Health Sciences Center;
Vice-Chairman and Director of Female Urology and
    Voiding Dysfunction,
Ochsner Clinic Foundation,
New Orleans, Louisiana
    Injection Therapy for Urinary Incontinence

John R. Woodard, MD
Formerly: Clinical Professor of Urology,
Director of Pediatric Urology,
Emory University School of Medicine;
Formerly: Chief of Urology,
Henrietta Egleston Hospital for Children,
Atlanta, Georgia
    Prune Belly Syndrome

Subbarao V. Yalla, MD
Professor of Surgery (Urology),
Harvard Medical School;
Chief, Urology Division,
Boston Veterans Affairs Medical Center,
Boston, Massachusetts
    Geriatric Incontinence and Voiding Dysfunction

**C. K. Yeung, MBBS, MD, FRCSE, FRCSG, FRACS, FACS,
FHKAM(Surg), DCH(Lond)**
Clinical Professor in Pediatric Surgery and
    Pediatric Urology,
Chinese University of Hong Kong,
Prince of Wales Hospital,
Hong Kong, China
    *Voiding Dysfunction in Children: Non-Neurogenic
    and Neurogenic*

Naoki Yoshimura, MD, PhD
Associate Professor of Urology and Pharmacology,
University of Pittsburgh School of Medicine,
Pittsburgh, Pennsylvania
    Physiology and Pharmacology of the Bladder and Urethra

PREFACE

For each discipline in medicine and surgery, there is generally an acknowledged authoritative text, otherwise known as "the bible." For virtually every urologist in current practice, *Campbell's Urology* has had that distinction. The text, first published in 1954 with Meredith Campbell as its sole editor, has seen the editor-in-chief position pass to J. Hartwell Harrison, and then to Patrick Walsh. Under Dr. Walsh's leadership as editor-in-chief for the past 20 years (4 editions), *Campbell's Urology* has changed as much as the field itself—in virtually every way possible except for its preeminence. The current editorial board felt strongly that Pat's contributions to urologic education through his continuing improvements and innovations to *Campbell's* should be recognized in perpetuity by renaming the text in his honor; thus the new title—*Campbell-Walsh Urology.*

Aside from the name, the 9th edition is quite different from its predecessors, continuing the tradition of a constant evolution paralleling the changing nature of the field and its relevant pertinent information. We have changed the editorial board and increased it by one. Louis Kavoussi, Andrew Novick, Alan Partin, and Craig Peters all have moved up from their associate editor positions. From the standpoint of organization, Volume 1 now covers anatomy; molecular and cellular biology, including tissue engineering; the essentials of clinical decision-making; the basics of instrumentation, endoscopy, and laparoscopy; infection and inflammation; male reproductive function and dysfunction; and sexual function and dysfunction in both men and women. Volume 2 covers all aspects of the upper urinary tract and adrenal, including physiology, obstruction, trauma, stone disease, and neoplasia. Volume 3 includes all topics related to lower urinary tract function and dysfunction, including calculi; trauma, bladder, and prostate disease; and all aspects of urine transport, storage, and emptying. Volume 4 remains a 900-page textbook of pediatric urology. There are 24 totally new chapters; an additional 19 chapters have new authors; and the remaining 89 chapters have all undergone substantial revision. All chapters contain the latest concepts, data, and controversies. Illustrations, algorithms (extensively used), and tables are now in color, as are clinical photographs. Extensive highlighting is utilized, as well as key point boxes. The complete reference list is now online and bound on a CD; a list of suggested key references appears at the end of each chapter. An **e**-dition includes a fully searchable online version with downloadable images (for powerpoint, papers, etc.) and video clips of the key portions of certain procedures, and it will include weekly content updates (summaries of key journal articles in all areas) for the life of the edition. The *Review*, with questions, answers, and explanations, will continue as a separate publication.

Each of us is grateful for the opportunity to be a part of the continuing tradition of *Campbell-Walsh Urology* and wish to express our immense appreciation to all of our superb authors and to those at Elsevier who facilitated our efforts in bringing the 9th edition to publication: Rebecca Schmidt Gaertner, Senior Acquisitions Editor, and Anne Snyder, Senior Developmental Editor.

ALAN J. WEIN, MD, PhD (Hon)
For the Editors

CONTENTS

VOLUME 3

VOLUME 4

SECTION XVII
PEDIATRIC UROLOGY

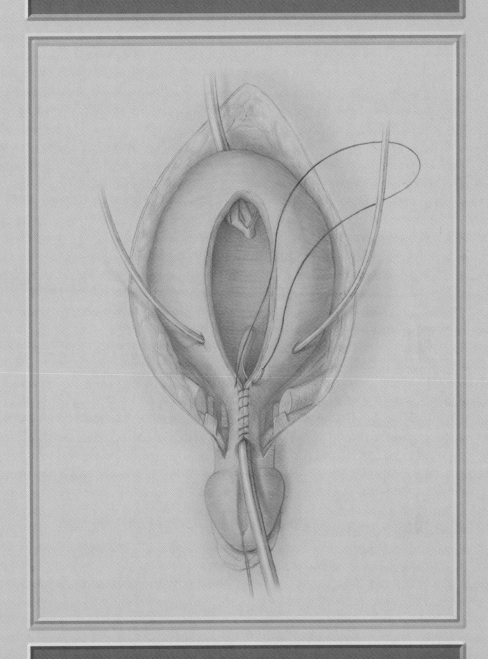

PEDIATRIC
UROLOGY

106 Normal Development of the Urogenital System

JOHN M. PARK, MD

The study of embryology provides a useful foundation for the understanding of definitive human anatomy and various congenital disease processes. During the past few decades, a torrent of molecular information and novel experimental techniques has revolutionized the field of embryology, and the knowledge base continues to expand at an exponential rate. From the urologic surgeon's perspective, however, the classical, descriptive aspects of anatomic embryology continue to serve as an important reference point from which various congenital problems are solved clinically. The aim of this chapter is to provide a concise presentation of the essential facts of normal urogenital system development, clarifying the important anatomic features and supplementing them with updated molecular information. Deliberate efforts have been made to separate the ever-expanding molecular information from that of the descriptive, anatomic embryology in order to keep the main "story" of urogenital system development clear and understandable from a surgical point of view (Fig. 106–1). To help with visualization of the key events, various schematic drawings have been added, and these illustrations have been supplemented with summarizing legends to help with easy review later on. The goal of this chapter is not to provide potential explanations for every congenital defect that might occur in the urogenital system, but selected, pertinent examples highlighting the fundamental concepts and principles are discussed.

KIDNEY DEVELOPMENT
Early Events

Mammals develop three kidneys in the course of intrauterine life. The embryonic kidneys are, in order of their appearance, the pronephros, the mesonephros, and the metanephros. The first two kidneys regress in utero, and the third becomes the permanent kidney. **Embryologically, all three kidneys develop from the intermediate mesoderm.** As the notochord and neural tube develop, the mesoderm located on either side of the midline differentiates into three subdivisions: paraxial (somite), intermediate, and lateral mesoderm (Fig. 106–2). As the embryo undergoes transverse folding, the intermediate mesoderm separates away from the paraxial mesoderm and migrates toward the intraembryonic coelom (the future peritoneum). At this time, there is a progressive craniocaudal development of the bilateral longitudinal mesodermal masses, called nephrogenic cords. Each cord is seen bulging from the posterior wall of the coelomic cavity, producing the urogenital ridge.

Pronephros and Mesonephros

The mammalian pronephros is a transitory, nonfunctional kidney, analogous to that of primitive fish. In humans, the first evidence of pronephros is seen late in the 3rd week, and it completely degenerates by the start of the 5th week. The pronephros develops as five to seven paired segments in the region of the future neck and thorax (Fig. 106–3A). Development of the pronephric tubules starts at the cranial end of the nephrogenic cord and progresses caudally. As each tubule matures, it immediately begins to degenerate along with the segment of the nephric duct to which the tubules are attached.

The second kidney, the mesonephros, is also transient, but in mammals it serves as an excretory organ for the embryo while the definitive kidney, the metanephros, begins its development (Fig. 106–3B and C). There is a gradual transition from the pronephros to the mesonephros at about the 9th and 10th somite levels. Development of the nephric ducts (also called the wolffian ducts) precedes the development of the mesonephric tubules. The nephric ducts can be seen as a pair of solid longitudinal tissue condensations at about the 24th day, developing parallel to the nephrogenic cords in the dorsolateral aspect of the embryo. Its blind distal ends grow toward the primitive cloaca and soon fuse with it at about the 28th day. This fused region later becomes a part of the trigone and posterior wall of the bladder. As the ducts fuse with the cloaca, they begin to form a lumen at the caudal end. This process of canalization then progresses cranially in a reverse direction, transforming the solid tissue condensations into the definitive nephric ducts with excretory capability. Soon after the appearance of the nephric ducts during the 4th week, mesonephric vesicles begin to form. Initially, several spherical

SECTION XVII

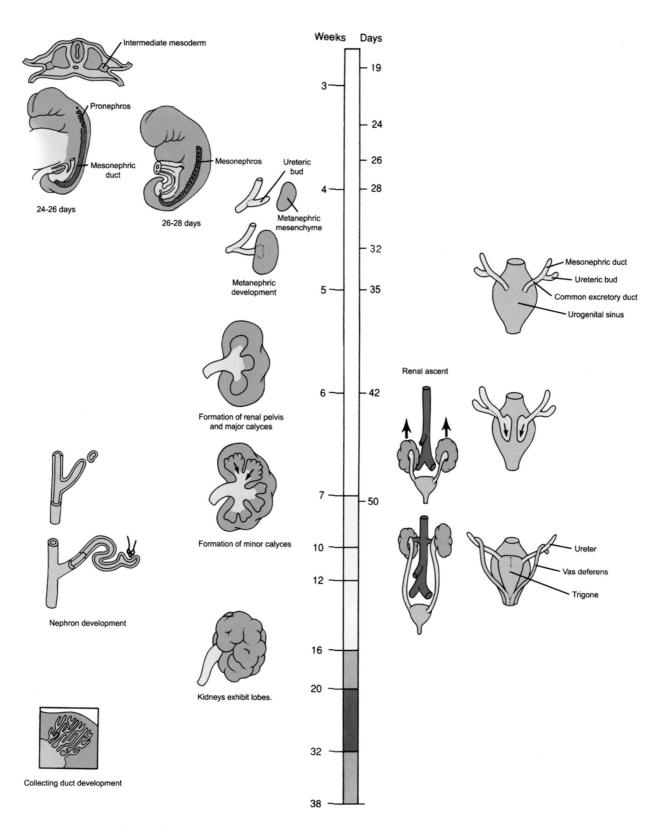

A. Kidney development

B. Ureter and bladder development

Figure 106–1. Time line and overview of urogenital system development. (Modified from Larsen WJ: Human Embryology. New York, Churchill Livingstone, 1997.)

Continued

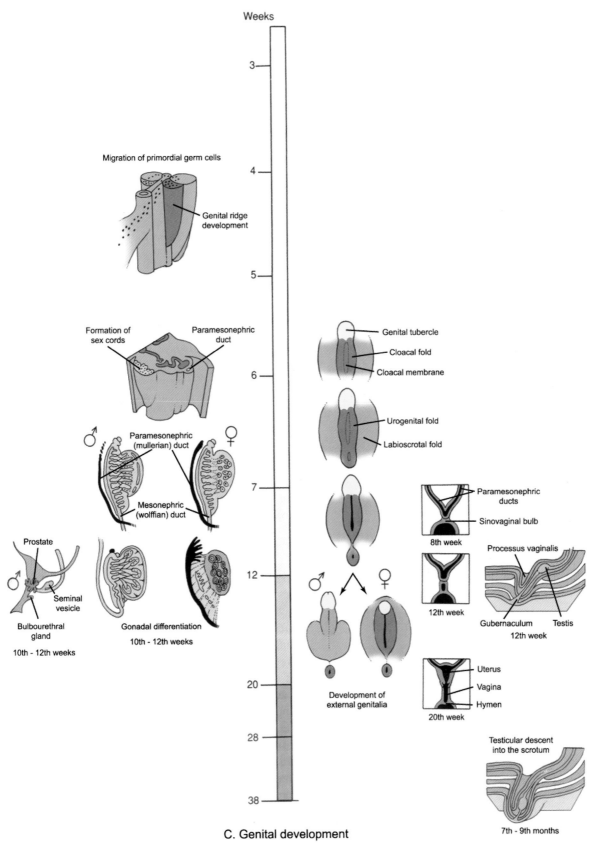

C. Genital development

Figure 106–1, cont'd.

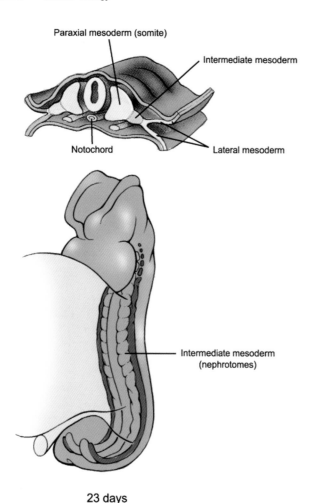

Paraxial mesoderm (somite)

Intermediate mesoderm

Notochord

Lateral mesoderm

Intermediate mesoderm
(nephrotomes)

23 days

Figure 106–2. The intermediate mesoderm gives rise to paired, segmentally organized nephrotomes from cervical to sacral region. Cervical nephrotomes are formed early during the 4th week and are collectively referred to as the pronephros. (Modified from Larsen WJ: Human Embryology. New York, Churchill Livingstone, 1997.)

masses of cells are found along the medial side of the nephrogenic cords at the cranial end. This differentiation progresses caudally and results in the formation of 40 to 42 pairs of mesonephric tubules, but only about 30 pairs are seen at any one time because the cranially located tubules start to degenerate starting at about the 5th week. By the 4th month, the human mesonephros has almost completely disappeared, except for a few elements that persist into maturity as part of the reproductive tract. **In males, some of the cranially located mesonephric tubules become the efferent ductules of the testes. The epididymis and vas deferens are also formed from the nephric (wolffian) ducts. In females, remnants of cranial and caudal mesonephric tubules form small, nonfunctional mesosalpingeal structures called *epoöphoron* and *paroöphoron*.**

The mesonephric tubules differentiate into excretory units that resemble an abbreviated version of an adult nephron. Shortly after the cell clusters are formed, they develop lumens and take the shape of vesicles. As the vesicle elongates, each end curves in an opposite direction to form an S-shaped tubule. The lateral end forms a bud that connects with the nephric duct. The medial end lengthens and enlarges to form a cup-shaped sac, which eventually wraps around a knot of glomerular capillaries to form a renal corpuscle. The tuft of glomerular capillaries originating from a branch of the dorsal aorta invades the developing glomerulus, while an efferent arteriole empties into a subcardinal sinus.

Metanephros

The definitive kidney, or the metanephros, forms in the sacral region as a pair of new structures, called the ureteric bud, sprouts from the distal portion of the nephric duct, and comes in contact with the condensing blastema of metanephric mesenchyme at about the 28th day (Fig. 106–4). The ureteric bud penetrates the metanephric mesenchyme and begins to divide dichotomously. The tip of the

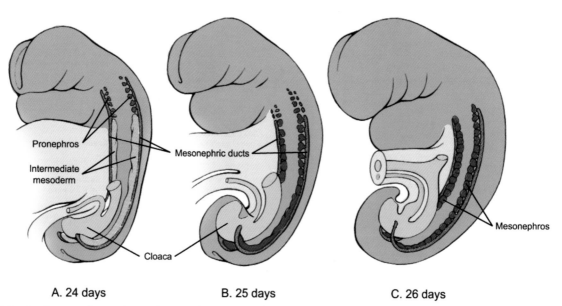

Pronephros

Intermediate mesoderm

Mesonephric ducts

Cloaca

Mesonephros

A. 24 days   **B. 25 days**   **C. 26 days**

Figure 106–3. Development of pronephros and mesonephros. **A,** Pronephros develops in each of five to seven cervical segments, but this primitive renal structure degenerates quickly during the 4th week. The (meso)nephric ducts first appear on day 24. **B** and **C,** Mesonephric vesicles and tubules form in a craniocaudal direction throughout the thoracic and lumbar regions. The cranial pairs degenerate as caudal pairs develop, and the definitive mesonephros contains about 20 pairs confined to the first three lumbar segments. (Modified from Larsen WJ: Human Embryology. New York, Churchill Livingstone, 1997.)

to derive from the metanephric mesenchyme; and the collecting system, consisting of collecting ducts, calyces, pelvis, and ureter, is formed from the ureteric bud (Fig. 106–6).

In principle, all nephrons are formed in the same way and can be classified into fairly well-defined developmental stages (Larsson et al, 1983) (Fig. 106–7). The first identifiable precursors of the nephron are cells of metanephric mesenchyme that have formed a vesicle completely separate from the ureteric bud ampulla (stage I). Cells of the stage I renal vesicle are tall and columnar in shape and are stabilized by their attachments to the newly formed basement membrane. It has not yet established a contact with the ampulla of the ureteric bud. The stage I renal vesicle then differentiates into an S-shaped stage II nephron that connects to the ureteric bud. At this stage, the cup-shaped glomerular capsule is recognized in the lowest limb of the S-shaped tubule. The rest of the S-shaped tubule develops into the proximal tubule, the loop of Henle, and the distal tubule. When the cup-shaped glomerular capsule matures into an oval structure, the nephron has now passed into stage III of development. Now the nephron can be divided into identifiable proximal and distal tubules.

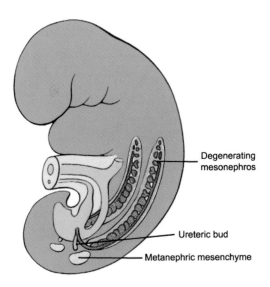

28 days

Figure 106–4. Metanephric mesenchyme condenses from the intermediate mesoderm during the early part of the 5th week and comes into contact with the ureteric bud, an outgrowth of the nephric duct, while the cranial mesonephros continues to degenerate. (Modified from Larsen WJ: Human Embryology. New York, Churchill Livingstone, 1997.)

dividing ureteric bud, called ampulla, interacts with the metanephric mesenchyme to induce formation of future nephrons through mesenchymal-epithelial interaction (see Fig. 106–4). As the ureteric bud divides and branches, each new ampulla acquires a caplike condensation of metanephric mesenchyme, thereby giving the metanephros a lobulated appearance (Fig. 106–5).

The ureteric bud and metanephric mesenchyme exert reciprocal inductive effects toward each other, and the proper differentiation of these primordial structures depends on these inductive signals. (See section on "Molecular Mechanism of Kidney Development.") The metanephric mesenchyme induces the ureteric bud to branch and divide, and, in turn, the ureteric bud induces the metanephric mesenchyme to condense and undergo mesenchymal-epithelial conversion. **The nephron, which consists of the glomerulus, proximal tubule, loop of Henle, and distal tubule, is thought**

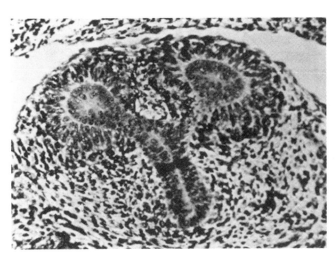

Figure 106–5. The ureteric bud divides to form enlarged tips, called ampulla, around which the metanephric mesenchyme condenses and begins nephron differentiation. The remaining mesenchymal cells remain stromal in nature and continue to interact with tubular mesenchymal cells and dividing ureteric bud epithelial cells. (From Potter EL: Normal and Abnormal Development of the Kidney. Chicago, Yearbook Medical Publishers, 1972.)

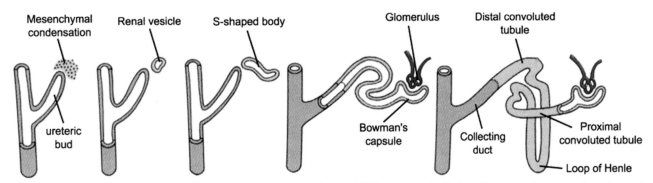

Figure 106–6. Development of the renal collecting ducts and nephrons. The tip of dividing ureteric bud induces the metanephric mesenchyme (pink color) to condense, which then differentiates into a renal vesicle. This vesicle coils into an S-shaped tubule and ultimately forms Bowman's capsule as well as the proximal convoluted tubules, distal convoluted tubules, and loops of Henle. The ureteric bud (purple color) contributes to the formation of collecting ducts. (Modified from Larsen WJ: Human Embryology. New York, Churchill Livingstone, 1997.)

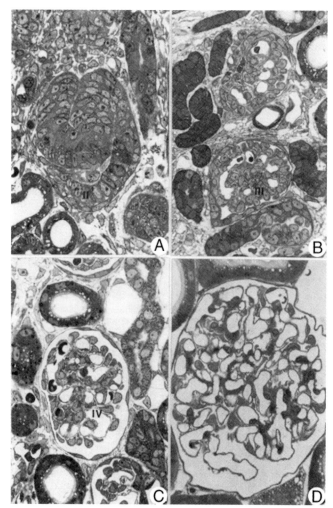

Figure 106–7. Nephron development as seen from a renal cortex of a 3-day-old rat. **A,** A developing nephron with S-shaped body (II). **B,** An oval-shaped glomerulus (III). **C,** Nephron now resembles that of mature tubules and glomeruli (IV). (D) Mature superficial glomerulus from adult rat kidney. (From Larsson L, Maunsbach AB: The ultrastructural development of the glomerular filtration barrier in the rat kidney: A morphometric analysis. J Ultrastruct Res 1980;72:392-406.)

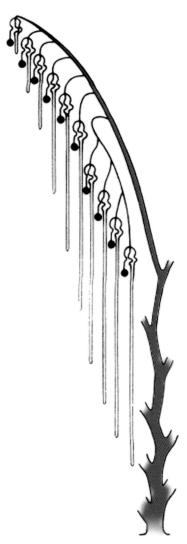

Figure 106–8. Schematic representation of progressive nephron differentiation. Older, more differentiated nephrons are located in the inner part of the kidney near the juxtamedullary region and newer, less differentiated nephrons are found at the periphery. (From Potter EL: Normal and Abnormal Development of the Kidney. Chicago, Yearbook Medical Publishers, 1972.)

The stage IV nephron is characterized by a round glomerulus that closely resembles the mature renal corpuscle. The morphology of the proximal tubule resembles that of a mature nephron, whereas the distal segments are still primitive. In some species (e.g., the rodents) all stages of nephron development are present at birth, whereas in others (e.g., the humans) all nephrons at birth are in varying steps of stage IV. Initially, vessels are seen in the cleft between the lower and middle portion of the S-shaped tubule, and they quickly branch into a portal system. Mesenchymal cells that do not become tubular epithelium either give rise to interstitial mesenchyme or undergo programmed cell death. **Overall, these events are reiterated throughout the growing kidney, so that older, more differentiated nephrons are located in the inner part of the kidney near the juxtamedullary region and newer, less differentiated nephrons are found at the periphery** (Fig. 106–8). **In humans, although renal maturation continues to take place postnatally, nephrogenesis is completed before birth.**

Collecting System

The dichotomous branching of the ureteric bud determines the eventual pelvicalyceal patterns and their corresponding renal lobules (Fig. 106–9). The first few divisions of the ureteric bud give rise to the renal pelvis, major and minor calyces, and collecting ducts. Thereafter, the first generations of collecting tubules are formed. When the ureteric bud first invades the metanephric mesenchyme, its tip expands to form an ampulla that eventually gives rise to the renal pelvis. By the 6th week, the ureteric bud has bifurcated at least four times, yielding approximately 16 branches. These branches then coalesce to form two to four major calyces extending from the renal pelvis. By the 7th week, the next four generations of branches also fuse, forming the minor calyces. By the 32nd week, approximately 11 additional generations of bifurcation have resulted in approximately 1 million to 3 million branches, which become the collecting duct tubules.

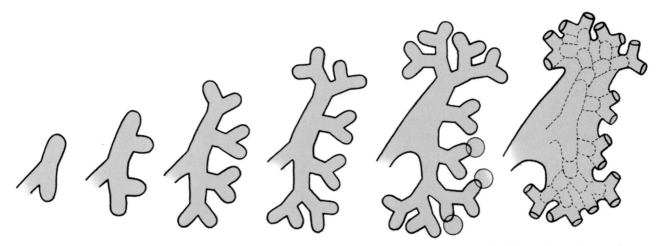

Figure 106–9. Dichotomous branching of the ureteric bud and subsequent fusion of the ampulla to form the renal pelvis and calyces. Circles indicate possible sites of infundibular development between the third, fourth, or fifth generations of branches and their subsequent expansions to give rise to the calyces. (From Potter EL: Normal and Abnormal Development of the Kidney. Chicago, Yearbook Medical Publishers, 1972.)

Renal Ascent

Between the 6th and 9th weeks, the kidneys ascend to a lumbar site just below the adrenal glands (Fig. 106–10). The precise mechanism responsible for renal ascent is not known, but it is speculated that the differential growth of the lumbar and sacral regions of the embryo plays a major role. As the kidneys migrate, they are vascularized by a succession of transient aortic sprouts that arise at progressively higher levels. These arteries do not elongate to follow the ascending kidneys but instead degenerate and are replaced by successive new arteries. The final pair of arteries forms in the upper lumbar region and becomes the definitive renal arteries. Occasionally, a more inferior pair of arteries persists as accessory lower pole arteries. When the kidney fails to ascend properly, its location becomes ectopic. If its ascent fails completely, it remains as a pelvic kidney. **The inferior poles of the kidneys may also fuse, forming a horseshoe kidney that crosses over the ventral side of the aorta. During ascent, the fused lower pole becomes trapped under the inferior mesenteric artery and thus does not reach its normal site.** Rarely, the kidney fuses to the contralateral one and ascends to the opposite side, resulting in a cross-fused ectopy.

Molecular Mechanism of Kidney Development

The details of inductive interactions among metanephric mesenchyme, ureteric bud epithelia, and, more recently, the stroma are becoming clearer and provide insights into the complex regulatory mechanisms underlying renal development. **Formation of renal tubules and collecting system occurs sequentially and requires dynamic interactions among epithelial, mesenchymal, and stromal cells.** Many of the early events in embryonic kidney development were first elucidated by manipulating lower vertebrate embryos and by utilizing a mammalian in vitro organ culture system. Clifford Grobstein's pioneering work in the 1950s led to an organ culture technique (Grobstein, 1956) whereby the metanephric mesenchyme is separated from the ureteric bud during the early part of kidney development and grown in vitro on a filter. An inducer tissue, such as ureter or spinal cord, cultured on the opposite side of the filter then provides the inductive signal (Fig. 106–11). This ingenious experimental approach has established the kidney as a model system for studying the role of epithelial-mesenchymal interaction in organ development. The development of many other organs, including lung, salivary glands, gonads, prostate, and bladder, also requires epithelial-mesenchymal interaction for the controlled differentiation and proliferation of tissues.

Formation of Nephric Ducts

The first recognizable event in renal development may be the formation of nephric ducts within the region of the intermediate mesoderm. The molecular signals responsible for this early event, in which seemingly unorganized mesenchymal cells aggregate to become an epithelial duct, remain essentially unknown, but details are beginning to emerge. The early intermediate mesoderm destined to become nephric ducts is distinguished by expression of the transcription factors Lim1, Pax2, and Sim1, but only Lim1 appears to be absolutely essential for nephric duct formation (Shawlot and Behringer, 1995). Pax2 may be important for maintaining other marker gene expression in the nephric ducts (Torres et al, 1995). Available data suggest a model in which few opposing secreted factors from the surrounding tissues cumulatively restrict Lim1 expression to the intermediate mesoderm. Lim1 then activates Pax2 expression to orchestrate further the formation of nephric ducts.

Ureteric Bud Outgrowth toward Metanephric Mesenchyme

The outgrowth of the ureteric bud from the nephric duct and its invasion into the condensing blastema of metanephric mesenchyme is a crucial initiating event in the development of the adult kidney (metanephros). Many candidate genes have been identified to play a critical role in this process (see http://www.ana.ed.ac.uk/anatomy/database/kidbase/kidhome.html). In particular, **several lines of experimental evidence have revealed a crucial role of the**

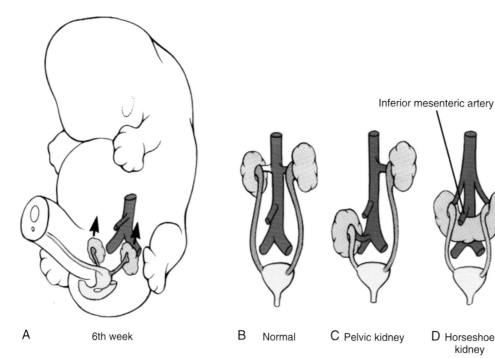

A 6th week **B** Normal **C** Pelvic kidney **D** Horseshoe kidney

Figure 106–10. Normal and abnormal ascent of the kidneys. **A** and **B,** The metanephros normally ascends from the sacral region to its definitive lumbar location between the 6th and 9th weeks. **C,** Rarely, a kidney may fail to ascend, resulting in a pelvic kidney. **D,** If the inferior poles of the kidneys fuse before ascent, the resulting horseshoe kidney does not ascend to a normal position because of entrapment by the inferior mesenteric artery. (Modified from Larsen WJ: Human Embryology. New York, Churchill Livingstone, 1997.)

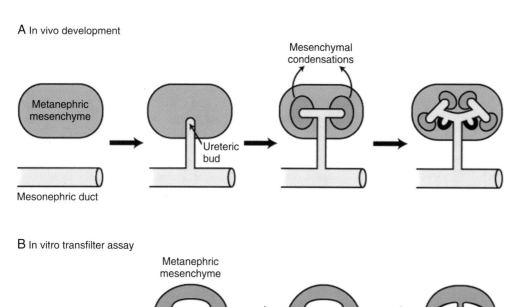

Figure 106–11. Schematic representation of in vivo kidney development (**A**) and an in vitro transfilter organ culture system of Grobstein (**B**). At an early stage of renal development, the metanephric mesenchyme is separated from the ureteric bud and cultured on a filter. If there is an inducer tissue grown on the opposite side of the filter, such as ureter and spinal cord, the metanephric mesenchyme continues to differentiate into nephron structures. In the absence of inducer tissue, the metanephric mesenchyme degenerates by apoptosis. (Modified from Vainio S, Muller U: Inductive tissue interactions, cell signaling, and the control of kidney organogenesis. Cell 1997;90:975-978.)

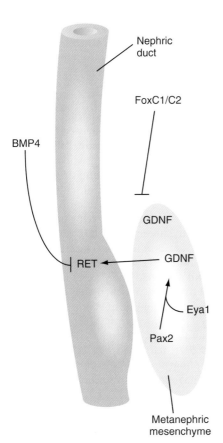

Nephric
duct

FoxC1/C2

BMP4

GDNF

RET

GDNF

Eya1

Pax2

Metanephric
mesenchyme

Figure 106–12. Inductive interactions during early kidney development. Glial cell line–derived neurotrophic factor (GDNF) is secreted from the metanephric mesenchyme and activates the RET receptor tyrosine kinase in the ureteric bud epithelium. The expression and localization of GDNF are positively regulated by Eya1 and Pax2 and negatively by FoxC transcription factors. The inducibility of nephric ducts to GDNF signaling is restricted by the action of BMP4. (Modified from Dressler GR: Tubulogenesis in the developing mammalian kidney. Trends Cell Biol 2002;12:390-395.)

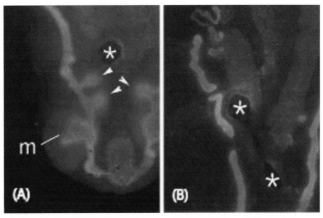

Figure 106–13. A, Stimulation of ectopic ureteric buds by glial cell line–derived neurotrophic factor (GDNF). To determine whether GDNF is sufficient to promote outgrowth of nephric duct epithelial cells, heparin acrylamide beads preadsorbed with recombinant GDNF (*) were placed between two nephric duct organ cultures. The native metanephros (m) is seen anteriorly. GDNF alone induces multiple ectopic ureteric buds in the posterior nephric ducts *(arrowheads).* **B,** However, the effect of GDNF is suppressed when Bmp4 is also added to the beads (*). Cultures were stained with anticytokeratin (green) and anti-Pax2 (red) antibodies. (From Dressler GR: Tubulogenesis in the developing mammalian kidney. Trends Cell Biol 2002;12:390-395.)

RET-GDNF-GFRα1 pathway in ureteric bud outgrowth

(Fig. 106–12). Glial cell line–derived neurotrophic factor (GDNF) is a secreted peptide expressed in the metanephric mesenchyme that activates the RET receptor, which is expressed along the nephric duct. GDNF activation of RET requires the glycosylphosphatidylinositol (GPI)-linked protein GFRα1, which is expressed in both metanephric mesenchyme and nephric duct. Gene knockout mutations in *ret*, *GDNF* (Moore et al, 1996; Pichel et al, 1996; Sanchez et al, 1996), and *GFRα1* (Cacalano et al, 1998) inhibit ureteric bud outgrowth. In organ culture systems, recombinant GDNF is sufficient to induce ectopic ureteric bud outgrowth (Sainio et al, 1997) (Fig. 106–13). However, the competence of the nephric duct to respond to GDNF is restricted along the anterior-posterior (A-P) axis. This A-P restriction might be mediated by suppressors of RET signaling within the surrounding tissue, such as BMP4. Mice that are deficient for BMP4 show more broadened ureteric buds or secondary anterior buds, suggesting that full BMP4 activity is required to limit RET signaling to the caudal aspect adjacent to the developing metanephric mesenchyme (Miyazaki, 2000). Similarly, in organ culture, BMP4 can suppress the activity of GDNF to induce ectopic ureteric bud formation (Brophy et al, 2001).

Proper positioning of the ureteric bud is also controlled by the localized expression of GDNF within the metanephric mesenchyme. Both positive and negative regulators have been described for GDNF localization. Homozygous mutation of a transcription factor, Eya1, causes failure of ureteric bud outgrowth, and their metanephric mesenchyme lacks *GDNF* expression, suggesting that Eya1 regulates *GDNF* expression (Xu et al, 1999). In humans, haploinsufficiency of Eya1 results in a dominantly inherited disorder called branchio-oto-renal (BOR) syndrome, which involves kidney and urinary tract anomalies (Abdelhak et al, 1997). Expression of Pax2 in the metanephric mesenchyme is also required for GDNF activation (Brophy et al, 2001), whereas GDNF expression is suppressed at the anterior boundary of the metanephric mesenchyme through the concerted action of the FoxC1 and FoxC2 transcription factors (Kume et al, 2000). Mutations in either *Fox* gene result in an expansion of GDNF expression and the formation of ectopic ureteric buds. Most *FoxC1* homozygous mutants have duplex kidneys, in which upper ureter is dilated and connects aberrantly to nephric duct derivatives in males such as seminal vesicles and vas deferens. The data therefore suggest that multiple factors regulate, both positively and negatively, the precise timing and localization of GDNF, which then functions as a guidance cue to activate RET. This signaling pathway then promotes migration and proliferation (ureteric bud outgrowth) of nephric duct to invade the metanephric mesenchyme.

Ureteric Bud Branching

Once the ureteric bud has reached the condensing metanephric mesenchyme, it undergoes a dichotomous branching morphogenesis. Many of the same factors that regulate the initial outgrowth of the ureteric bud also appear to be essential for the subsequent branching of the ureteric bud. As a first step toward branching, the leading edge of the ureteric bud grows into the metanephric mesenchyme and then dilates to form an *ampulla*. This ballooning of the bud tip might be necessary for the positioning of the branching point. Certain markers such as Wnt11 might already be compartmentalized to opposing poles of the dilated bud tips, even before a morphologic branch point is evident (Pepicelli et al, 1997). In mice deficient for the homeobox gene *Emx2* (Miyamoto et al, 1997), ureteric bud outgrowth into the metanephric mesenchyme appears normal, but the leading edge never dilates and branching is suppressed. Thus, ureteric development is arrested before the first branching event, and the resulting metanephric mesenchyme does not express any markers for induction. Similarly, mice with mutation of *Sall1* exhibit developmental arrest just after ureteric bud outgrowth and before dilation of the leading edge (Nishinakamura et al, 2001). In normal murine embryos, *Sall1* is expressed in the metanephric mesenchyme. Thus, *Sall1* might control mesenchyme-derived signals that are necessary for ureteric bud dilation and the early branch point determination. Clearly, the pattern of ureteric bud branching and the expression of ureteric bud–specific genes are influenced by the metanephric mesenchyme. Indeed, the heterologous mesenchyme derived from lung primordia can not only change the pattern of ureteric bud branching to that of lung epithelia but also induce the ureteric bud tissues to express lung-specific genes (Lin et al, 2001). **Thus, ureteric bud epithelial branching morphogenesis is controlled by both intrinsic and extrinsic factors working in concert to generate a kidney-specific branching pattern.**

Tubulogenesis

Classic tissue recombination experiments focused almost exclusively on the relationship between metanephric mesenchymal cells and ureteric bud epithelial cells. **It is now clear that at least three cell types are involved in the control of renal development: the ureteric bud tip cells, the condensed mesenchymal cells, and the stromal or interstitial mesenchymal cells** (Fig. 106–14). It is not known whether the mesenchyme is a homogeneous cell population prior to its interaction with the ureteric bud. It is clear, however, that once induced by the ureteric bud, the metanephric mesenchyme patterns itself into at least two different cell populations, a tubular one and a stromal one. The tubular cell population is thought to derive from mesenchymal cells in direct contact with the ureteric bud ampulla (Vainio et al, 1989; Stark et al, 1994; Torres et al, 1995), and the stromal cell population surrounds the tubular cells (Hatini et al, 1996). Once the mesenchyme has been patterned, the cells in the tubular zone undergo morphogenesis to become renal tubular epithelial cells. There is evidence that this process is dependent not only

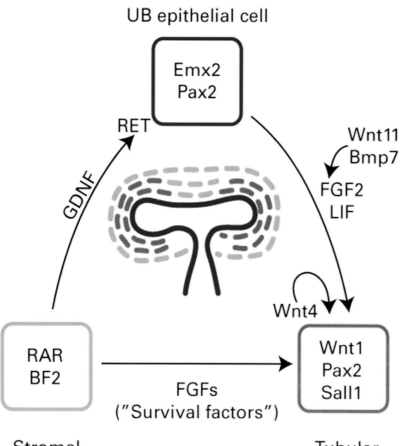

Figure 106–14. Cell-cell interactions promote nephrogenesis. Three major cell types—ureteric bud (UB) epithelial cells, condensing tubular mesenchymal cells, and stromal mesenchymal cells—are thought to play a critical role. At the UB tips, cells express unique markers such as Emx2 and Pax2. The stromal cell lineage is marked by expression of retinoic acid receptors (RAR) and BF2. Presence of Pax2, WT1, and Sall1 appears to be important for continued branching morphogenesis of the UB. Wnt4 is activated in the tubular mesenchymal cells by the invading UB and stimulates the development of polarized epithelium in an autocrine fashion. Finally, fibroblast growth factors (FGFs), such as FGF2, along with LIF, may be critical as survival factors for the developing renal tubular epithelial cells. (Modified from Dressler GR: Tubulogenesis in the developing mammalian kidney. Trends Cell Biol 2002;12:390-395.)

upon signals from the ureteric bud but also upon signals from the mesenchyme itself. One of these autocrine signals may be Wnt4, whose expression is induced in cells of the tubular zone upon interaction with the ureteric bud. In *Wnt4* gene knock-out mice, the ureteric bud forms and invades the metanephric mesenchyme, but subsequent development of epithelial tubules is abolished (Stark et al, 1994). This suggests that two signals are essential for renal tubule formation—initial ureteric bud–derived signals activating Wnt4 expression in the metanephric mesenchyme and Wnt4 itself as a mesenchymal autocrine signal. Signals from the stromal cell population also contribute to tubule formation because tubulogenesis is perturbed in *BF2* gene knockout mice (Hatini et al, 1996).

The discovery that Wnt4 acts as a downstream signal during the induction cascade leading to renal tubulogenesis leads to the question regarding the nature of the initial ureteric bud–derived signals. In vitro data suggest a role for fibroblast growth factor 2 (FGF2) and other uncharacterized factors secreted by the ureteric bud (Karavanova et al, 1996). Candidate molecules that may cooperate with FGF2 are Wnt11 and BMP7 (Kispert et al, 1996; Vukicevic et al, 1996). Localization of RET protein to the ureteric bud tips is reinforced by both GDNF (Pepicelli et al, 1997) and signals emanating from surrounding stromal cells. For example, retinoic acid receptors are expressed in the stromal cells and are required for stromal cell–mediated signaling to maintain high levels of RET expression in the bud tips (Mendelsohn et al, 1999; Batourina et al, 2001). Consistent with the role of retinoic acid receptors in maintaining RET expression in the dividing ureteric bud, rats suffering from vitamin A deficiency have smaller kidneys and fewer nephrons (Lelievre-Pegorier et al, 1999). The cellular crosstalk among stromal, mesenchymal, and ureteric bud cells is further highlighted by gain- and loss-of-function experiments involving FGFs and BMPs. *Fgf7* null mutant mice have fewer branch points and correspondingly fewer nephrons, whereas ectopic FGF7 in organ culture can stimulate branching (Qiao et al, 1999). FGF1 and FGF10 affect elongation of the ureteric bud stalk before the branch point decision is made (Qiao et al, 2001). Null mutations in *Bmp7* are even more severe, exhibiting limited branching morphogenesis and complete renal developmental arrest. Yet, it is difficult to assess how FGFs and BMPs exert their collective effects on branching given the interplay among all the cell types present in the early kidney (Dudley et al, 1999).

In addition to the proteins already mentioned, a growing list of growth factors, secreted peptides, and their receptors have been implicated in the control of branching morphogenesis, most by using a variety of in vitro model systems (Pohl et al, 2000; Davies, 2001). For many of these factors, however, genetic studies have not proved conclusive in assigning functional roles during ureteric bud branching in vivo, because of either potential redundancies or embryonic lethalities before the onset of kidney development. Nevertheless, the role of these factors in renal development must be considered.

Mesenchymal-Epithelial Conversion

The inductive signals emanating from the ureteric bud promote condensation of the metanephric mesenchymal cells around the ureteric bud tips and subsequent tubulogenesis. The ability to respond to inductive signals from the ureteric bud depends on at least two transcription factors expressed in

the uninduced mesenchyme: Wt1 and Pax2. Mice with null mutations of *Pax2* or *Wt1* fail to exhibit ureteric bud outgrowth and, in both cases, the metanephric mesenchyme does not respond to induction even when recombined with strong inducers in vitro (Kreidberg et al, 1993; Brophy et al, 2001). Evidence in support of Wnt proteins as mesenchyme inducers has been gained from in vitro induction assays using Wnt-expressing cell lines (Herzlinger et al, 1994; Kispert et al, 1998). Of the *Wnt* mutants examined to date, only *Wnt4*, which is expressed in the mesenchyme and not the ureteric bud, is crucial for propagation of the inductive signals. Although *Wnt4* mutant mesenchyme is able to aggregate in response to ureteric bud contact, these mutant aggregates do not form polarized epithelia. Rat ureteric bud cells secrete tubulogenic factors such as LIF, which, together with FGF2, appears to stimulate growth and tubulogenesis in vitro (Plisov et al, 2001). Once induced to form aggregates, metanephric mesenchyme becomes polarized into an early renal vesicle. This vesicle is closely associated with the branching ureteric bud and eventually connects to the ureteric bud epithelium to form a continuous tubule. Profound changes take place in the expression of cell adhesion molecules such as cadherins. Shortly after induction, metanephric mesenchyme expresses R-cadherin, cadherin-6, and E-cadherin, along with suppression of the mesenchyme-specific cadherin-11. Both R-cadherin and cadherin-6 mutants show defects in the rate of mesenchymal condensation and polarization (Mah et al, 2000; Dahl et al, 2002). Some renal vesicles in cadherin-6 mutants also fail to fuse to the ureteric bud epithelia, resulting in "dead-end" tubules and a subsequent loss of nephrons.

Renal Vascular Development

The origin of intrarenal vasculature is not completely understood. Until recently, it was thought that renal vasculature derived exclusively from branches off the aorta and other pre-existing extrarenal vessels ("angiogenic" hypothesis). There is evidence, however, that the renal vessels may originate in situ, within the embryonic kidney from vascular progenitor cells ("vasculogenic" hypothesis) (Loughna et al, 1996; Tufro et al, 1999). Using antibodies to Flk-1, a vascular endothelial growth factor (VEGF) receptor present in angioblasts and mature endothelial cells, it was demonstrated that endothelial cell precursors were already present in the prevascular rodent kidneys before any vessels were discernible from a morphologic standpoint. When embryonic kidneys are cultured at the usual atmospheric oxygen concentration, vessels do not develop. However, if the explants are cultured in a hypoxic atmosphere containing 5% oxygen, capillary sprouts develop within and outside the glomeruli, an effect that is inhibited by anti-VEGF antibodies (Tufro-McReddie et al, 1997). Depending on the developmental potential of the cells involved, both angiogenesis and vasculogenesis may play a role in the development of renal vasculature (Abrahamson et al, 1998).

BLADDER AND URETER DEVELOPMENT
Formation of Urogenital Sinus

At the 3rd week of gestation, the cloacal membrane remains a bilaminar structure composed of endoderm and ectoderm. During the 4th week, the neural tube and the tail of the embryo grow dorsally and caudally, projecting themselves over the cloacal membrane, and this differential growth of the body results in embryo folding. The cloacal membrane is now turned to the ventral aspect of the embryo, and the terminal portion of the endoderm-lined yolk sac dilates and becomes the cloaca (Fig. 106–15). According to the embryonic theories of Rathke and Tourneux, the partition of cloaca into an anterior urogenital sinus and a posterior anorectal canal occurs by the midline fusion of two lateral ridges of the cloacal wall and by a descending urorectal septum. This process is thought to occur during the 5th and 6th weeks, and it is culminated by the fusion of this urorectal septum with the cloacal mem-

brane. More recently, however, some investigators have challenged this classic view with evidence that there is neither a descending septum nor fusing lateral ridges of the cloacal wall (van der Putte, 1986; Kluth et al, 1995). There is further evidence that the urorectal septum never fuses with the cloacal membrane (Nievelstein et al, 1998). According to these new observations, the congenital cloacal and anorectal malformations, which were previously thought to be due to a failure of septum formation and its fusion with the cloacal membrane, may in fact result from an abnormal development of the cloacal membrane itself (Nievelstein et al, 1998) (Fig. 106–16).

The nephric (wolffian) duct fuses with the cloaca by the 24th day and remains with the urogenital sinus during the cloacal separation. **The entrance of the nephric duct into the primitive urogenital sinus serves as a landmark distinguishing the cephalad vesicourethral canal from the caudal urogenital sinus. The vesicourethral canal gives rise to the bladder and pelvic urethra, and the caudal urogenital sinus forms the phallic urethra for males and distal vaginal vestibule for females.**

Formation of Trigone

By day 33 of gestation, the common excretory ducts (the portion of nephric ducts distal to the origin of ureteric buds) dilate and become absorbed into the urogenital sinus. **The right and left common excretory ducts fuse in the midline as a triangular area, forming the primitive trigone.** The ureteric orifice exstrophies and evaginates into the bladder by day 37 and begins to migrate in a cranial and lateral direction within the floor of the bladder. During this process, the nephric duct orifice diverges away from the ureteric orifice and migrates caudally, flanking the paramesonephric (müllerian) duct at the level of the urogenital sinus. This is the site of the future verumontanum in males and vaginal canal in females (Fig. 106–17).

The embryonic pattern of ureteric orifice incorporation into the developing bladder is inferred primarily from clinical observations of duplex kidneys. The upper pole ureteric orifice rotates posteriorly relative to the lower pole orifice and assumes a more caudal and medial position. Weigert and Meyer recognized the regularity of this relationship between upper and lower pole ureteric orifices, which has come to be known as the Weigert-Meyer rule. **According to this concept, an abnormally lateral lower pole ureteric orifice may result from a ureteric bud arising too low on the nephric duct, resulting in premature incorporation and migration within the developing bladder.** In such a ureteric orifice, vesicoureteral reflux is more likely to occur because of an inadequate intramural tunnel. In contrast, an abnormally caudal upper pole ureteric orifice may result from a ureteric bud arising too high on the nephric duct. It may drain at the bladder neck and verumontanum or remain connected to the nephric (wolffian) duct derivatives such as the vas deferens (Mackie and Stephens, 1977; Schwarz and Stephens, 1978). In females, the ectopic upper pole ureter may insert into the remnants of the nephric ducts (such as a Gärtner's duct cyst) or vaginal vestibule (Fig. 106–18).

Anomalous development of the common excretory duct may lead to an ectopic vas deferens. In certain clinical situations, the vas deferens is connected to the ureter rather than

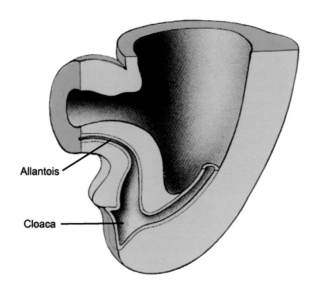

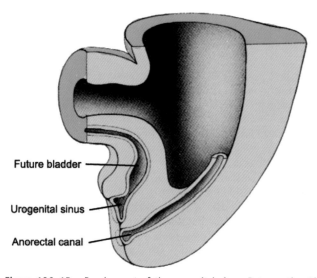

Allantois

Cloaca

Future bladder

Urogenital sinus

Anorectal canal

Figure 106–15. Development of the urogenital sinus. Between the 4th and 6th weeks, the cloaca is divided into an anterior urogenital sinus and a posterior anorectal canal. The superior part of the urogenital sinus, continuous with allantois, forms the bladder. The constricted narrowing at the base of the urogenital sinus forms the pelvic urethra. The distal expansion of the urogenital sinus forms the vestibule of the vagina in females and the penile urethra in males. (Modified from Larsen WJ: Human Embryology. New York, Churchill Livingstone, 1997.)

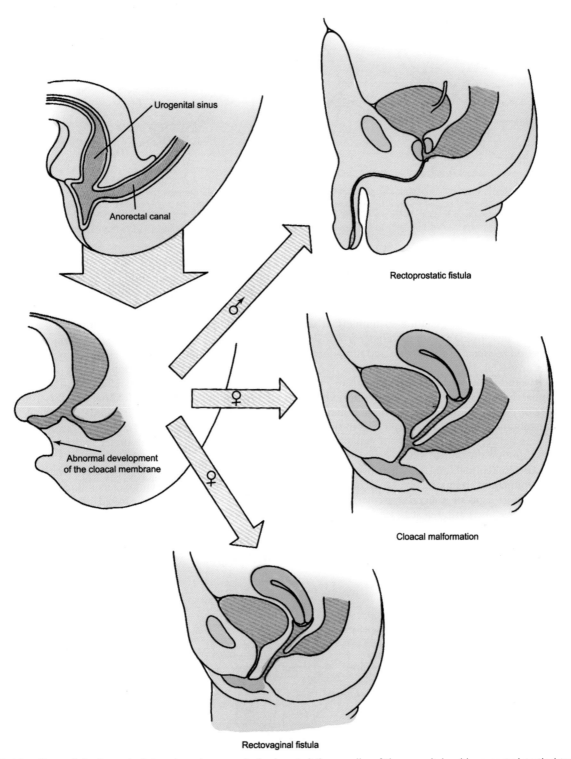

Figure 106–16. Abnormal development of cloacal membrane results in characteristic anomalies of the urogenital and lower gastrointestinal tract. (Modified from Larsen WJ: Human Embryology. New York, Churchill Livingstone, 1997.)

the verumontanum, so that both the ureter and vas drain into a common duct. This situation may occur when the ureteric bud arises too high on the nephric duct and the subsequent common excretory duct becomes too long, resulting in incomplete absorption into the developing bladder. This anomaly, although rare, should be kept in mind when evaluating males with epididymitis and ipsilateral hydronephrosis.

Development of the Ureter

In contrast to the previous discussion regarding the molecular aspects of renal development, little is understood at the molecular level concerning the events of ureter development. There is only a small amount of descriptive information and speculative theories regarding the molecular mechanism of

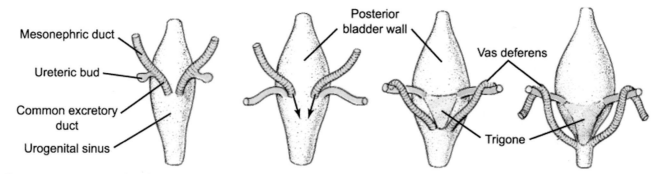

Figure 106–17. Incorporation of the mesonephric ducts and ureteric buds into the bladder wall. Between the 4th and 6th weeks, common excretory ducts, the terminal portion of the mesonephric ducts caudal to the ureteric bud formation, exstrophy into the posterior wall of the developing bladder. The triangular region of exstrophied mesonephric ducts forms the trigone of the bladder. This process brings the ureteric bud openings into the bladder wall, while the mesonephric duct openings are carried inferiorly to the level of pelvic urethra. (Modified from Sadler TW: Langman's Medical Embryology. Baltimore, Williams & Wilkins, 1985.)

smooth muscle cell and urothelial differentiation. Morphologically, the ureter begins as a simple cuboidal epithelial tube surrounded by loose mesenchymal cells, which acquires a complete lumen at 28 days of gestation in humans. It was suggested that the developing ureter undergoes a transient luminal obstruction between 37 and 40 days and subsequently recanalizes (Alcaraz et al, 1991). It appears that this recanalization process begins in the midureter and extends in a bidirectional manner both cranially and caudally. In addition, another source of physiologic ureteral obstruction may exist as Chwalla's membrane, a two-cell-thick layer over the ureteric orifice that is seen between 37 and 39 days of gestation.

In humans, urine production is followed by proliferative changes in the ureteral epithelium (bilaminar by 10 weeks of gestation). The epithelium attains a transitional configuration by 14 weeks. The first signs of ureteral muscularization and development of elastic fibers are seen at 12 weeks of gestation. In both rat and human, the ureteral smooth muscle phenotype appears later than that of the bladder. Smooth muscle differentiation is first detected in the subserosal region of

the bladder dome and extends toward the bladder base and urethra, whereas smooth muscle differentiation of the ureter occurs later within the subepithelial region in the ureterovesical junction, ascending toward the intrarenal collecting system (Baker and Gomez, 1998). In the embryonic ureter and bladder, it is likely that epithelial-mesenchymal interactions are important in the development of urothelium, lamina propria, and muscular compartments, but the exact nature of this induction process is unknown at this time. Before 10 weeks, elastic fibers are few in number, poorly developed, and randomly arranged. After 12 weeks, these fibers become more numerous throughout the ureter and are seen with specific orientation (Escala et al, 1989).

Although more than 30 genes are found to be involved in the development of mammalian kidneys, only a few *genes* have been thus far demonstrated to cause both kidney and ureteral anomalies concurrently—*Agtr2, Bmp4, FoxC1, Pax2,* and *Eya1* (see section on "Molecular Mechanism of Kidney Development"). A mutation of the *PAX2* gene has been identified in a human family carrying the renal-coloboma syn-

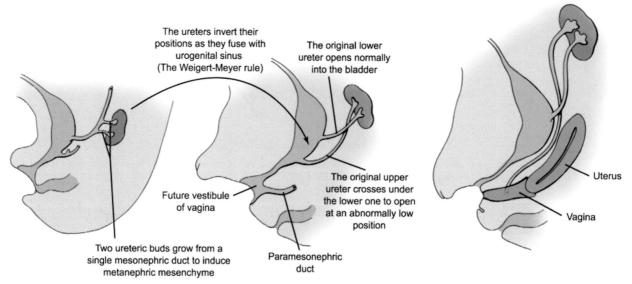

Figure 106–18. Development of an ectopic upper pole ureter draining into the vagina. (Modified from Larsen WJ: Human Embryology. New York, Churchill Livingstone, 1997.)

drome, a rare autosomal dominant syndrome characterized by optic nerve coloboma, renal anomalies, and vesicoureteral reflux (Sanyanusin et al, 1996). *EYA1* is mutated in patients with a dominantly inherited disorder, BOR syndrome, which includes duplex collecting system, renal hypoplasia/dysplasia, and renal agenesis (Abdelhak et al, 1997). Pax2 is required for the growth and elongation of nephric ducts prior to ureteric bud formation, whereas Eya1 appears to regulate GDNF expression, which is a prerequisite for ureteric bud outgrowth. Bmp4 and FoxC1 appear to play a suppressive role in ureteric bud outgrowth.

The renin-angiotensin system (RAS) is present and active during fetal life. It is generally thought that the major role of RAS in the fetus is to maintain fetal glomerular filtration and to ensure adequate urine production (Lumbers, 1995). There is growing evidence, however, that the RAS is also important for normal growth and development of the kidney and ureter. The kidney is able to produce all components of the RAS, and thus the local (intrarenal) production of angiotensin II may play a critical role in this regard. Renin messenger RNA is detectable in the human mesonephros at about 30 days of gestation and in the metanephros at about 56 days (Schutz et al, 1996). A similar profile of expression is seen for angiotensinogen and angiotensin-converting enzyme (ACE). Ten- to 12-month-old mutant mice lacking ACE are found to have abnormal renal vasculature and tubules as well as increased renin synthesis in interstitial and perivascular cells (Hilgers et al, 1997). Pharmacologic inhibition of ACE in the neonatal rat produces irreversible abnormalities in renal function and morphology (Guron et al, 1997), supporting the concept that an intact RAS is crucial for normal kidney development and maturation. In addition to the high rate of fetal loss, infants born to mothers treated with ACE inhibitors during pregnancy have increased rates of oligohydramnios, hypotension, and anuria (Shotan et al, 1994; Sedman et al, 1995).

Both subtypes of angiotensin II receptors, AT_1 and AT_2, are expressed in the developing mesonephros and metanephros. AT_2 expression predominates in the undifferentiated mesenchymal cells that surround the nephric duct at the time of ureteric bud outgrowth and declines with maturation, and this pattern of expression suggests AT_2's role in embryonic renal development. AT_1 is expressed in more differentiated structures and may be involved in modulating later stages of renal vascular development and acquisition of classical angiotensin II–mediated effects of vasoconstriction and sodium reabsorption. The function of AT_2 receptor is not defined completely, but when its gene, *Agtr2*, was inactivated genetically in mice, these mutants demonstrated a significant incidence of anomalies in the kidney and urinary tract. The abnormal phenotype in these mice mimicked all the key features of human congenital anomalies of the kidney and urinary tract (CAKUT), such as ureteropelvic junction obstruction, hypoplastic kidney, vesicoureteral reflux, megaureter, and duplicated collecting system (Nishimura et al, 1999).

Because of its embryonic expression pattern, it was initially speculated that AT_2 may play a role in regulating the initial outgrowth of the ureteric bud. Analysis of whole tissue sections showed that ectopic ureteric budding occurred in *Agtr2*-deficient mutant mice (Oshima et al, 2001). It was thus postulated that similarly to Bmp4, AT_2 may have a role in directing the site of ureteric bud outgrowth through its inhibitory effect. In other words, a defect in this process may lead to an abnormal timing and location of the ureteric bud outgrowth, resulting in congenital anomalies.

Development of Bladder and Continence Mechanisms

By the 10th week, the bladder is a cylindrical tube lined by a single layer of cuboidal cells surrounded by loose connective tissue. The apex tapers as the urachus, which is contiguous with the allantois. By the 12th week, the urachus involutes to become a fibrous cord, which becomes the median umbilical ligament. The bladder epithelium consists of bilayered cuboidal cells between the 7th and 12th weeks, and it begins to acquire mature urothelial characteristics between the 13th and 17th weeks. By the 21st week, it becomes four or five cell layers thick and demonstrates ultrastructural features similar to those of the fully differentiated urothelium. Between the 7th and 12th weeks, the surrounding connective tissues condense and smooth muscle fibers begin to appear, first at the region of the bladder dome and later proceeding toward the bladder base. Collagen fibers first appear in the lamina propria and later extend into the deeper wall between the muscle fibers (Newman and Antonakopoulos, 1989). **Embryologically, the bladder is composed of two regions: the trigone and the bladder body. The bladder body is derived from the endoderm-lined vesicourethral canal and the surrounding mesenchyme. The trigone has a different embryologic origin (mesodermal) in that it develops from the incorporation of the common excretory ducts (the portion of nephric ducts caudal to the origin of the ureteric bud) into the base of the developing bladder.**

Bladder compliance is thought to change during development. When studied in whole-organ preparation using fetal sheep bladders, bladder compliance is very low during early gestation and increases gradually thereafter (Coplen et al, 1994). The mechanism of these changes in bladder compliance is not known but may involve alterations in both smooth muscle tone and connective tissue composition. This phenomenon is also observed in developing human bladders (Kim et al, 1991). During gestation, the bladder wall muscle thickness increases and the relative collagen content decreases. The ratio of thick to thin collagen fibers also decreases, whereas the amount of elastic fibers increases. These changes in compliance seem to coincide with the time of fetal urine production, suggesting a possible role for mechanical distention (Baskin et al, 1994). Using fetal mouse bladders as organ culture explants, bladder distention promoted a more orderly development of collagen fiber bundles within the lamina propria in comparison with decompressed bladder explants, suggesting that mechanical factors from accumulating urine may play a role during bladder development (Beauboeuf et al, 1998).

As with other organ development, the epithelial-mesenchymal inductive interactions appear to be necessary for orderly differentiation and proper development of the bladder. A modified Grobstein technique was applied to study the mechanism of bladder smooth muscle cell differentiation (Baskin et al, 1996). Undifferentiated rat bladder epithelial and mesenchymal rudiments were separated prior to bladder smooth muscle cell differentiation and then recombined to grow within the immunologically compromised host (athymic nude mouse). In the presence of epithelial cells, the mesenchymal cells differentiated into smooth muscle cells with sequential expression of appropriate smooth muscle markers, whereas in the absence of epithelial cells, they involuted with evidence of apoptosis.

No functional study has been done to assess fetal continence mechanisms. Only a handful of ontogenic descriptions are available using human fetal specimens, providing a basis for speculative theories. A mesenchymal condensation forms around the caudal end of the urogenital sinus after the division of the cloaca and the rupture of the cloacal membrane. Striated muscle fibers can be seen clearly by the 15th week. At this time, the smooth muscle layer becomes thicker at the level of bladder neck and forms the inner part of the urethral musculature. The urethral sphincter, composed of central smooth muscle fibers and peripheral striated muscle fibers, develops in the anterior wall of the urethra (Bourdelat et al, 1992). Beyond this point, sexual dimorphism develops in conjunction with the formation of the prostate in males and the vagina in females (Tichy, 1989). The urethral sphincter muscle fibers extend to the posterior wall of the urethra. In males, these fibers project to the lateral wall of the prostate, whereas in females, the muscle fibers attach to the lateral wall of the vagina.

GENITAL DEVELOPMENT
Formation of Genital Ridges and Paramesonephric Ducts

During the 5th week, primordial germ cells migrate from the yolk sac along the dorsal mesentery to populate the mesenchyme of the posterior body wall near the 10th thoracic level (Fig. 106–19). **In both sexes, the arrival of primordial germ cells in the area of future gonads serves as the signal for the existing cells of the mesonephros and the adjacent coelomic epithelium to proliferate and form a pair of genital ridges just medial to the developing mesonephros** (Fig. 106–20). During the 6th week, the cells of the genital ridge invade the mesenchyme in the region of future gonads to form aggregates of supporting cells called the primitive sex cords. The primitive sex cords subsequently invest the germ cells and support their development. The genital ridge mesenchyme containing the primitive sex cords is divided into the cortical and medullary regions. Both regions develop in all embryos, but after the 6th week, they pursue different fates in the male and female.

During this time, a new pair of ducts, called the paramesonephric (müllerian) ducts, begins to form just lateral to the nephric ducts in both male and female embryos (Fig. 106–21). These ducts arise by the craniocaudal invagination of thickened coelomic epithelium, extending all the way from the third thoracic segment to the posterior wall of the developing urogenital sinus. The caudal tips of the paramesonephric ducts are adherent to each other as they connect with the urogenital sinus between the openings of the right and left nephric ducts. The cranial ends of the paramesonephric ducts form funnel-shaped openings into the coelomic cavity, which is the future peritoneum.

Development of Male Genital Structures

Under the influence of SRY (the sex-determining region of the Y chromosome), cells in the medullary region of the primitive sex cords begin to differentiate into *Sertoli cells*, while the cells of the cortical sex cords degenerate. Sex cord cells differentiate into Sertoli cells only if they contain the SRY protein; otherwise, the sex cords differentiate into ovarian follicles. During the 7th week, the differentiating Sertoli cells organize to form the *testis cords*. At puberty these testis cords

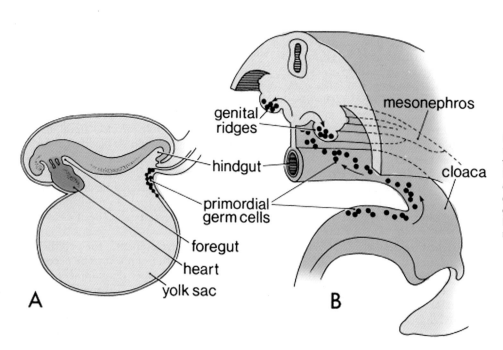

Figure 106–19. **A,** The site of the primordial germ cell origin in the wall of the yolk sac in a 3-week-old embryo. **B,** Migratory path of the primordial germ cells along the wall of the yolk sac and dorsal mesentery into the developing genital ridges. (Modified from Sadler TW: Langman's Medical Embryology. Baltimore, Williams & Wilkins, 1985.)

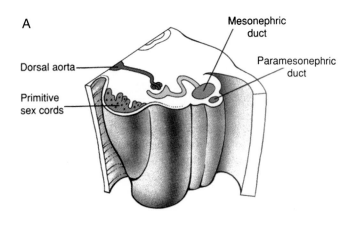

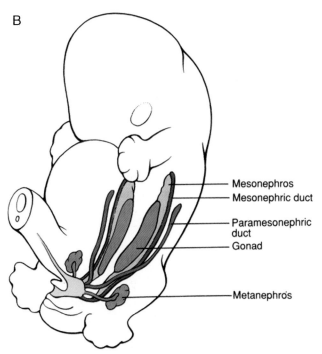

Figure 106–20. Formation of genital ridges and paramesonephric ducts. **A,** During the 5th and 6th weeks, the genital ridges form in the posterior abdominal wall just medial to the developing mesonephros. The primordial germ cells induce the coelomic epithelial cells lining the peritoneal cavity and the cells of the mesonephros to proliferate and form the primitive sex cords. **B,** During the 6th week, the paramesonephric ducts develop lateral to the mesonephros. The caudal tips of the paramesonephric ducts fuse with each other as they connect with the urogenital sinus. (Modified from Larsen WJ: Human Embryology. New York, Churchill Livingstone, 1997.)

associated with germ cells undergo canalization and differentiate into seminiferous tubules. Direct cell-to-cell contact between developing Sertoli cells and primordial germ cells is thought to play a key role in the proper development of male gametes. This interaction occurs shortly after the arrival of the primordial germ cells in the presumptive genital ridge. The testis cords distal to the presumptive seminiferous tubules also develop lumen and differentiate into a set of thin-walled ducts called the *rete testis*. Just medial to the developing gonad, the tubules of rete testis connect with 5 to 12 residual tubules of nephric ducts, called *efferent ductules*. The vas deferens also

develops from the nephric duct. At this time, the testicle begins to round up, reducing its area of contact with the surrounding mesonephros. As the testicle continues to develop, the degenerating cortical sex cords become separated from the coelomic (peritoneal) epithelium by an intervening layer of connective tissue called the *tunica albuginea* (see Fig. 106–21).

As the developing Sertoli cells begin their differentiation in response to the SRY, they also begin to secrete a glycoprotein hormone called *müllerian-inhibiting substance* (MIS). MIS causes the paramesonephric (müllerian) ducts to regress rapidly between the 8th and 10th weeks. **Small müllerian duct remnants can be detected in the developed male as a small tissue protrusion at the superior pole of the testicle, called the appendix testis, and as a posterior expansion of the prostatic urethra, called the** *prostatic utricle.* In female embryos, MIS is absent; therefore, the müllerian ducts do not regress. Occasionally, genetic males have persistent müllerian duct structures (uterus and fallopian tubes), the condition known as *hernia uteri inguinale*. In these individuals, either MIS production by Sertoli cells is deficient or the müllerian ducts do not respond to normal MIS levels.

During the 9th and 10th weeks, Leydig cells differentiate from mesenchymal cells of the genital ridge in response to the SRY protein. These endocrine cells produce testosterone. At an early stage of development, testosterone secretion is regulated by placental chorionic gonadotropin, but eventually the pituitary gonadotropins assume control of androgen production. Between the 8th and 12th weeks, testosterone secretion by Leydig cells stimulates the nephric (wolffian) ducts to transform into the vas deferens. The cranial portions of the nephric ducts degenerate, leaving a small remnant of tissue protrusion called the *appendix epididymis*, and the region of nephric ducts adjacent to the presumptive testicle differentiates into the epididymis. During the 9th week, 5 to 12 nephric ducts in the region of the epididymis make contact with the sex cords of the future rete testis. It is not until the 3rd month, however, that these tubules actually establish communication with the rete testis as the efferent ductules. Meanwhile, the nephric duct–derived tubules near the inferior pole of the developing testicle degenerate, sometimes leaving a remnant of tissue protrusion called the *paradidymis*.

Prostate and Seminal Vesicle Development

The seminal vesicles sprout from the distal nephric ducts, whereas the prostate and bulbourethral glands develop from the urogenital sinus (Fig. 106–22). They therefore have different embryologic origins. **The initial event in prostatic development is an outgrowth of solid epithelial cords from the urogenital sinus epithelium into the surrounding mesenchyme during 10 to 12 weeks of gestation.** This prostatic bud growth and subsequent branching morphogenesis occur in a specific spatial pattern that eventually establishes the lobar subdivisions of the mature prostate gland (Sugimura et al, 1986; Timms et al, 1994). The solid prostatic ducts are subsequently canalized from their urethral connections, proceeding distally toward the ductal tips. As the solid epithelial cords canalize, the epithelium organizes itself into two distinct cell types—luminal and basal cells (Hayward et al, 1996a). At this

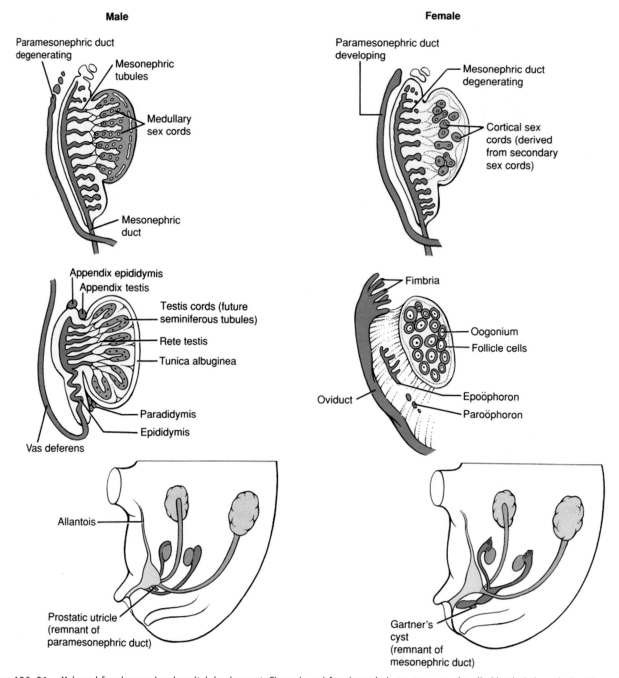

Figure 106–21. Male and female gonad and genital development. The male and female genital structures are virtually identical through the 7th week. In males, SRY protein produced by the Sertoli cells causes the medullary sex cords to become presumptive seminiferous tubules and causes the cortical sex cords to regress. Müllerian inhibiting substance (MIS) hormone produced by the Sertoli cells then causes the paramesonephric ducts to regress, leaving behind appendix testis and prostatic utricle as remnants. Appendix epididymis and paradidymis arise from the mesonephric ducts. In females, cortical sex cords invest the primordial germ cells and become the ovarian follicles. In the absence of MIS hormone, the mesonephric ducts degenerate and the paramesonephric ducts give rise to the fallopian tubes, uterus, and upper vagina. The remnants of the mesonephric ducts are found in the ovarian mesentery as the epoöphoron and paroöphoron and in the anterolateral vaginal wall as the Gartner's duct cysts. (Modified from Larsen WJ: Human Embryology. New York, Churchill Livingstone, 1997.)

time, the prostatic mesenchyme differentiates into a layer of smooth muscle cells that surround the prostatic ducts (Hayward et al, 1996b). At puberty, corresponding to a rise in circulating testosterone, the prostate size increases rapidly, along with functional cytodifferentiation of luminal cells, as evidenced by the expression of prostate-specific secretory proteins (Hayward et al, 1996a).

Circulating androgens produced by fetal testicles play a critical role in the development of prostate. Cellular responses to circulating androgens are mediated by nuclear androgen receptors that are activated by testosterone or dihydrotestosterone (DHT). The evidence for the requirement of androgens in establishing the prostate specificity of the urogenital sinus comes primarily from the absence of prostate

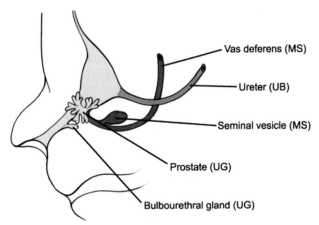

Figure 106–22. Development of male accessory sex glands. During the 10th week, the seminal vesicles sprout from the distal mesonephric ducts in response to testosterone, whereas the prostate and bulbourethral glands develop from the urethra in response to dihydrotestosterone. Thus, vas deferens and seminal vesicle derive from the mesonephric ducts (MS), and prostate and bulbourethral glands develop from the urogenital sinus (UG). UB, ureteric bud. (Modified from Larsen WJ: Human Embryology. New York, Churchill Livingstone, 1997.)

development in mice and humans that lack functional androgen receptors (Lubahn et al, 1989; He et al, 1991), as well as the development of prostate in the female urogenital sinus exposed to androgens (Takeda et al, 1986). In the urogenital sinus, testosterone could activate androgen receptors by directly binding to the receptor and also through a local conversion of circulating testosterone into the more potent DHT by the enzyme 5α-reductase (Russell and Wilson, 1994). DHT has a 10-fold greater affinity for the androgen receptor than testosterone (Deslypere et al, 1992). When 5α-reductase is deficient, the urogenital sinus is specified to become the prostate, but overall prostatic growth and development are severely compromised (Andersson et al, 1991). Tissue recombination and grafting experiments using testicular feminization mice that lack functional androgen receptor have shown that **the presence of androgen receptors in the urogenital sinus mesenchyme is required for prostate specification and differentiation** (Cunha and Lung, 1978). The fact that mesenchymal but not epithelial androgen receptors are required for prostate-specific ductal growth and branching suggests that paracrine signals from the urogenital sinus mesenchyme mediate the action of androgens on the epithelium. Prostate development appears to be affected by the levels of estrogenic compounds as well (vom Saal et al, 1997; Timms et al, 1999), but its specific role has not been fully elucidated.

Prostate development requires inductive and reciprocal interactions between the urogenital sinus epithelium and mesenchyme. In addition to mediating the effect of androgens on the developing prostatic epithelium, paracrine signals from the urogenital sinus mesenchyme appear to direct lobe-specific patterning of juxtaposed epithelium (Timms et al, 1995). The urogenital sinus mesenchyme, when combined with either embryonic or adult bladder epithelium (also a derivative of endodermal cloaca), stimulates formation of prostatic ducts. In contrast, the urogenital sinus mesenchyme combined with epithelia of other anatomic origins, such as seminal vesicle (a mesodermal derivative), salivary gland, or

esophagus, forms tissues with epithelial characteristics that resemble the anatomic origin of the partnering epithelium (Cunha et al, 1987). **These observations suggest that prostate development is spatially restricted by prostate-inducing paracrine signals from the urogenital sinus mesenchyme and that epithelial potential to respond to signals from the urogenital sinus mesenchyme is restricted to the endodermal epithelia of similar embryonic origin as the prostate.** The interactions between epithelium and mesenchyme are reciprocal. The presence of prostate epithelium plays a critical role in the differentiation of mesenchymal cells into the periductal smooth muscle cells (Hayward et al, 1998).

Several candidate genes have been implicated in prostate development, but the nature of paracrine mesenchymal factors that drive urogenital sinus epithelial transformation into prostatic ducts remains unknown. Furthermore, the precise relationship and the embryologic sequence of these candidate molecules have not been clearly defined. The Hox family of homeobox genes may be involved in the proper differentiation of male accessory sex glands including prostate (Podlasek et al, 1997, 1999b). In particular, Hoxa-13 and Hoxd-13 transcription factors are expressed in both urogenital sinus and nephric ducts, and the loss-of-function mutation of these genes in mice results in agenesis of bulbourethral glands and defective morphogenesis of the prostate and seminal vesicles. Two members of the FGF family of secreted proteins, FGF7 and FGF10, are expressed in the urogenital sinus mesenchyme. In vitro organ culture experiments have shown that exogenous FGF7 and FGF10 can stimulate proliferation and branching of developing prostate tissue, but these factors do not appear to be androgen responsive (Thomson and Cunha, 1999). There is also evidence that secreted factor activin A and its antagonistic binding protein follistatin may be important in the regulation of prostate epithelial development (Cancilla et al, 2001). Activin A is expressed in both urogenital sinus epithelium and mesenchyme, whereas its receptors are found in the epithelium. Follistatin, an activin A antagonist, is expressed in the urogenital sinus epithelium. Prostatic ductal growth and branching might therefore be a result of balanced interplay between activin A and follistatin. Other molecules implicated in prostate development include Bmp4 (Lamm et al, 2001), growth hormone receptor (Ruan et al, 1999), insulin-like growth factor 1 (Ruan et al, 1999), Nkx3.1 (Bhatia-Gaur et al, 1999), sonic hedgehog (Podlasek et al, 1999a), p63 (Signoretti et al, 2000), prolactin (Steger et al, 1998), hyaluronan (Gakunga et al, 1997), fucosyltransferase 1 (Marker et al, 2001), and urokinase plasminogen activator (Elfman et al, 2001).

Development of Female Genital Structures

In female embryos, the primitive sex cords do not contain the Y chromosome, do not elaborate SRY protein, and therefore do not differentiate into Sertoli cells. In the absence of Sertoli cells and SRY protein, therefore, MIS synthesis, Leydig cell differentiation, and androgen production do not occur. Consequently, male development of the genital ducts and accessory glands is not stimulated, and female development ensues. In females, the primitive sex cords degenerate, and the mesothelium of the genital ridge forms the secondary cortical sex cords. These secondary sex cords invest the primordial germ cells to form the ovarian follicles. The germ cells differentiate into oogonia and enter the first meiotic division as primary oocytes. The follicle cells then arrest further germ cell development until puberty, at which point individual oocytes resume gametogenesis in response to a monthly surge of gonadotropins.

In the absence of MIS and androgens, the nephric (wolffian) ducts degenerate, and the paramesonephric (müllerian) ducts give rise to the fallopian tubes, uterus, and upper two thirds of the vagina. The remnants of nephric ducts are found in the mesentery of the ovary as the epoöphoron and paroöphoron and near the vaginal introitus and anterolateral vaginal wall as Gartner's duct cysts. The distal tips of the paramesonephric ducts adhere to each other just before they make contact with the posterior wall of the urogenital sinus. The wall of the urogenital sinus at this point forms a small thickening called the sinusal tubercle. As soon as the fused tips of the paramesonephric ducts connect with the sinusal tubercle, the paramesonephric ducts begin to fuse in a caudal to cranial direction, forming a tube with a single lumen. This tube, called the uterovaginal canal, becomes the superior portion of the vagina and the uterus. The unfused, superior portions of the paramesonephric ducts become the fallopian tubes (oviducts), and the funnel-shaped superior openings of the paramesonephric ducts become the infundibula.

While the uterovaginal canal is forming during the 3rd month, the endodermal tissue of the sinusal tubercle in the posterior urogenital sinus continues to thicken, forming a pair of swellings called the sinovaginal bulbs. These structures give rise to the lower third of the vagina. The most inferior portion of the uterovaginal canal becomes occluded transiently by a block of tissue called the vaginal plate. The origin of the vaginal plate is not clear; it may arise from the sinovaginal bulbs, from the walls of the paramesonephric ducts, from the nearby mesonephric ducts, or from a combination of these tissues. The vaginal plate elongates between the 3rd and 5th month and subsequently becomes canalized to form the inferior vaginal lumen (Fig. 106–23).

As the vaginal plate forms, the lower end of the vagina lengthens, and its junction with the urogenital sinus migrates caudally until it comes to rest on the posterior wall of definitive urogenital sinus (future vestibule of the vagina) during the 4th month. An endodermal membrane temporarily separates the vaginal lumen from the cavity of the definitive urogenital sinus. This barrier degenerates partially after the 5th month, but its remnant persists as the vaginal hymen. The mucous membrane that lines the vagina and cervix may also derive from the endodermal epithelium of the definitive urogenital sinus.

Development of External Genitalia

Unlike the rest of the developing embryo, the cloacal membrane, along with the oropharyngeal membrane (future oral cavity), is a bilayered structure in which the outer ectoderm remains in close contact with the underlying endoderm

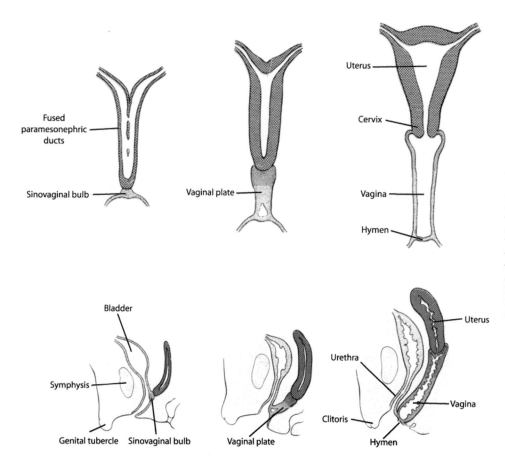

Figure 106–23. Development of uterus and vagina. During the 10th week, the paramesonephric ducts fuse at their caudal ends to establish a common channel and come into contact with a thickened portion of the posterior urogenital sinus called the sinovaginal bulb. This is followed by development of the vaginal plate, which elongates between the 3rd and 5th months and becomes canalized to form the inferior vaginal lumen. (Modified from Sadler TW: Langman's Medical Embryology. Baltimore, Williams & Wilkins, 1985.)

without the intervening mesoderm. Initially, the cloacal membrane represents an elongated midline structure that extends from the root of the umbilical cord to the future site of perineum distally. During the subsequent development, **this bilayered cloacal membrane "retracts" into the perineum as a result of cranial and medial migration of mesodermal cells into the anterior body wall between the ectoderm and the endoderm layers of the cloacal membrane.** This mesenchymal migration brings about the closure of the inferior part of the anterior abdominal wall and causes the caudal portion of the cloacal membrane to position itself in the perineal region. These migrating mesodermal cells give rise to the musculature of the medial portion of the anterior abdominal wall, the mesenchymal portion of the anterior bladder wall, the pubic symphysis, and the rudiments of the external genitalia (Vermeij-Keers et al, 1996). Failure of migration of these mesodermal cells into the midline results in bladder exstrophy and other associated genital defects (Langer, 1993; Vermeij-Keers et al, 1996).

The early development of the external genitalia is similar in both sexes. Migrating mesenchymal cells spread themselves around the cloacal membrane and pile up to form swellings. Early in the 5th week, a pair of swellings called *cloacal folds* develops on either side of the cloacal membrane. These folds meet just anterior to the cloacal membrane to form a midline swelling called the *genital tubercle* (Fig. 106–24). During the cloacal division into the anterior urogenital sinus and the posterior anorectal canal, the portion of the cloacal folds flanking the opening of the urogenital sinus becomes the *urogenital folds*, and the portion flanking the opening of the anorectal canal becomes the *anal folds*. A new pair of swellings, called the labioscrotal folds, then appear on either side of the urogenital folds.

The most popular hypothesis of external genital and urethral development is based upon work performed in the early part of the 20th century. Most embryology texts today quote the mechanism of urethral development proposed by Glenister (1954). As the genital tubercle elongates in males, a groove appears on its ventral aspect (called the *urethral groove*) during the 6th week. In both sexes, an ectodermal epithelial tag is present at the tip of the genital tubercle. The urethral groove is defined laterally by urethral folds, which are continuations of the previous urogenital folds surrounding the urogenital membrane. Initially, the urethral groove extends only part of the way distally along the shaft of the elongating genital tubercle. The distal portion of the urethral groove terminates in a solid epithelial plate called the *urethral plate* that extends into the glans penis. The solid urethral plate canalizes and thus extends the urethral groove distally toward the glans. The urethral groove is thought to be lined by endoderm. Likewise, the solid urethral plate, the distal precursor of the urethral groove, is also believed to derive from the endodermal source. **Clearly, fusion of the urethral folds is the key step in the formation of the penile urethra.** A prerequisite of urethral fold fusion is the canalization of the solid urethral plate and formation of the urethral groove bounded on each side by the urethral folds. If the urethral groove and urethral fold formations are abnormal, the urethral fold fusion is likely to be impaired as well (Figs. 106–25 and 106–26).

The formation of the distal glanular urethra may occur by a combination of two separate processes—the fusion of urethral folds proximally and the ingrowth of ectodermal cells distally. It is generally thought that the stratified squamous epithelium of the fossa navicularis results from an ingrowth of surface ectoderm as far proximally as the valve of Guérin. The lacuna magna (also known as the sinus of Guérin), which can give symptoms of hematuria and dysuria in some boys, may form as a result of dorsal extension of this ectodermal ingrowth. It was suggested that the entire penile urethra might differentiate from the fusion of the endodermal urethral groove through the mechanism of epithelial-mesenchymal interactions (Kurzrock et al, 1999).

The molecular basis of the sexual dimorphism in genital development is based upon the presence or absence of the signaling through the androgen receptor. As the fetal testicle produces testosterone, cells within the fetal external genitalia express the enzyme 5α–reductase, which converts testosterone to DHT. Androgen receptors are present in cells of the developing external genitalia and prominently expressed in the genital tubercle mesenchymal cells. The action of DHT through androgen receptors masculinizes the developing external genitalia. The key role of androgen in sexually dimorphic development of the external genitalia has been corroborated through many experimental studies. In utero exposure of rodents to antiandrogenic compounds reduces the size of the genital tubercle and prevents the development of the scrotum. Likewise, in utero exposure of rats to 5α–reductase inhibitors leads to the development of hypospadias. Mice and humans with functional loss of androgen receptors by mutations demonstrate complete feminization of the external genitalia.

The elongating phallus is covered externally by ectoderm that gives rise to the penile skin, and most of the substance of the penis is derived from mesodermal cells forming the

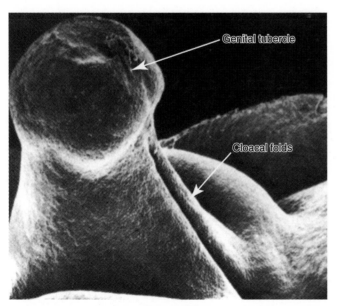

Figure 106–24. The early stages of cloacal fold development. (From Hamilton WJ, Mossman HW: Human Embryology Prenatal Development of Form and Function. New York, McMillan, 1976; Waterman RE: Human embryo and fetus. In Hafez ESE, Kenemans P [eds]: Atlas of Human Reproduction. Hinghman, Mass, Kluwer Boston, 1982.)

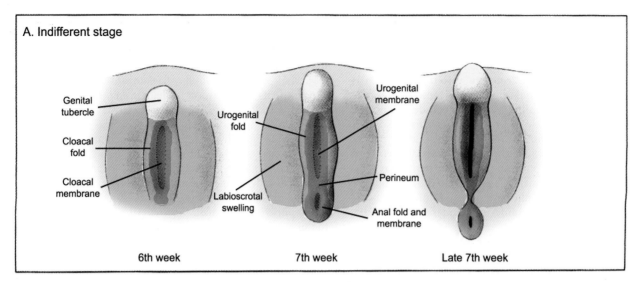

A. Indifferent stage

Genital tubercle

Cloacal fold

Cloacal membrane

Urogenital fold

Labioscrotal swelling

Urogenital membrane

Perineum

Anal fold and membrane

6th week

7th week

Late 7th week

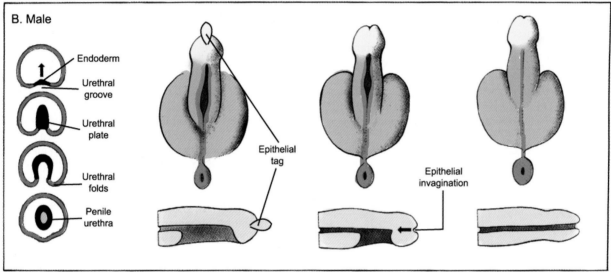

B. Male

Endoderm

Urethral groove

Urethral plate

Urethral folds

Penile urethra

Epithelial tag

Epithelial invagination

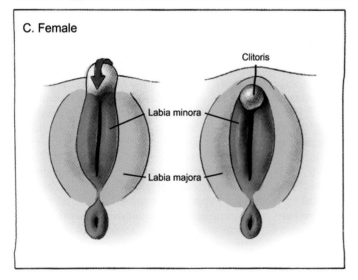

C. Female

Clitoris

Labia minora

Labia majora

Figure 106–25. Development of external genitalia in male and female. **A,** The external genitalia derive from a pair of labioscrotal swellings, a pair of urogenital folds, and an anterior genital tubercle. Male and female genitalia are morphologically indistinguishable until the 7th week. **B,** In males, the urogenital folds fuse, and the genital tubercle elongates to form the penile shaft and glans. A small region of the distal urethra in the glans is formed by the invagination of surface epithelial tag. The fused labioscrotal folds give rise to the scrotum. **C,** In females, the genital tubercle bends inferiorly to form the clitoris, and the urogenital folds remain separate to become the labia minora. The unfused labioscrotal folds form the labia majora. (Modified from Larsen WJ: Human Embryology. New York, Churchill Livingstone, 1997.)

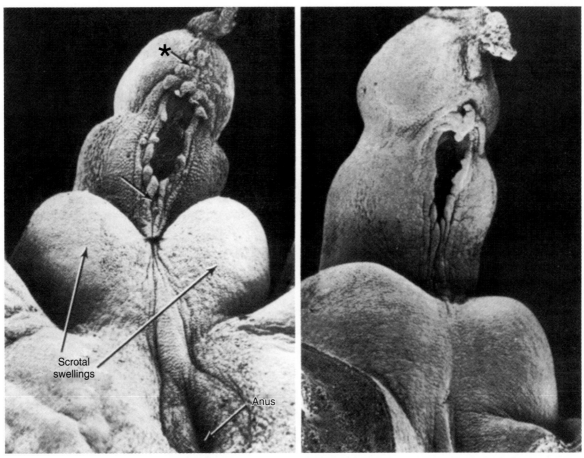

Figure 106–26. The epithelial tag and fusing urethral folds in the developing male external genital. (From Waterman RE: Human embryo and fetus. In Hafez ESE, Kenemans P [eds]: Atlas of Human Reproduction. Hingham, Mass, Kluwer Boston, 1982.)

corporal bodies, connective tissue, and dermis. Corporal tissue is first recognized as distinct dense mesenchymal condensations within the shaft of the developing penis. Little is known regarding the molecular regulatory mechanisms of the differentiation of penile mesenchyme into its various derivatives, but it is likely that this process is dependent upon epithelial-mesenchymal interactions.

In the female, because of absence of androgen receptor signaling through DHT, the primitive perineum does not lengthen, and the labioscrotal and urethral folds do not fuse across the midline. The phallus bends inferiorly, becoming the clitoris, and the ostium of the urogenital membrane becomes the vestibule of the vagina. The urethral folds become the labia minora, and the labioscrotal folds become the labia majora. The external genitalia develop in a similar manner in genetic males who are deficient in 5α-reductase and therefore lack DHT.

Gonadal Descent

Morphologically, the human urogenital ridge is identical in both sexes at 7 to 8 weeks of gestation. **Prior to gonadal differentiation, the testicle lies near the developing kidney, loosely held in place by two ligamentous structures. The dorsal ligament is referred to as the cranial suspensory ligament (CSL), whereas the ventral ligament later develops** into the gubernaculum (Fig. 106–27). Between 10 and 15 weeks, the testicle remains close to the future inguinal region during the enlargement of the abdominal cavity, and the ovary moves more cranially. **The testicle is anchored near the inguinal region by both enlargement of the gubernaculum and regression of the CSL.** As early as the 1700s, enlargement of the gubernaculum in males was observed to tether the testicle near the groin while the kidney migrated cranially (Wyndham, 1943; van der Schoot, 1993). In females, the CSL continues to develop, keeping the ovary close to the kidney, while the gubernaculum involutes. In males, androgen induces resorption of CSL, while the gubernaculum enlarges to become a plump ligamentous body, "holding" the testicle close to the inguinal region. Starting in the 7th month, the gubernaculum begins to bulge beyond the external inguinal ring and descends to the scrotal location, while, simultaneously, it is hollowed out by the evaginating peritoneal diverticulum called the processus vaginalis (Heyns, 1987). The processus vaginalis allows the intra-abdominal testicle to exit the abdominal cavity. The bulky distal end of the gubernaculum (known as the bulb) is resorbed in humans after completion of inguinoscrotal migration.

Caudal enlargement of the gubernaculum during the early relative transabdominal movement of the testicle is known as the "swelling reaction" or "gubernacular outgrowth." The proximal gubernacular cord appears to shorten

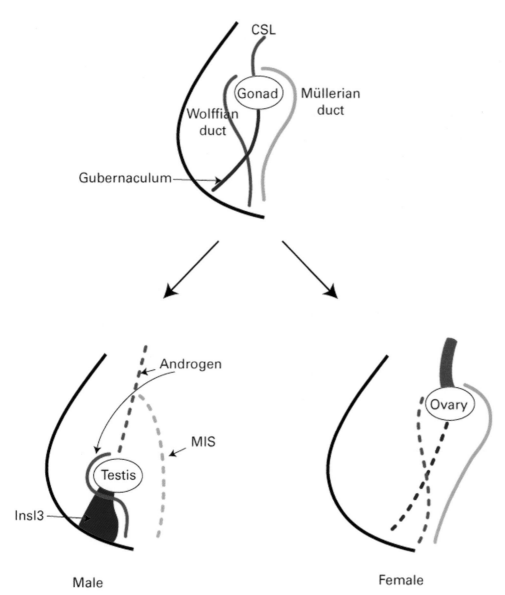

Male

Female

Figure 106–27. Mechanism of gonadal descent. The undifferentiated gonad is initially located high in the abdomen, anchored by the cranial suspensory ligament (CSL). In males, Insl3 causes the swelling and enlargement of gubernaculum to pull the developing testicle toward the inguinal region, and androgens cause an involution of CSL. Because of the action of müllerian inhibiting substance (MIS), müllerian ducts regress, while androgens continue to stimulate the development of wolffian ducts into male genital ductal structures. In females, CSL persists because of the absence of androgens, and gubernaculum remains thin because of the absence of Insl3 activity, thereby keeping the ovary well within the pelvis.

during this process as it becomes incorporated into the enlarging bulb (Wensing, 1986). Shortening of the cord may be an important mechanism to position the testicle over the inguinal ring to permit abdominal pressure to push the testicle out of the abdomen (Quinlan et al, 1988; Attah and Hutson, 1993; Husmann and Levy, 1995). Transection of the gubernacular cord can lead to either accidental testicular descent into the contralateral inguinal canal or aberrant intra-abdominal location (Frey and Rajfer, 1984; Beasley and Hutson, 1988; Attah and Hutson, 1993).

Although intra-abdominal pressure may not be a factor during the initial transabdominal descent, it is thought to be important during transit through the inguinal canal and the subsequent scrotal migration. Inguinoscrotal descent requires migration of the gubernaculum over a considerable distance, along with an increase in the length of the processus vaginalis. The force for movement may come from intra-abdominal pressure, transmitted directly and indirectly to the testicle by the lumen of the processus vaginalis and the gubernacular cord, respectively.

Although patients with defective androgen production or metabolism show varied manifestations of cryptorchidism, the exact role of androgen in testicular descent still remains unclear. During intra-abdominal testicular descent, androgen appears to play a role in the regression of CSL (van der Schoot, 1992). Gubernacular enlargement, in contrast, seems to be independent of androgen activity because it occurs in androgen-resistant mice and humans normally, being able to keep the testicle close to the inguinal region (Hutson, 1985). The second migratory step—the inguinoscrotal phase—is thought to be more androgen dependent. Migration of the gubernaculum beyond the inguinal region is absent in gonadotropin-deficient mice (Grocock et al, 1988) and those with complete androgen resistance (Hutson, 1986). Regression of the gubernacular bulb after completion of scrotal descent also appears to be androgen dependent because in humans with androgen resistance the gubernaculum remains enlarged (Hutson, 1986).

MIS is a glycoprotein produced and secreted by Sertoli cells and is responsible for regression of the müllerian ducts

(Josso et al, 1993; Lee and Donahoe, 1993). Evidence for the role of MIS in testicular descent is conflicting. Some clinical observations support the role of MIS, including patients with persistent müllerian duct syndrome caused by genetic defects of MIS or its receptor gene (Josso et al, 1983). In this clinical scenario, the testicles are undescended, and the gubernaculum is thin and elongated. Transgenic mice with MIS deficiency show a variable testicular position depending on their androgenic status: those with normal androgen receptors have normally descended testicles whereas those with androgen resistance have completely undescended testicles (Behringer et al, 1994). A study of MIS receptor knockout mice, however, failed to show any defect in gubernacular development and testicular positions (Bartlett et al, 2002).

INSL3 was identified as a novel gene product of the Leydig cells in 1993 (Adham et al, 1993). INSL3 is similar in structure to the peptide hormones relaxin and insulin and is expressed in both fetal and adult Leydig cells in a differentiation-dependent manner (Balvers et al, 1998). **Mice lacking a functional *Insl3* gene demonstrate intra-abdominal cryptorchidism but otherwise no obvious defects in other male reproductive organs. More important, early surgical correction of cryptorchidism in these mice can restore normal fertility potential** (Nef and Parada, 1999; Zimmermann et al, 1999). These are important findings because they reflect a phenotype most commonly observed in classical cryptorchidism in humans. A G protein–coupled receptor, LGR8, has been cloned with binding and functional response to INSL3 in transfected cells (Hsu et al, 2002; Kumagai et al, 2002). Moreover, mutations in this receptor in mice can lead to the development of cryptorchidism and have been linked to a cryptorchidism case in a human (Overbeek et al, 2001; Gorlov et al, 2002). Treatment of rat gubernacular explant with exogenous INSL3 led to rapid growth of the ligament, an effect that synergized with androgen treatment (Kubota et al, 2002). It was also demonstrated that LGR8 was expressed in the rat gubernaculum (Kubota et al, 2002). Although INSL3 appears to be a good candidate for a gene responsible for cryptorchidism, to date no causative mutations have been identified in the human INSL3 gene. Furthermore, because INSL3 is expressed in a differentiated testicle, any factor that influences Leydig cell differentiation may also affect INSL3 expression and thereby cause cryptorchidism.

Treatment of pregnant mothers with diethylstilbestrol as a hormonal support during pregnancy was abandoned because of a high rate of cryptorchidism and other genital defects (Stillman, 1982). The effect of environmental xenoestrogenic compounds has also been linked to the reported rise in cryptorchidism in humans (Toppari and Skakkebaek, 1998). In a more recent study, mice were treated with diethylstilbestrol to induce cryptorchidism in male newborns (Emmen et al, 2000; Nef et al, 2000). Interestingly, the treated animals demonstrated complete suppression of testicular *Insl3* expression on embryonic days 16 and 18.

The male knockout mice for the transcription factor Hoxa-10 gene are viable but infertile. Although they are normally virilized, they are bilaterally cryptorchid with severely underdeveloped gubernaculum. Fetal localization studies have shown that Hoxa-10 is expressed in the gubernaculum as well as in the kidneys but not in other reproductive tissues.

Although its function and role are not yet established, it appears to be another candidate regulatory gene for gubernacular development and testicular descent.

The spinal nucleus of the genitofemoral nerve (GFN) is located at L1-2 in the spinal cord and is sexually dimorphic (Goh et al, 1994). Transection of GFN produced cryptorchidism (Lewis, 1948), and the initial thought—now proved faulty—was that the cremasteric muscle paralysis caused by denervation led to abnormal traction of the testicle through the inguinal canal. When this observation was revisited many years later, it was speculated that androgens may act through the GFN nerve (Beasley and Hutson, 1987). The GFN innervates the gubernaculum from its posterior and caudal surface, so that distal transection would cause denervation of the gubernaculum (Tayakkanonta, 1963). Additional supporting evidence for the role of GFN comes from the analysis of patients with spina bifida and animals with spinal cord transection (Hutson et al, 1988). Of more than 300 boys with spina bifida, 23% had cryptorchidism, with a higher incidence found in those whose defect was higher than L4. In rats with neonatal spinal cord transection, approximately 40% had cryptorchidism when the lesions were midlumbar. Anatomic studies of the GFN identified calcitonin gene–related peptide (CGRP) as the primary neurotransmitter (Goh et al, 1994). The effect of CGRP on the rodent gubernaculum has been studied extensively. In male neonatal rats under anesthesia, the gubernaculum, which has not yet reached the scrotum, contracts rhythmically, and this is enhanced by increased intra-abdominal pressure and direct application of exogenous CGRP (Park and Hutson, 1991). In organ culture, neonatal rat gubernaculum responds to CGRP in a dose-dependent manner but not to other neuropeptides (Park and Hutson, 1991). Although these findings are raising a strong speculation for the role of CGRP, its significance in human testicular descent remains uncertain.

The ovaries also descend and become suspended within the broad ligaments of the uterus. As in males, the female embryos develop a gubernaculum-like structure extending initially from the inferior pole of the gonad to the subcutaneous fascia of the presumptive labioscrotal folds. This "female gubernaculum" later penetrates the abdominal wall as part of a fully formed inguinal canal and becomes the *round ligament*. In females, although the gubernaculum does not shorten like that in males, it still causes the ovaries to descend during the 3rd month (by anchoring the ovaries in the pelvis) and places them into a peritoneal fold (the *broad ligament of the uterus*). This translocation of ovaries appears to occur during the 7th week when the gubernaculum becomes attached to the developing paramesonephric (müllerian) ducts. As the paramesonephric ducts fuse together in their caudal ends, they sweep out the broad ligaments and simultaneously pull the ovaries into these peritoneal folds. In the absence of androgens, the female gubernaculum remains intact and grows in step with the rest of the body. The inferior gubernaculum becomes the round ligament of the uterus and attaches the fascia of the labia majora to the uterus, and the superior gubernaculum becomes the ligament of the ovary, connecting the uterus to the ovary. As in males, the processus vaginalis of the inguinal canal is normally obliterated, but occasionally it remains patent to become an indirect inguinal hernia.

Molecular Mechanism of Sexual Differentiation

Mammalian sexual development involves a complex interplay of multiple cell types, all occurring in a narrow window of time. Thus, it is important to understand the temporal and spatial pattern of gene expression as well as the anatomic sequence of tissue movement and differentiation. In both sexes, before the expression of male-determining gene *SRY*, a number of factors appear to play a role in urogenital ridge specification (Fig. 106–28). Because the urogenital ridge is the primordium for gonad, kidney, and reproductive tract, multiples organs are affected simultaneously by mutations of these genes.

In the mouse gonad, *Wt1* (Wilms' tumor 1) is expressed early, suggesting a role in specifying coelomic epithelial cells in the development of urogenital ridge. *Wt1* homozygous knockout mice do not form kidney, adrenal, or gonad (Kreidberg et al, 1993). Humans heterozygous for mutations in the *WT-1* gene exhibit abnormalities of the genital system in addition to abnormalities in renal development, including WAGR syndrome, Denys-Drash syndrome, and Frasier syndrome. Wt1 appears to function upstream of Sf1 (steroidogenic factor 1) and Dax1 (dosage-sensitive sex reversal, adrenal hypopla-

sia congenita, X chromosome) (Wilhelm and Englert, 2002). Wt1 and Sf1 enhance transcription of mouse MIS gene, whereas Dax1 appears to suppress this interaction (Nachtigal et al, 1998). Sf1 also regulates the expression of other genes involved in male differentiation, steroidogenesis, and reproduction (Achermann et al, 2001). While Sf1 stimulates Dax1 transcription (Ikeda et al, 1996), Dax1 in turn acts as a transcriptional repressor of Sf1-regulated genes (Ito et al, 1997). In Sf1 knockout mice, neither XX nor XY animals form gonads, and cells in the gonadal remnant undergo apoptosis, suggesting that Sf1 is a necessary survival factor for early progenitors of the developing gonad (Luo et al, 1994). Data suggest that Sf1 and Dax1 are both independently important for normal male gonadal differentiation. Other candidate genes have also emerged based on mouse gene deletion models and embryonic expression studies, although their functional significance in gonadal development is not fully elucidated yet, and they include M33, Lhx9, Pod1, Dmrt1, Mro, Pn1, and Vn1 (Park and Jameson, 2005).

Mammalian embryos remain sexually undifferentiated until the time of sex determination. When the Y-linked master regulatory gene called *SRY* is expressed in the male, the epithelial cells of the primitive sex cords differentiate into Sertoli cells, and this critical morphogenetic event

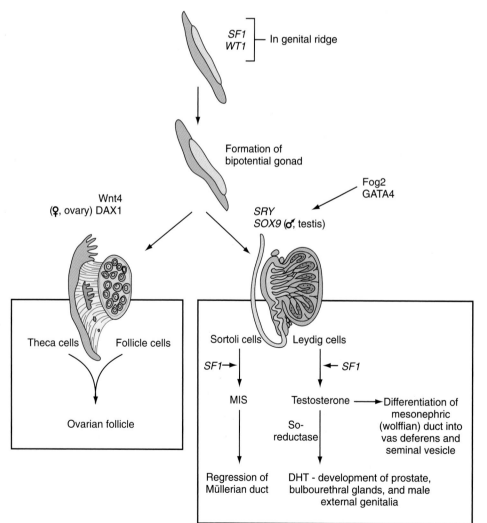

Figure 106–28. Molecular mechanism of male and female genital development. SF1 and WT1 expression is critical for genital ridge specification. SRY and SOX9, influenced by GATA4 and Fog2, are important factors for specifying the differentiation of Sertoli cells. SF1 is also critical in the regulation of MIS and other genes involved in androgen synthesis. No specific female factors have been identified, but Wnt4 and DAX1 are expressed with unique female patterns.

triggers subsequent testicular development. Once the testicles are established, they produce androgens to give rise to the male phenotype. In the female gonads, no morphologic change is observable at the time of SRY expression. It follows from this general picture that in mammals, sex determination is synonymous with testicle development, with the differentiation of Sertoli cells being the key event (McLaren, 1991). After three decades of search for the elusive mammalian testicle-determining gene, the *SRY* gene was discovered in 1990 by Sinclair and colleagues (see Fig. 106–28). Since then, research has focused on identifying the putative regulatory mechanisms operating downstream of *SRY* and the genetic control of SRY expression.

Although it has been known since 1921 that human males have an X and a Y chromosome, the role of these "sex" chromosomes in human sexual determination was not elucidated until 1959. This question was answered by the examination of two individuals with unique chromosome abnormalities: one female with Turner syndrome (45,X0 karyotype) and one male with Klinefelter syndrome (47,XXY karyotype). By 1966, analysis of many structurally aberrant Y chromosomes in humans led to the conclusion that the information necessary to initiate male phenotypic development was present on the short arm of the Y chromosome. The identity of the protein encoded by the testis-determining region of the Y chromosome proved elusive. In the mid-1980s, the DNA of sex-reversed males with 46,XX karyotype was examined. The genome in these individuals was found to contain small amounts of Y chromosome that had been translocated onto the X chromosome. Analysis of this DNA narrowed the location of the SRY to a relatively small region within the short arm.

The role of SRY in human sex determination has been further supported by studies using mice (Greenfield and Koopman, 1996). The comparable genetic locus in mice (*Sry*) is activated and expressed in the genital ridge 11.5 days after coitus, just before the initiation of testicular development. Moreover, when the DNA of female XY mouse chromosomes was analyzed with specific DNA probes for *Sry*, this locus was absent. Most important, it has been demonstrated that insertion of *Sry* into one of the X chromosomes of genetically female mouse embryos converted these mice to phenotypic males. These transgenic "female" mice exhibited testicles, vas deferens, and absence of the female reproductive tract. It was thought that identification of the SRY protein would rapidly lead to the identity of downstream elements regulating male sexual development. However, the binding of SRY protein to other genes or factors has not been demonstrated, and the molecular mechanism by which genes interact to determine sex remains speculative. Deletions of the *SRY* gene in humans cause XY male-to-female sex reversal, whereas *SRY* translocations to the X chromosome lead to XX female-to-male sex reversal (Harley et al, 2003). In mice, transgenic expression of *Sry* is sufficient to induce male differentiation in an XX background (Koopman et al, 1991). In the mouse, *Sry* expression occurs in a narrow temporal window in the developing Sertoli cells. The central region of the gonad demonstrates *Sry* expression first, followed by cephalad to caudal progression along the entire length of the gonad (Bullejos and Koopman, 2001).

A closely related gene, *Sox9*, is one other definitive male-determining gene identified thus far. *Sry* expression and *Sox9*

expression overlap in cells of the Sertoli lineage. As the *Sry* expression diminishes, *Sox9* expression increases in the male. *Sox9*, which is weakly expressed in the undifferentiated gonad, is downregulated in the female (Sekido et al, 2004). Transgenic expression of *Sox9* in XX mice is sufficient to induce female-to-male sex reversal and male differentiation (Vidal et al, 2001). Heterozygous human SOX9 mutation leads to camptomelic dysplasia, a severe skeletal disorder with defective cartilage development, and many of these patients have dysgenetic gonads (Foster et al, 1994). These individuals possess a normal SRY but may exhibit completely feminized genital structures. *Sox9* knockout embryos have elevated levels of *Sry* expression, suggesting a possible negative feedback regulatory loop that downregulates *Sry* (Chaboissier et al, 2004). GATA4 and Fog2 are important in cardiac development but also appear to affect gonadal development. GATA4 mutation eliminates expression of male differentiation markers Sox9 and MIS. Fog2 knockout mice have decreased expression of Sry, loss of Sox9, MIS, and desert hedgehog but persistence of the female gonad marker Wnt4 (Tevosian et al, 2002). Similarly, triple mutants for insulin receptor, insulin-related receptor, and Igf1 receptor have low *Sry* and *Sox9* expression and exhibit male-to-female sex reversal, implicating a role for the insulin signaling pathway (Nef et al, 2003).

Proliferation of Sertoli progenitor cells is an important event in male gonad development, a process driven by SRY expression (Schmahl et al, 2000). One paracrine factor linked to this proliferation is FGF9. *Fgf9* knockout mice demonstrate varying degrees of male-to-female sex reversal (Colvin et al, 2001). In addition, FGF9 is a candidate male gonad-specific chemoattractant paracrine signal that induces migration of cells from the mesonephros (endothelial and peritubular myoid cells) into the gonad (Martineau et al, 1997). Migration of these cells is critical for the development of testis cord formation (Buehr et al,1993) as well as *Sox9* expression (Tilmann and Capel, 1999). Such migration is absent in females, presumably because of absence of chemoattractants.

Once sex determination has occurred, the subsequent phenotypic differentiation depends mostly on the production of androgens. As bipotential gonad differentiates into testicle, *Sf1* expression becomes restricted to Leydig cells and mediates expression of several genes encoding enzymes that are required for testosterone biosynthesis, including StAR, Cyp11a1, Cyp17, and 3βHSD. Factors for Leydig cell determination are not known, and Leydig cell origin, whether from immigrant mesonephric cells or progenitors within gonad, remains speculative. There is evidence that Leydig cell fate is dependent on paracrine signals (Yao et al, 2002; Brennan et al, 2003).

Relatively few genes have been shown to exhibit a female-specific pattern of gene expression early in gonadal development. Thus far, no female determining gene has been identified. The *Dax1* gene was initially suggested as a pro-ovarian (or antitesticle) candidate gene because its duplication on an XY background was associated with impaired testicular development (Bardoni et al, 1994; Swain et al, 1998). However, loss of *Dax1* in an XX background does not prevent ovary development (Yu et al, 1998). A growing list of genes demonstrate ovary-specific expression patterns, including Fst and Stra8 (Park and Jameson, 2005). There has been a postulate of a "Z-factor" that suppresses protesticular events in both XX and XY backgrounds (McElreavey et al, 1993). According to this hypothesis, the Z-factor, which normally suppresses testicle determination, is repressed by SRY in males, and in females, because of the absence of SRY, it inhibits testicle development. Loss of Z-factor in an XX background results in female-to-male sex reversal, but gain of function in an XY background may or may not result in male-to-female sex reversal depending upon whether the Z-factor can override the suppression effect of SRY-driven signaling. One candidate for such a Z-factor is Wnt4. XX mice deficient for *Wnt4* develop testicle-like differentiation and wolffian duct derivatives (Vainio et al, 1999). Curiously, their external genitalia remain female. Furthermore, Wnt4 is downregulated in males, whereas its expression remains strong in females (Yao et al, 2004).

KEY POINTS: NORMAL DEVELOPMENT OF THE UROGENITAL SYSTEM

- The urogenital system develops from three embryonic sources—intermediate mesoderm, mesothelium of coelomic (future peritoneum) cavity, and endoderm of the urogenital sinus.

- The urinary system begins its development before the genital system development becomes evident. With the formation of nephric ducts, embryonic kidneys develop sequentially in the order of pronephros, mesonephros, and metanephros.

- The permanent kidney, metanephros, develops as a result of inductive interactions involving ureteric bud (an outgrowth of nephric duct), condensing blastema of metanephric mesenchyme, and stromal cells. The renal tubulogenesis occurs through mesenchymal-epithelial conversion, and dichotomous branching of the ureteric bud leads to the formation of collecting system.

- The nephric ducts, also known as the wolffian ducts, establish and maintain contacts with the developing bladder, and their terminal portion, along with the origin of ureteric bud, becomes incorporated to become the trigone of the bladder.

- The bladder and urethra develop from the endodermal urogenital sinus, which is an anterior portion of the cloaca after it becomes separated from the posterior anorectal canal.

- Morphologically, the genital development takes place about 3 weeks after the start of the urinary system development. Sexual dimorphism begins to take shape at about the 7th week. Primordial germ cells migrate from the wall of the yolk sac to invade the posterior mesenchyme to establish the gonadal ridge.

- In males, driven by the SRY gene of the Y chromosome, mesenchymal cells of developing testicle differentiate to become the Sertoli cells. Sertoli cells produce müllerian inhibitory substance (MIS) to cause degeneration of female müllerian ductal structures, while stimulating the development of testosterone-producing Leydig cells. Under the influence of testosterone, male external genitalia develop, as well as prostate and other male accessory sex glands.

- Both gonads descend to pelvic location by the 3rd month, but the testicle descends into the scrotum with the aid of gubernaculum at about the 7th month.

SUGGESTED READINGS

Dressler GR: Tubulogenesis in the developing mammalian kidney. Trends Cell Biol 2002;12:390-395.

Ichikawa I, Kuwayama F, Pope JC IV, et al: Paradigm shift from classic anatomic theories to contemporary cell biological views of CAKUT. Kidney Int 2002;61:889-898.

Baskin LS, Hayward SW, Young P, et al: Role of mesenchymal-epithelial interactions in normal bladder development. J Urol 1996;156:1820-1827.

Park SY, Jameson JL: Transcriptional regulation of gonadal development and differentiation. Endocrinology 2005;146:1035-1042.

Hutson JM, Hasthorpe S, Heyns CF: Anatomical and functional aspects of testicular descent and cryptorchidism. Endocr Rev 1997;18:259-280.

Marker PC, Donjacour AA, Dahiya R, et al: Hormonal, cellular, and molecular control of prostatic development. Dev Biol 2003;253:165-174.

107 Renal Function in the Fetus, Neonate, and Child

ROBERT L. CHEVALIER, MD • JONATHAN A. ROTH, MD

The development of renal function in the fetus and neonate can be viewed as a continuing evolution of interdependent morphologic and physiologic stages. During gestation, the functional changes are determined by increases in nephron number, growth, and maturation while homeostasis of the fetus is maintained predominantly by the placenta. At birth, the kidney must suddenly assume this previously maternal role. The kidney's response to this demand is governed to a great extent by its anatomic development (gestational age at delivery), and thus important functional differences are seen in the premature and term neonate.

In this chapter we review the anatomic and functional aspects of fetal renal development, postnatal functional development, the evaluation of postnatal renal function, and the hormonal control of renal function during development through childhood.

ANATOMIC STAGES OF DEVELOPMENT

The major morphogenic stages of the human kidney appear quite early in development and, except for the last one, are transitory (Fig. 107–1). **The pronephros appears at 3 weeks, never progresses beyond a rudimentary stage, and involutes by 5 weeks. The mesonephros is seen at 5 weeks of gestation,** appears to have transitory function, and degenerates by 11 to 12 weeks. Its major role in renal development is related to the fact that its ductal system gives rise to the ureteric bud. The ureteric bud is critical for development of the metanephric or definitive kidney. Recent studies have revealed that apoptosis is a primary mechanism responsible for the sequential development of the mammalian kidney. Apoptosis is a physiologic, programmed cell death that normally mediates the deletion of "unwanted" cells, such as the disappearance of uninduced metanephric mesenchyme (Koseki et al, 1992). **The metanephros begins its inductive phase after 5 weeks of gestation; and, in the human, nephrogenesis follows a sigmoidal curve, with most rapid increase in mid gestation, and is completed by 34 to 36 weeks** (see Fig. 107–1). In the developing metanephric kidney there is a centrifugal pattern of nephrogenesis and maturation, with the outer cortical nephrons being the last to complete development.

FUNCTIONAL DEVELOPMENT IN THE FETUS

Information regarding the functional development of the metanephric kidney is gained primarily through animal studies. One must be careful in extrapolating such data from species in which there is dissimilarity of structural maturation at comparable gestational ages. **Urine production in the human kidney is known to begin around 10 to 12 weeks.** The placenta throughout gestation, however, primarily handles salt and water homeostasis.

Fetal renal blood flow increases gradually during the second half of pregnancy (Veille et al, 1993). The ratio of renal blood flow to cardiac output at 20 weeks is 0.03 compared with the postnatal ratio of 0.2 to 0.3 (Rudolph and Heymann, 1976). This diminished renal blood flow is probably related to several different factors. The number of vascular channels is low early in gestation, and there is increased arteriolar resistance in these channels (Ichikawa et al, 1979; Robillard et al, 1987). Studies in animals have demonstrated a role for renal innervation as well as the renin-angiotensin system as chronic modulators of this effect (Robillard et al, 1987). This will be discussed in greater detail later.

Glomerular filtration rate (GFR) in the fetus is theoretically equal to the single nephron GFR times the number of functioning glomeruli. This is difficult to determine however,

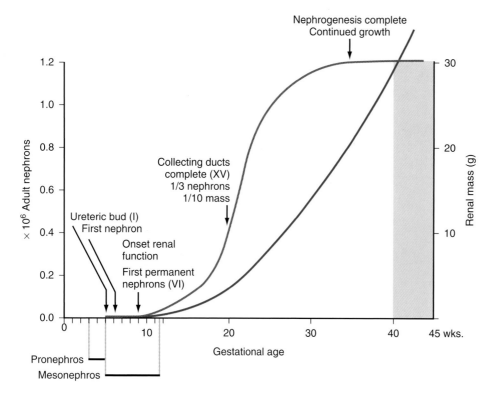

Figure 107–1. Human fetal renal development. The most rapid period of nephrogenesis occurs between 20 and 30 weeks' gestation *(red line)*. This is also the period of exponential increase in renal mass *(blue line)*. (From Harrison MR, Golbus MS, Filly RA, et al: Management of the fetus with congenital hydronephrosis. J Pediatr Surg 1982;17:739.)

because **GFR is much higher in juxtamedullary compared with subcortical glomeruli** (Spitzer and Brandis, 1974). GFR parallels renal mass and correlates with gestational age (Haycock, 1998).

Fractional excretion of sodium (FENa) shows a negative correlation with gestational age. **The fetus produces hypotonic urine with high sodium content and in large volumes.** Potassium excretion increases with gestation, which may be related to rises in fetal plasma aldosterone concentration. There is a maturational increase in glucose transport of the fetal kidneys. Other tubular functions such as bicarbonate reabsorption and acid production are low in the fetus. They are, however, responsive to parathyroid excretion, intravascular volume, and acid infusion, respectively.

KEY POINTS: FETAL RENAL DEVELOPMENT

- Nephrogenesis is complete by 34 weeks' gestational age in the fetus.

- Fetal urine production is normally 10 to 20 mL/kg/hr by the end of gestation.

- Regardless of gestational age, all infants normally void within the first 24 hours of birth.

- Neonatal GFR is dependent on gestational age and doubles in the first 2 weeks of life.

- In very low birth weight infants, GFR at birth is normally below 10 mL/min/1.73 m².

- Renal concentrating and acidifying capacity are reduced in the first 2 months of life.

EVALUATION OF FETAL RENAL FUNCTION

Human fetal renal blood flow can be measured by color-pulsed Doppler studies, which indicate that blood flow increases from approximately 20 mL/min at 25 weeks' gestation to more than 60 mL/min at 40 weeks' gestation (Veille et al, 1993). **Hourly human fetal urine production (determined by serial real-time bladder ultrasonography at 2- to 5-minute intervals) increases from 5 mL/hr at 20 weeks' gestation to 50 mL/hr at 40 weeks' gestation** (Fig. 107–2) (Rabinowitz et al, 1989). This extraordinary rate of diuresis would extrapolate to approximately 1 L/hr in the adult.

Owing to urinary dilution, the level of human fetal urine sodium is normally below 100 mEq/L, that of chloride is less than 90 mEq/L, and osmolality is less than 200 mOsm/L (Crombleholme et al, 1990). Although urine values greater than these in fetuses with obstructive nephropathy have been correlated with a poor prognosis, sequential fetal urine samples must be obtained, both before and after intrauterine bladder shunting, to improve the predictive value (Evans et al, 1991; Johnson et al, 1994).

More recently, urine total protein less than 20 mg/dL and β₂-microglobulin less than 4 mg/L have been shown to correlate with a favorable prognosis (Johnson et al, 1994). Other indices of tubular function include the measurement of amniotic fluid N-acetyl-β-D-glucosaminidase (NAG), which is an enzyme present in high concentration in proximal tubular cells, and fetal urine cystatin C, which is a marker of tubular damage in the fetus (Muller et al, 1999). Alterations of specific amino acids in fetal urine have also been used to identify fetuses with poor renal outcome (Pachi et al, 1993; Eugene et al, 1994). Increased amniotic fluid NAG has been correlated with renal impairment of intrauterine growth retardation

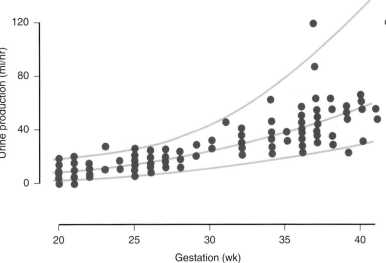

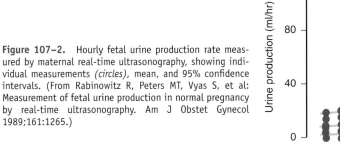

Figure 107–2. Hourly fetal urine production rate measured by maternal real-time ultrasonography, showing individual measurements *(circles)*, mean, and 95% confidence intervals. (From Rabinowitz R, Peters MT, Vyas S, et al: Measurement of fetal urine production in normal pregnancy by real-time ultrasonography. Am J Obstet Gynecol 1989;161:1265.)

(Pachi et al, 1993), and fetal urine valine concentration is increased in fetuses with bilateral renal dysplasia and fetal or neonatal death (Eugene et al, 1994).

POSTNATAL FUNCTIONAL DEVELOPMENT

At birth, several dramatic events occur that alter renal function. The kidney's response to the changing milieu and its success at maintaining homeostasis are heavily influenced by the gestational age at delivery. Intrauterine factors can also significantly affect postnatal renal functional development: intrauterine growth retardation can permanently reduce the number of functioning nephrons (Merlet-Benichou et al, 1994). This may lead to renal failure presenting at birth (Steele et al, 1988). Although nephrogenesis was presumed to progress after birth in extremely preterm infants, a recent report suggests that the formation of new nephrons ceases after 40 days and is further inhibited by renal failure (Rodriguez et al, 2004). These observations imply that long-term renal maturation is impaired in very low birth weight infants, even if there are no urinary tract anomalies or additional insults to the kidneys.

In a study of 500 normal neonates, Clark (1977) found that **every infant voided within the first 24 hours of life regardless of gestational age.** After the first 2 days of life, oliguria is generally defined as a urine flow rate less than 1 mL/kg/hr (Anand, 1982). However, infants receiving a restricted solute intake can remain in solute balance with urine flow rates as low as 0.5 mL/kg/hr.

The definition of polyuria is somewhat arbitrary, but any infant or child excreting more than 2000 mL/1.73 m² daily urine output should be evaluated further. It is important to distinguish pollakuria (urinary frequency) from polyuria in the child, because the former can be a sign of emotional stress rather than a pathologic process (Asnes and Mones, 1973; Zoubek et al, 1990).

Renal blood flow in the neonate is directly dependent on gestational age (Fig. 107–3) (Visser et al, 1992). Renal blood flow increases sharply at birth with a 5- to 18-fold rise in

different animal studies (Gruskin et al, 1970; Aperia and Herin, 1975). This reflects several factors. There is a redistribution of flow from the inner to the outer cortex (Aperia et al, 1977a) and a drop in renal vascular resistance associated with increased intrarenal levels of prostaglandins (Gruskin et al, 1970).

At birth, the GFR is below 10 mL/min/1.73 m² for infants with gestational age less than 34 weeks (the time for completion of nephrogenesis) and increases with gestational age to 40 weeks (Fig. 107–4) (Siegel and Oh, 1976). Because of the dependence of GFR on gestational age, for infants born before 34 weeks' gestation the GFR rises slowly. After reaching a post-conceptual age of 34 weeks, a rapid rise is then observed. After birth, GFR doubles during the first 2 weeks regardless of gestational age (Fig. 107–5) (Bueva and Guignard, 1994). Factors responsible for this rapid rise include diminished renal vascular resistance (Gruskin et al, 1970); increasing perfusion pressure, glomerular permeability, and filtration surface (John et al, 1981). In experimental animals, the increase in surface area for filtration accounts for most of the maturational increase in GFR (Spitzer and Brandis, 1974). Serum creatinine, which reflects maternal levels at birth, also decreases by 50% in the first week of life in term or near-term infants. Moreover, in very low birth weight infants, GFR does not catch up to that of age-matched term infants of the same postconceptional age until after 9 months of age (Vanpee et al, 1992).

In the neonate, tubular function changes inversely with the rise in GFR. At birth, FENa can be 2% in very low birth weight infants but is below 1% in term infants (Fig. 107–6) (Bueva and Guignard, 1994). **There remains a blunted response to sodium loading however, owing to a lack of increase in fractional excretion of sodium** (Kim and Mandell, 1988; Chevalier, 2001). This appears to be related to the high circulating renin, angiotensin, and aldosterone levels and to a diminished renal response to atrial natriuretic peptide (see later). Conversely, **premature infants less than 35 weeks' gestation, subject to sodium deprivation, may develop hyponatremia due to tubular immaturity and sodium wasting** (Roy et al, 1976; Engelke et al, 1978). **Thus, sodium supplementation is frequently required in premature infants.**

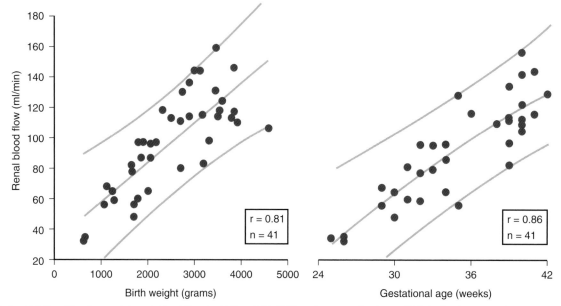

Figure 107-3. Relationship of neonatal renal blood flow to birth weight *(left)* and to gestational age *(right)*, showing regression ± 2 SD. (From Visser MO, Leighton JO, van de Bor M, Walther FJ: Renal blood flow in neonates: Quantification with color flow and pulsed Doppler US. Radiology 1992;183:443.)

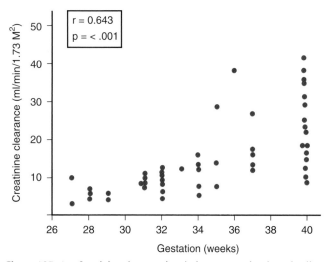

Figure 107-4. Creatinine clearance in relation to gestational age in clinically well infants studied from 24 to 40 hours after birth. (Reproduced from Siegel SR, Oh W: Renal function as a marker of human fetal maturation. Acta Paediatr Scand 1976;65:481-485.)

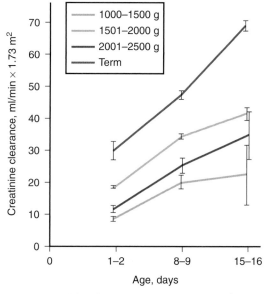

Figure 107-5. Creatinine clearance (corrected for 1.73 m² surface area) during the first 2 weeks of life for preterm and term neonates. (From Bueva A, Guignard JP: Renal function in preterm neonates. Pediatr Res 1994;36:574.)

In terms of concentrating ability, **the neonate can dilute urine fairly well (25 to 35 mOsm/L) but has limited concentrating capacity (600 to 700 mOsm/L)** (Hansen and Smith, 1953). The latter is even more restricted in the premature infant (500 mOsm/L). The factors responsible for this include anatomic immaturity of the renal medulla, decreased medullary concentration of sodium chloride and urea, and diminished responsiveness of the collecting ducts to antidiuretic hormone (Stanier, 1972; Schlondorff et al, 1978). By 2 months of age, term infants can generate urine concentrations exceeding 1000 mOsm/kg (Polacek, 1965); and by 9 years of age, maximal-concentrating ability of very low birth weight infants is not different from that of age-matched term infants (Vanpee et al, 1992).

Acid-base regulation in the neonate is characterized by a reduced threshold for bicarbonate reabsorption (Svenningsen, 1974). Bicarbonate reabsorption is gradually increased with increasing GFR. There is also an inability to respond to an acid load. This improves by 4 to 6 weeks postnatally and is accentuated in the premature infant who tends to be slightly acidotic when compared with the adult.

Glucose transport matures with the rising GFR in the neonate. This is more readily observed in the premature infant because fractional excretion of glucose is higher before 34 weeks of gestation (Arant, 1978).

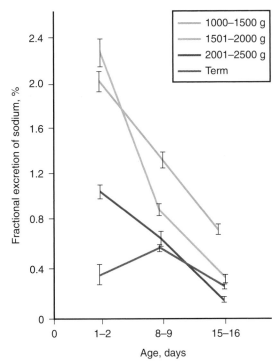

Figure 107–6. Fractional sodium excretion during the first 2 weeks of life for preterm and term neonates. (From Bueva A, Guignard JP: Renal function in preterm neonates. Pediatr Res 1994;36:575.)

Calcium and phosphate metabolism also changes shortly after birth. Parathyroid hormone (PTH) is suppressed at birth, and the serum calcium level falls. This secondarily causes an increase in PTH release. Initially, tubular reabsorption of phosphate is high in the premature infant and remains so until regular feedings commence at term (Arant, 1978).

Although not generally recognized, the renal interstitium also undergoes developmental changes. After the differentiation of the interstitial mesenchyme and apoptotic destruction of unwanted undifferentiated interstitial cells, interstitial fibroblasts undergo changes, with decreasing expression of α-smooth muscle actin and vimentin (Marxer-Meier et al, 1998). There is increasing evidence that the renal interstitium plays a crucial role in the maintenance of normal homeostasis, mediating crosstalk between tubular epithelial cells, extracellular matrix, fibroblasts, and endothelial cells (Fine et al, 1995; Zhuo et al, 1998). **Disruption of the interstitium by renal maldevelopment or injury (e.g., obstructive nephropathy) would clearly be expected to impair ongoing renal development and tubular transport** (Wolf, 1999).

EVALUATION OF RENAL FUNCTION IN THE INFANT AND CHILD
Glomerular Function

Measurement of GFR in the infant is problematic for a number of reasons. The primary difficulty is obtaining an accurately timed urine collection in the incontinent patient without bladder catheterization. The second is the inherent inaccuracy in measurement of the most readily available index of GFR, plasma creatinine concentration (PCr), because pre-

cision of the assay in most clinical laboratories is ± 0.3 mg/dL. Thus, calculated GFR in the infant can be overestimated or underestimated by 100% under the best circumstances of sample collections. The third is enhanced tubular creatinine reabsorption by the neonatal kidney (Guignard and Drukker, 1999). The fourth is the rapidly changing GFR with normal growth: GFR factored for adult surface area (1.73 m²) increases severalfold during the first 2 months of life. Within the first 2 days of life, PCr reflects maternal levels and may not reflect GFR of the infant. **By 7 days in the term infant, PCr concentration is normally less than 0.5 mg/dL, whereas in preterm infants levels can remain as high as 1.0 mg/dL for the first month of life** (Trompeter et al, 1983). In view of these considerations, it is important to obtain serial values of serum creatinine. A progressive increase in serum creatinine during the neonatal period suggests renal insufficiency regardless of gestational age.

Long-term monitoring of GFR in children with urologic abnormalities should account for increasing muscle mass, which results in increasing serum creatinine concentration with age. A simple and reliable estimate of creatinine clearance (CCr) can be derived from the serum creatinine concentration and the patient's height using the empirical formula developed by Schwartz and associates (1987):

$$CCr = k \times L/PCr$$

where CCr = creatinine concentration (mL/min/1.73 m²), k = a constant (0.33 for preterm, 0.45 for full-term infants, 0.55 for children), and L = body length (cm). **Although CCr is constant at 80 to 140 mL/min/1.73 m² after 2 years of age, the marked increase during the first 2 years of life should be taken into account when interpreting values for young infants. Estimation of GFR at 6 months of age is useful in predicting the long-term outcome of infants with renal dysplasia. Infants with GFR less than 15 mL/min/1.73 m² are at risk for early renal failure, whereas those with higher GFR have a more favorable prognosis** (Ismaili et al, 2001).

A more accurate determination of GFR can be obtained by creatinine clearance based on a 24-hour urine collection. As with the estimated CCr described earlier, the value should be corrected for adult surface area by multiplying by 1.73 and dividing by the patient's surface area (S.A., derived from a nomogram [Cole, 1984]) or using web-based calculators (available at either http://www.halls.md/body-surface -area/bsa.htm or http://www.ultradrive.com/bsac.htm). Thus,

CCr (mL/min/1.73 m²) = "uncorrected" CCr (mL/min)
$$\times 1.73/S.A.$$

Expression of all pediatric CCr in this fashion should reduce confusion and ambiguity in comparing the result to expected normal ranges. *Accuracy of the calculated CCr depends on adequacy of the timed urine collection.*

For more precise measurement of GFR, and to determine the relative contribution of each kidney to total GFR, a radiolabeled tracer that is cleared solely by glomerular filtration can be infused intravenously and plasma concentration of the isotope can be measured sequentially with concurrent scintigraphy. An agent frequently used for this purpose is ⁹⁹ᵐTc-diethylenetriaminepentaacetic acid (Tc-DTPA). As with CCr, measurement of GFR by Tc-DTPA clearance should be corrected for adult surface area as described earlier.

Tubular Function

Sodium Excretion

In the fetus and neonate, external sodium balance is positive as a consequence of sodium accretion necessary for rapid growth (Chevalier, 2001). In older infants and children, however, urinary sodium excretion is generally equivalent to sodium intake as long as the patient is in a steady state. **The 24-hour urine sodium excretion, therefore, reflects the quantity of sodium ingested over the previous day and is normally 1 to 3 mEq/kg/day.** Patients with obligatory renal sodium losses ("salt wasting") must increase sodium intake to compensate for these ongoing losses. A diagnosis of salt-wasting nephropathy must be made while the patient is maintained on a restricted sodium intake (less than 1 mEq/kg/day) for 3 to 5 days. To prevent dangerous volume depletion or hyponatremia, the patient's blood pressure, weight, urine output, and serum sodium concentration should be closely monitored during the study. The 24-hour urine sodium excretion can also be helpful in monitoring compliance of patients on a restricted sodium intake (e.g., patients with hypertension, nephrogenic diabetes insipidus, or nephrotic syndrome). Those with sodium excretion greater than 3 mEq/kg/day may be counseled to improve their diets.

Of even greater clinical utility, the FENa can be used to isolate the tubular from the glomerular contribution to sodium excretion. This may be used to distinguish "prerenal" causes of oliguria from "renal parenchymal" or "postrenal" causes. A timed urine collection is not necessary, because sodium and creatinine concentration can be measured in a random urine sample (UNa, UCr) and concurrent plasma sample (PNa, PCr):

$$FENa = 100\%(UNa \times PCr)/(PNa \times UCr)$$

In the oliguric neonate (urine flow < 1 mL/kg/hr), FENa less than 2.5% suggests a prerenal condition (Mathew et al, 1980), **whereas in the older infant or child, a value below 1% is consistent with prerenal oliguria.** Similar criteria can be used to differentiate causes of hyponatremia: FENa is increased in renal sodium wasting, adrenal insufficiency, and the syndrome of inappropriate antidiuretic hormone secretion (SIADH). In each case, the urine sample must be obtained (by bladder catheterization if necessary) before administration of any drugs affecting urine sodium excretion, such as diuretics.

Urinary Acidification

Although renal insufficiency can interfere with urinary acidification, retention of organic acids due to decreased GFR results in an increase in unmeasured anions. In renal tubular acidosis (RTA), this "anion gap" is in the normal range (5 to 15 mEq/L) and is defined as:

$$Anion\ gap = Na^+_s - [Cl^-_s + HCO_{3\ s}^-]$$

The diagnosis of RTA should be considered in any infant or child with failure to thrive, because chronic systemic acidosis impairs growth. In addition, RTA can lead to nephrocalcinosis or nephrolithiasis (see later).

A classification of RTA has been developed based on the nephron segment affected and the transport defect involved. Thus, RTA can result from defective distal tubular acidification (type I), decreased threshold for proximal tubular bicarbonate reabsorption (type II), or a distal defect involving impaired potassium secretion (type IV). **During the first 3 weeks of life, the threshold for bicarbonate reabsorption can be as low as 14.5 mEq/L in the normal infant** (Brown et al, 1978). This should *not* be regarded as RTA, because treatment with alkali has been shown not to alter growth and development (Brown et al, 1978). Congenital hydronephrosis can result in type I or type IV RTA in the infant or child (Hutcheon et al, 1976; Rodriguez-Soriano et al, 1983). **Appropriate evaluation and treatment are important to prevent the sequelae of RTA, which include growth retardation, osteodystrophy, nephrocalcinosis or nephrolithiasis, and polyuria.**

The approach to the infant or child with suspected RTA is shown in Figure 107–7. The presence of metabolic acidosis in the infant can be difficult to ascertain on the basis of serum total CO_2, because problems in obtaining the sample (venous access, small sample volume) can result in spuriously low values. It is therefore important to obtain the sample from a vein with good blood flow and to transfer it expeditiously to the laboratory in a capped syringe on ice (as with arterial blood for blood gas analysis). Accurate measurement of urine pH is also crucial to making the diagnosis, and a urine sample should be obtained at the time of the blood sample from a freshly voided or bagged specimen. Urine should be withdrawn into a syringe, the air should be expressed, and the sample should be transferred immediately to the laboratory for measurement by pH meter (dipsticks are not sufficiently accurate). **A urine pH below 5.5 in the presence of a total CO_2 below normal for the patient's age suggests gastrointestinal bicarbonate loss or a defect in proximal tubular bicarbonate reabsorption with intact distal acidification (type II), whereas inappropriately high urine pH is consistent with distal or type I RTA. Elevated serum potassium concentration in the presence of normal renal function suggests type IV RTA.**

Because of the difficulty in infants in pursuing bicarbonate infusion to rule out type II or acid infusion to rule out type I, alternate approaches have been developed to define the type of RTA. The simplest is to initiate alkali therapy with sodium bicarbonate or sodium citrate (Shohl's solution or Bicitra) at a dose of 3 mEq/kg/day divided in four doses. The aim is to increase serum total CO_2 to the normal range (generally greater than 20 mEq/L) and to raise urine pH above 7.8. Patients with type II RTA or infants with type I may require much greater doses of alkali (10 or more mEq/kg/day) to maintain a normal plasma total CO_2 concentration and to allow a normal growth rate. The fractional excretion of bicarbonate can then be calculated from random paired blood and urine samples as for FENa (see earlier). In contrast to types I and IV, in which the fractional bicarbonate excretion is less than 15%, the value in type II is greater than 15% owing to the reduced threshold for bicarbonate reabsorption (Chan, 1983). An alternate means to distinguish type II from other forms of RTA is to measure blood and urine PCO_2 after correction of acidosis with alkali therapy. In patients with type II the difference between urine and blood PCO_2 is greater than 20 mm Hg, whereas in those with type I the difference is less than 15 mm Hg (Donckerwolke et al, 1983). A third option to identify patients with a distal tubular acidification defect (types I or IV) is to calculate the urinary anion gap:

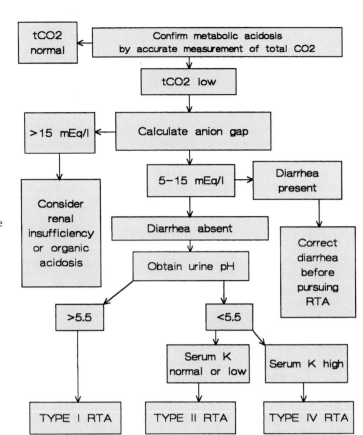

Figure 107–7. Evaluation of suspected renal tubular acidosis in the infant. See text for details.

$$\text{Urinary anion gap (mEq/L)} = Na^+ + K^+ - Cl^-$$

Normal patients and those with intact distal urinary acidification have a negative urinary anion gap, whereas those with types I or IV RTA have a positive gap (Batlle et al, 1988).

Although the just described studies should permit separation of type II from types I and IV, the latter two forms are usually distinguishable (before treatment with alkali) by the presence of hyperkalemia in type IV but not type I. In addition, infusion of furosemide, 1 mg/kg, should result in acidification of urine in patients with type IV but not in those with type I (Stine and Linshaw, 1985).

Although there are a number of causes of RTA in children (Chan, 1983), congenital obstructive nephropathy (Hutcheon et al, 1976; Rodriguez-Soriano et al, 1983) and Fanconi's syndrome should always be considered (see later). Serum levels of electrolytes, calcium, phosphorus, and parathyroid hormone and thyroid function tests should be obtained. A urinalysis should be performed to screen for glucosuria. In addition, the urine amino acid pattern may reveal diffuse aminoaciduria. A 24-hour urine collection should be obtained for calculation of creatinine clearance, protein excretion, calcium excretion, and tubular reabsorption of phosphorus (see later). Sonographic examination of the urinary tract should be performed not only to identify hydronephrosis but also to reveal nephrocalcinosis or nephrolithiasis that can develop in children with type I RTA.

As described earlier, most infants and children with RTA respond well to alkali therapy (sodium bicarbonate or Shohl's solution). Some patients with type IV, however, may have persistent hyperkalemia despite correction of acidosis. This can be managed by administration of chlorothiazide, 10 to 20 mg/kg/day, or polystyrene sodium sulfonate (Kayexalate), 1 g/kg/day. Patients receiving diuretics need to be monitored closely for development of volume contraction, which can actually reduce potassium excretion. Infants receiving Kayexalate may undergo volume expansion from exchange of sodium for potassium and may develop bowel obstruction from inspissated resin in the intestinal tract. As long as adequate GFR is maintained, most children with RTA due to urologic abnormalities will need indefinite treatment to ensure normal growth and to prevent complications such as nephrocalcinosis. **The dose of alkali may need to be adjusted every 3 to 6 months in the rapidly growing infant.**

Urinary Concentration

Most disorders of urinary concentration in infants and children are due to renal maldevelopment (renal dysplasia and obstructive nephropathy), interstitial nephritis (pyelonephritis), or renal insufficiency. Additional causes include renal tubular acidosis, sickle cell nephropathy, and medullary cystic disease. These generally result in a mild to moderate impairment in concentration, such that the urine specific gravity is greater than 1.005. Evaluation should include serum electrolytes, blood urea nitrogen (BUN), creatinine, urinalysis and urine culture, renal ultrasonography, and possibly voiding cystourethrography. Infants with diabetes insipidus usually have urine specific gravity consistently less than 1.005.

There is no physiologic definition of polyuria, and screening of urinary concentrating ability may be initiated based on parental concern over excessive voiding frequency. Measurement of urine output and interpretation of thirst in the infant is problematic. For these reasons, the infant with unexplained dehydration or hypernatremia should be screened for a urine concentrating defect.

A urine specific gravity greater than 1.020 generally rules out a serious abnormality of urinary concentration. In the young infant, overnight fluid restriction can result in dangerous volume depletion and hypernatremia. Such patients should undergo a formal water deprivation test in hospital. This should begin with fluid restriction starting in the morning, with close monitoring of body weight and vital signs until loss of 3% body weight or until the urine osmolality exceeds 600 mOsm in neonates (800 mOsm in older infants or children). If tachycardia or hypotension develops at any time, the test should be terminated.

In patients failing to produce a concentrated urine during water deprivation, fluid should be restricted on a separate day, and desmopressin (10 µg for infants or 20 µg for children) is instilled into the nostrils. Urine osmolality should be measured at 2-hour intervals for 4 to 6 hours. Renal response to desmopressin should be considered normal if the urine osmolality exceeds 600 mOsm for neonates or 800 mOsm for older infants and children. Such patients should be evaluated for central diabetes insipidus by a neurologist or endocrinologist.

Calcium Excretion

Urinary calcium excretion in the neonate is most easily assessed by determination of the calcium/creatinine ratio (mg/mg) in a random urine sample. In contrast to the older child, in whom a ratio exceeding 0.2 should be considered abnormal (Moore et al, 1978), **the ratio in the infant receiving breast milk can rise to 0.4 in the term infant and to 0.8 in the preterm neonate** (Karlen et al, 1985). **The most common cause of hypercalciuria in neonates is administration of calciuric drugs, such as furosemide and glucocorticoids, which are used in the management of bronchopulmonary dysplasia.** Such patients may be at risk for development of nephrocalcinosis or nephrolithiasis (Jacinto et al, 1988). This, in turn, may lead to renal dysfunction later in childhood (Downing et al, 1992). Although it may not be feasible to discontinue glucocorticoids, substitution of chlorothiazide for furosemide may reduce urinary calcium excretion.

Phosphorus, Glucose, and Amino Acid Excretion

Because serum phosphorus concentration is higher in the neonate than in the older infant or child, **any neonate with a serum phosphorus value below 4 mg/dL should be evaluated for renal phosphorus wasting.** This can be accomplished in the neonate by measurement of phosphate and creatinine concentration in urine (UCr, UPO$_4$) and plasma (PCr, PPO$_4$), and calculation of the fractional tubular reabsorption of phosphorus (TRP):

$$TRP = 100\%[1 - (UPO_4 \times PCr)/(PPO_4 \times UCr)]$$

After the first week of life in the neonate, the TRP should be greater than 95% in term infants and greater than 75% in preterm infants (Karlen et al, 1985). **After the neonatal period, the TRP should be greater than 85%.** Values below these ranges suggest a proximal tubular disorder or hyperparathyroidism.

In preterm infants, the threshold for tubular glucose reabsorption is lower than in the term infant or older child. **The most common cause of glucosuria in hospitalized infants is intravenous infusion of dextrose at rates exceeding the tubular reabsorptive threshold.** Percent glucose reabsorption (µmol/mL) is normally greater than 99% (Rossi et al, 1994).

Similar to glucose handling, the proximal tubule of the neonate is limited in its ability to reabsorb amino acids when compared with the older infant. This results in a generalized aminoaciduria that is normal during the neonatal period. Thus, **in the evaluation of aminoaciduria, it is important to compare results to those of age-matched normal infants** (Brodehl, 1978). Normal values for fractional amino acid reabsorption have been determined for neonates, infants, and children (Rossi et al, 1994).

Fluid and Electrolyte Management in the Neonate

Fluid and electrolyte management of the neonate, particularly of the preterm infant, requires knowledge of functional renal maturation, as described earlier, and strict attention to detail. **There are significant hazards to overhydration of the neonate, including the opening of a symptomatic patent ductus arteriosus, cerebral intraventricular hemorrhage, and necrotizing enterocolitis. Severe underhydration, on the other hand, may lead to hypoglycemia, hyperbilirubinemia, and hyperosmolality. To replace the usual urinary losses, 50 to 80 mL/100 kcal of formula is a reasonable starting point.** Insensible water losses can be large, particularly in the very low birth weight infant (El-Dahr and Chevalier, 1990). As shown in Figure 107–8, **initial parenteral fluid requirements in preterm infants are largely dependent on the infant's environment in the neonatal care unit.** Moreover, the requirements (relative to body weight) decrease with increasing body weight.

In monitoring infants with urinary tract disorders, serial body weight measurements are extremely useful, as are repeated assessments of the cardiopulmonary status (El-Dahr and Chevalier, 1990). Blood urea nitrogen and hematocrit values are not as useful in preterm infants as in older infants and children in view of the relatively low nitrogen intake and frequent blood sampling. **Once the physiologic postnatal diuresis has begun, 2 to 3 mEq/kg/day of sodium can be prescribed.** Neonates have a higher plasma potassium concentration than older infants and children (Chevalier, 1998). However, infants with high urine flow rates may have increased potassium losses. If the GFR is not significantly decreased, **potassium chloride, 2 mEq/kg/day, can be added to the fluid prescription once urine output is established.** Hypernatremia in neonates is more often the result of insufficient water intake than excessive sodium intake. In general, hyponatremia is more common than hypernatremia and is often due to excessive water intake, sometimes aggravated by increased antidiuretic hormone secretion (SIADH). The latter may result from perinatal asphyxia, intracranial hemorrhage, or pneumothorax. If SIADH is suspected, a trial of fluid restriction is appropriate.

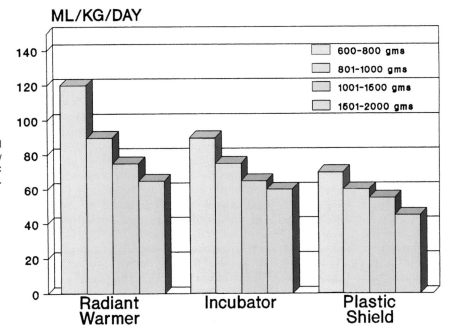

ML/KG/DAY

600-800 gms
801-1000 gms
1001-1500 gms
1501-2000 gms

Radiant Warmer   Incubator   Plastic Shield

Figure 107–8. Initial (day 1 to 3) parenteral fluid requirements in preterm infants according to body weight. (Reproduced from El-Dahr SS, Chevalier RL: Special needs of the newborn infant in fluid therapy. Pediatr Clin North Am 1990;37:323-336.)

KEY POINTS: SODIUM HOMEOSTASIS

■ Sodium balance in the neonate is negative immediately after birth and then becomes positive (sodium accumulation is necessary for growth).

■ There is a blunted natriuresis and sodium retention in response to sodium loading in the term neonate.

■ Preterm infants may develop hyponatremia through renal sodium losses due to immature tubular sodium reabsorption.

HORMONAL CONTROL OF RENAL FUNCTION DURING DEVELOPMENT
Renin-Angiotensin System

Fetal and neonatal renal function is significantly modulated by a number of circulating hormones. The best studied is the renin-angiotensin system (RAS). Inasmuch as angiotensin II receptors have been identified in the fetal rat by the 10th day of gestation (term = 21 days) (Jones et al, 1989) and renin appears in the mesonephric and renal arteries by the 15th day (Richoux et al, 1987), a role for the RAS has been postulated in the process of angiogenesis. In the human fetus, renin is present in the transient mesonephros and can be identified as early as the 8th week of gestation in the metanephros (Celio et al, 1985). By the 19th day of gestation in the rat, renin mRNA (demonstrated by in-situ hybridization histochemistry) as well as the renin protein (demonstrated by immunocytochemistry) are distributed along arcuate and interlobular arteries (Gomez et al, 1986, 1989). However, **in the early postnatal period, renin becomes localized to the juxtaglomerular apparatus, which persists to adulthood** (Gomez et al,

1986). **In addition to these developmental changes in distribution of renin, there is an eightfold decrease in the renal renin mRNA content during early development in the rat** (Gomez et al, 1988a). These developmental changes are not irreversible: inhibition of angiotensin II formation by chronic intake of enalapril in the adult rat causes a redistribution of renin upstream along afferent arterioles and an increase in renal renin mRNA content reminiscent of the fetal pattern (Gomez et al, 1988b, 1990). In view of these findings, it is possible that, as a result of normal maturation, the sensitivity of the renal vasculature to angiotensin II increases, with secondary inhibition of renin gene expression.

Not only is the renal RAS activated during fetal renal development but interference with this system also impairs fetal renal development. **Exposure of the fetus to maternal administration of angiotensin-converting enzyme (ACE) inhibitors results in abnormal fetal renal vasculature and tubules and leads to neonatal renal insufficiency** (Sedman et al, 1995).

Although plasma renin activity (PRA) remains low during fetal life (Pernollet et al, 1979), there is a marked increase in the perinatal period in most mammalian species, including humans (Osborn et al, 1980; Siegel and Fisher, 1980; Wallace et al, 1980; Fiselier et al, 1984). The mechanism underlying this increase in PRA, which is triggered by vaginal delivery (Jelinek et al, 1986), may relate to a rise in prostaglandin synthesis (Joppich and Hauser, 1982) or increased sympathetic nervous activity (Vincent et al, 1980). However, studies in piglets failed to support the latter (Osborn et al, 1980). It is likely that contraction of the extracellular space resulting from physiologic postnatal natriuresis contributes to the perinatal increase in PRA (Aperia et al, 1977b).

In addition to developmental changes in renin synthesis, **the adrenal response to angiotensin increases during fetal and early postnatal life.** In the fetal lamb, furosemide infusion does not increase either PRA or plasma aldosterone concentration (Siegel and Fisher, 1980). In late gestation, however, PRA increases without a mineralocorticoid response while in the neonate both PRA and aldosterone concentration increase after furosemide infusion (Siegel and Fisher, 1980). Maturation of the mineralocorticoid response can also be demonstrated by angiotensin II infusion, which results in greater plasma aldosterone concentrations in adults than in fetal sheep (Robillard et al, 1983). The physiologic significance of these events may rest in the response to hemorrhage, which causes a greater increase in PRA, plasma angiotensin II, and aldosterone in late than early gestation in the ovine fetus (Robillard et al, 1982). Because blood pressure is maintained during moderate hemorrhage in late but not earlier gestation (Robillard et al, 1982), the RAS may play a critical role in modulation of hemodynamics in the perinatal period. **Because of the critical dependence of the fetal and neonatal glomerular capillary pressure on angiotensin-mediated efferent arteriolar tone, fetal or neonatal GFR can fall precipitously after exposure to ACE inhibitors** (Fig. 107–9) (Martin et al, 1992). Both the potency and duration of action of captopril are significantly greater in the neonate than in older children (O'Dea et al, 1988). Moreover, in response to a reduction in renal mass, the remaining hyperfiltering immature nephrons are even more susceptible to the action of ACE inhibitors, which can induce renal failure and further nephron injury.

Atrial Natriuretic Peptide

Atrial natriuretic peptide (ANP), secreted by cardiac myocytes, has been shown to possess a number of systemic hemodynamic and renal effects, including an increase in GFR, natriuresis, diuresis, inhibition of renin and aldosterone release, vasorelaxation, and increase in vascular permeability (Goetz, 1988). Circulating ANP binds to specific receptors coupled to particulate guanylate cyclase, resulting in formation of cyclic guanosine monophosphate (GMP), a second messenger responsible for the physiologic effects of ANP (Inagami, 1989). In addition, ANP binds to an even greater number of receptors not coupled to guanylate cyclase. Classified as "clearance" receptors, these are believed to contribute to the regulation of plasma ANP levels by removal of ANP from the circulation (Inagami, 1989). The precise role of

ANP in regulation of sodium and fluid homeostasis remains unclear. However, evidence has accumulated to suggest that ANP plays a role in the physiologic adaptation of the fetus and neonate to its changing environment. ANP is present in the fetal rat heart shortly after completion of organogenesis (Dolan and Dobrozsi, 1987; Toshimori et al, 1987), and ANP mRNA first appears in the ventricles before becoming localized to the atria in the perinatal period (Wei et al, 1987). Compared with the mother, plasma ANP concentration is significantly higher in the fetus (Castro et al, 1988; Yamaji et al, 1988). Because metabolic clearance of ANP by the fetus exceeds that of the adult (Ervin et al, 1988), release of ANP from fetal cardiac myocytes must be far greater than in adults.

A number of stimuli have been shown to increase fetal plasma ANP levels. Acute volume expansion in the ovine fetus (Ross et al, 1987) and intrauterine blood transfusion in the human fetus (Robillard and Weiner, 1988) raise plasma ANP concentration. Induction of atrial tachycardia in the fetal lamb results in hydrops and an increase in plasma ANP concentration (Nimrod et al, 1988). Fetal hypoxia has also been shown to result in contraction of circulating volume as well as an increase in ANP levels (Cheung and Brace, 1988). By increasing vascular permeability, ANP may therefore contribute to regulation of blood volume in these pathologic states.

Atrial ANP content decreases in the perinatal period, with subsequent increase during the first 15 days of postnatal life in the rat (Dolan et al, 1989). **This pattern is the opposite of that observed for plasma ANP concentration, which is elevated in the first several days of life and then decreases with maturation** (Weil et al, 1986; Kikuchi et al, 1988). It is likely that reduction in atrial ANP during the perinatal period results from increased release into the circulation. In preterm infants, plasma ANP levels are initially even higher than in full-term infants, and the ensuing postnatal decrease in levels is correlated with decreasing atrial size and decreasing body weight (Bierd et al, 1990). It is therefore likely that ANP plays a role in physiologic postnatal natriuresis and diuresis. After the initial postnatal diuresis, however, the neonate enters a state of positive sodium balance necessary for rapid somatic growth (Chevalier, 2001).

The renal effects of infused ANP are reduced in the fetus compared with the adult (Brace et al, 1989; Hargrave et al, 1989). The natriuretic effect of ANP in the neonate is also

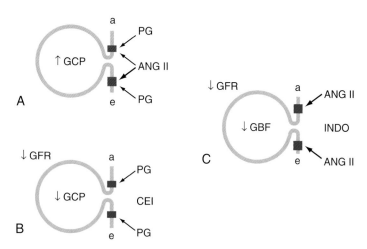

Figure 107–9. Regulation of glomerular filtration rate (GFR) in the neonate and its disturbance by the administration of angiotensin-converting enzyme inhibitors (CEI) and prostaglandin inhibitors such as indomethacin (INDO). **A,** Glomerular capillary pressure (GCP) is maintained by greater angiotensin II (ANG II) vasoconstriction at efferent (e) than afferent (a) arteriole but these effects are countered by vasodilation mediated by prostaglandins (PG). **B,** Angiotensin-converting enzyme inhibitors (CEI) allow unopposed vasodilation by prostaglandins, reducing glomerular capillary pressure and GFR. **C,** Indomethacin (INDO) reduces prostaglandin synthesis, allowing unopposed angiotensin II–mediated vasoconstriction, resulting in reduced glomerular blood flow (GBF) and decreased GFR. (From Chevalier RL: Developmental renal physiology of the low birth weight pre-term newborn. J Urol 1996;156:716.)

reduced (Braunlich, 1987; Chevalier et al, 1988b), and systemic clearance of ANP is increased compared with the adult (Chevalier et al, 1988b). Moreover, compared with the adult, the neonatal renal natriuretic and diuretic response to acute volume expansion is attenuated (Schoeneman and Spitzer, 1980). However, chronic sodium loading of artificially reared preweaned rat pups increases the renal response to acute volume expansion, with an increase in the urinary excretion of cyclic GMP (Muchant et al, 1995). It therefore appears that, rather than reflecting functional immaturity, the renal response to ANP in the neonate reflects an adaptation to the requirement for sodium conservation during this period (Chevalier, 2001).

Vasopressin

Similar to the adult, fetal and newborn sheep have been shown to respond to both osmolar and nonosmolar stimuli for release of arginine vasopressin (AVP) (Leake et al, 1979; Robillard et al, 1979). Despite circulating levels of AVP that can be significantly higher than in the adult (Pohjavuori and Fyhrquist, 1980), **the fetal collecting duct appears to be less sensitive than the adult to AVP** (Robillard and Weitzman, 1980). This may be due to a reduced density of AVP receptors, which increase during early development (Rajerison et al, 1982). In addition, the tubular effects of vasopressin may be antagonized by increased prostanoid synthesis in early development (Melendez et al, 1990). Whereas an immature medullary architecture, low sodium transport, and adaptations in urea transport contribute to low tonicity of the developing medullary interstitium, reduced expression of aquaporins does not appear to be a limiting factor (Bonilla-Felix, 2004).

In the postnatal period, during which the collecting ducts develop full responsiveness to AVP, excessive or "inappropriate" AVP secretion due to birth asphyxia, intracerebral hemorrhage, or respiratory distress syndrome can result in severe hyponatremia (Kaplan and Feigin, 1978; Moylan et al, 1978; Stern et al, 1979). Conversely, infants born with nephrogenic diabetes insipidus do not respond to circulating AVP and may develop life-threatening hypernatremia.

Prostaglandins

Maternal serum prostaglandin concentration increases progressively during pregnancy (Reyes and Melendez, 1990). Because prostaglandins cross the placenta, blood levels are also elevated in the fetus and neonate (Reyes and Melendez, 1990). **Maternal administration of nonsteroidal anti-inflammatory drugs (NSAIDs), such as indomethacin, can result in prolonged renal insufficiency and oliguria in the neonate. This is the result of increased activity of the RAS and enhanced renal vasoconstriction due to inhibition of vasodilating prostaglandins** (see Fig. 107–9) (Buderus et al, 1993; Kaplan et al, 1994). Prolonged intrauterine exposure to prostaglandin inhibitors can also impair fetal renal development (Kaplan et al, 1994). Administration of indomethacin to neonates with patent ductus arteriosus also frequently results in decreased GFR and oliguria (Reyes and Melendez, 1990). Caution should be exercised in the administration of NSAIDs to any infant or child with a single functioning kidney or with

renal impairment, because such patients are at increased risk for additional nephron injury and deterioration of GFR.

Nitric Oxide

Nitric oxide, a potent endothelium-derived relaxing factor (EDRF), has multiple effects on renal function, including renal vasodilatation, regulation of tubuloglomerular feedback, and natriuresis (Bachmann and Mundel, 1994). Basal production of nitric oxide in the third-trimester sheep fetus maintains baseline renal blood flow (Bogaert et al, 1993). In the neonatal pig, endogenous nitric oxide synthesis is also responsible for basal vasoconstrictor tone, and this effect is proportionately greater than that in the adult (Solhaug et al, 1993). Renal endothelial nitric oxide production may be increased in early development as a response to increased vasoconstrictor influences described earlier. A counter-regulatory function of renal nitric oxide production has been proposed also following unilateral ureteral obstruction in the adult rat in which endogenous renal nitric oxide activity parallels increased renal vascular resistance (Chevalier et al, 1992).

THE FUNCTIONAL RESPONSE OF THE DEVELOPING KIDNEYS TO MALFORMATION OR INJURY
Reduced Functioning Renal Mass

A reduction in the number of functioning nephrons in early development is most often the result of a congenital malformation or a perinatal vascular accident such as a renal embolus or renal vein thrombosis (Table 107–1). Unilateral ureteral occlusion in the fetal lamb at mid trimester results in a 50% increase in contralateral kidney weight by 1 month (Peters et al, 1993). These findings are corroborated by two prenatal ultrasound studies of human fetuses with unilateral renal agenesis or multicystic kidney. In both reports, the single functioning kidneys were significantly longer than those in the control patients (Glazebrook et al, 1993; Mandell et al, 1993). **Such studies demonstrate unequivocally that compensatory renal growth can begin prenatally.** Because the placenta provides the excretory function for the fetus, an increased excretory burden on the kidney is not required to initiate compensatory growth. Rather, alterations in growth factors or inhibitors presumably modulate the prenatal changes.

Perhaps not surprising in view of the rapid growth of the normal kidney in the early postnatal period, **compensatory renal growth in the neonate greatly exceeds that in the adult** (Dicker and Shirley, 1973; Shirley, 1976; Hayslett, 1979). Whereas compensatory increase in renal mass in the adult is largely due to cellular hypertrophy, hyperplasia is also stimulated in the uninephrectomized weanling rat

Table 107–1. Causes of Impaired Renal Function in the Neonate
Congenital anomalies of the kidneys and urinary tract
Circulatory disorders (including asphyxia, septicemia)
Iatrogenic/toxic nephropathy

(Phillips and Leong, 1967; Karp et al, 1971). Neonatal glomerular hypertrophy results also from increased glomerular basement membrane surface area and proliferation of mesangial matrix (Olivetti et al, 1980). Although previous reports concluded that compensatory renal growth in the uninephrectomized neonatal rat does not involve an increase in nephrogenesis of the remaining kidney (Kaufman et al, 1975; Larsson et al, 1980), a recent study suggests that uninephrectomy in the fetal sheep can stimulate an increase in nephron number (Douglas-Denton et al, 2002). Of note, glomerular volume was lower in the remaining fetal kidney compared with age-matched sham-operated controls (Douglas-Denton et al, 2002).

As in the adult, the majority of the compensatory increase in renal mass in the neonate is due to an increase in tubular volume (Hayslett et al, 1968; Horster et al, 1971). Although contralateral compensatory renal growth is robust after unilateral nephrectomy or complete ureteral obstruction, compensatory renal growth due to partial unilateral ureteral obstruction in the neonate may be far more gradual (Thornhill et al, 2005). This calls into question the proposal to monitor the adaptive growth of the contralateral kidney as an index of critical partial ureteral obstruction in the infant with ureteropelvic junction obstruction (Koff et al, 1994). Sonography permits serial measurement of renal size in the fetus and after birth. Such "tracking" of renal size reflects the function of an abnormal contralateral kidney in infants with two functioning kidneys: an exaggerated rate of increase in renal size is correlated with contralateral renal function contributing less than 15% of total function (O'Sullivan et al, 1992). **By the time compensatory renal growth can be detected, there may be significant progression of renal dysfunction in the contralateral kidney.**

As with the enhanced increase in compensatory renal growth observed in the neonate with reduced renal mass, **the functional adaptation by remaining nephrons is greater in early development than in the adult.** In dogs subjected to 75% renal ablation at birth, GFR increased markedly such that at 6 weeks of age it was not different from that of sham-operated littermates (Aschinberg et al, 1978). However, dogs undergoing renal ablation at 8 weeks of age had a GFR 6 weeks later that was less than 50% that of sham-operated controls (Aschinberg et al, 1978). Reduced renal mass in the neonatal guinea pig or rat results in acceleration of the normal "centrifugal" functional nephron maturation, such that the compensatory increase in single nephron GFR is greater in superficial than in deep nephrons (Chevalier, 1982a; Ikoma et al, 1990). These studies indicate that functional as well as morphologic correlates of compensatory renal growth are augmented in early postnatal development compared with the adult.

Congenital Urinary Tract Obstruction

The response of the developing kidney to ureteral obstruction differs from that of the adult. **Complete unilateral ureteral obstruction (UUO) during mid gestation in the fetal sheep results in dysplastic development of the ipsilateral kidney** (Beck, 1971). When subjected to UUO later in gestation, however, dysplastic changes do not develop (Glick et al, 1983). In the human infant, ureteral atresia in early gestation results

in irreversible multicystic dysplasia of the ipsilateral kidney (Griscom et al, 1975). Ureteropelvic junction obstruction presumably develops later in gestation and causes less severe functional renal impairment, which may be minimized by early release of obstruction postnatally (King et al, 1984). These studies illustrate both the critical importance of the timing of urinary tract obstruction with respect to renal development and the greater susceptibility to injury of the fetal kidney.

Even in the early postnatal period, the maturing kidney appears to be more susceptible to injury resulting from UUO than the adult kidney. As for uninephrectomy (see earlier), partial UUO in the neonatal guinea pig results in a greater early adaptive increase in GFR of the intact opposite kidney than UUO in older animals (Taki et al, 1983). However, despite lower intraureteral hydrostatic pressure in neonatal than adult guinea pigs (Chevalier, 1984), the decrement in GFR due to ipsilateral UUO is more severe in younger than older animals (Taki et al, 1983), and renal growth of kidneys with partial UUO since birth is arrested by 3 weeks of age (Chevalier et al, 1988). Partial UUO in the neonatal rat also impairs renal growth, with a critical threshold occurring with ureteral constriction exceeding 60% of the ureteral diameter (Thornhill et al, 2005).

Morphologically, the neonatal guinea pig with ipsilateral partial UUO develops contraction of glomerular volume, glomerular sclerosis, and tubular atrophy (Chevalier et al, 1987). Most importantly, growth arrest could not be prevented and function is not restored by release of obstruction after 10 days even though intraureteral pressure is normalized (Chevalier et al, 1988). In contrast, release of obstruction after a similar period in the adult animal does not cause renal atrophy and allows restoration of a normal glomerular perfusion pattern and renal blood flow (Chevalier et al, 1987). Relief of temporary complete UUO in the neonatal rat allows recovery of normal GFR in the postobstructed kidney 1 month later, despite a 40% reduction in the number of nephrons (Chevalier et al, 1999a). However, the significant hyperfiltration of the remaining nephrons leads to progressive glomerular sclerosis, tubular atrophy, interstitial fibrosis, and deterioration of GFR (Chevalier et al, 1999b). These studies suggest that **after surgical relief of congenital urinary tract obstruction, postoperative measurements of individual kidney GFR using radionuclide scans may be misleading because functional adaptation by a population of nephrons may mask the deterioration of other nephrons. Follow-up studies extending well into adulthood are essential in defining the natural history of these patients.**

As with UUO in the adult, chronic partial UUO in the neonatal guinea pig results in a marked increase in vascular resistance of the ipsilateral kidney. Whereas normal renal development in the guinea pig is characterized by a progressive increase in renal blood flow and recruitment of perfused glomeruli (Chevalier, 1982b, 1983), these events are prevented by ipsilateral UUO at birth (Chevalier et al, 1987; Chevalier and Gomez, 1989). Normal renal growth and hemodynamic maturation can be restored, however, by removal of the intact opposite kidney at the time of ureteral obstruction (Chevalier and Kaiser, 1984). This suggests that growth factors regulated by total functional renal mass can modulate the response of the developing kidney to ipsilateral UUO.

The greater hemodynamic impairment of the neonatal kidney subjected to UUO may relate to the increased renal vascular resistance of the immature kidney and increased activity of the RAS (see earlier). Renin content of the neonatal guinea pig kidney with ipsilateral UUO is increased compared with sham-operated controls, and release of obstruction returns renin content to normal levels (Chevalier and Gomez, 1989). Inhibition of endogenous angiotensin II formation by chronic administration of enalapril to neonatal guinea pigs with UUO restores the normal maturational rise in renal blood flow, the number of perfused glomeruli, and the increase in glomerular volume of the ipsilateral kidney (Chevalier and Peach, 1985; Chevalier et al, 1987). Although administration of enalapril does not restore the renal blood flow of the neonatal guinea pig kidney after release of 5 or 10 days of ipsilateral UUO, enalapril reduces renal vascular resistance of the intact opposite kidney by 40% after release of contralateral UUO (Chevalier and Gomez, 1989). Moreover, the vasoconstrictor response of the intact kidney to exogenous angiotensin II is increased after release of contralateral UUO (Chevalier and Gomez, 1989). These studies indicate a dynamic functional balance between the two kidneys, which appears to be mediated or modulated by the intrarenal RAS.

As discussed earlier, the intrarenal distribution of renin changes dramatically during development. In the fetus and early postnatal period, microvascular renin extends along interlobular and afferent arterioles, becoming localized to the juxtaglomerular region by the 20th postnatal day in the rat (Gomez et al, 1986). **In 4-week-old rats subjected to complete UUO during the first 2 days of life, renal renin content is increased in the obstructed kidney and immunoreactive renin extends along the afferent arteriole** (El-Dahr et al, 1990). Thus, UUO from birth results in persistence of the fetal or early neonatal pattern even after the time of weaning (21 days). Furthermore, the proportion of juxtaglomerular apparatuses with renin gene expression (identified by in-situ hybridization histochemistry) is increased in the obstructed kidney of 4-week-old rats (El-Dahr et al, 1990). In addition to increased renin production and storage, neonatal UUO results in recruitment of renin-secreting cells by the renal cortex (Norwood et al, 1994). Four weeks of UUO in adult rats, however, did not alter the juxtaglomerular localization of renin (El Dahr et al, 1990). These studies indicate that the renal response to UUO is age dependent, with the neonate manifesting a greater activity of the RAS. Although inhibition of angiotensin receptors may have a salutary renal effect in the weanling rat with partial UUO (Beharrie et al, 2004), caution must be exercised in blocking angiotensin during nephrogenesis or renal maturation (Guron et al, 1999). **The use of ACE inhibitors or angiotensin receptor blockers should be avoided in the first several months of life unless indicated for significant hypertension or cardiovascular disorders.**

Perinatal Ischemia and Hypoxia

Renal dysfunction in the fetus and neonate is often the result of circulatory disturbances in the perinatal period (see Table 107–1). In response to hemorrhage or hypoxia, renal vascular resistance in the ovine fetus is increased while GFR is maintained, suggesting predominant efferent arteriolar vaso-

constriction (Robillard et al, 1981; Gomez et al, 1984). This may be mediated at least in part by angiotensin (Robillard et al, 1982). Catecholamine release may be more important in mediating renal vascular resistance in early fetal life, whereas vasopressin appears to play a greater role in the more mature ovine fetus (Gomez et al, 1984). In the neonatal lamb, hypoxia increases plasma renin activity, aldosterone, and vasopressin (Weismann and Clarke, 1981). Although GFR is reduced during hypoxia, the effect does not change during the first month of life (Weismann and Clarke, 1981). The preterm infant, however, may have renal responses to ischemia and hypoxia that are more similar to the fetus than neonate.

One of the homeostatic mechanisms for preservation of renal perfusion in the presence of hypotension is autoregulation of renal blood flow. Compared with adult rats, **young rats manifest autoregulation of renal blood flow at lower perfusion pressures, commensurate with the lower mean arterial pressure during early development** (Chevalier and Kaiser, 1983). Interestingly, whereas adult rats with prior uninephrectomy maintain autoregulation (albeit at higher levels of renal blood flow), **uninephrectomy at birth impairs autoregulation in young rats** (Chevalier and Kaiser, 1983). These observations raise the possibility that following reduction in functioning renal mass, the neonatal kidney may be at greater risk for renal ischemia in the presence of superimposed hypotension. After temporary complete occlusion of the renal artery, however, mortality has been shown to be greater in adult than young rats (Kunes et al, 1978). Although this study suggests that the neonatal kidney may be more resistant than the adult kidney to certain insults, **perinatal circulatory disorders can result in a variety of persistent glomerular and tubular functional abnormalities** (Dauber et al, 1976; Stark and Geiger, 1990).

Toxic Nephropathy

Neonates are increasingly exposed to a variety of potentially nephrotoxic agents (see Table 107–1). Fortunately, the developing kidney appears to be more resistant than the adult to some toxic agents. Sodium dichromate and uranyl nitrate, both experimental models of toxic acute renal failure, cause less renal injury in young than in adult animals (Pelayo et al, 1983; Appenroth and Braunlich, 1988). More relevant clinically, renal concentrations of aminoglycosides (Marre et al, 1980; Lelievre-Pegorier et al, 1985; Provoost et al, 1985) and cisplatin (Jongejan et al, 1986) are lower in young than adult animals receiving high doses. This may be due to the normally reduced perfusion of superficial cortical nephrons in the developing kidney, such that these nephrons receive a lower dose of toxin. Another possibility is the proportionately greater renal mass compared with body weight in early development. Few studies have addressed the potential long-term impact of toxic renal injury, however. After uninephrectomy for Wilms' tumor, for example, irradiation and chemotherapy cause greater impairment of compensatory renal growth in younger than older infants and children (Mitus et al, 1969; Luttenegger et al, 1975). As discussed earlier, exposure of the fetus to maternal administration of ACE inhibitors or NSAIDs can significantly impair normal renal development, with major postnatal consequences.

Recovery from Renal Injury: Relationship to Normal Development

Recent studies suggest that recovery from renal injury in the adult involves "recapitulation of phylogeny by ontogeny" (Hammerman, 2000). Thus, insulin growth factor-1 plays a role in determining nephron number and nephron size and also can alter the course of recovery from ischemic acute renal failure or temporary ureteral obstruction (Chevalier et al, 2000; Hammerman, 2000). **Temporary ureteral obstruction in the neonatal rat delays maturation of the renal microvasculature, glomeruli, tubules, and interstitium** (Chevalier et al, 1999a). After relief of obstruction, some aspects of renal maturation proceed whereas others are permanently impaired (Chevalier et al, 1999a). Identification of the timing of expression of various genes involved in normal development may therefore lead to insight into the reparative process and to new therapeutic interventions.

Unfortunately, without aggressive medical management, the development of chronic renal insufficiency in infancy can impair long-term somatic growth and neurologic development. Impaired growth due to congenital renal disorders appears to begin in fetal life (Karlberg et al, 1996). Mortality in infants with chronic renal failure occurs primarily in the first year of life. However, with early intensive nutritional supplementation, the mean height standard deviation score can normalize (Van Dyck et al, 1998; Warady et al, 1999; Kari et al, 2000), although psychosocial development is often delayed (Madden et al, 2003).

Implications of Congenital Renal Disease for Adult Function

Glomerular hyperfiltration and glomerular hypertrophy have been implicated in the progression of most forms of renal insufficiency (Brenner et al, 1982; Fogo and Ichikawa, 1989). **In view of the greater response by remaining nephrons, the neonate with reduced renal mass is theoretically at greater risk than the adult for long-term renal dysfunction.** In this regard, reduced renal mass causes greater proteinuria and glomerular sclerosis in the immature than in the adult (Celsi et al, 1987; Okuda et al, 1987; Ikoma et al, 1990). There is circumstantial evidence that intrauterine growth retardation is also accompanied by a nephron deficit and that in addition to renal insufficiency it may lead to the development of hypertension in adulthood (Brenner and Chertow, 1994; Barker, 1999). Likewise, congenital unilateral renal agenesis in humans has been associated with focal glomerular sclerosis and progression to renal insufficiency in adulthood (Kiprov et al, 1982; Bhathena et al, 1985; Wikstad et al, 1988). A significant fraction of preterm infants with neonatal acute renal failure develop proteinuria and decreasing renal function (Abitbol et al, 2003). The critical question is what is the number of functioning nephrons below which progression is inevitable. In oligomeganephronia, a form of renal hypoplasia in which the number of nephrons is reduced to less than 50%, glomeruli develop marked hypertrophy and sclerosis leading to renal failure in later childhood (Elema, 1976; Bhathena et al, 1985). These considerations underscore the importance of attempting to maximize functional renal mass in the neonate or infant with renal impairment of any etiology.

KEY POINTS: INJURY RESPONSES

- Overhydration of the preterm neonate can lead to opening of the ductus arteriosus, cerebral hemorrhage, or necrotizing enterocolitis.

- Underhydration can lead to hypoglycemia, hyperbilirubinemia, and hyperosmolality.

- The fetal and neonatal kidney are exquisitely susceptible to injury from exposure to angiotensin inhibitors or nonsteroidal anti-inflammatory drugs.

SUMMARY

Renal functional development spans a continuum from fetal through perinatal and postnatal periods. The gestational age at birth has a profound influence on the evolution and outcome of renal function. Whereas nephrogenesis is normally complete by the 34th fetal week, abnormal renal morphogenesis, intrauterine stresses, preterm birth, and perinatal insults may interfere with this process, resulting in long-term consequences. In the neonate, GFR is low and doubles in the first 2 weeks of life. Renal concentrating capacity is less than 1000 mOsm/kg in the first 2 months of life and remains decreased for longer periods in preterm infants. After perinatal natriuresis, neonates remain in positive sodium balance for a number of months, which is necessary for normal growth. The threshold for renal bicarbonate reabsorption is diminished in the neonate, and net acid excretion matures by the second month of life. Evidence is accumulating to suggest that, regardless of etiology, a reduction in nephron number in early life leads to significant morbidity in adulthood. Compensatory mechanisms may prove to be maladaptive, leading to impaired somatic growth and neurologic development. The urologist caring for the infant and child should therefore seek to preserve functional renal mass as early as possible and to ensure long-term follow-up.

Acknowledgment

Original studies by Dr. Chevalier were supported by NIH grants AM25727, HL40209, DK40558, DK45179, DK52612, and DK62328.

SUGGESTED READINGS

Bueva A, Guignard JP: Renal function in preterm neonates. Pediatr Res 1994;36:572-577.

Chevalier RL: Developmental renal physiology of the low birth weight preterm newborn. J Urol 1996;156:714-719.

Chevalier RL: The moth and the aspen tree: Sodium in early postnatal development. Kidney Int 2001;59:1617-1625.

El-Dahr SS, Chevalier RL: Special needs of the newborn infant in fluid therapy. Pediatr Clin North Am 1990;37:323-336.

Haycock GB: Development of glomerular filtration and tubular sodium reabsorption in the human fetus and newborn. Br J Urol 1998;81(Suppl 2):33-38.

Schwartz GJ, Brion LP, Spitzer A: The use of plasma creatinine concentration for estimating glomerular filtration rate in infants, children, and adolescents. Pediatr Clin North Am 1987;34:571-590.

108 Congenital Urinary Obstruction: Pathophysiology

CRAIG A. PETERS, MD • ROBERT L. CHEVALIER, MD

INTRODUCTION
Clinical Context

Obstruction is one of the most common conditions affecting the urinary tract in children and has substantial health consequences. **Obstructive nephrouropathy is the single largest entity leading to renal insufficiency in boys younger than 1 year and the largest single cause of renal failure requiring transplantation, with about 23% of such children undergoing transplantation** (Seikaly et al, 2003). Because a large number of children are also affected by lesser degrees of obstruction, ongoing imaging to monitor renal function and the status of the obstruction is necessary.

The wide spectrum of obstructive changes is one of the major challenges in the clinical management of these conditions in that there is no definitive dividing line between obstruction warranting intervention and obstruction not warranting intervention (Peters, 1995), The presence of an obstructive lesion is readily determined with current imaging, but the criteria for intervention are highly controversial, largely because of a lack of information regarding the natural history of differing degrees of obstruction and the absence of effective markers of the pattern and progression of obstruction (Chevalier, 2004a). We are left with few guideposts along the spectrum of obstruction by which clinical decisions may be made.

This chapter reviews the current state of knowledge regarding the pathophysiology of congenital urinary obstruction, its distinction from postnatal obstruction, and how it may be correlated with clinical scenarios. It is anticipated that with progressive understanding of the mechanisms of congenital urinary obstruction, we will become better able to discriminate between children requiring therapeutic intervention and those in whom intervention would be unnecessary.

Clinical Manifestations of Obstruction

Prenatal ultrasonographic diagnosis has radically altered the clinical manifestations of obstructive conditions, and today, most are detected before birth, with many having no apparent clinical signs. Those with clinical manifestations are often severe obstructive conditions such as posterior urethral valves or massive hydronephrosis. Children are still found with clinical signs of obstruction, usually infection or pain and rarely hypertension. In a child with obstruction of the entire urinary tract, even when the obstruction is relieved, the functional abnormalities present inform us of the effects of obstruction on developing kidneys. **Reduced filtration function as manifested by a rising serum creatinine concentration is associated with glomerular injury, acidosis is due to tubular injury, and nephrogenic diabetes insipidus is secondary to collecting duct abnormalities. In extreme cases, all of these abnormalities may be present, but on occasion they are found in isolation and usually persist after correction of the obstruction** (Hutcheon et al, 1976; Chandar et al, 1996). Obstructive hypertension is often mediated by renin and associated with glomerular sclerosis.

The pathologic correlates of these functional alterations have been described in congenitally obstructed kidney to varying degrees (Elder et al, 1995; Stock et al, 1995; Han et al, 1998; Poucell-Hatton et al, 2000; Zhang et al, 2000;

Weei-Yuarn et al, 2005). The pathologic changes associated with lesser degrees of obstruction have been less thoroughly investigated, and a spectrum of qualitatively similar alterations have been described. **In the absence of overt functional alterations and in patients with unilateral conditions, determining the state of the affected kidney becomes a clinical challenge.** This challenge is often tied to the question of whether surgical intervention is appropriate, and much controversy has emerged from this issue. Clinical imaging studies are currently the only widely used modality to make such an assessment, and their interpretation is not uniform. The natural history of many conditions in the spectrum of obstruction is not well described, yet it is the essence of the question. It should be clearly seen that the spectrum of obstruction is wide, involves conditions that do not require intervention, as well as others that produce profound renal injury, and may change with age and persistence of the condition.

Progressive Renal Dysfunction

One of the concerns regarding obstructive conditions in the urinary tract is the potential for a progressive situation to lead to ever more loss of renal function. **Progression may be seen in two forms, one with an uncorrected, partially obstructive lesion (e.g., ureteropelvic junction [UPJ] obstruction) and the other with a previously obstructed, but corrected lesion that has produced some degree of renal damage (e.g., posterior urethral valves).** In the first, renal function may initially appear intact on imaging tests, yet in time there will be progressive loss of absolute and relative function of the kidney affected by the obstruction. If this impending loss were known prospectively, intervention would be appropriate and should be performed early. The challenge in predicting progressive loss of function is that few markers are available. In general, this situation is less common, yet it cannot be neglected because every prospective study of obstructive conditions has documented the potential for progressive loss (Parkhouse et al, 1988; Koff and Campbell, 1992; Palmer et al, 1998; Koff, 2000).

The second situation reflects the fact that the damaged kidney does not have the functional reserve of a normal kidney by which it may maintain its absolute function over time. These kidneys demonstrate a steady decline in function over time, and this deterioration is usually manifested as bilateral obstruction. The mechanism may be hyperfiltration of remnant renal units, which is most often seen clinically with posterior urethral valves (Parkhouse et al, 1988; Nguyen and Peters, 1999). These children may have very adequate renal function early in life but demonstrate delayed and inexorable progression to renal failure in adolescence. As shown in Figure 108–1, most infants in whom posterior urethral valves are diagnosed in the perinatal period suffer progressive renal insufficiency by 10 years of age despite relief of the obstruction (Roth et al, 2001). Whether earlier intervention would have protected their renal function is uncertain, but that possibility cannot be neglected.

Predictors of continuing progression of renal injury secondary to either ongoing or previous renal obstruction are of critical importance, yet there are few to rely on. **The most evident predictor is altered absolute renal function as indi-

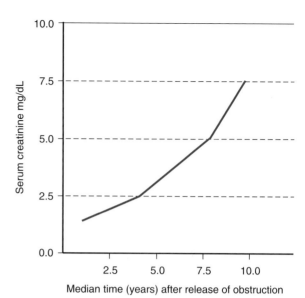

Figure 108–1. Graph depicting the progressive deterioration in renal function as indicated by a rising serum creatinine in patients with posterior urethral valves despite surgical relief of obstruction. (From Roth KS, Carter WH Jr, Chan JCM: Obstructive nephropathy in children: Long-term progression after relief of posterior urethral valve. Pediatrics 107:1004-1010, 2001).

cated clinically by creatinine clearance or serum creatinine. However, these findings are relatively insensitive in the early stages of progression.** Radionuclide imaging may be helpful in some cases, but there is no gold standard for the best interpretation of potentially progressive disease.

KEY POINTS: CLINICAL CONTEXT

- Obstruction is the single largest entity leading to renal insufficiency in boys younger than 1 year and the largest single cause of renal failure requiring transplantation.

- Progression of obstructive renal dysfunction may be seen in two forms, one with an uncorrected, partially obstructive lesion and the other with a previously obstructed, but corrected lesion that has produced some degree of renal damage.

- The second situation reflects the fact that the damaged kidney does not have the functional reserve of a normal kidney by which it may maintain its absolute function over time.

- Elevated creatinine indicates altered absolute renal function but is relatively insensitive in the early stages of progression.

Definition of Obstruction

Although it may not be difficult to diagnose a potentially obstructed urinary tract, usually by ultrasonographic identification of hydronephrosis, determination of whether this particular condition requires surgical intervention to preserve renal function and development is much more diffi-

cult. The frequently quoted definition of congenital obstruction (Koff, 1987)—"any condition producing a restriction of urinary flow that will lead to deterioration in renal function"—is too limited. In a growing child, renal function is expected to increase markedly, initially in excess of body mass and subsequently parallel to it. If this increase in function does not occur, renal functional potential is lost, which may be of greater consequence than losing absolute function. Therefore, impairment of renal functional development should be considered an aspect of obstruction that warrants intervention (Peters, 1995).

If such is the case, an obstructive or hydronephrotic condition that has already resulted in a reduction in anticipated normal function should be considered justification for intervention. A child who has significant hydronephrosis with a kidney contributing significantly less than the anticipated 50% on a radionuclide renal scan has already suffered a loss in functional potential and should perhaps be considered as having sufficient obstruction to warrant intervention so that further injury may be limited.

A critical element of congenital obstructive uropathy (COU) is the recognition that it is distinct from acquired obstruction in a mature animal (or mature kidney). The fact that the obstruction develops simultaneously with formation of the kidney creates an entirely different paradigm for COU than for obstruction of a mature kidney (Peters, 1997). **The patterns of renal development are affected by obstruction, and these alterations produce the ultimate functional effects.** The mechanisms for these changes are therefore wholly distinct from those for mature obstruction. Although there is likely to be some overlap in the critical mechanisms of change, many will be different. It cannot be assumed that the principles relevant to mature obstruction are applicable to congenital obstruction. These differences will clearly have an impact on our interpretation of experimental data in postnatal and mature animals, as well as the selection and application of experimental systems.

One of the frustrations in the clinical management of congenital obstruction is the dichotomy between therapeutic options, which are currently limited to either observation or surgery. Although surgical options have expanded somewhat, the large gap between these divergent options has created a great deal of tension in the minds of the patient and family, as well as physicians. The absence of any medical or pharmacologic therapy to ameliorate or prevent the complications of obstruction has been a major factor in the controversy between those who choose to correct a problem and those who believe that it is better to await spontaneous resolution or unambiguous evidence of obstructive injury. The horizon holds promise for medical therapies that might prevent renal injury in various ways, but it will be essential to more completely understand the nature of COU to permit such specific treatment.

PATTERNS OF CONGENITAL OBSTRUCTIVE NEPHROPATHY

In an attempt to understand the pathophysiology of COU, examination of obstructed renal tissue has shown disorganization of structure with primitive forms of renal tissue, or dysplasia. **Although the definition of dysplasia is not universally agreed on, evidence of altered renal development in association with obstruction is frequently reported** (Bernstein, 1971; Matsell, 1998). Dysplasia is often considered to be an embryonic process and irreversible, yet this has not been proved. It is clear that some cases of dysplasia are due to very early abnormalities in renal development, unrelated to obstruction; nonetheless, it is equally clear that obstructive processes can produce dysplasia. Whether there are subtle differences between these patterns is unclear, but it should not be difficult to understand that several underlying causes may produce similar outcomes when renal developmental patterns are disrupted.

In some cases, however, usually in patients with lesser degrees of obstruction, there is no dysplasia (Bonsib, 1998; Zhang et al, 2000). In such cases, the mechanisms of the obstructive effect may be similar, but present in various degrees, or they may be entirely different. It is important to recognize the variability in patterns of response to obstruction.

If obstruction can produce dysplasia or abnormal developmental patterns, the particular mechanisms of the obstructive effects may be identifiable. These include the fundamental processes of development, and by examining them specifically, we may be able to understand the critical mechanisms of obstructive nephropathy. Development is the controlled process of growth and differentiation of tissues in the formation of an organ or tissue. The forces that regulate these processes are the probable targets of obstructive effects.

Structural alterations caused by obstruction are obviously evident in the case of hydronephrosis, but this is largely a distortion of normal architecture and relative alteration in the amount of renal tissue elements. There may, however, be subtle changes that are functionally important. Other alterations include fibrosis and increased interstitial tissue, as well as the presence of abnormal tubules and glomeruli. The normal layered organization of the kidney—cortical and medullary areas with inner and outer stripes—is often distorted or absent (Zhang et al, 2000). Less obvious will be changes in differentiation of the individual renal cell types that make up nephrons. Cells are unlikely to perform their normal functions, including communication with neighboring cells in an integrated fashion. Function will therefore be disrupted.

Closely tied with these altered patterns of structure are distortions in normal regulation of growth, with either increased or decreased growth of specific structures. In some cases, obstructed kidneys are markedly smaller than normal, and in a developmental context this does not represent atrophy, but hypoplasia. The distinction is important in that renal tissue mass has not been lost; it has just never formed. **This is growth failure, not atrophy, and the mechanisms are probably distinct.**

These observations are supported by both clinical and experimental work. Several biopsy studies have shown patterns indicative of altered differentiation and growth at various levels of obstruction, including both upper (UPJ obstruction) (Elder et al, 1995; Stock et al, 1995; Zhang et al, 2000) and lower (posterior urethral valves) (Poucell-Hatton et al, 2000; Haecker et al, 2002). These variations are not well explained, and correlation with clinical parameters is often imperfect. Experimental studies, however, have shown similarly that obstruction during development will produce changes in patterns of renal differentiation and growth regulation (Steinhardt et al, 1988; Gonzalez et al, 1990; Peters et al, 1992; Wen et al, 2002a; Cachat et al, 2003). **Chronic ureteral obstruction in the neonatal rodent delays the maturation of all components of the nephron, from the glomerulus to the collecting duct, as well as the interstitial cells and microvasculature** (Chung and Chevalier, 1996; Chevalier, 1996). **The effects of obstruction on the developing kidney vary with the time of onset in experimental models, as well as the severity of obstruction** (Chevalier et al, 1988; Chevalier et al, 1999c; Thornhill et al, 2005). Severe (but not mild) chronic partial UPJ obstruction in the neonatal rat impairs growth of the kidney (Thornhill et al, 2005). As shown in Figure 108–2, the reduction in renal growth is not a linear function of the severity of ureteral obstruction; rather, there is a critical reduction in ureteral diameter (about 65%), which if exceeded, compromises renal growth (Thornhill et al, 2005). **Although the validity of any of these model systems may be challenged until we have more definite correlations, it is clear that induced obstruction will produce such severe abnormalities in differentiation that they are considered dysplasia and will lead to disruptions in regulation of growth** (Peters et al, 1992). It is therefore reasonable to examine the specific patterns observed and the potential mechanisms of these changes, all of which are probably contributing factors in the development of obstructive nephropathy.

PATTERNS OF EFFECT

The effects of obstruction on a developing kidney may be summarized as producing alterations in the regulation of growth, tissue differentiation, and ECM and fibrosis, as well as alterations in functional integration of the kidney. The

KEY POINTS: PATTERNS OF CONGENITAL OBSTRUCTIVE NEPHROPATHY

- Impairment of renal functional development should be considered a determinant of obstruction that warrants intervention.
- Congenital obstructive uropathy is distinct from acquired obstruction in a mature kidney.
- Obstructed renal tissues show disorganization of structure with primitive forms of renal tissues, called dysplasia.
- Structural alterations caused by obstruction are evident in hydronephrosis as a distortion in normal architecture and relative alterations in the amount of renal tissue elements. Subtle changes are functionally important and include fibrosis and increased interstitial tissue, as well as abnormal tubules and glomeruli.
- The effects of obstruction on the developing kidney vary with the time of onset, as well as the severity of obstruction.
- Models of obstruction produce severe abnormalities in differentiation that are considered to be dysplasia and disruptions in growth regulation.
- Obstruction of a developing kidney produces alterations in the regulation of growth, tissue differentiation, and extracellular matrix (ECM) and fibrosis, as well as alterations in functional integration of the kidney.

latter is largely a result of the first three major factors and refers to the mechanisms producing vascular, neural, and humoral homeostasis and regulation of the inflammatory cascades. Understanding the mechanisms by which these systems are dysregulated by obstruction will permit a better understanding of the outcomes of obstruction and should improve our diagnostic, prognostic, and therapeutic ability.

GROWTH

Growth regulation is a critical part of development, and an obstructed kidney may show evidence of impaired or accelerated growth. It is important to recognize that a small obstructed kidney is not atrophic, as might be seen in an adult, but is hypoplastic. The growth that it should have experienced never occurred. This can be readily seen by prenatal ultrasound (Mandell et al, 1994) and has been shown repeatedly in experimental models (Peters et al, 1992; Chevalier et al, 1999c; Thornhill et al, 2005). It seems to usually be a generalized impairment in all parts of the kidney, with both reduced numbers of nephrons and smaller nephrons. **Differential growth impairment within the nephron segments may be present as well** (Cachat et al, 2003; Weei-Yuarn et al, 2005).

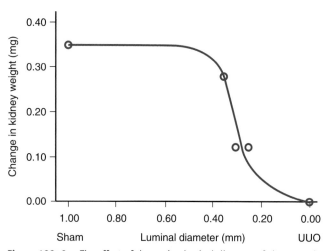

Figure 108–2. The effect of decreasing luminal diameter of the ureter in experimental models of partial ureteral obstruction on renal weight. The sharp drop in weight suggests a threshold effect on the obstructive effects on renal growth regulation. (From Thornhill BA, Burt LE, Chen C, et al: Variable chronic partial ureteral obstruction in the neonatal rat: A new model of ureteropelvic junction obstruction. Kidney Int 67:42-52, 2005.)

The functional effects of significant growth impairment are obvious inasmuch as there are fewer nephron units and nephron maturation is delayed. After relief of complete temporary ureteral obstruction in the neonatal rat, function of the postobstructed kidney is initially normal despite a marked reduction in nephron number (Chevalier et al, 1999b). However, after prolonged recovery, function of the remaining nephrons deteriorates, most likely because of long-standing hyperfiltration injury (Chevalier et al, 2000c). Reduced renal mass can be associated with hypertension, as well as reduced filtration function, and loss of tubular mass will affect electrolyte and acid-base homeostasis, in addition to water balance.

Growth acceleration can be seen in larger than normal hydronephrotic kidneys, although this is difficult to prove in humans because few of these kidneys are removed. In fetal animal experiments, it is clear that partial obstruction will increase renal mass (Gobet et al, 1999a; Ayan et al, 2001). This increase in renal mass is not seen with dysplastic changes and is not a product of edema because total protein and DNA are increased as well. Factors that predict altered growth appear to be the severity of obstruction and probably timing, although the latter is difficult to ascertain in human situations. The functional consequences of accelerated growth are not known, and this may correlate with the occasional hyperfunction measured on renal scans that is seen in some patients with hydronephrosis (Inanir et al, 2005). Growth enhancement of the glomeruli will occur in early diabetes and is later associated with glomerular sclerosis, thus suggesting that similar effects with obstruction may not be benign.

Regulation of Growth of the Kidney

Regulation of renal growth is extremely complex and dynamic through development. A variety of growth factors are known to influence kidney growth at various stages of renal development and act at different loci of the nephron. Obstructive conditions have been shown to alter the expression of growth regulatory genes, as well as the presence of proteins coded by these genes (Chevalier, 1996; Yoo et al, 1998; Kiley et al, 2003). Microarray analysis has shown a remarkable alteration in the expression of a number of regulatory and structural genes in neonatal rats subjected to ureteral obstruction, as well as in rats with spontaneous ureteral obstruction (Silverstein et al, 2003; Seseke et al, 2004). Epidermal growth factor (EGF) has been studied more closely than others and has also been used to alleviate some of the growth effects of obstruction when administered exogenously (Kennedy et al, 1997; Chevalier et al, 1998; Chevalier et al, 1999a; Kiley et al, 2003). However, the complexity of renal development and growth regulation clearly indicates that no single growth factor is the key element in obstructive changes and multiple cytokines are likely to play significant roles in the response to obstruction.

Regulation of Apoptosis

A critical component of growth in the developing kidney is apoptosis, or regulated cell death. The early kidney is extremely active in terms of new cell formation, as well as turnover (Carr et al, 1995). Such activity permits remodeling during development, in addition to providing a control system over unregulated growth. Small increases in the rate of apoptosis, even with normal ongoing growth, would lead to significant reductions in renal mass over time. Evidence of increased apoptotic activity has been shown in congenital obstruction, including cellular patterns characteristic of apoptosis and enhanced expression of apoptosis-regulating molecules (Chevalier et al, 2000b; Liapis et al, 2000; Malik et al, 2001; Cachat et al, 2003; Lama et al, 2003; Nguyen et al, 2000; Thornhill et al, 2005). It is important to recognize that the fate of individual cells depends on an interplay between survival signals and death signals (Fig. 108–3). Thus, stimuli for apoptosis may include mechanical stretching of tubular epithelial cells, infiltration of macrophages, or production of the sphingolipid ceramide (already upregulated in the developing kidney) (Malik et al, 2001; Lange-Sperandio, 2002; Kiley et al, 2003; Lange-Sperandio, 2003). The ultimate cellular effects of such stimuli, however, depend on the summation of competing pro-apoptotic signals (such as transforming growth factor β1 [TGF-β1], p53, and BAD) and anti-apoptotic signals (such as EGF, insulin-like growth factor type I [IGF-I], and catalase) (Chevalier et al, 2000a; Miyajima et al, 2000b; Choi et al, 2001; Kiley et al, 2003; Sunami et al, 2004). The changes may be seen heterogeneously (Chevalier et al, 2000b), but the precise mechanisms by which these alterations occur remain unclear. An important aspect of understanding the role of apoptosis in congenital obstruction is that the mediators may be measurable in urine or blood, which may permit therapeutic manipulation.

REGULATION OF APOPTOSIS IN THE HYDRONEPHROTIC KIDNEY

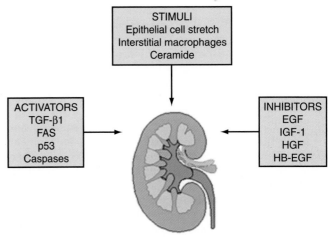

Figure 108–3. Regulation of apoptosis in a hydronephrotic kidney. Renal tubular cell apoptosis is enhanced by a variety of stimuli in the immature hydronephrotic kidney, including mechanical stretch of dilated tubular segments, release of pro-apoptotic molecules by infiltrating macrophages, and increased renal generation of ceramide. The ultimate fate of the cell is decided by the balance of signals mediating cell death [transforming growth factor β1 (TGF-β1), FAS, p53, caspases] and those acting as survival factors [epidermal growth factor (EGF), insulin-like growth factor type 1 (IGF-1), hepatocyte growth factor (HGF), and heparin-bound epidermal growth factor (HB-EGF)]. (From Chevalier RL, Roth JA: Obstructive Uropathy. In: Avner ED, Harmon WE, Niaudet P (eds): Pediatric Nephrology, 5th ed. Philadelphia, Lippincott, Williams & Wilkins; 2004: chap 55.)

KEY POINTS: GROWTH AND DIFFERENTIATION

- The functional effects of growth impairment are fewer nephron units and delay in nephron maturation.

- Obstructive conditions have been shown to alter the expression of growth-regulating genes, as well as the presence of proteins coded by these genes.

- Congenital obstruction increases apoptosis and cellular patterns characteristic of apoptosis, with enhanced expression of apoptosis-regulating molecules.

- The ultimate cellular effects of such stimuli, however, depend on the summation of competing pro-apoptotic signals and anti-apoptotic signals.

- Alteration in the differentiation of cells is unique to congenital obstruction and does not occur in a major way in adult obstruction.

- The critical determinant of dysplasia in animal studies has been complete obstruction early in gestation.

DIFFERENTIATION

Differentiation is the complex process of cells attaining specific functional traits to permit specialized functions and organization into tissues. It is the basis for renal function in its many aspects. Obstruction affects these finely tuned patterns, as can be seen histologically in a severely obstructed kidney with dysplasia. More subtle effects may require assessment of tubular or glomerular function, but all are a result of altered differentiation. Disruption of differentiation may begin as early as induction of the nephron or later in development with injury to renal collecting duct cells, which regulate urinary concentrating ability. Some of these changes may be reversible, but it is usually presumed that many are not because some cells will undergo terminal differentiation, and if it does not occur at a particular time point in development, there will not be another opportunity for it to occur. **Alteration in differentiation of cells is unique to congenital obstruction and does not occur in a major way in adult obstruction.** Cells may be injured and lose their differentiated capacity, but the cell types are not thought to actually change their behavior once differentiated. Understanding the patterns of altered differentiation and its regulators is critical to understanding congenital obstructive nephropathy.

Induction Process

Renal differentiation begins with co-induction of the ureteral bud and metanephric mesenchyme and is exquisitely sensitive to various outside effects that may disrupt the normal sequence of cellular changes that result in a kidney. When in time these changes may be disturbed by obstruction is unclear,

but it can be presumed that some of the variation in the spectrum of obstruction is due to different times of onset of the obstructive effect and different degrees of severity. The pattern of effect is likely to reflect the time of onset and be reflected in the number of nephron generations and the degree of dysplastic transformation. Controversy remains regarding whether obstruction can produce dysplasia, and it is often stated that if dysplasia is present, it was due to abnormal induction and not obstruction. Abnormal induction and nephronogenesis may be produced by various factors, including genetic ones, or be due to cellular disruption from mechanical forces. The studies of Maizels indicate that obstruction alone is insufficient to produce dysplasia (Berman and Maizels, 1982) and that mechanical disruption of the metanephric mesenchyme is needed to produce histologic dysplasia (Maizels and Simpson, 1983). This elegant work in the chick kidney (a mesonephric kidney) may not have produced sufficient obstruction given the small size of the model, however, and several of the preparations were not obstructed. It is unclear whether they all were to a sufficient degree. It also suggests that mechanical forces can in fact disrupt nephronogenesis sufficiently to produce dysplasia, and there is no inherent reason to believe that disruption of nephronogenesis cannot result from obstruction as well. **Studies in fetal rabbits** (Fetterman et al, 1974), **neonatal rodents** (Wen et al, 2002a), **fetal sheep** (Glick et al, 1983; Gonzalez et al, 1990; Peters et al, 1992; Matsell et al, 1996; Medjebeur et al, 1997; Kitagawa et al, 1999), **and primates** (Tarantal et al, 2001) **have shown dysplastic changes produced by obstruction.**

The critical determinant of dysplasia in animal studies has been complete obstruction early in gestation. In the fetal sheep this was seen only when the obstruction was induced before 50% of gestation had elapsed (70 days in most sheep species, which have a gestation of 140 to 145 days) (Peters et al, 1992; Gobet et al, 1999a). Obstruction induced after that point produced only hydronephrotic changes, albeit severe. Partial obstructions produced only hydronephrosis, without apparent disruption of the renal architecture. The reason is presumably altered sensitivity of the developing nephrons to obstructive effects at this point. It is also possible that by this point in gestation, most nephrons have been formed. The time course of nephronogenesis is not linear, and there is some evidence that although new nephron formation continues until term, the vast majority have formed by midgestation. This might explain the particular sensitivity to obstruction before that time point. Alternatively, the particular signaling systems that are active in the early phases of renal development begin to fade away with ongoing development. It is possible that the pathways sensitive to obstruction that would inherently alter the pattern of development have run their course of expression and activity by midgestation.

One of the histologic hallmarks of renal dysplasia is the presence of fibromuscular collars around tubular structures, so-called primitive ducts. These structures have a characteristic appearance, and the smooth muscle surrounding the tubules stains for alpha smooth muscle actin (α-SMA) (Daiekha-Dahmane et al, 1997). This pattern indicates an abnormality in the regulation of epithelial-mesenchymal transformation (EMT), an important ongoing process in early kidney development in which the mesenchymal structures of the primitive nephrogenic blastema and the epithelium of the ureteral bud processes interact with bidirectional differentiation from epithelial to mesenchymal phenotypes (Herzlinger et al, 1993; Herzlinger, 1995; Hatini et al, 1996). It is uncertain whether the presence of primitive tubules suggests persistence of mesenchyme that should have transformed to epithelium or inappropriate epithelial to mesenchymal transformation. Understanding the signaling pathways involved in these processes will have a direct impact on our understanding of obstructive processes. In dysplastic human kidneys, TGF-β1 mRNA and protein are upregulated in epithelia and surrounding mesenchymal cells, which suggests that EMT may play a role in abnormal renal development (Yang et al, 2000). Expression of α-SMA is regulated in part by TGF-β (Kondo et al, 2004), thus linking mediators of both growth and fibrosis. Persistent expression of α-SMA can be seen in partial obstruction without dysplastic patterns and may therefore be important at several levels of obstructive severity (Gobet et al, 1999a).

Development of the glomerulus is a tightly regulated process that involves interaction of the mesenchyme and epithelium with a very specific pattern of growth and the formation of intermediate structures such as the S-shaped body. In general, primitive glomeruli are not evident in obstructive changes, but reduced numbers (McVary and Maizels, 1989; Chevalier et al, 2002; Eskild-Jensen et al, 2002) and abnormal or hypoplastic glomeruli are seen (Thornhill et al, 2005). In some cases, glomeruli may be enlarged in obstruction, suggestive of the changes seen in the hyperfiltration that leads to glomerulosclerosis.

FIBROSIS

A universal characteristic of obstructive nephropathy appears to be renal fibrosis, although it is a nonspecific pattern found in a variety of pathologic conditions affecting the kidney. It is seen as infiltration of the interstitium with abnormal amounts of ECM, including collagens, fibronectin, and other connective tissue proteins. The presence of these proteins disrupts the normal interconnections between cells that permit functional integration of renal tissues. Tubular cells may be disrupted and inadequately regulated. Cell-to-cell signaling by direct connection or paracrine messengers may be disrupted. Tissue oxygenation may be impaired. Fibrosis is a histopathologic hallmark of many renal diseases (Eddy, 2000).

The ECM is also essential to normal function of the kidney in that it provides structural integrity and contributes to normal signaling systems. When abnormally expressed, however, it becomes detrimental. ECM homeostasis is a complex balance of synthesis and breakdown. Synthetic regulation is controlled by various mechanisms, including growth factors and signaling systems, which are just being discerned. Mechanical forces contribute to these signals in various conditions, including hypertension and hydronephrosis. **ECM breakdown is tightly regulated and represents the product of degradative enzymes (i.e., matrix metalloproteinases [MMPs] and their endogenous inhibitors (i.e., tissue inhibitors of metalloproteinases [TIMPs]). This product is the proteolytic balance and is regulated by various cytokines, hormones, and mechanical forces** (Engelmyer et al, 1995; Diamond et al, 1998). This balance has been studied

vigorously in renal disease and to a limited degree in congenital obstruction (Gobet et al, 1999a).

Modulation of renal fibrosis may be a significant potential target for managing obstructive nephropathy, but the delicate balance of these factors needs to be understood to a greater degree than at present.

KEY POINTS: FIBROSIS

- One of the histologic hallmarks of renal dysplasia is the presence of fibromuscular collars around tubular structures, so-called primitive ducts.

- A universal characteristic of obstructive nephropathy appears to be renal fibrosis.

- Breakdown of ECM is tightly regulated and represents the product of degradative enzymes (matrix metalloproteinases [MMPs] and their endogenous inhibitors (tissue inhibitors of metalloproteinases [TIMPs]).

Evidence and Patterns

Increased interstitial connective tissue is a hallmark of various renal pathologic processes, including obstruction (Eddy, 1996; Diamond et al, 1998; Eddy, 2000). Although it is unclear whether the mechanisms of fibrotic change are universal, they are believed to interfere with intercellular signaling and therefore with functional integration. The most likely causes of excessive connective tissue include abnormal accumulation as a result of an imbalance in synthesis and breakdown. It may also represent abnormal inductive signaling that produces excessive conversion of epithelium to mesenchymal and connective tissue (Herzlinger, 2002; Yang and Liu, 2002). These processes may be normal developmental sequences that persist because of the obstructive effect.

Abnormal accumulation may represent simply excessive synthesis with no change in ECM breakdown. Increased collagen synthesis may be due to upregulation of collagen gene expression in obstructive models (Liapis et al, 1994). Collagen synthesis is regulated in part by various cytokines, including TGF-β (Yokoi et al, 2004), platelet-derived growth factor (PDGF), and the renin-angiotensin system (RAS) (Klahr et al, 1995). Reduced fibrosis has been reported when angiotensinogen activity is downregulated in an obstructed system (Fern et al, 1999) or with inhibition of angiotensin II type 1 (AT1) receptor blockade (Ishidoya et al, 1995). This effect may be countered by activity of the AT2 receptor, whereas absence of this receptor exacerbates obstructive lesions (Ma et al, 1998). Somewhat paradoxically, however, the renal lesions produced with angiotensin blockade are similar to those seen with obstruction, perhaps because of inhibition of ureteral function (Miyazaki et al, 1999). **It is important to recall that the administration of angiotensin-converting enzyme (ACE) or angiotensin receptor inhibitors during pregnancy or in the neonatal period can markedly interfere with normal renal development and function** (Guron et al, 1999; Guron and Friberg, 2000). **Thus, renal development and renal function may be compromised in the setting of either too much or too**

little angiotensin (Chevalier, 2004b), Similar therapeutic approaches to reduce the action of endogenous angiotensin have been demonstrated in nonobstructive fibrosis as well (Weber, 1997; Sharma et al, 1999; Toblli et al, 2004).

The role of TGF-β is complex and dependent on the context, yet inhibition of its activity will produce less fibrosis as well (Isaka et al, 2000). There is evidence that TGF-β is tightly regulated with the RAS (Chung et al, 1995; Miyajima et al, 2000a), in addition to regulating cellular growth dynamics. Fetal obstruction induces increased expression of TGF-β1 (Medjebeur et al, 1997; Ayan et al, 2001). As reviewed earlier, TGF-β1 regulates EMT, thereby contributing to renal dysplasia (Yang et al, 2000), There is considerable interest in the role of TGF-β1 in promoting EMT of differentiated renal tubular epithelial cells in response to chronic ureteral obstruction. As shown in Figure 108–4, renal interstitial fibroblasts, through transformation to myofibroblasts, play a pivotal role in the deposition of ECM in a hydronephrotic kidney. There is growing evidence that in addition to proliferation of resident interstitial fibroblasts and transformation of hematopoietic stem cells, renal tubular epithelial cells can undergo EMT and migrate to the interstitium to contribute to the pool of fibroblasts (Iwano et al, 2002). Many of the steps involved in the transformation of tubular epithelial cells are regulated by TGF-β1; these steps include loss of cell adhesion, expression of α-SMA, disruption of tubular basement membrane, and cell migration to the interstitium (Liu, 2004), Signaling by TGF-β1 is mediated in part by Smads, which are both pro-fibrotic (Smad2 and Smad3) and inhibitory (Smad7). Thus, targeted deletion of Smad3 reduces apoptosis and fibrosis in mice with ureteral obstruction, whereas gene therapy with Smad7 also reduces fibrosis (Lan et al, 2003; Sato et al, 2003). In contrast, hepatocyte growth factor (HGF) blocks EMT by blocking Smad2 and Smad3, and gene therapy with HGF reduces fibrosis in rats with ureteral obstruction (Yang et al, 2003; Gao et al, 2002). These complex networks of counterbalancing factors provide many potential opportunities for therapeutic intervention to prevent the progression—or even promote the reversal—of interstitial fibrosis resulting from obstructive nephropathy (Fogo, 2003).

Nitric oxide (NO) has also been shown to regulate the development of obstructive fibrosis in postnatal animals and may play a similar role prenatally. Increased NO generation reduces the degree of interstitial fibrosis, and in animals without the gene to produce NO synthase, unilateral ureteral obstruction (UUO) produces a greater degree of fibrosis than in animals with this enzyme intact (Hochberg et al, 2000; Miyajima et al, 2001).

Altered regulation of ECM breakdown, the proteolytic balance, is also a potential mechanism for the interstitial fibrosis associated with obstruction, though less explored. Connective tissue breakdown is controlled by the MMPs, at least 15 of which have specific activity against particular connective tissue proteins. MMP-1, for instance, is a collagenase (Pardo and Selman, 2005), whereas MMP-2 specifically degrades gelatin. Their expression and activity are both subject to close regulation because it is crucial to appropriate ECM homeostasis. Too much activity will degrade tissues, and too little permits accumulation of abnormal amounts of ECM. These pathologic alterations have been described in a variety of disease states, including arthritis and pulmonary fibrosis (Corbel et al, 2002; Vincenti and Brinckerhoff, 2002). One of the means by which their activity is regulated is through endogenous TIMPs. These enzymes are less varied and may have less specific activity over the MMPs in their environment, and they serve to check the degradative activity of MMPs. The role of proteolytic balance in a wide variety of disease states has been the subject of active research (Diamond et al, 1998; Vincenti, 2001).

Altered activity and regulation of MMPs and TIMPs have been studied in the kidney (Eddy, 1996) in several conditions, and it is clear that they are important regulators of the state of the ECM. Their expression has been shown in the developing kidney as well, and in postnatal obstruction (Engelmyer

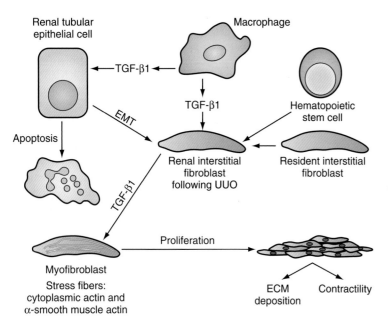

Figure 108–4. Diagram depicting the possible origin, fate, and regulatory factors of renal interstitial fibroblasts in the setting of obstruction. Factors mediating epithelial to mesenchymal transformation (EMT) would clearly be important in determining the myofibroblast population, which thereby determines extracellular matrix deposition (fibrosis) and the mechanical properties of the renal interstitium. (From Chevalier, RL: Obstructive nephropathy: Towards biomarker discovery and gene therapy. Nat Clin Prac Nephrol 2:157-168, 2006.)

et al, 1995), they are altered in activity. The complexity of this interaction is suggested by the finding that TIMP-1 knockout mice with obstruction have unchanged fibrosis, probably because of other TIMPs being activated (Kim et al, 2001). Proteolytic dysregulation has been demonstrated in prenatal obstruction (Gobet et al, 1999a). The precise regulators of MMPs and TIMPs in development and obstruction are not well defined but are likely to be an important element in the development of pathologic fibrosis. There is evidence of regulation by the RAS and TGF-β as well (Diamond et al, 1998; Zaoui et al, 2000).

Fibrosis is clearly a major component of the pathophysiology of congenital obstruction. Understanding the role and activities of the various components of this system may permit more specific diagnosis through urinary biomarkers reflecting the elements of the system. These elements may also be relevant targets of therapeutic intervention to modulate ECM homeostasis.

FUNCTIONAL INTEGRATION

Renal function is regulated at numerous levels, including neural, vascular, and endocrine, and such regulation may be significantly affected by inflammatory processes. Congenital obstruction alters both ongoing functional integration of the kidney and development of the mechanisms that are intrinsic to this regulation. It can change the regulatory mechanisms themselves. For example, hypertension is well recognized as a potential consequence of obstruction and may have effects beyond the kidney. More subtle effects on the normal regulatory systems of the kidney may be more difficult to detect.

Inflammation

Inflammation appears to be a common consequence of obstruction in the postnatal human or animal model (Diamond et al, 1994; Diamond, 1995). **Much attention has been paid to inflammation in acquired obstruction, but it is surprisingly absent in congenital obstruction.** Biopsies of human kidneys with obstruction but no history of infection have sparse inflammatory infiltrates (Weei-Yuarn et al, 2005), whereas models of fetal obstruction have little evidence of inflammation (Peters et al, 1992). The reason for this marked difference is unclear but suggests fundamentally distinct mechanisms. It is another indication that congenital obstruction is distinct in many ways from postnatal acquired obstruction.

Although inflammatory changes do not appear to be a major factor in early postnatal COU, it is likely that they begin to play a greater role with age. It will be necessary to confirm the pattern and role of these factors in COU in humans inasmuch as many animal systems demonstrate significant inflammation postnatally although fetal systems do not. Human pathologic material has not shown large amounts of inflammation, except when complicated by infection. If there is a subset of patients with inflammatory changes in the face of obstruction, it would seem an important target for investigation to improve both diagnosis and therapy. The various inflammatory cascades that have been investigated postnatally

can be manipulated pharmacologically, which may permit important therapeutic regulation of renal injury. These mediators will be measurable in urine as well, as has been shown in experimental systems (el-Dahr et al, 1993; Diamond et al, 1994; Stephan et al, 2002; Silverstein et al, 2003).

Many of the inflammatory responses to ureteral obstruction are mediated or modulated by angiotensin (Chevalier and Cachat, 2001). **A variety of cytokines and chemokines play a role, including monocyte chemoattractant protein (MCP-1), which promotes the recruitment of interstitial macrophages.** Gene therapy with injection of a mutant MCP-1 gene (*CCL2*) can block macrophage recruitment and reduces interstitial fibrosis in experimental obstructive nephropathy (Wada et al, 2004). Urinary MCP-1 is increased in children with UPJ obstruction, and renal tissue MCP-1 is increased in rats with ureteral obstruction (Grandaliano et al, 2000; Stephan et al, 2002), which suggests that this cytokine may be useful as a biomarker of obstructive nephropathy.

Vascular

The developing vascular tree plays a critical role in renal development (Gomez and Norwood, 1995; Tufro-McReddie et al, 1995), and any alteration could be associated with a wide variety of abnormalities ranging from lack of development of the glomerulus to aberrant regulation of renal blood flow. Sensitivity to humoral and neural regulation of blood flow may be altered as well, and this effect may be permanent.

Expression of renal renin is increased in the obstructed kidney and decreased in the contralateral one (el Dahr et al, 1990). **Renin-secreting renal cortical cells appear to be recruited with obstruction as well** (Norwood et al, 1994). Expression of receptors for the RAS is altered in specific patterns in neonatal obstruction (Yoo et al, 1997). AT1, which mediates vasoconstriction (as well as growth alterations), increases, whereas levels of AT2, which acts in a contrary manner, are decreased. These alterations suggest a role for a local renal RAS in obstruction-mediated vasoconstriction and are independent of the systemic RAS (Gobet et al, 1999b).

Altered sensitivity of both kidneys to renin-mediated vasoconstriction has been shown to occur with unilateral obstruction. After release of the obstruction, sensitivity to angiotensin II–mediated vasoconstriction was reduced in the obstructed kidney but increased in the contralateral one (Chevalier and Gomez, 1988). These observations indicate the sensitivity of renal vascular regulation to obstruction, as well as the importance of recognizing the interaction of the two developing kidneys. **The role of renal counterbalance in obstruction has been recognized but investigated to a limited degree.** A possible mechanism for these observations is neural regulation of renin expression.

Neural

Renal innervation is an important regulator of vascularity and perfusion and is associated with expression of renin in the kidney (el Dahr et al, 1991). Sympathetic pharmacologic denervation has been shown to reduce the expected increase in renin expression in the setting of obstruction. **A more primitive pattern of renin gene expression appears to persist with congenital obstruction and may cause persistence of the fetal patterns of vascular regulation. Although renin-expressing cells of the juxtaglomerular apparatus had long been thought to represent highly specialized terminally differentiated cells, it is now recognized that renin expression represents an immature phenotype.** This immature pattern can be re-expressed by vascular cells when stressed by urinary tract obstruction or other threats to homeostasis (Lopez et al, 2001; Lopez et al, 2004).

Hormonal

The major hormones regulating renal functional development are in the RAS and have clearly been shown to be affected by COU. This has a variety of effects, including growth alteration, fibrosis, and altered blood flow. The sensitivity of the kidney to elements of the RAS changes during development, presumably to permit transition from the fetal state to the postnatal environment. Postnatally, all filtration must take place through the kidneys rather than the placenta, as it did prenatally. This transition is likely to be related to the shift in expression of angiotensin receptors as one aspect of this system. In fetal life, AT2 is predominant in expression, has a vasodilating effect, and may promote growth, whereas AT1 is less active until after birth and permits regulation of renal perfusion in the postnatal environment (Robillard et al, 1995; Gimonet et al, 1998). **Altered developmental regulation of these receptors has been induced with fetal obstruction** (Gobet et al, 1999b; Ayan et al, 2001). Targeting these specific alterations may provide information about the impact of obstruction, as well as have therapeutic value. Improved diagnostics may be developed if imaging can be linked to hormonal activity that has distinct patterns in obstruction. For example, if COU induces a fetal pattern of RAS receptor subtypes, perfusion renography or imaging coupled with pharmacologic inhibition or stimulation of this system, as in a captopril renogram, may permit identification of this specific pattern (Bajpai et al, 2002).

Another target may be aldosterone, an element of the RAS that has been shown to contribute to cardiac and renal fibrosis in various pathologic situations (Weber et al, 1994). Inhibition with spironolactone, a receptor antagonist, has been demonstrated experimentally to limit the amount of interstitial fibrosis in a juvenile rodent model of complete obstruction (Trachtman et al, 2004). This finding raises the potential for therapeutic interventions with familiar pharmacologic tools, yet it also indicates the complexity of interaction in the kidney's responses to obstruction.

Tubular Function

Although glomerular filtration and renal plasma flow are the most commonly measured aspect of renal function, renal tubular function is equally important but often ignored in obstructive uropathy. Tubular function regulates acid-base homeostasis, electrolyte balance, and urinary concentration, as well as vitamin D homeostasis. When bilateral,

---

KEY POINTS: FUNCTIONAL INTEGRATION

- Angiotensin is a key modulator of many of the inflammatory responses to ureteral obstruction.

- Expression of renal renin is increased in the obstructed kidney and decreased in the contralateral one. Renin-secreting renal cortical cells appear to be recruited with obstruction as well.

- The activity of the RAS is altered with obstruction, which affects renal functional development by a variety of changes, including growth, fibrosis, and blood flow.

- Tubuloglomerular feedback, the mechanism for regulating the amount of fluid delivered to the tubules by the glomerulus, is altered in the face of obstruction.

---

defects in these various functions are major clinical problems. When unilateral, they are often compensated for by the contralateral kidney and are therefore difficult to measure accurately and noninvasively. **There are reports of persisting tubular dysfunction in various unilateral congenital obstructions** (Hutcheon et al, 1976; Chandar et al, 1996), **but it is uncommon for such dysfunction to be a clinical problem.**

Congenital obstruction can be shown experimentally to produce several functional effects on the renal tubules, including sodium and water homeostasis. Specific downregulation of sodium transporters in the tubules, as well as a reduction in expression and protein levels of the aquaporins, has been demonstrated in neonatal obstruction in rats (Frokiaer et al, 1996; Frokiaer et al, 1997; Li et al, 2001; Li et al, 2003; Shi et al, 2004a), Although these defects may be compensated for by a contralateral kidney and thus be limited in their clinical impact, alterations in urinary levels of these proteins may serve as markers for significant obstructive effects.

Tubuloglomerular feedback, the mechanism for regulating the amount of fluid delivered to the tubules by the glomerulus, has been shown to be specifically altered in the face of obstruction, perhaps as a protective response. This has not been studied in congenital obstruction but in juvenile animals (Morsing et al, 1987; Morsing and Persson, 1991a; Morsing and Persson, 1991b; Morsing et al, 1995).

The obstructive mechanisms of injury are likely to be a combination of the effects just described, and therapeutic interventions targeted to these mechanisms may limit tubular dysfunction. Measuring abnormal tubular function may be possible with more sensitive measures and imaging technology (Wen et al, 2002b; Pedersen et al, 2003).

REVERSAL OF CONGENITAL RENAL OBSTRUCTION

An important element in the understanding of congenital obstruction is the potential for reversal of renal functional and developmental impairment with correction of the obstructive lesion. This is clinically relevant when making decisions regarding the utility of intervention either postnatally or prenatally. In the latter, the potential for reversal has great significance in determining whether the risks associated with fetal intervention are warranted. Improvement in function is also important in the expectation of response to relief of obstruction.

In the fetal obstructed kidney, Glick and colleagues showed that the functional salvageability of a unilaterally obstructed kidney was dependent on the duration of obstruction and gestational age (Glick et al, 1984). A direct relationship between progression of nephronogenesis and reversibility can be demonstrated (Edouga et al, 2001). Similar observations have been made in early postnatal models, with the recognition that complete reversal of the damage is seldom achieved (Claesson et al, 1987; Chevalier et al, 1988; Chevalier et al, 1999b; Chevalier et al, 2002; Eskild-Jensen et al, 2003; Shi et al, 2004b). Mediators of improvement have not been explored. The severity of obstruction is also a critical determinant (Bussieres et al, 1993), but it is challenging to measure in any meaningful way. Biomarkers of salvageability have been developed and were first used clinically in accordance with the work of Glick and Adzick in obstructed fetal sheep (Adzick et al, 1985). From these basic parameters emerged the clinical prognostic factors currently used, with modification, in fetal obstruction (Harrison et al, 1982; Glick et al, 1985). **Measures of urinary sodium, chloride, osmolarity, and calcium have correlated with fetal renal functional potential** (Muller et al, 1993; Johnson et al, 1995; Dommergues et al, 2000). **When fetal urine approaches the character of serum, irreversible damage appears to have been done to the developing kidney.** Other markers have been explored in the fetus, including α_1-microglobulin in amniotic fluid and β_2-microglobulin in urine and serum (Burghard et al, 1987; Freedman et al, 1997; Nicolini and Spelzini, 2001).

The mechanisms of functional recovery may be similar to the mechanisms of injury, but they may also be unique and the potential may exist for enhancing recovery if these mechanisms can be understood and used. In part, the pathway of recovery includes normal developmental pathways that had been impaired because of obstruction (Chevalier et al, 1988). **As a consequence of urinary tract obstruction, nephron injury is heterogeneous, with some nephrons undergoing adaptive growth and hyperfiltration and others being destroyed. Thus, 1 month after relief of 5 days of UUO in the neonatal rat, the glomerular filtration rate (GFR) of the postobstructed kidney was normal despite a 40% reduction in the number of glomeruli** (Chevalier, 1999b). **However, 1 year after relief of the obstruction, the GFR of the postobstructed kidney had decreased by 80%** (Chevalier et al, 2000c). Even though there had been no further loss of nephrons during this interval, the remaining glomeruli had undergone progressive sclerosis (Chevalier et al, 2000c), Although relief of temporary UUO did not lead to nephron loss in the adult rat, there was a reduction in glomeruli after relief of temporary UUO in the period immediately following nephrogenesis, as well as during nephrogenesis (Chevalier et al, 2002). This underscores the susceptibility of the developing kidney to obstructive injury not only during nephrogenesis but also during subsequent nephron maturation.

KEY POINTS: REVERSAL OF CONGENITAL RENAL OBSTRUCTION

- The functional salvageability of a unilateral obstructed fetal kidney is dependent on the duration of obstruction and gestational age.

- Measures of urinary sodium, chloride, osmolarity, and calcium have been correlated with fetal renal functional potential.

- When fetal urine approaches the character of serum, irreversible damage appears to have been done to the developing kidney.

HUMAN RELEVANCE
Approach to Clinical Cases

The clinical challenge of COU is due to the clinical spectrum of the condition itself. On the one hand, we are challenged in determining which patients may need intervention to preserve renal functional development. Some will clearly need such intervention, whereas many others will do well without it. Given the wide spectrum, it is extremely difficult to determine a clinically practical dividing line between those in whom intervention is appropriate and those in whom it is not needed. This question is relevant to the largest number of patients with some form of COU. Ultimate determination of the need for intervention may come as a single diagnostic test or be based on a pattern of change or lack thereof over time. In this situation we wish to be sensitive but will accept being less specific. We would rather not miss a large number of patients with COU who need intervention while recognizing that some patients may undergo further evaluation or intervention when they might not have needed it.

The second challenge in COU concerns patients at the extreme end of the spectrum in whom renal functional impairment has already occurred and poses a threat of permanent renal insufficiency. In the face of obstruction, what is our best approach to preserve the maximal amount of renal function? Even with successful surgical intervention, we are often confronted with an inexorable progression to renal failure in these children, yet it would seem reasonable to ask whether we can prevent this renal demise. Thus far, there has been no clinically applicable approach, but as our understanding of the pathophysiologic mechanisms of COU improves, we may be able to specifically affect a critical component of the system to better regulate the mechanisms affecting the renal response to obstruction.

Diagnosis

The challenge to be able to diagnose "obstruction" has been made more difficult because of disagreement regarding the definition of obstruction in the first place. **Although the concept that obstruction is an "impairment of urine flow that will produce a reduction in function if left uncorrected" is logical** (Koff, 1987), **it misses several important elements in the context of congenital obstruction.** One is that the developing kidney should be increasing its function, not remaining static. It also does not provide any insight into the interpretation of a kidney that has reduced function when diagnosed. Strictly interpreted, this kidney is already affected and by definition is "obstructed." This interpretation has not been used clinically, however, and it is only on prospective follow-up that a decrease from normal is considered by many to be indicative of "obstruction." **A more useful definition might be that any condition that has or will limit ultimate functional potential should be considered clinically significant obstruction** (Peters, 1995). It should also be recognized that "obstruction" does not mean that surgical therapy is required. The obstruction may be mild and clinically insignificant. Exclusion of these patients from the diagnosis of "obstruction" has tended to force people to create convoluted descriptions of hydronephrotic kidneys.

Ultimately, a determination of the potential risk to a kidney will have to be made clinically and a judgment made regarding whether a particular child would benefit from intervention. It would seem reasonable and cautious to assume that any hydronephrotic kidney is obstructed until proved otherwise and assess the degree of risk. Understanding the pathologic mechanisms of obstructive nephropathy will permit more specific examination of the kidney to determine its response. It should be the renal response primarily that is used to make a determination of the obstructive effect. The fluid dynamics of the upper urinary tract, though obviously relevant to the renal effect, should not be the primary focus. This may be why many drainage studies, including diuretic renography and pressure perfusion tests, are imperfect predictors of the renal response. **We have seen that an obstructed kidney is undergoing altered growth regulation, abnormal differentiation, and increased fibrosis, all mediated through a variety of molecular, cellular, and renal homeostatic mechanisms. These patterns of change are likely to be reflected in altered expression of proteins and chemicals, which may be assayed in urine.** There may be systemic alterations that are detectable in blood as well. The search for these biomarkers has been active, yet few have been firmly linked to the pathologic progression of obstructive nephropathy.

Biomarkers of renal obstruction may reflect the response of the kidney in a direct manner, such as expression of growth factors that contribute to fibrosis or that are associated with increased apoptosis in renal epithelium (Chevalier, 2004a). They may also be downstream effects reflecting specific alterations mediated by other cytokines and in themselves not directly relevant, but indicative of the level and pattern of the obstructive effect. A broad approach that is emerging uses assessment of changes in overall protein expression in urine, or proteomics. Normal kidneys will have a somewhat consistent urinary protein fingerprint, which is altered with obstruction. If particular elements of the alteration can be identified and associated with clinical outcomes, these patterns may be diagnostic of functionally significant obstruction. Such patterns may reflect a single protein, which may be an element of a response pattern or a downstream consequence. It may be that a particular pattern of protein expression involving several factors will be the best indicator of obstruction. Such studies will require development in animal systems and validation in humans. It will be necessary to set limits for what is

and is not "obstruction" and correlate this with clinical and functional outcomes of relevance.

An alternative approach to diagnosis may be to assess response to a stimulus. This is the basis of the captopril renogram, in which radionuclide uptake in the face of obstruction is reduced when the RAS is inhibited by the ACE inhibitor captopril, but not in the dilated, nonobstructed system. The underlying rationale for this test, which remains poorly defined, is that in an obstructed kidney, function is dependent on increased activity of the RAS, as suggested earlier. By reducing the capacity of this system to support function, a drop is detected in the postcaptopril study. The concept is reasonable, but problems with definitions of true "obstruction" continue to thwart its wide applicability. Alternative pharmacologic manipulations may be needed to more specifically address one or more functional factors in a potentially obstructed kidney. The production of various cytokines in the face of a stimulus may be able to distinguish a kidney at risk for injury from a kidney not at risk.

Prognosis

Assessment of possible outcome for an obstructed kidney is important in terms of determining the value of an intervention and providing clinical prediction of possible failure of the kidney. These predictions will serve to guide therapy and assessment of the risk-benefit balance in treatment. As yet, there are few studies that suggest any accuracy in either unilateral or bilateral obstruction. The use of renal biopsies in obstruction has shown some correlations, but none that are clinically practical (Weei-Yuarn et al, 2005). It is likely that this ability will follow from more accurate diagnostic testing.

Management Strategies

Can any of our current incomplete understanding of COU be used to develop a clinical management strategy for these patients? Several factors seem to emerge from the many conflicting and incomplete studies of congenital obstruction. Obstruction can be very harmful to a developing kidney, to an extent far beyond that seen in a mature kidney. The effects of obstruction may not be reversible because of alteration of the actual structure and functional characteristics of the kidney, which does not occur in a mature kidney. There seems to be a limited time window to permit reversal of obstruction and anticipate clinically relevant recovery of functional potential. It is clear that a developing kidney, as with a mature kidney, is able to compensate for obstruction and can appear to be healthy. However, most biologic compensation mechanisms are ultimately limited in their ability to maintain homeostasis and may mask eventual significant functional derangements. The clinical threshold for intervention may therefore be better set lower than in a mature patient.

The response to obstruction in a developing kidney is extremely complex, and multiple factors are involved in various aspects of this response. Although this may seem to be a significant impediment to understanding and clinically managing these problems, it should be seen as providing multiple opportunities to develop biomarkers of these responses that may eventually facilitate our decision-making.

It is clear that not all children with dilated kidneys will suffer ill effects from this condition; it is equally evident that the potential for obstructive nephropathy is significant and has severe clinical implications. As our understanding of these conditions and the mechanisms of the renal response to obstruction in development improves, determination of kidneys at risk for developmental impairment will become more accurate.

SELECTED READINGS

Bernstein J: The morphogenesis of renal parenchymal maldevelopment (renal dysplasia). Pediatr Clin North Am 1971;18:395-407.

Chevalier RL: Pathophysiology of obstructive nephropathy in the newborn. Semin Nephrol 1998;18:585-593.

Chevalier RL: Biomarkers of congenital obstructive nephropathy: Past, present and future. J Urol 2004;172:852-857.

Chevalier RL, Goyal S, Wolstenholme JT, et al: Obstructive nephropathy in the neonatal rat is attenuated by epidermal growth factor. Kidney Int 1998;54:38-47.

Chevalier RL, Thornhill BA, Wolstenholme JT, et al: Unilateral ureteral obstruction in early development alters renal growth: Dependence on the duration of obstruction. J Urol 1999;161:309-313.

Daiekha-Dahmane F, Dommergues M, Muller F, et al: Development of human fetal kidney in obstructive uropathy: Correlations with ultrasonography and urine biochemistry. Kidney Int 1997;52:21-32.

Eskild-Jensen A, Munch Jorgensen T, Olsen LH, et al: Renal function may not be restored when using decreasing differential function as the criterion for surgery in unilateral hydronephrosis. BJU Int 2003;92:779-782.

Glick PL, Harrison MR, Adzick NS, et al: Correction of congenital hydronephrosis in utero IV: In utero decompression prevents renal dysplasia. J Pediatr Surg 1984;19:649-657.

Gobet R, Park JM, Nguyen HT, et al: Renal renin-angiotensin system dysregulation caused by partial bladder outlet obstruction in fetal sheep. Kidney Int 1999;56:1654-1661.

Kennedy WA 2nd, Buttyan R, Garcia-Montes E, et al: Epidermal growth factor suppresses renal tubular apoptosis following ureteral obstruction. Urology 1997;49:973-980.

Koff SA: Postnatal management of antenatal hydronephrosis using an observational approach. Urology 2000;55:609-611.

Matsell DG: Renal dysplasia: New approaches to an old problem. Am J Kidney Dis 1998;32:535-543.

Miyazaki Y, Tsuchida S, Fogo A, et al: The renal lesions that develop in neonatal mice during angiotensin inhibition mimic obstructive nephropathy. Kidney Int 1999;55:1683-1695.

Muller F, Dommergues M, Mandelbrot L, et al: Fetal urinary biochemistry predicts postnatal renal function in children with bilateral obstructive uropathies. Obstet Gynecol 1993;82:813-820.

Peters CA: Obstruction of the fetal urinary tract. J Am Soc Nephrol 1997;8:653-663.

Peters CA, Carr MC, Lais A, et al: The response of the fetal kidney to obstruction. J Urol 1992;148:503.

Steinhardt GF, Vogler G, Salinas ML, et al: Induced renal dysplasia in the young pouch opossum. J Pediatr Surg 1988;23:1127-1130.

Thornhill BA, Burt LE, Chen C, et al: Variable chronic partial ureteral obstruction in the neonatal rat: A new model of ureteropelvic junction obstruction. Kidney Int 2005;67:42-52.

Weei-Yuarn H, Peters CA, Zurakowski D, et al: Renal biopsy in congenital ureteropelvic junction obstruction: Evidence for parenchymal maldevelopment. Kidney Int 2005;69:137-143.

109 Perinatal Urology

CRAIG A. PETERS, MD

FETAL DIAGNOSIS

The impact of prenatal ultrasonographic (US) diagnosis on pediatric urology continues to be significant, effectively creating a new class of disorders that require unique management approaches. Many of these patients are helped greatly with early diagnosis and prevention of secondary complications, particularly infection. Others, however, may be seen as being subjected to needless interventions because of prenatal findings of uncertain long-term clinical significance. The debate will continue until a more practical understanding of the pathophysiology and an accurate assessment of these conditions' natural history is obtained. For now, we are obliged to make clinical decisions based upon the patient's condition and parents' wishes. The chapter reviews the principles of prenatal urologic diagnosis and management and immediate care of the neonate with urologic problems.

Diagnostic Findings

Interpretation of any prenatal US image is based upon a synthesis of specific findings to generate a differential diagnosis, exactly as is done postnatally. As with any one test, a definitive diagnosis may not always be made with certainty, and the ability to make a definitive diagnosis depends upon the interpreter. The need for diagnostic accuracy, particularly when there is a spectrum of involvement, is also relative to the clinical situation. There are several essential elements to any prenatal US examination of the urinary tract that are used to define the possible diagnoses and they are illustrated in Table 109–1. Recognizing these specific findings and their variations and knowing the patterns of association that suggest specific diagnostic entities usually permit the perinatal urologist to make an accurate diagnosis, adequate for the immediate perinatal period.

The **normal kidney** (Fig. 109–1) has an elliptical shape with distinctive internal echoes defined by the medullary pyramids and peripelvic echo complex. The renal cortex should be of uniform echogenicity, slightly less than that of the spleen or liver. **The echolucent pyramids should not be confused for dilated calyces and first become evident at about 20 weeks. Their absence later in gestation is abnormal.** The size of the normal kidney is important as it may reflect the condition of the contralateral kidney.

The renal parenchyma may be abnormally echogenic without having frank cysts. In some children this has been seen as an isolated finding without apparent negative sequelae, but it has also been associated with renal parenchymal disorders (Brenbridge et al, 1986; Estroff et al, 1991; Carr et al, 1995; Tsatsaris et al, 2002). When associated with hydronephrosis, increased renal echogenicity suggests dysplastic changes, but this is not invariable unless there is profound hydronephrosis, often with decreasing amniotic fluid (Kaefer et al, 1997b). The thickness of the parenchyma in the setting of hydronephrosis is important to note but does not clearly predict decreased function. Often this thinning is simply due to stretching of the parenchyma around a dilated collecting system. The label "cortical atrophy" should be discouraged.

Hydronephrosis is the most common abnormality found on prenatal ultrasonography and is seen in a wide spectrum, from pelvic dilation that is barely noticeable to massive dilation taking up much of the fetal abdomen (Figs. 109–2, 109–3, and 109–4). **Hydronephrosis is not a specific diagnosis but a finding or sign. The cause of the hydronephrosis is the diagnosis and indicates the appropriate treatment.** The character of the hydronephrosis, however, is extremely important to permit a diagnosis and prognosis. A variety of grading systems have been used in the literature, all of which have similar strengths and limitations. Numerical grading systems convey a sense of quantification, as do renal pelvic anterior-posterior (AP) diameter measurements (Fernbach et al, 1993). The correlation between degree of hydronephrosis and postnatal outcome, as discussed in the following, remains poor, which limits the value of an overprecise grading system. We have used the descriptive scale shown, with specific comment on the nature of calyceal dilation. AP diameter measurements are useful in a comparative sense, but there is variability in the reliability of these numbers. Practical thresholds have been developed from these measurements but should be used only as rough guidelines (Corteville et al, 1991; Clautice-Engle

Table 109-1. Elements of Prenatal Urologic Ultrasonographic Diagnosis

Parameter	Comment	Possible Causes
Hydronephrosis	Variable severity; may include pelviectasis and/or caliectasis	Obstruction, reflux
Caliectasis	Intrarenal dilation; more indicative of significant pathologic process	Obstruction, reflux
Pelvic AP diameter	Measured in the coronal plane, variable; in extremes may predict clinical outcome; caution should be exercised in overreliance on these measurements	Increased in obstruction, reflux
Renal parenchyma	Echogenicity should be less than that of liver or spleen; lucent medullary pyramids should be seen	Increased echogenicity in dysplasia, obstruction, ARPKD
Urothelial thickening	Increased thickness of pelvic lining	Variable dilation as with reflux or occasionally obstruction
Duplication	Separation of renal pelvic sinus echoes when no hydronephrosis seen	Possible associated reflux or obstruction; look for dilated ureter and ureterocele
Cystic structures, renal	Simple cysts rare	MCDK, ADPKD
Cystic structures, intravesical	May be very large and fill bladder; thin walled	Ureterocele
Urinoma	Fluid collection around kidney; perinephric or subcapsular	Obstruction
Bladder filling	Fill and void cycles may be demonstrated over time	Urine production
Bladder wall thickness	Must be interpreted in context of bladder filling	Obstruction, neurogenic dysfunction
Keyhole sign	Dilated posterior urethral; difficult to image	Posterior urethral valves
Oligohydramnios	Markedly reduced amniotic fluid; usually considered as no pocket of fluid > 2 cm	Poor urine output because of obstruction and/or renal failure

AP, anterior-posterior; ADPKD, autosomal dominant polycystic kidney disease; ARPKD, autosomal recessive polycystic kidney disease; MCDK, multicystic dysplastic kidney.

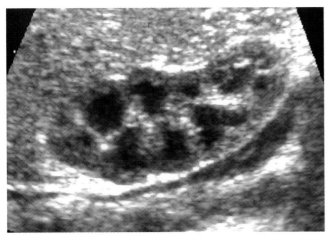

Figure 109-1. Ultrasound appearance of normal fetal kidney with echolucent medullary pyramids distinguishable from the more echogenic cortical parenchyma. The cortical parenchyma should be of lower echogenicity than adjacent liver or spleen.

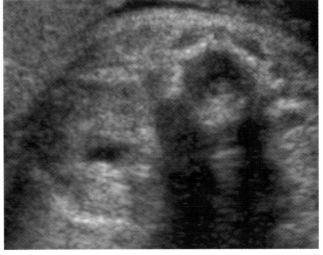

Figure 109-2. Mild fetal hydronephrosis seen in a transverse view. The bright area to the right of the kidney is the spine. The anterior-posterior pelvic diameter is best measured in this view; however, calyceal configuration is not well seen.

et al, 1995; Scott and Renwick, 2001). **When describing hydronephrosis, the pelvic and calyceal configuration must be included, as well as whether it is unilateral or bilateral.** It is best if the side of involvement is known as this does not always correlate with postnatal findings and might suggest variability, perhaps related to reflux. Any variation in the degree of hydronephrosis during one examination is an important finding that is strongly suggestive of reflux.

Hydroureter may be more difficult to detect, but if it is present, the appearance is characteristic. The markedly dilated ureter is seen in multiple adjacent cross sections, giving it a folded sausage look between the kidney and bladder (Fig. 109-5). **In less severe cases, a dilated ureter is best detected**

behind a full bladder. Ureteral peristalsis may be recognized as well. Confusion may occur if a duplex system has both ureters dilated, as resolution of these structures may not be possible.

Renal cysts may be seen in a variety of disorders and are usually multiple and heterogeneous in size. Multiple small cysts not resolved on US appear as a very bright, large, and echogenic kidney, as seen with autosomal recessive polycystic kidney disease (ARPKD), and the large macrocysts of a multicystic dysplastic kidney (MCDK) are readily apparent. **Cysts do not communicate visibly with each other, in contrast to**

dilated calyces. **A single upper pole cyst is probably not a cyst but a dilated upper pole.** A single cyst in the renal fossa may be an unusual MCDK, severe hydronephrosis without recognizable parenchyma, or a nonrenal structure, including intestinal duplications, cystic tumors of the adrenal, or a loop of bowel.

KEY POINTS: PRENATAL URINARY TRACT ULTRASONOGRAPHY

- The echolucent pyramids of the normal fetal and neonatal kidney should not be confused for dilated calyces and first become evident at about 20 weeks. Their absence later in gestation is abnormal.

- Hydronephrosis is not a specific diagnosis but a finding. The cause of the hydronephrosis is the diagnosis and indicates the appropriate treatment.

- When describing hydronephrosis, the pelvic and calyceal configuration must be included, as well as whether it is unilateral or bilateral.

- Cysts do not communicate visibly with each other, in contrast to dilated calyces. A single upper pole cyst is probably not a cyst but a dilated upper pole.

- Dilation of the posterior urethral, the "keyhole" sign, is strongly suggestive of posterior urethral valves.

- The time of onset of changes in the AF is critical and reflects a normal shift from where most of the AF is a placental transudate to where it becomes predominantly a product of fetal urine. This occurs after 16 weeks, and by 20 or 22 weeks most AF is fetal urine.

- Concurrent with any fetal diagnosis of a urinary tract anomaly must be a thorough fetal survey, including all major systems, an estimate of fetal growth, AF, and the placenta.

The **bladder** is often neglected in fetal studies, as it is often difficult to image well. The bladder should be seen in a filled state on a fetal US and, occasionally, voiding may be detected. If there is a question regarding renal function, bladder filling may be a useful sign of urine output. **The inability to identify a bladder on several studies should raise the question of bladder exstrophy.** The appearance of the bladder wall should be assessed as it may be a clue to bladder outlet obstruction such as posterior urethral valves or neurogenic dysfunction. This is a subjective observation, but, if present, is likely to be a real phenomenon, particularly if associated with hydronephrosis. **Dilation of the posterior urethral, the "keyhole" sign, is strongly suggestive of posterior urethral valves (PUV)** (Figs. 109–6 and 109–7). Intravesical structures, which are always abnormal, should be sought, particularly if a ureterocele may be present in association with a duplex system and upper pole hydronephrosis. An ectopic ureter, also associated with a dilated upper pole, may give the false appearance of an intravesical ureterocele, but the ureterovesical wall is much thicker.

In some obstructive conditions, a **perirenal urinoma** may be present, indicating a significant obstructive effect (Yerkes et al, 2001) (Fig. 109–8). These usually appear as an anechoic structure around the kidney, at times with a thick outer rim that fuses with the kidney cortex, indicating a subcapsular urinoma. Urinary ascites may also be noted in the fetus with severe bladder outlet obstruction. The significance of a urinoma depends on the time of appearance and the anatomic basis. We have reported on perinephric urinomata associated with gradual involution of a previously hydronephrotic kidney, with no detectable function postnatally (Mandell et al, 1994). This probably indicates a high degree of unilateral obstruction, sufficient to induce a pop-off, but also permanent and severe injury to normal development. The pop-off effect may also serve to protect the kidney, but this is more often seen with posterior urethral valves (Adzick et al, 1985b).

A less commonly considered element of fetal US diagnosis is the characterization of the **external genitalia.** In cases in which PUV is a diagnostic possibility, male gender is a required part of the diagnosis, but other conditions may depend on this determination. In situations where there is uncertainty about the development of the external genitalia, careful examination may reveal particular aspects, such as phallic length, chordee, and the presence of scrotal testes. **Care must be exercised in this determination, as a virilized clitoris may appear as a small phallus and without the presence of scrotal testes one cannot finalize a male assignment** (Benacerraf et al, 1989; Bromley et al, 1994; Mandell et al, 1995). The appearance of a dilated, elongated penile urethra may be consistent with megalourethra, which is associated with the prune belly syndrome, although isolated cases have been reported (Dillon et al, 1994) (Fig. 109–9). Bilateral renal obstruction in the setting of a female fetus should suggest the possibility of a cloacal anomaly and bladder outlet obstruction (Cilento et al, 1994; Ohno et al, 2000; Taipale et al, 2004) (Fig. 109–10).

Any assessment of the fetal urinary tract must include a comment on the **amniotic fluid** (AF) volume. Although it is difficult to quantitate AF volume and several systems exist to do so, some indication of whether there is a noticeable reduction and what the time course of any change has been are important indicators of the health of the urinary tract (Queenan et al, 1972; Manning et al, 1981). **The time of onset of changes in the AF is critical and reflects a normal shift from where most of the AF is a placental transudate to where it becomes predominantly a product of fetal urine** (Takeuchi et al, 1994). **This occurs after 16 weeks, and by 20 or 22 weeks most AF is fetal urine.** Oligohydramnios, the condition of reduced AF, may therefore be due to urinary tract obstruction and may become evident only after 18 or 20 weeks of gestation. It may also be the product of abnormal renal development without obstruction, such as bilateral MCDK or ARPKD (Stiller et al, 1988).

Concurrent with any fetal diagnosis of a urinary tract anomaly must be a thorough fetal survey, including all major systems, an estimate of fetal growth, AF, and the placenta. If a major anomaly is identified, and particularly if any consideration for intervention is present, amniocentesis and karyotype are considered essential elements of the evaluation. The incidence of concurrent chromosomal anomalies is relatively high in fetuses with urologic anomalies (Callan et al, 1990; Nicolaides et al, 1992a, 1992b; Snijders et al, 1995).

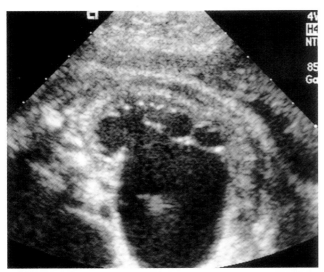

Figure 109–3. Severe fetal hydronephrosis with diffuse calyceal dilation arrayed around the markedly dilated renal pelvis. The renal parenchyma is stretched over the dilated collecting system, but this does not mean loss of functional potential. Corticomedullary differentiation is difficult to see in this configuration.

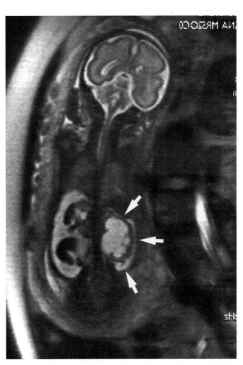

Figure 109–4. Fetal magnetic resonance image of severe hydronephrosis with diffuse calyceal dilation indicated by the *arrows*. The fluid-filled dilated renal pelvis is bright on this imaging sequence.

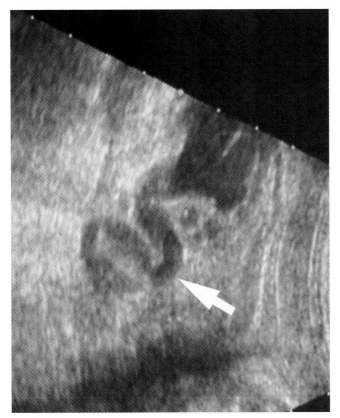

Figure 109–5. Fetal ultrasonography showing a dilated, tortuous ureter *(arrow)*. These may be associated with reflux, valves, ectopic ureters, ureteroceles, and ureterovesical junction obstruction. In this case the ureter is associated with a dilated upper pole indicating an ectopic ureter or ureterocele.

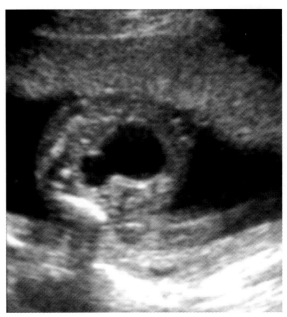

Figure 109–6. Fetal ultrasonography at 22 weeks of a male with posterior urethral valves. The bladder is thick walled and has a dilated posterior urethra (keyhole). There was also bilateral hydronephrosis, echogenic renal parenchyma, and a perinephric urinoma.

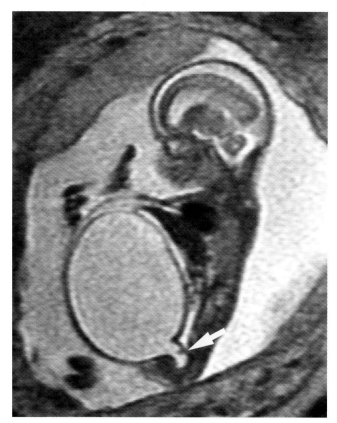

Figure 109-7. Fetal magnetic resonance image showing massive bladder distention from posterior urethral valves. The dilated posterior urethra is seen below the bladder and indicated by the *arrow*.

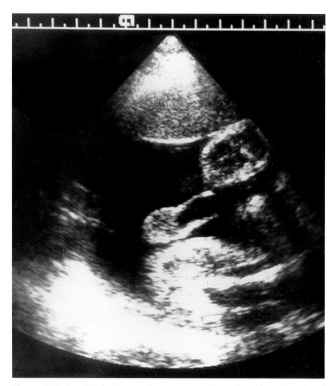

Figure 109-9. Fetal ultrasound appearance of a male with a dilated and patulous urethra typical of a megalourethra. This may be seen in the prune belly syndrome as well as in isolation. This child also had marked vesicoureteral reflux.

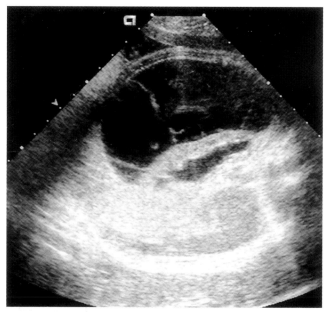

Figure 109-8. Appearance of a fetal perinephric urinoma associated with posterior urethral valves.

Appearance of Major Diagnoses

A tentative fetal diagnosis may be made with US evaluation based on the association of the various elements noted earlier. Although a precise diagnosis may not always be made because of fetal imaging or overlap of some conditions, the differential diagnosis may be refined. Changes over time may also assist in making the ultimate diagnosis. The severity of certain conditions must be considered as well. It is difficult to make a firm prediction of outcome with postnatal imaging studies in many conditions, and in the fetus this is even more restricted.

The usual appearance of a ureteropelvic junction obstruction (UPJO) is limited to some degree of pelvic and calyceal dilation, without any evidence of ureteral dilation. It is usually unilateral, but lesser degrees of dilation may at times be seen on the opposite side. Whether these dilations are all actually due to a functional obstruction at the UPJ remains unclear, largely because of the wide spectrum of severity and the fact that surgery is rarely done for mild to moderate degrees of dilation. It is possible that some component of these cases is secondary to bladder hypertonicity, which is suggested by the extremely high proportion of males with these conditions. There is no postnatally validated degree of hydronephrosis that is truly "normal" or "physiologic." Mild degrees of dilation may reflect significant reflux, even without a dilated ureter.

Ureterovesical junction obstruction is characterized prenatally by dilation of the renal pelvis and ureter to the level of the bladder. The degree is also highly variable, and the amount of renal pelvic and calyceal dilation may be significant (Dorenbaum et al, 1986). The amount of dilation in the ureter may be greater distally than proximally. The ureters may be best seen at the level of the bladder, and some authors have used postnatal ureteral diameter measurements to attempt to prognosticate clinical outcome (Liu et al, 1994; McLellan et al, 2002). The causes of ureterovesical junction obstruction may be several, including primary obstruction of a normally positioned ureter or an ectopic ureter inserting into the bladder neck. Reflux may also produce a very similar pattern.

Vesicoureteral reflux (VUR) may be evident by a variable degree of collecting system dilation; however, there is no reliable way to predict the presence of reflux or its grade on the basis of fetal ultrasonography. Variable hydronephrosis during one examination or between examinations should always raise the suspicion of reflux and prompt postnatal evaluation (Scott, 1987; Scott and Renwick, 2001). Reflux may occasionally be suspected on the basis of increased renal parenchymal echogenicity, which should prompt a postnatal voiding cystourethrogram (VCUG). Massive bilateral hydro-ureteronephrosis may be due to reflux in the megacystis-megaureter association, yet appear similar to bladder outlet obstruction (Mandell et al, 1992a).

One of the most important, although at times challenging, fetal diagnoses is that of **posterior urethral valves.** The wide spectrum of severity seen in postnatal valves gives sufficient indication of the range of possible fetal appearances of this condition. In some situations, the diagnosis is obvious, but in most this suggests a dismal prognosis. In others, the suspicion may be present, but it remains unclear how aggressively to evaluate the patient in the postnatal period. The most severe manifestation of the condition may be seen early in gestation (even as early as 13 weeks) with bladder distention and bilateral hydronephrosis, associated with increased renal echogenicity (Bellinger et al, 1983; Reuter and Lebowitz, 1985;

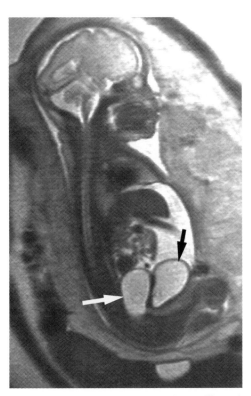

Figure 109–10. Fetal magnetic resonance image illustrating severe bladder dilation *(black arrow)* and a separate dilated pelvic structure behind the bladder *(white arrow)* in a female fetus at 22 weeks. The kidneys were bilaterally and symmetrically dilated with ureteral distention. This pattern can be seen with oligohydramnios and represents a urogenital sinus malformation with bladder outlet obstruction caused by vaginal distention from urine flowing into the urogenital sinus.

Barakat et al, 1991; Dinneen et al, 1993; Hutton et al, 1994; Gunn et al, 1995; Kaefer et al, 1997b; Abbott et al, 1998). The latter may be indicative of renal dysplasia. On occasion, bladder dilation may be massive, taking up most of the fetal abdomen (see Fig. 109–7). With gestational progression, the bladder may become thick walled and the posterior urethra may be recognized by its dilation (see Fig. 109–6). By the mid-second trimester (18 weeks) AF volume may begin to decrease because of the decreasing contribution of the placenta to fluid volume and the increasing contribution of fetal urine, which is obstructed.

Second-trimester oligohydramnios (minimal AF) is usually associated with a lethal outcome in the immediate postnatal period because of pulmonary hypoplasia (Barss et al, 1984). Oligohydramnios may develop later in gestation with a very different prognosis. **Late-onset oligohydramnios (after 30 weeks) is usually not associated with pulmonary insufficiency but may pose obstetric risks** (Mandell et al, 1992c). Valves may also present with a less obvious clinical picture, which may make it indistinguishable from other entities. In the setting of a distended bladder and dilated upper tracts, posterior urethral valves, bilateral megaureters, and bilateral reflux are real possibilities (Abbott et al, 1998). On occasion, the dilated posterior urethra may be noted, and this is strongly suggestive of valves. Other elements that might suggest the presence of valves include perinephric urinomata, increased renal parenchymal echogenicity, and occasionally a thick-walled bladder. In the setting of a dilated fetal bladder, bilateral hydroureteronephrosis with increased parenchymal echogenicity is suggestive of valves, and if oligohydramnios is seen at any time, the diagnosis becomes almost certain (Kaefer et al, 1997a; Oliveira et al, 2000; Oliveira et al, 2002). Significant reflux, however, may appear very similar in male fetuses and only postnatal imaging differentiates the two.

In the female fetus, the appearance of bladder outlet obstruction with bilateral hydroureteronephrosis and a dilated bladder should suggest the presence of the cloacal anomaly or a urogenital sinus causing vaginal distention and bladder obstruction. There is usually a retrovesical fluid-filled structure representing the dilated vagina (see Fig. 109–10).

An unusual cause of fetal bladder outlet obstruction is apparent neurogenic dysfunction with bladder sphincter dyssynergy. This can produce a dilated, thick-walled bladder with hydroureteronephrosis. In a small group of patients, a neurogenic cause was hypothesized, but no clear neurologic lesion could be identified postnatally and the true underlying etiology was speculative (Bauer et al, 1989).

Ureterocele is one of the most definitive diagnoses that may be made in the fetal period, although one of the more challenging (Schoenecker et al, 1985; Fitzsimons et al, 1986; Sherer et al, 1989; Kang et al, 1998; Vergani et al, 1999; Sozubir et al, 2003). **The usual indication of the possibility of a uretero-cele is the presence of upper pole hydronephrosis and a dilated ureter that may be traced to the bladder. Careful inspection of the bladder then usually demonstrates an intravesical, thin-walled cystic structure associated with the base of the bladder** (Fig. 109–11). Communication with the dilated ureter may be seen as well. An alternative appearance is the association of an intravesical cystic structure with a cystic dysplastic upper pole without obvious hydronephrosis. This appearance may evolve to where the

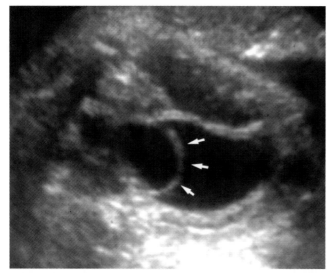

Figure 109–11. Fetal ultrasonography showing an intravesical ureterocele. The ureterocele is indicated by the *arrows* and partially fills the bladder. With this finding, the ultrasonographer should examine the upper tracts to determine whether there is hydronephrosis in the entire affected kidney or only the upper pole, as shown in Figure 109–5.

upper pole is no longer apparent and only the ureterocele is seen. This pattern is termed ureterocele disproportion in which there is little ureteral dilation and a small dysplastic upper pole (Share et al, 1989). **The absence of upper pole dilation should therefore not preclude the diagnosis of a ureterocele when the characteristic intravesical findings are noted.** Single system ureteroceles, seen more frequently in boys, usually have associated hydronephrosis of the entire kidney of variable degree.

In the setting of a ureterocele, it is important to assess the contralateral renal unit as well as the ipsilateral lower pole. Lower pole reflux may produce ipsilateral hydronephrosis, which may occasionally be massive. Contralateral reflux may be present as well, in either a single or a duplex system with lower pole reflux. **Bilateral hydronephrosis may imply bilateral reflux but may also indicate an element of bladder outlet obstruction related to bladder neck prolapse of the ureterocele** (Sozubir et al, 2003). This has occasionally caused oligohydramnios from bladder outlet obstruction (Ashmead et al, 2004).

Upper pole hydronephrosis in the fetus also suggests an ectopic ureter in the absence of an intravesical cystic structure; ureteral ectopia with obstruction is the presumed diagnosis (Abuhamad et al, 1996). The dilated ureter may create a large impression on the back wall of the bladder, mimicking the appearance of a ureterocele. Although it is not always possible to differentiate these accurately, **the wall thickness of the ectopic ureter is much greater than that of the ureterocele, as the latter is made up only of attenuated ureteral wall and the ectopic ureter impression includes both the ureter and bladder walls.** The appearance of bilateral single system ectopic ureters is quite distinct from that of the more common duplex ectopic ureters. Bilateral single ectopic ureters are usually associated with significant renal abnormality manifest by echogenic parenchyma and cysts as well as minimal to no bladder filling. Reduced AF may be associated with severe renal impairment, as is frequently seen.

KEY POINTS: MAJOR DIAGNOSES IN PRENATAL ULTRASONOGRAPHY

- The usual appearance of a ureteropelvic junction obstruction (UPJO) is limited to some degree of pelvic and calyceal dilation, without any evidence of ureteral dilation. It is usually unilateral, but lesser degrees of dilation may at times be seen on the opposite side.

- Vesicoureteral reflux may be evident by a variable degree of collecting system dilation; however, there is no reliable way to predict the presence of reflux or its grade on the basis of fetal ultrasonography.

- Second-trimester oligohydramnios (minimal amniotic fluid) is usually associated with a lethal outcome in the immediate postnatal period related to pulmonary hypoplasia.

- The usual indication of the possibility of a ureterocele is the presence of upper pole hydronephrosis and a dilated ureter that may be traced to the bladder.

- Upper pole hydronephrosis in the fetus also suggests an ectopic ureter in the absence of an intravesical cystic structure.

- The classical US appearance of an MCDK is that of a nonreniform structure, with multiple noncommunicating fluid-filled cystic spaces, no central large cyst, and minimal to no recognizable renal parenchyma.

- The principal diagnostic confusion with MCDK is severe hydronephrosis.

- Autosomal recessive polycystic kidney disease (ARPKD; infantile polycystic kidney disease) does not appear cystic but is characterized by markedly enlarged, brightly echogenic kidneys.

- Classical bladder exstrophy is characterized by the absence of bladder filling on repeated examinations, low-set umbilical cord, and abnormal-appearing external genitalia.

- Clues that the diagnosis is obstruction, rather than VUR, include bladder wall thickening, echogenic renal parenchyma, and a dilated posterior urethra.

One of the most characteristic fetal US appearances is that of the MCDK. The classic US appearance of an MCDK was initially defined by Sanders as being a nonreniform structure, with multiple noncommunicating fluid-filled cystic spaces, no central large cyst, and minimal to no recognizable renal parenchyma (Bearman et al, 1976; Sanders et al, 1984). The overall size of the cyst complex is quite variable, but its appearance is quite characteristic and immediately recognizable (Fig. 109–12). The absence of communication of the cystic structures, which is an essential part of the imaging diagnosis, is apparent on real-time imaging. In the severely hydronephrotic kidney, dilated calyces may appear to be noncommunicating on a static image, but the communications may be seen in

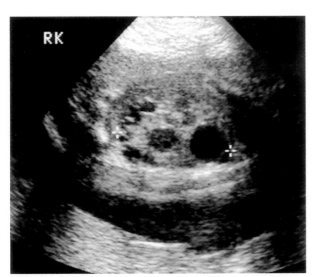

Figure 109–12. Multicystic dysplastic kidney with large, multiple, variable-sized cysts without a central large cystic area. As here, most cases show virtually no parenchyma.

dynamic views. The absence of US communication is in distinction to anatomic communication, usually through fine channels (Peters et al, 1989; Borer et al, 1994). The amount of parenchyma is also variable, and there are examples of MCDKs that have a more substantial amount of parenchyma visible (Felson and Cussen, 1975). It is invariably echogenic and may be seen to contain small cysts. It is not oriented in any particular aspect of the cystic complex.

The **location of the MCDK**, although typically in the usual renal position, may be seen in any position of an ectopic kidney, including the pelvis or as a crossed ectopic renal unit. In these locations, of course, the diagnosis may be more difficult in that other cystic anomalies may also be found in those positions.

Duplex systems may include a multicystic dysplastic moiety, usually the upper pole and rarely the lower. Associated ureteral pathology should then be sought, including ureteroceles or ureteral ectopia. This is best performed with a careful examination of the bladder.

The **principal diagnostic confusion with MCDK is severe hydronephrosis.** In such severe cases, the renal parenchyma is markedly attenuated, echogenic, and distorted by the dilated collecting system. The characteristic of most severely hydronephrotic kidneys is the presence of a central cystic structure that is medial and has multiple calyces arrayed about its lateral aspect. These are usually of similar size and with real-time examination may be seen to communicate with the central cystic structure. There are some cases in which this typical appearance is not evident, probably in the more severely affected kidneys in which the dividing line between the hydronephrotic and MCDK becomes unclear (Felson and Cussen, 1975). Use of Doppler US assessment of the renal vascular pulse pattern has been reported to aid in the distinction between these entities (Kaminopetros et al, 1991). When such ambiguity is present postnatally, it is best to assume that a salvageable kidney is present and direct the postnatal evaluation in that light.

The prenatal natural history of MCDK may be reflected in the varying appearance of the kidney with gradual involution (Avni et al, 1986). In some instances, the kidney becomes undetectable by US, either prenatally or in the postnatal period (Mandell et al, 1994). This observation raises the question of how many cases of absent kidneys are actually the endpoint of an MCDK that is nondetectable on US imaging. The functional consequences of this may not be relevant, but it is clear that some renal parenchyma, albeit dysplastic, is present.

Other diagnostic entities that may appear similar to an MCDK include any renal cystic disease with large cysts. This is in distinct contrast to the other common congenital cystic renal disease, ARPKD, which is characterized by large uniformly echogenic kidneys without recognizable cysts (Smedley and Bailey, 1987; Townsend et al, 1988). The cysts are too small to be resolved by US. In contrast, congenital multilocular cystic nephroma has macrocysts detectable on US. This is a rare entity, characterized by segmental involvement of the kidney with variably sized macrocysts (Eble et al, 1998). It is considered a neoplasm by many but is also viewed as a hamartomatous malformation. Other elements of this spectrum of congenital cystic malformations that include cystic Wilms' tumor may also have a macrocystic appearance on US. These are rare, typically have larger amounts of parenchyma, and ultimately demonstrate function on postnatal imaging.

Nonrenal cystic lesions may also be confused for MCDK, although these are typically not in the renal fossa (Rubenstein et al, 1995), and they may be confirmed to be nonrenal by the presence of two normal kidneys. These may include **mesenteric duplication cysts** (Barr et al, 1990), **neurenteric cysts** (Uludag et al, 2001), **bronchogenic cysts** (Bagolan et al, 2000), **extrathoracic pulmonary sequestration** (Carpentieri et al, 2000), **and the occasional cystic neuroblastoma** (Kozakewich et al, 1998; Hamada et al, 1999; Granata et al, 2000). It is unlikely that these should be confused for an MCDK, but in the event of ambiguity, postnatal evaluation should permit resolution of any of these entities.

ARPKD (infantile polycystic kidney disease) does not appear cystic but is characterized by markedly enlarged, brightly echogenic kidneys (Lonergan et al, 2000) (Fig. 109–13). This appearance begins to develop prior to 20 weeks in most affected fetuses, but late development has been reported, making an early diagnosis difficult in affected families (Zerres et al, 1988; Edwards et al, 1989; Mandell et al, 1991). ARPKD is associated with various mutations on the *PKHD1* gene on chromosome 6p12 and can be identified prenatally in some cases (Wilson, 2004; Zerres et al, 2004) This would permit early diagnosis and the option for termination as the neonatal mortality is so high and those surviving progress to renal and liver morbidity and mortality. As the condition progresses in utero, oligohydramnios develops and most of these infants die of pulmonary insufficiency with Potter's syndrome. Postnatal mutational analysis can permit efficient diagnosis (Bergmann et al, 2005a). Macrocystic disease associated with ADPKD has also been reported in the fetus, although with a very different prognosis (Reeders et al, 1986; McHugo et al, 1988; Ceccherini et al, 1989; Edwards and Baldinger, 1989; Novelli et al, 1989). The cysts are heterogeneous in size and location and may be few in number. It may be important to assess the family when this finding is noted, in order to confirm the diagnosis and identify affected members. The health insurance ramifications of this must be considered, however.

Bilateral renal agenesis is evidenced by the progressive absence of AF after 16 to 18 weeks, the time when fetal urine

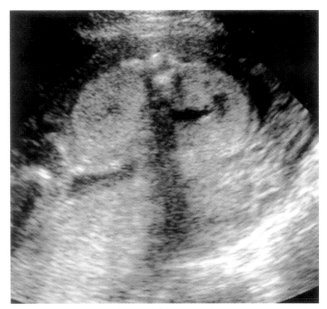

Figure 109–13. Bilaterally enlarged, echogenic kidneys without grossly apparent cysts are typical of autosomal recessive polycystic kidneys. This appearance usually, but not always, becomes apparent by 22 weeks of gestation. In early-onset cases, oligohydramnios is seen.

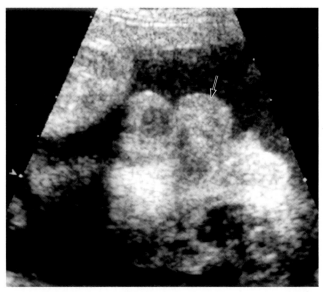

Figure 109–14. Fetal ultrasonography showing a low-set umbilical insertion, no evidence of bladder filling, normal kidneys, and a protuberance of tissue from the lower abdomen *(arrow)*. The scrotum may be seen below the tissue protuberance. This pattern is typical of classic bladder exstrophy.

begins to constitute the bulk of the AF (Cardwell, 1988; Holmes, 1989; Sherer et al, 1990). The kidneys are not detectable and no bladder filling is seen. The adrenal glands may be visible in their normal position but with a linear appearance, the so-called lying down adrenal (Hoffman et al, 1992). A small thorax is evident later in gestation. These children represent the classical appearance of Potter's syndrome with oligohydramnios, pulmonary hypoplasia, skeletal defects, low-set ears, and lethal neonatal pulmonary insufficiency.

An important and difficult diagnosis is that of the **exstrophy** conditions. **Classical bladder exstrophy is characterized by the absence of bladder filling on repeated examinations, low-set umbilical cord, and abnormal-appearing external genitalia** (Barth et al, 1990; Gearhart et al, 1995; Evangelidis et al, 2004; Wu et al, 2004). The protrusion of the bladder plate may be apparent just below the umbilical cord (Fig. 109–14). The kidneys are normal, and associated extraurinary abnormalities are uncommon. A prenatal diagnosis of exstrophy permits appropriate parental education and preparation for delivery. This can be of enormous value in facilitating the family in dealing with this major anomaly. Planned delivery is possible with subsequent planned surgical intervention. In sharp contrast, cloacal exstrophy is often associated with myelomeningocele, lower extremity abnormalities, and cardiac defects (Meglin et al, 1990; Kaya et al, 2000; Della Monica et al, 2005). Its lower abdominal appearance is often confused with an isolated omphalocele. Intestinal protrusion, as seen postnatally, may or may not be evident on prenatal ultrasonography (Austin et al, 1998). The diagnosis of either of these conditions requires careful counseling of the prospective parents about the postnatal implications of these conditions, and many families choose termination of the pregnancy. As a result, the diagnostic accuracy must be high in early gestation. The ability to make these complex diagnoses has been associated with a large proportion of terminations (Cromie et al, 2001).

Genital abnormalities are occasionally detected in utero, usually as penile anomalies such as hypospadias or severe chordee (Benacerraf et al, 1989; Mandell et al, 1995). Isolated epispadias is rarely detected in utero. The presence of a penile anomaly in utero should prompt a search for the testes to determine whether the fetus may be a male or female (Carr et al, 1994). Karyotyping by way of amniocentesis may be appropriate as well. In the absence of testes in the inguinal canals or scrotum, the diagnosis of a male fetus should not be made. Severe virilization of females with congenital adrenal hyperplasia (CAH) may produce a markedly enlarged clitoris. Inappropriate, prenatal sex assignment has been made in this context (Bromley et al, 1994).

Imperforate anus (Mandell et al, 1992b) and its extreme manifestation, cloacal malformation (Cilento et al, 1994; Ohno et al, 2000; Taipale et al, 2004), have been specifically detected prenatally through identification of various elements of these complex abnormalities. The association of bilateral hydroureteronephrosis, an enlarged bladder with a fluid-filled retrovesical structure, should suggest the possibility of the cloacal anomaly with vaginal distention producing bladder outlet obstruction (see Fig. 109–10).

Certain genitourinary (GU) abnormalities have been shown to be associated with other particular anomalies in other systems. **The finding of hydronephrosis has an association with Down's syndrome with an incidence of 3.3% in fetuses with hydronephrosis** (Benacerraf et al, 1990). Although the incidence of Down's with isolated hydronephrosis is low, consideration of further evaluation may be appropriate, including searching for increased nuchal fold thickness on ultrasonography (Benacerraf and Frigoletto, 1987) and amniocentesis for karyotyping. Certain extraurinary diagnoses should prompt consideration of more careful urinary evaluation. Oligohydramnios has many etiologies, several of which are directly related to the urinary tract, including bladder outlet obstruction, dysplasia, and cystic kidneys. **The** finding of a cardiac mass (rhabdomyosarcoma) is frequently associated with tuberous sclerosis and possible renal masses (Becker, 2000).

Renal masses are unusual in the fetal urinary tract (Leclair et al, 2005), and **the most common is congenital mesoblastic nephroma. This benign tumor typically replaces the entire kidney with a homogeneous round mass** (Fung et al, 1995; Shibahara et al, 1999; Irsutti et al, 2000; Won et al, 2002; Chen et al, 2003). **It may be associated with polyhydramnios** (Geirsson et al, 1985). Because of the possibility of a malignant renal mass, however, these masses must be considered potentially malignant and early postnatal removal is recommended. There is little justification for early delivery, however. Wilms' tumor has rarely been described prenatally (Applegate et al, 1999; Beckwith, 1999; Vadeyar et al, 2000; Leclair et al, 2005). **Neuroblastoma has been detected prenatally and may appear as a renal mass** (Ho et al, 1993; Acharya et al, 1997; Kesrouani et al, 1999; Granata et al, 2000). **They have also been seen as cystic suprarenal masses** (Kozakewich et al, 1998; Hamada et al, 1999; Merrot et al, 2004; Athanassiadou et al, 2005). Magnetic resonance imaging has shown some added benefit in characterizing these lesions (Kozakewich et al, 1998; Hamada et al, 1999; Aslan et al, 2004; Houlihan et al, 2004). **Metastatic neuroblastoma may also be present, and careful total body examination is needed** (Toma et al, 1994). Metabolic effects of excessive norepinephrine secretion by a neuroblastoma have been documented in fetuses, including maternal tachycardia and hypertension (Newton et al, 1985).

It is important to consider several **potential diagnostic pitfalls.** The severity of hydronephrosis may be variable. This often reflects reflux, and the complete resolution of significant hydronephrosis in a short period of time is a strong indicator of VUR. This should prompt appropriate postnatal evaluation. Hydronephrosis may vary in the short term, as well, reflecting peristalsis of the pelvis and ureter (Persutte et al, 2000), but this is not seen with severe degrees of dilation. **A very difficult differentiation is that between posterior urethral valves and severe VUR in male fetuses.** In the absence of oligohydramnios, there is little prenatal clinical impact of an ambiguous diagnosis, and a VCUG is needed in either case. In this situation, the VCUG should be performed early, on the assumption that PUV is the diagnosis. **Clues that the diagnosis is obstruction, rather than VUR, include bladder wall thickening, echogenic renal parenchyma, and a dilated posterior urethra** (Kaefer et al, 1997b; Oliveira et al, 2002). All of these are subjective features of a prenatal ultrasound study but, if present, indicate PUV. **The diagnosis of an upper pole renal cyst in a fetus indicates the presence of a duplication anomaly with hydronephrosis rather than a cyst.** Examination for a dilated upper pole ureter and possible ureterocele or ectopic ureter usually reveals the actual diagnosis.

PATHOPHYSIOLOGY OF CONGENITAL OBSTRUCTION

The largest component of prenatally detected uropathies is manifest by hydronephrosis and represents the spectrum of congenital obstruction. This categorization deserves some analysis. Hydronephrosis is a manifestation or sign of obstruc-

tion in its broadest sense and exists in a wide spectrum. Any "threshold" of hydronephrosis that is considered diagnostic of obstruction is arbitrary and serves to confuse our thinking about congenital obstructive processes. Not all obstruction is clinically significant, but obstruction of the urinary tract produces hydronephrosis and, as noted previously, all primary hydronephrosis not related to reflux indicates some degree of obstruction. The term physiologic hydronephrosis has emerged in reference to the degrees of mild dilation that resolves spontaneously and whose etiology is unclear. A lack of understanding of etiology and spontaneous resolution should not imply a "physiologic" process. **Furthermore, the term "physiologic hydronephrosis" begs the question of when it becomes nonphysiologic** (Adra et al, 1995). This produces attempts to set absolute divisions within an entity that is present as a spectrum and probably represents multiple underlying causes. The spectrum of hydronephrosis ranges from simple minimal pelvic dilation to extreme dilation of the pelvis and calyces. These issues become critical when clinical, yes or no, decisions must be made because they cannot truly reflect the character of the spectrum. Those decisions should therefore be based upon the potential negative effects of a particular condition. A detailed discussion of the pathophysiology of congenital urinary obstruction is presented in Chapter 108, "Congenital Urinary Obstruction: Pathophysiology." Three basic concepts must be recognized in the context of congenital obstructive uropathy that affect interpretation and decision-making related to prenatally detected urinary abnormalities.

First, congenital obstruction is different from postnatal obstruction. The affected kidney not only is undergoing rapid growth and differentiation (development) but also is not acting as the essential filtration system of the fetus (Peters, 1995, 1997). **That function is taken up by the maternal placenta and urinary tract. Broadly viewed, the patterns of fetal renal response may be seen as altered growth, differentiation, and induction of injury responses.**

Second, when renal function in utero is impaired the consequences of this are unique to the fetal environment. Potter first identified the association between renal agenesis, oligohydramnios, and pulmonary hypoplasia in the syndrome that bears her name (Potter, 1972). The pathophysiology of pulmonary hypoplasia in the setting of severe renal impairment and oligohydramnios remains incompletely defined, but several clues have emerged. Reid characterized the pathologic basis of pulmonary hypoplasia and defined it as reflecting a developmental insult of the lung (Hislop et al, 1979). This is evidenced by impairment of the normal orderly sequence of lung development in which the patterns of bronchial branching are established by 16 to 18 weeks of gestation in humans. This branching is the foundation for all subsequent lung development. If this is abnormal, all future development is affected and a small, insufficient lung is the product. As with renal nephron development, if normal branching has not occurred, there is little likelihood of reversing the process to permit catch-up. After bronchial branching, canalicular development occurs prior to actual alveolar development. Reduced canalicular growth precludes adequate alveolar development as well. It was further shown that pulmonary hypoplasia reflected both abnormal growth and immaturity (Docimo et al, 1989).

The role of the kidney in lung development is difficult to define, and it remains unclear how the lung and kidney interact. It seems that early in gestation, normal kidney function is needed, independent of AF volume, and later the role of the AF is to provide a mechanical stenting force for later alveolar development (Peters et al, 1991). There is some evidence of a kidney-lung axis that regulates growth of each, although this remains speculative (Glick et al, 1990, 1991; Hosoda et al, 1993). It is clear that mechanical forces play a role in normal lung development, and perhaps normal AF volume is important to permit this (Wilson et al, 1993; DiFiore et al, 1994; Nobuhara et al, 1998). The mechanism is somewhat counterintuitive, however. It had long been thought that with oligohydramnios, there would be elevated intrauterine pressures that compressed the fetal thorax, causing poor lung growth. Intrauterine pressures measured in humans with oligohydramnios were lower than normal, presumably related to tenting effects of the fetus and its limbs on the uterine wall (Nicolini et al, 1989). Consequently, with reduced external pressures, lung fluid would drain more freely into the amniotic space, reducing the stenting pressure in the lung and impairing normal growth. Experimental data support this concept (Moessinger et al, 1986). When lung fluid is retained by tracheal ligation, even in the absence of the kidneys, lung growth is maintained and actually accelerated (Wilson et al, 1993). This has become the basis for fetal interventions to prevent pulmonary hypoplasia associated with diaphragmatic hernia (DiFiore et al, 1994; Harrison et al, 1996).

The timing of the onset of oligohydramnios is therefore important in assessing its potential consequences. As would be predicted from an understanding of the pathophysiology, late-onset oligohydramnios was not associated with pulmonary insufficiency, with a threshold at about 30 weeks (Mandell et al, 1992c). Consequently, in the setting of presumed severe bladder outlet obstruction, if oligohydramnios has developed by 22 or 24 weeks, pulmonary insufficiency is highly likely. This has become the basis for in utero interventions for bladder obstruction. In contrast, if oligohydramnios develops after 30 weeks, there is little likelihood of pulmonary complications and therefore no rationale to intervene or deliver the child early on a pulmonary basis. If the lungs have been able to develop adequately up to that point, they do not reverse themselves and become hypoplastic.

Third, the incidence of certain prenatally detected uropathies is markedly sex specific. Hydronephrosis of all etiologies is four to five times more common in males. VUR indicated by prenatal hydronephrosis is four times more common in boys than girls (Elder, 1992). These observations are well recognized, although there is no definite explanation. A variety of data suggest the possibility that these differences reflect elevated male bladder pressure related to higher bladder outlet resistance. Kokoua and colleagues (1993) have examined different developmental patterns of the male rhabdosphincter and noted variation in the development of the normal omega shape from a circular form. Persistence of the circular sphincter may produce more resistance. This would lead to higher bladder pressures and upper tract dilation or reflux. Postnatal human studies have shown that boys tend to have higher grades of reflux, elevated voiding pressures, and more bladder instability (Sillen et al, 1996b; Yeung et al, 1997). The latter are characteristic of an obstructed bladder.

Experimental data support this hypothesis; it was shown that in fetal sheep urachal ligation without any bladder neck manipulation caused upper tract dilation in males only (Gobet et al, 1998a). Experimental fetal reflux is of higher grade in males, and its persistence seems to be related to bladder dynamics (Gobet et al, 1999). This suggests that the developing male sphincter-urethral complex is of higher resistance than the female. This may be due to urethral length but may also be due to differences in the sphincter or prostate, an organ with a large component of smooth muscle. In the sheep, the urachus remains patent until term to maintain normal pressures, which does not seem to be needed in humans. However, a certain fraction of children have evidence of upper tract dilation in the absence of any other pathology. In most cases this mild hydronephrosis resolves spontaneously, just as the altered patterns of bladder activity resolve. Why this occurs in only some children remains unclear, yet raises the question of differences in sphincteric maturation as a basis for the male predominance in transient congenital uropathies.

MANAGEMENT OF FETAL UROPATHIES
Incidence

Fetal urinary tract anomalies are a common finding, occurring in 0.2% to 1.5% of all pregnancies, based upon larger population studies (Helin et al, 1986; Scott et al, 1987; Scott et al, 1993; Ismaili et al, 2003). Well over half of these are due to some form of hydronephrosis. UPJ obstruction is the largest single entity producing hydronephrosis, followed by reflux, valves, and megaureter (Mandell et al, 1991). Evidence of severe obstruction that might warrant fetal intervention is uncommon, representing about 5% of all prenatally detected uropathies. Their clinical impact is out of proportion to their incidence because of the severity of potential outcomes in these patients.

Indications

The principal role of the perinatal urologist is to act as an educator for prospective parents. The need for prenatal intervention is rare and its precise role remains undefined. It is important to recognize the anxiety of prospective parents who have been told that there is something wrong with their future child's kidneys. There is little appreciation for the wide spectrum of severity and the likelihood of minimal postnatal complications. Often, the initial diagnosis is by someone with little perspective on the natural history, necessary urologic evaluation, and appropriate interventions. Some have already been given recommendations about management that may not reflect reasonable practice. These recommendations may reflect a defensive attitude among obstetricians concerned about the ramifications of a serious congenital defect. Many parents have used the Internet to try to learn about their child's condition, often drawing erroneous conclusions. Although it is seldom possible to provide an exact prediction of the natural history of a particular condition, it is usually possible to give a detailed description of what may need to be done to define the condition and to determine a management plan. In cases with severe obstruction or the risk for serious postnatal problems, the perinatal urologist is often in the best position to provide a detailed discussion of the pros and cons of various management approaches in utero.

In cases of mild hydronephrosis with normal-appearing renal parenchyma, further prenatal follow-up is seldom useful, although it is usually recommended by obstetricians. In the rare case of rapid increases in the severity of hydronephrosis, prompt evaluation may be appropriate but is unlikely to change acute postnatal management. It should be recognized that increases in the absolute dilation of the renal pelvis usually reflect normal fetal and renal growth and not increasing obstructive severity (Mandell et al, 1991). There are no data to correlate strictly the US appearance or course of mild to moderate hydronephrosis in utero with postnatal outcomes sufficient to define management (Toivi-ainen-Salo et al, 2004). **For the parents, however, a follow-up study can be very reassuring that there has been no worsening, and perhaps improvement may be noted.** Whether this should alter postnatal evaluation is controversial, as reviewed in the following. In the setting of more severe unilateral hydronephrosis or bilateral hydronephrosis, prenatal follow-up is reasonable and may be helpful. **When severe bilateral hydronephrosis is present, with a suspicion of bladder outlet obstruction, regular follow-up is needed. The particular parameters to be followed include AF volume, renal echogenicity, and the presence of any extrarenal fluid collections.** Fetal growth is monitored as well. Changes in these factors may provide useful information on prognosis and on the need for in utero intervention.

KEY POINTS: MANAGING FETAL UROPATHIES

- Fetal urinary tract anomalies are a common finding, occurring in 0.2% to 1.5% of all pregnancies

- The principal role of the perinatal urologist is to act as an educator for prospective parents. The need for prenatal intervention is rare and its precise role remains undefined.

- When severe bilateral hydronephrosis is present, with the suspicion of bladder outlet obstruction, regular follow-up is needed. The particular parameters to be followed include amniotic fluid volume, renal echogenicity, and the presence of any extrarenal fluid collections.

- At present, fetal intervention for obstructive uropathy is indicated when the life of the neonate is at risk. This is the case when oligohydramnios is present in the setting of presumed bladder outlet obstruction.

Fetal Intervention

Recognition of the lethal outcome in neonates found to have severe bladder outlet obstruction in utero is a strong impetus to attempt to prevent neonatal demise through an in utero intervention. As maternal-fetal ultrasonography evolved and specific diagnoses were made, this association became evident. Initial animal experiments with models of bladder outlet obstruction provided encouragement to attempt in utero drainage procedures to salvage lung development (Adzick et al, 1985a). The first attempted intervention for obstructive uropathy was reported in 1982, when bilateral cutaneous ureterostomies were performed (Harrison et al, 1982a). The child did not survive, but subsequent attempts demonstrated proof of principle with surviving children who would otherwise have been predicted to die in the neonatal period. Initial reports of success prompted widespread interventions for a variety of conditions, but a review in 1986 of 73 fetal interventions for obstructive uropathy brought practitioners back to earth (Manning et al, 1986). Despite initial enthusiasm and less than stringent criteria for intervention, outcomes were less than encouraging with higher than expected mortality (59%) and high procedural complication rates (7% mortality). This report brought on a moratorium of activity for about 10 years, during which time slow progress in refining techniques and selection was made.

Part of the problem of early practice may be seen in the report. Seventy percent of the cases were from institutions reporting only one intervention. A large fraction (45%) of patients had no specific etiology identified for their hydronephrosis. More recently, however, there has been a reexploration of fetal interventions for obstructive uropathy. Some of the same questions about selection, techniques, and outcomes persist; however, long-term follow-up has improved our understanding of the consequences of in utero interventions.

At present, fetal intervention for obstructive uropathy is indicated when the life of the neonate is at risk. This is when oligohydramnios is present in the setting of presumed bladder outlet obstruction. It is also essential that no other life-threatening conditions, particularly cardiovascular or neurologic, exist. It is essential that there is a reasonable chance that the fetus will benefit from in utero decompression of the bladder. This is the difficult issue at present, and several means of assessing the fetal kidneys are in use. Other factors that must be present include a singleton pregnancy, normal karyotype, and informed consent (Table 109–2). There is an emerging view that fetal intervention for renal

Table 109–2. Indications and Conditions for In Utero Urinary Decompression

Indices	Comment
Evidence of bladder outlet obstruction	Dilated bladder, hydroureteronephrosis
Normal karyotype	By amniocentesis
No systemic anomalies	For example, central nervous system, cardiovascular
Male fetus	
Singleton	
Oligohydramnios	Early onset: <25 weeks
Noncystic kidneys	Degree of echogenicity is subjective; cysts are poor prognostic sign
Favorable urinary indices	Na < 100, Cl < 110, Osm < 210; or serial samplings trending toward normal; β_2-microglobulin in <10 to 20
Informed consent	Risks of partial treatment must be included

salvage alone is reasonable and may actually be more useful, but data are limited.

Early studies recognized that fetal bladder decompression provided no benefit in some fetuses. In these cases, there was no return of AF and neonatal death. The pathology was usually consistent with renal dysplasia and correlated with severely echogenic and cystic kidneys in utero. Biochemical analysis of the fetal urine was performed to assess potential renal function, and parameters of a "good" prognosis were established (Glick et al, 1985; Mandelbrot et al, 1991; Nicolini et al, 1992; Muller et al, 1993). These reflected fetal renal function in which there was sodium retention and free water excretion. Clinical assessment of these parameters was not always encouraging about their validity, and false positives and negatives have been reported (Elder et al, 1990). Part of the explanation for these inconsistencies is the lack of standardization of the gestational age at sampling in many cases. Normal ranges for various components of fetal urine depend upon gestational age.

A further refinement of this approach employed serial sampling of the bladder urine over 3 days (Johnson et al, 1995). **This provides a dynamic assessment of the response of the fetal kidneys to decompression and offered a better indication of the ability of the kidneys to continue to produce urine, essential for correction of pulmonary hypoplasia and postnatal renal function.** The long-term accuracy of these indicators remains imperfect, but they are the best available. Long-term postnatal prognostication has been attempted with a range of obstructive severity, and using an index of several urinary parameters, identification of neonates with normal, moderate, and severe renal impairment can be made with some reliability (Muller et al, 1993). These indicators use urinary electrolytes as well as proteins (Muller et al, 1999) as indicators of glomerular and tubular function. Reports of serum indicators of fetal renal function hold further promise of improved prognostic precision (Muller et al, 2004). Because β_2-microglobulin is excreted by the kidney and does not cross the placenta, fetal serum levels reflect fetal renal capacity; they are elevated in renal dysplasia, and the elevation correlates with postnatal serum creatinine levels in obstructive uropathy (Dommergues et al, 2000).

There has been a trend to consider intervention for the fetus without oligohydramnios but in whom chronic renal insufficiency is likely. Although this requires greater accuracy in prognostication, the potential gain is significant. The neonate with early renal failure is extremely difficult to manage and early renal transplantation is challenging. If intervention would delay the need for renal replacement for 2 or 3 years or perhaps eliminate the need, the benefit would be enormous. This group of children would perhaps benefit even more than those at risk for pulmonary hypoplasia. As yet, however, there are no data on such interventions.

The technique of fetal intervention for bladder outlet obstruction emerged from the University of California, San Francisco (UCSF) group and is based upon placement of a double pigtail vesicoamniotic shunt (Harrison et al, 1982b). **Placed under ultrasound guidance over an introducing needle, these shunts bypass the obstructed urethra.** The initial shunts were limited by frequent dislodgement, clogging with debris, and the need for replacement. Subsequently, a larger shunt was developed that was positioned within a

large-bore trocar and held in position by a pigtail oriented flat against the abdomen, limiting the possibility of the fetus pulling the shunt out. These shunts (Rodeck shunt; Rocket, London) drained well and remained in position but were complicated because of their large size (Nicolini et al, 1987). Several cases of intestinal herniation through the shunt site were reported (Robichaux et al, 1991; Gehring et al, 2000).

Current practice for vesicoamniotic shunt placement uses the Rodeck shunt placed under ultrasound guidance. It is occasionally necessary to perform amnioinfusion to permit fetal visualization. This is limited in amount, as too much permits excessive fetal movement. Occasionally the fetus must be paralyzed to facilitate shunt placement. The large-bore trocar needle is placed and the shunt passed within it until seen in the bladder (Fig. 109–15). A persistent problem with all vesicoamniotic shunts has been accurate placement. In the setting of a markedly enlarged bladder, the shunt may be placed high in the abdomen. As the bladder decompresses, it pulls away from the shunt. Some authors have investigated endoscopically controlled placement of the shunt to prevent this problem, although none have been used in a clinical context (Luks et al, 1994a, 1994b, 1996; Skarsgard et al, 1995; Calvano et al, 1997; Fowler et al, 2002).

Endoscopic fetal intervention has emerged as a new element in the management of fetal disease. Reports have described fetal cystoscopy and valve ablation using endoscopic

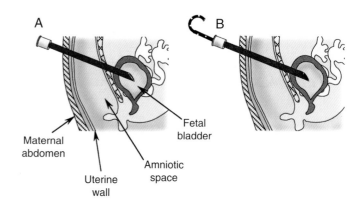

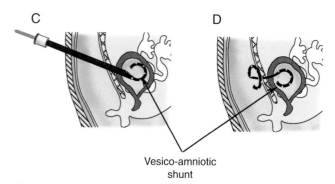

Figure 109–15. Diagram showing technique of fetal vesicoamniotic shunt placement. The fetal bladder is initially reached by needle and a large-bore introducing sheath is passed into the bladder (**A**). Within this sheath, the shunt is passed (**B** and **C**). It is a double pigtail shunt with holes at each end allowing free drainage between the bladder and amniotic space (**D**). (From Peters CA: Surgical Management of Fetal Uropathies. In Marshall FF: Textbook of Operative Urology. Philadelphia, WB Saunders, 1996, p 1063.)

techniques (Quintero et al, 1995; Quintero et al, 2000a, 2000b). This method is being used in a small number of centers. The rationale is to ablate the valves, as would be done postnatally, and maintain "normal" bladder filling and emptying. Antegrade and retrograde methods have been attempted using rigid and flexible instrumentation with laser ablation or hydroablation (Welsh et al, 2003). Limited reporting of results has occurred to date, but there has been limited success in the technique with a high mortality rate of the fetus. Although it may be attractive to maintain near-normal anatomy, **it is very uncertain that this approach would provide the degree of decompression needed in a fetus with sufficiently severe urinary compromise to require intervention.** Normal neonatal male bladder pressures are high without valves and would be high in the fetus whose bladder has been so severely obstructed. This condition, even with complete valve ablation, may not permit adequate renal recovery to allow continued **optimal** development of the kidneys or lungs. **At present, in utero endoscopic valve ablation can be considered only experimental, and only anecdotal cases have been reported.**

The only outcome data available are for vesicoamniotic shunting, and this remains limited by variability in diagnosis, inadequate reporting as correlated with diagnosis, and short-term postnatal follow-up. Most series include patients with the prune belly syndrome, in whom the presence of obstruction is controversial. Whether they benefit from in utero decompression is unclear. However, when all recent reports are considered, there is evidence to support the benefits of fetal intervention for severe bladder outlet obstruction, although the benefit must be assessed carefully (Crombleholme et al, 1990; Johnson et al, 1994; Coplen et al, 1996; Freedman et al, 1996; Shimada et al, 1998; Holmes et al, 2001; McLorie et al, 2001; Clark et al, 2003; Biard et al, 2005).

Several aspects of the outcome assessment are important. Because the first priority is to save the life of the neonate, early survival is important, yet long-term renal function is critical as well. The duration of follow-up is very important in considerations of renal functional outcome, as renal failure may take months or years to develop. In children with a poor prognosis at fetal urinary evaluation, the outcome is poor. Survival is increased, yet most of those children have renal insufficiency and may have pulmonary impairment as well. These patients may be alive, but the benefit of intervention is not certain. Three studies have reported long-term outcomes of patients undergoing in utero shunting and echo the results of the initial reports (Freedman et al, 2000; Holmes et al, 2001; Biard et al, 2005). A substantial fraction of children have renal insufficiency (57%) and many have growth impairment (86%). It is difficult to assess the real impact in this small series, however, as it includes patients with both valves and prune belly syndrome. In a study of patients with confirmed posterior urethral valves, the prenatal mortality was high (43%) and five of eight surviving children had chronic renal insufficiency with a mean of 11 years of follow-up. It must be recognized that this series from UCSF includes the first cases in which in utero relief of urinary obstruction was attempted and therefore reflects the early learning curve (Holmes et al, 2001).

In a long-term follow-up study of patients undergoing and surviving in utero shunting, renal functional outcomes were good with a mean of 5.8 years follow-up (1 to 14 years) (Biard et al, 2005). Forty-five percent of patients had acceptable renal function, 22% had mild impairment, and 33% had renal failure. Patients with the prune belly syndrome had the best chance of adequate function (57%), valves second at 43%, and those with urethral atresia had the least chance of adequate function (25%). There was some correlation of the patterns of prognostic urinary electrolytes with renal outcomes (M. Johnson, personal communication). Biard and colleagues (2005) reported on bladder outcomes as well, with 61% of patients voiding spontaneously and the others requiring some degree of catheterization. Unique to this report was an assessment of quality of life outcomes by parent proxy and child, and these patients were surprisingly well adjusted, with overall scores similar to those of the healthy population and better than those of a chronically ill group. Although it must be recognized that this report is selective in that more than 33% of shunted patients were lost to assessment, it nonetheless indicates the potential benefits of carefully selected in utero shunting in terms of overall health and renal survival.

A large meta-analysis of prenatal drainage procedures showed a statistically significant advantage in terms of perinatal survival with in utero shunting. In patients with a poor prognosis, based upon urinary electrolytes and imaging criteria, shunting afforded an improvement with an odds ratio of 8.1 (95% confidence interval [CI]: 1.2 to 52.9; $P < .03$), and in those with a good prognosis, the improvement was an odds ratio of 2.8 (95% CI: 0.7 to 10.8; $P = .13$). This analysis included the outcomes of 147 fetuses (Clark et al, 2003).

At present, the data suggest that the potential exists for in utero intervention to be effective in reducing the risk of a lethal neonatal outcome because of in utero bladder outlet obstruction and to improve long-term renal and bladder functional outcomes. It is clear that the ability to identify patients with posterior urethral valves who will benefit from in utero intervention has improved but remains incomplete.

The horizon of fetal intervention holds promise. It is anticipated that with improved understanding of the pathophysiology of congenital obstruction, there will be increased ability to predict outcomes through biomarkers of the relevant pathophysiologic processes. New technologies for in utero visualization, perhaps combining ultrasonography and endoscopy, will facilitate placement of shunts or creation of a vesicostomy. Further refinements may permit rational shunting for children at risk for renal failure in the early years of life and thereby prevention of the multitude of complications associated with renal replacement in infancy.

POSTNATAL EVALUATION AND MANAGEMENT

The presumed diagnosis and severity of prenatally detected uropathies determine the postnatal evaluation and management of fetal uropathies. This must account for the likely risk to the child from the specific condition and the nature of the postnatal evaluation needed. Structural conditions, such as bladder exstrophy, are self-evident. When a specific diagnosis has been made that must be confirmed using imaging studies, the timing and intensity are the critical issue, and this decision-making must be made in the context of the child's condition. A practical scheme to guide this process is shown in Table 109–3 and divides patients depending upon risk of complications.

KEY POINT: POSTNATAL EVALUATION AND MANAGEMENT

■ The presumed diagnosis and severity of prenatally detected uropathies determine the postnatal evaluation and management of fetal uropathies. This must account for the likely risk to the child from the specific condition and the nature of the postnatal evaluation needed.

Bilateral Hydronephrosis

Children at risk for severe bilateral obstruction, including valves, should have early evaluation and initiation of treatment. Prenatally, these children have had bilateral moderately severe to severe hydronephrosis, often with ureteral dilation and bladder distention or thickening. Evaluation should begin with ultrasonography on the first day of life, recognizing that this may underestimate the severity of the hydronephrosis because of neonatal dehydration. In the presence of severe bilateral hydroureteronephrosis (HUN) in a boy, early VCUG is appropriate.

Posterior Urethral Valves (see also Chapter 122)

Bladder outlet obstruction from valves in the newborn is now usually detected prenatally but may also be identified in a boy with a palpable mass from a distended bladder, neonatal ascites in the setting of oligohydramnios and pulmonary insufficiency, or neonatal sepsis. The finding of a diminished urinary stream, although suggestive of valves, is not common. In any of these situations in which a question of valves is present, immediate US evaluation is needed to identify bladder distention, bladder wall thickening, hydroureteronephrosis, and evidence of renal dysplasia. The bladder in boys with valves is often not massively distended, which is more often seen with massive VUR. Wall thickening is,

however, a consistent finding. The dilated posterior urethra may also be visible when specifically sought. A voiding cystogram establishes the diagnosis.

Immediate care of the neonate with valves is dictated by the severity of the presentation and overall clinical status. A bladder catheter is left in place until a decision is made about appropriate initial therapy, usually valve ablation. A 5 French feeding tube is preferred over a Foley catheter. The retention balloon of the Foley catheter may be compressed against the ureteral orifices with bladder spasm and cause ureteral obstruction. Bladder drainage usually permits upper urinary tract decompression and facilitates medical stabilization in the case of a child with respiratory compromise or acidosis. Antibiotics should be initiated as well. Initial creatinine levels reflect maternal levels but serve as an important baseline. In boys who are clinically stable, valve ablation may be performed as the initial procedure, followed by careful assessment of any remnant valvular obstruction and the condition of the upper tracts.

Management of the infant with persisting hydronephrosis or azotemia after catheter placement or valve ablation remains controversial. Total early reconstruction is an option when the bladder is such that one may expect to be able to reimplant two ureters and achieve closure (Hendren 1970). Cutaneous vesicostomy is reserved for boys in whom primary valve ablation may not be achieved because of prematurity. Proximal diversion, in the appropriate patient, offers efficient urinary drainage and does not necessarily hamper subsequent surgical reconstruction (Krueger et al, 1980). Although this may be condemned by some, it is in large part due to a long history of misapplication. In children with severe renal compromise, any slight benefit that might be obtained from better renal drainage is of value in prolonging renal survival. In performing any such diversion, however, plans for reconstruction should be made and followed up. Controversy remains about the long-term effects of early valve ablation in contrast to upper diversion on bladder function (Jayanthi et al, 1995; Kim et al, 1996; Smith et al, 1996; Close et al, 1997; Jaureguizar et al, 2000; Podesta et al, 2000).

Diligent follow-up of renal and bladder function is critical in all these boys, including assessment of somatic growth, measured creatinine clearances, and imaging studies of the urinary tract. Aggressive early treatment may best serve to

---

Table 109–3. Postnatal Management Scheme for Hydronephrosis

Prenatal Findings	Early Antibiotics	Imaging	Timing	Possible Diagnoses	Surgery
Mild hydronephrosis	No	RUS VCUG (controversial)	2 to 3 months	Mild UPJO Mild UVJO Reflux	Unlikely
Moderate to severe hydronephrosis	Yes	RUS VCUG	1 to 2 months	Moderate UPJO Moderate UVJO Reflux Valves, mild	Unlikely
Severe unilateral hydronephrosis	Yes	RUS VCUG IVP/MAG3	1 month	UPJO UVJO Reflux Valves (unusual)	Possible
Severe bilateral hydronephrosis	Yes	RUS VCUG	<1 week	Reflux Valves Bilat UPJO Bilat UVJO	Probable
Intravesical cystic structure	Yes	RUS VCUG	<1 month	Ureterocele	Likely

MAG3, mercaptoacetyltriglycine diuretic renogram; UPJO, ureteropelvic junction obstruction; UVJO, ureterovesical junction obstruction; RUS, renal ultrasound; VCUG, voiding cystourethrogram; IVP, intravenous pyelogram.

prevent the slow, often subtle progression of renal damage that may lead to end-stage renal failure (Merguerian et al, 1992).

Vesicoureteral Reflux and Megacystis-Megaureter
(see also Chapter 117)

Some boys with bilateral hydroureteronephrosis in utero have VUR only and do not need catheter drainage but only antibiotics. The ability to differentiate between valves and reflux in the fetus, however, remains limited, except in the extremes (Kaefer et al, 1997b).

The association of a massively dilated bladder, hydroureteronephrosis, and bilateral VUR has been termed the megacystis-megaureter association (Willi et al, 1979; Burbige et al, 1984). **The constant recycling of bladder urine into the upper tracts effectively prevents true bladder emptying.** The US appearance, both prenatally and postnatally, may mimic that of PUV, yet the bladders in these children are typically thin walled and smooth. The association occurs most commonly in males. Although prenatal diagnosis is common, boys may present early in life with sepsis. They may even present with a clinical picture consistent with adrenal crisis, mimicking CAH with a salt-losing nephropathy, considered to be due to renal aldosterone resistance caused by bacterial toxins (Vaid et al, 1989).

In either presentation, antibiotic treatment or prophylaxis is needed and is often sufficient to stabilize the child. Although it may be of some merit to observe these children to permit spontaneous resolution of their reflux, many have ultimately required surgery because of recurrent infection or deteriorating renal function (Farhat et al, 2000; Upadhyay et al, 2003). Surgical repair typically requires formal excisional megaureter tailoring and ureteral reimplantation. There seems to be little indication for cutaneous vesicostomy.

With bilateral HUN in the absence of reflux or valves, bilateral obstructive megaureters are present. Evaluation for a neurogenic cause should be considered. If this is not present, management is usually elective with prophylactic antibiotics and delayed functional evaluation. If there is no ureteral dilation present, the diagnosis is presumed bilateral UPJO, and timing of evaluation can also be more elective. In the absence of a prenatal history of oligohydramnios, very few of these patients have acute renal insufficiency. When the initial ultrasound examination shows profound hydronephrosis and renal parenchymal echogenicity, follow-up needs to be more aggressive. In girls, bilateral HUN suggests reflux or obstructive megaureters, but bilateral single system ectopic ureters should be considered as well. Each of these can be managed more electively with prophylactic antibiotics and delayed VCUG.

Mild to moderate bilateral hydronephrosis may be managed more electively in boys and girls. Whether this is obstructive or refluxing, it is rarely necessary to intervene early in life as long as infection is prevented with prophylactic antibiotics. Postnatal US evaluation is deferred until 1 or 2 months and may be planned in combination with a VCUG. The decision regarding selection of patients for cystography is a difficult one, with conflicting recommendations in the literature (Anderson et al, 1991; Elder, 1992; Zerin et al, 1993; Walsh et al, 1996; Horowitz et al, 1999; Herndon et al, 2000; Arena et al, 2001; Brophy et al, 2002). The same analysis applies to unilateral mild to moderate hydronephrosis.

Unilateral Hydronephrosis

There is rarely any indication to obtain urgent postnatal studies when unilateral hydronephrosis has been identified prenatally (in a child with a normal contralateral kidney). Even with the most severe unilateral obstruction, intervention is deferred for at least several weeks in current practice. There is often great pressure to obtain an early ultrasound study, but this seldom prompts early intervention and, more important, the **normal oliguria of the neonate may underrepresent the degree of obstruction or the likelihood of reflux.** Figure 109–16 illustrates the normal US examination on day 2 of the life of a child with prenatal unilateral moderately severe hydronephrosis. At this point, we have seen parents and pediatricians determine that the condition had resolved and resist recommendations for further evaluation. In this example, follow-up ultrasonography demonstrated marked caliectasis related to significant UPJ obstruction. Docimo has shown that an early ultrasonography does not miss significant pathology in most cases, but it may cloud the issue and inappropriately guide follow-up (Docimo et al, 1997; Wiener et al, 2002). In cases in which the perinatal urologist is not yet involved, this may cause neglect of a significant condition. We would actively recommend against early ultrasonography in these cases, as it plays little role in management but may induce unnecessary confusion.

The decision about selecting patients in whom VCUG is appropriate continues to evolve. Several studies have addressed this issue, and the conclusion seems to be that if there has been any degree of prenatal hydronephrosis, reflux is present in about 20% to 30% of the patients. Even when there is no hydronephrosis at birth, patients have a 23% chance of showing some degree of VUR (Zerin et al, 1993). In contrast, the study of Mandell and colleagues (1991) concluded that routine cystography was not indicated if hydronephrosis was less than moderate (i.e., with calyceal dilation). In part, this was in recognition of the need to reduce the enormous number of cystograms being performed as progressively greater numbers of infants with prenatal hydronephrosis were being identified. Ismaili and coauthors (2002) have reported that in neonates with prenatally detected hydronephrosis, a normal US examination at 5 days and 1 month eliminates the need for VCUG, as only 6.7% of those children have an abnormal study. Other **studies have identified thresholds of renal pelvic dilation as indicating the need for postnatal evaluation. Each threshold selects a level of tolerance for missing certain conditions** (McIlroy et al, 2000). **Most do not clearly separate between refluxing and nonrefluxing conditions, however.**

Although it has been assumed that it is important to detect reflux in neonates, it is not established that all reflux is clinically significant (Yerkes et al, 1999). Moorthy and associates (2003) reported on two groups of patients, one with prenatal hydronephrosis, postnatal follow-up, and discharge. Of these 425 patients, 284 had only US imaging. In a similar time period in the same geographic region, 230 infants with urinary tract infection (UTI) were assessed and only 3 were from the discharged group, indicating that any missed reflux was unlikely to permit infectious problems during the first year of life. Whether more children would develop infections in the toilet training years is unknown.

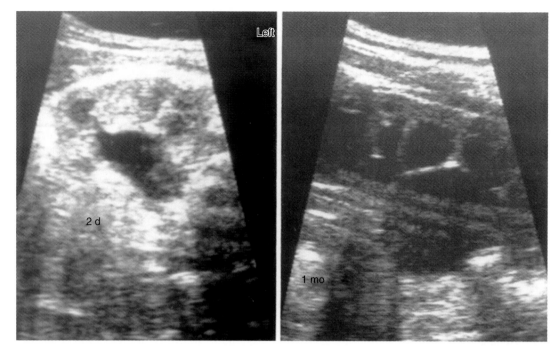

Figure 109–16. Postnatal renal ultrasonography in the same baby at 2 days of life and then again at 30 days. The baby had moderate hydronephrosis in utero. Early postnatal ultrasound examinations may miss significant dilation and, more important, may lead to misguided recommendations regarding further evaluation. There is seldom a benefit to performing these studies early in life.

The experience at our institution has also raised this question. We have followed up a group of 357 patients with mild and mild-moderate hydronephrosis in whom no VCUG was performed and antibiotic prophylaxis was not used. Most have shown resolution of their hydronephrosis as expected. On the basis of reported data, as well as our own recent experience wherein cystography has been performed in similar degrees of hydronephrosis, 28% of these patients may be presumed to have reflux (Zerin et al, 1993). Of 1156 patients in our group having a VCUG, 325 (28.1%) were found to have VUR. In the first years, there were few infections in the group without prior VCUG; however, with late follow-up, the incidence of febrile UTI was significantly increased in this population. Of an estimated 98 patients with VUR, 12.2% developed febrile UTI and had reflux on evaluation. This rate is in contrast to a 1.5% incidence in the group of patient with documented VUR and receiving prophylactic antibiotics. Dimercaptosuccinic acid (DMSA) imaging revealed parenchymal abnormalities consistent with pyelonephritis in some of the patients not receiving prophylaxis (Estrada et al, 2005). Several studies have shown the value of early diagnosis with lower rates of DMSA abnormality in the children diagnosed prenatally than those presenting with infection in the early years (Assael et al, 1998; Lama et al, 2000; Ylinen et al, 2003).

We have subsequently examined patients with mild to moderate hydronephrosis and attempted to select thresholds for cystography on the basis of the incidence of reflux. **In order to identify 95% of patients with grade 3 and higher, all levels of hydronephrosis would need to be evaluated with cystography.** Other groups have reported a similar inability to correlate hydronephrosis severity with reflux risk or grade (Scott and Renwick, 2001; Phan et al, 2003). Current practice varies. Some centers choose to evaluate all patients with any history

of prenatal hydronephrosis, whereas others use a cutoff at calyceal dilation or between 7 and 10 mm of AP pelvic diameter at term or immediately after birth. **The important issue in making any recommendation is that any cutoff is arbitrary and some patients with reflux are not diagnosed. The clinical significance of that misdiagnosis is not known and is unlikely to be so distinctly different as to make any one threshold clinically useful. This information must be available to parents as they make their decisions regarding evaluation, with a large measure dependent upon their level of risk aversion.**

Similar issues related to selecting thresholds of risk are relevant to the selection of patients for renal functional evaluation of obstructive conditions. In profound bilateral obstruction, serum creatinine reflects renal functional impairment and is useful in managing patients with valves. It is seldom useful in patients with bilateral megaureter or UPJO. In boys with valves, in whom it is apparent that renal function may be compromised on the basis of the ultrasound appearance, it is useful to obtain a baseline creatinine at day 1 or 2 of life. Although this reflects maternal creatinine, it is the starting point, and the significance of subsequent changes can be interpreted only with this knowledge. A creatinine value of 1.0 mg/dL at day 5 suggests very different degrees of functional impairment depending upon whether maternal creatinine at birth was 1.0 or 1.5 mg/dL. The rate of decline of neonatal creatinine is a useful guide to both renal function and efficacy of drainage.

For unilateral obstructive processes, functional imaging serves the purpose of determining the need for and timing of intervention. As is made clear in the discussion on the evaluation and management of UPJO in Chapter 115, Anomalies and Surgery of the Ureteropelvic Junction in Children, there is significant controversy about the interpretation of functional imaging studies in UPJO in infants. Therefore, it is impossible to establish absolute guidelines to selection of patients for these studies. All of the reports attempting to do this create arbitrary definitions of postnatal "obstruction" to permit creation of selection criteria. The study of Mandell and colleagues (1991) identified levels of AP diameter as indicating risk of having surgery. More recent studies have made similar attempts to define thresholds for evaluation on the basis of imaging outcomes rather than any clinical outcomes (Langer, 2000; Toiviainen-Salo et al, 2004). The selection criteria for postnatal surgery are controversial, and any threshold based upon them is of limited value. AP pelvic diameter is a commonly used criterion for setting thresholds for what is often called pathologic dilation; however, the criteria are unclear and may not be clinically useful.

A practical way to deal with this difficulty is to select a threshold that is reproducible and identifies all patients in whom some consideration for surgery might be appropriate. Even if early surgery is not recommended, a baseline study is appropriate because these children need to be followed closely. The specific functional study used is also controversial, although intravenous pyelography is falling away from use in this context, being replaced by diuretic renography. The advantage of the latter is that it makes longitudinal comparison more practical using numerical parameters. Caution must be exercised, however, in the overinterpretation of those numbers (Connolly et al, 2000). In our practice, the presence of generalized calyceal dilation is the selection threshold for a diuretic renogram. When patients with less dilation than this were studied, there was no evidence of any functional impairment and the washout times were uniformly within normal ranges (i.e., less than 20 minutes). The degree of pelvic or ureteral dilation has been reported by other groups as the most important predictor of outcome (Ransley et al, 1990; Liu et al, 1994).

When reflux is present, functional imaging as a baseline may be useful as there is a high incidence of abnormal renal scans in the absence of any infection (Lama et al, 2000; Nguyen et al, 2000). Renal scan abnormalities in the absence of infection suggests either a prenatal effect of reflux on renal development or an underlying developmental defect that causes both reflux and abnormal renal development. Although this controversy is unresolved, it raises significant questions regarding the potential for ongoing postnatal renal impairment from uncorrected sterile reflux. **Several studies have identified markedly abnormal patterns of renal function in infants with dilating reflux, predominantly in males** (Marra et al, 1994; Assael et al, 1998; Stock et al, 1998; Lama et al, 2000; Nguyen et al, 2000; Polito et al, 2000). The incidence of renal abnormalities is heavily weighted toward males and to higher grades of reflux, approaching 85% in males (Lama et al, 2000). Histologic studies of kidneys removed for nonfunction associated with reflux show heterogeneous patterns of structural abnormalities consistent with "dysplasia."(Risdon et al, 1993) The patterns reported appear to echo the focal nature of reflux-induced pyelonephritic changes with infection. Experimental studies have shown renal abnormalities induced by fetal reflux in the absence of infection, particularly in males, and without the induction of bladder outlet obstruction (Gobet et al, 1998b, 1999).

Associated with these observations have been several studies demonstrating markedly abnormal urodynamic patterns in boys with dilating reflux. These have generally shown a high incidence of bladder hypertonicity and instability. This raises the question of whether the high grades of reflux are a product of bladder dysfunction or just associated with it (Sillen et al, 1992, 1996a, 1996b; Yeung et al, 1997). Some centers have suggested temporary vesicostomy or early reimplantation. Although this debate continues, the frequency of renal abnormalities associated with neonatal reflux is high and obtaining baseline data to permit interpretation of later studies is recommended. The association of abnormal bladder function with abnormal kidneys has been reported to be predictive of lack of resolution by 16 months, and conversely, normal bladder dynamics with normal kidneys predict likely resolution within that time period (Godley et al, 2001). In some cases, therefore, severe reduction in function may prompt consideration of earlier intervention. The natural history of neonatally detected VUR indicates a moderate likelihood of resolution with high-grade VUR and high probability of low-grade resolution (Farhat et al, 2000; Upadhyay et al, 2003). In general, these patients do not show progressive scarring while receiving prophylaxis (McIlroy et al, 2000; Nguyen et al, 2000; Ylinen et al, 2003).

Renal Cystic Diseases (see also Chapter 114)

Multicystic dysplastic kidney and autosomal recessive polycystic kidney disease are the two principal cystic conditions identified prenatally. MCDK is usually a unilateral, isolated finding with a good prognosis; the second is typically bilateral and lethal. It is important that the clinician be able to distinguish these two entities with certainty.

MCDK is usually detected prenatally as described previously, having a typical US appearance characterized by multiple fluid-filled spaces of varying size, without interconnection or a central large cyst, and minimal associated parenchyma (Sanders and Hartman, 1984). Occasionally, MCDK is detected as an abdominal mass in an otherwise healthy newborn. Some are massive and impair pulmonary or gastrointestinal function. The principal responsibility of the urologist is to ensure that the contralateral kidney is entirely normal. An increased frequency of VUR and UPJO has been reported in association with contralateral MCDK (Kaneko et al, 1995; Miller et al, 2004), although not all agree that VCUG is needed (Ismaili et al, 2005). Appropriate evaluation and management of those conditions, if present, are of primary concern as they put the functionally solitary kidney at risk. Rarely, bilateral MCDK is identified, often prenatally, with a uniformly dismal postnatal outlook (Feldenberg and Siegel, 2000). These children die from the pulmonary hypoplasia associated with bilateral renal dysplasia.

When the diagnosis of MCDK is uncertain and severe hydronephrosis may be present, a DMSA renal scan is the most effective means of confirming the diagnosis. MCDK can be expected to demonstrate no uptake on DMSA scanning.

Urgent management of a patient with MCDK is seldom necessary. Controversy persists regarding the need for surgical removal; this should be a carefully considered decision between the clinician and parents (Strife et al, 1993; Wacksman et al, 1993; Minevich et al, 1997; Eckoldt et al, 2003; Kuwertz-Broeking et al, 2004; Narchi, 2005; Rabelo et al, 2004, 2005).

ARPKD is now being identified prenatally, particularly in affected families. As noted earlier, screening for the affected gene (*PKHD1*) and its various mutations can permit more specific prenatal diagnosis (Zerres et al, 2004; Bergmann et al, 2005a, 2005b). These children usually have a lethal outcome in the newborn period because of pulmonary failure. If diagnosis is sufficiently early, prenatal termination is an option to some. **In the newborn, the classical ultrasonographic constellation of symmetrically large kidneys with a reniform shape, multiple small cysts giving a uniformly bright echogenic sonotexture, and poor pulmonary and renal function is highly suggestive of ARPKD** (Traubici et al, 2005). Little specific therapy may be offered, although some centers have begun peritoneal dialysis in children with sufficient pulmonary capacity (Munding et al, 1999) A small number of children with ARPKD present with large echogenic cystic kidneys yet show slower renal functional deterioration. They live long enough to develop evidence of hepatic and pancreatic cystic disease (Caroli's disease) (Cole et al, 1987; Hussman et al, 1991; Parfrey 2005). It remains difficult to prognosticate about these children in the newborn period, although genetic analysis may be useful (Bergmann et al, 2005a).

NEONATAL UROLOGIC EMERGENCIES

This section reviews the major and minor emergencies and urgencies that may be seen in the perinatal period, based on the presenting signs and symptoms, not covered in other chapters in this book (Table 109–4). Although an anatomic organization has been imposed upon this review, it is important to maintain a clear awareness of the fact that disorders of one particular part of the urogenital system may affect the entire system and the entire well-being of the child. They may also be heralds of other aspects of congenital or acquired conditions. Therefore, it is often necessary to evaluate, to various degrees of intensity, the remainder of the GU system. In this way, associated or secondary problems are not neglected.

Perineal Mass in a Female

The appearance of a protuberant mass in the perineum of a newborn girl should suggest four principal diagnoses. The appearance usually indicates the most likely diagnosis. The most common entity producing this general finding in a newborn is a periurethral cyst. These are whitish in appearance and covered by a delicate but normal epithelium. The urethral meatus is adjacent but uninvolved. Incision and drainage are usually curative. **Imperforate hymen with resulting hydrocolpos may arise with a midline bulging of whitish tissue symmetrically between the labia and behind the urethra.** A palpable abdominal mass may be present because of uterine distention, and occasionally hydronephrosis is found on ultrasonography. A separate fluid-filled cavity in the pelvis should be distinguishable from the bladder, yet may also be confused for the bladder. Management of an imperforate hymen is incision and drainage, which is also

Table 109–4. Presenting Signs of Neonatal Urologic Emergencies		
Sign	**Etiologies**	**Evaluation**
Sepsis	Bladder outlet obstruction—valves, neurogenic	Urine and blood cultures
	Vesicoureteral reflux	Ultrasound
	Megaureter	VCUG
	Ectopic ureter	
	Ureterocele	
	UPJ obstruction	
	Fungal infection with secondary obstruction	
Hematuria	Urinary infection	Urine culture
	Renal vein thrombosis	Ultrasound
Hypertension	Renal vein thrombosis	Ultrasound
	Renal artery thrombosis	DMSA scan
Renal mass	Hydronephrosis	Ultrasound
	ARPKD	CT/DMSA/MRI
	MCDK	
	CMN	
	Neuroblastoma	
	Wilms' tumor	
Renal failure	Urinary obstruction	Urine culture
	Sepsis	Urine electrolytes
	Renal cortical necrosis	Ultrasound
	Renal dysplasia/agenesis	DMSA/MAG3
Urinary ascites	Urinary obstruction	Ultrasound
Scrotal mass	Neonatal torsion	Examination
	Hydrocele	Ultrasound
	Tumor	

ARPKD, autosomal recessive polycystic kidney disease; CT, computed tomography; DMSA, dimercaptosuccinic acid; MAG3, mercaptoacetyltriglycine; MCDK, multicystic dysplastic kidney; MRI, magnetic resonance imaging; UPJ, ureteropelvic junction; CMN, congenital mesoblastic nephroma; VCUG, voiding cystourethrogram.

appropriate for the less common vaginal stenosis. The substance drained is often milky white and may be of surprising volume. Subsequent intervention is seldom needed. **Prolapse of an ectopic ureterocele may have a similar appearance, distinguished by its often edematous, congested, or frankly necrotic appearance. With close examination, it may be seen emerging from the urethra in an eccentric fashion, usually posteriorly.** A distended bladder may be palpable and less often a palpable hydronephrotic kidney.

Ultrasonography usually provides the diagnosis, which should be supplemented with voiding cystography and functional renal imaging. The most useful option is to incise the ureterocele sufficiently to allow reduction into the bladder and temporary catheter drainage. Further management of the ureterocele is dictated by the response of the bladder outlet obstruction and any associated obstruction of functional renal elements. **Urethral prolapse is uncommon in newborns but may be seen as a circumferential collar of edematous and ecchymotic tissue at the urethral meatus** (Lowe et al, 1986). **Topical measures such as skin moisturizers, hot compresses, and relief of aggravating factors (urethral catheter, prolonged coughing, or straining) may relieve the prolapse.** If tissue necrosis is evident, surgical resection is appropriate. Although uncommon in the neonatal period, botryoid sarcomata of the vagina may arise as a protuberant vaginal mass, usually with a distinctive, multilobulated appearance. Evidence of a solid pelvic mass is present on examination and ultrasonography. This should prompt thorough evaluation based on imaging, tissue diagnosis, and assessment of regional involvement.

Abdominal Mass

The diagnosis of an abdominal mass in a neonate has become greatly simplified with the availability of US imaging. In many cases the identity of the mass will have been suggested prenatally. **The principal entities to be considered include hydronephrosis, cystic renal disease, adrenal hemorrhage, a dilated bladder, gastrointestinal duplications, or tumor** (Hartman et al, 1989; Schwartz and Shaul, 1989; McVicar et al, 1991; Chandler et al, 2004) (Table 109–5). Physical examination should consider the location, size, texture, and mobility of the mass, as well as other abnormalities on examination, including limb, cardiac, and central nervous system findings. Ultrasonography is usually able to identify the organ of origin, the cystic or solid nature of the mass, and the condition of the uninvolved elements of the GU tract and permit a more focused and detailed subsequent evaluation. It cannot be overemphasized that care must be taken to examine the entire abdomen rather than immediately focusing attention on the usually obvious anomaly. In all instances, as with more specific GU conditions, the aim of evaluation is to provide a detailed picture of the anatomy with an associated functional assessment.

The likelihood of any abdominal mass being of urinary tract origin is high, over 60%, with hydronephrosis and MCDK being the most frequent (Schwartz and Shaul, 1989).

Imperforate Anus

The pediatric urologist should be familiar with the presentation and management of imperforate anus in light of the high frequency of associated GU anomalies and the potential for functionally significant neurologic bladder dysfunction in these children. **Prenatally, the presence of imperforate anus may be suggested by punctate calcifications in the intestinal lumen related to formation of meconium calcifications from exposure to urine** (Mandell et al, 1992b). At initial presentation a routine ultrasound study should be obtained to assess the urinary tract, as well as a voiding cystourethrogram. The latter may be of particular importance in assessing the level of the rectourethral/vesical fistula in boys. Complications related to the confluence of the gastrointestinal and urinary tracts may occur, including infection and metabolic derangements. Initial management is usually with a diverting colostomy, which should be constructed using the transverse colon and with separation of the proximal and distal limbs. This limits the risk of fecal contamination of the urinary tract in boys in whom a rectourethral fistula is present.

Many children with imperforate anus have associated spinal cord abnormalities, particularly spinal cord tethering (Warf et al, 1993; De Gennaro et al, 1994; Golonka et al, 2002). This may be readily identified in the newborn using ultrasonography of the distal spine before the vertebral column is fully ossified.

Oligohydramnios/Potter's Syndrome/Renal Agenesis

The anatomic features of Potter's syndrome should be familiar to all urologists. These include oligohydramnios; limb contractures, particularly clubfeet; and compressed facies with low-set ears. If it is suspected, immediate ultrasonography permits confirmation of the diagnosis, as evidenced by absent, or bilaterally dysplastic, or cystic kidneys. These children usually die from respiratory failure in the first hours of life, although survival for several days has been reported. The role of the urologist is largely one of confirming the diagnosis and providing counseling to parents and staff in these tragic cases. Little specific therapy is available to the urologist.

Single Umbilical Artery

The presence of a single umbilical artery, occurring in about 0.3% to 0.55% of live births, has been associated with an increased incidence of GU anomalies in the past (Vlietinck et al, 1972). Many of these early studies included stillborn fetuses in which the incidence of renal anomalies was about 60% (Thummala et al, 1998). More recent examination of the incidence has suggested that the degree of increase is relatively minimal, about 7.1% for all renal anomalies, including reflux with an incidence of 4.5% (Bourke et al, 1993). Those authors recommended routine screening for single umbilical artery, although the clinical significance of the anomalies identified is unclear. **A meta-analysis of 37 studies of single umbilical arteries indicated that it would require screening of 14 children with a single umbilical artery to identify 1 child with a renal anomaly, and these are of minimal significance** (Thummala et al, 1998; Cristina et al, 2005). The authors did not recommend routine screening. If there is suspicion, a renal ultrasound examination is an adequate screening tool.

Table 109–5.	Causes of Abdominal Mass in Newborns		
Etiology		*Number*	*%*
Urinary Tract		186	68
MCDK		65	35
Hydronephrosis (nonspecified)		38	20
UPJO		20	11
PUVs		18	10
UDEC		11	6
ARPKD		12	6
Wilms' tumor (also CMN)		8	4
RVT		5	3
Miscellaneous		9	5
Other Causes		88	32
Neuroblastoma		22	25
GI duplication		16	18
Hydrometrocolpos		13	15
Ovarian cysts		9	10
Miscellaneous		28	32

ARPKD, autosomal recessive polycystic kidney disease; GI, gastrointestinal; MCDK, multicystic dysplastic kidney; UPJO, ureteropelvic junction obstruction; PUV, posterior urethral values; UDEC, urinary duplication and ectopia; CMN, congenital mesoblastic nephroma; RVT, renal vein thrombosis.
From McVicar and colleagues (1991), summarizing Griscom (1965) and Raffensperger and Abouseleiman (1968).

Sepsis

The infant presenting with sepsis should be evaluated for a possible urinary source. A catheterized or suprapubically aspirated urine specimen for culture must be obtained prior to antibiotic therapy. If pyuria is present, urosepsis should be strongly considered. A screening ultrasound study is an excellent means to assess the urinary tract quickly and accurately. Most cases of urosepsis are found to have some sonographic abnormality. This permits directed evaluation. The most common causes include obstructive uropathy with anatomic abnormalities or massive VUR. A normal ultrasound study does not rule out reflux, and in the presence of urosepsis, a VCUG is essential. This should probably be obtained during the acute hospital admission. Further workup should be tailored to the findings of the initial examinations.

Infant boys with intact foreskins have a higher risk of urosepsis and may not have specific anatomic findings (Wiswell and Hachey, 1993; Wiswell, 2000). **These boys should undergo the usual evaluation in any event, with a US examination and VCUG to rule out obstruction and reflux.**

Absence of Voiding

The pediatric urologist is often called to evaluate a newborn who has not voided. The normal time for the first postnatal void extends to 24 hours, and some healthy children wait even longer (Clark, 1977). The most useful physical finding to determine is whether the bladder is distended. Physical examination may precipitate voiding. Ultrasound examination may be obtained when there has been no void after 24 hours, the bladder is distended, or parental concern is high. Specific findings dictate management. The time to void after circumcision is predictable and depends in part upon feeding times. Within 8 hours of circumcision, 75% of breast-fed and 100% of formula-fed infants had voided (Narchi and Kulayat, 1998).

A common cause of concern is the pinpoint meatus often seen with hypospadias in conjunction with delayed first void. These are virtually never obstructed, and this may be readily demonstrated with a feeding tube.

Hematuria

Hematuria in the newborn provokes expected anxiety yet often does not represent a significant process. One possible explanation is maternal hormonal withdrawal producing urethral bleeding through an as yet unspecified mechanism. Urine cultures, examination, and US evaluation are usually sufficient. The appearance of hematuria may occasionally be noted in the diaper, produced by urate crystals that have a characteristic rusty red color. Other etiologies include renal vein thrombosis, which is identified on US examination, dependent upon the duration of the process, with an enlarged, echogenic kidney and occasionally with a visible inferior vena cava thrombus (Hibbert et al, 1997).

Hypertension

Neonatal hypertension is rare and should prompt a careful evaluation of the infant's urinary tract. Iatrogenic renal injury from umbilical artery lines has been described to produce hypertension. Radioisotope renal scanning may be confirmatory by demonstrating focal or diffuse renal nonperfusion.

Urinary Ascites

The differential diagnosis of neonatal ascites includes urinary obstruction, which should be specifically sought, most efficiently with an ultrasound examination (Checkley et al, 2003). Posterior urethral valves are probably the most common underlying etiology (Misra et al, 1987; Ahmed and LeQuesne 1988; Huang and Cheng, 1990; Sakai et al, 1998; Merrot et al, 2003; Patil, 2003). Unusually, other obstructive processes may cause urinary ascites (Chun and Ferguson, 1997; Adams et al, 1998; Cimador et al, 2003; Beetz et al, 2004). Electrolyte analysis of the ascitic fluid may reveal high creatinine indicative of urine, but it may also have equilibrated with the serum across the peritoneum.

SPECIFIC DIAGNOSES
Renal Vein Thrombosis

Renal vein thrombosis (RVT) is suggested in the neonate with enlarged kidneys, hematuria, anemia, and thrombocytopenia, often with a history of a prolonged delivery and prematurity (Keating et al, 1985). Approximately 20% of infants with gross hematuria are found to have RVT, and about 20% of neonates with RVT have bilateral involvement. The presumed etiology is impaired renal blood flow in the setting of a neonate with normally low blood pressure, polycythemia, and dehydration, including adrenal hyperplasia and salt wasting (Glassock et al, 1983; Sharma et al, 2001). Conditions that may exacerbate those factors may predispose to RVT. Up to 50% of neonates with RVT are found to have prothrombotic abnormalities and should be screened (Kuhle et al, 2004; Marks et al, 2005). Thrombosis is peripheral and does not usually propagate centrally.

The diagnosis of RVT is best made using ultrasonography, in which an enlarged kidney is evident and the thrombus may be visualized directly (Hibbert et al, 1997). Management of RVT is directed initially at reversing any predisposing factors such as dehydration and secondary electrolyte imbalances. Specific treatment remains controversial but may include anticoagulation with heparin or fibrinolytic therapy with streptokinase. Each of these modalities can be associated with significant complications (Chevalier 1991; Nuss et al, 1994; Bokenkamp et al, 2000). When treated with heparin, fewer patients are left with renal functional abnormalities (Zigman et al, 2000). Bilateral RVT requires more aggressive therapy to prevent end-stage renal failure (Cozzolino and Cendron, 1997; Marks et al, 2005).

Adrenal Hemorrhage

Adrenal hemorrhage is a relatively common condition, estimated to occur in about 1% to 2% of healthy infants. More small adrenal hemorrhages are being detected with routine perinatal ultrasonography. **Predisposing factors include prolonged labor, birth trauma, and large birth weight. RVT may be associated** (Suga et al, 2000). An association with the Beckwith-Weidemann syndrome has been reported in several cases (Anoop and Anjay, 2004; Merrot et al, 2004; Gocmen et al, 2005). Clinically, the neonate with adrenal hemorrhage may have anemia, shock, and an abdominal mass. Gross hematuria is unusual. Ultrasonography is the most efficient diagnostic measure and usually reveals an echogenic suprarenal mass (Rubenstein et al, 1995; Schwarzler et al, 1999; Lee and Lin, 2000; Velaphi and Perlman, 2001). This may appear similar to a neuroblastoma, and further evaluation, particularly with magnetic resonance imaging, may be necessary. Scrotal hemorrhage may also be a presenting sign of adrenal hemorrhage (Avolio et al, 2002; Duman et al, 2004). The imaging characteristics of an adrenal hemorrhage evolve with time, often providing a definitive diagnosis as the mass is seen to involute. Calcifications may later develop, reportedly as soon as 1 week (Smith and Middleton, 1979). **The late appearance of an adrenal hemorrhage is that of peripheral eggshell calcifications in contrast to stippled calcifications of neuroblastoma.** Management is almost always supportive and expectant, with rare need for intervention.

Renal Artery Thrombosis

Hypertension and hematuria in a neonate should suggest the possibility of renal artery thrombosis (Roth et al, 2003). The clinical setting is usually suggestive in that umbilical artery catheterization is the most common cause of this condition. Renal insufficiency may be a clinical feature of this condition, as well as proteinuria and congestive heart failure (Andreoli, 2004; Cachat et al, 2004). Thrombotic involvement of the aorta may be present as well. US examination usually reveals the diagnosis and the extent of the thrombus. Management is dependent upon the clinical setting, and unilateral involvement is best managed expectantly, although thrombolytic therapy may be appropriate (Ellis et al, 1997; Kavaler and Hensle, 1997). Control of hypertension is the most important aspect of management and occasionally requires removal of a nonfunctional kidney.

Acknowledgment

Fetal imaging was generously provided by Drs. Beryl R. Benacerraf, Bryann Bromley, Carol E. Barnewolt, and Judy A. Estroff.

SUGGESTED READINGS

Benacerraf BR, Mandell J, Estroff JA et al: Fetal pyelectasis: A possible association with Down syndrome. Obstet Gynecol 1990;76:58-60.

Biard JM, Johnson MP, Carr MC, et al: Long-term outcomes in children treated by prenatal vesicoamniotic shunting for lower urinary tract obstruction. Obstet Gynecol 2005;106:503-508.

Cromie WJ, Lee K, Houde K, et al: Implications of prenatal ultrasound screening in the incidence of major genitourinary malformations. J Urol 2001;165:1677-1680.

Dommergues M, Muller F, Ngo S, et al: Fetal serum beta2-microglobulin predicts postnatal renal function in bilateral uropathies. Kidney Int 2000;58:312-316.

Fernbach SK, Maizels M, Conway JJ: Ultrasound grading of hydronephrosis: Introduction to the system used by the Society for Fetal Urology. Pediatr Radiol 1993;23:478-480.

Freedman AL, Bukowski TP, Smith CA, et al: Fetal therapy for obstructive uropathy: Diagnosis specific outcomes. J Urol 1996;156:720-723; discussion 723-724.

Glick PL, Harrison MR, Golbus MS, et al: Management of the fetus with congenital hydronephrosis II: Prognostic criteria and selection for treatment. J Pediatr Surg 1985;20:376-387.

Harrison MR, Golbus MS, Filly RA, et al: Fetal surgery for congenital hydronephrosis. N Engl J Med 1982;306:591-593.

Johnson MP, Bukowski TP, Reitleman C, et al: In utero surgical treatment of fetal obstructive uropathy: A new comprehensive approach to identify appropriate candidates for vesicoamniotic shunt therapy. Am J Obstet Gynecol 1994;170:1770-1776; discussion 1776-1779.

Kaefer M, Peters CA, Retik AB, et al: Increased renal echogenicity: A sonographic sign for differentiating between obstructive and nonobstructive etiologies of in utero bladder distension. J Urol 1997;158:1026-1029.

Mandell J, Blyth BR, Peters CA, et al: Structural genitourinary defects detected in utero. Radiology 1991;178:193-196.

Mandell J, Peters CA, Estroff JA, et al: Late onset severe oligohydramnios associated with genitourinary abnormalities. J Urol 1992;148:515-518.

Manning FA, Harrison MR, Rodeck C: Catheter shunts for fetal hydronephrosis and hydrocephalus. Report of the International Fetal Surgery Registry. N Engl J Med 1986;315:336-340.

Peters CA: Obstruction of the fetal urinary tract. J Am Soc Nephrol 1997;8:653-663.

Ransley PG, Dhillon HK, Gordon I, et al: The postnatal management of hydronephrosis diagnosed by prenatal ultrasound. J Urol 1990;144:584.

Zerin JM, Ritchey ML, Chang AC: Incidental vesicoureteral reflux in neonates with antenatally detected hydronephrosis and other renal abnormalities. Radiology 1993;187:157-160.

TRIAGE OF THE PEDIATRIC UROLOGIC PATIENT

THE PEDIATRIC UROLOGY OFFICE VISIT

SUMMARY

Pediatric urology encompasses a spectrum of disorders from complex reconstructive puzzles such as the repair of bladder or cloacal exstrophy to more routine but often pressing difficulties such as daytime wetting in a school-aged child. Due to the pioneers of the past generation of pediatric urologists, most of these problems are readily identified and treated. Despite the dramatic progress made over the past 50 years, new discoveries are made each year that continue to streamline care. More than 80% of our patients now can be cared for expediently with outpatient office visits or in outpatient surgical centers (Hoebeke et al, 1997; Valero Puerta et al, 1999). These impressive figures underscore the importance of rapid diagnosis and treatment in the child with a congenital or acquired pediatric urologic problem.

TRIAGE OF THE PEDIATRIC UROLOGIC PATIENT

In most cases, the initial contact with the child and family will be through a referring phone call from the parent, pediatrician, family practitioner, or, if prenatal evaluation is desired, the obstetrician. In many cases, the family is calling from a distance and the urologist will need to decide with the referring clinician whether the child is healthy enough to be transferred or must first have his or her condition stabilized. Usually, even in remote areas, skilled general pediatric support is available. With coaching from the accepting team, most clinicians will be able to manage even complex problems in the stabilization phase of the triage process.

We try to triage all children into categories (Table 110–1): **those who need to be seen immediately (emergent), those who can be seen in the next 24 hours (urgent), those who must be seen in the next 72 hours (semi-urgent), and those who require more routine evaluation (routine).**

Emergent Evaluations

Children with acute problems related to recent surgical procedures, certain patients with neonatal hydronephrosis or hydronephrosis in a solitary kidney, acutely ill infants with urinary tract infection (UTI), and infants with gross hematuria, ambiguous genitalia, major abdominal defects, imperforate anus, or spina bifida may suffer further injury if not immediately evaluated. Children of all ages with acute abdominal pain, genitourinary trauma including spermatic cord torsion or evidence of physical abuse, and priapism should also be seen as soon as possible. In most cases, these children should be evaluated initially in the emergency department.

Patients who have developed acute problems such as pain, fever, or bleeding after a surgical procedure should be evaluated immediately. Many problems that threaten success of the procedure can be averted if the child is evaluated and treated quickly.

Infants with bilateral hydronephrosis or hydronephrosis in a solitary kidney should be evaluated immediately after delivery. Boys with an abnormally thickened bladder wall or dilated bladder outlet on the newborn ultrasound examination may have posterior urethral valves or the prune-belly syndrome or urethral atresia. Many will develop compromised renal function. A few will need a direct admission to the newborn intensive care unit or to a similar inpatient stepdown unit. One third of infants with prune-belly syndrome or posterior urethral valves develop pulmonary insufficiency. Care for these newborns may require intubation with assisted ventilation or extensive pulmonary therapy (Freedman et al, 1999; Noh et al, 1999). Surgical procedures to decompress the urinary tract or to reconstruct the urinary tract in these infants must follow the initial stabilization in these infants. A few girls with urethral atresia will need similar therapy.

Febrile UTIs in the newborn are treated emergently because newborns are particularly susceptible to significant renal damage if the infection is not treated promptly. A urine culture should be obtained, and these infants need intravenous antibiotics as early as possible after the diagnosis is made because they have a higher prevalence of concomitant bacteremia (10% to 22%) (Pitteti and Choi, 2002). Appropriate antibiotic therapy administered without delay has been shown to reduce the incidence of scarring (Ransley and Risdon, 1981).

Table 110–1. Triage Categories

Category	Diagnosis
Emergent (as soon as possible)	Trauma
	Suspected child abuse
	Acute postoperative problem
	Newborns with bilateral hydronephrosis or a solitary kidney
	Newborns with gross hematuria, urinary tract infections
	Newborns with ambiguous genitalia, bladder or cloacal exstrophy, posterior urethral valves, prune-belly syndrome, spina bifida
	Children with acute abdominal or scrotal pain
	Boys with priapism
Urgent (in 24 hr)	Gross hematuria outside newborn period
	Nephrolithiasis
	Febrile urinary tract infections outside newborn period
Semi-urgent (in 48 to 72 hr)	Postnatal evaluation of prenatal hydronephrosis
	Symptomatic hernia or hydrocele
	Failure to thrive
	Amenorrhea in the adolescent female
Routine (at family's convenience)	Asymptomatic hernia or hydrocele
	Circumcision evaluation
	Hypospadias
	Undescended testes
	Varicocele
	Vesicoureteral reflux
	Microscopic hematuria
	Enuresis

Gross hematuria in the newborn is also an emergency because it may indicate renal venous thrombosis or renal arterial thrombosis. Both may be life threatening. Renal vein thrombosis affects males twice as often as females, with a left-sided predominance. These infants require resuscitation and, occasionally, anticoagulant or operative therapy (Kuhle et al, 2004).

Infants with ambiguous genitalia also require immediate evaluation. Many will require direct transfer from a referring hospital. **Because congenital adrenal hyperplasia (CAH) may result in salt wasting, which may be life threatening, infants with ambiguous genitalia must be evaluated quickly and stabilized** (Forest, 2004). **If CAH is suspected, the infant should not be discharged home from the nursery before appropriate testing is complete.** In some cases, a genotypic female with CAH may be incorrectly identified as a male. The correct diagnosis should be made as quickly as possible to establish the appropriate sex of rearing. Infants with ambiguous genitalia may also have other syndromes and may require further evaluation (Tables 110–2 and 110–3).

Patients with major abdominal defects such as bladder or cloacal exstrophy require direct admission to the neonatal nursery for stabilization and surgical planning. Patients with imperforate anus and variants such as a cloacal anomaly require decompression of the intestinal tract, usually within the first 24 to 48 hours (Chen, 1999). At the time of the colostomy, the urologist may evaluate the perineum and perform endoscopy to further assess the urinary anomalies. Procedures to correct these major defects must be planned by

surgeons who are familiar with the potential risks and complications associated with the reconstruction of the urethra, vagina, and colon. In many cases, a team is assembled and provides orthopedic, general surgical, and urologic care during the surgery (Jeffs, 1978; Lattimer et al, 1979; Gearhart, 1999). The anesthesia team must be skillful in the management of the complex metabolic changes that may occur in infants who are under anesthesia for long periods. The neonatologists must be expert in the management of infants who have undergone major surgical procedures.

Today, **many newborns with spinal dysraphisms are diagnosed in utero** (Babcook et al, 1995). These infants are referred by direct admission to the neonatal intensive care nursery. Most of these children are not in urinary retention initially, but a few develop spinal shock after neurosurgery in the newborn period and have a transient period of overflow urinary drainage. As soon as possible after closure of the back defect, baseline investigations include renal/bladder ultrasound and voiding cystourethrography (VCUG) to evaluate for evidence of bladder dysfunction or vesicoureteral reflux. Initial urodynamics investigation is performed after resolution of the spinal shock to ensure that bladder storage pressures are not excessive (McGuire et al, 1977, 1983; Bauer, 1998). High-risk infants (those with a detrusor leak-point pressure greater than 40 cm H_2O or detrusor-sphincter dyssynergia) are started on anticholinergic therapy and intermittent catheterization (Snodgrass and Adams, 2004).

Children with acute abdominal pain should be seen immediately. In addition to a thorough abdominal examination designed to rule out surgical abdominal disease, these children should be evaluated for UTI, constipation, and spermatic cord torsion. Usually an acute abdominal series is ordered, which will show considerable amounts of stool throughout the colon if constipation is the problem. Other, more unusual causes for abdominal pain should also be considered (Table 110–4). Occasionally, some children with spermatic cord torsion complain of abdominal pain and have surprisingly few complaints referring to the scrotum. Acute renal colic from obstruction at the ureteropelvic junction or from urolithiasis may also present as abdominal pain and should be a part of the differential diagnosis of abdominal pain.

Most abdominal masses originate in genitourinary organs and should be evaluated immediately (Chandler et al, 2004) (Table 110–5). The most common malignant abdominal tumor in infants is neuroblastoma, followed by Wilms' tumor (Golden and Feusner, 2002). If an abdominal mass is suspected, an abdominal ultrasound evaluation should be ordered. If the mass is solid, computed tomography (CT) is almost always required. Testicular masses should be evaluated immediately. Testicular tumors occur in the newborn and in early childhood as well as after adolescence. The peak incidence of childhood testicular tumor is at age 2, and approximately 75% are malignant (Levy et al, 1994; Ciftci et al, 2001).

Vaginal masses may be palpable or may protrude from the introitus. The differential diagnosis of these masses includes benign periurethral cysts, skin tags, prolapsed urethra, or malignancies such as a rhabdomyosarcoma. **Bladder outlet obstruction may result from a prolapsed ureterocele.**

Sexual abuse victims will sometimes suffer trauma and initially be evaluated in the emergency department, but they may

Table 110–2. Syndromes Associated with Multisystemic Disease

Syndrome	Inheritance	Renal Anomaly	Genital Anomaly	Anomalies in Other Systems
Aarskog-Scott			Shawl scrotum, cryptorchidism	Broad facies, short stature
Beckwith-Wiedemann		Wilms' tumor		Macroglossia, gigantism, hepatoblastoma
Carpenter	AR		Small genitalia	Acrocephaly, polydactyly
Caudal regression		Hydronephrosis, renal agenesis	Vaginal and uterine agenesis	Imperforate anus, LS spine abnormality
Cerebro-oculo-facial	AR	Renal agenesis	Cryptorchidism	Arthrogryposis, microcephaly, cataracts
CHARGE			Small genitalia	Coloboma, heart defects, ear anomalies
Cornelia de Lange			Small genitalia, cryptorchidism	Micromelia, bushy eyebrows
Curran		Renal agenesis		Acral anomalies
Donohue			Enlarged penis or clitoris	Hirsutism, elfin face, thick lips, low-set ears
Drash		Wilms' tumor, glomerulonephritis	Mixed gonadal dysgenesis	
Dubowitz	AR		Hypospadias, cryptorchidism	Eczema, small stature, peculiar facies
Ehlers-Danlos	AR	Hydroureter		Skin hyperextensibility, poor wound healing
Fraser			Hypospadias, cryptorchidism	Cryptophthalmos
G			Hypospadias	Esophageal defect, low-set ears, abnormal facies
Holt-Oram		Renal anomalies		Defects of upper limb
Laurence-Moon-Biedl			Small genitalia	Obesity, retinal pigmentation, polydactyly
Marfan	AD	Renal duplication, hydroureter	Cryptorchidism	Aortic aneurysm, arachnodactyly
Mayer-Rokitansky		Renal agenesis	Duplex uterus, vaginal atresia	
Meckel-Gruber	AR	Renal cysts	Ambiguous genitalia, cryptorchidism	Microcephaly, polydactyly
Menkes		Hydronephrosis, reflux	Cryptorchidism	Kinky hair, CNS abnormality
Ochoa		Neurogenic bladder, hydronephrosis	Cryptorchidism	Aortic aneurysm, arachnodactyly
Opitz	AR		Hypospadias, cryptorchidism	Hypertelorism, mental retardation
Prader-Willi			Cryptorchidism	Hypotonia, obesity, mental retardation
Prune-belly		Hydronephrosis	Cryptorchidism	Hypoplastic abdominal muscle
Robert	AR	Hydroureter	Hypospadias, large penis, cryptorchidism	Hypomelia, growth retardation
Robinow	AD		Small genitalia, cryptorchidism	Flat face, short forearms
Rubenstein-Taybi	AR		Chordee	Hypoplastic maxilla, broad thumbs and toes
Rudiger	AR	Hydroureter	Small penis	Bicornuate uterus, coarse facies, stub nose
Russell-Silver	AR	Nonspecific renal anomalies	Small penis, hypospadias, cryptorchidism	Short stature, café-au-lait spots, skeletal asymmetry
Seckel	AR		Small genitalia, cryptorchidism	Small head, beak nose
Smith-Lemli-Opitz	AR		Hypospadias, cryptorchidism	Pernicious anemia, mental retardatic syndactyly, microcephaly
VATER		Hydronephrosis, renal dysplasia	Hypospadias	Vertebral anomalies, anal atresia, VSD, TE fistula, radial dysplasia
von Hippel-Lindau		Renal cyst, renal tumor		Pancreatic cyst, cerebral tumor, ichthyosis
Wolfram	AR	Hydroureter		Optic atrophy, deafness, diabetes
Zellweger	AR	Hydroureter	Hypospadias, cryptorchidism	Hypotonia, hepatomegaly

AD, autosomal dominant; AR, autosomal recessive; CHARGE, coloboma, heart anomaly, choanal atresia, retardation, and genetic and ear anomalies; CNS, central nervous system; LS, lumbosacral; TE, tracheoesophageal; VATER, vertebral, anal atresia, tracheoesophageal, renal; VSD, ventriculospetal defect.

Data from Barakat AY, Seikaly MG, Perkaloustian VM: Urogenital abnormalities in genetic disease. J Urol 1987;136:778-785; Walker RD: Familial and genetic urologic disorders in childhood. AUA Update Series 1987;6:1-6; and Mininberg D: The genetic basis of urologic disease. AUA Update Series 1992;9:218-223.

Table 110–3. Chromosomal Syndromes Associated with Genitourinary Anomalies

Chromosome Number	Clinical Features	Renal Anomalies	Genital Anomalies
4 Autosome Wolf-Hirschhorn syndrome 4p Trisomy 4q	Microcephaly Hemangiomas Hypertelorism Cleft lip/palate Low-set ears	Hydronephrosis	Hypospadias Undescended testis
8 Autosome Trisomy 8	Large, square head Prominent forehead Widely spaced eyes Slender body and limbs	Hydronephrosis Horseshoe kidney Reflux	Hypospadias Undescended testis
9 Autosome 9p Trisomy, 9p tetrasomy 9p Monosomy	Small cranium Strabismus Large nose Webbed neck	Renal hypoplasia Pancake kidney	Hypospadias Undescended testis Infantile male genitalia
10 Autosome 10q Syndrome 10p Syndrome	Microcephaly Oval, flat face Microphthalmia Short neck	Cystic kidney Hydronephrosis	Undescended testis Small penis
11 Autosome 11q Syndrome	 Flat nose Wide glabella Cleft lip/palate	High forehead Micropenis	
13 Autosome Patau's syndrome Trisomy 13	Microcephaly Hypertelorism Polydactyly Congenital heart disease	Horseshoe kidney Hydronephrosis Cystic kidney	Undescended testis
15 Autosome Monosomy 15q Prader-Willi syndrome	Obesity Hypotonia Retardation		Hypogonadism Cryptorchidism
18 Autosome Trisomy 18 Edwards' syndrome	Micrognathia Hypertonia Congenital heart disease	Horseshoe kidney Hydronephrosis	Undescended testis Small penis
20 Autosome 20p Syndrome	Round face Short nose Dental abnormalities Vertebral abnormalities	Hydronephrosis Polycystic kidney	Hypospadias
21 Autosome Trisomy 21 Down syndrome	Brachycephalic skull Congenital heart disease Nasal hypoplasia Broad, short hands		Undescended testis Small penis
22 Autosome Trisomy 22	Microcephaly Preauricular skin tags Low-set ears Beaked nose Cleft palate		Undescended testis Small penis
Cat's eye syndrome Possibly from both 13 and 22 autosomes	Coloboma Anal atresia Low-set ears Hemivertebrae Congenital heart disease	Renal agenesis Horseshoe kidney Reflux	
Sex chromosome Y Klinefelter's syndrome XXY, XXXY XXXXY	Elongated legs Gynecomastia Eunuchoid body build Sparse body hair		Small penis Small testes
Sex chromosome X Turner's syndrome XO	Short stature Primary amenorrhea Webbed neck Broad chest Coarctation of aorta	Horseshoe kidney	Infantile genitalia

Data from Barakat AY, Seikaly MG, Derkaloustian VM: Urogenital anomalies in genetic diseases. J Urol 1986;136:778-785; Walker RD: Familial and genetic urologic disorders in childhood. AUA Update Series 1987;6:1-6; and Mininberg D: The genetic basis of urologic disease. AUA Update Series 1992;9:218-223.

Table 110–4. Recurrent Abdominal Pain in Children

Disorder	Characteristics	Key Evaluations
Nonorganic		
Recurrent abdominal pain syndrome (functional abdominal pain)	Nonspecific pain, often periumbilical	History and PE; tests as indicated
Irritable bowel syndrome	Intermittent cramps, diarrhea, and constipation	History and PE
Nonulcer dyspepsia	Peptic ulcer–like symptoms without abnormalities on evaluation of the upper GI tract	History; esophagogastroduodenoscopy
Gastrointestinal Tract		
Chronic constipation	History of stool retention, evidence of constipation on examination	History and PE; plain radiograph of abdomen
Lactose intolerance	Symptoms may be associated with lactose ingestion: bloating, gas, cramps, and diarrhea	Trial of lactose-free diet; lactose breath hydrogen test
Parasite infection (especially *Giardia*)	Bloating, gas, cramps, and diarrhea	Stool evaluation for ova and parasites; specific immunoassays for *Giardia*
Excess fructose or sorbitol ingestion, Crohn's disease	Nonspecific abdominal pain, bloating, gas, and diarrhea	Large intake of apples, fruit juice, candy, or chewing gum sweetened with sorbitol
Peptic ulcer	Burning or gnawing epigastric pain; worse on awakening or before meals; relieved with antacids	Esophagogastroduodenoscopy or upper contrast radiographs
Esophagitis	Epigastric pain with substernal burning	Esophagogastroduodenoscopy
Meckel's diverticulum	Periumbilical or lower abdominal pain; may have blood in stool	Meckel scan or enteroclysis
Recurrent intussusception	Paroxysmal severe cramping abdominal pain; blood may be present in stool with episode	Identify intussusception during episode or lead point in intestine between episodes with contrast studies of GI tract
Internal, inguinal, or abdominal wall hernia	Dull abdomen or abdominal wall pain	PE, CT of abdominal wall
Chronic appendicitis or appendiceal mucocele	Recurrent RLQ pain; often incorrectly diagnosed, may be rare cause of abdominal pain	Barium enema, CT
Gallbladder and Pancreas		
Cholelithiasis	RUQ pain, may worsen with meals	Ultrasound of gallbladder
Choledochal cyst	RUQ pain ± elevated bilirubin	Ultrasound or CT of RUQ
Recurrent pancreatitis	Persistent boring pain, may radiate to back, vomiting	Serum amylase and lipase ± serum trypsinogen; ultrasound of pancreas
Genitourinary Tract		
Urinary tract infection	Dull suprapubic pain, flank pain	Urinalysis and urine culture; renal scan
Hydronephrosis	Unilateral abdominal or flank pain	Ultrasound of kidneys
Urolithiasis	Progressive, severe pain: flank to inguinal region to testis	Urinalysis, ultrasound, IVP, spinal CT
Other genitourinary disorders	Suprapubic or lower abdominal pain; genitourinary symptoms	Ultrasound of kidneys and pelvis; gynecologic evaluation
Miscellaneous Causes		
Abdominal migraine	Nausea, family history of migraine	History
Abdominal epilepsy	May have seizure prodrome	EEG (may require more than one study, including sleep-deprived EEG)
Gilbert's syndrome	Mild abdominal pain (causal or coincidental?); slightly elevated unconjugated bilirubin	Serum bilirubin
Familial Mediterranean fever	Paroxysmal episodes of fever, severe abdominal pain, and tenderness with other evidence of polyserositis	History and PE during an episode, DNA diagnosis
Sickle cell crisis	Anemia	Hematologic evaluation
Lead poisoning	Vague abdominal pain ± constipation	Serum lead level
Henoch-Schönlein purpura	Recurrent, severe crampy abdominal pain, occult blood in stool, characteristic rash, arthritis	History, PE, urinalysis
Angioneurotic edema	Swelling of face or airway, crampy pain	History, PE, upper GI contrast radiographs, serum C1 esterase inhibitor
Acute intermittent porphyria	Severe pain precipitated by drugs, fasting, or infections	Spot urine for porphyrins

CT, computed tomography; EEG, electroencephalogram; GI, gastrointestinal; IVP, intravenous pyelography; PE, physical examinations; RLQ, right lower quadrant; RUQ, right upper quadrant.
From Ulshen M: Major symptoms and signs of digestive tract disorders. In Behrman R, Kliegman R, Jenson H (eds): Nelson Textbook of Pediatrics, 16th ed. Philadelphia, WB Saunders, 2000, p 1106.

Table 110-5. **Distribution of Abdominal Masses of 280 Patients in the Neonatal Period***

Type	No.
Kidney (65%)	
Hydronephrosis (UPJ obstruction, UVJ obstruction, ureterocele, etc.)	80 (28%)
Multicystic kidney	63 (22%)
Polycystic kidney disease	18
Renal vein thrombosis	5
Solid tumor	13
Ectopy	4
Total	183
Retroperitoneum (9%)	
Neuroblastoma	17
Teratoma	3
Hemangioma	1
Abscess	4
Total	25
Bladder (1%)	
Posterior urethral valves	2
Female genital system (10%)	
Hydrocolpos	16
Ovarian cyst	13
Total	31
Gastrointestinal (12%)	
Duplication	17
Giant cystic meconium ileus	4
Mesenteric cyst	3
Ileal atresia	2
Volvulus (ileum)	2
Teratoma (stomach)	1
Leiomyosarcoma (colon)	1
Meconium peritonitis with ascites	1
Ascites	1
Total	32
Hepatic or biliary (3%)	
Hemangioma (liver)	3
Solitary cyst (liver)	2
Hepatoma	1
Distended gallbladder	1
Choledochal cyst	1
Adenomatoid malformation of the lung	1
Total	9

*Distended bladder, hepatomegaly, and splenomegaly were excluded in most series.
UPJ, ureteropelvic junction; UVJ, ureterovesical junction.
Data from Griscom, 1965; Raffensperger and Abousleiman, 1968; Wedge et al, 1971; Wilson, 1982; and Emanuel and White, 1968.

also present in the urologist's office with symptoms of urinary frequency or urgency, dysfunctional voiding, or constipation. In a recent review, the peak incidence of sexually transmitted diseases was seen in the 10- to 14-year age group (Pandhi et al, 2003). Pelvic inflammatory disease rates are highest in females age 15 to 25. Thirty-three percent of those infections are in females younger than age 19 (Jenkins, 2000).

Boys with painful priapism must be evaluated immediately. Pain may suggest ischemia of the corporeal bodies, which may progress to corporeal fibrosis if untreated. **Children with sickle cell anemia are especially at risk for priapism,** with 75% of patients experiencing their first episode by the age of 20 years (Mantadakis et al, 1999; Adeyoju et al, 2002). Outpatient treatment with penile aspiration and epinephrine irrigation has successfully been used in the treatment of this condition (Mantadakis et al, 2000).

Urgent Evaluations

Gross hematuria outside the newborn period, although not life threatening, should be evaluated without delay. Many children have an easy-to-recognize source such as UTI, urethral prolapse, trauma, and meatal stenosis with ulceration, coagulation abnormalities, or urinary tract stones. Less obvious sources include acute nephritis, ureteropelvic junction obstruction, cystitis cystica, epididymitis, or tumor (Diven and Travis, 2000; Meyers, 2004).

Febrile UTIs in children older than newborns should be treated acutely. Children of all ages with a severe urinary tract infection may be subject to renal scarring (Ransley and Risdon, 1981; van der Voort et al, 1997) and should be seen within 24 hours or sooner.

Infants and children with an inguinal hernia or a hydrocele that changes in volume should be seen within 24 hours and sooner if there is history of inguinal or scrotal pain. Not all of these children will need emergency surgery, but a few will need surgery within a short period. If there is a history of scrotal or inguinal pain, the child's parents should be taught to recognize the signs of an incarcerated inguinal hernia and instructed to go to the emergency department if symptoms occur before the planned surgical correction.

Semi-urgent Evaluations

In neonates with prenatally detected hydronephrosis and a normal bladder, we begin the postnatal evaluation of the hydronephrosis within the first few days of life. Families are concerned about the diagnosis and are anxious to make a management plan.

Children older than newborns with nonfebrile UTI should be seen semi-urgently. In practice, many of these patients are seen by their pediatrician and are seen in follow-up by the pediatric urologist. Nearly all children with culture-proven UTI should be evaluated with ultrasound and VCUG, although some groups are reevaluating the role of renal nuclear scans in these children.

A few infants undergoing evaluation for failure to thrive will be referred for suspected renal and ureteral disease. The child's pediatrician coordinates the diagnostic plan. The process is extensive and may require a complicated sequence of examinations that may be time consuming and frustrating for the family. These children should be scheduled quickly to expedite the workup and minimize the inconvenience to the child and the family.

We see adolescents who have not menstruated and in whom there is concern about ureteral or vaginal anomaly within 3 days. Many of these patients have an imperforate hymen or uterine anomaly that results in poor uterine drainage that may be uncomfortable. If left untreated, retrograde drainage of the uterus may place these patients at risk of endometriosis and infertility (Rock et al, 1982).

Routine Evaluations

The remaining children are scheduled at their convenience. These include infants with history of prenatal hydronephrosis who are not suspected of having bladder outlet obstruction on the postnatal ultrasound. The ultrasound must not show bilateral hydronephrosis or a thickened bladder wall. The infant must be thriving and have normal electrolytes and normal blood urea nitrogen and creatinine levels. The additional tests include a repeat ultrasound, a renal scan, or a voiding cystourethrogram to evaluate the relative drainage and percentage of function of the kidneys as well as to evaluate for vesicoureteral reflux.

An increasing number of **pregnant mothers carrying a fetus with hydronephrosis seek prenatal evaluation with the urologist. These visits are scheduled within the week unless the following conditions exist: (1) there is bilateral hydronephrosis or hydronephrosis in a single system kidney, (2) there is oligohydramnios, and (3) there is evidence of significant cystic renal disease in a fetus younger than 22 weeks' gestation.** In a few, termination of pregnancy may be considered. In these cases, fetal intervention may be indicated. Because the decision for discontinuation of the pregnancy may be dependent on gestational age of the fetus, prompt evaluation may be required.

Infants with asymptomatic hydrocele rarely require surgery initially. In most cases the hydrocele will resolve in the first year of life. An exception is if the hydrocele is particularly large or palpable in the inguinal region. A large hydrocele with a palpable inguinal component or one that is enlarging may indicate the presence of an abdominoscrotal hydrocele. These do not spontaneously resolve and usually enlarge and should be corrected, usually at 6 to 12 months (Luks et al, 1993; Belman, 2001). **We operate on patients with undescended or absent testes at about 6 months of age. Very few of these testes will descend after 3 months of age** (Berkowitz et al, 1993). Some infants with impalpable testes may require laparoscopic evaluation, and this examination may be done at 6 months as well.

As long as there is no active bleeding, if the child is voiding normally, and if the infant has not suffered injury to the penile shaft or shaft skin, we evaluate children who have developed a complication after circumcision at the convenience of the family. Narrowing of the preputial ring after circumcision may result in a trapped penis (Casale et al, 1999; Gillett et al, 2005). These infants can usually be managed with application of petroleum jelly to the penis for 4 to 6 weeks as healing continues. As long as voiding remains normal during this period, the revision of the circumcision may be postponed until age 4 to 6 months when an outpatient surgical procedure can be performed. A more common complication, urethral meatal stenosis, may be present as early as 6 months of age in circumcised infants (Upadhyay et al, 1998; Ahmed et al, 1999). This problem may be easily corrected in the office (Smith and Smith, 2000).

Boys with hypospadias are seen routinely. Normally, we initiate the evaluation as a newborn because most parents of a child with a birth defect, even a relatively minor one such as hypospadias, desire an early opportunity to speak with a specialist.

Varicoceles are uncommon in prepubertal boys and increase in incidence to around 15% by 15 years of age (Schiff et al, 2005). We normally try to document the size of the varicocele with an ultrasound examination. From the three-dimensional measurements on ultrasound, the relative testicular volumes may be calculated and used to guide further treatment (Diamond et al, 2000).

The completion of the evaluation for UTI is done at the parent's convenience after the initial infection has been treated. In most cases, radiologic studies after UTI in a child include VCUG to detect vesicoureteral reflux. However, a substantial number of cortical defects on DMSA scan occur in the absence of reflux (62% to 82%) that is not identifiable on ultrasound (Majd et al 1992; Benador et al, 1997; Ditchfield and Nadel, 1998; Biggi et al, 2001; Ditchfield et al, 2002). This has led us to reevaluate the role of VCUG as the initial investigation in a child with a UTI.

Microscopic hematuria in the absence of other symptoms is not an emergency in children. In more than 30% of cases, the source is never definitively identified. Our algorithm for a practical evaluation is discussed further in this chapter.

Children with daytime or night-time wetting are evaluated routinely in the absence of other complicating problems. The care of children with nocturnal enuresis is individualized. Although some recommend treatment in children after age 5, we often wait to treat until the child seems bothered by the problem. If the child does not perceive night-time wetting as a problem, there is usually little gained by treatment with medications or alarms. In our experience, only a few children younger than age 6 or 7 are bothered emotionally by nocturnal enuresis. Wetting during the day causes more concern and may indicate incomplete or infrequent voiding. Incomplete or infrequent voiding may lead to UTI, which may exacerbate wetting.

KEY POINTS: TRIAGE OF THE PEDIATRIC UROLOGY PATIENT

- Pediatric diagnoses can be triaged into categories: emergent, urgent, semi-urgent, and routine.

- Infants with bilateral hydronephrosis or hydronephrosis in a solitary kidney should be evaluated immediately after delivery.

- If congenital adrenal hyperplasia is suspected, testing should be completed before hospital discharge.

- Surgical exploration should be performed when spermatic cord torsion cannot be definitively excluded with the physical examination.

- Children with daytime or night-time wetting are evaluated routinely in the absence of other complicating problems.

THE PEDIATRIC UROLOGY OFFICE VISIT
The Pediatric Urology Team

In our practice, primary care providers make an initial referral to a physician who triages the patient and then refers the child, if appropriate, to an outpatient coordinator. The coordinator schedules the appointment based on the child's level of acuity. Before the clinic visit, our file room team gathers any appropriate medical records and radiologic studies. At the clinic visit, dedicated registrars at the front desk initially meet the patient and caretakers. Medical assistants review our intake forms and obtain vital signs in preparation for the medical team. If the child requires surgery, surgical coordinators assist in financial counseling as well as scheduling the surgery date. Dedicated urology operating room nurses and assistants help ensure that the surgery runs as smoothly as possible.

The child born with or acquiring a urologic disorder may present with symptoms vastly different from an adult with a similar condition. As the subspecialty of pediatric urology has evolved, teams dedicated to children have become increasingly common. With this increased interest in the care of children with urologic problems, pediatricians have referred more and more patients with lower acuity. This has provided us an opportunity to link with pediatricians to help provide front-line care for children with dysfunctional voiding, enuresis, and UTIs. To help contend with this increasing patient load, a number of practices have collaborated with physician extenders such as nurses, nurse practitioners, or physician's assistants to help provide improved teaching and treatment. The roles of these physician extenders include first assisting in the operating room, assisting physicians in the general pediatric urology or dysfunctional voiding clinics, and performing urodynamics.

History

In most cases the primary care provider has identified a problem that requires review by the pediatric urologist. However, because other processes may coexist, the urologist must be alert for evidence of disease in other organ systems. Although few children are severely ill when evaluated in the urologist's office, it is important to develop the skills to recognize an infant or child that requires hospitalization. The ability to determine when an infant requires an inpatient admission is particularly important because the metabolic reserve is less abundant in the newborn (Park, 2000).

Observation of the child and a careful history from the parent may be more important than the vital signs or the physical examination when attempting to determine the severity of illness, particularly in the infant or small child. The child's color (pale or cyanotic), level of alertness, response to the parent's comforting, quality of interaction with the examiner, and the quantity of tearing while crying may provide considerable information about mental status and level of hydration. If the child's response in any of these areas suggests severe illness, the child should be transferred to the emergency department, where appropriate resuscitation can be delivered while the diagnostic evaluation continues.

An important first question when taking the history in the pediatric patient with a urologic problem is **"why is the child here?"** In some cases, the child can begin to answer these questions, and it is worthwhile early in the interview to ask the child a few questions directly. This shows respect for the child, who may be an excellent historian despite young age. As soon as the child realizes that the interview is directed to him or her, rather than to the parent, he or she will concentrate harder. If future therapy requires behavioral training that involves cooperation from the child, he or she may be more receptive. **What goals do the patient and family have?** Do the parents expect treatment at the facility, or do they seek a second opinion to confirm or refute another treatment plan? Do they prefer a reconstructive surgical procedure or the most appropriate nonsurgical therapy? In many children, the treat-

ment must be tailored to the family's social condition or to the family's geographic location. Citizens of other countries or children from military families who may be mobile may require a different approach to a surgical problem than families who live near a major center. In some cases there is more than one therapy for a given problem, and the clinician should be prepared to offer more than one approach to provide the most appropriate care.

Voiding Symptoms

A large number of children are referred with voiding complaints. **The ability to place children in categories based on the voiding history will help to focus the rest of the evaluation and guide further therapy.** The time and duration of the voiding disorder must be identified early in the interview. Did symptoms begin before or after potty training? Is wetting associated with pain, urgency, or frequency? What is the character of the voiding? Is the urinary stream steady from beginning to end or is it a "staccato" or stop and start pattern suggestive of dysfunctional voiding? Are the symptoms worse at a particular time of the day? Does the child void frequently during the day yet sleep through the night without wetting? Is wetting confined to the night time, suggestive of primary nocturnal enuresis?

The voiding history is incomplete without a record of the child's eating and drinking pattern. Does the child consume small amounts of water during the day and large amounts of alternative liquids such as soft drinks and juices, which tend to be laden with salt and sugar and low on free water? What is the stooling pattern? Does the child have firm, chunky, or pebble-like bowel movements, which are suggestive of a retentive pattern of stooling, or does the child have soft, well-formed bowel movements more suggestive of a normal stooling pattern? Very few children hold the urine and not the stool. Conversely, children who retain stool nearly always retain urine. All of these are indicators of a dysfunctional voiding pattern, which may lead to UTI.

Signs of Illness in the Pediatric Urologic Patient—The Physical Examination

Generalized Signs in the Pediatric Patient

The term "failure to thrive (FTT)" may be used to describe children whose physical growth is significantly less than that of his or her peers. Often associated with poor developmental and socioemotional functioning, the prevalence of FTT depends on the population sampled (Wright et al, 2000). From 5% to 10% of low-birth-weight children and children living in poverty may have FTT. Family discord, maternal depression, and neonatal problems other than low birth weight are also associated with FTT. In the United States, nonorganic causes are far more common than organic FTT. Psychosocial FTT is usually due to poverty or poor child-parent interaction that sometimes occurs with severe stress such as child abuse. **The causes of insufficient growth include (1) failure of a parent to offer adequate calories, (2) failure of the child to take sufficient calories in, and (3) failure of the child to retain sufficient calories.** Major organic causes of

FTT and an approach to the workup based on age are listed in Tables 110–6 and 110–7. As urologists, we must be alert to common urologic sources of FTT such as UTI, renal tubular acidosis, diabetes insipidus, and chronic renal insufficiency. But we must also be wary of psychosocial or abusive issues that may exist and be ready to help to alert the pediatrician and to play a supportive role in the analysis of this problem (Bauchner, 2000).

In children, as in adults, normal body temperature varies in a regular pattern each day. This circadian temperature rhythm results in lower body temperatures in the early morning and temperatures approximately 1°C higher in the later afternoon or early evening. Fevers with temperatures less than 39°C (102.2°F) in healthy children generally do not require treatment. If temperatures become higher, administration of antipyretics will usually make the child more comfortable. Other than providing symptomatic relief, antipyretic therapy does not change the course of infectious diseases in normal children. Antipyretic therapy can be beneficial, however, in higher-risk patients with chronic pulmonary disease, metabolic disorders, or neurologic diseases. **Temperatures greater than 41°C (105.8°F) place patients at higher risk than do normal temperature responses.** This high temperature elevation is associated with severe infection, hypothalamic disorders, or central nervous system hemorrhage and always requires antipyretic therapy (Powell, 2000). **Aspirin has been associated with Reye's syndrome in children and adolescents and is not recommended for the treatment of fever in children.** Acetaminophen (10 to 15 mg/kg every 4 hours) or ibuprofen (5 to 10 mg/kg every 6 hours) is not associated with significant adverse effects. However, massive overdoses of acetaminophen can lead to hepatic failure. Although focus must be on urologic sources for fever, the urologist should be aware of other causes of fever, particularly in compromised or at-risk groups (Table 110–8).

Table 110–6. Major Organic Causes of Failure to Thrive

System	Cause
Gastrointestinal	Gastroesophageal reflux, celiac disease, pyloric stenosis, cleft palate/cleft lip, lactose intolerence, Hirschsprung's disease, milk protein intolerance, hepatitis, cirrhosis, pancreatic insufficiency, biliary disease, inflammatory bowel disease, malabsorption
Renal	Urinary tract infection, renal tubular acidosis, diabetes insipidus, chronic renal insufficiency
Cardiopulmonary	Cardiac diseases leading to congestive heart failure, asthma, bronchopulmonary dysplasia, cystic fibrosis, anatomic abnormalities of the upper airway, obstructive sleep apnea
Endocrine	Hypothyroidism, diabetes mellitus, adrenal insufficiency or excess, parathyroid disorders, pituitary disorders, growth hormone deficiency
Neurologic	Mental retardation, cerebral hemorrhages, degenerative disorders
Infectious	Parasitic or bacterial infections of the gastrointestinal tract, tuberculosis, human immunodeficiency virus disease
Metabolic	Inborn errors of metabolism
Congenital	Chromosomal abnormalities, congenital syndromes (fetal alcohol syndrome), perinatal infections
Miscellaneous	Lead poisoning, malignancy, collagen vascular disease, recurrently infected adenoids and tonsils

From Bachner H: Failure to thrive. In Behrman R, Kliegman R, Jenson HB (eds): Nelson Textbook of Pediatrics. Philadelphia, WB Saunders, 2000, p 120.

Table 110–7. Approach to Failure to Thrive Based on Age

Age at Onset	Major Diagnostic Consideration
Birth to 3 mo	Psychosocial failure to thrive, perinatal infections, gastroesophageal reflux, inborn errors of metabolism, cystic fibrosis
3-6 mo	Psychosocial failure to thrive, human immunodeficiency virus infection, gastroesophageal reflux, inborn errors of metabolism, milk protein intolerance, cystic fibrosis, renal tubular acidosis
7-12 mo	Psychosocial failure to thrive (autonomy struggles), delayed introduction of solids, gastroesophageal reflux, intestinal parasites, renal tubular acidosis
12+ mo	Psychosocial failure to thrive (coercive feeding, new psychological stressor), gastroesophageal reflux

Adapted from Frank D, Silva M, Needlman R: Failure to thrive: Mystery, myth and method. Contemp Pediatr 1993;10:114.

Table 110–8. Febrile Patients at Increased Risk for Serious Bacterial Infections

Condition	Comment
Immunocompetent Patients	
Neonates (<28 days)	Sepsis and meningitis caused by group B streptococci, *Escherichia coli*, *Listeria monocytogenes*, herpes simplex virus
Infants <3 mo	Serious bacterial disease (10-15%); bacteremia in 5% of febrile infants
Infants and children 3-36 mo	Occult bacteremia in 4%; increased risk with temperature >39°C and white blood cell count >15,000/μL
Hyperpyrexia (>41°C)	Meningitis, bacteremia, pneumonia, heatstroke, hemorrhagic shock–encephalopathy syndrome
Fever with petechiae	Bacteremia and meningitis caused by *Neisseria meningitidis*, *Haemophilus influenzae* type b, *Streptococcus pneumoniae*
Immunocompromised Patients	
Sickle cell anemia	Pneumococcal sepsis, meningitis
Asplenia	Encapsulated bacteria
Complement/properdin deficiency	Meningococcal sepsis
Agammaglobulinemia	Bacteremia, sinopulmonary infection
Acquired immunodeficiency syndrome	*S. pneumoniae*, *H. influenzae* type b, *Salmonella*
Congenital heart disease	Increased risk of endocarditis
Central venous line	*Staphylococcus aureus*, coagulase-negative staphylococci, *Candida*
Malignancy	Gram-negative enteric bacteria, *S. aureus* coagulase-negative staphylococci, *Candida*

From Powell KR: Fever. In Behrman R, Kliegman R, Jenson H (eds): Nelson Textbook of Pediatries, 16th ed. Philadelphia, WB Saunders, 2000, p 74.

Table 110–9. Distinguishing Features of Acute Gastrointestinal Tract Pain in Children

Disease	Onset	Location	Referral	Quality	Comments
Pancreatitis	Acute	Epigastric, left upper quadrant	Back	Constant, sharp, boring	Nausea, emesis, tenderness
Intestinal obstruction	Acute or gradual	Periumbilical—lower abdomen	Back	Alternating cramping (colic) and painless periods	Distention, obstipation, emesis, increased bowel sounds
Appendicitis	Acute	Periumbilical, localized to lower right quadrant; generalized with peritonitis	Back or pelvis if retrocecal	Sharp, steady	Anorexia, nausea, emesis, local tenderness, fever with peritonitis
Intussusception	Acute	Periumbilical—lower abdomen	None	Cramping, with painless periods	Hematochezia, knees in pulled-up position
Urolithiasis	Acute, sudden	Back (unilateral)	Groin	Sharp, intermittent, cramping	Hematuria
Urinary tract infection	Acute, sudden	Back	Bladder	Dull to sharp	Fever, costochondral tenderness, dysuria, urinary frequency

From Ulshen M: Major symptoms and signs of digestive tract disorders. In Behrman R, Kliegman R, Jenson H (eds): Nelson Textbook of Pediatrics, 16th ed. Philadelphia, WB Saunders, 2000, p 1107.

The evaluation and relief of pain is as old as the profession of medicine. As primarily abdominal and retroperitoneal surgeons, we focus on abdominal and perineal sources of pain. **Abdominal pain** commonly suggests pyelonephritis, hydronephrosis, or constipation but may also be due to sickle cell crisis. **An accurate history of the character of the pain may be the best indicator of the source of the pain.** Details about the character of the pain, time and acuteness of onset, radiation, or migration are important and should, if possible, be elicited directly from the child. Associated loss of appetite, nausea, vomiting, or a change in bowel pattern may help to distinguish gastrointestinal from genitourinary sources (Table 110–9).

A child with acute scrotal pain must be presumed to have spermatic cord torsion regardless of age until proven otherwise. However, in some cases, an accurate history may save the child an unnecessary surgical exploration. It is particularly important to interview the child as well as the parent. Gradual onset of the pain is more consistent with epididymitis, whereas abrupt pain suggests spermatic cord torsion or torsion of one of the testicular appendices. Associated scrotal wall swelling, erythema, or superior displacement of the testis is suggestive of spermatic cord torsion.

Perineal or rectal pain may be associated with chronic constipation or bladder spasm. We have also observed girls with chronic constipation presenting with vaginal pain. The pain of constipation or of bladder spasm may be referred to the penis, testes, scrotum, or perineum, as well as to the groin (Fein et al, 2001).

We record vital signs on every new patient, and in children with history of renal anomalies or vesicoureteral reflux, on all subsequent visits. **Because the blood pressure and heart rate change as a function of age,** reference ranges for blood pressure and pulse rates for boys and girls should be posted in the clinic near where the vital signs are taken (Bernstein, 2000). Assistants taking the blood pressure should all be aware of the variation with age and should notify the team of blood pressure readings greater than the 90th percentile.

In the infant, generalized edema may occur with prematurity or hypoproteinemia. Localized edema suggests a congenital malformation of the lymphatic system. **When confined to one or more extremities, edema may be a presenting sign of coarctation of the aorta in association with Turner's syndrome.** Vasomotor instability and decreased peripheral circulation are revealed by red or purple color in a crying infant. Scattered petechiae in the infant may be present in the scalp and face after a difficult delivery. Café-au-lait spots are uniformly hyperpigmented sharply demarcated macular lesions, the hues of which vary within the normal degree of pigmentation of the individual. These may be dark brown in African American children. They may vary in size and may be large, covering a significant proportion of the trunk or limb. One to three lesions are common in normal children. Approximately 10% of normal children have café-au-lait macules. They may be present at birth or develop during childhood. **If there are five or more spots each more than 5 mm in diameter in prepubertal patients or six or more spots more than 15 mm in postpubertal children, neurofibromatosis type 1 (von Recklinghausen's disease) should be suspected.**

The skin, hair, and nails should be evaluated with special focus on congenital or metabolic problems that may be associated with brittle or abnormal hair and nails or abnormal skin dryness (see Tables 110–2 and 110–3). Supernumerary nipples may occur in a unilateral or bilateral distribution along a line from the anterior axillary fold to the inguinal area. They are more common in African American infants (3.5%) than white (0.6%) children. Accessory nipples may not have an associated areola and may be mistaken for congenital nevi. They may be excised if desired to improve appearance. Renal or urinary tract anomalies may be present.

An exceptionally large head suggests hydrocephaly, a storage disease, achondroplasia, cerebral gigantism, neurocutaneous syndromes, or inborn errors of metabolism; or it may be familial. Dysmorphic features such as **broadened epicanthal folds, widely spaced eyes, micrognathia, and low-set ears are often associated with congenital syndromes that may suggest a genitourinary problem.** Preauricular sinuses and pits may be the result of imperfect fusion of the tubercles of the first and second branchial arches. These anomalies may be unilateral or bilateral, may be familial, are more common in females and blacks, and at times are associated with other anomalies of the ears and face. Preauricular pits are present in bronchio-oto-renal dysplasia, an autosomal dominant disorder that consists of external ear malformations, bronchial fistulas, hearing loss, and renal anomalies. **Macroglossia can be associated with the Beckwith-Wiedemann syndrome, which also includes hepatosplenomegaly, nephromegaly, and hypoglycemia secondary to pancreatic beta cell hyperplasia in a large gestational age infant.** These children are predisposed to a specific subset of childhood neoplasms, including Wilms' tumor and adrenocortical carcinoma. Webbing of the neck in a female infant suggests intrauterine lymphedema in Turner's syndrome, as do the widely spaced nipples with a shield-shaped chest (Stoll and Kliegman, 2000).

The abdomen is protuberant in boys with the prune-belly syndrome. Occasionally, children with other types of bladder outlet obstruction or profound antenatal hydronephrosis will also have considerable laxity of the abdominal muscles. The abdomen should be inspected for other abnormalities, such as ventral hernia, flaring of the rib cage, umbilical leakage, mass, or hernia. When examining the abdomen, the examiner's hand should be placed behind the flank to help palpate the kidney on either side. If the abdomen is supple, the approximate size and location of each kidney may be determined with deep palpation. An attempt should be made to feel the liver edge and spleen as well as the colon, particularly the descending colon. In the newborn, the liver may be palpable, sometimes as much as 2 cm below the ribs on the left. When examining the left lower quadrant, an estimate should be made of the volume of stool in the descending colon. In infants, a large amount of gas may be present within the gastrointestinal tract. The abdominal wall is normally weak, especially in premature infants. Separation of the rectus muscles and umbilical hernias are common in the newborn. Unusual masses should be investigated immediately with ultrasonography. **Renal pathology is the source of up to two thirds of neonatal abdominal masses** (Pinto and Guignard, 1995). **Cystic abdominal masses include hydronephrosis, multicystic dysplastic kidneys, adrenal hemorrhage, hydrometrocolpos, intestinal duplication, and choledochal ovarian omental or pancreatic cysts. Solid masses include neuroblastoma, congenital mesoblastic nephroma, hepatoblastoma, and teratoma.** A solid flank mass may be due to renal venous thrombosis, which becomes apparent with signs of hematuria, hypertension, and thrombocytopenia. Renal venous thrombosis in infants is associated with polycythemia, dehydration, diabetic mothers, asphyxia, sepsis, and coagulopathies such as antithrombin-3 or protein C deficiencies. **Abdominal distention at birth or shortly afterward suggests either obstruction or perforation of the gastrointestinal tract often due to meconium ileus. Later distention suggests bowel obstruction, sepsis, or peritonitis.** Abdominal wall defects may be present either through the umbilicus (omphalocele) or lateral wall (gastroschisis). Omphaloceles are associated with other anomalies and syndromes such as the Beckwith-Wiedemann syndrome, conjoined twins, trisomy 18, meningomyelocele, and imperforate anus (Hassink et al, 1996; Chen et al, 1997; Kallen et al, 2000).

The inguinal canal should be inspected on each side for signs of asymmetry or mass. To begin the examination, the examiner's left hand closes the internal inguinal ring (Fig. 110–1). This maneuver prevents an intracanalicular testis from migrating into the abdomen. The inguinal canal is then palpated to identify a fullness or mass suggestive of a hernia

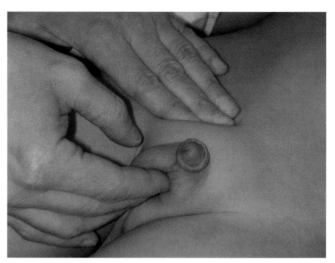

Figure 110–1. Clinical examination of male groin.

or hydrocele of the spermatic cord. The examiner may feel a "silk glove" sign suggestive of a thickened patent processus vaginalis that may be present if a hernia is intermittent. The examiner's right hand is then brought down to the scrotal area, and the testis is then palpated. The testis should be examined with consideration of the anatomy of the testis, the epididymis, and the vas deferens, which can be palpated even in some newborns. Particular attention to the symmetry of the examination is important if intersex conditions are thought to exist. **In the infant with a possible intersex condition, a symmetrical gonadal examination (gonads palpable on each side or impalpable on both sides) suggests a global disorder such as CAH or androgen insensitivity. Asymmetry in the gonadal examination suggests a localized problem such as mixed gonadal dysgenesis or true hermaphroditism.**

Undescended testes can be palpated if they are in the scrotum or outside the external inguinal ring. Occasionally, the testis in a newborn can be palpated if it is in the inguinal canal, but in many cases, the testis will move in and out of the canal into the abdomen, which makes palpation of the testis inconsistent. Retractile testes may in some cases be difficult to distinguish from a low, undescended testis. Pressure on the femoral artery may sometimes help to relax the cremasteric reflex in boys older than age 2. Placing the child in a squatting or legs-crossed position will sometimes relax the reflex and facilitate palpation of the testis. A testis is descended if it can be manipulated to the base of the scrotum and remains there after release, at least for a moment. Testes that feel tethered during manipulation and cannot be manipulated to the base of the scrotum are at risk for becoming ascending testes. If doubt exists, a second examination 6 to 18 months later may be helpful to distinguish a retractile testis from a tethered testis. As the child ages, an ascending or tethered testis (both cryptorchid testes) will be more and more difficult to manipulate into the bottom of the scrotum (Eardley et al, 1994; Clarnette and Hutson, 1997; Davey, 1997).

The normal newborn scrotum is relatively large. Its size may be increased with the trauma of breech delivery or by a newborn hydrocele that can be distinguished from hernia by palpation and transillumination as well as from the absence of a mass in the inguinal canal. In the absence of volume changes within the hydrocele, the processus vaginalis is usually not patent and the newborn hydrocele resolves by age 1 year without surgery. Persistence of a hydrocele beyond 12 to 18 months even in the absence of volume changes usually indicates a patent processus vaginalis and is an indication for surgical ligation of the processus vaginalis and incision of the scrotal component of the hydrocele.

Varicoceles (varicosities of the internal spermatic vein) almost always occur on the left side and are bilateral in about 10%. Varicoceles are palpable when the boy is standing but drain when supine. If only the right side is involved or if the varicocele does not decompress when the boy is supine, there exists a possibility that a retroperitoneal tumor is present and compressing the vein.

In the newborn, the foreskin is adherent to the glans. These glanular adhesions should not be separated, and the glans need not be inspected if the parents do not desire a circumcision. Glanular preputial adhesions usually separate before the age of 4 but may persist in some boys for longer periods. **In the absence of balanitis or UTI, the prepuce should not be retracted but allowed to separate naturally** (Imamura, 1997). If symptoms do develop, topical corticosteroids have successfully been used as an alternative to circumcision in some boys with adherent foreskin (Monsour et al, 1999; Chu et al, 1999; Orsola et al, 2000; Elmore et al, 2002).

The position of the urethral meatus is almost never abnormal in the uncircumcised penis with a circumferential foreskin. If the ventral foreskin is short, or absent, or if there is a ventral or dorsal curvature, the boy should not be circumcised and should be reexamined at a later date when hypospadias or epispadias correction may be performed. The presence of a midline dimple on the ventral penile shaft should lead one to suspect a diagnosis of hypospadias, despite a normal-appearing foreskin. The severity of hypospadias is based on the position of the urethral meatus, the presence or absence of penile curvature, and the degree of ventral penile shaft skin coverage. Occasionally, when the foreskin is pulled back before a circumcision, the distal urethra and urethral meatus are enlarged. If a megameatus is identified before a newborn circumcision, the circumcision should be cancelled. The foreskin may be removed at the time of the urethral repair. However, because normal spongiosum is present on the ventral surface of the penis, repair of the urethra is not usually difficult even after a circumcision has been performed (Duckett and Keating, 1989).

Stretched penile length and girth should be measured. If the penis in a term infant is less than 1.9 cm, micropenis should be suspected and a karyotype should be performed and the hypothalamic-pituitary-testicular axis should be assayed. **The penis should be examined in relation to the scrotum for evidence of penile concealment, buried penis, or webbed penis.** In these conditions, the penis is of normal size but buried or concealed beneath a prominent pubic fat pad; trapped by a narrowed, more proximal preputial ring; or tethered to the scrotum. If the penile shaft skin is shortened, correction may require a rotational flap of inner preputial skin to provide additional coverage for the ventrum of the penis after release of the narrowed preputial ring. If a newborn clamp circumcision is performed, more penile shaft than indicated is often removed, resulting in a scar and sometimes a secondary trapped penis. If there is encroachment of the scrotum onto

the penile shaft, circumcision should be deferred until it can be done free hand in the main operating room under a general anesthetic usually at 4 to 6 months (Casale et al, 1999; Williams et al, 2000).

The perineal examination in the female is similar to that of the male. In a teenaged girl, the examination may be performed with the mother present as long as the adolescent agrees. In general, bimanual examination in an adolescent is best performed in the operating room. The girl is placed in a frog-leg position or in a knee-chest position (Fig. 110–2). The clitoris is examined for evidence of hypertrophy that may be suggestive of an intersex condition. Gently spreading the labia majora in an inferior direction will allow for inspection of the clitoral area and usually of the introitus. The vestibule is assessed for any evidence of discharge. An easy way of examining the perineum is to gently grasp the labia majora and pull inferiorly. This maneuver tends to better define the various perineal folds and provide for a consistent examination in nearly all cases (Redman, 1982). The hymen should be inspected as well as the introitus. **An imperforate hymen may result in hydrometrocolpos and a lower abdominal mass.** In older girls, a small speculum may be used to evaluate the cervix and interior of the vagina. Palpation of the vaginal walls and cervix and bimanual examination of the uterus completes the examination. A Valsalva maneuver may allow adequate assessment of the introital vaginal area. Vaginal discharge is frequently associated with vaginal voiding and is particularly common in children who hold the urine and subsequently dribble urine into the vagina. Treatment of dysfunctional voiding results in reduced vaginal drainage. Vaginal bleeding in the preadolescent may result from foreign bodies such as wadded toilet paper trapped in the vagina. Occasionally other foreign bodies may have been inserted intentionally or accidentally.

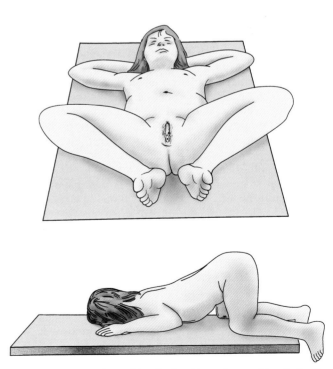

Figure 110–2.   Frog-leg position *(top)* and knee-chest position *(bottom)*.

Although genital injuries may be accidental, the possibility of physical or sexual abuse must be considered in all cases of genital trauma in females or males. **Sexual abuse is surprisingly common and includes any activity with a child before the age of legal consent that is for sexual gratification of an adult or a significantly older child.** Sexual intercourse includes vaginal, oral, or rectal penetration, which is defined as entry into an orifice with or without tissue damage. Sex acts perpetrated by young children are learned behaviors and are associated with experiencing sexual abuse or exposure to adult sex or pornography. In 1999, there were more than 93,000 reported victims of sexual abuse in the United States (U.S. Department of Health and Human Services, 1999). Twelve to 38 percent of adult women were sexually abused by age 18. The incidence of sexual abuse of males ranges from 3% to 9% of the population. About one third of sexual abuse victims are younger than 6 years of age, one third are 6 to 12 years of age, and one third are 12 to 18 years of age. Reported offenders are 97% male (Johnson, 2000). In one study, of women presenting to an urban sexual assault clinic, 43% were adolescents (Jones et al, 2003).

The possibility of sexual abuse should be considered as a result of associated physical symptoms, including (1) vaginal, penile, or rectal pain, discharge, or bleeding or (2) chronic dysuria, enuresis, constipation, or encopresis. In one study, 74% of pediatric patients with documented sexually transmitted diseases had histories or signs of abuse (Pandhi et al, 2003). Investigating the possibility of sexual abuse requires supportive, sensitive, and detailed history taking. Many hospitals have a sexual abuse team that can be readily consulted if sexual abuse is suspected. The key is to be aware of the possibilities when they might exist and to invite the team in early. The pediatric urologist will likely be asked to evaluate the abdomen and perineum (Johnson, 2000).

Sexual abuse should be considered when the vaginal mucosa is bruised or injected, the vaginal opening is dilated, or the hymen is damaged, showing a V-shaped notch or cleft (Walker, 1998). Despite these guidelines, the diagnosis of sexual abuse is often made by the history and not by the physical examination. In a review of 157 children referred to a sexual abuse clinic with only a physical complaint without a history of abuse, only 16% had examination findings suggestive of sexual abuse (Kellogg et al, 1998). If abuse is suspected, it must be reported to the police. Furthermore, if the perpetrator is a caregiver of the child, or a parent, the state child welfare team must be contacted.

Benign and malignant tumors of the vaginal area should be considered when vaginal bleeding occurs in young girls. A broad spectrum of entities ranging from capillary hemangioma, rhabdomyosarcoma, or carcinoma may be associated with vaginal bleeding. Labial masses may be associated with hernia or hydrocele of the canal of Nuck (Kizer et al, 1995). **Adhesions of the labia minora are common.** In most cases, they are not symptomatic. Occasionally, a girl with labial adhesions will complain of vaginal irritation from pooled urine. If not separated, the irritation may progress to irregular voiding that may exacerbate the problem. In some girls, a short course of estrogen cream applied to the labia may be effective. In many, however, separation of the adhesions in the office with local anesthetic cream may be required. Labial fusion may be associated with CAH, gonadal dysgenesis, or

cloaca (Powell et al, 1995). A genitosinogram is indicated in cases where the urethra cannot be distinguished from the vaginal orifice.

Urethral prolapse is relatively common, particularly in African American females. The prolapse is through the meatus, forming a hemorrhagic, often sensitive mass that bleeds with palpation or with contact of the undergarments. Girls may have difficulty with urination depending on the size of the prolapse and whether it includes the urethral meatus. Urethral prolapse may respond to topical application of estrogen and may be managed expectantly as long as voiding is normal (Redman, 1982).

Passage of meconium usually occurs within the first 12 hours after birth; 99% of term infants and 95% of premature infants pass meconium within 48 hours of birth. The presence of an imperforate anus is not always obvious. Gentle insertion of the small finger or a rectal tube to the anal dimple may be necessary to confirm the diagnosis. Any child with an early and consistent history of constipation must be suspected to have imperforate anus or a variant (Kim et al, 2000).

The lower back should be examined for any evidence of presacral dimpling or other cutaneous markers of occult spinal dysraphisms. **An "atypical" presacral dimple may indicate spina bifida or cord tethering if the dimple is off center, more than 2.5 cm from the anal verge at birth or deeper than 0.5 cm** (Soonawala et al, 1999). In a series of 207 neonates with sacral and presacral cutaneous stigmata, 40% of patients with atypical dimples were found to have occult spinal dysraphism (Kriss and Desai, 1998). Other skin markers to suggest occult spinal abnormalities include subcutaneous lipomas, dermal sinuses, tails, and localized hypertrichosis (Fig. 110–3). A combination of two or more of these congenital midline skin lesions is the strongest marker of occult spinal dysraphism (Guggisberg et al, 2004). We recommend an ultrasound of the lumbosacral spine in the newborn if any of these conditions exists (Unsinn et al, 2000; Hughes et al, 2003). For equivocal ultrasound studies and in older children, we order magnetic resonance imaging (MRI) for complete evaluation. A brief evaluation of the upper and lower extremities and of the back is performed for any evidence of asymmetry, length discrepancy, or misalignment of the spine.

The neurologic examination begins with observation of the child at the outset of the visit. Often, delays in development (Table 110–10) are identified by simple observation. A note is made of the level of alertness of the pediatric patient. Factors affecting the alertness of a newborn include the time of the last feeding, room temperature, and the gestational age. One should suspect an underlying metabolic or infectious cause in cases of decreased alertness.

Identification of a sensory level in association with a spinal cord lesion can be very difficult in the infant. Differences in color or temperature can sometimes be observed, with the skin drier and cooler below the level of the cord lesion. Children older than 4 to 5 years of age are often capable of detailed sensory testing; however, success depends on the ingenuity and patience of the examiner. A child with a low spinal cord lesion may have a patulous anus and absence of contraction of the anal sphincter when stimulated in the anal region by a sharp object (anal wink). Changes in bladder function, such as new-onset urinary incontinence, may indicate a spinal cord lesion.

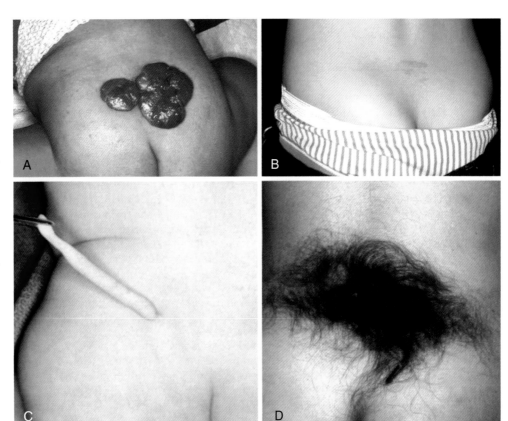

Figure 110–3. Clinical aspects of congenital median lumbosacral cutaneous lesions. **A,** Ulcerated hemangioma centered on a dermal sinus and deviation of the gluteal furrow. **B,** Isolated port-wine stain. **C,** Human tail. **D,** Faun tail. (From Guggisberg D, Hadj-Rabia S, Viney C, et al: Skin markers in occult spinal dysraphism: A review of 54 cases. Arch Dermatol 2004;140:1109-1115.)

Table 110–10.	**Developmental Milestones**			
Age (mo)	*Gross Motor*	*Fine Motor*	*Social Skills*	*Language*
3	Supports weight on forearms	Opens hands spontaneously	Smiles appropriately	Coos, laughs
6	Sits momentarily	Transfers objects	Shows likes and dislikes	Babbles
9	Pulls to stand	Pincer grasp	Plays pat-a-cake, peek-a-boo	Imitates sounds
12	Walks with one hand held	Releases an object on command	Comes when called	1-2 meaningful words
18	Walks upstairs with assistance	Feeds from a spoon	Mimics actions of others	At least 6 words
24	Runs	Builds a tower of six blocks	Plays with others	2-3 word sentences

From Haslam RHA: Neurological examination. In Behrman R, Kliegman R, Jenson H (eds): Nelson Textbook of Pediatrics, 16th ed. Philadelphia, Elsevier, 2000.

KEY POINTS: THE PEDIATRIC UROLOGY OFFICE VISIT

■ An important first question when taking the history in the pediatric patient with a urologic problem is **"why is the child here?"**

■ Renal pathology is the source of up to two thirds of neonatal abdominal masses.

■ Sexual abuse is surprisingly common and requires supportive, sensitive, and detailed history taking.

■ The lower back should be examined for evidence of cutaneous markers suggestive of occult spinal dysraphisms.

Laboratory Examination in the Pediatric Urology Patient

The urine specimen may be obtained in a number of different ways. In the child who is not potty trained, a bagged specimen, although the most susceptible to contamination, is the easiest and least invasive to obtain. To minimize contamination with fecal or skin flora, a hole is cut in the diaper and the perineal bag is brought through the hole in the diaper. A parent is instructed to watch the bag and as soon as urine is noted (which can be easily seen since the bag is visible coming through a hole in the diaper), the bag should then be removed. If the specimen is collected in the office, the bag is immediately drained and the urine plated and sent to the laboratory for culture. In this way, the skin contamination of the urine specimen is minimized and the trauma of catheterization is avoided (Falcao et al, 1999).

Older children generally provide a clean midstream urine. Most studies have failed to show any benefit to formally cleansing the introitus before obtaining the specimen. Only a midstream urine specimen is collected and sent to the laboratory for urinalysis and culture. **Pyuria is defined as more than 5 white blood cells per high-powered field for girls and more than 3 white blood cells per high-powered field for boys.** Infection can occur without pyuria and, conversely, pyuria may be present without UTI. Consequently, pyuria as an isolated finding is more confirmatory than diagnostic for UTI. Nitrate and leukocyte esterase assays are usually positive in infected urine. However, if the urine has not remained in the bladder for more than 1 hour, the conversion of nitrates to nitrites may not be complete and the chemical strip may read negative despite the presence of nitrogen-splitting bacteria in the bladder. If the culture grows greater than 100,000 colonies of a single pathogen or if there are 10,000 colonies and the child is symptomatic, we consider a UTI to be present. **White blood cell casts and urinary sediment suggest renal involvement,** but these are rarely identified. If the child is not symptomatic and the urinalysis is normal, it is unlikely that the urine is infected. However, if the child is symptomatic, a UTI is possible regardless of the results of the urinalysis (Bonadio, 1987). Microscopic hematuria is common in acute bacterial as well as viral cystitis. Gross hematuria may be present in viral cystitis but is less common in acute bacterial cystitis.

If the child is symptomatic, the urinalysis is suggestive of UTI, and the culture grows more than one organism or fewer than 100,000 colonies, the clinician has the option of treating with an antibiotic that is effective based on the sensitivities or repeating the culture. We repeat the culture but start the child on a treatment dose of antibiotic at that time. If a second catheterized culture is negative, then the antibiotics are discontinued and close follow-up is provided. This is particularly important in infants who may not demonstrate the usual signs and symptoms of infection that would be present in an older child.

Hematuria

Microscopic hematuria is common in children. Routine office screening with urinalysis for urinary abnormalities is no longer recommended. Thus the actual time of onset for microscopic hematuria is often unknown. Normally, the first indicator is a positive urine strip test for blood. Most strips can detect concentrations of 5 to 10 intact red blood cells/mL. This corresponds to 2 to 5 red blood cells per high-powered field. Improper interpretation of the dipstick such as delayed reading or cross-contamination of urine from other chemically impregnated pads may result in false-positive results. The urine should be dipped, the excess urine tapped off, and the strips should be read immediately at the recommended time. **Confirmation of microscopic hematuria after a positive dipstick examination requires a microscopic examination of the urine for the presence of red blood cells.** Microscopic hematuria may be defined as more than 5 red blood cells per high-powered field in at least two of three urinalyses over 2 to 3 weeks. An absence of red blood cells in the urine with a positive dipstick result suggests hemoglobinuria or myoglobinuria. A positive dipstick on a single specimen with micro-

scopic confirmation should be viewed as an indication for further urine testing rather than as diagnostic until persistence is confirmed on subsequent studies. A practical approach to the evaluation of hematuria in children is presented in Chapter 111, "Renal Disease in Childhood." **Our recommendation in patients with microscopic hematuria with unrelated clinical symptoms is to treat the affiliated illness (pulmonary or immunologic conditions, glomerular and interstitial disease, lower urinary tract disease, stones, tumors, vascular disease, or acute abdominal conditions) and ignore hematuria until the treatment for the underlying illness is underway. The large majority of children with microscopic hematuria are evaluated, and the source of the hematuria is never identified** (Diven and Travis, 2000).

Gross hematuria in children is less common than microscopic hematuria, with an estimated prevalence of 1.3 per 1000 (Ingelfinger et al, 1977). The most common diagnoses are UTI (26%), perineal irritation (11%), trauma (7%), meatal stenosis with ulceration (7%), coagulation abnormalities (3%), and urinary tract stones (2%). The most common glomerular causes of gross hematuria in children are poststreptococcal glomerulonephritis and IgA nephropathy. An antecedent sore throat, pyoderma, edema, or red blood cell casts suggest glomerulonephritis. IgA nephropathy can cause recurrent gross hematuria with flank or abdominal pain and may be preceded by an upper respiratory tract infection (Meyers, 2004). Adenoviral infection, hypercalciuria, and hyperuricosuria are other sources to consider. We perform an ultrasound of the kidneys, ureters, and bladder in children with gross hematuria, although the yield is low (Fernbach, 1992). Contrary to the adult patient, cystoscopic examination in children rarely reveals a cause for hematuria but should be performed when bladder pathology is a consideration.

Radiologic Examination in the Pediatric Urology Patient

Ultrasound

The ultrasound of the kidneys, ureters, and bladder is an extension of the physical examination. Palpable masses within the abdomen can be localized and even diagnosed with the aid of ultrasonography performed by a uroradiologist with an interest in pediatrics. The examination should evaluate not only the genitourinary system but also adjacent organs such as the adrenal gland, liver, and spleen. The image of the parenchyma of the liver and spleen should be used as a comparison to assess the parenchyma of the right and left kidney, respectively. The density of the kidney and of the renal medullary pyramids as well as the wall thickness and configuration of the collecting system, the presence or absence of caliectasis, pelviectasis, or ureterectasis are all important indicators of renal and ureteral pathophysiology (Hulbert et al, 1992). The luminal diameter of the ureters, thickness of the bladder wall, and the volume of the bladder both before and after voiding should be recorded. If hydronephrosis or ureterectasis is present before voiding, the kidneys and ureters should be rescanned after voiding. A skillful ultrasonographer can provide anatomic detail about the insertion of the ureters and the degree of dilation of the ureter and can identify the jet of urine as it enters the bladder (Kirby and Rosenberg,

1992). **Ultrasound in the absence of comparison studies or appropriate history cannot by itself distinguish obstructive from nonobstructive hydronephrosis.** Therefore, a functional study such as a renal scan is usually required for diagnosis.

Ultrasound is sensitive in detecting solid renal masses, particularly those that measure at least 1.5 cm in largest dimension. For smaller renal masses, the ultrasound findings should be considered preliminary and should be confirmed with CT or MRI (Jamis-Dow et al, 1996). Ultrasonography may also be used to accurately measure postvoid residual urine (Coombes and Millard, 1994). Increased thickness of the bladder wall may be suggestive of bladder outlet obstruction from posterior urethral valves or urethral atresia. Trabeculation within the bladder, bladder diverticulum, and ureteral duplication or ureterocele are all easily identified with ultrasound.

Ultrasound is also frequently used to examine the scrotum, such as in cases of boys with varicoceles (Diamond et al, 2000). It may also be used to assess blood flow if spermatic cord torsion is suspected, as well as to distinguish between epididymitis and torsion of the appendix testis in cases in which tenderness is localized to the upper pole of the testis. We have also found it useful in distinguishing hernia from hydrocele or identifying abdominoperineal hydroceles (Finkelstein et al, 1986).

When used as a first-line test in suspected occult spinal dysraphism, optimal timing of the spinal ultrasound is before 6 months of age. Ossification of the posterior elements after 6 months of age prevents an acoustic window. Agreement between ultrasound and MRI is good, particularly for the detection of the low-lying cord (90%) (Hughes et al, 2003).

Voiding Cystourethrography

VCUG is used to identify vesicoureteral reflux (VUR), to evaluate the anatomy of the bladder outlet during bladder filling and voiding, and to assess the presence of residual urine after micturition. Additional information regarding trabeculation of the bladder, bladder diverticula, and presence or absence of urachal abnormalities may be identified with a fluoroscopic VCUG (Fernbach, 2000; Goldman et al, 2000; McDonald et al, 2000). The VCUG begins with a plain film, followed by placement of a feeding tube rather than a Foley catheter. The balloon on a Foley catheter may obscure the anatomy of the bladder neck and trigone, particularly at the beginning of the study. On the plain film, abnormalities of the spine, ribs, and pelvis and the presence or absence of stones within the kidney, ureter, or bladder should be noted. The gas pattern and volume of stool is particularly important in infants and in children with dysfunctional voiding in whom constipation may be an important part of the clinical pattern. Gas should normally be present in the rectum on plain film by 24 hours of age. The bladder should be drained, and contrast medium should be gently infused. In children in whom a ureterocele is suspected, the first few images during filling of the bladder best demonstrate the ureterocele. The bladder is then filled slowly, and the child voids.

Voiding views must be obtained in all cases, but particularly if bladder outlet obstruction such as a posterior urethral valve is suspected. In children in whom VUR is suspected or in patients with an ectopic ureter, cyclic VCUG must be performed in which at least two voiding cycles are completed. In some cases, the ectopic ureter that is draining to the bladder neck must empty for additional contrast material to reflux. If a second voiding cycle is not performed, one might miss reflux into the ectopic system (Hellstrom and Jacobsson, 1999; Polito et al, 2000a). It is important to image the bladder neck during voiding in the female as well as the male. The presence of a "spinning top urethra" in a school-aged girl may be an important indicator of dysfunctional voiding (Saxton et al, 1988; Soygur et al, 2004). Vaginal voiding should also be noted, which may be seen on the postvoid views.

In patients with a urogenital sinus, contrast VCUG is modified to image the urethra and vagina simultaneously. In this study, the urogenital sinus is intubated with a blunt-tipped catheter (which can be made by trimming the cone-shaped end of a feeding tube) and placed against the perineal opening. Contrast medium is injected retrograde to identify the point where the vaginal introitus meets the urethra to form the urogenital sinus. The study will also aid in differentiating a cervical dimple from a prostatic utricle. If a cloaca is present, the sinogram will provide detail about the position of the rectum, vagina, and urethra and about the point of confluence and the distance to the perineum (Shaul et al, 1997; De Filippo et al, 1999). The distances of these structures will help determine the approach required during surgery (Pena et al, 2004).

We use the nuclear cystogram as part of the follow-up examinations in children with VUR. Some studies report the sensitivity to be higher than in conventional contrast VCUG (Polito et al, 2000b). We also use it as the first examination to screen for VUR in sisters of children with VUR. Measuring the percentage of the bladder volume refluxing into the ureters during bladder filling may quantitate the nuclear cystogram. The percentage of bladder filling when the reflux is first identified may also be an indicator of potential resolution of VUR. On subsequent examinations, improvement in VUR may be assumed if a smaller percentage of total bladder volume is refluxing into the ureter or if the reflux occurs at a greater percentage of total bladder filling (Mozley et al, 1994).

Nuclear Medicine Renal Scan

A radionuclide renal scan is measured in two phases: the cortical imaging and tubular imaging phase. Most radionuclide agents will demonstrate renal tubular as well as renal cortical binding. Radionuclide studies are best suited to demonstrate changes in tubular or cortical transit that result from abnormalities of renal perfusion, secretion, and filtration. In most cases, the radionuclide study is inferior to CT, MRI, or ultrasound for demonstration of morphologic alterations. When a glomerular filtration excreted agent such as **technetium-99m diethylenetriaminepentaacetic acid (DTPA)** is given, an approximate estimation of glomerular filtration rate (GFR) may be calculated either in vivo by computer-aided scanning or in vitro with the collection of one or two blood samples at predetermined time intervals. In addition, an "extraction factor" can be calculated that estimates the single-kidney GFR during minutes 1 and 2 of the clearance of the radiotracer (Heyman and Duckett, 1988). **Technetium-99m mercaptoacetyltriglycine (MAG-3)** is secreted in part by renal tubular function and may also be used to approximate relative renal plasma flow. If detailed imaging of the renal cortex is required to identify renal scarring, **technetium-99m dimer-**

captosuccinic acid (DMSA) may be given and the kidneys imaged 3 to 4 hours after the injection.

Renal scintigraphy scans using gallium-67– or indium-111–labeled leukocytes may be helpful to diagnose and localize the site of urinary tract infections (Yen et al, 1999; Velasco et al, 2004). These techniques may be used to identify and guide therapy for children with focal segmental bacterial pyelonephritis in whom the duration of therapy is uncertain. In a prospective study by Yen and associates (1999), gallium-67 renal scans were more sensitive than DMSA scans in the diagnosis of acute pyelonephritis, especially in differentiating new lesions from old ones. These are particularly useful in patients with abnormal renal anatomy or in patients with diminished renal function in whom the DMSA scan may be less specific.

Intravenous Pyelography

Despite the newer imaging techniques that are now available, the intravenous pyelogram (IVP) is useful in selected cases. The plain film of the abdomen should be inspected for calculi, spinal abnormalities, and an abnormal intestinal gas pattern. The nephrogram phase of the IVP identifies mass effects within the kidney and the presence or absence of scarring after pyelonephritis. Subsequent views can sequentially assess the anatomy of the renal cortex, calyces, fornices, renal pelvis, ureters bladder, and urethra (Smellie, 1995). Subtle anatomic variations in normal anatomy of the renal calyces or of the ureteropelvic junction that may be confusing on ultrasound or CT may be clarified with the IVP.

Computed Tomography

Spiral CT has in most cases replaced the IVP as the first-line study in children in whom stone disease is suspected. In addition, CT with or without contrast medium enhancement is particularly important as an adjunct in children with suspected focal segmental bacterial pyelonephritis. CT is also particularly important in the diagnosis and staging of solid tumors of the chest and abdomen. Contrast medium–enhanced CT is particularly useful in cases of nephroblastomatosis, in which ultrasound shows little displacement of the renal capsule. One must be reminded that radiation doses from CT are cumulative over the life of an individual (Frush et al, 2003). With sufficient clinical information, the radiologist may be able to recommend other imaging modalities (e.g., ultrasonography, MRI) that do not use ionizing radiation.

Magnetic Resonance Imaging

Although still expensive as an individual radiologic study, **magnetic resonance urography (MRU) may provide the best information of the anatomy and function of the genitourinary tract from a single study.** Advantages of MRU include the avoidance of ionizing radiation, its use in patients with impaired renal function, and higher quality contrast and spatial resolution in any plane relative to other imaging modalities (Fig. 110–4) (Grattan-Smith et al, 2003; Wille et al, 2003). If obstruction of the urinary tract is suspected, gadolinium followed by furosemide can be administered. MRU has been utilized to diagnose ureteropelvic junction obstruction, ectopic ureter draining into seminal vesicle cyst, ureteral buds associated with renal agenesis, and cloacal exstrophy in utero

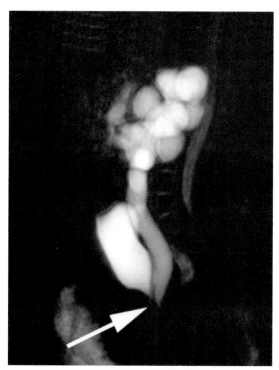

Figure 110–4. Magnetic resonance urogram of a megaureter on the left side in the sagittal plane with narrowing of the distal ureter *(arrow).* (From Wille S, Knobloch R, Klose KJ, et al: Magnetic resonance urography in pediatric urology. Scand J Urol Nephrol 2003;37:16-21.)

(Maas et al, 1997; Matsuki et al, 1998; Wille et al, 2003). Limitations of MRU at this time include its high costs and the requirement for sedation/anesthesia in some patients. Although not routine, MRI is used more frequently now in the evaluation and identification of the impalpable testis (Yeung et al, 1999; Lam et al, 2001). In the workup of suspected renovascular hypertension, gadolinium-enhanced MR angiography (MRA) is a noninvasive modality with comparable accuracy to digital subtraction angiography (Hacklander et al, 2004).

Outpatient Procedures in the Pediatric Urologic Patient

The well-equipped urology office will have a urodynamic suite as part of the overall complex. Modern urodynamic systems allow accurate measurements of the intravesical pressures before, during, and after bladder contraction. From these measurements, estimates of bladder compliance as well as the bladder outlet resistance may be made. With this information, the pediatric urologist may assess whether the bladder stores at pressures low enough to prevent renal damage and empties well enough to prevent UTI. The addition of fluoroscopic monitoring of the bladder and upper tracts during urodynamics greatly adds to the information garnered from the urodynamic study. However, the videourodynamic suites require being located within a lead-lined room, which may preclude its placement in every office.

Biofeedback training designed to help the child to improve bladder emptying may also be performed in the

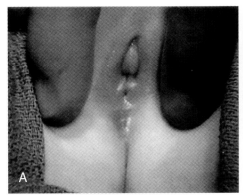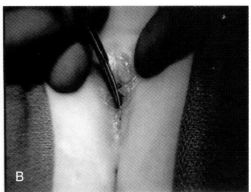

Figure 110–5. Outpatient lysis of labial adhesions. **A,** Dense labial adhesions. **B,** Adhesions clamped and incised. (From Nurzia MJ, Eickhorst KM, Ankem MK, Barone JG: The surgical treatment of labial adhesions in prepubertal girls. J Pediatr Adolesc Gynecol 2003;16:21-23.)

office. Biofeedback sessions should be done in a room that is separate from the urodynamic suite, because in most cases a different population of patients requires biofeedback training than will undergo urodynamic study (Yamanishi et al, 2000; Schulman, 2004). Biofeedback, if done properly, is time consuming. The child must be relaxed and motivated for the session to be effective. Awareness of the pelvic floor muscle and urinary sphincter is a key factor to achieve successful biofeedback treatment. Biofeedback incorporating interactive computer games is available, with success rates approaching 90% after a mean of 4.9 sessions (Herndon et al, 2001).

Office Surgical Procedures

Successful outpatient surgery with local anesthetic depends on cooperation from the parent as well as the child. Parents must believe that the convenience of having the procedure in the office outweighs the advantages of a general anesthetic in the main operating room. We believe many infants weighing less than 10 pounds may easily undergo an office circumcision with an anesthetic cream combined with injected local anesthetic (Hoebeke et al, 1997). However, in a recent meta-analysis by Brady-Fryer and colleagues (2004), dorsal penile nerve block was the most effective at reducing circumcision pain compared with EMLA and placebo. We rarely provide for office circumcision in older children. Infants older than 3 months are too big to be easily restrained, and the risk of bleeding postoperatively if the skin edges are not sutured is considerable.

A number of techniques may be used in the clinic for circumcision, including a Plastibell, Mogen clamp, and GOMCO clamp. We use the GOMCO clamp, which is a three-component device that includes a bell that fits over the glans of the penis and separates the glans from the inner preputial skin (Guazzo, 1999; Amir et al, 2000; Wan 2002). The clamp is applied, and the foreskin is trimmed away from the clamp. If the clamp is left in place for a considerable amount of time (usually about 10 minutes), then there is very little separation of the skin postoperatively. If desired, a small nonstick bandage is placed beneath a transparent adhesive dressing. The bandage is removed the next day. The boy's parents are instructed to apply petroleum jelly to the incision during the healing period.

Complications after neonatal circumcision include bleeding, wound infection, meatal stenosis, and secondary phi- mosis resulting from removal of insufficient foreskin or removal of insufficient inner preputial skin.** Potentially serious complications include death, sepsis, amputation of distal part of the glans, removal of excessive foreskin, and urethrocutaneous fistula (Baskin et al, 1997; Hutcheson, 2004). After a circumcision, the cut edge of the preputial surface may occasionally graft to the inflamed glans tissue forming a preputial-glanular bridge that may be incised in the office with application of local anesthetic cream and subsequent injection of local anesthetic. After injection, the skin bridge is clamped, the clamp is removed, and the skin bridge is sharply incised. No suturing is required in most cases. This procedure is easy and virtually painless. After the procedure, the parents apply petroleum jelly to the incised edges to prevent them from readhering.

Meatal stenosis is common after circumcision. It may result from contraction of the meatus after healing of the inflamed, denuded glans tissue that occurs after retraction of the foreskin or from damage to the frenular artery at the time of circumcision (Persad et al, 1995; Upadhyay et al, 1998). If the narrowing is pronounced enough to cause deflection of the urinary stream or dysuria, a meatotomy is indicated.

To perform a meatotomy in the office, an anesthetic cream is applied. After 45 minutes, lidocaine with 1% epinephrine is injected with a 26-gauge needle to provide a small wheal at the ventrum of the urethral meatus. The ventral edge of the urethral meatus is clamped, and a small wedge of the scarred tissue is crushed with a straight hemostat and sharply excised. After the procedure, the parents are advised to apply a fine petrolatum ointment to the cut edges of the urethral meatus. A small meatal dilator is used twice a day for 4 to 6 weeks. Postoperatively, these children are seen 2 to 3 months later to assess the result.

If a VCUG is required, or if dysuria associated with vaginal pooling of urine contributes to a dysfunctional voiding pattern, we have occasionally separated labial adhesions in the office. These membranous adhesions are easy to separate on the midline with a probe or the tip of a curved hemostat (Fig. 110–5). A local anesthetic cream is applied to the labia in hopes of easing the discomfort, which is minimal. After lysis of the adhesions, the child's parent must separate the labia and apply a barrier cream such as petroleum jelly at least twice a day for 4 to 6 weeks while the labial tissue matures. With diligent postoperative care, recurrence is rare.

KEY POINTS: OUTPATIENT PROCEDURES IN THE PEDIATRIC PATIENT

■ A well-equipped urology office will have a urodynamics and biofeedback training suite.

■ Most infants weighing less than 10 pounds may easily undergo an office circumcision with an anesthetic cream combined with injected local anesthesia.

■ Petroleum jelly is applied after circumcision, urethral meatotomy, or lysis of labial adhesions to prevent complications.

SUMMARY

The final goal of the surgical care of children is to assure as normal an adult life as possible. The pediatric urologist should continue to act as consultant even after the child enters adulthood for boys with prune-belly syndrome or posterior urethral valves and for children of either sex born with bladder or cloacal exstrophy. **As the children grow into adults, the** pediatric team must develop a liaison with a skilled, interested adult team. In this way, a lifetime plan of care may be designed and carried out to ensure well-coordinated urologic therapy that is capable of addressing the complicated problems unique to this special group of patients.

SUGGESTED READINGS

American Academy of Pediatrics, Committee on Quality Improvement, Subcommittee on Urinary Tract Infection: Practice parameter: The diagnosis, treatment, and evaluation of the initial urinary tract infection in febrile infants and young children. Pediatrics 1999;103(4 pt 1):843-852.

Bonadio WA: Urine culturing technique in febrile infants. Pediatr Emerg Care 1987;3:75-78.

Hoebeke P, Depauw P, Van Laecke E, Oosterlinck W: The use of EMLA cream as anaesthetic for minor urological surgery in children. Acta Urol Belg 1997;65:25-28.

Jeffs RD: Exstrophy and cloacal exstrophy. Urol Clin North Am 1978;5:127-140.

McGuire EJ, Woodside JR, Borden TA: Upper urinary tract deterioration in patients with myelodysplasia and detrusor hypertonia: A follow-up study. J Urol 1983;129:823-826.

Meyers KE: Evaluation of hematuria in children. Urol Clin North Am 2004;31:559-573.

Pena A, Levitt MA, Hong A, Midulla P: Surgical management of cloacal malformations: A review of 339 patients. J Pediatr Surg 2004;39:470-479.

Pinto E, Guignard JP: Renal masses in the neonate. Biol Neonate 1995;68:175-184.

Ransley PG, Risdon RA: Reflux nephropathy: Effects of antimicrobial therapy on the evolution of the early pyelonephritic scar. Kidney Int 1981;20:733-742.

Schulman SL: Voiding dysfunction in children. Urol Clin North Am 2004;31:481-490.

111 Renal Disease in Childhood

H. NORMAN NOE, MD • DEBORAH P. JONES, MD

This chapter discusses the most common renal disorders seen in children. The primary goal is to familiarize the reader with fundamental knowledge regarding the epidemiology of hematuria and proteinuria, characteristics and treatment of the more common glomerular and tubular diseases of childhood, the approach to the child with nephrolithiasis, and care of the child with chronic renal failure.

HEMATURIA

Hematuria may be divided into several categories based on characteristics at presentation: it may be macroscopic or microscopic; by the associated symptoms it may be symptomatic or asymptomatic (implies incidental discovery usually on well-child examination); or it may be isolated, which implies that proteinuria and/or pyuria are absent. Among children, hematuria is probably the most commonly identified urinary abnormality leading to referral to a nephrologist or urologist for evaluation. Like most discussions of hematuria in children, we will delineate the common clinical syndromes, provide a list of possible causes, as well as provide diagnostic algorithms. In addition, the present discussion will also review the major case series of childhood hematuria published over the past 25 years.

Hematuria is defined as the presence of 5 or more red blood cells per high-power microscope field (Fitzwater and Wyatt, 1994). Although its presence is typically detected by dipstick via a reaction of a peroxidase with hemoglobin, hematuria must be differentiated from pigmenturia—either hemoglobinuria or myoglobinuria—by microscopic examination of the urinary sediment. Enough emphasis cannot be placed on this vital component of the patient's evaluation.

It is helpful to classify the type of hematuria. Hematuria may be characterized as macroscopic (gross) or microscopic. It is not unusual for the parent or child to report red or brown color but the urine be normal in appearance at the time of evaluation. This may pose a challenge to the precise characterization until gross hematuria can be documented. Hematuria may occur with or without clinical symptoms that would help to localize the source of the hematuria. These include symptoms of lower urinary tract irritation such as dysuria, frequency, enuresis, bladder spasms, presence of clots, or end-micturition bleeding. Alternatively, symptoms and signs of glomerular disease may include edema, hypertension, abnormal creatinine level, arthralgia, rash, anemia, or hypoalbuminemia. Hematuria may occur with or without proteinuria. As much as 2+ protein by dipstick may be found during episodes of gross hematuria, just from the presence of a generous number of red blood cells. Quantitation of urinary protein aids in the delineation of isolated hematuria versus hematuria with proteinuria. Thus, four categories of hematuria have been proposed: gross hematuria, microscopic hematuria with clinical symptoms, asymptomatic isolated hematuria, and asymptomatic hematuria with proteinuria. In addition, hematuria can be intermittent (also known as recurrent) or persistent.

Epidemiology of Hematuria in Children

Studies of hematuria in children have been conducted by screening apparently healthy children or by retrospective analyses of children with hematuria comprising cases usually from a single center. Many of these include children with both macrohematuria and microhematuria. Vehaskari and co-workers (1979) used the "screening approach" to estimate the prevalence of hematuria among school-aged children (age 8 to 15 years) to be 1.1% after excluding children who had only transient hematuria. Of 10,268 children screened, 8,954 participated in the study; 74% had blood detected in only one sample. Of the remaining 131 who continued to have hematuria, 83 children had isolated hematuria, whereas 59 also had associated proteinuria. Further evaluation revealed that of the children with isolated microhematuria, urinary tract infection was the most common identified cause (7%). Other causes included urinary tract malformations in 2, IgA nephritis in 2, and Alport's syndrome in 1 child. However, it is important to note that this study was conducted before the identification of hypercalciuria as a relatively common cause of hematuria in children.

A screening study for hematuria conducted by Hisano and associates (1991) in Fukuoka, Japan, in 160,000 junior high children found that 251 had isolated microscopic hematuria. A cause for hematuria was identified in 115: menses (35%), urinary tract infection (5.6%), hypercalciuria (2%), Henoch-Schönlein purpura (1.2%), hydronephrosis (1.2%), and polycystic kidney disease (0.4%). After exclusion of identifiable causes among theses children, 136 children were considered to have idiopathic, isolated hematuria and were observed along with their parents over a mean of 7.4 years. Nineteen underwent renal biopsy because of abnormalities among family members. IgA nephropathy was the most commonly identified pathologic lesion, occurring in 37%, followed by other glomerular diseases. Minor lesions were found in 21%. Examination of clinical status at follow-up revealed that approximately 25% of children had resolution of hematuria whereas 75% had persistent hematuria, less than 1% had proteinuria, and none developed renal insufficiency. The findings of these two studies support the concept that **isolated asymptomatic hematuria is a relatively benign condition after exclusion of children with easily identifiable causes by history and physical examination, family history, urine microscopy, renal imaging, urine culture, urinary calcium excretion, and renal biopsy, if indicated.**

Retrospective analyses of hematuria were reported by Turi and colleagues (1989): a multicenter study of 341 Hungarian children with persistent, isolated hematuria for a minimum of 6 months' duration observed children ages 2 to 12 years for 2 to 17 years. Before inclusion, children underwent evaluation to exclude urinary tract infection, urinary tract malformations, vesicoureteral reflux, proteinuria (>250 mg/24 hr), hypertension, renal dysfunction, or systemic disease. Categorization of hematuria revealed isolated microscopic in 31%, macroscopic in 28%, or a combination of microscopic and macroscopic in 41%. The group was composed of equal proportions of girls and boys. Persistent hematuria was documented by monthly urine examinations in 40%, whereas 60% were characterized as having recurrent (intermittent) hematuria. Forty-seven children underwent renal biopsy a mean of 12 months after initial detection of hematuria, usually because of a nephritic urine sediment or development of significant proteinuria. In this subgroup, mesangial proliferative glomerulonephritis and hereditary nephritis were the most common pathologic diagnoses. Twenty percent of subjects were found to have hypercalciuria and/or nephrolithiasis. The

remaining two thirds had isolated hematuria. Of these 226 children, 163 had resolution of hematuria. Again, this large series supports the concept that after exclusion of commonly identifiable causes of hematuria, those with idiopathic hematuria follow a benign course. Unfortunately, the authors did not distinguish long-term outcome based on the presence or absence of macroscopic hematuria.

A second retrospective study included patients from two centers in North America and included only those children referred for evaluation of asymptomatic, microscopic hematuria (Feld and coworkers, 1998). After children were excluded because of proteinuria (>1+ or a urine protein:creatinine ratio >0.2), history of renal stones, presence of urinary tract infection, presence of systemic illness, or evidence of glomerulonephritis, sickle cell disease, or bleeding disorder based on the diagnostic evaluation of the referring physician, 325 children were identified. The diagnostic studies performed on these were reviewed. Not all studies were performed on all children. Hypercalciuria was found in 11%, and minor renal structural abnormalities were found in 9 of 81 (11%) on voiding cystourethrography (VCUG) (grade I or II vesicoureteral reflux), and in 18 of 265 (7%) renal ultrasounds detected each of the following: ureteric duplication (3), increased echogenicity (5), ectopic kidney, discrepant renal size (6), bifid collecting system, and extrarenal pelvis (2). The authors concluded that the initial evaluation of microscopic hematuria should include a first morning voided urine sample with microscopic examination. In the absence of proteinuria or cellular casts, serum chemistries and imaging are not necessary. In addition, they concluded that renal biopsy and cystoscopy are not indicated in children with isolated microscopic hematuria.

A single-center study reported by Wyatt and colleagues (1977) described 164 children with macroscopic or microscopic hematuria seen in Lexington, Kentucky, over 5 years. Initial diagnoses included glomerular disease in 71 (41%); extraglomerular, renal sources in 19 (12%); and lower tract sources in 6 (4%). Isolated microhematuria without a clear etiology at presentation was diagnosed in 68 children (41%). Eventual diagnoses among the latter group included glomerular disease in 40 and idiopathic hematuria in 28, or 17% of the original cohort.

Another single-center report addressed the etiology of gross hematuria in children presenting over a 2-year period to an emergency department clinic in Boston, Massachusetts (Ingelfinger et al, 1977). Of 169 children who presented with a chief complaint of red urine, 158 had documented macrohematuria. Identifiable sources were found in 84 children (56%), not including the 8 children who suffered postoperative hematuria. Sources of hematuria identified included local perineal irritation (16 children), meatal stenosis (11 children), trauma (10 children), urinary tract infection (39 children), coagulopathy (5 children), and renal stones (3 children). Of those children who did not have a source identified after the initial diagnostic evaluation, causes included acute glomerulonephritis (6 children), ureteropelvic junction obstruction (2 children), cystitis cystica (1 child), epididymitis (1 child), and tumor (1 child). Twenty children had not received a diagnosis, of whom 7 had recurrent gross hematuria. **Thus, sources for gross hematuria are generally**

more readily identifiable as compared with microhematuria. Cystoscopy is seldom required to identify the source of macroscopic hematuria in children with hematuria. However, cystoscopy may be beneficial in the setting of persistent, idiopathic gross hematuria. If bloody effluent is observed from both ureteral orifices, one is directed to the possibility of renal parenchymal disease; if bloody urine is observed from only one ureteral orifice, unilateral urinary tract or vascular disease may be present.

Both of the previous single-center series were reported before the description of hypercalciuria-associated hematuria. Several centers reported the association of hypercalciuria with hematuria in the early 1980s. Roy and associates (1981) identified hypercalciuria in 30% of children with isolated hematuria, an estimate that was later supported by a multicenter study (Stapleton and the Southwest Pediatric Nephrology Study Group, 1990). Some of the children went on to form renal stones, particularly those who had a family history of nephrolithiasis or who had gross hematuria (see section on hypercalciuria).

Clues from the History and Physical Examination

As mentioned previously, clinical symptoms and signs in a child with hematuria may provide important clues to the underlying diagnosis (Meyers, 2004). Signs of systemic illness such as weight loss, fever, rash, pallor, anemia, arthralgias, or even respiratory symptoms often accompany glomerular disease. Edema is an important finding and usually indicates glomerular involvement. The importance of hypertension cannot be overemphasized, and its presence should make one consider diagnostic evaluation as an inpatient, particularly if it accompanies edema (acute glomerulonephritis). Certain clinical patterns are often indicative of a chronic glomerular disease, usually either IgA or hereditary nephritis. Alternatively, symptoms such as flank pain or those indicative of lower tract irritation, such as dysuria, frequency, passage of clots, end-micturition blood, and enuresis point to the urinary tract as the source of hematuria. Figure 111–1 outlines one approach to the management of the child with hematuria.

PROTEINURIA

Proteinuria is the second most commonly identified urinary abnormality in children referred to pediatric nephrology centers. Isolated proteinuria may be a transient event or may indicate urinary tract inflammation or glomerular disease. Rarely, proteinuria is indicative of renal tubular disease. Postural (or orthostatic) proteinuria is a benign, idiopathic cause of isolated proteinuria commonly found in older children (Hogg et al, 2000).

Proteinuria is first detected by urinary dipstick, which primarily detects albumin. The colorimetric reaction between albumin and tetrabromophenol blue results in variable shades of green depending on the approximate concentration of protein in the urine: trace indicates approximately 15 mg/dL; 1+, 30 mg/dL; 2+, 100 mg/dL; 3+, 300 mg/dL; and 4+, 2000 mg/dL or more. Confirmation of the level of proteinuria may be performed using sulfosalicylic acid, which uses protein pre-

---

KEY POINTS: HEMATURIA

- Isolated microhematuria in children is usually a benign condition.

- Hematuria in the presence of significant proteinuria often indicates glomerular disease requiring percutaneous renal biopsy.

- Gross hematuria in children with normal urinary tract imaging rarely indicates cystoscopic examination unless it is persistent and nonglomerular in origin.

- Hypercalciuria is a common cause of both macroscopic and microscopic hematuria in children.

- A family history of renal disease or renal stones may help to guide the diagnostic evaluation of hematuria in children.

---

cipitation and turbidity to estimate the level of proteinuria. This is usually reserved for clinical laboratories. False-positive urine protein levels may be caused by an alkaline urine, antiseptic cleanser, radiocontrast agents, or a highly concentrated sample. Alternatively, children with very dilute urine may have significant proteinuria, which may not be detected by dipstick alone. Finding of protein in the urine prompts the clinician to consider any other signs or symptoms of renal or urinary tract disease, including systemic disease. If absent, then the urinalysis may be repeated in several weeks to confirm that the proteinuria is persistent.

Quantitation of Urinary Protein Excretion

Proteinuria may be quantitated by use of timed urine collection, which is the classic method to establish the degree of proteinuria (Hogg et al, 2000). More recently, the random urine protein:creatinine ratio has been substituted for timed collections. In children, proteinuria is best expressed as milligrams per hour per square meter of body surface area. Normal urine protein excretion in children is less than 4 mg/m^2/hr, or alternatively less than 100 mg/m^2/24 hr. To avoid errors related to collection of too much or too little, the urinary creatinine value should also be measured. In females the urinary creatinine excretion is 15 to 20 mg/kg/day, and it is 20 to 25 mg/kg/day for males. Calculation of the random urine protein:creatinine ratio can be performed on urine collected at a single point in time. Creatinine and protein measured in milligrams per deciliter are then expressed as a ratio of protein divided by creatinine concentration. A value of less than 0.2 is normal for children older than 2 years, and a value of less than 0.5 is considered normal for children 6 to 24 months of age. In normal individuals, small amounts of protein are present in the urine but not usually detected by dipstick. Proteins normally present in the urine include Tamm-Horsfall protein, which is secreted by the loop of Henle, and smaller molecular weight proteins, which are filtered by the glomerulus and then reabsorbed by the proximal tubule.

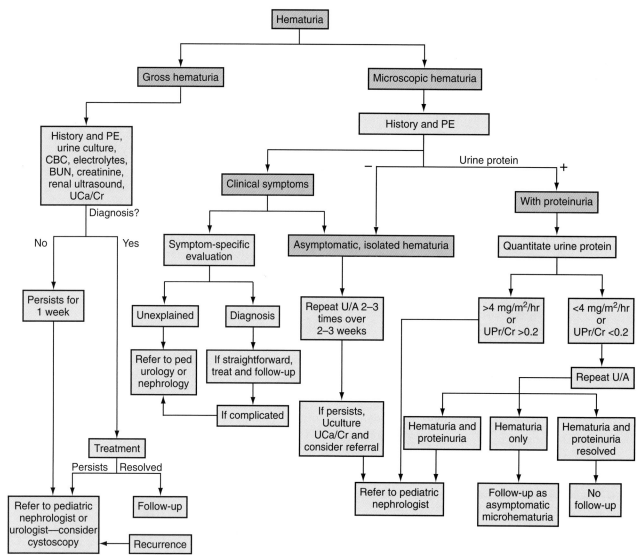

Figure 111–1. Algorithm for the treatment of hematuria. BUN, blood urea nitrogen; CBC, complete blood count; PE, physical examination; U/A, urinalyses; UCa/Cr, urinary calcium:creatinine ratio; UPr/Cr, urinary protein:creatinine ratio.

Investigation of Proteinuria in Children

Proteinuria may be transient, orthostatic, or fixed/persistent. Transient proteinuria is poorly characterized but may be associated with fever, stress, dehydration, and exercise and does not require extensive evaluation. Orthostatic proteinuria is also poorly characterized but appears to have a benign prognosis. Theories as to the origin of the proteinuria include changes in renal venous pressure with position. Orthostatic proteinuria may be documented by collection of two timed urine samples: one while the child is recumbent (sleeping) and one while the child is ambulatory (awake). Alternatively, our practice evaluates postural protein excretion by collection of the first morning urine and a separate urine specimen later in the day on 3 days; the samples are returned for dipstick testing for protein. The recumbent urine specimen should have a normal urine protein level. Children must be instructed to empty their bladder immediately before going to bed so as to avoid contamination of the morning urine from urine produced when upright. The 24-hour urinary protein excretion in children with orthostatic proteinuria should not exceed 1000 mg/day because there may be diurnal variation in protein excretion even in children with renal disease.

Children with 1+ or more protein by dipstick on more than one occasion have persistent proteinuria and deserve further evaluation (Fig. 111–2). The finding of isolated proteinuria on a single urine sample is not uncommon in children with prevalence estimates of 5% to 15%. However, persistence of proteinuria is much less common. Vehaskari and Rapola (1982) screened school-aged children for proteinuria, which was present in at least one of four samples obtained in 10% of children, while only 0.1% had protein detected in all four samples. As mentioned previously, other signs and symptoms of kidney disease may prompt a sooner rather than later approach. These include edema, polyuria, dysuria, incontinence, growth failure, hypertension, or pres-

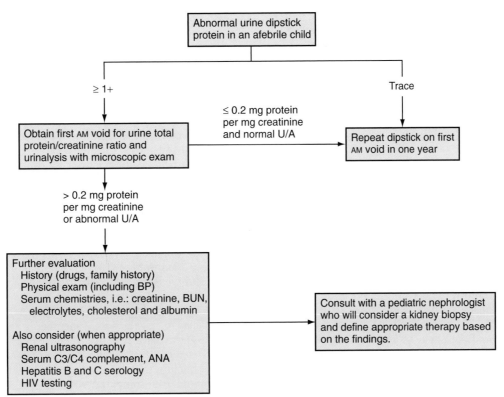

Figure 111–2. Evaluation of persistent proteinuria in children/adolescents.

ence of systemic disease. Excess urinary protein may be the result of increased glomerular permeability to protein or decreased tubular reabsorption of protein.

After documentation of persistent proteinuria, comprehensive evaluation for possible renal diseases should be done. This includes a careful history to look for previous urinary tract infections, family history of renal diseases, history of bladder function, and medications. Physical examination should include measurement of height and weight with calculation of age-appropriate percentiles and measurement of blood pressure. The presence of hypertension would increase the likelihood of finding renal pathology. Normative data for blood pressure are available and are classified by gender, age, and height percentile (National High Blood Pressure Education Program, 2004). Serum chemistries should be done, including creatinine, blood urea nitrogen, and albumin values. Further studies may include renal imaging by ultrasound or serology aimed at detection of secondary glomerular diseases (C3, C4, fluorescent antinuclear antibody, anti–streptolysin O, and hepatitis B or C titers).

Mass urinary screening of school-aged children has been performed in Taiwan over the past decade (Lin et al, 2001). The identifiable causes for persistent hematuria, proteinuria, or the combination of hematuria and proteinuria were described. Of the children found to have abnormal urinalyses, 5% had isolated proteinuria of 1 to 2+. Sixty percent of these children were identified as having some type of glomerular disease, 8% had urinary tract disorders, and 29% had orthostatic proteinuria. **Those children with heavier proteinuria, with or without hematuria, were more likely to have glomerular disease** (86%). Of nonglomerular causes, orthostatic proteinuria was found in 4% and urinary tract disease

was found in 4% (including one child with polycystic kidney disease). Only one child had chronic kidney failure and presented with heavy proteinuria.

NEPHROLITHIASIS

The true incidence of renal stones among children is unknown. The only estimate is based on the number of hospital admissions related to renal stones reported by Stapleton

---

KEY POINTS: PROTEINURIA

- Asymptomatic, isolated proteinuria is a common finding on urinalysis screening examinations in children.

- Quantitation of urinary protein excretion is the most important diagnostic test.

- Presence of hematuria, edema, hypertension, or systemic disease increases the suspicion of glomerular disease and makes the diagnostic evaluation more urgent.

- Postural (orthostatic) proteinuria may be observed in adolescence as benign disease if protein is absent from the first morning voided urine specimen and the urinary protein excretion is less than 1 g/24 hr.

- Proteinuria, with or without hypertension, may also be a sign of renal scarring as a result of vesicoureteral reflux even after the reflux has resolved.

(2002): 1 in 1000 to 1 in 7600 hospital admissions. Symptoms and signs at the time of presentation differ among children depending on age. Milliner (2004) reported clinical features at the time of presentation of renal stones in 221 children. Children were grouped by age: birth to 5, 6 to 11, and 12 to 16 years. Hematuria was the primary finding at presentation in 32%, 27%, and 30%, respectively, whereas pain was the primary symptom in 18%, 36%, and 55%, respectively. Identification of calculi after radiographic study indicated by another reason or urinary tract infections was more common in the younger children. As in adults, the most sensitive radiographic technique for diagnosis of renal stone disease is helical computed tomography (CT) (Milliner, 2004).

When a stone is available for analysis, calcium-containing stones are much more common in North American children. Based on work by Stapleton (1996) and Milliner and Murphy (1993), calcium oxalate comprises 45% to 65%; calcium phosphate, 14% to 30%; struvite, 13%; cystine, 5%; uric acid, 4%; and other/mixed, 4%. Identification of the stone composition can be helpful in refining the diagnostic evaluation for underlying metabolic causes. We believe that the metabolic evaluation and treatment of children with nephrolithiasis is more aggressive compared with that in adults. Unfortunately, no multicenter, prospective studies have been performed in children to assess stone composition prevalence, underlying metabolic disorder, or the most effective method for prevention of renal stones regardless of the etiology. **Therefore, the recommendations for evaluation and management of urolithiasis in children follow good clinical judgment based on observational, single-center case series.**

Hypercalciuria

Hypercalciuria is the underlying metabolic cause in approximately one third of childhood stones (Bartosh, 2004). Hypercalciuria, which is an important cause of isolated hematuria in children, may be present before the formation of renal calculi. These children tend to have a positive family history of calcium stones, a trait suspected to be inherited in an autosomal dominant pattern. Hypercalciuria is defined as a urinary calcium excretion greater than 4 mg/kg/day while the child is well and ingesting a normal diet. Most children with hypercalciuria as the underlying cause of renal stone formation have primary, idiopathic hypercalciuria. Secondary causes of hypercalciuria include metabolic bone disease, distal renal tubular acidosis (RTA), loop diuretics, Bartter's syndromes, chloride shunt disorders (Dent disease), and any

condition causing hypercalcemia or following immobilization. In addition to the risk for renal stone formation, hypercalciuria may also increase the risk for undermineralization of bone in children (Table 111–1).

Idiopathic Hypercalciuria

The clinical diagnosis of idiopathic hypercalciuria in children is usually made when the child presents with hematuria or during the metabolic evaluation of a child with nephrolithiasis or nephrocalcinosis. In a single-center, prospective study of children with isolated hematuria, 22 of 83 children, or 27%, had hypercalciuria (Stapleton et al, 1984). Furthermore, many of these children, particularly those with gross hematuria and a family history of nephrolithiasis, went on to form renal stones (Roy et al, 1981). In a prospective, multicenter study of children aged 3 to 18 years over a period of 30 months with idiopathic, isolated hematuria, 76 of 215 (35%) children had a urinary calcium excretion of more than 4 mg/kg/day (Stapleton and the Southwest Pediatric Nephrology Study Group, 1990). Compared with those with normal urinary calcium excretion, the children with idiopathic hypercalciuria were more likely to have a family member with nephrolithiasis, more likely to have had macroscopic hematuria, and more likely to demonstrate calcium oxalate crystalluria. The mean urinary calcium excretion among those with hypercalciuria was 6.46 ± 0.48 compared with 1.7 ± 0.09 among those without idiopathic hypercalciuria. The mean ages of the groups were similar: 7.1 ± 0.6 year for those with idiopathic hypercalciuria and 8.4 ± 0.5 year in the group without idiopathic hypercalciuria. The mechanism of hematuria associated with hypercalciuria is speculated to be mechanical irritation of the uroepithelium from microaggregates of calcium oxalate crystals.

Hypercalciuria in children with hematuria is believed to be a precursor of renal stone formation. Approximately 15% of children with hypercalciuria develop renal stones over a period of 3 years, but the incidence rate varies among the single-center series. Of 184 children in the original cohort reported by Stapleton and the Southwest Pediatric Nephrology Study Group (1990) (60 with idiopathic hypercalciuria after exclusion of those on hydrochlorothiazide treatment) in whom follow-up data were available, documented renal stones occurred in 6 of the hypercalciuric children and 2 of the children with normal urinary calcium excretion. Two hypercalciuric children had renal colic but no documented stones. Using these data, the relative risk for renal stones among children with isolated hematuria and idiopathic hypercalciuria is 9.5 compared with those children with isolated hematuria and normal urinary calcium excretion. Among children with isolated hematuria with duration of at least 6 months, 20% were identified with idiopathic hypercalciuria; and of those 68 children, 49 (or 72%) later developed nephrolithiasis (Turi et al, 1989). Garcia and colleagues (1991) provided follow-up ranging from 1 to 6 years, or a mean of 3 years, in 58 children with hematuria and found that 10 later developed documented renal stones. The interval between diagnosis of idiopathic hypercalciuria/hematuria and nephrolithiasis averaged 13 months (range: 1 to 41 months). In another single-center case series of children with idiopathic hypercalciuria not as many children with renal stones as the previous groups were found: of 33 children 8 to 17 years of age at follow-up, none

Table 111–1. **Identifiable Causes for Renal Stones in Children**		
Cause	*Medical Centers*	*Surgical Centers*
Hypercalciuria	23–42%	9–27%
Infection	13–19%	2–30%
Urinary tract anomalies	35–44%	
Uric acid	3.6%	0.5–2%
Hyperoxaluria	3–11%	0–1%
Cystinuria	4–7%	0–2%
Idiopathic	19–25%	14–26%
Others	12–15%	0–8%

had symptomatic nephrolithiasis and 1 had a renal calculus identified on renal ultrasonography (Alon and Berenbom, 2000). However, in another single-center report, microcalculi as identified by ultrasonography were identified in 57% of children with idiopathic hypercalciuria at the time of diagnosis, whereas calculi were identified in 4% (Polito et al, 2000). Of note, these children did not necessarily have hematuria along with idiopathic hypercalciuria. During follow-up, 4 of 30 children (13%) developed renal stones 1 to 3 years after the diagnosis of idiopathic hypercalciuria. However, one concern about the identification of microcalculi by ultrasonography is its specificity. Therefore, the impressive prevalence of microcalculi in this series of children with idiopathic hypercalciuria may not represent the true occurrence rate.

Treatment of Idiopathic Hypercalciuria

Approaches can be divided into dietary interventions, mineral supplements, and pharmacologic treatment (Stapleton et al, 1982). Currently, treatments for idiopathic hypercalciuria include dietary sodium restriction with increase in dietary potassium intake, administration of thiazide diuretics, which reduce urinary calcium excretion, and potassium citrate, which provides a natural inhibitor for stone formation (citrate) while the potassium decreases urinary calcium excretion. No prospective studies are available regarding treatment to prevent renal stones in children with hypercalciuria.

Hyperuricosuria

Increased uric acid excretion accounts for approximately 8% of the identifiable metabolic causes for renal stones in children. Hyperuricosuria not only increases the risk for uric acid calculi but also that for calcium oxalate stones. In children, gout is uncommon and uric acid stones are more often associated with underlying inborn errors of metabolism such as Lesch-Nyhan syndrome or glycogen storage disease type I or due to myeloproliferative disorders. In addition, uric acid stones occur in 5% to 10% of children placed on a ketogenic diet for control of severe seizure disorders. In this specific population the factors predisposing to stone formation are low fluid intake, hypercalciuria, acidic urine, and low urinary citrate excretion.

Hyperoxaluria

Hyperoxaluria is found as the underlying metabolic alteration in childhood nephrolithiasis in 3% to 11%. Hyperoxaluria may be mild and idiopathic, may be associated with hyperabsorption of oxalate from the intestinal tract in association with malabsorptive disorders of the gastrointestinal tract, or may be primary (type 1 and 2) due to a genetically transmitted inborn error of metabolism involving oxalate. Primary hyperoxaluria, although rare, is associated with nephrolithiasis (calcium oxalate) in the majority of affected individuals. Both types are inherited in an autosomal recessive pattern. Three separate phenotypes have been described for primary hyperoxaluria type I, which is the more common of the two types. There is a severe infantile form with systemic oxalate deposition and renal failure; adult-onset disease, which is characterized by occasional renal stones; and the most common phenotype, which presents during childhood with nephrocalcinosis or nephrolithiasis and progressive renal insufficiency. Primary hyperoxaluria type I results from alterations in oxalate metabolism by the liver due to mutations in the gene for alanine:glyoxylate aminotransferase (AGT), leading to either reduced enzyme activity or abnormal cellular targeting of the enzyme to the mitochondria instead of the peroxisomes. Urinary excretion of oxalate is markedly increased (also the excretion of glycolate) to levels well over the upper limit of normal (<0.5 mmol/1.73 m^2/day or <45 mg/1.73 m^2/day). The mean oxalate excretion reported by Milliner and colleagues (2001) in children with primary hyperoxaluria type I was 2.19 ± 0.6 mmol/1.73 m^2/day. The presumptive diagnosis in the more common phenotype is made after demonstrating markedly elevated urinary oxalate excretion in children or adolescents with nephrolithiasis. Stones are typically composed of calcium oxalate monohydrate crystals (whewellite $CaC_2O_4:H_2O$). Treatment consists of high fluid intake to reduce urinary oxalate to a concentration less than 0.4 mmol/L, provision of stone inhibitors (sodium/potassium citrate), and occasionally use of diuretics. Pyridoxine, a cofactor for the enzyme, may reduce oxalate production in about one third of affected individuals; a trial of pyridoxine starting at 3 to 5 mg/kg/day up to a maximum of 15 mg/kg/day should be given with measurement of urinary oxalate before and after to determine individual response (Cochat and Basmaison, 2000).

Cystinuria

Cystinuria is identified as the underlying metabolic abnormality in 4% to 7% of children. The disorder results from an inherited defect in the proximal tubular brush border transporter responsible for reabsorption of cystine and the dibasic amino acids ornithine, lysine, and arginine (mnemonic: COLA). Owing to relatively poor solubility of cystine, the amino acid precipitates in the urinary space, leading to cystine stone formation. Alkalinization of the urine and increased fluid intake to reduce the concentration of cystine is the first line of treatment. Second, a class of compounds that bind to cystine by thiol groups may also be beneficial in prevention of stone disease: penicillamine or tiopronin (Thiola) lower the urinary supersaturation of cystine. The inheritance patterns of cystinuria are complex: three types have been identified, with type I being the most common (70%). Type I is an autosomal recessive mutation of the *SLC3A1* gene located on chromosome 2p, which encodes the dibasic amino acid transporter rBAT. Stone formation is common within the first decade of life; as many as 50% of known type I children developed nephrolithiasis in one case series from Quebec (Goodyear et al, 1998). The degree of hypercystinuria varies, with each subtype being the greatest in type I. The other forms of cystinuria (type II and III) are composed of various combinations, resulting in a compound heterozygous state for mutations of the gene *SLC7A9* on chromosome 19.

Other Causes

Struvite stones comprise 2% to 14% of stones in North American children and are more likely to occur in association with obstruction or malformations of the urinary tract.

Children with acute lymphoblastic leukemia are at risk for developing calcium renal stones during chemotherapy, with increased risk if corticosteroids are included in the continuation chemotherapy (Howard et al, 2003). In addition, the antimicrobial ceftriaxone, which is commonly used in acute febrile illnesses in children, has been associated with small asymptomatic renal stones (incidence of 8% after a 7-day course) (Avci et al, 2004). In addition, nephrolithiasis is not uncommon in children after kidney transplantation (Khositseth et al, 2004). A retrospective analysis of 399 children from a single center found occurrence of renal stones in 5%. Retention of suture material, recurrent urinary tract infection, hypercalciuria, and urinary stasis were identified with increased risk for post-transplant stones.

Diagnostic Approach Including Metabolic Evaluations

An algorithm for the evaluation of renal stones in children is found in Figure 111–3. History including family history and dietary history as well as physical examination with attention to growth serves as the starting point for the investigation of children with urinary calculi. Examination of the urinary sediment with attention to the presence of crystals is also recommended. A 24-hour urine collection while the child is well, infection free, and on routine diet serves as the starting point for laboratory investigation. Urinary evaluation of creatinine, calcium, oxalate, citrate, uric acid, sodium, and cystine is usually ordered. Often more than one collection is required to confirm the underlying metabolic abnormality. Normal values for urinary excretion of calcium, uric acid, and oxalate are age dependent and can be found in Table 111–2.

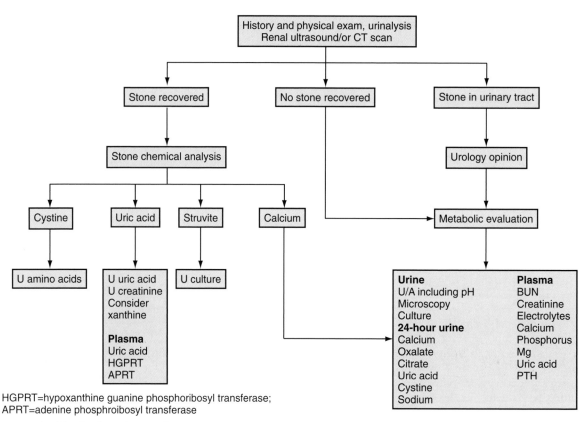

HGPRT=hypoxanthine guanine phosphoribosyl transferase;
APRT=adenine phosphroibosyl transferase

Figure 111–3. Algorithm for the evaluation of renal stones in children. APRT, adenine phosphoribosyl transferase; HGPRT, hypoxanthine guanine phosphoribosyl transferase; PTH, parathroid hormone.

Table 111-2. Normal Urinary Values for School-Aged Children

Calcium	<4 mg/kg/day (or alternative–random urine Ca/Cr <0.21)
Uric acid	<0.56 mg/dL glomerular filtration rate [(urine uric acid/urine creatinine)/plasma creatinine]
Oxalate	<50 mg/1.73 m^2/day
Citrate	>300 mg/g creatinine
Cystine	<60 mg/1.73 m^2/day
Creatinine	15-25 mg/kg/day (higher for males compared to females)
Volume	>20 mL/kg/day

RENAL PARENCHYMAL DISEASES COMMON IN CHILDHOOD
Nephrotic Syndrome

Nephrotic syndrome **is defined as edema, hypoalbuminemia, hyperlipidemia, and heavy proteinuria.** Nephrotic-range proteinuria is defined as a protein excretion greater than 40 mg/m^2/hr or, alternatively, as a random urine protein:creatinine ratio of greater than 3.0 (Hogg et al, 2000). Nephrotic syndrome may be subdivided into congenital, primary, or secondary. In general, nephrotic syndrome is a disease of the glomerular podocyte. Marked advances have been made in the past decade to elucidate the functional role of many podocyte proteins. The identification of genetic disorders of podocyte proteins has provided the basis for this understanding, starting with the Finnish-type congenital nephrotic syndrome, which is a mutation in the protein nephrin.

The most common cause of primary nephrotic syndrome in children is minimal change disease, also referred to as steroid-responsive nephrotic syndrome. Most children between the ages of 1 and 10 years of age who respond to oral corticosteroids have minimal change disease. Because most children who respond to corticosteroids with resolution of proteinuria do not undergo biopsy, the actual pathologic diagnosis is often unknown. However, the most important prognostic feature is remission of the disease with corticosteroids. Children 11 years of age or older undergo renal biopsy at the initiation of therapy in our center because they are more likely to have pathologic diagnoses other than minimal change disease.

Most children with steroid-responsive nephrotic syndrome present with edema, which is commonly mistaken for an allergic reaction until the child has generalized edema or a urinalysis is performed. Marked edema may be present with significant ascites and/or genital edema. In the absence of systemic infection, most children otherwise appear well. Diagnosis of the disease is made by demonstrating a serum albumin value of 2.5 g/dL or less, elevated plasma cholesterol and/or triglyceride levels, and nephrotic-range proteinuria (>40 mg/m^2/hr or a random urine protein:creatinine ratio >3.0) in a child with edema. The blood pressure and renal function are usually normal, and the urinalysis has minimal hematuria and no cellular casts. Fatty casts and oval fat bodies are often seen on microscopy.

Once the presumptive diagnosis is made, oral prednisone or prednisolone is started at a dosage of 60 mg/m^2/day (Mendoza and Tune, 1992). Dietary salt restriction is another important component of treatment. This high-dose daily treatment is continued for a minimum of 4 weeks after the initial diagnosis, followed by 4 weeks of 40 mg/m^2/day on alternate days and then a gradual taper using alternate-day dosing. Most children respond with remission of proteinuria (defined as negative or trace for 3 consecutive days by urinary Albustix) within 4 weeks. Approximately two thirds of children have a relapse. Relapses are treated with high daily doses of corticosteroids until remission and then tapered. Some children require additional therapy if relapses are frequent or corticosteroids cannot be tapered without relapse. Cytotoxic agents (cyclophosphamide or chlorambucil) or cyclosporine are the most frequently used immunosuppressive agents after corticosteroids.

Associated complications of steroid-responsive nephrotic syndrome are increased risk for infections due to the urinary loss of opsonins, with particular risk for spontaneous bacterial peritonitis. In addition, the acute nephrotic syndrome is characterized by a relatively hypercoagulable state because urinary loss of protein favors the anticoagulant factors. Although rare, children with nephrotic syndrome may have venous thromboses during relapse. Therefore, placement of central venous catheters or femoral venipuncture is to be avoided. Renal insufficiency as an acute or late complication of this type of nephrotic syndrome is rare.

Focal Segmental Glomerulosclerosis

Focal segmental glomerulosclerosis is the second most common cause of primary nephrotic syndrome in children (Bonilla-Felix et al, 1999). The name describes the most striking pathologic feature—that of segmental sclerosis of some glomeruli. The cause of the condition is unknown and is likely to be multifactorial. **Focal segmental glomerulosclerosis is more common among older children and African American children and is much less likely to respond to corticosteroids.** In addition, focal segmental glomerulosclerosis may not present as all of the features of nephrotic syndrome but rather with isolated proteinuria, normal serum albumin, or only a few features of the nephrotic syndrome. The diagnosis is made in (1) children who either present with nephrotic syndrome but fail to respond to corticosteroids (and undergo renal biopsy), (2) children older than the age of 10 who present with nephrotic syndrome (most pediatric centers perform renal biopsy in older children with nephrotic syndrome), or (3) children with moderate to heavy proteinuria without all of the features of nephrotic syndrome. Only 20% to 25% of children with focal segmental glomerulosclerosis–associated nephrotic syndrome have favorable response to prednisone. Despite the less than optimal response to corticosteroids, evidence-based analyses still recommend them as the initial therapy. Some favor the use of high doses of intravenously administered methylprednisolone (Mendoza protocol) (Mendoza and Tune, 1992). However, the efficacy of this protocol is questioned by some; therefore, it has not been universally accepted. It seems to be more efficacious in younger, non–African American children. If there is failure to respond after 2 months, cyclosporine has the most promise to induce remission, if only partial in nature. Diseases such as focal segmental glomerulosclerosis often lead to end-stage renal disease if heavy proteinuria persists. Nonimmunosuppressive agents such as angiotensin-converting enzyme (ACE) inhibitors or angiotensin receptor blockers, as well as lipid-lowering agents, are used in combination in an attempt to slow the progressive nature of the disease. **Unfortunately, focal segmental glomerulosclerosis may recur after renal allograft in as many as 50% of patients.**

Membranous Nephropathy

The diagnosis of membranous nephropathy is made after renal biopsy, because the diagnosis is dependent on demonstration of thickening of the glomerular basement membrane as a result of immune deposits in a subepithelial location (Makker, 2004). Children may present with proteinuria or nephrotic syndrome. Membranous nephropathy may be primary, in which an underlying disorder is not identified, or secondary, in which a condition resulting in immune complex formation is present. Secondary forms include hepatitis B, congenital syphilis, systemic lupus erythematosus, and some malignancies. Membranous nephropathy is more likely to be secondary in children but is a much less common cause of nephrotic syndrome in children (2% to 6%) compared with adults (25% to 40%). Microscopic hematuria is common, yet hypertension is rare in children with membranous nephropathy. Outcome is variable: approximately 20% will progress to end-stage renal disease, 40% achieve remission, and 40% have continued active disease. Treatment is similar to that described for focal segmental glomerulosclerosis: immunosuppressive drugs in combination with renoprotective agents.

Congenital Nephrotic Syndrome

Congenital nephrotic syndrome is usually defined as the onset of symptoms either before or shortly after birth. There are several pathologic subtypes (Holmberg et al, 2004). This discussion will focus on the Finnish type, which is an autosomal recessive condition with common occurrence in Finland (1 in 8200 live births). Premature birth and large placental weight are characteristic of the disorder. Massive protein loss occurs, leading to the severe hypoalbuminemia (often <1 g/dL), hypogammaglobulinemia, and severe hyperlipidemia. Mutations of the gene *NPHS1*, the gene for the protein nephrin, have been identified in infants with congenital nephrotic syndrome, with two major variants, one in 90% of Finnish patients with the disorder: Fin-major and Fin-minor. Nephrin is a protein component of the podocyte slit diaphragm, and its absence leads to alterations in the pores that impede filtration of protein. Initial treatment of congenital nephrotic syndrome of the Finnish type includes aggressive replacement of albumin and immunoglobulins, nutritional support, and early unilateral or bilateral nephrectomy, followed by dialysis and transplantation. Post-transplant nephrotic syndrome may occur as a result of antinephrin antibodies. Other causes of congenital nephrotic syndrome include diffuse mesangial sclerosis and Denys-Drash syndrome (triad of male pseudohermaphroditism, Wilms' tumor, and progressive glomerulopathy).

Nephritic Syndromes

Glomerulonephritis is usually divided into acute and chronic forms, although at presentation it may be difficult to differentiate acute presentation of a chronic disorder from an acute, more self-limited one. **Nephritic diseases as opposed to the nephrotic disorders are more likely to have (1) gross hematuria, the classically tea-colored urine; (2) hypertension and other signs of excess intravascular volume; and (3) renal dysfunction at presentation, with signs of immune activation, such as hypocomplementemia.** Glomerulonephritis involves all three cellular components of the glomerulus; however, the endothelial and mesangial cells are the primary sites of injury. The major diseases of childhood are briefly discussed.

Postinfectious Glomerulonephritis

Postinfectious glomerulonephritis, usually occurring after group A β-hemolytic streptococcal pharyngitis or pyoderma, is the most common cause of acute glomerulonephritis in children. There is a latency period of 7 to 21 days after a group A β-hemolytic streptococcal infection and the acute phase of glomerulonephritis, with common presenting symptoms of edema and cola-colored urine. **The diagnostic studies include a positive antistreptolysin-O or streptozyme titer and a decreased serum complement (C3) concentration.** The acute phase lasts approximately 2 weeks and is characterized by fluid retention, hypertension, significant hematuria (often macroscopic), and proteinuria. Varying degrees of acute renal insufficiency with oliguria, even anuria requiring intermittent dialysis, may be seen. Control of hypertension, management of electrolyte and fluid balance, and treatment of renal functional impairment are necessary during the acute phase of the illness. Complete recovery of renal function can be expected in more than 90% of cases, even in those that have a protracted clinical course requiring dialysis. Microscopic hematuria and minimal proteinuria may persist for 3 to 6 months. C3 concentrations usually become normal within 2 months after disease onset. Proteinuria that persists for 12 months after disease onset may require a renal biopsy to assess the degree of renal histologic damage. Biopsy is not required for diagnosis if the clinical picture is consistent and the previously mentioned serologic abnormalities are present. The characteristic findings on biopsy are marked cellular proliferation within the glomerulus due to infiltration of polymorphonuclear leukocytes and monocytes and the associated stimulation and proliferation of endothelial and mesangial cells. Electron microscopy in classic cases demonstrates humplike dense deposits.

It is worth mentioning in this section that some cases of poststreptococcal glomerulonephritis could present after the acute phase with asymptomatic microhematuria because it may persist for up to 12 months; unless the onset was within 6 weeks, the associated hypocomplementemia is no longer present.

IgA Nephropathy/Henoch-Schönlein Purpura

Although IgA nephropathy is a chronic glomerular disease and Henoch-Schönlein purpura is an acute glomerulonephritis, they are discussed together because of (1) the potential for there to be affected members with both within the same family and for an individual with Henoch-Schönlein purpura to evolve into IgA nephropathy; (2) the similar nature of their pathologic appearance (predominant deposition of IgA and mesangial proliferation); and (3) their presumed common etiology: abnormal glycosylation of the IgA molecule (Delos Santos and Wyatt, 2004).

IgA nephropathy (also referred to as Berger's disease) most often presents as hematuria with evidence of a glomerular source of the hematuria (red blood cell casts or dysmorphic red blood cells) (Davin and Weening, 1999). Proteinuria may or may not be present. The classic childhood presentation of IgA nephropathy is macroscopic hematuria (77% of children) in association with a respiratory tract infection or pharyngitis. Although anti-streptococcal titers may be elevated, the C3 levels are normal. In addition, the hematuria occurs during but not after the respiratory infection. The diagnosis of IgA nephropathy is based on renal biopsy: variable degrees of mesangial cell proliferation along with deposition of IgA as the predominant immunoglobulin are typical. Progression to end-stage renal disease is not uncommon. From a series of children reported by Wyatt and associates (1995) from two pediatric referral centers, 15% will reach end-stage renal disease after 10 years and 30% after 20 years. Alternatively, nearly half will experience apparent remission of the disease at some point, but the silent nature of the disease in adults warrants long-term follow-up. Treatment is usually based on the severity of disease at diagnosis and includes renoprotective agents such as ACE inhibitors or fish oil, corticosteroids, and, more recently, mycophenolate mofetil.

Henoch-Schönlein purpura is a systemic vasculitis that involves the skin, gastrointestinal tract, and joints and may also involve the kidney (Rai et al, 1999). A palpable purpuric rash is the most often identifiable physical finding. Children also present with abdominal pain and refusal to bear weight due to arthralgias of the knees or ankles. Renal involvement, if present, is usually not evident until several weeks after the initial symptoms. Whereas IgA nephropathy is more common in the second and third decades of life, the peak age for presentation of Henoch-Schönlein purpura is 4 to 6 years of age. Henoch-Schönlein purpura is considered an acute glomerulonephritis. Renal biopsy may demonstrate segmental necrosis of glomeruli or crescent formation. Treatment has not been rigorously studied but typically includes renoprotective agents and, in more aggressive Henoch-Schönlein purpura nephritis, immunosuppressive drugs.

Lupus Nephritis

The major renal manifestation of systemic lupus erythematosus (SLE) is glomerular disease. **The primary symptoms leading to the diagnosis of renal disease in children with SLE are proteinuria, microscopic hematuria, hypertension, and mild renal insufficiency** (Cameron, 1994). SLE is an autoimmune disease that has the potential to affect numerous organ systems, the kidney being one of the most important with respect to long-term prognosis. Children with SLE are more likely than adults to have renal involvement. The peak age at onset is 14 years, around the time of puberty, and females are more likely to be affected than males (M:F = 4.4:1) Half of children with lupus nephritis have nephrotic syndrome and/or renal insufficiency at diagnosis. SLE is divided into classes based on histopathology (the prevalence of each from several biopsy series in children is given in parentheses): class I, normal (6%); class II, mesangial proliferative (19%); class III, focal endocapillary proliferative (23%); class IV, diffuse endocapillary proliferative (43%); and class V, membranous (9%).

Both C3 and C4 are commonly decreased during acute illness. Abnormalities common at presentation in children with lupus nephritis are fever (78%), arthralgia (75%), rash (68%), weight loss (40%), Coombs' positive anemia (48%), leukopenia (47%), thrombocytopenia (25%), coagulopathy (27%), and renal disease (82%).

Primary therapy for lupus nephritis is based on the class or severity at diagnosis and usually consists of corticosteroids plus additional cytotoxic therapy. Although no clinical trials have been performed in children, therapy is based on adult data, which show that the best long-term renal preservation for class IV nephritis is achieved with cyclophosphamide plus corticosteroids. Monthly pulses of cyclophosphamide are given during the 6-month induction phase followed by every-3-month doses up to 2 years. More recently, mycophenolate mofetil has been shown to have equal efficacy at 2 years compared with cyclophosphamide. Renoprotective therapy is a common adjunct in lupus nephritis, and many children require more than one antihypertensive medication during therapy. Long-term follow-up studies of childhood-onset lupus nephritis are lacking. From the case series at Guy's Hospital in London, of 78 children, 15% had progressed to end-stage renal disease, 6% were dead, 27% had remission of renal disease (some still on treatment), and 36% continued to have signs of renal disease on therapy (follow-up ranged from 1 to 26 years).

Hemolytic-Uremic Syndrome

Hemolytic-uremic syndrome is defined by the triad of (1) hemolytic microangiopathic anemia in association with (2) thrombocytopenia and (3) renal insufficiency. In children, hemolytic-uremic syndrome may be the typical form, which is associated with diarrhea, or an atypical form (Pickering et al, 1994; Loirat and Taylor, 2004). This discussion will focus on the typical diarrhea-associated hemolytic-uremic syndrome, which in North America is secondary to primary infection with enterotoxic *Escherichia coli*. The enteropathic *E. coli* are usually contracted through ingestion of food contaminated with bovine feces: ground beef, water supplies, or vegetables/fruits. Person-to-person spread is also possible. Specific serotypes of *E. coli* (O157:H7) produce a verotoxin that binds to enterocytes and gains access to the microcirculation. After endocytosis into vessels, the toxin causes endothelial injury, particularly in the kidney, by inhibition of protein synthesis by the endothelial cell. The diagnosis of hemolytic-uremic syndrome is based on clinical features at presentation, because renal biopsies are not usually performed in the classic, diarrhea-associated hemolytic-uremic syndrome. Platelet-fibrin thrombi within glomeruli cause ischemia of glomerular capillaries associated with mesangiolysis. Severe forms are also characterized by cortical necrosis as larger arterioles may become involved.

The prodrome of diarrhea-associated hemolytic-uremic syndrome is enterocolitis, typically bloody diarrhea (70% of cases), followed by transient improvement and then 4 to 7 days later the onset of pallor (anemia), general malaise, oligoanuria, fluid overload, and hypertension. Serious neurologic involvement, characterized by seizures, encephalopathy, and coma, may be present in 20% of cases. Although the severity of renal involvement is not related to the severity of anemia, it does appear to be related to the severity of the gastrointestinal prodrome. Efforts to isolate *E. coli* O157:H7 from stool of affected children should be made, and recovery is better when samples are obtained within 6 days from onset of diarrhea. Cases are reported to the state health department.

Treatment of diarrhea-associated hemolytic-uremic syndrome is supportive. Antibiotic therapy for *E. coli*–associated enterocolitis is discouraged because there may be increased risk to develop hemolytic-uremic syndrome possibly owing to release of the bacterial toxin. A potential new therapy based on binding of gut toxin, a novel approach to prevention of hemolytic-uremic syndrome, has yet to be clinically proven to prevent hemolytic-uremic syndrome. Careful attention must be paid to fluid balance and electrolyte disturbances. Hyperkalemia, which occurs because of increased release of potassium during red blood cell lysis, is further complicated by acidosis and decreased GFR. Packed red blood cell transfusions are indicated when the hemoglobin drops to less than 7 g/dL, but platelet transfusions are discouraged. Dialysis may be required during the oliguric phase, but early dialysis does not appear to improve outcome. Mortality associated with hemolytic-uremic syndrome is 1% to 2%, and irreversible renal failure occurs in 5%. Late sequelae of hemolytic-uremic syndrome including proteinuria, hypertension, and renal insufficiency have been reported in as many as 30% of survivors. Late sequelae are more likely in individuals with anuria for more than 1 week or who require more than 2 weeks of dialysis.

Other, non–diarrhea-associated forms of hemolytic-uremic syndrome that may occur in children but are not discussed in this brief review include (1) *Streptococcus pneumoniae*–associated hemolytic-uremic syndrome, (2) complement factor H deficiency, (3) abnormal von Willebrand protease inhibitor, (4) abnormalities of vitamin B_{12} metabolism, (5) calcineurin inhibitor–associated hemolytic-uremic syndrome, and (6) post–bone marrow transplant associated hemolytic-uremic syndrome.

RENAL TUBULAR DISORDERS

Disorders of tubular function may be genetic (or congenital) or acquired. They are organized according to the portion of the renal tubule most affected (Gregory and Schwartz, 1998).

Proximal Tubular Disorders

The proximal tubule is responsible for reabsorption of the bulk of filtrate presented to the tubule for processing. Water, sodium, potassium, bicarbonate, glucose, phosphate, amino acids, uric acid, and small molecular weight proteins are all reabsorbed in this segment. The transport of the majority of solute depends on a favorable sodium gradient created by the basolateral Na^+-K^+-ATPase, which consumes adenosine triphosphate, and is the major energy requiring process in the proximal tubule. **Disorders that interfere with energy production by the proximal tubule may result in generalized dysfunction, called Fanconi syndrome. Isolated transport disorders of the proximal tubule are less common.**

Fanconi syndrome is not a specific disorder but the combination of tubular loss of numerous substrates and may be caused by inherited disorders or acquired diseases. Patients usually present with polyuria, signs of dehydration, or

Table 111–3.	Causes of Fanconi Syndrome

Inborn errors of metabolism
    Cystinosis
    Galactosemia
    Hereditary fructose intolerance
    Tyrosinemia
    Wilson's disease
    Lowe's syndrome
    Cytochrome C deficiency
    Glycogen storage disease type I
Intoxications
    Heavy metals: lead, cadmium
    Glue sniffing
Medications
    Ifosfamide
    Gentamicin
Other
    Multiple myeloma
    Sjögren's syndrome

symptoms of electrolyte depletion. These include rickets (hypophosphatemia, calcitriol deficiency), muscle weakness (hypokalemia), growth failure (acidosis), or constipation (dehydration). Hypouricemia is also commonly found in children with Fanconi syndrome. A list of causes of the Fanconi syndrome is presented in Table 111–3.

Treatment consists of replacement of electrolytes lost, such as Na^+/K^+ citrate, Na^+/K^+ phosphate, and active vitamin D (calcitriol) since 1α-hydroxylation takes place in the proximal tubule. Other treatments to reduce urinary losses such as indomethacin may also be added. Children who present during infancy or early childhood are more likely to have an inborn error of metabolism. Great effort should be undertaken to identify the underlying cause because many of the metabolic disorders have specific treatments available to prevent further renal damage or serious sequelae. For example, cystinosis, a defect of the lysosomal cysteine transporter, may be treated with cysteamine, which allows the digress of the accumulated amino acid via the disulfide cotransporter. If provided within the first 2 years of life, early renal failure may be prevented.

Disorders of the Distal Tubule

Distal Renal Tubular Acidosis

Distal RTA usually presents in infancy with polyuria, vomiting, dehydration, failure to thrive, hypokalemia, normal anion gap acidosis, and inappropriately alkaline urine during systemic acidosis. Distal RTA may be inherited as autosomal dominant, which is the less severe form, or autosomal recessive, the more severe, infantile form, which is often accompanied by nephrocalcinosis and may progress to renal insufficiency. The infantile form is also often associated with sensorineural hearing loss (Karet, 2002).

Distal RTA is characterized by hypercalciuria and hypocitraturia, which likely explains the high prevalence of nephrocalcinosis and renal stones among individuals with the disorder. In the α-intercalated cell of the cortical collecting duct, hydrogen ions are actively secreted by the H^+-ATPase, which is a multimeric pump in the superfamily of proton ATPases. To maintain intracellular pH, bicarbonate is exchanged for chloride at the basolateral cell membrane. Mutations in the anion exchanger have been reported to account for both autosomal dominant and recessive distal RTA (Nicoletta and Schwartz, 2004). Recently mutations in the β subunit and the noncatalytic subunit of the proton ATPase have been described in individuals with distal RTA (Karet, 2002).

Treatment of RTA consists of supplementation of base in the form of sodium bicarbonate or a combination of sodium and potassium citrate divided into three to four daily doses. Patients with type I typically require 2 to 3 mEq/kg/day, whereas those with proximal RTA usually need in excess of 10 mEq/kg/day.

Bartter's Syndromes

This syndrome, which was first described in 1962 in children with hypokalemia, metabolic alkalosis, polyuria, and growth failure, is now known to consist of a group of transport disorders (Rodriquez-Soriano, 1998). A Bartter-like syndrome, known originally as Gitelman's syndrome, typically presents later in life with less severe systemic effects. The advances in molecular biology of renal transporters over the past 2 decades have allowed nephrologists to understand the basics of this group of disorders. First, they may be compared and contrasted according to their clinical features and, second, by the membrane transporter mutation most often associated with the clinical syndrome. Unfortunately, there is some overlap, because affected individuals within the same kindred have variable degrees of clinical expression. The primary defect is potassium and chloride loss. Hypercalciuria, which is found in the classic Bartter's syndrome, may result in nephrocalcinosis.

Neonatal Bartter's Syndrome

Neonatal Bartter's syndrome is the most severe and may present prior to birth with polyhydramnios, resulting in preterm delivery. Polyuria is usually severe. Defects causing the neonatal form include mutations in the loop $Na^+/K^+/2Cl^-$ cotransporter and a renal potassium channel (ROMK). The disorder is similar to that encountered with use of loop diuretics. Early nephrocalcinosis is also found as a result of significant hypercalciuria.

Bartter's Syndrome

Symptoms are usually present within the first 2 years of life, but not necessarily from birth. They include polyuria, salt craving, constipation (sign of dehydration), and muscle weakness/cramping. Hypokalemia and hypochloremic metabolic alkalosis are usually present. Hypomagnesemia may be observed in 20% to 50% of patients. Increased urinary losses of sodium, potassium, and chloride are demonstrated. Treatment is supplementation with potassium chloride in the range of 5 mEq/kg/day and sometimes use of prostaglandin synthetase inhibitors (indomethacin) to reduce urinary losses of fluid and electrolytes.

Gitelman's Syndrome

This syndrome usually presents as muscle weakness or tetany, often with vomiting, abdominal pain, and fever. Hypokalemia, hypomagnesemia, and alkalosis are seen. Hypocalciuria is a unique feature distinguishing this syndrome from the Bartter's syndromes. Gitelman's syndrome results from mutations in the distal tubule and resembles the effects of thiazide-like diuretics. Mutations in the distal tubular Na^+-Cl^- cotransporter have been described. Treatment consists of magnesium repletion and occasionally supplementation with potassium chloride.

KEY POINTS: TUBULAR DISORDERS

■ Polyuria, polydipsia, and poor growth are common presenting complaints in children with tubular diseases.

■ Hypokalemia is common to both Bartter's syndrome and RTA; however, Bartter's syndrome is characterized by alkalosis.

■ Hypernatremia is typically the presenting electrolyte disturbance in nephrogenic diabetes insipidus.

■ Nephrocalcinosis may complicate RTA and Bartter's syndrome.

NEPHROGENIC DIABETES INSIPIDUS

Nephrogenic diabetes insipidus is characterized by polyuria, excessive thirst, hypernatremia, and the inability to concentrate the urine due to a defect in the renal tubular response to vasopressin. The most common form is X-linked recessive mutation of the vasopressin receptor. A less common autosomal form (both recessive and dominant) is caused by mutations of the aquaporin-2 water channel gene (Van Lieburg et al, 1999).

Diagnosis of nephrogenic diabetes insipidus occurs at a median age of 9 months and mean age of 25 months; however, the majority of cases are diagnosed in the first year of life. The most common signs and symptoms are vomiting/anorexia, failure to thrive, fever, constipation, polydipsia, and developmental delay. Demonstration of insufficiently concentrated urine (UOsm < 300) in the presence of hypernatremic dehydration is sufficient for diagnosis in most children. Treatment with a combination of hydrochlorothiazide and the potassium-sparing diuretic amiloride reduces urinary volume and results in improved polydipsia and food intake. Urologic complications related to the massive urinary flow rate include severe hydronephrosis, urinary retention, nocturnal enuresis, or transient ureteric dilation.

CARE OF THE CHILD WITH CHRONIC RENAL INSUFFICIENCY AND END-STAGE RENAL DISEASE

Chronic renal insufficiency is defined as having a decreased GFR up to the time that renal replacement therapy is initiated (defined as end-stage renal disease). Most centers caring for children with chronic renal insufficiency are unable to measure true GFR; therefore they estimate creatinine clearance with the Schwartz formula. The method for estimation

Table 111–4. **Estimation of the Glomerular Filtration Rate by Creatinine Clearance Using the Schwartz Formula**

Age <18 mo	$\dfrac{\text{Height (cm)} \times 0.45}{\text{Creatinine (mg/dL)}}$
Age >18 mo and weight <70 kg	$\dfrac{\text{Height (cm)} \times 0.55}{\text{Creatinine (mg/dL)}}$
Male with weight >70 kg	$\dfrac{\text{Height (cm)} \times 0.70}{\text{Creatinine (mg/dL)}}$

Table 111–5. **Causes of Renal Insufficiency in Children**

Cause	%
Obstructive uropathy	23
Hypoplasia/dysplasia	18
Chronic glomerulonephritis	9.7
Reflux nephropathy	8.7
Focal segmental glomerulosclerosis	7.7
Polycystic kidney disease	4.1
Eagle-Barrett	3.2
Hemolytic-uremic syndrome	2.3
Cystinosis	1.5
Wilms' tumor	0.4
Diabetes	0.2

From Seikaly MG, Ho PL, Emmett L, et al: Chronic renal insufficiency in children: The 2001 annual report of the NAPRTCS. Pediatr Nephrol 2003;18:796-804.

is contained in Table 111–4. In children, the stages of chronic renal insufficiency were defined 2 decades ago as mild, moderate, or severe. Unfortunately, these do not coincide with the new stages of chronic kidney failure recently outlined for adults. A recent position paper proposes that the newer adult classification be adopted for use in children: stage 1: GFR greater than or equal to 90 (kidney damage with normal or increased GFR); stage 2: GFR 60 to 89 (kidney damage with mild decrease in GFR); stage 3: GFR 30 to 59 (moderate reduction of GFR); stage 4: GFR 15 to 29 (severe reduction in GFR); and stage 5: GFR < 15 (kidney failure) Hogg et al, 2003). The incidence of chronic renal insufficiency among children less than 16 years of age is estimated to be 1.5 to 3 per million.

Causes of Chronic Renal Insufficiency in Children

The primary causes of kidney failure in children aged birth to 18 years are listed in Table 111–5. Unlike in adults, congenital diseases are a very common cause of kidney failure in children, particularly if the child reaches end-stage renal disease within the first decade of life (Andredi et al, 2005). Care of the child with chronic renal insufficiency includes (1) renoprotective efforts to slow the progression of kidney failure, (2) correction of the metabolic disturbances associated with chronic renal insufficiency, (3) provision of nutritional/hormonal support for growth failure, and (4) preparation for renal replacement therapy, preferably renal transplantation.

In the setting of reduced nephron mass, the tendency for renal function to decline as a child grows involves factors independent of the initiating disease. Mechanisms for progressive renal damage include hemodynamic factors, such as hypertension, and metabolic factors such as hyperlipidemia. Clinical factors that influence progression include the severity of initial renal damage, age at the onset of disease, and the presence of hypertension. Treatment with renoprotective agents such as ACE inhibitors or angiotensin receptor blockers and lipid-lowering agents has become common in children with chronic renal insufficiency.

Correction of underlying metabolic disturbances requires monitoring electrolytes, calcium, phosphorus, parathyroid hormone, hemoglobin, and iron levels (Warady et al, 1999). The earliest detectable abnormality in chronic renal insufficiency is hyperparathyroidism. This results from phosphate retention and insufficient calcitriol synthesis. Plasma calcium and phosphorus levels are usually normal in early chronic renal insufficiency. Treatment includes provision of calcitriol or reduction of dietary phosphorus intake. Metabolic acidosis is treated with sodium bicarbonate or sodium citrate (2 to 3 mEq/kg/day) to maintain normal serum bicarbonate levels, which impact growth and bone health. Once hyperphosphatemia occurs, dietary phosphate restriction and provision of phosphate binders (calcium carbonate, calcium acetate, or sevelamer) is begun. Correction of anemia with iron supplementation along with erythropoietin administration is recommended once the hemoglobin is less than 11 g/dL.

Linear growth failure is common in children with chronic renal insufficiency and is related to numerous factors. Nutrition assessment is necessary to ensure adequate intake of calories, because appetite may be affected. In younger children, supplemental tube feedings are often needed. When all other metabolic and nutritional needs have been corrected, initiation of recombinant human growth hormone injections has become the standard for children whose height percentile is 2 or more standard deviations from the mean or in children who have dropped two height percentile categories.

Preparation for renal replacement therapy should be considered once the estimated clearance is 25 mL/min/1.73 m^2 or less. This includes consideration of bladder issues or potential need for nephrectomy before the time of transplantation. Other factors to be addressed are provision of necessary immunizations, the family's ability to comply with treatments, potential living donors, cardiovascular health, and examination for other risk factors. Although the indications for initiation of dialysis are not concrete, they include inability to maintain metabolic control with medical treatments, symptomatic uremia, and renal clearance less than 10 mL/min/1.73 m^2.

Initiation of dialysis in children involves counseling the family on the choice of modality—either peritoneal dialysis or hemodialysis—including the potential complications of these therapies. In children, transplantation is the preferred renal replacement option, but for some children it may not be the immediate option because of the acute nature of their presentation, social issues, medical contraindications, and, occasionally, urologic issues. In contrast to adult end-stage renal disease, children are much more likely to receive peritoneal dialysis, with 60% of the current dialysis cohort of the North American Pediatric Renal Transplant Cooperative Study (NAPRTCS) database on peritoneal dialysis. In the pediatric patient on dialysis, school attendance, growth and development, and impact on the family are major issues that differentiate them from adults.

SUMMARY

In this chapter we have discussed some of the more common renal conditions encountered during childhood, with emphasis on how they compare with those seen in adulthood. Because hematuria, proteinuria, and nephrolithiasis commonly pose diagnostic dilemmas, their presentation and diagnostic evaluation have been discussed in detail. Glomerular and tubular disorders were briefly discussed. Because of the limited space, hypertension and polycystic kidney disease were not discussed. Often, adult diseases have their origin in childhood and many childhood diseases continue into young adult life. Preservation of renal function in the child with renal disease is a primary goal of pediatric nephrologists and urologists.

SUGGESTED READINGS

Bartosh SM: Medical management of pediatric stone disease. Urol Clin North Am 2004;31:575-587.

Cameron JS: Lupus nephritis in childhood and adolescence. Pediatr Nephrol 1994;8:230-249.

Delos Santos NM, Wyatt RJ: Pediatric IgA nephropathies: Clinical aspects and therapeutic approaches. Am J Kidney Dis 2004;24:269-286.

Gregory MJ, Schwartz GJ: Diagnosis and treatment of renal tubular disorders. Am J Kidney Dis 1998;18:317-329.

Hogg RJ, Portman RJ, Milliner D, et al: Evaluation and management of proteinuria and the nephritic syndrome in children: Recommendations from the Pediatric Nephrology Panel established at the National Kidney Foundation Conference on Proteinuria, Albuminuria, Risk, Assessment, Detection and Elimination (PARADE). Pediatrics 2000;105:1242-1249.

Loirat C, Taylor CM: Hemolytic uremic syndromes. In Avner ED, Harmon WE, Niaudet P (eds): Pediatric Nephrology, 5th ed. Philadelphia, Lippincott Williams & Wilkins, 2004, pp 887-915.

Mendoza SA, Tune BM: Treatment of childhood nephrotic syndrome. J Am Soc Nephrol 1992;3:889-894.

Meyers KEC: Evaluation of hematuria in children. Urol Clin North Am 2004;31:559-573.

Rodriquez-Soriano J: Bartter and related syndromes: The puzzle is almost solved. Pediatr Nephrol 1998;12:315-327.

Van Lieburg AF, Knoers AM, Monnen LAH: Clinical presentation and follow-up of 30 patients with congenital nephrogenic diabetes insipidus. J Am Soc Nephrol 1999;10:1958-1964.

Warady BA, Alexander SA, Watkins S, et al: Optimal care of the pediatric end-stage renal disease patient on dialysis. Am J Kidney Dis 1999;33:567-583.

112 Infection and Inflammation of the Pediatric Genitourinary Tract

LINDA M. DAIRIKI SHORTLIFFE, MD

Inflammation of many kinds may occur in the urinary tract of a child, but the most common is bacterial. In this era as we manage urinary tract inflammation and infection we should be mindful of the scientific advances that have improved our management of infections, but we must also understand issues of (1) prenatal fetal anatomy, (2) issues of infection prevention versus treatment, and (3) medical globalism.

Recognition that bacteriuria may cause renal parenchymal and functional loss has prompted recommendations for rapid diagnosis and evaluation of urinary tract infection (UTI) and the use of new genitourinary imaging techniques and tests. In infants, UTI is a common cause of fever and may be the most common cause of renal parenchymal loss. For this reason, the goal of managing UTIs in children is based upon identifying and modifying, if possible, factors that may increase risk of renal parenchymal and functional loss from the time of the index infection forward. This chapter focuses upon host and bacterial mechanisms by which bacteria gain access to the bladder and kidney, the management and evaluation of first and recurrent UTIs, the possible short- and long-term complications of UTI, and potential factors that may identify a child with risk for bacteriuria or its potential complications. Possible means of preventing or limiting morbidity from UTI and the importance of understanding socially responsible management of UTI risk are discussed.

EPIDEMIOLOGY OF PEDIATRIC URINARY TRACT INFECTIONS

Only during the first year of life do males contract more UTIs than females (Asscher et al, 1973; Winberg et al, 1974), and during that period **uncircumcised boys have up to 10 times the risk of circumcised boys of having a UTI** (Rushton and Majd, 1992; Wiswell and Hachey, 1993). By age 1, 2.7% of boys and 0.7% of girls have had bacteriuria (Wettergren et al, 1980). Although this incidence declines below 1% in school-age boys (ranging between 0.03% and 1.2%), it rises to 1% to 3% in school-age girls (Asscher, 1975; Savage, 1975; Bailey, 1979), and sexually active females have even more UTIs than sexually inactive females (Kunin and McCormack, 1968).

Data from the U.S. Healthcare Cost and Utilization Project (HCUP) show that approximately 51 per 100,000 children and 174 per 100,000 infants (children younger than 3 months) are hospitalized annually with UTI; about 18 to 20 per 100,000 of these are coded for pyelonephritis (Freedman, 2004). Overall, girls were hospitalized 2.5 times more than boys. UTIs accounted for 2.4% to 2.8% of physician visits for children with commercial insurance or Medicaid, and National Ambulatory Medical Care Survey data suggest that UTIs account for

Table 112-1. Criteria for the Diagnosis of Urinary Tract Infection

Method of Collection	Colony Count (Pure Culture)	Probability of Infection (%)
Suprapubic aspiration	Gram-negative bacilli: any number	>99%
	Gram-positive cocci: more than a few thousand	
Transurethral catheterization	>10^6	95%; Infection likely suspicious; repeat infection unlikely
	10^4-10^6	
	10^3-10^4	
	<10^3	
Clean void		
Boy	>10^4	Infection likely
Girl	3 Specimens ≥ 10^6	95%
	2 Specimens ≥ 10^6	90%
	1 Specimen ≥ 10^6	80%
	$5 \times 10^4 - 10^6$	Suspicious, repeat
	$10^4 - 5 \times 10^4$	Symptomatic: suspicious, repeat
		Asymptomatic: infection unlikely
	<10^4	Infection unlikely

From American Academy of Pediatrics. Committee on Quality Improvement. Subcommittee on Urinary Tract Infection: Practice parameter: The diagnosis, treatment, and evaluation of the initial urinary tract infection in febrile infants and young children. Pediatrics 1999;103:847, Table 2.

0.7% of all pediatric office visits, thus documenting the heavy burden of visits related to UTI (Freedman, 2004).

Given an average of 40,000 admissions for UTI per year (HCUP data) and a mean cost of $4500 per child for each UTI admission (National Association of Children's Hospitals and Related Institutions [NACHRI] data, 1999, 2001), the financial cost for hospitalization of children with UTI alone is $180 million a year without the ambulatory visits that account for the majority of UTI treatment in this country (Freedman, 2004).

Definition of Infection

What is a "significant" clinical UTI is controversial. The urinary tract is normally sterile. Whether "colonization" of the urinary tract occurs (benign bacteriuria) and whether colonization is true infection are debatable. Specimen contamination can occur, and specimens are often difficult to interpret.

The collection technique by which the urinary specimen is obtained is related to the reliability for UTI diagnosis (Table 112–1) (Hellerstein, 1982).

Classification of Urinary Infections

UTIs have been classified in many ways: complicated versus uncomplicated, upper versus lower tract, persistent infections versus reinfections, and symptomatic versus asymptomatic. For practical purposes, pediatric UTIs are most simply cate-gorized into two types: first infections and recurrent or other infections (Fig. 112–1). These recurrent infections may then be categorized as (1) unresolved bacteriuria during therapy, (2) bacterial persistence at an anatomic site, and (3) reinfections (Stamey, 1975). Categorizing pediatric UTIs in this way can be justified on a clinical basis. As discussed here, first childhood UTIs are considered complicated because of the evaluation and management implications.

A UTI may be unresolved because it is treated inadequately because the bacteria are resistant to the antimicrobial agent, the antimicrobial urinary concentration is too low because of poor renal concentrating ability or gastrointestinal malabsorption, or the infection is caused by multiple organisms. Most unresolved infections are treated successfully when proper culture and antimicrobial sensitivity patterns are available.

Sources of urinary tract bacterial persistence are usually found early in children because imaging is performed after the first UTI. The discovery of surgically correctable sources of bacterial persistence is obviously important (Table 112–2). The majority of recurrent UTI is, however, reinfection with the same organism or a different organism that ascends from the bowel and is not surgically correctable.

"Asymptomatic" or "covert" UTI (Savage, 1975) that is found on a screening urinary culture only when a child is being examined for reasons unrelated to urinary infection is also classified and managed as either a first or recurrent UTI.

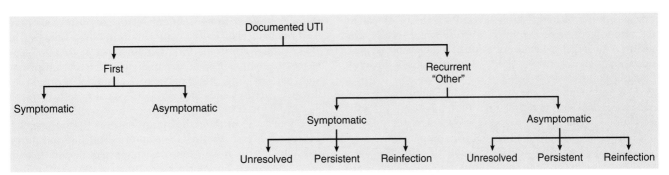

Figure 112–1. Functional classification of urinary tract infections (UTIs) in children.

Table 112-2. Surgically Correctable Causes of Bacterial Persistence in Children

Infection stones
Infected nonfunctioning or poorly functioning kidneys or renal segments
Infected ureteral stumps after nephrectomy
Vesicointestinal or urethrorectal fistula
Vesicovaginal fistula
Infected necrotic papillae in papillary necrosis
Unilateral medullary sponge kidney
Infected urachal cyst
Infected urethral diverticulum or periurethral gland

Bacteria

Although some bacteria appear to have special affinity for the urinary tract, not all share these characteristics. The most common bacteria infecting the urinary tract are the gram-negative Enterobacteriaceae, usually *Escherichia coli* (Kunin et al, 1964; Bergström, 1972; Winberg et al, 1974). Specific cell wall O-antigens that are identified by serotyping such as *E. coli* serotypes O1, O2, O4, O6, O7, and O75 commonly cause pediatric UTI (Kunin et al, 1964; Winberg et al, 1974). Experimental findings suggest that *Enterococcus faecalis* that is increasingly difficult to treat because of multidrug resistance may have specific affinity for the kidney (Kau et al, 2005b).

Bacterial surface structures, pili or fimbriae, may increase uropathogenicity. The bacterial fimbriae mediate bacterial adherence to uroepithelial cells and red blood cell agglutination, both of which are used to characterize virulence. Red blood cell agglutinating characteristics of the *E. coli*, called hemagglutination, can be blocked by different sugars (Duguid et al, 1978; Svanborg Edén and Hanson, 1978). Using this characteristic, Källenius and associates (1981) discovered that pyelonephritic *E. coli* cause mannose-resistant hemagglutination (MRHA) of human red blood cells. The terminal glycolipid of the human red cell P blood group antigen is a receptor that binds the P fimbriae on these *E. coli*. Therefore, **two important markers for *E. coli* virulence are MRHA characteristics and P blood group–specific adhesins** (P fimbriae or P pili) (Källenius et al, 1981; Väisänen et al, 1981).

These two virulence markers are associated with bacteria that cause clinical pyelonephritis and cystitis. In one study, most *E. coli* strains causing pediatric clinical pyelonephritis had both MRHA and P fimbriae (MRHA 91% [29 of 32], P fimbriae 81%) (Väisänen et al, 1981), and P fimbriae were absent on less virulent strains. In another study, Kallenius and associates (1981) found P fimbriae on 94% (33 of 35) of *E. coli* causing acute pyelonephritis, 19% (5 of 26) of *E. coli* causing acute cystitis, 14% (5 of 6) of *E. coli* causing asymptomatic bacteriuria, and 7% (6 of 82) of *E. coli* from the feces of healthy children.

When pyelonephritis and cystitis are defined by findings of renal inflammation (the technetium-99m dimercaptosuccinic acid [DMSA] renal scan shows decreased activity in areas of inflammation), the distinctions between upper and lower UTIs are less clear. Although P-fimbriated *E. coli* are more likely to cause fever than non–P-fimbriated *E. coli*, renal inflammation observed on DMSA scan correlates less well

(Majd et al, 1991; Jantausch et al, 1992). This characteristic of P fimbriation causing fever is supported by the finding that the urinary interleukin 6 (IL-6) response is higher in children infected with P-fimbriated *E. coli* than children infected by non–P-fimbriated *E. coli* (Benson et al, 1994). IL-8 receptor–deficient mice have increased susceptibility to acute UTI caused by uropathogenic *E. coli* (Frendeus et al, 2001). It is suggested, moreover, that UTIs caused by P-fimbriated strains need longer antimicrobial courses than those caused by other strains (Tambic et al, 1992).

Other less well characterized virulence factors are hydrophobic *E. coli* properties and the iron-binding capability of the bacteria associated with aerobactin production (Jacobson et al, 1988, 1989). Genetic epidemiology has associated three putative *E. coli* genes with three specific uropathogenic proteins (usp, a *Vibrio cholerae* zot gene homolog; IrgA homolog adhesin iha, a nonhemagglutinating adhesin; and iron $_{E.coli}$, a catechol siderophore receptor homolog) and found that these are associated with *E. coli* isolates that cause UTI and pyelonephritis (Bauer et al, 2002).

Organisms that cause covert or asymptomatic UTIs may lack such virulence characteristics, be self-agglutinating, and lack fimbriae.

PATHOGENESIS OF URINARY TRACT INFECTION IN CHILDREN

The natural course of UTIs in children may be unpredictable. Although risk factors and bacterial virulence may influence this course, these factors alone are not useful in predicting that an individual will develop pyelonephritis, renal scarring, or parenchymal and functional loss from a single or recurrent UTI. Of the 3% of girls and 1% of boys who contract a prepubertal UTI (Winberg et al, 1974), 17% or more have infection-related renal scarring. Of those with scarring, 10% to 20% may become hypertensive, but only a rare child has progressive renal dysfunction culminating in end-stage renal disease.

The course of UTIs in adults and that in children differs, but the epidemiology of UTIs in children is often reported without regard for age and other specific pediatric factors (Shortliffe and McCue, 2002). For this reason, much about the course of pediatric UTI is still elusive.

Cystitis and Pyelonephritis

Bacterial genetic clonal studies confirm that entry into the urinary tract occurs through the suspected fecal-perineal-urethral route with subsequent retrograde ascent of periurethral bacteria (Kaijser and Larsson, 1982; Tullus et al, 1984; Mitsumori et al, 1997; Yamamoto et al, 1997). These bacteria overcome urethral defenses such as urethral washout, epithelial shedding, and paraurethral glandular secretion, all of which vary by gender, age, and individual to cause variable likelihood for bacterial ascent (Kunin et al, 2002). At the molecular level, **microbial proteins such as lipopolysaccharides may trigger urothelial receptors (Toll-like receptors) that activate the local immune system** (Akira and Takeda, 2004). Moreover, Tamm-Horsfall protein, a common urinary protein, adheres specifically to type 1 fimbriated uropathogenic *E. coli* to participate in the host defense by helping to wash out bacteria during voiding (Bates et al, 2004).

Rodent and murine models have revealed the potential bacterial and uroepithelial interaction through which UTI occurs and explain a new paradigm for acute and recurrent UTI. Bladder surface umbrella cells are unique, slowly cycling cells that renew only every few months. These cells contain special two-dimensional hexagonal crystals of 16-nm uroplakin particles that normally allow these superficial cells to flatten and expand and allow normal bladder surface activity (Kong et al, 2004). The genetically altered uroplakin-deficient mouse has major urinary tract abnormalities.

Although the **initial event in infection is known to be attachment between the uroepithelial cell and bacteria through factors such as type 1 and P pili and fimbriae, it was discovered more recently that this attachment initiates a molecular interaction in which the adhesin receptor complexes to trigger a series of events that causes uptake of the bacteria into the bladder surface umbrella cells** (Kau et al, 2005a). The host response rapidly sheds the uroepithelial cells (Mulvey et al, 1998). The bacteria then enter the bladder epithelial cells and interact with lipid rafts and uroplakins, forming intracellular bacterial communities. These bacterial communities develop and the organisms transform into an organized biofilm with a more coccoid form. As these communities enlarge, they form cellular "pods" that protrude from the surface and may detach. These may then retransform into their rodlike motile form and disseminate through the urinary tract (Anderson et al, 2003). The intracellular bacterial pod may be protected from the usual host cellular immune

response and antimicrobial effects (Justice et al, 2004). **These biofilms appear to allow microbial adaptation to variable environments and aggregate detachment that causes systemic infection, antimicrobial resistance through plasmid exchange, endotoxin production, and overall increased resistance to host immune systems** (Donlan, 2002) (Fig. 112–2).

When bacteria have reached the bladder, ascent to the kidneys is affected by host immunity, impaired ureteral peristalsis, vesicoureteral reflux, or the specific organism uropathogenicity. Under normal circumstances, nonspecific mechanisms such as cytokine release may play a role (Davidoff et al, 1997).

Although hematogenous dissemination of bacteria through other routes may occur, this appears to be relatively uncommon and may primarily involve infants with incompletely developed immunity, staphylococcal skin or systemic infections with organism dissemination, or systemic infection, such as tuberculosis. In these situations, renal, perirenal, or epididymal abscesses can occur.

Pyelonephritis is important because of the clinical severity of the illness and the potential renal damage that may occur. Bacterial infection of the urinary tract also causes bladder and ureteral inflammation with tissue changes that alter dynamics of the entire urinary tract (Hinman, 1971; Boyarsky and Labay, 1972; Issa and Shortliffe, 1992; Johnson et al, 1992). Animal studies have shown that UTIs cause abnormally elevated renal pelvic pressures even if (or especially if) vesicoureteral reflux is absent (Issa and Shortliffe, 1992; Angell et al, 1998), thus implicating increased pressure and poor

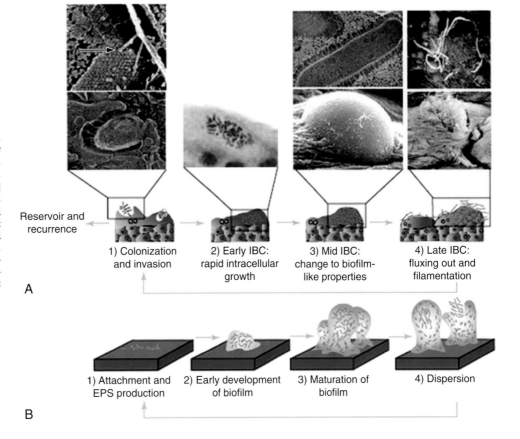

Figure 112–2. **A,** The stages of bacterial invasion of uropathogenic *E. coli* attaching to uroepithelial cell and subsequent formation of pod and dispersion. **B,** The similar stages compared with previously known biofilm formation on inert surfaces such as urethral catheters. EPS, extracellular polymeric substances; IBC, intracellular bacterial communities. (From Kau A, Hunstad D, Hultgren SJ: Interaction of uropathogenic *Escherichia coli* with host uroepithelium. Curr Opin Microbiol 2005;8: 54, Fig. 2.)

smooth muscle compliance as a further explanation for ureteral dilation observed in patients with acute pyelonephritis and otherwise normal upper collecting systems (Mårild et al, 1989a).

Determining the point of clinical progression from cystitis to pyelonephritis or differentiating between these entities is impossible because simple techniques with which to localize the level and extent of urinary tract bacteria are lacking. Although ureteral catheterization with sequential cultures is the "gold standard" for localizing upper and lower tract bacteriuria, this requires cystoscopy and is an impractical invasive means of following the course of infection (Stamey, 1980). Localizing the site of bacteria cannot, moreover, show the extent of renal inflammation. The Fairley bladder washout localization technique requires urethral catheterization during acute infection and subsequent bladder irrigation and washing with sterile water to attempt to localize the source of bacteria as the bladder (found in the first bladder culture) or as supravesical (found in cultures taken after the washing). **Clinical symptoms correlate poorly with the results of localization studies using the Fairley or ureteral catheterization techniques. In one study comparing clinical symptoms with Fairley results, fewer than half of the patients (the majority children) with fever and flank pain had upper tract bacteria (34 of 73) on the Fairley test and almost 20% (83 of 473) who were asymptomatic had upper tract bacteria** (Busch and Huland, 1984).

KEY POINTS: URINARY TRACT INFECTION PATHOGENESIS

- The first year of life is the only year during which males have more UTIs than females.

- Each year about 50 per 100,000 children are hospitalized for UTI; the rate is greater than three times this number in infants (children younger than 3 months).

- In children, discovering surgically correctable sources of bacterial persistence is important.

- Bacterial pili or fimbriae increase uropathogenicity.

- Approximately 17% or more of children who have pyelonephritis acquire renal scarring.

- Clinical symptoms correlate poorly with bacterial localization within the urinary tract.

- Bacterial clonal studies confirm the fecal-perineal-urethral retrograde ascent of periurethral bacteria causing UTI.

- Microbial lipopolysaccharides (Toll-like receptors) may trigger urothelial receptors to activate the local immune system.

- Intracellular bacterial biofilms allow microbial adaptation to variable environments and allow aggregate detachment causing systemic infection in a way that increases bacterial resistance to the host immune system.

Risk Factors for Bacteriuria and Renal Damage

It is clear that various factors exist that may make bacteriuria or renal scarring more or less likely for any individual, and these risks appear to be distinct for each individual. Although we are unable to alter bacterial pathogenicity at this time, it is worthwhile reviewing specific host characteristics that alter the risk of bacteriuria and others that may alter the risk of renal damage when bacteriuria occurs to understand those that may or may not be therapeutically altered (Table 112–3). Some of these host characteristics are discussed even though they are interactive (Fig. 112–3).

Age

The prevalence of bacteriuria or UTI is age dependent. **Bacteriuria is more common at the extremes of life—in neonates and in elderly people** (Shortliffe and McCue, 2002). As already discussed, the prevalence of bacteriuria for both males and females younger than age 1 is higher than at other times during childhood. There may be many factors causing this age-dependent relationship, some of which involve interactions with other host factors, such as periurethral colonization, breast-feeding, or immature immune status. Although none of these factors appears to be independent, the importance of the various factors may be age related. Others have discussed major factors creating risk for UTI in females, for instance sexual intercourse, contraceptive usage (diaphragm or spermicidal), antimicrobial usage, prior UTI, previous history of UTI, estrogen status, and postvoid residual (Stamm and Raz, 1999). The importance of these factors is more or less dependent upon the subject's age and previous history.

Genetics

Genetic factors that may affect risk of bacteriuria and others that affect subsequent morbidity are multifactorial and incompletely investigated. Follow-up studies document that individuals who have childhood UTIs continue to be at risk for adult UTIs whether or not they have vesicoureteral reflux (Beetz et al, 2002). Issues related to gender, race, or ethnicity are specific genetic links and are discussed separately.

Factors that increase bacterial-epithelial adherence and bacteriuria are inherent host risk factors, as increased periurethral colonization precedes UTI. Children who originally had

Table 112–3. **Host Factors Affecting Bacteriuria**
Age
Gender
Colonization
Periurethral
Preputial
Fecal
Genetics (uroepithelial receptors)
Renal scarring
Native immunity
Sexual activity
Genitourinary abnormalities
Vesicoureteral reflux
Pregnancy
Neurogenic bladder
Iatrogenic factors

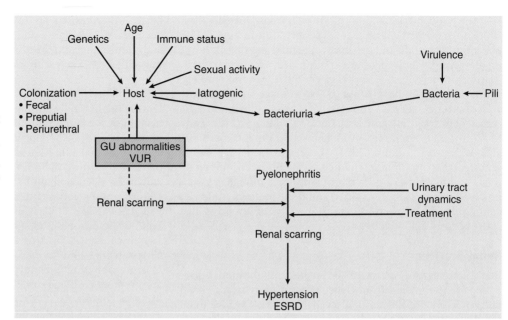

Figure 112–3. Factors that affect the development of bacteriuria and subsequent pyelonephritis, renal scarring, hypertension, and end-stage renal disease (ESRD). Urinary tract urodynamics reflect urinary tract pressures and related factors. GU, genitourinary; VUR, vesicoureteral reflux.

primary vesicoureteral reflux but no longer have reflux as adults are commonly still susceptible to recurrent UTIs with symptoms confined to the lower tract (Mansfield et al, 1995; Beetz et al, 2002).

Host receptors to uropathogens have been identified. When bacterial P fimbriae were identified as a virulence factor, glycolipids characterizing the P blood group system were found on host uroepithelial cells and found to act as bacterial receptors. Because hosts with these receptors (i.e., P blood group phenotype) would be suspected to have increased susceptibility to infection, children with recurrent infections were tested for this P blood group phenotype (Lomberg et al, 1983). The **P1 blood group phenotype was found in 97% (35 of 36) of girls with recurrent pyelonephritis with minimal (grade I) or no reflux;** it was found in 75% (63 of 84) of control subjects without UTI. Eighty-four percent (27 of 32) of girls with pyelonephritis and reflux (grades II to V) had the P1 blood group phenotype, not a significantly different incidence from that in individuals without UTI. They found, moreover, that bacteria binding to glycolipid receptors (bacteria with P fimbriae) were more likely to be found in the girls with the P1 blood group without reflux than those with the P1 blood group having reflux. This suggests that vesicoureteral reflux may contribute more to the pathogenesis of pyelonephritis than bacterial virulence. Thus, in children with minimal or no reflux, P-fimbriated uropathogens may be more important in causing pyelonephritis, but vesicoureteral reflux is an overwhelming factor in those with higher grade reflux.

Other blood group antigens on the urothelial surface (ABO, Lewis, and secretor phenotypes) also influence UTI susceptibility. Adult women with Le (a–b–) and Le (a+b–) blood phenotypes are three times more likely to have a recurrent UTI than Le (a–b+) women, and epithelial cells from nonsecretors have more bacterial receptors than cells from secretors (Sheinfeld et al, 1989). Similarly, in children with UTI, the frequency of Le (a–b–) phenotype is higher and the relative risk of infection in these children is 3.2 (Jantausch et al, 1994).

Immunohistochemical analysis to characterize H, A, B, Le^a, and Le^b was performed in 72 children with various anatomic abnormalities (ureteropelvic junction obstruction, vesicoureteral reflux, ureteroceles, and primary obstructive disease) (Sheinfeld et al, 1990). These data suggest that children with anatomic abnormalities and presumed nonsecretor phenotype (minimal or undetectable ABO and Le^b immunoreactivity) were more likely to have had a history of UTIs (16 of 17, 94.1%) than secretors (16 of 30, 53.3%) whose tissue had intense ABO and Le^b staining. Twenty-three of 24 (95.8%) children without UTIs were secretors and had intense ABO and Le^b immunoreactivity. In summary, nonsecretor status may allow structures that serve as bacterial receptors to be more available for binding and result in greater susceptibility to UTI.

Clinical histories support a familial risk for UTI. Sisters of girls who have recurrent UTIs have a higher incidence of significant bacteriuria on screening cultures than expected for the normal population (Fennell et al, 1977; Stauffer et al, 2004). **Notably, two distinct risks for recurrent UTI in young women (18 to 30 years) are age at first UTI (UTI before age 15; odds ratio [OR] 3.9) and UTI in the mother (OR 2.3)** (Scholes et al, 2000). The possible genetic relationship of renal scarring and UTI is discussed with renal scarring.

Gender

As discussed before, the ratio of UTI in the white population by sex shows a preponderance of UTI in boys during the first year of life, but, thereafter, more girls than boys have UTI. Although many factors, including urethral length, prostate, and foreskin, have been hypothesized to account for this finding, the complete explanation is unclear.

Race and Ethnicity

UTIs occur in all races, but epidemiologic studies show varying prevalence and complications of UTI in different races. These factors are incompletely studied. In one comparative study of children younger than 2 years, including white,

Hispanic, and black children, UTIs were most prevalent in white, then Hispanic, and then black girls, but in boys UTIs were most common in Hispanic, white, and then black boys in that order. These data are confounded by circumcision status, however (Bachur and Harper, 2001). **Several studies show that blacks have fewer UTIs, a lower incidence of vesicoureteral reflux, and perhaps less likelihood of reflux nephropathy than Hispanics or whites** (Kunin and McCormack, 1968; Kunin, 1970; Lohr et al, 1994; Hoberman and Wald, 1997; Pinto, 2004). Interestingly, it has been reported that in Chinese children, UTIs and vesicoureteral reflux and renal scarring are more common in boys than girls; however, the ages are unreported and these findings could be confounded by age and circumcision status (Howard et al, 2001; Lee and Chow, 2001).

Renal Scarring

Renal scarring is a risk factor for further complications such as hypertension, renal insufficiency, progressive renal scarring, and renal functional deterioration (Berg, 1992). **The idea that renal scarring begets renal scarring is supported by clinical studies that examined the association of recurrent bacteriuria and new renal scarring or progressive renal scarring** (Newcastle Asymptomatic Bacteriuria Research Group, 1975; Savage, 1975; Cardiff Oxford Bacteriuria Study Group, 1978; Newcastle Covert Bacteriuria Research Group, 1981). Long-term follow-up has also shown that kidneys that were initially normal after UTI tend to remain normal and those that were initially scarred appear to be more likely to suffer subsequent damage (Smellie, 1991; Smellie et al, 1998).

Angiotensin-converting enzyme (ACE) gene polymorphisms have been implicated in renal scarring. The ACE gene is located on chromosome 17, and a specific 287-base-pair deletion (D) polymorphism is associated with increased renin-angiotensin system activity and increased angiotensin II levels. Increased DD genotype has been associated with increased risk of progressive renal failure in immunoglobulin A (IgA) nephropathy, diabetic nephropathy, autosomal dominant polycystic kidney disease, and focal glomerulosclerosis (Brock et al, 1998). **Several series suggest that the DD genotype may also be associated with patients with congenital urologic abnormalities who have evidence of renal parenchymal damage and reflux nephropathy** (Brock et al, 1997; Ozen et al, 1999).

Colonization

Periurethral Colonization

Host factors causing susceptibility to UTIs have also been examined (see Fig. 112–3). From epidemiologic data, it is known that the **incidence of UTI for all infants is higher during the first few weeks to months of their life than at any subsequent time in their next few years.** During this time, the periurethral area of healthy girls and boys is massively colonized with aerobic bacteria (especially *E. coli*, enterococci, and staphylococci) (Bollgren and Winberg, 1976a). **This colonization decreases during the first year and is unusual in children who do not have recurrent infections after age 5.** After this period, women and children who suffer repeated UTIs remain more colonized by periurethral gram-negative

bacteria than those who do not have infections (Stamey and Sexton, 1975; Bollgren and Winberg, 1976a, 1976b). Times and conditions of increased periurethral colonization are, therefore, associated with increased risk of UTI.

Preputial Skin

During the first few months of life there appears to be a connection between the foreskin, periurethral and preputial colonization, and UTIs. During the past decade, however, the association of the foreskin and neonatal UTIs has caused controversy regarding the advantages and disadvantages of circumcision (Hallett et al, 1976). This has resulted in numerous editorials and recommendations by the American Academy of Pediatrics (King, 1982; Cunningham, 1986; Roberts, 1986; Lohr, 1989; Schoen et al, 1989; Winberg et al, 1989; Poland, 1990; Schoen, 1990; American Academy of Pediatrics and Circumcision, 1999).

In a group of mainly uncircumcised healthy boys, Bollgren and Winberg (1976a) documented that preputial aerobic bacterial colonization is highest during the first months after birth, decreases after 6 months, and is uncommon after age 5. Subsequently, **Wiswell and associates (1988) compared the periurethral bacterial flora (using intraurethral and glanular cultures) during the first year of life in circumcised and uncircumcised boys and found that for the first 6 months periurethral uropathogenic organisms were cultured more frequently from the uncircumcised than circumcised boys.** They and others have concluded that the foreskin is responsible for this finding (Hallett et al, 1976; Glennon et al, 1988; Wiswell et al, 1988).

Neonatal bacterial colonization of the foreskin is related to multiple factors, including immature immune status, unusual nosocomial colonization, breast-feeding (Winberg et al, 1989), and other characteristics mediating bacterial adherence (Fussell et al, 1988). This higher colonization is associated with a greater number of neonatal UTIs. In a series of retrospective reviews of 55 worldwide U.S. Army hospitals, Wiswell and associates (Wiswell and Roscelli, 1986) examined the incidence of UTIs diagnosed by catheterization or suprapubic aspirate in infants hospitalized during 1974 to 1983. **They found that the incidence of infections in circumcised male infants was 0.11% (193 of 175,317), that in uncircumcised male infants was 1.12% (468 of 41,799), and that in female infants was 0.57% (1164 of 205,212).** These data included only hospitalized children in Hawaii and may have underestimated these numbers; others report a higher overall incidence of UTI in infant boys of 2.2% to 4.1% with the majority (70% to 86%) occurring in uncircumcised infants (Wiswell et al, 1985; Schoen et al, 2000; Wiswell, 2000).

Uncircumcised male infants, moreover, have an increased relative risk of UTI of 3.12 compared with circumcised boys, but this risk decreases from 3.7 at 1 year to 3.0 at 3 years (Wiswell and Hachey, 1993; To et al, 1998; Wiswell, 2000). The majority of infections occurred during the first 3 months of life. When the incidences of infections during the first and the final years of the study were compared, the total number of UTIs increased as the circumcision rate decreased (Wiswell and Roscelli, 1986; Wiswell et al, 1987), and Wiswell concluded that UTIs are more frequent in uncircumcised boys. A case-control methodology was used to compare circumcised and uncircumcised boys in a population with a high rate of uncircumcised boys (Australia). It was concluded that circumcision was still associated with a lower rate of UTIs before and past the first year of life (Craig et al, 1996). Although there may be difficulties with these data related to retrospective analysis and selection bias, periurethral colonization is also associated with increased risk of UTI in girls and women.

Others have examined the rate of UTI in young boys before and after vesicoureteral reimplantation in which circumcision was performed or not performed at the time of reimplantation surgery; no difference between the rates was found for any of the groups (Kwak et al, 2004).

At this time, there is no way to predict whether a male infant with a normal urinary tract who contracts a UTI has a genetic or familial predisposition for infection. Because few infant boys who suffer a neonatal UTI risk a recurrent UTI after a year if they remain clear in the interim, prophylactic antibiotics for 6 months may be helpful in these boys. **There is some evidence that circumcision in hospitalized (neonatal intensive care) premature boys may decrease the risk of recurrent UTI during this period** (Cason et al, 2000). UTI in uncircumcised infant boys also tends to be more expensive to treat because these children are more likely to be hospitalized, especially during the first 3 months of life (Schoen et al, 2000). The reason for this is unknown, but it has been reported that the organisms involved in these uncircumcised boys are more virulent and appear more similar to the strains causing pyelonephritis and urosepsis in adults (Bonacorsi et al, 2005).

Present data do not support routine neonatal circumcision to prevent UTI in neonates or to prevent future infection (American Academy of Pediatrics and Circumcision, 1999), although opinions on this differ (Thiruchelvam and Cuckow, 2005). Some reports document a slightly higher UTI incidence following ritual circumcision that may be related to circumcision technique (Liora et al, 2002).

Fecal Colonization

Because most UTIs result from fecal-perineal-urethral ascent of bacteria, fecal colonization is an important consideration. The human fecal flora is dependent upon the surrounding microbial ecology, native immunity, and microbial altering drugs and foods. The importance of abnormal fecal colonization in neonates is emphasized by studies showing that fecal colonization with specific pyelonephritic bacteria may occur in a neonatal nursery or hospital with subsequent bacteriuria or pyelonephritis occurring several months later (Tullus, 1986).

The creation of and selection for multiply antimicrobial agent resistant organisms in the gut by antimicrobial usage is well recognized. **Because the fecal flora is commonly responsible for perineal and periurethral colonization, the importance of responsible antimicrobial usage cannot be overestimated.** In one study, antibiotic treatment of schoolgirls with phenoxymethylpenicillin for intercurrent nonbladder infections, usually otitis media, caused colonization and bacteriuria with strains more likely to be symptomatic (Hansson et al, 1989b).

Immune Status and Infancy

The complete influence of host cellular and humoral immunity on risk of UTI is unknown, but in all human disease, compromised native immunity is associated with increased risk of infection. In children, the immune status varies during normal development, transmission either natural or acquired (vaccination, breast-feeding, illness), and congenital or acquired states of immunodeficiency.

UTIs are common in infants and children while their immune system is immature. For instance, serum IgG is lowest between age 1 and 3 months (Robbins, 1972), when periurethral colonization is high in normal children. Secretory IgA, moreover, is an important human immunoglobulin at the secretory and mucosal surfaces and may be transferred to the newborn in colostrum if the child is breast-fed. Serum IgA is found in diminished concentrations for the first several months and is absent or almost absent at the secretory surfaces of the nasopharynx, gut, and urothelium during this time (Svanborg Edén et al, 1985; Fliedner et al, 1986; Yoder and Polin, 1986) and undetectable in the urine at birth (James-Ellison et al, 1997). Urinary secretory IgA and total IgA increase during the first year and are higher in children who are breast-fed (James-Ellison et al, 1997).

The role that urinary IgA plays in children with UTIs has not been investigated extensively. In children with acute UTI or pyelonephritis, urinary excretion of IgA is higher than in those without UTI, and these levels are still far exceeded in normal adults (Svanborg Edén et al, 1985; James-Ellison et al, 1997). Urinary IgA in infants, moreover, is in the monomeric rather than the secretory form normally found in adults, suggesting that urinary IgA in infants may be systemic immunoglobulin excreted as a result of infection-related tubular dysfunction rather than secretory (Svanborg Edén et al, 1985). Children with recurrent UTIs have lower urinary secretory IgA concentrations than those without (Fliedner et al, 1986).

The benefits of breast milk in preventing infection in infancy are expounded by many, but whether its effect is related to colostrum IgA or other factors is unclear (Hanson, 1998; Gartner et al, 2005). **Case-control studies suggest that the duration of breast-feeding confers a protective effect against UTI during the first 6 months of life.** These studies show duration of breast-feeding to be shorter in children who have UTIs (9 versus 16 weeks in children who had exclusive breast-feeding) (Mårild et al, 1989b), but full or partial breast-feeding may confer a protective effect against UTI for the first 6 months of life (Pisacane et al, 1990, 1992). Although the mechanism of the protective effect is unknown, the oligosaccharide content of the mother's breast milk and urine is the same as that in the breast-fed infant's. Perhaps these oligosaccharides inhibit the adherence of pathogenic E. coli to the uroepithelium (Coppa et al, 1990). Other **studies show that exclusive breast-feeding for 4 or more months protects against single or recurrent otitis media in children** (Duncan et al, 1993) or infants with cleft palate (Paradise et al, 1994).

As expected, children with specific immune deficiency syndromes have altered immunity and commonly have an increased risk for infection and its dissemination. About 20% of human immunodeficiency virus (HIV)-infected children have bacterial UTIs with both common and opportunistic organisms (Grattan-Smith et al, 1992), and others have associated UTI and HIV; specifically in HIV-seropositive women, UTI was associated with high viral load (OR 1.82) (Park et al, 2002).

Sexual Activity

Epidemiologic studies have shown that sexual activity may also be a risk factor for UTI. Sexually active females have more UTIs than inactive females (nuns) (Kunin and McCormack, 1968). This association has caused some to suggest that **UTI is a marker for teenage sexual activity** (Nguyen and Weir, 2002). Whether this relationship stems from colonization or other factors is unclear.

Genitourinary Anatomic Abnormalities

Historically, UTI is a marker for pediatric genitourinary tract anatomic abnormalities; hence, UTI evaluation consists of imaging. Specific genitourinary abnormalities, in particular, nonfunctioning segments, can serve as a nidus of bacterial infection, causing bacterial persistence because of the inability to achieve urinary antimicrobial concentrations adequate to eradicate bacteria in the poorly concentrating renal segment (see Table 112–2). Similarly, genitourinary partial obstruction or renal functional impairment may create increased risk of renal damage because of poor or inadequate antimicrobial penetration. The severe sequela of chronic UTI and inflammation, xanthogranulomatous pyelonephritis, may occur in young children with obstruction and UTI in renal segments associated with genitourinary abnormalities and poor function (Stamey et al, 1977; Zafaranloo et al, 1990; Cousins, et al, 1994; Hammadeh et al, 1994). The importance of specific situations is discussed in the following.

Vesicoureteral Reflux

Vesicoureteral reflux is discussed fully in Chapter 117. Reflux is common in children with UTI, but no correlation between reflux and susceptibility to UTI is known (Winberg et al, 1974). Epidemiologic surveys show that 21% to 57% of children who have bacteriuria have vesicoureteral reflux if evaluated (Kunin et al, 1964; Abbott, 1972; Asscher et al, 1973; Newcastle Asymptomatic Bacteriuria Research Group, 1975). Reflux may resolve spontaneously (Bellinger and Duckett, 1984; Skoog et al, 1987). In one study, when UTIs were prevented, 87% of grade I reflux, 63% of grade II, 53% of grade III, and 33% of grade IV resolved over about 3 years (Bellinger and Duckett, 1984). When it resolves, the rate of spontaneous resolution is about 30% to 35% each year (Skoog et al, 1987).

Peripubertal Girls with Persistent Vesicoureteral Reflux (Pregnancy)

The question of whether girls approaching puberty who have persistent vesicoureteral reflux should have the reflux corrected because of the potential for future pregnancy is problematic. If primary vesicoureteral reflux persists as a girl approaches puberty, it becomes statistically less likely each year to resolve spontaneously. For this reason, some advocate that all girls approaching puberty undergo surgical correction of reflux to avoid the risks of pyelonephritis during future pregnancies. Whether a female with persistent vesicoureteral reflux who has never had a UTI and demonstrated no increased susceptibility for UTI should undergo routine correction of reflux is controversial; moreover, whether a female with persistent vesicoureteral reflux who has demonstrated increased susceptibility for UTI should undergo correction is also controversial.

Although the prevalence of bacteriuria in pregnant women is the same as that in nonpregnant women (Shortliffe and Stamey, 1986b; Shortliffe, 1991), **the likelihood that the bacteriuria may progress to pyelonephritis is greatly increased. From 13.5% to 65% of pregnant women who are bacteriuric on a screening urinary culture develop subsequent pyelonephritis during pregnancy if untreated** (Sweet, 1977), **whereas pyelonephritis is rarely the consequence of uncomplicated cystitis in a nonpregnant woman.** The reason for this increased likelihood of pyelonephritis during pregnancy is unknown, but it may be related to hormonal and hydrodynamic changes of pregnancy. There is increased bladder and urinary tract compliance and bladder enlargement; an enlarging uterus may cause anatomic displacement of the bladder and ureters (Hsia and Shortliffe, 1995).

There are no data to suggest that pregnancy causes vesicoureteral reflux (Shortliffe and Stamey, 1986b). When 321 women had a single-film voiding cystourethrogram during the third trimester of pregnancy or in the immediate postpartum period, only 9 (2.8%) had vesicoureteral reflux (Heidrick et al, 1967). Although 6.2% (20 of 321) of these women had asymptomatic bacteriuria, only 1 of these 20 had vesicoureteral reflux. Therefore, as opposed to the pediatric situation, few bacteriuric pregnant women who develop pyelonephritis have reflux. Of the nine women who had reflux, three developed pyelonephritis during a pregnancy.

In another series, 21 of 100 pregnant women (27 refluxing renal units in 21 patients) with asymptomatic bacteriuria evaluated postpartum had vesicoureteral reflux, mostly low grade (67% into the ureter only), and 17% of these women had renal scarring (Williams et al, 1968). Although some use these data to justify correction of all pubertal reflux in girls, this renal scarring is unlikely to be the result of bacteriuria during pregnancy. This rate of scarring is similar to that found in children with screening bacteriuria and renal scarring (Asscher et al, 1973; Newcastle Asymptomatic Bacteriuria Research Group, 1975; Savage, 1975). These women were not imaged before pregnancy, and it is most likely that any renal scarring found postpartum was present beforehand and occurred in childhood. These data suggest that postpubertal females who have vesicoureteral reflux and a predisposition for frequent UTIs continue to have this predisposition for infections into adulthood and pregnancy. Moreover, the women who were susceptible to UTIs before pregnancy continue to be more likely to develop UTI during and after pregnancy whether or not they have vesicoureteral reflux (Mansfield et al, 1995; Bukowski et al, 1998; Beetz et al, 2002).

Even though correction of vesicoureteral reflux, spontaneously or surgically, may decrease the likelihood of ascending pyelonephritis from bacteriuria under normal circumstances, under the physiologic changes of pregnancy the nonrefluxing orifice does not appear to offer the expected protection from pyelonephritis. Unless a surgically corrected ureterovesical junction is better at protecting against the pyelonephritis of pregnancy than nature's normal nonrefluxing ureteral junction, reflux correction cannot be justified only by these data. Therefore, both persistent reflux and a patient's susceptibility to UTI should be assessed before surgical correction of reflux is considered. **If vesicoureteral reflux is** surgically corrected, these patients should not be assured that pyelonephritis during pregnancy is impossible or even unlikely. The urine of these pregnant women must still be screened routinely for bacteriuria.

Pregnant Women with Renal Insufficiency

Before a woman with known reflux nephropathy and renal insufficiency is counseled about pregnancy, her renal function must be evaluated. Although outcome data for pregnancy are sparse, when there is moderate or severe renal insufficiency (moderate, initial serum creatinine 1.4 to 2.4 mg/dL; severe, 2.5 mg/dL or greater), even though infant survival may be greater than 90%, maternal and obstetric complications are high (Bear, 1976; Davison and Lindheimer, 1978; Jones and Hayslett, 1996). In these high-risk women 43% had a pregnancy-related deterioration in creatinine clearance of at least 25% that occurred during pregnancy (20%) or immediately postpartum (23%), and in the majority this was irreversible (Epstein, 1996; Jones and Hayslett, 1996). This accelerated renal insufficiency was associated with increased hypertension and high-grade proteinuria (Jones and Hayslett, 1996). Almost 60% of these pregnancies ended in preterm delivery with cesarean section, and the majority of infants were below the 50th percentile in birth weight (Jones and Hayslett, 1996). These data have been interpreted to indicate that when the serum creatinine exceeds 2.0 mg/dL in a pregnant woman, she has a 1 in 3 risk of progressing to end-stage renal disease either during or just after delivery (Epstein, 1996).

The effect of a maternal UTI on the fetus has been controversial. Analyses of National Collaborative Perinatal Project (NCPP) data from the 1970s and Medicaid data from the 1990s (both representative of women of low socioeconomic status) show an association between third-trimester maternal UTI and fetal mental retardation or developmental delay; and NCPP data, furthermore, associate third-trimester UTI with increased chance of fetal death (McDermott et al, 2001). Others have documented infant low birth weight and prematurity (Naeye, 1979).

Neurogenic and Bowel-Augmented Bladders

Children who have neurogenic bladders with abnormally elevated bladder pressures risk increased renal damage from the elevated urinary tract pressures. The risk of UTI is also increased secondary to the increased instrumentation common with neurogenic bladder (intermittent catheterization). Increased pressure within the neurogenic system combined with the physiologic effects of UTI that create increased pressure creates an even more likely situation for subsequent renal parenchymal damage (Hansen et al, 2002). Chronically or intermittently elevated bladder pressures may cause secondary vesicoureteral reflux because of decompensation of the ureterovesical junction from the elevated pressure (Hutch, 1952). If this does not occur, the elevated bladder pressures associated with a neurogenic bladder may also cause effective ureterovesical obstruction. This obstruction increases the risk

of renal damage associated with UTIs (Cowan and Shortliffe, 1998), and, as discussed earlier in this chapter, intermittent elevations in bladder pressure associated with physiologic bladder dynamics in the immature bladder may exacerbate the effects of vesicoureteral reflux and UTI.

Children with neurogenic bladder are more likely to risk the effects of bacteriuria and renal damage because of inability to clear bacteria spontaneously. Clean intermittent catheterization programs are useful for emptying the neurogenic bladder, but these catheterizations introduce bacteria. Although conclusions from previous studies involving clean intermittent catheterization in children are limited because they combined sexes, wide age ranges, different types of neurogenic bladders, short follow-up, different prophylactic regimens, and different definitions of bacteriuria, they all agree that bacteriuria and even pyuria occur in most children. Forty percent to 80% of the urinary specimens sampled had bacteriuria or pyuria or both (Taylor et al, 1985; de la Hunt et al, 1989; Joseph et al, 1989; Gribble and Puterman, 1993; Johnson et al, 1994; Schlager et al, 1995, 1998), and most were asymptomatic (Geraniotis et al, 1988; Joseph et al, 1989; Schlager et al, 1995).

Even though prophylactic antibiotics administered during clean intermittent catheterization may delay and possibly decrease bacteriuria in the short term (Johnson et al, 1994), the actual efficacy of such antibiotic usage is unproved. The costly usage of sterile catheters in intermittent catheterization programs for neurogenic bladder does not reduce bacteriuria and appears to have no proven benefits (Schlager et al, 2001). One study with more than 5 years of follow-up noted complications such as episodes of urinary calculi and epididymitis (de la Hunt et al, 1989); the long-term natural history of clean intermittent catheterization programs deserves further study.

Little investigation of the bacteriuria of bowel-augmented bladders exists. In a prospective study, those who had bladder substitution were found to have greater bacteriuria than those without and there was a substantial local IgA antibody response to the resident bacteria and increased IgG response from the bladder or upper tracts (Iwakiri et al, 2002). Whether this local response contributes to asymptomatic UTI or is protective is unknown.

Iatrogenic Factors

The urinary tract is the most common site of nosocomial infection. Although there are no good data on risk of catheter-induced infections in children, in adult women the incidence of catheter-induced UTI ranges from 1% to 20% depending upon the circumstances of catheterization (Stamey, 1980). It has been documented that nosocomial UTIs frequently complicate hospitalization in children, especially when urethral catheterization is performed (Dele Davies et al, 1992; Lohr et al, 1994). This may be a reason to consider giving antimicrobial prophylaxis whenever urethral manipulation is performed. It is on this basis that children who contract hospital-acquired UTI, who have urinary tract abnormalities, who have recently been instrumented, or have had recent antimicrobial treatment are more likely to have infections caused by unusual and more antibiotic-resistant organisms (Ashkenazi et al, 1991b).

Table 112–4. Bacterial Endocarditis Prophylaxis for Pediatric Genitourinary Procedures

Oral	
Amoxicillin*	50 mg/kg 1 hr before procedure
Parenteral	
Ampicillin†	50 mg/kg IM or IV within 30 min before procedure
±Gentamicin	1.5 mg/kg IM or IV within 30 min before procedure
Penicillin allergy	
Vancomycin	20 mg/kg IV infused slowly over 1 hr beginning 60-120 min before procedure
±Gentamicin‡	1.5 mg/kg IM or IV within 30 min before procedure

*Risk of endocarditis is high in patients with previous endocarditis, prosthetic heart valves, complex cyanotic congenital heart disease such as tetralogy of Fallot, or surgically constructed systemic pulmonary shunts or conduits. High risk of endocarditis is also seen in other forms of congenital heart disease (but not uncomplicated secundum atrial septal defect), acquired (such as rheumatic) valvular disease, hypertrophic cardiomyopathy, and mitral valve prolapse with regurgitation of thickened leaflets. Enterococci are the most common cause after genitourinary procedures.
†High-risk patients given parenteral ampicillin before the procedure should receive a dose of ampicillin 1 g IN or IV or a dose of amoxicillin 1 g orally 6 hr afterward.
‡Gentamicin should be added for patients with a high risk of endocarditis.
Modified from Abramowicz M: Prevention of bacterial endocarditis. Med Lett 2001;43:98-99.

When urethral catheters remain indwelling for longer than 4 days, bacteriuria is almost inevitable, as bacteria attach to the device surface and form biofilms of extracellular polymers, making these bound organisms resistant to routine antimicrobial treatment (Donlan, 2001).

As the urinary tract is second only to the mouth as the source of bacterial endocarditis, the American Heart Association recommends bacterial endocarditis antimicrobial prophylaxis before urethral catheterization in individuals with a known urinary infection (Table 112–4). Cost outcome analysis for bacterial endocarditis prophylaxis of febrile children with moderate cardiac lesions in an emergency room being evaluated for UTI showed no cost-benefit value (Caviness et al, 2004). Endocarditis antimicrobial prophylaxis is not recommended, however, when urine is sterile.

In school-age boys, urethral self-manipulation with water injection or self-instrumentation has been reported to cause UTI (Labbé, 1990). About 25% of children who are victims of sexual abuse may complain of dysuria and urinary frequency, but these children rarely have UTIs (Klevan and DeJong, 1990).

DIAGNOSIS OF URINARY TRACT INFECTION

Rapid diagnosis of UTI is essential to initiating rapid antimicrobial treatment and preventing renal damage. In children who have no alternative fever source on the basis of history or physical findings, greater than 5% are found to have UTIs (American Academy of Pediatrics, 1999). In febrile infants (younger than 8 weeks), the prevalence of UTIs has been found to be 13.6% with the majority occurring in males (Lin et al, 2000).

KEY POINTS: URINARY TRACT INFECTION RISK FACTORS

- Risk factors for bacteriuria and subsequent renal damage are distinct for individual hosts (see Table 112–3).

- Bacteriuria is most common at the extremes of life—infants and elderly people.

- Blood group phenotypes found on the urothelial surface influence risk of UTI.

- Two risks for recurrent UTI in young women are age at first UTI younger than 15 years and UTI in the mother.

- Renal scarring is a risk factor for future renal scarring.

Young children may show only signs of generalized illness—fever, irritability, poor feeding, vomiting, and diarrhea. In a busy children's hospital emergency room, the **overall prevalence of UTIs in febrile infants younger than 12 months and girls younger than 2 years with a temperature higher than 38.5° C without other cause was 3.3%,** with a higher prevalence in whites, girls, and uncircumcised boys; white girls had a UTI prevalence of 16.1% (Shaw et al, 1998a).

Symptoms

UTI is a common cause of pediatric bacterial infection (Bonadio et al, 1993; Crain and Gershel, 1990; Hoberman et al, 1993). Fever accounts for about 20% of pediatric office visits (Eggli and Tulchinsky, 1993), and UTI causes 4.1% to 7.5% of these febrile episodes (American Academy of Pediatrics, 1999).

Infants

In seriously ill infants and young children, one must suspect UTI and obtain a urinary specimen even if signs may point elsewhere (Hoberman and Wald, 1997; American Academy of Pediatrics, 1999). Specifically, in febrile infants from birth to 8 to 10 weeks, neither clinical symptoms nor laboratory tests can be used to predict a presumptive UTI or eliminate the likelihood of a UTI even if other sites of infection are suggested clinically (Crain and Gershel, 1990) (Table 112–5).

The prevalence of UTI in febrile infants (younger than 8 weeks) has been found to be about 13.6% with the majority occurring in males (Lin et al, 2000). **It is important to note that febrile infants unsuspected of having a urinary source of infection are as likely to have a urinary source as those who are suspected of having a urinary source (5.1% versus 5.9%); 3.5% of infants with another possible source, such as otitis media, also had a UTI** (Hoberman et al, 1993).

Young Children

As in infants, children younger than age 2 have UTI symptoms that are vague and generalized—fever, irritability, poor feeding, vomiting, diarrhea, and ill appearance (Ginsburg and

Table 112–5. **Symptoms of Urinary Tract Infection in 100 Infants with Acute Urinary Tract Infections**	
Symptom	**Percentage**
Fever	67
38° C	100
39° C	57
Irritable	55
Poor feeding	38
Vomiting	36
Diarrhea	36
Abdominal distention	8
Jaundice	7

Modified from Ginsburg CM, McCracken GHJ: Urinary tract infections in young infants. Pediatrics 1982;69:409-412.

McCracken, 1982) (see Table 112–5). **If one uses a clinical decision rule to decide which febrile young girls should be cultured for UTI, the presence of two of the following five variables may be useful: (1) younger than 12 months, (2) white race, (3) absence of other fever source, (4) temperature greater than 39° C, and (5) fever of 2 days or more. These parameters predict UTI with sensitivity of 95% and specificity of 0.31 and avoid 30% of unnecessary urine cultures** (Gorelick and Shaw, 2000).

Older Children

The older toilet-trained, talking child may indicate signs that better localize to the urinary tract, such as dysuria, suprapubic pain, voiding dysfunction, incontinence, or flank or abdominal pain. Many of these children still do not describe urinary tract symptoms, however. For children without localizing signs or with symptoms only vaguely referable to the urinary tract, suspicion must still be high to avoid missing the diagnosis.

Adolescents

In adolescents with dysuria and frequency, physicians must evaluate for both UTI and sexually transmitted diseases (STDs). **There are estimates that about 50% of high school students have had at least one sexual encounter. The prevalence of *Chlamydia* is 13% to 26% and *Neisseria gonorrhoeae* about 2% to 10% in this population.** For this reason, considering STDs in this group (16 to 24 years) may be as important as or more important than considering UTIs in the differential diagnosis (Claudius, 2000; Pimenta et al, 2000). Some also suggest UTI as a possible marker for teenage sexual activity (Nguyen and Weir, 2002).

In this group of teenagers, untreated STDs can progress to pelvic inflammatory disease in 10% to 40% with 12% infertility and an even greater possibility of chronic pelvic pain. One clinical report was unable to differentiate on the basis of symptoms between females with culture-proven UTI and those with SDT (Claudius, 2000).

Physical Examination

There are no signs specific for UTI in the infant. If there is a gross genitourinary anatomic abnormality, a renal mass may be palpable, as found in children with xanthogranulomatous pyelonephritis or infected severe hydronephrosis. Palpation in the suprapubic and flank areas may cause pain in the older child, but generalized abdominal or upper quadrant pain may also be present. Perineal examination rarely shows an ectopic ureteral opening, ureterocele, or urethral discharge in girls. Signs such as back scars, sacral fat pads, or sacral dimples or pits may suggest a neurogenic bladder and may require further investigation. In boys, the testes are abnormal if affected by epididymitis or epididymo-orchitis.

Diagnostic Tests

Urinary Specimens

Good urinary specimens with which to make the diagnosis of UTI are hard to obtain in children, and diagnostic reliability is related to the quality of the specimen. Routinely, there are four ways in which urinary specimens are obtained in children. **In order of least to most reliable for UTI diagnosis** (Hardy et al, 1976), **they are (1) plastic bag attached to the perineum, a "bagged specimen"; (2) midstream void; (3) catheterization; or (4) suprapubic bladder aspirate.**

Even after extensive skin cleansing, a plastic bag specimen usually reflects the perineal and rectal flora and often leads to indeterminate results. Although an individual midstream-voided specimen in a circumcised boy, older girl, or older uncircumcised boy who can retract his foreskin can be reliable, such specimens obtained in young girls and uncircumcised boys usually reflect periurethral and preputial organisms and cells. A catheterized specimen is reliable if the first portion of urine that may contain urethral organisms is discarded and the specimen is taken from later flow through the catheter. Catheterization has the disadvantages of being traumatic and potentially introducing urethral organisms into a sterile bladder (Dele Davies et al, 1992; Lohr et al, 1994).

The most reliable urinary specimen for culture is obtained by suprapubic bladder aspiration. This can be performed safely in children and even premature infants with a full bladder by cleansing the skin and percutaneously introducing a 21- or 22-gauge needle 1 to 2 cm above the pubic symphysis until urine is obtained by aspirating into a sterile syringe (Barkemeyer, 1994). Although unnecessary in most instances, in infants and young children suprapubic aspiration may be simplified with ultrasound guidance (Buys et al, 1994) and the use of topical and local anesthesia.

Because the urine does not cross the urethra in the aspirated specimen, urethral or periurethral organisms are absent; skin contamination should be nil. **Organisms present in a suprapubic aspirate are pathognomonic of bacteriuria and low bacterial counts are routine** (Buys et al, 1994). The main drawback of suprapubic aspiration is that needle aspiration may be distasteful or inconvenient to the older child, parent, or even physician, and these considerations are important (Kramer et al, 1994a).

Generally, if a UTI is suspected in a child who is not yet toilet trained, only a catheterized or needle-aspirated specimen is acceptable for diagnosis because bagged urinary specimens have an unacceptably high false-positive rate. Under special collection circumstances when the perineum is cleaned well and the bag removed and processed promptly after voiding, a bagged specimen or even a diaper specimen that shows no growth is useful in eliminating bacteriuria as a diagnosis (Ahmad et al, 1991). **Plastic bag specimens are unreliable and unacceptable for diagnosis of UTI in high-risk populations and infants younger than 2 months** (Crain and Gershel, 1990).

Urinalysis

Four determinations from the urinalysis have been advocated to support a diagnosis of UTI: (1) microscopic urinary examination for white blood cells (WBCs), "pyuria," usually defined as more than 5 WBCs per high-power field (HPF) in a centrifuged specimen; (2) microscopic urinary examination for bacteria defined as any bacteria per HPF in the unstained centrifuged urinary sediment; (3) urinary leukocyte esterase; and (4) urinary nitrite. The finding of red and white cell casts in the urinary sediment is unreliable.

Sensitivity of routine urinalysis for UTI has been calculated to be 82% and is independent of age in children younger than 2 years, and the probability of a UTI with a negative urinalysis is based upon the patient-specific prevalence of UTI (Shaw et al, 1998b; Bachur and Harper, 2001). The prevalence depends upon the child's age, race, sex, and temperature (Bachur and Harper, 2001). Urinalysis findings that do not support a UTI, however, decrease the likelihood of a UTI five-fold (Bachur and Harper, 2001).

Microscopic Examination

Although there are many confounding factors, the microscopic identification of bacteria in the urine is more sensitive and specific for diagnosing UTI than identification of pyuria (Hallender et al, 1986; Lohr, 1991). **Identification of bacteria under high dry magnification (magnification 450 to 570) represents about 30,000 bacteria per milliliter.** In a meta-analysis of screening tests, microscopic identification of any bacteria on Gram staining of uncentrifuged urine had the best combination of sensitivity and false-positive rates (Gorelick and Shaw, 1999). The use of either of these tests separately has such low sensitivity in this high-risk population, however, that neither can be relied upon.

In febrile children younger than 2 years, Hoberman and Wald (1997) found that catheter-collected specimens had a positive predictive value for UTI diagnosis of 84.6% if microscopic examination showed bacteria (any bacteria on 10 oil immersion fields in a Gram-stained specimen) and 10 WBC/mm^3 (on enhanced urinalysis; note that this is not per HPF). Although these two parameters may offer the best predictive value, the office practitioner cannot perform either of these tests easily and rapidly without further instruction (enhanced quantitative WBC count and Gram-stained bacteria on unspun specimen). **These investigators emphasized that UTI in these children is still best defined by a urinary leukocyte count of 10/mm^3 and 50,000 colony-forming units (CFU)/mL on culture** (Hoberman et al, 1994; Hoberman and Wald, 1997).

Urinary Leukocyte Esterase, Nitrite, and Other Chemical Tests

Several other "quick" tests that may be performed on urinalysis have been popular for trying to predict UTI. Urinary leukocyte esterase detects urinary enzymes produced by the breakdown of white cells in the urine and, as such, is dependent upon the presence of white cells, which may or may not be present with the infection. The test may be less reliable in infants (Hoberman et al, 1994). **Dietary nitrates that are reduced to nitrite by many gram-negative urinary bacteria are measured by the urinary nitrite test. The facts that first morning voided urinary specimens should be used for this test because bacterial reduction of nitrate can take several hours and that many gram-positive bacteria do not perform this reduction are serious drawbacks.** Urinary catalase, an enzyme commonly produced by bacteria infecting the urinary tract, is sensitive but has too high a false-positive rate to be reliable (Waisman et al, 1999). Although these tests are rapid and efficient, they are even less reliable when the bacterial count is below 100,000 CFU/mL.

In a general pediatric population, when urinary specimens are properly collected and promptly processed, **the combination of positive leukocyte esterase and nitrite testing and microscopic confirmation of bacteria has almost 100% sensitivity for detection of UTI, and when all (or leukocyte esterase and nitrite tests) are negative the negative predictive value approaches 100%** (Wiggelinkhuizen et al, 1988; Lohr et al, 1993). The arguments for and against relying upon urinalysis characteristics for presumptive diagnosis of a UTI have been well summarized (Lohr, 1991; American Academy of Pediatrics, 1999; Gorelick and Shaw, 1999). Moreover, presumptive treatment when the dipstick shows at least 2+ leukocyte esterase or positive nitrite while the culture is obtained appears to be most cost-effective as well (Shaw et al, 1998b).

Although there is no test or combination of urinary tests that meets the gold standard of culture, combinations of these tests may help suggest patients in whom culture will be positive and in whom presumptive treatment might be started, but the urinalysis cannot replace urinary culture (American Academy of Pediatrics, 1999) (Table 112–6). Interestingly, when a risk-benefit analysis based on the current literature on febrile children 3 to 24 months old was performed with the goal of preventing the majority of cases of end-stage renal disease and hypertension, both urinalysis and culture were needed to optimize prevention (Kramer et al, 1994b).

Table 112–6. **Sensitivity and Specificity of Components of the Urinalysis, Alone and in Combination (References in Text)**		
Test	Sensitivity % (Range)	Specificity % (Range)
Leukocyte esterase	83 (67-94)	78 (64-92)
Nitrite	53 (15-82)	98 (90-100)
Leukocyte esterase or nitrite positive	93 (90-100)	72 (58-91)
Microscopy: white blood cells	73 (32-100)	81 (45-98)
Microscopy: bacteria	81 (16-99)	83 (11-100)
Leukocyte esterase or nitrite or microcopy positive	99.8 (99-100)	70 (60-92)

From American Academy of Pediatrics. Committee on Quality Improvement. Subcommittee on Urinary Tract Infection: Practice parameter: The diagnosis, treatment, and evaluation of the initial urinary tract infection in febrile infants and young children. Pediatrics 1999;103:847, Table 1.

Serum Tests Indicating Urinary Tract Infection Severity

Complete blood counts (Kramer et al, 1993), erythrocyte sedimentation rates (ESRs), C-reactive protein (CRP), urinary concentrating ability (Åbyholm and Monn, 1979), urinary tubular enzymes (Johnson et al, 1990; Tomlinson et al, 1994), antibody-coated bacteria, urinary antibodies, and IL-6 (Benson et al, 1994) have been examined as possible simple and noninvasive markers of renal infection (Buyan et al, 1993), but none alone has been validated as definitive.

CRP greater than 7 mg/dL has been associated with serious bacterial infection in febrile children 1 to 36 months old (Pulliam et al, 2001). Although the host urinary tract responds to bacterial infection with the production of cytokines and IL-6 is secreted in response to *E. coli* attachment, it appears that this local response is followed by a systemic increase in CRP and fibrinogen, which suggests that fever, CRP, and ESR are part of the host response to bacterial attachment (de Man et al, 1991). Serum procalcitonin, a hormonally inactive propeptide of calcitonin, is elevated in sepsis. **Elevation of serum procalcitonin has also been reported to correlate with the severity of UTI and predict risk of renal scarring** (Pecile et al, 2004). Greater prospective numbers are needed to validate the use of this test.

Reduced urinary concentrating ability is associated with pyelonephritis, but this appears to be unassociated with the acute febrile response in pyelonephritis and probably not a reliable sign for early detection of pyelonephritis (de Man et al, 1991). Unfortunately, none of these tests is reliable enough for early UTI detection or to differentiate between upper and lower tract infections or severity of infection for routine use. These tests are being performed primarily on an investigational basis.

Urinary Culture

The gold standard for the diagnosis of UTI is quantitative urinary culture. This requires a known quantity of urine to be plated on a culture plate and the number of bacterial CFU that grow to be counted and determined as CFU/mL. The interpretation of the culture result defining a UTI diagnosis is, however, debatable and dependent upon specimen quality. Because it may take 24 or more hours before bacterial CFU grow and the culture is complete, indirect urinary tests that may be performed with routine urinalysis to detect the presence of bacteria or by-products have been sought for more rapid diagnosis.

Although 100,000 CFU/mL of voided urine is the traditional definition for a clinically significant UTI (Kass and Finland, 1956), other studies have shown that 10,000 or fewer organisms on a voided specimen may indicate a significant UTI (Stamm et al, 1982; Bollgren et al, 1984). In febrile children younger than 2 years, Hoberman and associates (1994) showed that 50,000 CFU/mL in catheterized specimens constitutes a significant UTI. Occasionally, even lower numbers of bacteria may justify diagnosis of a significant UTI, especially when the specimen is obtained by suprapubic needle aspiration, circumstances under which any number of organisms might be significant. Cultured CFU/mL may be low because of hydrational dilution, frequent voiding preventing bacterial multiplication in the bladder, and bacterial growth characteristics.

Acute and Focal Pyelonephritis (Lobar Nephronia or Focal Bacterial Nephritis)

Symptoms and Signs

Children with pyelonephritis have the classical symptoms of fever, chills, and unilateral or bilateral flank pain with or without accompanying lower tract symptoms of dysuria, frequency, and urgency. They may not localize symptoms to their flanks and complain of nonspecific abdominal discomfort. Physical examination reveals fever usually accompanied by abdominal discomfort and pain over the costovertebral area.

The urine is usually cloudy and malodorous. Urinary sediment usually shows pyuria, white blood cell casts, and red blood cells. Bacterial rods are often present. Bacterial infection of the urinary tract causes bladder, ureteral, renal pelvic, and renal inflammation that alters urinary tract urodynamics and causes ureterectasis, elevated renal pelvic pressures, and renal inflammatory changes that may be associated with renal swelling (Hinman, 1971; Boyarsky and Labay, 1972; Issa and Shortliffe, 1992; Johnson et al, 1992).

Radiologic Findings

The discoveries that early renal cortical lesions from pyelonephritis can be detected by 99mTc-DMSA nuclear scan and that these lesions correlate with histopathologic areas of acute renal inflammation in animal models have advanced knowledge of the natural history of urinary tract bacteriuria (Parkhouse et al, 1989; Wikstad et al, 1990; Rushton and Majd, 1992a; Giblin et al, 1993). Radiologic findings in acute pyelonephritis depend upon the imaging modality used. When intravenous urography was the main urinary tract imaging modality, the majority of patients had normal studies. Other modalities now show that findings commonly include renal enlargement related to inflammation and edema, focal renal enlargement (acute lobar nephronia or focal bacterial pyelonephritis), impaired or delayed excretion, and dilation of the urinary collecting system. These acute changes affect renal and collecting system dilation and size, making the interval between the UTI and imaging evaluation an important consideration when a clinician evaluates renal size or shape. What appears to be a kidney of normal or even enlarged size and shape may be a scarred small one at a later time (Hansen and Shortliffe, 1998).

Focal or general renal enlargement or swollen kidneys may be found in acute pyelonephritis. Renal ultrasonography, nuclear scans, and computed tomography (CT) may show generalized renal enlargement or focal hypoechoic or hyperechoic areas representing focal pyelonephritis (lobar nephronia). The latter represents a localized, severe nonliquefactive infection of one or more renal lobules (Greenfield and Montgomery, 1987; Klar et al, 1996; Wallin et al, 1997; Uehling et al, 2000). Other findings on ultrasonography include thickening of the renal pelvis, hypoechogenicity, and focal or diffuse hyperechogenicity and ureteral dilation (Mårild et al, 1989a; Morin et al, 1999). **CT or power Doppler may show areas of decreased perfusion** (Dacher et al, 1996). High-resolution renal ultrasonography has been suggested to be almost as sensitive as DMSA for diagnosing renal involvement in pyelonephritis (Dacher et al, 1996; Morin et al, 1999).

When DMSA lesions are used as the standard for diagnosing acute pyelonephritis, about 50% to 86% of children (about 60% of kidneys) with febrile UTIs and other clinical signs have renal involvement or pyelonephritis (Verber and Meller, 1989; Rushton and Majd, 1992b; Benador et al, 1994; Jakobsson et al, 1994). About half (38% to 75%) of these lesions persist on DMSA scans performed 2 months to 2 years later (Rushton and Majd, 1992b; Benador et al, 1994; Stokland et al, 1996) with fewer lesions persisting at longer intervals of follow-up. This suggests that as many as 40% to 50% of young children who have febrile UTIs suffer renal scarring. Of children older than age 1 with first time symptomatic UTI, 38% had DMSA evidence of renal damage after 1 year and almost half of these (47%) had reflux. **Children who had an elevated CRP, fever, and dilating reflux had a 10 times higher risk of renal damage than children with UTI who had a normal or slightly elevated CRP, no or mild fever, and no vesicoureteral reflux** (Stokland et al, 1996; Yen et al, 1999).

Pyonephrosis

Pyonephrosis is characterized by accumulation of purulent debris and sediment in the renal pelvis and urinary collecting system. Children with pyonephrosis have symptoms similar to those of acute pyelonephritis but have additional obstructive hydronephrosis. This situation usually implies bacterial infection and obstruction, and rapid diagnosis and treatment are essential to avoid sepsis and parenchymal loss.

Renal ultrasonography is usually diagnostic. The majority of obstructed pyonephrotic kidneys are either nonfunctioning or poorly functioning (Coleman et al, 1981). **The renal sonogram may show shifting fluid-debris levels with changes in the patient's position, persistent echoes from the lower collecting system, air in the collecting system, or weak echoes secondary to pus in a dilated poorly transonic renal collecting system** (Coleman et al, 1981). If performed, retrograde pyelography shows ureteral obstruction and irregular renal pelvic filling defects caused by purulent sediment. When it is possible to pass a ureteral catheter past the obstruction, drainage becomes both diagnostic and therapeutic.

Pyonephrosis is treated by administration of appropriate antimicrobial drugs and prompt drainage of the infected pelvis by either retrograde catheterization or nephrostomy placement. When the acute infection is treated and the patient is receiving appropriate antimicrobial agents, further evaluation to identify and treat the obstruction may be necessary.

Perinephric or Renal Abscess

Improvements in imaging of the genitourinary tract and widespread use of powerful antimicrobial agents have changed the evaluation and natural history of perinephric and renal abscesses (Shortliffe and Stamey, 1986a). In the past, the high mortality rate from perinephric abscesses was related in part to diagnostic delay. Perinephric and renal abscesses are uncommon in children.

These abscesses arise from either hematogenous seeding from extragenital sites of infection or renal extension of ascending urinary infections. **Since the introduction of broad-spectrum and powerful antimicrobial agents in the 1940s, the percentage of perirenal abscesses caused by staphylococci decreased from 45% before 1940 to 6% after 1940, and those attributed to E. coli and Proteus rose from 8% to 30% and 4% to 44%, respectively** (Thorley et al, 1974). This large decrease in perirenal and renal abscesses caused by staphylococci may be related to the advent of antimicrobial agents discovered to treat skin and wound abscesses (Thorley et al, 1974; Shortliffe and Stamey, 1986a).

Children with renal and perirenal abscesses have severe pyelonephritis—fever, flank pain, leukocytosis, and occasionally sepsis. With the frequent use of renal ultrasonography for evaluation of such symptoms and characteristic findings, diagnosis is now easier. Because most abscesses have a fluid component, perinephric collections usually appear sonolucent and diagnostic aspiration of this area is usually associated with minimal morbidity. Extent of the abscess can be more extensively assessed with CT, which may show perirenal fluid or gas, renal distortion, and involvement of the retroperitoneum (Hoddick et al, 1983).

Whereas Staphylococcus aureus with antecedent skin lesions may have been the most common cause of renal abscesses in children and adults over two decades ago (Rote et al, 1978), gram-negative organisms (E. coli) are now the most common cause. These are more likely to be associated with retrograde extension of ascending infection in relation to severe pyelonephritis and genitourinary anomalies (Rote et al, 1978; Steele et al, 1990; Barker and Ahmed, 1991; Vachvanichsanong et al, 1992). Anaerobic bacteria may cause perinephric or renal abscesses in association with previous abdominal surgery, renal transplantation, malignancy, and oral or dental infection (Brook, 1994).

The current systemic antimicrobial agents allow successful treatment of some abscesses with antimicrobial therapy alone without surgical drainage (Steele et al, 1990; Vachvanichsanong et al, 1992). In many cases, however, percutaneous or surgical drainage combined with appropriate antibiotic therapy is required (Rote et al, 1978; Steele et al, 1990; Vachvanichsanong et al, 1992).

MANAGEMENT OF PEDIATRIC URINARY TRACT INFECTIONS

The therapeutic strategy in managing pediatric UTIs is first to minimize renal damage during the acutely diagnosed UTI and second to minimize risk of future renal damage from subsequent infections. Rapid recognition of a UTI and rapid, appropriate antimicrobial treatment are keys to preventing renal damage. As discussed earlier, clinical and experimental data show that early antimicrobial treatment appears to be the most effective means of preventing renal scarring and subsequent complications.

Treatment of Acute Urinary Tract Infections

Infants (Children Younger than 90 Days)

When treatment of UTI is considered, infants or children younger than 90 days are usually treated separately from older children. Children younger than 90 days are more likely to have their course of disease change rapidly because of their physiology and incompletely developed immune system.

KEY POINTS: URINARY TRACT INFECTION DIAGNOSIS

- Febrile infants unsuspected of having a UTI are as likely to have a UTI as those who are suspected of having a UTI.

- In adolescents, UTI is a possible marker for teenage sexual activity and they should be evaluated for STD.

- Any organisms present in a suprapubic urine aspirate are pathognomonic of bacteriuria; low bacterial counts are routine.

- Plastic bag specimens are unreliable and unacceptable for UTI diagnosis in high-risk populations and infants.

- Identification of bacteria under high dry microscope field conditions represents about 30,000 bacteria per mL.

- C-reactive protein (CRP) greater than 7 mg/dL is likely to be associated with serious bacterial infection in febrile children to 3 years.

- In acute pyelonephritis, focal or general renal swelling may be found in imaging tests.

- Children with elevated CRP, fever, and dilating reflux are at 10 times greater risk for renal damage than those with these elements absent.

- Gram-negative organisms are now the most common cause of renal abscesses, whereas *S. aureus* was the most common cause three decades ago.

There have been documented studies that emphasize immune deficiencies or alterations in neonatal T, B, and antigen-presenting cells compared with adult cell behavior (Adkins et al, 2004). Moreover, infants have vague and nonspecific symptoms of illness that are difficult to interpret. Most commonly, children may be seen with growth failure, diarrhea, irritability, lethargy, malodorous urine, fever, oliguria, or polyuria.

As UTIs are a common cause of fever in infants with a prevalence of 5% to 11%, consideration of UTI diagnosis and management is important. In these children with "occult" serious bacterial infection, CRP (Pulliam et al, 2001), absolute neutrophil count greater than 10.6×10^9/L (Isaacman and Burke, 2002), and asymptomatic jaundice (Garcia and Nager, 2002) may be present. **It has been recommended that testing for UTI be part of the evaluation of asymptomatic jaundice that occurs in an infant younger than 8 weeks, especially with onset after 8 days of life** (Garcia and Nager, 2002). Other risks for infantile UTI are lack of circumcision, female sex, and fever lasting longer than 24 hours (Newman et al, 2002).

For febrile infants younger than 90 days, UTI (67%) is one of the common causes of serious bacterial infection (Byington et al, 2003). Although those younger than a month are most often hospitalized for treatment, those between 30 and 90 days have been managed as outpatients. Antibiotic prophylaxis against group B *Streptococcus* during pregnancy has decreased serious neonatal infections with this organism, but

in many communities increased pathogens are ampicillin resistant. In one study from Utah Children's Hospital, **ampicillin-resistant gram-negative bacteria were the most common cause of serious bacterial infection in infants younger than 3 months** (Byington et al, 2003). This resistance must be taken into consideration for judicious and effective treatment.

Treatment depends upon the child's age and severity of illness. In the child younger than 2 to 3 months, particularly 30 days or younger, with a presumptive serious bacterial infection and possibly a UTI, consideration must be given to antimicrobial coverage of *Listeria monocytogenes* (perinatally acquired) and enterococcus (usually considered postnatally acquired), in which ampicillin gives coverage, thus making ampicillin and gentamicin recommended in this age group (Brown et al, 2002).

Others have recommended that in children 60 days and younger a third-generation cephalosporin may replace ampicillin with or without gentamicin unless meningitis or gram-positive UTI is suspected because of the unlikelihood of *Listeria* and the high resistance rate of other gram-negative organisms; however, as enterococcus UTI still occurs in this group, this is not appropriate when UTI is suspected (Sadow et al, 1999). Other young children who are suspected to have UTI and are severely systemically ill, have a fever and flank or abdominal pain, or are unable to take fluids and immune-compromised children should be treated with parenteral broad-spectrum antimicrobial agents (e.g., aminoglycoside and ampicillin, third-generation cephalosporin, aminoglycoside, and cephalosporin) (Table 112–7). Whether the child requires hospitalization or outpatient parenteral or oral treatment depends upon the clinical status.

Children and Outpatient Therapy

In appropriate infants and young children with presumptive febrile UTI who are taking fluids, have cooperative and reliable parents, and with whom daily contact is possible, some of the newer third-generation cephalosporins, such as **ceftriaxone, allow once-daily outpatient parenteral therapy** (Gordon, 1991; Baskin et al, 1992). Most of these third-generation cephalosporins have a broad spectrum, treat *Enterobacter* species and some *Pseudomonas aeruginosa*, and conveniently require only once- or twice-daily dosing. It must be emphasized that *Enterococcus* is still resistant to most. **Meta-analysis of available randomized evidence recommends adoption of once-daily dosing of aminoglycosides in children; this minimizes cost, may improve efficacy and safety, and allows day or potentially outpatient treatment** (Contopoulos-Ioannidis et al, 2004). The efficacy of once-daily dosing for treatment of UTIs may stem from the fact that serum aminoglycoside levels, so often targeted in treatment of bacteremia, are unnecessary in the treatment of UTIs without associated sepsis because the drugs are concentrated during excretion in the kidney and urine to levels many times those achieved in the serum, This makes serum aminoglycoside levels less useful in treating UTIs. There is little evidence that gentamicin is likely to affect permanently those with reduced residual renal function (Baker et al, 2003).

Because the antimicrobial spectrum varies slightly for each of these drugs, the environment and local ecology (e.g., community-acquired outpatient versus hospital-acquired UTI)

Table 112–7. Useful Antibacterial Drugs for Urinary Tract Infection

Urinary Tract Infection Severity	Adult Dosage*	Pediatric Dosage*	Mode	Cost ($)†
Urinary Tract Sepsis				
Third-generation cephalosporin ± (aminoglycoside)				
Cefotaxime (Claforan)		50-180 mg/kg/day* (q4-6 h)		
Ceftriaxone (Rocephin)		50-75 mg/kg/day (q12-24 h)		
Cefepime (Maxipime)				
Ceftazidime (Fortaz, Tazicef, Tazidime)		90-150 mg/kg/day (q8-12 h)		
Cefpodoxime (Vantin)	200 mg q12 h	10 mg/kg q24 h or 5 mg/kg q12 h	PO	106
Ticarcillin/clavulanate (Timentin)		50-200 mg/kg/day (q4-8 h)		
Piperacillin/tazobactam (Zosyn)				
Imipenem (Primaxin)				
Meropenem (Merrem)				
Ampicillin ± aminoglycoside		50-100 mg/kg/day (q4-8 h)	PO	
Gentamicin		7.5 mg/kg/day* (q8 h)		
Tobramycin				
Amikacin		7.5 mg/kg/day* (q8 h)		
Acute Uncomplicated Pyelonephritis				
Fluoroquinolone				
Ciprofloxacin (Cipro)	500 mg q12 h	10-15 mg/kg q12 h	PO	
Amoxicillin/clavulanate (Augmentin)		20-40 mg/kg/day (q8 h)		
Third-generation cephalosporin				
Acute Uncomplicated UTI				
Trimethoprim-sulfamethoxazole				
Average generic (400 mg/80 mg)	1 tablet q6 h	4-5 mg/kg (TMP) q6 h	PO	16.00
Double strength (DS) (800 mg/160 mg)	1 DS tablet q12 h		PO	11.60
Penicillins				
Amoxacillin	500 mg q8 h	6.6-13.3 mg/kg q8 h or	PO	9.60
Amoxicillin/clavulanate (Augmentin)		15 mg/kg q12 h	PO	
Cephalosporin				
Cephalexin (average generic)	500 mg q6 h	6.25-25 mg/kg q6 h	PO	38.80
Cefuroxime axetil (Ceftin) (average generic cost)	500 mg bid	10-15 mg/kg q12 h	PO	135.40
Cefaclor (Ceclor)	500 mg q12 h	6.6-13.3 mg/kg q8 h	PO	89.90
Cefprozil (Cefzil)	500 mg q12 h	15 mg/kg q12 h	PO	173.60
Ceftibuten (Cedex)	400 mg daily	9 mg/kg q24 h	PO	86.30
Nalidixic acid		55 mg/kg/day (q6 h)	PO	
Fluoroquinolones				
Ciprofloxacin	500 mg q12 h	10-15 mg/kg bid‡	PO	109.20
Azithromycin (Zithromax)	500 mg day 1, then 250 mg days 2-5	5-12 mg/kg q24 h		
Nitrofurantoin				
Average generic	100 mg q6 h	1.25-1.75 mg/kg q6 h	PO	44.40
Macrodantin (macrocrystals)				81.20
Macrobid	100 mg q12 h		PO	42.80

*Dosage may need to be adjusted for renal or hepatic insufficiency and age. Checking for specific age-related dosing is recommended.
†Cost for 10 days' treatment (5 days with azithromycin and 1 day with fosfomycin) for an adult, according to data from NDCHealth, December 2003.
‡This agent is approved for children for postanthrax prophylaxis only as of this date; pediatric trials for UTI indications are ongoing.
Data from Abramowicz M: Choice of antibacterial drugs. Treat Guidelines Med Lett 2004;2:18-25; Shortliffe LMD: Infection and inflammation of the pediatric genitourinary tract. In Walsh PC, Refik AB, Vaughan ED Jr, Wein AJ (eds): Campbell's Urology, 8th ed. Philadelphia, WB Saunders, 2002, pp 1864-1865.

should determine drug selection. National and local antimicrobial resistance to common organisms that commonly infect the urinary tract must be considered in the selection of both the agent for initial treatment and that for prophylaxis. Generally, parenteral treatment is continued for 2 to 4 days until fever is gone, the child is able to take adequate fluids, and bacterial sensitivities are available to allow treatment with an oral drug with a narrow spectrum.

The clinical response to treatment also depends upon the severity and rapidity of treatment. Of children age 2 or younger (median 5.6 months) hospitalized with a diagnosis of febrile UTI, **89% (of 288 children) became afebrile by 48 hours after parenteral antimicrobial agents were started even if bacteremia or significant genitourinary abnormality was found** (Bachur, 2000). **The median time to attain a normal temperature was 13 to 16 hours.**

Although the duration of treatment is debatable, in most studies involving treatment of febrile UTIs in young children the total duration of therapy has extended from 7 to 10 days. When culture and sensitivity information is available, the antimicrobial agent should be reevaluated and changed if necessary, with treatment continuing for 7 to 10 days. In most cases an oral drug to which the organism is sensitive with a narrower spectrum can be selected. **Analysis has shown that no follow-up urinary culture after 48 hours is required if organisms are sensitive to the antibiotic selected** (Currie et al, 2003).

Less ill older infants and young children who have presumptive febrile UTIs and are capable of taking fluids and oral medicines may be treated with an antimicrobial agent that has a broad spectrum for genitourinary pathogens (see Table 112–7). Although the newer oral cephalosporins have good gram-positive and gram-negative treatment spectra and most often can be given only once or twice a day, many *Enterococcus*, *Pseudomonas*, and *Enterobacter* may be resistant to treatment (Fennell et al, 1980; Ginsburg et al, 1982; Dagan et al, 1992; Stutman, 1993). **In a multicenter randomized clinical trial, oral cefixime appeared as effective as initial intravenous cefotaxime in children 1 to 24 months of age with febrile UTI** (Hoberman et al, 1999).

In adults the newer quinolones are useful because of their broader antimicrobial spectrum and special activity against *P. aeruginosa*, but in children usage of this drug has been limited because of studies showing quinolone-induced cartilage toxicity in young animals. With careful monitoring, limited quinolone usage has shown no cartilage-related toxicities. In situations such as an abnormal urinary tract with upper tract *P. aeruginosa*, there may be a good indication for usage (Schaad, 1991). In 2005 the quinolones were not yet approved for the treatment of pediatric UTIs, but clinical trials are examining pediatric safety and efficacy issues, and they are more widely used in children. It is notable that in adult women amoxicillin-clavulanate is less effective than ciprofloxacin for treatment of uncomplicated cystitis for the possible reason that ciprofloxacin is more likely to eradicate vaginal *E. coli* (Hooton et al, 2005). As young children are less likely to be sexually active, vaginal colonization may be less important in the pathogenesis.

As with other effective antimicrobial agents, resistance to quinolones is on the horizon. In one report from Spain in 1995, 6.4% of *E. coli* UTIs were found to be resistant to ciprofloxacin (Ena et al, 1995). Risk for resistance was related to urinary tract abnormalities, previous quinolone treatment, urinary catheterization, and age of 65 or older. Quinolone resistance in other organisms unrelated to UTI has led to the withdrawal of approval for addition of these drugs in animal feed in 2005.

School-Age Children

In school-age children who do not appear systemically ill and have a "clinically uncomplicated" bladder infection, many oral broad-spectrum antimicrobial agents that are well tolerated cure the uncomplicated UTI in a course of 3 to 5 days; there are no clinical advantages of longer therapy (Lohr et al, 1981; Copenhagen Study Group of Urinary Tract Infections in Children, 1991; Jójárt, 1991; Gaudreault et al, 1992). In some of these children single-dose treatment, particularly with intra-

muscular aminoglycoside, may be curative and cause less fecal antimicrobial resistance (Grimwood, 1988; Khan, 1994), but **in unselected children single doses may not be quite as effective as 3 to 5 days of treatment** (Madrigal et al, 1988; Khan, 1994). Although these trials appear to show that shorter therapy of 3 to 5 days may be as effective as 7 to 14 days, a **meta-analysis of trials involving 3 to 5 versus 7 to 10 days of therapy has shown that longer therapy is more effective, attributing the findings to the fact that in children, unlike adults, there is more likely to be urinary tract abnormality or vesicoureteral reflux that may require longer treatment** (Keren and Chan, 2002).

"Switch" Therapy

Switch therapy, intravenous therapy followed by oral therapy, is commonplace in adults and becoming common in children. **A large series of children from 3 months to 5 years old had successful treatment of febrile UTI with intravenous gentamicin until afebrile (2 to 4 days) given in a day treatment center of a tertiary care hospital, followed by oral antibiotic for a total of 10 days** (Contopoulos-Ionnidis et al, 2004; Gauthier et al, 2004). Similar findings were reported in a randomized trial involving once-daily intravenous treatment with ceftriaxone for 3 or 10 days when followed by oral cefixime for 15 days (Benador et al, 2001).

Antimicrobial Agent Selection

Studies have shown that common uropathogens are increasingly resistant to trimethoprim-sulfamethoxazole and ampicillin. This should be considered when prescribing initial antimicrobial therapy for UTI. The prevalence of uropathogen resistance to trimethoprim-sulfamethoxazole increased from 8% in 1992 to greater than 16% in 1996 (Gupta et al, 1999) with *E. coli* resistance as high as 32% (range of 0% to 46%) in the western United States (Talan et al, 2000). Resistance to ampicillin has been reported to range from 25% to 45% (Dyer et al, 1998; Gupta et al, 1999). **Predictors of situations in which uropathogens are more likely to be resistant to commonly used agents are diabetes; recent hospitalization; recent use of antibiotics, especially trimethoprim-sulfamethoxazole** (Wright et al, 1999); **and presence of urinary malformations, urethral catheters, and antimicrobial prophylaxis** (Ashkenazi et al, 1991a).

Nitrofurantoin attains high urinary concentrations and low serum concentrations and is a poor choice to treat any severe systemic or renal infection, but it is ideal for treating a bladder UTI when there is a normal urinary tract. Resistance rates to nitrofurantoin have changed little over the past decade.

After the therapeutic regimen for acute UTI, the child should be started on a daily prophylactic antimicrobial agent until full radiologic evaluation of the urinary tract may be conveniently performed in the next days to weeks.

PROPHYLACTIC ANTIMICROBIAL AGENTS

Taking daily antimicrobial agents to prevent recurrent UTIs in individuals who may have a 30% to 40% chance of recurrence within a year may seem rational if this management prevents significant morbidity and renal damage. No definitive randomized trials to examine efficacy in the most common situations of vesicoureteral reflux and hydronephrosis have been performed, however. Nonetheless, retrospective data show that reflux nephropathy is less likely in children with high-grade vesicoureteral reflux who present without a UTI (Sweeney et al, 2001). Reviews of the few trials of randomized studies of children involving prophylactic antibiotics offer inadequate data to support prophylaxis definitively (Le Saux et al, 2000; Thompson et al, 2001; Williams et al, 2001; Wheeler et al, 2003; Fanos and Cataldi, 2004). In children, antimicrobial prophylaxis is most commonly used to prevent UTI in the situations listed in Table 112–8.

Although urinary tract prophylaxis has been accepted and shown to decrease infections over a limited period in some groups such as children with vesicoureteral reflux (Hanson et al, 1989), long-term efficacy compared with adequate supervision of patients (Cascio et al, 2001), surveillance, and education has not been studied with randomization and proper stratification of patients (Bollgren, 1999; Thompson et al, 2001). In some of these situations, such as partially obstructive hydronephrosis, the efficacy of prophylaxis has not been established.

The use of antimicrobial prophylaxis with clean intermittent catheterization is controversial, and some of the considerations are discussed in the section on neurogenic bladder. The use of nightly urinary tract antibiotic prophylaxis in children who suffer recurrent UTI without known urinary tract abnormalities is often successful in decreasing symptomatic UTI, as is postintercourse prophylaxis in teens who suffer apparent postcoital "induced" UTI (Pfau and Sacks, 1994; Vosti, 2002).

It has been suggested that circumcision be performed to remove bacterial colonization of the prepuce (uncircumcised penis) in infant boys with vesicoureteral reflux and severe hydronephrosis, as one report stated that antibiotic prophylaxis was ineffective as periurethral swabs grew uropathogens in 37% of boys (mean 2.5 years) taking prophylaxis (Cascio et al, 2001). Although periurethral colonization is a risk factor for UTI, it is unclear how prophylaxis was managed and unlikely that the only role of prophylaxis is in clearing the periurethral area of organisms (Cascio et al, 2001). Moreover, the benefits of prophylactic circumcision are controversial.

When urinary tract antimicrobial prophylaxis is initiated, the time for discontinuing prophylaxis is unclear. Prophylaxis is usually stopped when resolution of the urinary tract abnormality for which prophylaxis is being given occurs (e.g.,

spontaneous or surgical resolution of vesicoureteral reflux or obstruction).

When resolution does not occur within a few months to years, however, the time for stopping prophylaxis is indeterminate. Because evidence exists that renal scarring in girls with pyelonephritis may be less likely after 5 to 6 years of age and may occur less frequently until age 15 to 16, it may be reasonable to perform a trial of stopping prophylaxis when a patient reaches age 5 to 8 or older if the patient has no history of UTI and no renal scarring. Selected groups of children have been observed for a few years after stopping prophylaxis and have generally done well without evidence of UTIs or new scars, but these studies are limited by lack of randomization, short follow-up, or small numbers (Cooper et al, 2000).

Although many agents may be used for treatment of a UTI, the efficacy, microbiology, and pharmacology of few antimicrobial agents used for prophylactic effect have been examined in children (Table 112–9). **The ideal prophylactic agent should have low serum and high urinary concentrations, have minimal effect on the normal fecal flora, be easily administered and tolerated, and be cost-effective.** The potency of these antimicrobial agents is based upon the general susceptibility of most fecal Enterobacteriaceae to the agents at urinary levels. Because these agents are generally concentrated in the urine, the urinary drug levels should be much higher than the drug levels found simultaneously in serum, gut, or tissue, and, if sufficiently low, antimicrobial resistance patterns should not develop in the gut. In some instances this characteristic of the prophylactic antimicrobial agents may be dose related, so that inappropriately high dosing for prophylaxis is less effective rather than more effective because bacterial resistance is created (Martinez et al, 1985).

A difficulty in determining prophylaxis efficacy is dose selection. Adequate urinary levels are required for bactericidal activity, but how many hours per day these levels must be maintained is unknown. In one of the few pediatric studies of urinary drug bioassay in prophylaxis, after a single prophylactic evening dose, cotrimoxazole and cefixime sustained bactericidal effect for about 60% of a 24-hour day with much shorter effects for nalidixic acid and cephalexin (Pomeranz et al, 2000). From this study, however, it is unclear whether a shorter lived, lower urinary concentration may achieve better prophylaxis with less likelihood of creating bacterial resistance. There is evidence that commonly selected antibiotics

Table 112–8. Indications for Urinary Tract Antimicrobial Prophylaxis

Vesicoureteral reflux
Unstable urinary tract abnormality (e.g., partial urinary tract obstruction)
Normal urinary tract but frequent reinfections
After acute UTI awaiting radiologic evaluation
Urethral instrumentation
Immunosuppressed or immunocompromised status
Infants with first UTI before 8-12 weeks of age
Clean intermittent catheterization and vesicoureteral reflux (?)

UTI, urinary tract infection.

Table 112–9. Oral Antimicrobial Agents Useful for Pediatric Urinary Tract Prophylaxis

Drug	Daily Dosage	Age Limitations
Useful and Tested		
Nitrofurantoin	1-2 mg/kg/day	>1 mo
Trimethoprim-sulfamethoxazole	(trimethoprim) 1-2 mg/kg/day	>2 mo
Cephalexin	2-3 mg/kg/day	
Possibly Useful		
Amoxicillin	5 mg/kg/day	
Sulfisoxazole	20-30 mg/kg/day	>2 mo
Trimethoprim	2 mg/kg/day	>2 mo*

*?, little data.

may have different absorption and metabolism patterns in children than adults (Rylance et al, 1985; Hoppu, 1987; Pomeranz et al, 2000).

In any case, the parent who doubles or triples the dose of prophylactic antimicrobial agent each time the child develops the slightest symptom or cold may be losing the prophylactic value of the agent and creating greater numbers of resistant bacteria with greater likelihood of a breakthrough infection with a resistant organism. Another consideration is that long-term compliance of patients with daily prophylaxis may be difficult (Smyth and Judd, 1993).

Because urinary prophylaxis is usually initiated following treatment of an infection for which long-term (10 days) high-dose treatment was given, the fecal flora is usually resistant to the treating drug and many of the prophylactic agents. The child who is very susceptible to urinary infections is likely to become reinfected with an organism resistant to the prophylactic agent before the gut is repopulated with more normal flora. This accounts for frustrating breakthrough infections that occur soon after the child is prescribed prophylactic antimicrobial agents or after treatment of other frequent infections such as otitis media. **The period of greatest risk of recurrent infection is usually the first few weeks after any full-dose treatment. This is the reason that the therapeutic antimicrobial agent should not be the prophylactic agent.**

In children with normal urinary function, useful agents for urinary prophylaxis that have been studied are nitrofurantoin, cephalexin, and trimethoprim-sulfamethoxazole (Brendstrup et al, 1990). Amoxicillin, sulfisoxazole, and trimethoprim alone may also be useful urinary tract prophylactic antimicrobial agents, but they have not been as well studied in children. In toilet-trained children, urinary tract prophylactic antimicrobial drugs may be best given once nightly, when they will be excreted into and remain in the urine overnight.

The long-term effects of prophylactic agents on the child and their microbial ecology have not been completely examined. A literature review of nitrofurantoin and trimethoprim-sulfamethoxazole prophylaxis in children supports long-term safety (Karpman and Kurzrock, 2004). A question concerning antibiotic usage and breast cancer in women was raised following an epidemiologic study relating the two; however, data relating the two are equivocal and further exploration of this information is needed before a clear conclusion can be drawn (Sørensen et al, 2005; Velicer et al, 2004). Although there is some evidence that antibiotics that lack systemic absorption and are excreted only in the urine may result in less overall bacterial resistance and change to human microbial ecology than systemic agents, long-term studies are lacking (Gribble and Puterman, 1993; Johnson et al, 1994; Sandock et al, 1995; Schlager et al, 1998).

Nitrofurantoin

Nitrofurantoin is an effective urinary prophylactic agent because its serum levels are low, urinary levels are high, and it produces minimal effect upon the fecal flora (Winberg et al, 1973). Its effect is based upon urinary excretion of antimicrobial once a day, and it has been found to be effective in girls at doses of 1.0 to 2.4 mg/kg each evening (Lohr et al, 1977). When renal function is reduced to less than half normal, the efficacy of nitrofurantoin may be reduced.

Although the majority of nitrofurantoin drug reactions occur in adults, it has caused acute allergic pneumonitis, neuropathy, and liver damage (Holmberg et al, 1980). Long-term treatment has been associated with rare cases of pulmonary fibrosis. **It should not be used in children with glucose-6-phosphate dehydrogenase deficiencies because it is an oxidizing agent and can cause hemolysis.** About 10% of blacks in the United States, Sardinians, non-Ashkenazi Jews, Greeks, Eti-Turks, and Thais may have a glucose-6-phosphate deficiency, and in these people regeneration of glutathione, which is partially responsible for maintaining red blood cell integrity, is impaired by the enzyme deficiency. When nitrofurantoin is given it oxidizes the hemoglobin to methemoglobin, which is degraded (Thompson, 1969).

Cephalexin

Cephalexin has been studied in adults as a prophylactic agent (Martinez et al, 1985). **Although fecal Enterobacteriaceae resistance has developed in many patients taking full-dose cephalexin (500 mg four times daily), patients taking low doses (one quarter to one eighth the adult daily dose, 250 to 125 mg/day) do not appear to develop resistance.** Cephalexin at one quarter or less of the treatment dose per weight may then be a useful pediatric prophylactic agent.

Trimethoprim-Sulfamethoxazole

Trimethoprim-sulfamethoxazole has been a successful combination drug in the treatment of UTIs and useful for prophylaxis at a dose of approximately 2 mg/kg of trimethoprim (Grüneberg et al, 1976; Stamey et al, 1977). Trimethoprim has the unusual characteristic that it diffuses into the vaginal fluid and therefore decreases vaginal bacterial colonization in the female (Stamey and Condy, 1975). **Because trimethoprim-sulfamethoxazole contains a sulfonamide, it probably should not be used for the first few months of life because sulfonamides may compete for bilirubin binding sites on albumin and cause neonatal hyperbilirubinemia and kernicterus.** As previously mentioned, there has been a significant increase in bacterial resistance to this drug over the past decade (Table 112–10).

Table 112–10. Factors Associated with Trimethoprim-Sulfamethoxazole Resistance	
Factor	**Odds Ratio (OR)**
Antibiotics taken for >4 weeks in past 6 months	23.4
Genitourinary tract abnormality	2.4
Number of hospital admissions in past year	
0 (reference)	1.0
1	2.3
≥2	3.2
Age in years	
<2	0.3
2-6 (reference)	1.0
>6	0.5

Modified from Allen U, MacDonald N, Fuite L, et al. Risk factors for resistance to "first-line" antimicrobials among urinary tract isolates of *Escherichia coli* in children. Can Med Assoc J 1999;160:1436-1440, Table 4.

Trimethoprim

Initial studies performed in adult women found trimethoprim (dose approximately 2 mg/kg once nightly) to be as effective as trimethoprim-sulfamethoxazole and nitrofurantoin in preventing recurrent UTIs (Stamm et al, 1980), but other studies showed rapid emergence of significant trimethoprim-resistant *E. coli* during either treatment or prophylaxis (Huovinen and Toivanen, 1980; Brogden et al, 1982; Murray et al, 1982; Murray and Rensimer, 1983; Brumfitt et al, 1985; Brendstrup et al, 1990).

Studies examining emergence of resistance are controversial. In one study after 14 days of trimethoprim at 200 mg daily, 96% of the trimethoprim-resistant *E. coli* isolated from the fecal flora were resistant to at least four other antimicrobial agents (Murray et al, 1982), emphasizing the need for concern regarding resistance and spread of multidrug resistance. **A clinical trial in children examined the efficacy of nitrofurantoin and trimethoprim prophylaxis in preventing recurrent UTIs and showed nitrofurantoin to be more effective as prophylaxis when used in association with urinary tract abnormalities or vesicoureteral reflux** (Brendstrup et al, 1990). Nitrofurantoin prophylaxis did not change the resistance pattern in uropathogens causing subsequent UTIs, whereas those receiving trimethoprim prophylaxis developed a breakthrough UTI with an organism resistant to the drug in 76% (Brendstrup et al, 1990). With the distribution of liquid trimethoprim approved for treatment of acute otitis media in children and possible wider usage, the drug should be used judiciously to prevent a repetition of previous antimicrobial resistance.

Nalidixic Acid

Nalidixic acid was used to treat children before the advent of more powerful quinolones; however, testing of the newer quinolones (norfloxacin, cinoxacin, ciprofloxacin) has shown that these drugs may be contraindicated in prepubertal children because they have caused cartilage erosion in weight-bearing joints and arthropathy in immature animals. In limited groups of children treated with quinolones, no such effects have been noted (Schaad, 1991).

Probiotics

Concern for the patient's normal flora and the growing rate of bacterial resistance has created interest in probiotic and alternative therapies. **Probiotic therapy refers to a concept in which live organisms are given to patients for therapeutic benefit.** This is based upon the possible mechanism that competitive colonization may create a barrier to colonization with potential pathogens. Although several different organisms and strains have been used, most commonly the strains of gram-positive lactobacillus normally found in the intestinal and urogenital region have been used to colonize or recolonize the gut and urovaginal area.

There is some evidence that probiotic therapy may have efficacy in infants with necrotizing enterocolitis (Reid, 2002; Lin et al, 2005); the few randomized trials available show an equivocal protective effect from neonatal UTI (Dani et al, 2002; Kliegman and Willoughby, 2004). There has also been a report of lactobacillus sepsis, in a neonate and in circumstances of immune compromise, confirmed by DNA fingerprinting following deliberate colonization (Land et al, 2005); this does not negate potential value under the correct circumstances (Vanderhoof and Young, 2002).

Bladder colonization with nonpathogenic organisms has not been used routinely to prevent UTI. Public interest in cranberry products is not supported by study at this time (Schlager et al, 1999).

Future Treatments

At this time the most powerful therapies for UTI are antimicrobial agents. On the horizon are promising vaccine trials that have prevented mucosal adherence of uropathogenic *E. coli* in animals by using common bacterial antigens or the FimH subunit of type 1 pili (Langermann et al, 1997; Thankavel et al, 1997; Uehling et al, 1999). Future studies need to examine whether these vaccines will be clinically useful in children.

IMAGING EVALUATION

Imaging studies are basic to urinary tract evaluation for infection. The goal of management of UTIs is to minimize renal damage from the acute infection and minimize future risk of renal damage. With the multiple imaging modalities available, however, the most efficient and rational order and selection of studies must be made with this goal in mind. **Radiologic imaging can be used to (1) evaluate and localize the acute urinary infection, (2) detect renal damage from the acute infection, (3) identify genitourinary anatomy that increases risk of future renal damage from infection, and (4) evaluate change in the urinary tract over time.** Deciding which studies are necessary in a child with a presumptive or diagnosed UTI should depend on whether potential radiologic findings would change the child's clinical management (Lowe et al, 2004) (Fig. 112–4).

Acute Imaging

Early urinary tract imaging is important in a seriously ill or febrile child in whom the site of infection is unclear or who has unusual circumstances. Circumstances such as newly diagnosed azotemia, a poor response to appropriate antimicrobial drugs after 2 to 3 days, an unusual infecting organism (tuberculosis or urea-splitting organism such as *Proteus*), known partial obstruction such as a ureterocele, ureteropelvic junction obstruction, megaureters, nonfunctioning or poorly functioning renal units, or a history of diabetes, papillary necrosis, or a neuropathic bladder may warrant acute or early upper and lower tract urinary tract imaging.

If treatment depends upon localizing the infection to the kidney, an acute imaging study should be performed. This is particularly important in the severely ill hospitalized child who improves on initial parenteral treatment but whose urinary cultures are inadequate or indeterminate for bacterial infection. An acute DMSA scan may show whether acute renal inflammation is present and justify treatment or not. If, on the other hand, UTI appears highly likely and antimicrobial treatment will be started regardless of radiologic findings, early

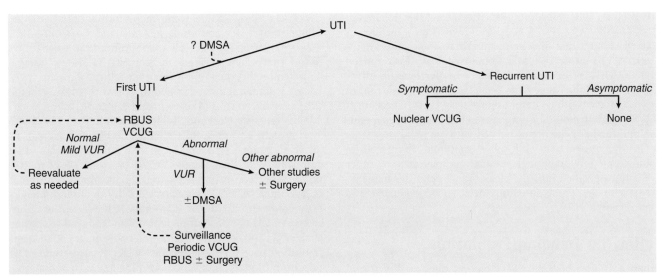

Figure 112–4. Flow diagram of imaging studies used to evaluate and manage urinary tract infections (UTIs) in infants and children using the functional classification of UTI from Figure 112–1. DMSA, technetium-99m dimercaptosuccinic acid renal scanning; RBUS, renal and bladder ultrasonography; VCUG, voiding cystourethrogram; VUR, vesicoureteral reflux.

DMSA scintigraphy is probably unnecessary. This has been confirmed by Hoberman and associates (2003).

Definition of Renal Morphology and Identification of Urinary Tract Abnormalities

Because UTIs in infants and young children may serve as a marker for anatomic abnormalities, after the initial UTI has been adequately treated, the child should be maintained with antimicrobial prophylaxis and radiologic studies performed to delineate the urinary tract. Although there is controversy about whether studies should be performed after the first or recurrent episode, if obstructive lesions are found in 5% to 10% of children and reflux occurs in 21% to 57% (Kunin et al, 1964; Abbott, 1972; Asscher et al, 1973; Newcastle Asymptomatic Bacteriuria Research Group, 1975), early detection of these abnormalities merits full radiologic urinary tract evaluation after the first documented UTI in all young children and infants. It is of interest that vesicoureteral reflux is diagnosed more frequently in children than neonates. One study of the first UTI in neonates showed that vesicoureteral reflux was detected at a rate of 20% in both girls and boys, yet the rate of UTI in the infant boys and girls was 6:1 (Cleper et al, 2004).

Urinary tract imaging evaluation consists of some form of renal and upper collecting system evaluation (usually renal and bladder ultrasonography) and a voiding cystourethrogram (VCUG). The need for evaluative renal ultrasonography has been questioned as the cited data related to obstructive lesions and gross hydronephrosis were obtained before the advent of routine prenatal ultrasonography. In one multicenter study examining children after their first UTI, however, no cases of grade V vesicoureteral reflux or obstructive lesions and few cases of grade IV reflux were detected, although 39% of children scanned had mild to moderate vesi-

coureteral reflux (Hoberman et al, 2003). If this recommendation is followed, knowledge of the results and quality of the prenatal ultrasonography must be known; furthermore, the decision to perform the VCUG is based upon the occurrence of UTI, and early detection before UTI is not planned.

On the other hand, need for the VCUG in children younger than 2 who have a UTI, renal ultrasonography without evidence of urinary tract dilation, and DMSA scan without scarring 3 months later has also been questioned (Hansson et al, 2004). In a retrospective study of children younger than 2 years with UTI in which children who had suspected obstruction were eliminated, vesicoureteral reflux grade III or higher correlated with the presence of renal lesions, and 26% of the children had evidence of renal scarring on DMSA. Although normal DMSA and dilating grade III vesicoureteral reflux were present in seven children, after 2 years five had vesicoureteral reflux resolve spontaneously, one improved, and one had developed a scarred kidney. Forty-six percent of infants without vesicoureteral reflux had DMSA scarring, and 20 of 44 (45%) of children with grade I or II vesicoureteral reflux had scarring (Hansson et al, 2004). Had the children with normal DMSA and grade I to III vesicoureteral reflux been undetected and untreated with prophylaxis, as suggested by these authors, the outcome is unclear.

As previously emphasized, the child's kidney is susceptible to renal scarring and evaluation of the renal morphology and documentation of any anomalies or scarring may be important to the child's management. Although the American Academy of Pediatrics practice parameter limited the recommendations for first UTI imaging evaluation of the upper and lower urinary tract to children between 2 months and 2 years (American Academy of Pediatrics, 1999), others support such evaluation in even younger infants (Goldman et al, 2000).

Acute studies of the kidney may cause overestimation of renal size because of initial edema or lack of appreciation of renal scarring, and mature renal scars may take up to 2 years to be seen by certain imaging techniques (Filly et al, 1974;

Troell et al, 1984; Gordon, 1986; Conway, 1988; Johansson et al, 1988b). As a result, later studies may show smaller or scarred kidneys that may be misinterpreted and cause inappropriate changes in the patient's management. **It is reported that the risks of missing renal scars by performing ultrasonography alone range from 0.4% (school-age children) to 11.1% (infants with recurrent upper tract UTI)** (Christian et al, 2000), but it should be emphasized that this is age dependent, and further evidence associated with the risk is needed.

Clearly, obstruction and other anatomic abnormalities demonstrated by radiologic evaluation may require other evaluation specific to the diagnosis before definitive management is made. These situations need to be evaluated and treated individually.

Follow-up Imaging Evaluation

When a child who has a UTI has no abnormality found after urinary tract radiologic evaluation, no routine further studies need be prescribed. If the collecting systems are normal but one or both kidneys show massive generalized or focal edema with areas of possible hypoperfusion during the acute infection, a subsequent study may be performed to examine the kidney for signs of renal scarring or shrinkage. In this way, a child who should be observed for potential recurrent infections, hypertension, and renal dysfunction may be identified.

If a child has recurrent symptomatic pyelonephritis and no reflux found on previous fluoroscopic VCUG, a nuclear VCUG may be more sensitive at revealing reflux although less likely to define it (Kogan et al, 1986; Macpherson and Gordon, 1986).

SPECIFIC IMAGING TECHNIQUES

Imaging techniques that are useful for evaluating children with UTIs consist of an upper tract modality and a lower tract one that evaluates for vesicoureteral reflux (see Fig. 112–4). The radiologic follow-up of children diagnosed with vesicoureteral reflux is discussed in Chapter 117, "Reflux and Megaureter." Details related to the use of each of these modalities are discussed in relation to the specific study.

Voiding Cystourethrography (Fluoroscopic versus Nuclear)

The VCUG is the most important examination in assessing vesicoureteral reflux in children and, as such, is important for assessing UTIs. The VCUG may be performed either with fluoroscopy and iodinated contrast material or with nuclear imaging agents (usually 99mTc-pertechnetate) using similar techniques (direct radionuclide cystography), but these studies give different information. The traditional fluoroscopic VCUG can show urethral and bladder abnormalities and vesicoureteral reflux.

The radionuclide VCUG may be more sensitive for reflux detection but offers poorer spatial resolution so that urethral lesions, degree of reflux, and details of the collecting system may not be realized. Both fluoroscopic and radionuclide VCUG detection of vesicoureteral reflux is dependent upon

the child voiding and the technical performance (e.g., bladder filling volume) of the study (Fairley and Roysmith, 1977; Lebowitz, 1986; Macpherson and Gordon, 1986). It has been found that when a single nuclear VCUG shows no vesicoureteral reflux when performed for reflux follow-up, a year later it still may show reflux about 30% of the time. Whether this is related to missed or recurrent reflux or technical variation is unclear (Neel and Shillinger, 2000).

The main advantage of radionuclide VCUG has been the lower radiation exposure of 1 to 5 mrad (ovarian dose) compared with fluoroscopic VCUG exposure of 27 to 1000 mrad (reported ovarian exposure depends upon equipment) (Cleveland et al, 1992; Lebowitz, 1992). With modern imaging technology and a tailored examination, however, the fluoroscopic VCUG has been done with 1.7 to 5.2 mrad (Kleinman et al, 1994) and, if available, may offer advantages of anatomic resolution over the radionuclide VCUG. Fluoroscopic radiation from modern equipment claiming low-dose radiation at four different children's hospitals may produce a wide exposure range from 34 to 2230 mrad/min, and pulsed fluoroscopy with optimization for pediatric imaging produces the best image quality to exposure (Brown et al, 2000).

The radionuclide VCUG may be most useful for periodic reflux reevaluation (Lebowitz, 1992) or for screening siblings who have a low risk of reflux. **The radionuclide VCUG should not be used to evaluate first infections in infants or young boys in whom risk of genitourinary abnormality is high and urethral visualization important or in any child in whom high-resolution imaging of the lower urinary tract is important.**

Indirect radionuclide VCUG is performed as part of a renal imaging study. The radionuclide is injected intravenously and the study performed when the kidneys and upper collecting systems are cleared of the radiopharmaceutical agent and bladder is filled maximally with it. The child is then asked to void. Although this method avoids catheterization, when compared with the direct radionuclide VCUG, there is increased radiation exposure and decreased resolution because of body radionuclide background. As it detects only about 60% of the reflux compared with direct VCUG, there are few reasons to perform this test (Eggli and Tulchinsky, 1993).

The VCUG may be performed as soon as the urine is sterile and voiding is normal; patients' compliance may be greater when performed within a week of the diagnosis (McDonald et al, 2000). **Studies have shown that UTI does not cause reflux and there is no reason to wait 3 to 6 weeks to perform the study as long as voiding and bladder volumes have returned to normal** (Lebowitz, 1986; McDonald et al, 2000). Whether the VCUG is done during antimicrobial therapy, immediately after, or a few weeks afterward is not important as long as the child has normal renal function, has normal voiding, responds rapidly to antimicrobial treatment with urinary sterilization, or is maintained on prophylactic antimicrobial treatment to keep urine sterile in the interval between the herald infection and the radiologic evaluation.

If the VCUG is performed as the initial radiologic study, subsequent imaging may be planned depending upon the VCUG results (Hellström et al, 1989). If the VCUG is normal or shows a ureterocele or vesicoureteral reflux, an ultrasound examination of the kidney and bladder will usually

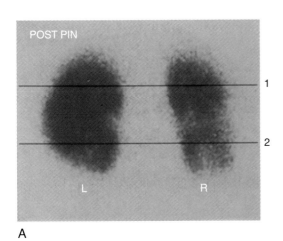

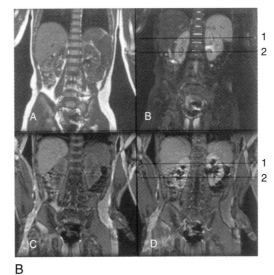

A   B

Figure 112–5. Dimercaptosuccinic acid (DMSA) renogram with single photon emission computed tomography (SPECT) (**A**) and magnetic resonance imaging (MRI) (**B**), showing renal scars in a 3-year-old girl with reflux nephropathy. Comparative coronal levels of DMSA (**A**) and MRI (**B**) are shown. (From Rodriguez L, Spielman D, Herfkens R, Shortliffe L: Magnetic resonance imaging (MRI) for the evaluation of hydronephrosis, reflux, and renal scarring in children. J Urol 2001;166:1023-1027.)

demonstrate other urinary tract structural abnormalities or anomalies, such as dysplasia or obstruction, should they exist. In general, renal and bladder ultrasonography detects children who may need urgent urologic surgery (Alon et al, 1986; Honkinen and Ruuskanen, 1986; Lindsell and Moncrieff, 1986; Macpherson and Gordon, 1986; Alon et al, 1989). If, however, vesicoureteral reflux appears to be the primary diagnosis, DMSA scintigraphy with single photon emission computed tomography (SPECT) or three-dimensional renal magnetic resonance imaging (MRI) may be the most useful studies with which to detect renal scars (Fig. 112–5).

Renal and Bladder Ultrasonography

Renal ultrasonography is the standard for evaluating the pediatric urinary tract after UTI and has replaced intravenous pyelography. Because this modality is not dependent upon renal function, ultrasonography detects both gross and subtler abnormalities of the urinary tract including those that involve poorly functioning or nonfunctioning renal units. **Routine renal ultrasonography is not as sensitive as DMSA at detecting the subtle changes associated with acute UTI** (Verboven et al, 1990; Björgvinsson et al, 1991; Eggli and Tulchinsky, 1993; MacKenzie et al, 1994; Mucci and Maguire, 1994).

When performed at the time of acute inflammation, ultrasonography may show enlarged swollen kidneys, focal enlargement from edema and inflammation that may create a masslike effect (focal pyelonephritis or lobar nephronia), and ureteral widening (Silver et al, 1976; Hellström et al, 1987; Conway, 1988; Johansson et al, 1988a). High-resolution power and color Doppler ultrasonography may also detect small areas of inflammation and resulting hypoperfusion that are on DMSA (Dacher et al, 1996; Morin et al, 1999). As noted previously, renal pelvic debris and sediment levels are diagnostic of pyonephrosis. Although renal inflammatory masses are usually differentiated from other masses easily by symptom context, sometimes imaging with CT or MRI is needed (Cheng, 2004).

Renal and bladder ultrasonography is, moreover, more likely to detect perinephric fluid collections or anatomic abnormalities, especially those involving urinary tract dilation, than either DMSA or intravenous urography (MacKenzie et al, 1994). Pediatric renal and bladder ultrasonography is probably more dependent upon the skill and experience of the ultrasonographer with children than DMSA scintigraphy (Patel et al, 1993). **Even with careful examination for vesicoureteral reflux, however, renal and bladder ultrasonography is notoriously poor at detecting or predicting vesicoureteral reflux** (Mahant et al, 2002).

Nuclear Renography

Because nuclear scintigraphy can detect areas of acute renal inflammation and chronic scarring, this test has improved detection of renal inflammation in pediatric UTI over the past 10 years. **Because approximately 60% of injected 99mTc-DMSA is bound to the proximal renal tubular cells and is excreted slowly in the urine, it is a good cortical imaging agent** (Jakobsson et al, 1992). Radionuclide technology using pinhole images and high-resolution computed tomography (SPECT) give greater renal anatomic detail, resolution, and scar detection (Eggli and Tulchinsky, 1993). DMSA imaging is the common agent when cortical definition alone is needed (Björgvinsson et al, 1991; Eggli and Tulchinsky, 1993).

As 99mTc-glucoheptonate, on the other hand, is partially concentrated and excreted and partially bound to the renal tubule, some collecting system visualization and cortical definition is observed. Similarly, 99mTc-mertiatide (MAG3), a tubular renal imaging agent that is primarily used to assess renal parenchymal flow and function and drainage, also has renal cortical imaging characteristics (planar or SPECT). MAG3 or 99mTc-glucoheptonate may be almost as effective as DMSA in detecting changes of acute pyelonephritis (Traisman et al, 1986; Sreenarasimhaiah and Alon, 1995; Sfakianakis and Georgiou, 1997; Laguna et al, 1998). MAG3 has the advantages over DMSA that it is more rapid, involves a lower radiation dose to most organs and to urinary bladder and gonads, and evaluates urinary tract drainage (Sfakianakis and Georgiou, 1997).

The findings of pyelonephritis detected by renal nuclear scintigraphy (i.e., DMSA with SPECT) differ depending upon the timing of the scan. Acutely, the renal studies usually show either uptake defects or renal swelling (Wallin and Bajc, 1993; Wallin et al, 1997). The uptake defects may appear as wedge-shaped polar or lateral renal defects or as scattered uptake defects within the kidney (Wallin and Bajc, 1993). For this reason DMSA may differentiate focal pyelonephritis or lobar nephronia, column of Bertin, and neoplasm, although CT and MRI are generally more detailed. **Later, after the acute episode heals, scans show (1) a normal pattern, (2) generally diminished uptake and small kidney volume, (3) diminished uptake in the medial kidney, or (4) polar defects with diminished uptake in the renal poles** (Wallin and Bajc, 1994).

DMSA is clearly more sensitive than routine renal ultrasonography or even intravenous urography at detecting renal scarring, but newer high-resolution ultrasonography is nearly as sensitive as DMSA in diagnosing acute renal involvement (Morin et al, 1999). Because recurrent pyelonephritis appears to occur in the same areas, however, it may be difficult to differentiate new and old or progressive renal scarring unless serial studies have been performed (Björgvinsson et al, 1991; Rushton and Majd, 1992b). **Attempts to distinguish between congenital and acquired reflux nephropathy cite generalized decreased renal uptake related to congenital changes and dysplastic changes, whereas focal defects are usually acquired** (Polito et al, 2000). These distinctions are important if one believes acquired lesions are preventable.

In children in whom severe renal scarring has occurred and the glomerular filtration rate (GFR) may need to be estimated, the radionuclide renogram has been found to give an accurate estimate of GFR even in young children (Gates, 1982; Shore et al, 1984; Rehling et al, 1989).

Intravenous Urography

Although the traditional means of evaluating the upper urinary tract and documenting renal scarring was intravenous urography with renal tomography, in most situations DMSA scintigraphy has replaced the role of intravenous urography. DMSA scintigraphy is more sensitive for detecting renal scars but shows less resolution in defining the scars. Intravenous urography still defines collecting system abnormalities in more detail than either DMSA or ultrasonography. It is probably most useful in defining the collecting system in patients with confusing situations or in whom calyceal detail may be important.

Computed Tomography and Magnetic Resonance Imaging

Although seldom used to evaluate acute renal inflammatory processes unless unusual or complicating anatomic configurations are seen on ultrasonography, CT and MRI reveal detailed and sensitive signs of acute renal inflammation. These modalities are often able to differentiate and distinguish between inflammatory, neoplastic, and other renal masses that are seen on other imaging techniques.

For CT evaluation, all four stages of renal enhancement following contrast delivery—renal vascular (10 to 15 seconds), corticomedullary nephrographic (20 to 5 seconds), parenchymal nephrographic (45 seconds to 2 minutes), and excretory phase when the contrast appears in the collecting system (2 to 3 minutes)—should be examined for changes related to inflammation. Acute inflammatory changes of the kidney may be described as (1) unilateral or bilateral, (2) focal or diffuse, (3) with or without focal swelling, and (4) with or without renal enlargement. Other features that may be seen during the various phases are cortical hypoattenuation, wedge defects, poor corticomedullary differentiation during the cortical and parenchymal nephrographic phases, and linear bands of alternating hyper- and hypoattenuation parallel to the tubules and collecting ducts creating a striated effect during the excretory phase. Scans delayed 3 or more hours may help in differentiating renal abscess from hypofunctioning parenchyma in severe pyelonephritis (Kawashima et al, 1997). It should be noted that acute focal pyelonephritis (or lobar nephronia) has been misinterpreted as renal abscess because of this appearance with acute decreased perfusion, and at times MRI- or CT-guided needle aspiration may be needed to clarify the clinical situation. As the mass effect of focal pyelonephritis may take months to resolve, in more remote times these may need to be differentiated from neoplasm.

No studies have compared directly the sensitivity and specificity of DMSA and CT or MRI for detecting renal lesions in acute or chronic pyelonephritis. For routine evaluation of UTI, neither CT nor MRI is cost-effective, but in children with complicated anatomy and UTI, either CT or MRI may be highly useful at defining renal abnormalities and extent of disease when other modalities are inconclusive. MRI and CT are probably as sensitive as or more sensitive than DMSA scintigraphy in detecting renal scars and outline complicated anatomy with greater accuracy (June et al, 1985; Montgomery et al, 1987; Rodriguez et al, 2001) (see Fig. 112–5). Reports of MRI studies that determine function, anatomy, and vesicoureteral reflux may make this modality more useful in the future (Rodriguez, 2000).

SEQUELAE OF URINARY TRACT INFECTION
Chronic Pyelonephritis—Renal Scarring and Dysfunction

Coarse renal scarring seen radiologically as calyceal deformity and renal parenchymal thinning over localized or multiple calyces has been called "reflux nephropathy." Now that it is clear that such scarring is as likely to occur with or without reflux, it would be better termed "pyelonephritic scarring."

The pediatric kidney appears to be at greater risk for scarring from bacterial pyelonephritis than the mature kidney. Many factors, such as intrarenal reflux, urinary tract pressures, host immunity, age, and treatment, appear to contribute to this risk.

In 1974, Rolleston and associates found that areas of renal scar were associated with intrarenal foci of reflux (pyelotubular backflow) observed on voiding cystourethrography in children younger than age 4 who had vesicoureteral reflux. Calyces allowing reflux contained papillae fused with adjacent papillae that caused the papillary ducts to open at right angles rather than at oblique angles more resistant to reflux (Ransley and Risdon, 1974). **These compound papillae are usually found at the renal poles, the areas in which clinical renal scarring is most commonly observed clinically** (Hannerz et al, 1987). Common patterns of scarring are seen in Figure 112–6.

In pigs with vesicoureteral reflux and even intrarenal reflux, however, renal scarring occurs only when both vesicoureteral reflux and bacteriuria are present (Ransley and Risdon, 1978). Reflux without bacteriuria resulted in renal scarring only when the urethra was partially obstructed causing abnormally high voiding pressures (Hodson et al, 1975; Ransley et al, 1984). Experimentally, therefore, the "water hammer" (back pressure) effect of vesicoureteral and intrarenal reflux alone causes renal scarring only when associated with abnormally high bladder and renal pressures.

In the neonate, however, the kidney may respond to urinary back pressure, the water hammer effect, at different thresholds and in different ways than the adult kidney. Autopsy studies on normal neonates (younger than 1 month old) reveal that intrarenal reflux into compound calyces may be created at low pressures of 2 mm Hg, whereas the same reflux in a child 1 year old occurs at 20 mm Hg. At autopsy, furthermore, at 50 mm Hg pressure intrarenal reflux occurs in all calyces, even simple ones, in children younger than 12 years (Funston and Cremin, 1978).

These findings suggest that physiologically normal urinary intrapelvic pressures in adults or older children could elicit a different response in neonates. This effect could be augmented by increases in renal pelvic pressures that may result from ureteral and pelvic smooth muscle dysfunction in infection (Issa and Shortliffe, 1992). Animal models with bacterial urinary infection show that infection elevates renal pelvic pressures whether or not reflux is present and, in fact, renal pelvic pressures may even be higher when reflux is absent; this may also account for further parenchymal damage with severe infection (Issa and Shortliffe, 1992; Angell et al, 1998).

Young children have incompletely developed immune and neurologic systems. A depressed or incompletely mature immune system may allow bacteria more easy colonization of the bladder and kidney because of decreased local and systemic defenses and eliminate bacteria even less efficiently when bacteriuria occurs. Immature bladder activity associated with increased contractions may also contribute to dynamic change in the upper tracts even in the apparently normal child (Koff and Murtagh, 1984). As a result, bacteriuria combined with reflux may result in greater susceptibility to renal damage.

Finally, neonatal symptoms of urinary infection and pyelonephritis are often vague and nonspecific, resulting in delayed or inadequate treatment. During this period of delay, bacterial invasion of the kidney creates an inflammatory response characterized by vascular granulocytic aggregation and hypoperfusion with subsequent scarring and loss of renal parenchyma (Winberg et al, 1974).

Small, scarred kidneys must not be confused with congenitally small, dysplastic, or poor or nonfunctioning kidneys. This distinction, one that is difficult and sometimes impossible to make radiologically, is important because dysplastic kidneys are histologically abnormal. Dysplastic kidneys and atrophic, scarred kidneys are histologically distinct. Although gross renal changes may be detected radiologically, lesser lesions that are related to infectious insult, such as cortical pitting, and mild global renal shrinkage may not be detected by imaging tests and yet may affect renal histology and function.

Using pyelographic techniques before DMSA, about 17% of schoolchildren with screening bacteriuria (bacteriuria found on cultures performed for screening rather than for symptoms) were diagnosed with renal scarring (Asscher et al, 1973; Newcastle Asymptomatic Bacteriuria Research Group, 1975; Savage, 1975). This correlates with Winberg's observation that 4.5% of children had radiologic renal scars after their first symptomatic UTI, and 17% had scars after the second symptomatic UTI (Winberg et al, 1974). Although the percentage of scars found using these earlier techniques may

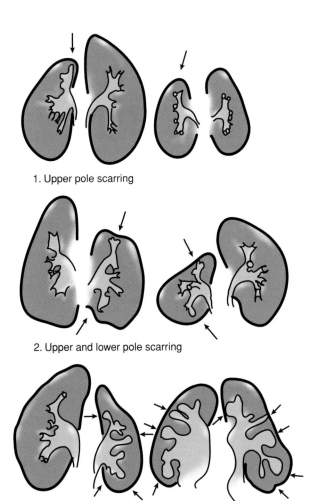

1. Upper pole scarring

2. Upper and lower pole scarring

3. Generalized scarring

Figure 112–6. The common areas of renal scarring, characterized by parenchymal thinning over a deformed calyx, as examined from intravenous pyelograms. The extent of scarring was related to single polar scars; multiple areas of upper, lower, and medial scars; or generalized scarring, as depicted. (From Hodson CJ: Natural history of chronic pyelonephritic scarring. Br Med J 1965;2:191-194.)

underestimate scarring, as some studies using DMSA scintigraphy suggest the incidence of scarring after symptomatic UTI could be almost twice this rate, these data emphasize that a child with both covert and symptomatic UTI has significant risk for renal scarring. Although, by definition, the natural history and pathogenesis of scarring in covert or asymptomatic bacteriuria is unknown, these scars probably reflect injury from previous undiagnosed bacteriuric episodes.

In most children with UTI in whom renal scars are found (and who have normal voiding), on the first set of imaging studies, the scarring does not improve or worsen irrespective of the child's future clinical course (Verber and Meller, 1989). It has been hypothesized that the young kidney may be more susceptible to damage, the initial UTI in the neonate or child younger than 4 or 5 years causes whatever renal damage will occur, and this initial response determines the kidney's future course ("big bang" theory). This theory is supported by the higher prevalence of early cortical DMSA defects observed in children younger than age 2 who have UTIs than in older children (Ditchfield et al, 1994b). One retrospective study linked individuals with scars found on DMSA with a greater likelihood of breakthrough UTI and less likely spontaneous resolution of their vesicoureteral reflux (Mingin et al, 2004).

Although older children appear to have less risk of scarring from UTI than those younger than 5 years, vulnerability for scarring persists until puberty (10 to 15 years old) (Smellie et al, 1985; Shimada et al, 1989). Early studies linked new or progressive renal scarring after early childhood diagnosis to uncontrolled recurrent UTIs and persistent vesicoureteral reflux (Filly et al, 1974; Smellie et al, 1985). Filly and associates (1974) found that in girls younger than age 10 who had recurrent UTIs and vesicoureteral reflux, renal scars progressed (developed clubbing or scarring in previously normal areas) in 43% of kidneys (17 of 40), and 2 of 16 normal kidneys developed new scars. Some of these scars took up to 2 years from the episode of pyelonephritis to evolve maximally.

Investigators who have used DMSA routinely to detect renal scars have also found that new or progressive renal scarring is more common than previously thought. Up to 7.3% of children with recurrent or persistent bacteriuria and reflux have progressive scarring (Shimada et al, 1989; Verber and Meller, 1989; Jakobsson et al, 1994), and almost all young children with recurrent pyelonephritis suffer renal scarring (Jakobsson et al, 1994).

Conversely, imaging evaluation of girls with reflux grades II to IV/V (international grading) without further UTI showed no progressive renal damage when observed up to 10 years (Holland et al, 1990). This supports earlier animal and clinical data showing that with normal urinary tract urodynamics, vesicoureteral reflux alone (sterile reflux) does not cause renal damage or impaired renal growth (Ransley and Risdon, 1978; Smellie et al, 1981; Ransley et al, 1984). If no infections occur, no association between the severity of vesicoureteral reflux and impaired renal growth has been demonstrated in an otherwise normal urinary tract (Smellie et al, 1981). Adults who have acute nonobstructive pyelonephritis and normal urinary tracts, furthermore, rarely develop focal renal cortical scarring and papillary or calyceal distortion or measurable generalized renal shrinkage (Davidson and Talner, 1978). Renal infection stimulates both humoral and cellular immune responses. In rat models of pyelonephritis, maximal renal suppuration and exudation with inflammatory infiltration occurred 3 to 5 days after the infection started, and collagen infiltration and scarring followed (Glauser et al, 1978; Miller et al, 1979; Miller and Phillips, 1981; Roberts et al, 1981; Shimamura, 1981; Slotki and Asscher, 1982). During the acute inflammatory infiltration, granulocytic aggregation may cause vascular occlusion and ischemia with elevation in renin (Kaack et al, 1986; Ivanyi and Thoenes, 1987). Bactericidal activity of the neutrophils and release of enzymes, superoxide, and oxygen radicals may cause the renal tubular damage observed in pyelonephritis (Roberts et al, 1982). The resulting proximal and distal tubular dysfunction causes reduced urinary concentrating ability (Walker, 1990) with increased fractional sodium excretion, decreased phosphate reabsorption, and increased low-molecular-weight protein excretion (Tulassy et al, 1986).

Decreased renal concentrating capacity has been correlated with severity of renal scarring (bilateral worse than unilateral) (Åbyholm and Monn, 1979). Other investigators correlated elevated urinary retinol-binding protein (a tubular protein giving evidence of tubular dysfunction) excretion with the type and severity of renal scarring and linked elevated N-acetyl-β-D-glucosaminidase (an excretory protein indicating tubular damage) and albumin excretion to bilateral scarring in children. These data suggest that tubular dysfunction occurs before glomerular dysfunction and commonly occurs in children with bilateral renal scarring (Tomlinson et al, 1994).

If antimicrobial treatment is started within the first days of infection, the acute suppurative response to the bacteria may be minimized and renal scarring may be decreased or prevented (Glauser et al, 1978; Miller and Phillips, 1981; Shimamura, 1981; Slotki and Asscher, 1982). Inhibition of superoxide production may decrease renal inflammation and tubular damage (Roberts et al, 1982). Other animal studies suggest that supplementing antimicrobial treatment with anti-inflammatory agents such as ibuprofen, which decreases neutrophil chemotaxis and blocks the cyclooxygenase pathways, or any other glucocorticoid anti-inflammatory agent may decrease renal scarring (Huang et al, 1999; Pohl et al, 1999). Clinically, larger cortical defects correlate with longer delay in treatment and longer length of illness (Jakobsson et al, 1992). The likelihood of renal scarring directly correlates, moreover, with the number of UTI occurrences (Jodal, 1987; American Academy of Pediatrics, 1999) (Fig. 112–7).

Xanthogranulomatous Pyelonephritis

Under certain circumstances, chronic bacterial pyelonephritis and obstruction are associated with a distinct severe inflammatory process known as xanthogranulomatous pyelonephritis (XGP). Although this occurs in only about 1% of cases (Malek and Elder, 1978), it is important because the entity has been confused with childhood renal tumors (Wilms' tumor, multilocular cystic nephroma, congenital mesoblastic nephroma, malignant rhabdoid, and clear cell sarcoma). Although the cause is unknown, the process is almost always associated with both infection and obstruction.

XGP affects mainly adults, but children have been reported to have the entity. Symptoms in children are similar to those in adults, with flank pain, fever, chills, and chronic bacteriuria

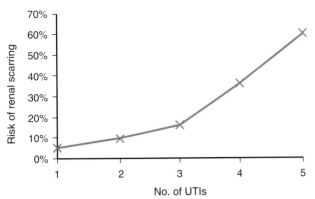

Figure 112-7. The relationship between risk of renal scarring and number of urinary tract infections (UTIs). (From American Academy of Pediatrics. Committee on Quality Improvement. Subcommittee on Urinary Tract Infection: Practice parameter: The diagnosis, treatment, and evaluation of the initial urinary tract infection in febrile infants and young children. Pediatrics 1999;103:845.)

(*E. coli* and *Proteus* most common), and associated with more vague symptoms of malaise, malnutrition, weight loss, and failure to thrive. Lower tract irritative symptoms are uncommon. Symptoms are often chronic, with the majority with XGP being symptomatic for more than a month (Brown et al, 1996). The most common infecting organisms are *Proteus* and *E. coli.* Urinalysis usually shows pus and protein, and blood counts often show anemia reflecting the chronic nature of the disease.

The process is usually unilateral and may involve pericalyceal tissue alone (focal) or the kidney diffusely (diffuse), with extension into the perinephric fat and even the retroperitoneum with encasement of the great vessels (Malek and Elder, 1978; Eastham et al, 1994). The clinical presentation in children differs from that in adults. **In children, XGP often affects those younger than 8 years and is of the focal renal rather than diffuse renal form (17% to 25% of cases in children). Boys are affected more frequently** (Brown et al, 1996), **and contralateral renal hypertrophy may occur** (Quinn et al, 1999). Although obstructive calculi are found in children as well as adults, obstruction in children may involve obstructive genitourinary abnormalities. It has also been noted that focal XGP is seldom associated with obstruction (Brown et al, 1996).

Radiologic findings include renal calculi in 38% to 70% of patients, nonfunctioning renal segments in 27% to 80%, and a mass in as many as 62% (Anhalt et al, 1971; Malek and Elder, 1978). Ultrasonography may show an enlarged kidney with hypoechoic areas that represent areas of necrosis and pus-filled calyces. CT with contrast shows areas of low attenuation that do not enhance and may show extension of the mass into the perinephric fat. The "bear paw" sign with areas of low-attenuation nonenhancing dilated calyces and abscesses within areas of high-attenuation enhancing renal parenchyma may be present (Cousins et al, 1994; Goodman et al, 1998). No radiologic feature of XGP is diagnostic, but CT has allowed correct preoperative diagnosis and planning in some patients (Cousins et al, 1994; Eastham et al, 1994; Goodman et al, 1998).

Grossly, the kidney shows yellow-white nodules and evidence of pyonephrosis. The histologic diagnostic feature is the xanthoma cell, a foamy lipid-laden histiocyte that may simulate the renal carcinoma cell. Xanthoma cells may also appear in other conditions of chronic inflammation and obstruction such as obstructive pneumonia (Moller and Kristensen, 1980).

If the diagnosis is made preoperatively, localized XGP may be treated with partial nephrectomy, but diffuse and extensive disease associated with a nonfunctioning kidney usually requires removal of the involved kidney and perinephric fat. Rare instances of successful medical treatment of focal XGP have been reported (Brown et al, 1996; Quinn et al, 1999). Amyloidosis has been reported as a remote complication in the remaining kidney (Brown et al, 1996; Quinn et al, 1999).

Pyelonephritic Hypertension

The incidence of hypertension in childhood depends upon age and sex and has been cited as between 1% and 11%. Renal-related hypertension is most common (Dillon, 1979). **Children with gross pyelonephritic nephropathy (reflux nephropathy) have at least a 10% to 20% risk of future hypertension** (Holland et al, 1975; Wallace et al, 1978; Smellie and Normand, 1979; Jacobson et al, 1989a) with risks of later progressive deterioration in renal function and other complications of hypertension.

Wallace and associates (1978) found that 12.8% of 141 patients with urinary infections and surgically corrected vesicoureteral reflux developed hypertension during the first 10 years of follow-up. Of those with renal scarring, 17% became hypertensive during follow-up. In another series, Smellie and Normand (1979) observed 83 children with scars of whom 11 had initial hypertension, 6 with malignant hypertension, and another 14 (19%) became hypertensive over the next 4 to 20 years, making a total of 30% who developed infection-related hypertension.

In Sweden, Jacobson and associates (1989a) found that 7 of 30 (23%) children with focal renal scarring developed hypertension after 27 years and of these, 10% developed end-stage renal disease. Eleven of the children observed by Smellie and Normand had hypertension initially and none of Wallace's or Jacobson's did, probably indicating that the group followed by Smellie and Normand had more severe initial renal damage. In both series, however, **hypertension occurred whether renal scarring was segmental, focal, unilateral, or bilateral and was, therefore, independent of the degree of scarring.** More recent examination of ambulatory blood pressure (24-hour ambulatory blood pressure measurement) suggests that hypertension obtained by ambulatory blood pressure measurement correlates directly with the degree of reflux nephropathy. Nocturnal hypertension was the most sensitive indicator, but whether this is predictive of daytime hypertension has not been validated (Patzer et al, 2003).

The etiology of pyelonephritic hypertension is poorly understood. It is likely that the renin-angiotensin system is involved. In 1978 at Great Ormond Street in London the plasma renin activity was measured in children with reflux nephropathy that had been corrected surgically 1 to 10 years before (Savage et al, 1978). In all 15 children who were hypertensive when studied, plasma renin activities were above the normal mean with 9 having levels above normal for their age, whereas in 8 of 100 children who were normotensive after the surgery the plasma renin levels were elevated above the normal range for their age. When 85 of these 100 children were traced 5 years later, 4 had developed serious hypertension and 4 others had borderline hypertension (Savage et al, 1987). A single elevated plasma renin activity level in 1978 did not, however, predict hypertension 5 years later, and by 1987 19% (16 of 85) of the children had elevated plasma renin activity. In this study, moreover, the normal tendency for the plasma renin activity to decrease with increasing age was not seen; instead, the opposite was observed; plasma renin activity increased with age and the standard deviation increased. Almost 10 years later the percentage of children with elevated peripheral plasma renin activity continued to increase in teenagers older than 15 years, but elevation appeared to level off by age 25 and blood pressure had leveled by age 15 (Goonasekera et al, 1996). Peripheral plasma renin elevation did not predict future hypertension during the 15 years of follow-up.

The value of selective renal vein renin measurements in the management of children with hypertension from reflux nephropathy is controversial (Holland et al, 1975; Stecker et al, 1977; Bailey et al, 1978, 1984a; Dillon et al, 1984) even though segmental renal vein renins have been useful in some for localizing sources of renin production (Dillon et al, 1984). Further indirect evidence of the role of renin in pyelonephritic nephropathy has been the successful treatment of hypertension with agents specifically aimed at blocking the renin-angiotensin system. In children who have been examined with renal arteriography, normal main renal arteries are found to proceed into scarred kidneys with vascular changes limited to small interlobular arterial branches (Holland et al, 1975; Stecker et al, 1977).

Progressive Renal Dysfunction

Although renal failure associated with acute pyelonephritis occurs rarely, after recurrent pyelonephritis, especially that associated with pyelonephritic nephropathy, some children develop delayed hypertension and progressive renal dysfunction without further known UTI. **Generally, when measured years after UTI, overall renal function is well preserved, but individual GFR of scarred kidneys is decreased; this decrease correlates inversely with the original degree of vesicoureteral reflux when associated with reflux (higher grade reflux, lower GFR)** (Jacobson et al, 1989a; Wennerström et al, 2000). As might be expected with long-term follow-up, those with small kidneys, whether scarred or not, had a lower GFR than those with normal kidneys, and those with bilaterally small or scarred kidneys had the lowest GFRs (Berg, 1992). **Most long-term studies emphasize that early detection of complications of renal scarring such as hypertension, renal insufficiency, and proteinuria is useful in minimizing progressive deterioration in renal function** (Jacobson et al, 1989a; Berg, 1992; Martinell et al, 1996; Smellie et al, 1998; Wennerström et al, 2000). When renal scarring is found in children or bilateral renal scarring is found in adults with a history of UTI, it seems to be a risk factor for further decreasing renal function (Smellie, 1991; Smellie et al, 1998; Wennerström et al, 2000).

Glomerular lesions and progressive proteinuria have been observed in patients who have renal scarring (Kincaid-Smith, 1975; Torres et al, 1980). Significant proteinuria (greater than 1 g per 24 hours) has been a routine finding in patients with vesicoureteral reflux and progressive deterioration in renal function (Torres et al, 1980). Certain investigators, moreover, have found glomerular sclerosis in the nonscarred, radiologically normal kidney in cases of unilateral reflux nephropathy (Kincaid-Smith, 1975; Bailey et al, 1984b; Kincaid-Smith, 1984). Two theories, one involving progressive renal damage from hyperfiltration of remaining nephrons and the other involving progressive immunologic damage to the kidney, have been postulated to explain this.

Micropuncture studies of rat renal tubules allow measurement of single-nephron GFRs. These investigations show that removal of a kidney or loss of a majority of functioning nephrons results in hyperfiltration in the remaining nephrons and increased glomerular plasma flow. In rat studies in which one kidney and two thirds of the other kidney are removed (a five-sixths nephrectomy model), increases in glomerular plasma flow, mean net glomerular transcapillary hydraulic pressure, and single-nephron GFRs are measured in the remnant nephrons. Later, as an apparent consequence, these rats develop focal segmental glomerulosclerosis (Hostetter et al, 1981, 1982). The glomerulosclerosis is thought to result from vascular injury caused by renal hyperfiltration. Rats maintained on a low-protein diet failed to show the pressure or pathologic changes, and rats maintained on a high-protein diet had greater degrees of glomerular sclerosis and more rapid renal death than those on normal diets (Brenner et al, 1982).

Focal segmental glomerulosclerosis has been found in children with reflux nephropathy and proteinuria even when renal function (measured by GFR) is relatively preserved. In these children glomerular involvement correlates with degree of proteinuria. Because most children who suffer renal scarring and loss of parenchyma have adequate renal function, the glomerular and vascular changes may be an evolving response to hyperfiltration injury (Morita et al, 1990).

Another explanation for the progressive renal dysfunction involves a chronic inflammatory response that develops into an autoimmune phenomenon. Tamm-Horsfall protein is produced in the renal tubular cells of the loop of Henle and distal convoluted tubules and is secreted into the urine. Whether it has any specific physiologic role is unknown, but it does appear to affect bacterial adherence to the mucosa and may play some protective role (Duncan, 1988). Although Tamm-Horsfall protein is usually found only in the urine and on the luminal side of the tubules, both clinically and experimentally the protein has been detected in interstitial deposits in kidneys that have been subject to infection or reflux and has been associated with mononuclear cell infiltrates and renal scarring (Andriole, 1985). Even though antibodies (autoantibodies) to Tamm-Horsfall protein are widespread, the immunologic response to Tamm-Horsfall protein after a UTI may be disturbed in children with renal scarring (Fasth et al, 1980). This protein may account for findings of renal dysfunction or scarring associated with urinary vesicoureteral reflux without known infections, and the autoimmune response related to it may also provide a reason why chronic or progressive renal damage occurs long after cessation of reflux or active infections (Andriole, 1985).

End-Stage Renal Disease

Although end-stage renal disease (ESRD) caused by UTI alone is rare, ESRD related to reflux nephropathy is commonly associated with UTI and is estimated to account for 7% to 17% of ESRD worldwide (Craig et al, 2000) but only about 2% in the United States. A retrospective analysis of ESRD caused by reflux nephropathy has been unable to show that treatment of vesicoureteral reflux with long-term antimicrobial prophylaxis or surgery has improved the natural history of reflux nephropathy (Craig et al, 2000). This finding may be related to the trend of diagnosing about one third of renal lesions as congenital renal dysplasia or hypoplasia possibly associated with antenatal vesicoureteral reflux rather than diagnosing these as postnatal pyelonephritic scarring (Craig et al, 2000). It is also notable that in Sweden no child has been registered to have had ESRD related to pyelonephritic scarring in at least a decade, and according to the Swedish registry of uremia, the incidence of end-stage renal failure related to pyelonephritic scarring is now only 6% to 7% (Wennerström et al, 2000). **The early identification and management of children with renal scarring have been associated with this decreased incidence of ESRD.**

MANAGEMENT OF SPECIAL URINARY TRACT INFECTIONS AND COMMON ASSOCIATED PROBLEMS
Urinary Tract Abnormalities

From epidemiologic data, 5% to 10% of children with UTIs have obstructive urinary tract lesions, and an additional 21% to 57% have vesicoureteral reflux (Kunin et al, 1964; Abbott, 1972; Asscher, 1973; Winberg et al, 1974; Newcastle Asymptomatic Bacteriuria Research Group, 1975). When children with pyelonephritis are diagnosed by DMSA criteria, 25% to 83% have vesicoureteral reflux, and reflux is absent in over half these children with pyelonephritis (Tappin et al, 1989; Jakobsson et al, 1992; Rushton and Majd, 1992b; Ditchfield et al, 1994a).

Children with febrile UTIs and reflux have a high incidence of acute DMSA defects. Which of these acute defects results in scar is still debatable, but the risk of scarring increases with grade of reflux (Jakobsson et al, 1992). Older investigations have documented scars in 5% to 20% of kidneys with grade I reflux and in 50% or more of kidneys in which reflux is grade V (Govan et al, 1975; Ozen and Whitaker, 1987; Skoog et al, 1987). **Conversely, when renal scarring is used as the index and children with renal scarring are evaluated, about 60% have vesicoureteral reflux** (Asscher et al, 1973; Newcastle Asymptomatic Bacteriuria Research Group, 1975; Savage, 1975). In at least 25%, except for the scar, the urinary tract is normal (Jodal, 1987). These data confirm that vesicoureteral reflux is only one factor involved in the ascent of bacteria into the kidney and the subsequent renal scarring. There is no documented association between vesicoureteral reflux and risk of UTI.

Recurrent Urinary Tract Infections with a Normal Genitourinary System

Children who have no anatomic genitourinary problems but have recurrent UTI are common and frustrating to parents and physician. Because host uroepithelial characteristics are independent of gross urinary tract abnormalities or reflux, **recurrent UTIs occur in about 20% of patients, the majority girls, regardless of whether the urinary tract is normal** (Bratslavsky et al, 2004). Recurrent UTIs are common and Winberg has nicely documented the natural history (Winberg et al, 1974). **Of boys who are infected before they are a year old, 18% have a recurrent infection, but recurrences more than a year after the initial infection are rare. In contrast, if the initial infection occurs in an older boy, 32% become reinfected, suggesting that risk for neonatal UTI differs from that in older children.**

About 26% of girls who have an initial neonatal infection have a recurrence, and, as with infant boys, recurrences after a year from the neonatal infection are less frequent. Girls who have their first infection after the neonatal period have a 40% recurrence rate, with the majority of recurrences occurring within the first 3 months after the hallmark UTI and two thirds occurring within the first year. Although the risk of recurrent infection in these girls drops with each subsequent infection-free year, 8% had their first recurrence over 4 years after their original UTI, so the risk never totally disappears.

For a girl who has a UTI, Winberg calculated the risk of another UTI occurring within a year of the previous UTI to be proportional to the number of previous infections (i.e., the more UTIs a girl has, the more likely she is to have another). His data show that this risk is greater than 25% with one previous UTI, greater than 50% with two previous UTIs, and almost 75% after three previous UTIs (Winberg et al, 1974). This rate did not change depending on whether the initial infection was symptomatic or asymptomatic or pyelonephritis or cystitis; in fact, about a third of the recurrences were asymptomatic. Data from polymerase chain reaction analysis of UTI *E. coli* isolates suggest that more recurrent UTIs in infants may be endogenous relapses (reinfection with same organism from bowel) rather than new organism reinfections (Jantunen et al, 2002).

The lower rate of recurrent UTI in neonates and young boys and higher rate in older girls support the importance of variable host and bacterial factors that create risk for bacteriuria in any individual. Unfortunately, there are no routinely available tests with which to predict children who have a normal urinary tract who may have a biologic predisposition for UTIs. Routine bacterial biotyping and sensitivity data obtained from culture, moreover, are not necessarily related to bacterial virulence. For this reason, management of the possibility of recurrences in these patients depends upon the child's age and severity of symptoms.

Children with urinary tract anatomic abnormalities or vesicoureteral reflux may be treated with prophylactic antimicrobial agents to try to minimize risk of infections (see Chapter 123, "Voiding Dysfunction in Children: Non-Neurogenic and Neurogenic"). In the majority of children with normal urinary tracts who have mainly bladder irritative symptoms with their UTIs (so-called uncomplicated infections), there is evidence that 3 to 5 days of an appropriate antimicrobial agent to which the organism is sensitive (Lohr et al, 1981; Madrigal et al, 1988; Copenhagen Study Group of Urinary Tract Infections in Children, 1991; Jójárt, 1991) or even a single dose of a parenteral antimicrobial agent (e.g., aminoglycoside) is effective treatment (Principi et al, 1977; Vigano et al, 1985; Grimwood, 1988). Longer antimicrobial courses of 10 to 14 days have not been proved to be more effective in these cases and may cause increased side effects and antimicrobial resistance in the fecal bacteria (Hansson et al, 1989b; Copenhagen Study Group of Urinary Tract Infections in Children, 1991).

If a child has frequent recurrent infections (two or more over a 6-month period), a urinary prophylactic antimicrobial treatment over a limited period may be worthwhile because the child then has an established biologic predisposition for infections. Antimicrobial agents taken at a prophylactic dosage usually successfully decrease the rate of infections during the period of prophylaxis. When the antimicrobial agent is stopped, however, the child may extend into a period of remission from infection but often eventually returns to an increased basic susceptibility to urinary infections (Winberg et al, 1974; Kraft and Stamey, 1977).

Voiding Dysfunction and Constipation

Symptoms of nocturnal and diurnal incontinence are common in children with recurrent UTIs. Epidemiologic investigations show that monosymptomatic nocturnal enuresis is unassociated with UTI, but diurnal enuresis or a combination of diurnal and nocturnal enuresis even if as infrequent as once a week may be associated with pediatric UTI (Hansson, 1992). Interestingly, **this study also revealed that 7-year-old girls who were older than 3 years when they had their first UTI were more likely to have voiding dysfunction symptoms than those who were younger than 3 years at the time of the first UTI** (Hansson, 1992); this may indicate an age-related phenomenon in this syndrome. Others who compared children younger than age 2 when they had their UTI with children who had no UTI were unable to associate dysfunctional elimination syndrome with either UTI or vesicoureteral reflux if the children were assessed again when they were 7 years old (Shaikh et al, 2003). **Of note, almost 20% of children who had a recurrent UTI developed new diurnal enuresis starting with the onset of the UTI and persisting as long as 12 months even when they remained free of UTI during the follow-up interval** (Sørensen et al, 1988).

Urodynamic testing in neurologically normal children with recurrent urinary infections and incontinence has shown abnormal cystometry and voiding patterns (Kass et al, 1979; Koff et al, 1979; Bauer et al, 1980; Koff, 1982; Kondo et al, 1983; Qvist et al, 1986; Hansson, 1992; Passerini-Glazel et al, 1992; vanGool et al, 1992a). In 35 such children, Bauer and associates (1980) found that 12 (34%) had normal filling cystometry, 9 (26%) had large hypotonic bladders, 9 (26%) had small-capacity hypertonic bladders with increased intravesical filling pressure and sustained uncontrolled detrusor contraction at a low volume, and 5 (14%) had hyperreflexic bladders showing uninhibited detrusor contractions during filling. Voiding dysfunction has also been described with staccato (interrupted) urinary flows during voiding, showing increased

pelvic floor activity during voiding with resulting incomplete bladder emptying (Bauer et al, 1980; Hansson, 1992; Passerini-Glazel et al, 1992; vanGool et al, 1992a; Kjølseth et al, 1993).

In addition to voiding dysfunction, children with recurrent UTIs have frequent constipation (O'Regan et al, 1985; Loening-Baucke, 1997). When 47 girls with normal urinary tracts but recurrent UTIs (with or without incontinence) and cystometry-proven bladder instability were studied by digital rectal examination and rectal manometry, all had signs of functional constipation (O'Regan et al, 1985). Diurnal and nocturnal urinary incontinence (29% and 34% respectively) and UTI (11%) were found in children older than 5 years with chronic constipation (as defined by stool retention on rectal examination) and encopresis at least once a week (Loening-Baucke, 1997). Notably, these findings were present even when constipation or encopresis was denied. Others have not found constipation or daytime incontinence to be predictive of recurrent UTI (Bratslavsky et al, 2004).

Although these findings do not establish causality between UTIs, constipation, and voiding dysfunction, it can be seen that UTIs may initiate symptoms of bladder and sphincter (urethral and rectal) dysfunction with variable persistence. **Girls with recurrent UTIs are more likely** (Stauffer et al, 2004) **to have a family history of UTI, infrequent voiding, poor fluid intake, and stool retention** (Stauffer et al, 2004). In some situations, treatment of constipation or voiding abnormalities, or both, has resulted in decreased UTIs (Kass et al, 1979; Koff et al, 1979; Bauer et al, 1980; Koff, 1982; O'Regan et al, 1985; vanGool et al, 1992a, 1992b; Kjølseth et al, 1993; Loening-Baucke, 1997), and this possible relationship should be considered in the management of vesicoureteral reflux as well (Koff et al, 1998; Upadhyay et al, 2003) even though the association is unclear (Chen et al, 2004). These data suggest that bacteriuria or constipation may provoke abnormal detrusor-sphincter activity or vice versa.

Covert or Asymptomatic Urinary Tract Infection

When covert or asymptomatic infections are diagnosed on screening urinary cultures, children often have symptoms related to the lower urinary tract when carefully interviewed. They may have nocturnal or diurnal enuresis, squatting, and urgency, and at least 20% have a history of previous UTI (Kunin et al, 1962; Savage et al, 1975); these symptoms were not the reason they had the urinalysis or culture, however.

About 50% of these children have normal urinary tracts defined by intravenous urography and VCUG (Kunin et al, 1962; Savage et al, 1975). A majority of infants who have covert bacteriuria may clear their bacteriuria without treatment (Jodal, 1987); others state that only about 30% of asymptomatic school-age girls with asymptomatic UTI clear spontaneously without treatment (Verrier-Jones et al, 1975; Lindberg et al, 1978). Whether treated or not, the majority of these girls acquire persistent infections or reinfections (Savage, 1975; Verrier-Jones et al, 1975; Jodal, 1987).

Whether the UTI is symptomatic or asymptomatic is not important for the first UTI; the UTI is marking host susceptibility. For this reason, the first UTI should have imaging evaluation and therapeutic management just as any other first

UTI. When the urinary tract has been evaluated and found to be normal or abnormal, however, treatment or screening for subsequent asymptomatic or covert UTI is debatable and probably unnecessary; obtaining routine cultures or urinary screening cultures is not supported (Shortliffe, 1995; Narchi, 2004).

Covert bacteriuria may not be totally asymptomatic in school-age children, and if associated symptoms such as incontinence are elicited they should be treated. Treatment of the infection alone, however, may not obviate symptoms of voiding dysfunction. **Controlled studies involving older children with treated and untreated covert bacteriuria showed that treatment makes little difference in the rate of future reinfections; over half have recurrent infections whether treated or not, and the risk of any renal damage in these older children is very low** (Savage, 1975; Verrier-Jones et al, 1975; Lindberg et al, 1978; Jodal, 1987).

Women with type 2 diabetes mellitus and asymptomatic bacteriuria, furthermore, have increased risk for a symptomatic UTI (Geerlings et al, 2001). There is little evidence, therefore, that the natural history of asymptomatic UTI is changed by therapy, and the UTI event, symptomatic or asymptomatic, marks a susceptible host. This is now supported by long-term follow-up of women with symptomatic bacteriuria and prospective studies of those with asymptomatic bacteriuria (Hooton et al, 2000; Vosti, 2002). Not all share this conclusion and management implications, however (Bensman, 2002).

In several series in which girls with UTIs were randomly assigned to antimicrobial treatment and no treatment, subsequent renal scars rarely occurred when the kidney was free of scars at first imaging; conversely, new or increased scarring usually occurred in previously scarred kidneys in which vesicoureteral reflux was present. This was independent of antimicrobial therapy (Newcastle Asymptomatic Bacteriuria Research Group, 1975; Savage, 1975; Cardiff Oxford Bacteriuria Study Group, 1978; Newcastle Covert Bacteriuria Research Group, 1981).

There is evidence that *E. coli* causing covert bacteriuria may belong to strains of *E. coli* that show self-agglutination, loss of surface antigens, and less overall pathogenicity (Lindberg et al, 1975; Hansson et al, 1989b). Some studies have suggested that urinary tract colonization with a strain of *E. coli* causing asymptomatic bacteriuria may prevent colonization with an *E. coli* causing symptoms and that treatment may actually lead to later acute symptomatic pyelonephritis (Hansson et al, 1989a, 1989b). For this reason, in difficult cases of recurrent asymptomatic infection without other urinary tract abnormalities, follow-up without further antimicrobial treatment should be considered seriously.

Incontinence Associated with Urinary Tract Infection and Normal Urinary Tracts

When symptoms of voiding dysfunction accompany recurrent UTIs, it is probably worth observing the child with prophylactic antimicrobial agents to observe any change in voiding pattern while the urine is sterile. If symptoms of incontinence persist, addition of an anticholinergic agent such as oxybu-

tynin or bladder rehabilitation that includes timed voiding and biofeedback techniques may help to improve incontinence and decrease the frequency of UTIs (Kass et al, 1979; Koff et al, 1979; Qvist et al, 1986; Passerini-Glazel et al, 1992; vanGool et al, 1992b; Kjølseth et al, 1993; Shortliffe, 1995).

In addition, if constipation is found or even suspected, there may be an improvement in voiding and reduction in UTIs if this is treated (O'Regan, et al, 1985; Loening-Baucke, 1997). With the acute onset of bowel and bladder dysfunction in a child, the possibility of tethered cord or other neurologic abnormalities must be eliminated.

OTHER GENITOURINARY TRACT INFECTIONS AND SYNDROMES

Inflammatory Acute Hemorrhagic Cystitis (Viral Cystitis)

Acute hemorrhagic cystitis accompanied by frequency, urgency, and dysuria in children has been associated with UTIs caused by adenovirus 11 (Numazaki et al, 1968, 1973; Manolo et al, 1971; Mufson et al, 1973) and occasionally *E. coli* (Loghman-Adham et al, 1988-89). **Adenovirus is the most common cause of viral acute hemorrhagic cystitis in children.** In a series of 69 infants and children with acute hemorrhagic cystitis, adenovirus 11 was recovered from the urine of 10 (14.5%), adenovirus 21 from the urine of 2 (2.9%), and *E. coli* from the urine of 12 (17.4%), but the remainder (over 60%) had no infectious agents isolated from the urine (Mufson et al, 1973). Polyomaviruses have caused both hemorrhagic and nonhemorrhagic cystitis in children.

Viral cystitis has been commonly associated with bone marrow transplantation and other states of immunosuppression. Severe adenovirus in these children has caused fatalities as high as 50% to 80% without successful treatment, although recent ribavirin usage has been reported (Gavin and Katz, 2002). **BK, a DNA virus of the polyomavirus genus, has been found in the urine of bone marrow transplantation and other immunosuppressed patients having hemorrhagic cystitis (0.5 to 5 months after transplantation), causing both symptomatic hematuria and dysuria and asymptomatic infections** (Apperley et al, 1987; Bedi et al, 1995). It is hypothesized that immunosuppression may be related to reactivation of BK virus. In several series, hemorrhagic cystitis was associated with persistent BK viruria the majority of the time and shedding of BK virus was usually correlated with onset of hemorrhagic cystitis (Bedi et al, 1995).

Because viral cultures are rarely done, children with symptoms of acute hemorrhagic cystitis most often have no growth on routine urinary culture. Although no antimicrobial treatment is indicated in healthy individuals with viral cystitis, radiologic evaluation should still be performed to eliminate other causes for hematuria. It has been suggested that ribavirin may be useful for adenovirus cystitis after bone marrow transplantation (Cassano, 1991). Chemically induced hemorrhagic cystitis is not discussed in this section.

Interstitial Cystitis

Although individuals with interstitial cystitis often have a history of possible UTI, there is no evidence that it results from infection. Initial symptoms of frequency, suprapubic pain, nocturia, and urgency may be confused with UTI but must be differentiated from those of children with either voiding dysfunction or urinary frequency syndrome. When strict diagnostic criteria for interstitial cystitis such as Hunner's ulcers, pain on bladder filling relieved with emptying, suprapubic pain, and urinary urgency or frequency are applied, this is a rare condition in children (Farkas et al, 1977; Close et al, 1996). This is primarily a diagnosis of exclusion, but the diagnosis is usually based upon finding bladder glomerulations on cystoscopy and decreased compliance on a cystometrogram. Urodynamic findings of instability and involuntary bladder contractions are incompatible with this diagnosis (Close et al, 1996). When culture and sensitivity information are available, the antimicrobial agent should be reevaluated and changed if necessary, with treatment continuing for 7 to 10 days.

Epididymitis, Epididymo-orchitis, and Orchitis

Epididymitis is an important clinical syndrome because of its differential diagnosis and management. Although in earlier series prepubertal epididymitis was diagnosed rarely (Anderson and Giacomantonio, 1985), more **recent series using newer imaging modalities have diagnosed epididymitis almost as frequently as acute testicular torsion.** In 2000, according to HCUP data, children were rarely hospitalized with orchitis—1.6 hospitalizations per 100,000 (Freedman 2004). **Epididymitis is often difficult to distinguish from other pediatric acute scrotal processes, especially acute testicular torsion, and occurs almost as frequently (15% to 45%)** (Caldamone et al, 1984; Knight and Vassy, 1984; Mendel et al, 1985; Yazbeck and Patriquin, 1994). Although the differential diagnosis and evaluation of the acute scrotum are discussed in Chapter 127, the etiology and evaluation of epididymitis are related to UTI in some of these cases.

Although there is overlap, pediatric epididymitis occurs in a somewhat bimodal age distribution. **It occurs in very young boys and postpubertally in greater numbers** (Gierup et al, 1975; Knight and Vassy, 1984; Likitnukul et al, 1987; Melekos et al, 1988; Siegel et al, 1987; Anderson and Giacomantonio, 1985). This is a useful distinction clinically because the etiologies and management differ.

Symptoms and Signs

The symptoms and signs of acute epididymitis cannot be differentiated from those of any acute scrotal condition and may also be the reactive result of early torsion of the testes or appendix testes. Characteristics that may be useful for comparison with acute torsion of the testes are history of more gradual onset, dysuria, urethral discharge, history of urethral manipulation, recent urinary tract surgery (hypospadias, ureteral reimplantation), catheterization, neurogenic bladder, imperforate anus, or known lower tract genitourinary anatomic abnormalities (ureteral or vasal ectopia, bladder exstrophy) (Mandell, 1981; Knight and Vassy, 1984; Umeyama et al, 1985; Siegel et al, 1987; de la Hunt, 1989; Stein and Stöckle, 1994).

The scrotum is usually inflamed and swollen, there may be localized epididymal pain, 18% to 33% of boys have fever (Doolittle et al, 1966; Gierup et al, 1975; Knight and Vassy, 1984; Siegel et al, 1987), 24% to 73% have pyuria (Doolittle et al, 1966; Siegel et al, 1987), and 17% to 73% have a peripheral leukocytosis (Doolittle et al, 1966; Gierup et al, 1975; Gislason et al, 1980; Knight and Vassy, 1984; Anderson and Giacomantonio, 1985; Siegel et al, 1987). Although these symptoms are more likely to be associated with epididymitis than acute testicular torsion or torsion of the appendix testes, none is diagnostic. Pyuria and bacteriuria are rarely found in torsion (Doolittle et al, 1966; Gierup et al, 1975; Knight and Vassy, 1984; Anderson and Giacomantonio, 1985; Siegel et al, 1987).

As discussed in Chapter 127, **scrotal color flow Doppler ultrasonography and testes scintigraphy are helpful to confirm or follow epididymitis and may at times confirm torsion of the appendix testes** (Mendel et al, 1985; Mueller et al, 1988; McAlistar and Sisler, 1990; Atkinson et al, 1992; Yazbeck and Patriquin, 1994). Ultrasonography may show an enlarged epididymis of mixed echogenicity surrounded by reactive fluid. Color flow Doppler sonography usually shows increased testicular flow except when there is such extensive swelling that ischemia may occur, but most changes including those from viral or mumps orchitis or epididymo-orchitis are nonspecific (Tarantino et al, 2001). Nuclear scintigraphy similarly usually shows increased perfusion and increased radiotracer deposition in the affected side of the scrotum. Although nuclear scintigraphy may be more sensitive in detecting flow, especially in prepubertal boys (Atkinson et al, 1992), sonography has better anatomic resolution and may reveal epididymal or testicular abscesses (McAlistar and Sisler, 1990).

Pathogenesis

In young boys and infants, epididymitis is more likely to be related to genitourinary abnormalities (abnormal connections) or systemic hematogenous dissemination than in older males (Williams et al, 1979). **Urethral and urinary cultures from the prepubertal male are likely to show either nothing or gram-negative organisms and thus be ascribed to "nonspecific epididymitis," whereas in postpubertal sexually active boys the cause may involve sexually transmitted organisms (*N. gonorrhoeae, Chlamydia trachomatis*).** As with the pathogenesis of renal abscess, data support two means of bacterial access to the epididymis and testes: hematogenous dissemination and urinary tract–related infection. In young boys and infants, hematogenous pathogenesis is supported by reports in which *Haemophilus influenzae* type b has been cultured from epididymal abscesses concurrent with other sites of infection, such as otitis media while the urinalysis remains normal, and findings of associated positive viral titers in others with acute findings (Weber, 1985; Greenfield, 1986; Lin et al, 1988; Somekh et al, 2004). Because organisms such as *H. influenzae* may require special culture techniques that may not ordinarily be used for urinary cultures, this may also account for the 40% to 84% of cultures from boys diagnosed to have epididymitis without an identifiable organism (Knight and Vassy, 1984; Cabral et al, 1985; Likitnukul et al, 1987). The fact that ascending UTI or bacteria sometimes causes epididymitis and epididymo-orchitis is supported by the observation that boys who have pyuria and bacteriuria are more likely to have a urinary tract abnormality and appear at a younger age (Siegel et al, 1987).

Management

Epididymitis should be treated for the presumptive causative organism. Specifically, in the young child who has pyuria and possible bacterial epididymitis, initial broad-spectrum antimicrobial coverage similar to that used to treat a UTI in an ill child should be used. When the culture results and antimicrobial sensitivities are available, the most specific, most cost-effective agent with few side effects that achieves good tissue and urinary levels should be selected. Clearly, children who are thought to have epididymitis on the basis of viral infection, reaction to torsion of the appendix testes, trauma, or other nonbacterial etiology should not be given antimicrobial agents, and treatment with analgesics and nonsteroidal anti-inflammatory agents is more appropriate.

During or after treatment of the acute bacterial urinary and epididymal infections, radiologic evaluation of the urinary tract should be performed as with any UTI. Two studies reported a high likelihood of genitourinary anatomic abnormalities, in particular abnormal connections between the urinary tract and bowel or genital duct system when a child has bacterial epididymitis and a UTI (Siegel et al, 1987; Anderson et al, 1989). In both studies, boys with negative urinary cultures had normal urinary tracts. Whether all boys with epididymitis, including those with negative urethral and urinary cultures, need a full radiologic evaluation of the urinary tract is unclear from current data. It does appear prudent, however, to perform a VCUG and renal and bladder ultrasonography for prepubertal boys with documented urinary infections and perhaps those in whom epididymal abscesses are found, although the latter may be related to hematogenous spread.

Epididymitis Associated with Unusual Organisms

Whenever scrotal masses are considered, tuberculous epididymitis must also be considered as the most common form of urogenital tuberculosis (Cabral et al, 1985). This form of epididymitis is more likely to be confused with a malignancy rather than a cause of an acute scrotal mass because it usually involves painless swelling, but this can be an important cause of epididymitis when dealing with patients from areas in which tuberculosis may be endemic. Although there is evidence for both local urinary spread and hematogenous spread of tuberculosis to the epididymis, in the reported pediatric cases of tuberculous epididymitis there were usually other signs of hematogenous involvement and the urine may or may not have been positive for the organism (Cabral et al, 1985).

Funguria

Fungal UTI is an increasing health care–associated infection, especially in individuals who have received antimicrobial agents and have urinary drainage catheters (Kauffman et al, 2000). **Candidemia in one neonatal intensive care unit increased more than 11 times between 1985 and 1995** (Kossoff et al, 1998). In children, predisposing factors may include antimicrobial therapy, prematurity, intravenous or umbilical artery catheterization, parenteral nutrition, and immunocompromised status (Keller et al, 1977). The urinary tract may serve both as a primary portal of entry and as a site of disseminated infection. **Prophylactic usage of oral nystatin or fluconazole in very low birth weight babies (less than 1000 to 1500 g) has been reported to be useful in preventing colonization and invasive fungal infection** (Sims et al, 1988; Kaufman et al, 2000; Kicklighter et al, 2001).

In children and adults with disseminated candidiasis, the kidney is the most commonly involved organ (Keller et al, 1977). *Candida* species are the most common cause of fungal UTI, with *C. albicans* the most likely of these and responsible for about a half of the infections. The second most common is *Torulopsis glabrata* (also known as *Candida glabrata*), an important species to recognize because of its common resistance to fluconazole (van't Wout, 1996; Kauffman et al, 2000).

Fungal bezoars may form in the renal pelvis, causing obstruction and anuria in infants with bilateral involvement (Keller et al, 1977; Eckstein and Kass, 1982; Robinson et al, 1987; Bartone et al, 1988; Rehan and Davidson, 1992; Hitchcock et al, 1995). For this reason, renal ultrasonography may be helpful in evaluating the extent of fungal infection when funguria is persistent (Bartone et al, 1988). Although urinary alkalinization and oral and intravenous antifungal chemotherapy may dissolve some of these fungus balls, in infants these balls may totally obstruct the small urinary tract, requiring percutaneous or surgical removal of the bezoars or drainage so that both local irrigation and systemic therapy can be given. Streptokinase was reported to dissolve a fungus ball rapidly in one infant (Kabaalioglu et al, 2001).

Deciding when asymptomatic funguria related to an indwelling urethral catheter should be treated remains controversial, and a surveillance study involving 861 patients has shown that progression to disseminated candidemia is relatively uncommon (Kauffman et al, 2000). When repeated cultures grow more than 10,000 to 15,000 CFU/mL, treatment is usually recommended (Wise, 1998).

Although stopping unnecessary antimicrobial agents, changing or removing indwelling catheters, and urinary alkalinization may be helpful, these means do not clear many cases of funguria. Prospective studies with intravesical amphotericin B bladder irrigation and oral fluconazole appear to show that both may clear funguria, although fungal recurrences are common (Gubbins et al, 1994, 1999). Optimal dosages, length of treatment, and, for amphotericin, delivery (intermittent versus continuous) are indeterminate and controversial, but amphotericin B (50 mg/L) infused continuously at 42 mL/hr for 72 hours is effective (Trinh et al, 1995; Nesbit et al, 1999). Fluconazole has been used successfully in children, although it is not approved for those younger than 6 months (Hitchcock et al, 1995; Zia-ul-Miraj, 1997).

Fungal bezoars in the collecting system require treating obstruction when present with a percutaneous nephrostomy tube for drainage and potential local irrigation. In these situations, both local and systemic therapy with amphotericin B or oral fluconazole may be useful for management (Keller et al, 1977; Eckstein and Kass, 1982; Robinson et al, 1987; Bartone et al, 1988; Rehan and Davidson, 1992; Hitchcock et al, 1995; Zia-ul-Miraj, 1997). Should the fungal balls persist, surgical removal is necessary.

GENITOURINARY TRACT AND NOSOCOMIAL INFECTIONS
Surgical Site Infections and Surgical Prophylaxis

There is scant literature on surgical site infection for the urinary tract in children (Grabe et al, 2001). In 1992, the Centers for Disease Control and Prevention (CDC) changed the term surgical procedure–associated infections to surgical site infections: incisional—superficial (skin and subcutaneous tissue) and deep (deep soft tissue, muscle, fascia); organ; and organs and spaces manipulated during an operation. The organisms associated with such infections are related to the organs and orifices entered. When the gastrointestinal, genitourinary, or respiratory tracts have not been entered, the most common pathogen is *S. aureus*.

Data from the U.S. National Nosocomial Infections Surveillance System show the **incidence of surgical site infections are higher in infants younger than 2 months than in older children** (Richards et al, 1999). Other data support that prepubertal children, excepting neonates, have a lower incidence of surgical site infections than older children and adults, but these data are difficult to compare. One report on genitourinary infections in children and adolescents stated that shaving of the surgical site in the operating room, rather than the night before, is associated with decreased wound infections (McCray et al, 1986).

The latest published CDC guidelines related to surgical site infections appeared in 1999 and were summarized by Nichols (2001). None are specific for children or include genitourinary operations (Bratzler et al, 2005). These **recommend (1) not removing hair unless it will interfere with the operation and, if it is removed, clipping immediately before operation; (2) identifying and treating all remote infections; (3) maintaining as short a hospitalization as possible; (4) administering antimicrobial agents only when indicated on the basis of published recommendations for a specific operation; (5) administering antimicrobial agents intravenously to ensure bactericidal serum and tissue levels when the incision is made (60 minutes before most and 120 minutes before vancomycin) and maintaining these levels for a few hours after closure with discontinuation no later than 24 hours after surgery, even if drainage catheters are left in place (Botto et al, 2001); (6) preparing bowel for elective operations with mechanical bowel preparation including enemas and cathartic agents and nonabsorbable oral antimicrobial agents the day before surgery in addition to the intravenous drugs; and (7) withholding routine vancomycin usage** (Zanetti et al, 2005). In situations in which the value of antibiotic prophylaxis is unproved, a single-dose systemic appropriate cephalosporin given during the immediate preoperative period may be indicated.

Nosocomial Urinary Tract Infection

Catheter-associated UTIs are the most common hospital-acquired infection usually associated with urethral instrumentation or chronic indwelling catheterization (Shortliffe, 1997). The risk of UTI increases with the duration of catheterization, and the acute nosocomial UTI is usually asymptomatic. **In one study, 20% of childhood bacteremia was caused by UTI or prior urinary tract manipulation with introduction of pathogens** (Dupont and Spink, 1969). Other infectious complications associated with catheterization and UTI are acute epididymitis-orchitis, pyelonephritis, periurethral abscesses, and struvite and renal calculi. Cultures taken from urethral catheter tips show little correlation with urine cultures (Gross et al, 1974).

When urethral catheters are placed, the patient risks urethral injury and bacteremia from catheter manipulation. As a result, **any individual with a cardiac problem who is at risk for endocarditis must receive antimicrobial prophylaxis before catheter manipulation** (see Table 112–4). The incidence of UTI is related directly to the duration of the indwelling catheterization. There are no studies examining the rate of bacteriuria in children, but adult studies show that **in open drainage systems, in 95% of systems bacteriuria occurs by 4 days** (Kass and Finland, 1956), **and with closed drainage systems 5% to 10% become bacteriuric each day** (Warren et al, 1978).

Catheter-associated UTI originates from (1) periurethral organisms, (2) organisms infecting the collecting bag or device, and (3) organisms entering the system with breaks in the closed drainage system or lack of a closed system. **Recommendations for indwelling catheter care are as follows: (1) genital washing once or twice daily with water and soap without antiseptics or antimicrobial agents, (2) regular emptying of the collection bag, and (3) ongoing prophylactic antimicrobial drug therapy to prevent infection during insertion or while indwelling is not recommended unless the patient is at risk for endocarditis or is neutropenic** (Daschner et al, 2001; Warren et al, 2001). There is no need for irrigation with antibacterial substances, antimicrobial agent instillation into the collecting bag, special antibacterial-coated catheters, or routine change of catheter. None of these can prevent catheter-associated UTI permanently.

Asymptomatic bacteriuria associated with catheter drainage needs to be treated only before any urinary tract manipulation or when the drainage tube is removed; the resident organisms should then be treated and the urine sterilized prior to removal (Botto et al, 2001; Warren et al, 2001). **If the catheter has been left in for 4 or more days, the practitioner should assume that the urine is infected.**

BACTERIOLOGIC ECOLOGY AND ANTIMICROBIAL RESISTANCE

The development of more powerful antimicrobial agents allows improved and less morbid treatment of UTI, specifically pyelonephritis. At the same time, however, infecting organisms are becoming more and more resistant to routine antimicrobial agents and more problematic to treat, with fewer agents from which to select. In 1993 Calvin Kunin referred to this problem as a "worldwide calamity" resulting from bacterial genetic change causing resistance and population mobility (Kunin, 1993). The situation has not improved.

The widespread usage of antimicrobial agents was thought to create the pressure that selects for most resistant organisms. On the basis of techniques of DNA fingerprinting, electrophoretic pattern characterization, serotyping, and virulence identification, however, **certain clones of multidrug-resistant E. coli behave with characteristics of an epidemic outbreak.** For instance, an outbreak of *E. coli* O15:K52:H1 caused community-acquired cystitis, pyelonephritis, and sepsis in London in 1987 to 1988 with epidemic-like spread and caused endemic *E. coli* urinary infections in Spain. In another instance, a single previously unidentified multidrug-resistant *E. coli* clonal group A (with resistance to trimethoprim-sulfamethoxazole) was discovered to cause 11% of community-acquired UTIs in women seen in a California university health service during a 4-month period and about 50% of the resistant isolates; the same clonal group appeared to cause almost 40% of resistant infections in cohort groups in Michigan and Minnesota (Manges et al, 2001). In another evaluation of this resistant clonal A *E. coli* in a large public health system in Denver, Colorado, **risk for having the resistant organism UTI was associated with those younger than 3, Hispanic ethnicity, recent travel outside the United States, and prior UTI.** Almost 15% of groups had trimethoprim-sulfamethoxazole–resistant organisms (Burman et al, 2003). The source of these clonal epidemic-like occurrences is unclear, but some evidence implicates food or contact with food sources that may have had antimicrobial agent contact (Drexler, 2002).

This resistance is global; in 1999 in Israel, community-acquired UTI organisms were resistant to trimethoprim-sulfamethoxazole (31%), to cephalexin (37%), and to ampicillin (70%) (Prais et al, 2003). In Canada in 1992 to 1994, in 1636 consecutive isolates of *E. coli* causing UTI, antimicrobial resistance was ampicillin 45%, trimethoprim-sulfamethoxazole 31.4%, and combined resistance to both 22.2%; 1.7% of organisms were resistant to both ampicillin and gentamicin. Case-control examination of those with resistant trimethoprim-sulfamethoxazole organisms showed that children who had antimicrobials for more than 4 weeks in the previous 6 months were 23 times more likely to have resistance and children with genitourinary abnormalities 2.4 times more likely (genitourinary tract abnormality, spina bifida, vesicoureteral reflux); also included were children who had one (OR 2.3) or more (OR 3.2) previous hospital admissions and those younger than 2 years compared with those 2 to 6 years old (OR 0.3) (Allen et al, 1999) (see Table 112–10).

To attempt any control of this global problem, we must prescribe antimicrobial agents in a socially conscious manner. Recommendations by the Infectious Diseases Society of America include **(1) optimal use of antimicrobial agents, (2) restriction of classes or specific agents, (3) rotational or cyclic usage, and (4) use of combination antimicrobial therapy to decrease resistance** (Shlaes et al, 1997).

CONSIDERATIONS IN TREATING CHILDREN WITH URINARY TRACT INFECTION

Rational treatment of infants and children with UTI is based upon an understanding of bacterial and host risk factors with rapid detection of UTI and evaluation of potential risks to modify them when possible. Moreover, judicious use of antimicrobial agents allows effective treatment and limits organism selection and bacterial resistance. We should consider the inevitable emergence of antimicrobial resistance with widespread usage of any antimicrobial agent and that future virulence targets for drugs are limited (Lee et al, 2003).

Antimicrobial usage should be limited to the shortest effective duration and narrowest spectrum. When a child with bacteriuria and renal scarring has been identified, the management should minimize the child's chances of future bacteriuria and assess potential risk factors to prevent further infection-related renal damage. In some instances, knowledge of predisposing risk factors may help select children for urinary tract antimicrobial prophylaxis or further evaluation. In others, anatomic knowledge may allow consideration of lack of antimicrobial treatment.

When renal scarring is identified, the child and parents should be educated about potential future hypertension, proteinuria, and progressive nephropathy. In moderate to severe renal scarring with renal insufficiency, early nephrologic consultation for evaluation and surveillance for hypertension, proteinuria, acid-base imbalance, and counseling and management may improve or stabilize renal function and improve growth. In particular, the young female with renal insufficiency from pyelonephritic nephropathy and recurrent UTI may desire pregnancy counseling related to future renal insufficiency.

KEY POINTS: URINARY TRACT INFECTION MANAGEMENT

- No follow-up urinary culture after 48 hours of treatment is required if organisms are sensitive to the antibiotic selected.

- Risks for antimicrobial-resistant uropathogens are diabetes, recent hospitalization, recent antibiotic usage (especially trimethoprim-sulfamethoxazole), urinary malformations, urethral catheters, and antimicrobial prophylaxis.

- Radionuclide VCUG should not be used to evaluate first infections in infants, young boys, or those in whom risk of genitourinary abnormality is high and urethral visualization is important.

- VCUG for purposes of UTI evaluation may be performed when the urine is sterile, bladder volume is normal, and bladder irritability is no longer present.

- The pediatric kidney is more likely to scar than the mature adult kidney.

- Focal segmental glomerulosclerosis is found in children with reflux nephropathy and proteinuria even when renal function is relatively preserved.

- Epididymitis in children is difficult to distinguish from testicular torsion and occurs almost as frequently.

- Antimicrobial agents must be prescribed in a responsible way to avoid and decrease antimicrobial agent resistance.

Although familial screening for vesicoureteral reflux may not be required in all situations, families in whom a member has vesicoureteral reflux or renal scarring must be made aware of familial risk for vesicoureteral reflux, consequences of UTI, and the need for early diagnosis, treatment, and evaluation of UTIs in family members.

SUGGESTED READINGS

Drexler M: Secret Agents: The Menace of Emerging Infections. Washington, DC, National Academies Press, 2002.

Hansson S, Dhamey M, Sigstrom O, et al: Dimercapto-succinic acid scintigraphy instead of voiding cystourethrography for infants with urinary tract infection. J Urol 2004;172:1071-1074.

Justice S, Hung C, Theriot JA, et al: Differentiation and developmental pathways of uropathogenic *Escherichia coli* in urinary tract pathogenesis. Proc Natl Acad Sci USA 2004;101:1333-1338.

Kau A, Hunstad D, Hultgren SJ: Interaction of uropathogenic *Escherichia coli* with host uroepithelium. Curr Opin Microbiol 2005;8:54-59.

Kawashima A, Sandler CM, Goldman SM, et al: CT of renal inflammatory disease. Radiographics 1997;17:851-866.

Manges A, Johnson J, Foxman B, et al: Widespread distribution of urinary tract infections caused by a multidrug-resistant *Escherichia coli* clonal group. N Engl J Med 2001;345:1007-1013.

Patzer L, Seeman T, Luck C, et al: Day- and night-time blood pressure elevation in children with higher grades of renal scarring. J Pediatr 2003;142:117-122.

Pomeranz A, El-Khayam A, Korzets Z, et al: A bioassay evaluation of the urinary antibacterial efficacy of low dose prophylactic antibiotics in children with vesicoureteral reflux. J Urol 2000;164:1070-1073.

Schlager T, Clark M, Anderson S: Effect of a single-use sterile catheter for each void on the frequency of bacteriuria in children with neurogenic bladder on intermittent catheterization for bladder emptying. Pediatrics 2001; 108:71-75.

Shaikh N, Hoberman A, Wise B, et al: Dysfunctional elimination syndrome: Is it related to urinary tract infection or vesicoureteral reflux diagnosed early in life? Pediatrics 2003;112:1134-1137.

Shaw K, Gorelick M, McGowan KL, et al: Prevalence of urinary tract infection in febrile young children in the emergency department. Pediatrics 1998;102:16-21.

Anomalies of the Upper Urinary Tract

STUART B. BAUER, MD

Congenital anomalies of the upper urinary tract comprise a diversity of abnormalities, ranging from complete absence to aberrant location, orientation, and shape of the kidney as well as aberrations of the collecting system and blood supply. This wide range of anomalies results from a multiplicity of factors that interact to influence renal development in a sequential and orderly manner. Abnormal maturation or inappropriate timing of these processes at critical points in development can produce any number of deviations in the development of the kidney and ureter.

The embryology of the urinary tract is described in Chapter 106, "Normal and Anomalous Development of the Urinary Tract." The reader is encouraged to review this material in order to appreciate the complexity of renal and ureteral development and the factors involved in the formation of an abnormality.

The classification of renal and ureteral anomalies used in this chapter is based on structure rather than function.

ANOMALIES OF NUMBER
Agenesis
Bilateral Renal Agenesis

Of all the anomalies of the upper urinary tract, **bilateral renal agenesis (BRA) has the most profound effect on the individual.** Fortunately, it occurs infrequently when compared with other renal abnormalities. Although BRA was first recognized in 1671 by Wolfstrigel, it was not until Potter's eloquent and extensive description of the constellation of associated defects that the full extent of the syndrome could be appreciated and easily recognized (Potter, 1946a, 1946b, 1952). Subsequently, many investigators have attempted to understand all of the facets of this syndrome and to explain them by employing a single unifying etiology (Fitch and Lachance, 1972). However, there is no unanimity regarding this topic, and controversy still exists concerning the exact mechanism of formation. More recently, **evidence has been gathering that a genetic and, consequently, a molecular basis may be the causative factor.** Deficient levels of several compounds that when present induce ureteral bud branching and invasion into the metanephric blastema are absent or markedly reduced in affected fetuses (Bullock et al, 1998; Froster et al, 2000; Kamba et al, 2001; Hartner and Dotsch, 2002; Hartner et al, 2002; Vrontou et al, 2003).

Incidence. The anomaly is quite rare, with only slightly more than 500 cases having been cited in the literature. Potter (1965) estimated that BRA occurs once in 4800 births, but in British Columbia the incidence is 1 in 10,000 births (Wilson and Baird, 1985). Davidson and Ross (1954) noted a 0.28% incidence in autopsies of infants and children, whereas Stroup and associates (1990) detected an incidence of 3.5 per 100,000 in the Centers for Disease Control (CDC) Birth Defects Monitoring Program. A recent study using prenatal ultrasound in 8500 pregnancies in Poland denoted an incidence of 0.25% (Forys et al, 2003). As with most anomalies there is significant male predominance (almost 75%). Increasing maternal age appears to be a risk factor (Bianca et al, 2003), but specific complications of pregnancy or any maternal disease do not appear to influence its development (Davidson and Ross, 1954; Ruhland et al, 1998). The anomaly was reported in three infants of an insulin-dependent diabetic mother (Novak and Robinson, 1994). It has been observed in several sets of siblings (Rizza and Downing, 1971; Dicker et al, 1984) and even in monozygotic twins (Thomas and Smith, 1974; Cilento et al, 1994). In four pairs of monozygotic twins, one sibling was anephric while the other had normal kidneys (Kohler, 1972; Mauer et al, 1974; Cilento et al, 1994; Klinger et al, 1997). It has been suggested that an autosomal recessive inheritance pattern exists (Dicker et al, 1984). There is a genetic predisposition to this syndrome with a high level of penetrance (Stella, 1998): when siblings and parents of an index child with BRA were screened, 4.5% had unilateral renal agenesis (Roodhooft et al, 1984) and 3.5% had BRA (McPherson et al, 1987). This is 1000 times higher than what has been reported in the general population (Stroup et al,

1990). Other investigators have suggested this is an autosomal dominant trait with variable penetrance (Kovacs et al, 1991; Murugasu et al, 1991; Moerman et al, 1994; Stella, 1998).

Embryology. Complete differentiation of the metanephric blastema into adult renal parenchyma requires the presence and orderly branching of a ureteral bud. This occurs normally between the 5th and 7th weeks of gestation, after the ureteral bud arises from the mesonephric or wolffian duct. It is theorized that induction of ureteral branching into major and minor calyces depends on the presence of a normal metanephric blastema (Davidson and Ross, 1954). The absence of a nephrogenic ridge on the dorsolateral aspect of the coelomic cavity or the failure of a ureteral bud to develop from the wolffian duct will lead to agenesis of the kidney. The absence of both kidneys, therefore, requires a common factor causing renal or ureteral maldevelopment on both sides of the midline.

It is impossible to say which of these two factors is most important. Certainly no kidney can form in the absence of a metanephric blastema, but the presence of a ureteral bud and orderly branching are also necessary for the renal anlage to attain its potential. In an extensive autopsy analysis, Ashley and Mostofi (1960) found many clues to the multifactorial nature of this developmental process and shed some light on the causes of BRA. Most anephric children in their series had at least a blind-ending ureteral bud of varying length. Therefore, the embryologic insult in such cases was thought to affect the ureteral bud just as or shortly after it arose from the mesonephric duct. Recent studies implicate a genetic defect that limits or prevents production of certain molecules responsible for ureteral bud induction into the metanephric blastema (Froster et al, 2000; Kamba et al, 2001; Hartner and Dotsch, 2002; Hartner et al, 2002). Even with complete ureteral atresia, structures of wolffian duct origin (vas deferens, seminal vesicle, and epididymis) were usually present and normally formed, suggesting that the injury occurred at about the time the ureteral bud formed (the 5th or 6th week of gestation). With complete absence of the ureter, a rudimentary kidney was discovered in only a few instances, supporting the concept of the interdependency of the two processes. Conversely, in some instances, the ureter was normal in appearance up to the level of the ureteropelvic junction (UPJ), where it ended abruptly. In those cases, no recognizable renal parenchyma could be identified. In a small number of autopsies the gonads were absent as well, indicating an abnormality or insult that took place before the 5th week and involved the entire urogenital ridge (Carpentier and Potter, 1959). Although the nephric and genital portions of the urogenital ridge are closely aligned on the dorsal aspect of the coelomic cavity, an extensive lesion affecting the entire area is necessary to produce both conditions in the developing fetus. **Therefore, absence of one or both kidneys may result from any of several causes.**

Description. The kidneys are completely absent on gross inspection of the entire retroperitoneum. Occasionally, there may be a small mass of poorly organized mesenchymal tissue containing primitive glomerular elements. Tiny vascular branches from the aorta penetrate this structure, but no identifiable major renal artery is present (Ashley and Mostofi, 1960).

KEY POINTS: BILATERAL RENAL AGENESIS

- Forty percent of the affected infants are stillborn.

- Most of the children who are born alive do not survive beyond 48 hours because of respiratory distress associated with pulmonary hypoplasia.

- The adrenal glands are usually normally positioned.

- The characteristic Potter facies and the presence of oligohydramnios are pathognomonic.

Besides the absence of functioning kidneys, each ureter may be either wholly or partially absent. **Complete ureteral atresia is observed in slightly more than 50% of affected individuals** (Ashley and Mostofi, 1960). The trigone, if developed, is poorly formed owing to failure of mesonephric duct structures to be incorporated into the base of the bladder. The bladder, when present (about 50% of cases), is usually hypoplastic from the lack of stimulation by fetal urine production. Alternatively, it has been postulated that ureteral bud and wolffian duct structures migrating into the ventral cloacal region are needed to initiate bladder development; their absence, and not the *lack* of urine, is the cause of arrested development (Katz and Chatten, 1974; Levin, 1952). With increasing use of prenatal ultrasound, affected fetuses are being detected before birth. Absence of kidneys and/or renal vasculature, small lung volumes and chest diameter, and abnormal adrenal gland appearance are additional diagnostic clues on prenatal screening (Latini et al, 1998; Sepulveda et al, 1998; Heling et al, 2001; Strouse et al, 2002).

Associated Anomalies. Other findings associated with BRA were extensively described by Potter. **The infants have low birth weights,** ranging from 1000 to 2500 g, and intrauterine growth retardation due in part to low iron stores in the liver (Georgieff et al, 1996). At birth, oligohydramnios (absent or minimal amniotic fluid) is present. In addition, the characteristic facial appearance and deformity of the extremities sets these children apart from normal newborns. The infants generally look prematurely senile and have "a prominent fold of skin that begins over each eye, swings down in a semi-circle over the inner canthus and extends onto the cheek" (Potter, 1946a, 1946b). It is Potter's contention that this facial feature is a sine qua non of nonfunctioning renal parenchyma. She even suggests that its absence confirms the presence of kidneys (Fig. 113–1A). In addition to this finding, the nose is blunted and a prominent depression between the lower lip and chin is evident. The ears appear to be somewhat low set, are drawn forward, and are often pressed against the side of the head, making the lobes seem unusually broad and exceedingly large (see Fig. 113–1B). The ear canals are not dislocated, but the appearance of the ear lobes gives the impression that the ears are displaced downward. Periauricular pits and tags have been noted as well (Wang et al, 2001). The legs are often bowed and clubbed, with excessive flexion at the hip and knee joints. Occasionally, the lower extremities are completely fused as well (sirenomelia) (Bain et al, 1960).

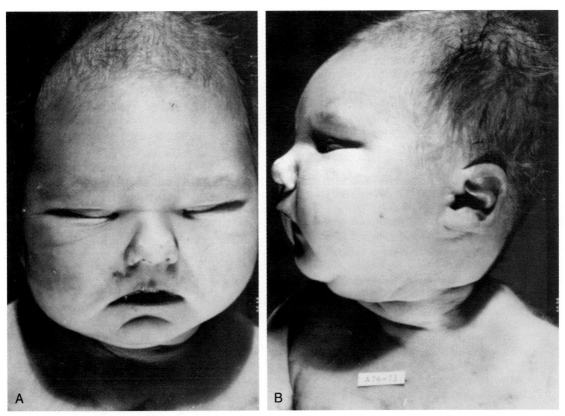

Figure 113–1. An anephric child who lived 2 days has typical Potter's facial appearance. **A,** Note the prominent fold and skin crease beneath each eye, blunted nose, and depression between lower lip and chin. **B,** The ears give an impression of being low set because lobes are broad and drawn forward, but actually the ear canals are located normally.

The skin can be excessively dry and appears too loose for the body. This may be secondary to severe dehydration or loss of subcutaneous fat. The hands are relatively large and clawlike.

It is thought that these characteristic facial abnormalities and limb features are caused by the effects of oligohydramnios rather than by multiple organ system defects (Fitch and Lachance, 1972; Thomas and Smith, 1974). This observation was confirmed by an experiment in nature in which one twin with bilateral agenesis did not have the characteristic Potter facies because it shared the same amniotic sac, containing adequate amniotic fluid, with the second twin (Klinger et al, 1997). Therefore, compression of the fetus against the internal uterine walls without any cushioning effect from amniotic fluid could explain all of the findings of this syndrome. Urine from the developing kidney is the major source of amniotic fluid, accounting for more than 90% of its volume by the third trimester (Thomas and Smith, 1974), but the skin, gastrointestinal tract, and central nervous system also contribute small amounts, particularly before urine production begins at 14 weeks. Therefore, the absence of kidneys reduces severely the amount of amniotic fluid produced during the latter stages of pregnancy.

Pulmonary hypoplasia and a bell-shaped chest are common associated conditions. Originally, these findings were thought to be secondary to uterine wall compression of the thoracic cage as a result of the oligohydramniotic state (Bain and Scott, 1960). Subsequently, it was thought that the amniotic fluid itself is responsible for pulmonary development (Fitch and Lachance, 1972). However, this theory was discounted when it was discovered there is a significant reduction in the number of airway generations as well as a decrease in acini formation in these fetuses (Hislop et al, 1979). Pulmonary airway divisioning occurs between the 12th and 16th weeks of gestation (Reid, 1977). A reduction in the number of divisions implies an interference with this process before the 16th week of gestation. The contribution from the kidneys to the amniotic fluid volume before that time is small, if any. Therefore, the oligohydramnios seen in cases of BRA is a later finding in pregnancy, occurring after the structural groundwork of the lung has been laid out. Hislop and colleagues (1979) suggested that the anephric fetus fails to produce proline, which is needed for collagen formation in the bronchiolar tree. The kidney is the primary source of proline (Clemmons, 1977). Thus, pulmonary hypoplasia may result from the absence of renal parenchyma and not from diminished amniotic fluid. This hypothesis is supported by the finding of normal lungs in two infants with prolonged leakage of amniotic fluid beginning at a time when pulmonary hypoplasia would have been expected if the amniotic fluid alone were responsible for the defect (Perlman et al, 1976; Cilento et al, 1994).

In the male, **penile development is usually normal** but a few cases of penile agenesis have occurred (O'Connor et al, 1993). Hypospadias is rare, but its occurrence is not related to the presence or absence of the testes. In 43% of the cases, however, the testes are undescended (Carpentier and Potter, 1959). They did not find any infants without testes, but Ashley and Mostofi (1960) noted testicular agenesis in 10%. The vas deferens is normal in most cases. The presence of vasa implies that whatever caused the renal agenesis influenced the ureteral bud only after it formed or that the insult affected just the nephrogenic ridge.

Although this syndrome occurs uncommonly in females, they have a relatively high incidence of genitourinary anomalies (Carpentier and Potter, 1959). The ovaries are frequently hypoplastic or absent. The uterus is usually either rudimentary or bicornuate; occasionally, it is absent entirely, as in sirenomelia. Finally, the vagina is either a short, blind pouch or completely absent.

The adrenal glands are rarely malpositioned or absent (Davidson and Ross, 1954), but they can appear flattened or "lying down" on ultrasonography (Hoffman et al, 1992), and fused and/or horseshoe-shaped glands have been noted on prenatal ultrasound screening (Strouse et al, 2002). Anomalies of other organ systems are not unusual. The legs are frequently abnormal, with clubbed or even fused feet producing sirenomelia (Saing et al, 1998; Das et al, 2002; Carbillon et al, 2001). A lumbar meningocele with or without the Arnold-Chiari malformation is not infrequently observed (Davidson and Ross, 1954; Ashley and Mostofi, 1960). Other malformations include abnormalities of the cardiovascular and gastrointestinal systems, which are present in up to 50% of infants.

Diagnosis. **The characteristic Potter facies and the presence of oligohydramnios are pathognomonic** and should alert the practitioner to this severe urinary malformation. Amnion nodosum—small white, keratinized nodules found on the surface of the amniotic sac—may also suggest this anomaly (Bain et al, 1960; Thompson, 1960). Ninety percent of newborns void during the first day of life (Sherry and Kramer, 1955; Clarke, 1977). Failure to urinate in the first 24 hours is not uncommon and should not arouse suspicion. Anuria after the first 24 hours without distention of the bladder should suggest renal agenesis (Williams, 1974). However, most infants who are born alive experience severe respiratory distress within the first 24 hours of life. When this becomes the focus of attention, the anuria may go unnoticed, with the renal anomaly being thought of only secondarily. BRA has been detected in higher than expected proportions in several syndromes: cryptophthalmos or Frazer's syndrome (Fryns et al, 1997), Klinefelter's syndrome (Barroeta et al, 2004), Kallmann's syndrome (Colquhoun-Kerr et al, 1999), and esophageal atresia (Saing et al, 1998).

Renal ultrasonography is probably the easiest way to identify the kidneys and bladder to confirm the presence or absence of urine within these structures. The advent of power Doppler ultrasonography to diagnose renal agenesis when renal arteries are not detectable has been highly accurate, even in fetuses with oligohydramnios and suspected BRA (Sepulveda et al, 1998). A clue to an absent kidney (or kidneys) is a flattened adrenal gland that lies in its normal location (Hoffman et al, 1992). If abdominal ultrasonography is inconclusive, a renal scan can be performed. The absence of uptake of the radionuclide in the renal fossa above background activity confirms the diagnosis of BRA. Umbilical artery catheterization and an aortogram can be undertaken if other modalities are unavailable or not diagnostic. This defines the absence of renal arteries and kidneys.

As the use of maternal ultrasonic screening becomes more pervasive, infants with this condition are being diagnosed in the second and third trimesters, when severe oligohydramnios is noted and no kidney tissue can be detected (Forys et al, 2003). Termination of the pregnancy has been considered when the clinician is certain of the diagnosis (Rayburn and Laferla, 1986).

Prognosis. **Almost 40% of the affected infants are stillborn. Most of the children who are born alive do not survive beyond the first 24 to 48 hours because of respiratory distress associated with pulmonary hypoplasia.** Those infants who do not succumb early remain alive for a variable period, depending on the rate at which renal failure develops. The longest-surviving child lived 39 days (Davidson and Ross, 1954).

Unilateral Renal Agenesis

Complete absence of one kidney occurs more commonly than does BRA. In general, **there are no telltale signs** (as with BRA) that suggest an absent kidney (Campbell, 1928). The diagnosis usually is not suspected, and the condition remains undetected unless careful examination of the external and internal genitalia uncovers an abnormality that is associated with renal agenesis or an imaging study done for other reasons reveals only one kidney. In the past 15 years prenatal ultrasonography and more recently fetal magnetic resonance imaging (MRI) have increased the detection rate of this condition. These imaging studies have revealed that a substantial number of cases are caused by involution of a multicystic or dysplastic kidney before birth (Mesrobian et al, 1993; Hitchcock and Burge, 1994; Dell'Acqua et al, 2002; Hiraoka et al, 2002).

Incidence. The clinically silent nature of this anomaly precludes a completely accurate account of its incidence. Most autopsy series, however, suggest that **unilateral agenesis occurs once in 1100 births** (Doroshow and Abeshouse, 1961). In a survey of excretory urograms performed at the Mayo Clinic, the clinical incidence approached 1 in 1500 (Longo and Thompson, 1952), but Wilson and Baird (1985) noted a 1 in 5000 occurrence rate in British Columbia. With the increased use of prenatal and postnatal ultrasonic screening, the incidence of unilateral renal agenesis (URA) may actually be higher than previously reported. Ultrasonic screening of 280,000 schoolchildren in Taipei revealed the incidence of unilateral agenesis to be 1 in 1200 (Shieh et al, 1990), and in the Czech Republic a similar incidence was found on prenatal screening (Sipek et al, 1997).

The higher incidence of BRA noted in male children is not nearly as striking in the unilateral condition, but **males still predominate in a ratio of 1.8:1** (Doroshow and Abeshouse, 1961). This is not surprising considering the timing of embryologic events. Wolffian duct differentiation occurs earlier in the male fetus than does müllerian duct development in the female, taking place closer to the time of ureteral bud formation. Therefore, it is postulated that the ureteral bud is influenced more by abnormalities of the wolffian duct than by those of the müllerian duct.

Absence of one kidney occurs somewhat more frequently on the left side. A familial tendency has been noted (Arfeen et al, 1993; Selig et al, 1993; Cascio et al, 1999). Siblings within a single family and even monozygotic twins have been affected (Kohn and Borns, 1973; Uchida et al, 1990). In a study of several families, McPherson and associates (1987) noted a familial pattern of inheritance and concluded in this study group that an autosomal dominant transmission with a 50% to 90% penetrance exists. This inheritance pattern has been confirmed by others who evaluated families with more than one affected individual (Biedel et al, 1984; Roodhooft et al, 1984; Battin et al, 1993). An absent kidney has been noted in a number of genetic disorders in which there is a deletion of several chromosomal loci: 8q13.3 (Pierides et al, 2002), 18q22.2 (Dowton et al, 1997), 22q11 (Stewart et al, 1999; Anonymous, 1998), as well as in X-linked and sporadic cases of Kallmann's syndrome (Colquhoun-Kerr et al, 1999; Zenteno et al, 1999; Quinton et al, 2001). Absence of several proteins such as ALL1 and certain oncogenes have also been associated with URA (Salerno et al, 2000; Lore et al, 2001; Nishinakamura et al, 2001; Sato et al, 2004).

Embryology. The embryologic basis for URA does not differ significantly from that described for the bilateral type. **The fault lies most probably with the ureteral bud.** Complete absence of a bud or aborted ureteral development prevents maturation of the metanephric blastema into adult kidney tissue.

It is unlikely that the metanephros is responsible, because the ipsilateral gonad (derived from adjacent mesenchymal tissue) is rarely absent, malpositioned, or nonfunctioning (Ashley and Mostofi, 1960). The high incidence of absent or malformed proximal mesonephric duct structures in the male and müllerian duct structures in the female strengthens the argument that the embryologic insult affects the ureteral bud primarily early in its development and even influences its precursor, the mesonephric duct. The abnormality most likely occurs no later than the 4th or 5th week of gestation, when the ureteral bud forms and the mesonephric or wolffian duct in the male begins to develop into the seminal vesicle, prostate, and vas deferens. The müllerian duct in the female fetus at this time starts its medial migration, crossing over the degenerating wolffian duct (6th week) on its way to differentiating into the fallopian tube, uterine horn and body, and proximal vagina (Woolf and Allen, 1953; Yoder and Pfister, 1976).

Magee and coworkers (1979) **proposed an embryologic classification based on the timing of the faulty differentiation.** If the insult occurs before the 4th week (type I URA, Fig. 113–2A), nondifferentiation of the nephrogenic ridge with retardation of the mesonephric and müllerian components results, leading to complete unilateral agenesis of genitourinary structures. The individual has a solitary kidney and a unicornuate uterus. In type II anomalies (see Fig. 113–2B), the defect occurs early in the 4th week of gestation, affecting both the mesonephric duct and the ureteral buds. The maldeveloped mesonephric duct prevents crossover of the müllerian duct and subsequent fusion. As a consequence, a didelphys uterus with obstruction of the ipsilateral horn and the vagina is produced. If the insult occurs after the 4th week (type III, see Fig. 113–2C), the mesonephric and müllerian ducts develop normally; only the ureteral bud and metanephric blastema are affected. Normal genital architecture is present despite the absence of one kidney.

With the discovery that multicystic and dysgenetic kidneys can involute completely before birth (Hiraoka et al, 2002), it is clear that **the cause of every case of URA cannot be attributed to one of the mechanisms cited previously.** In fact, the presence of the splenic flexure of the bowel in its normal location and not in the left renal fossa suggests that a dysplastic or multicystic kidney may have started to form in the proper location but involuted before delivery.

Associated Anomalies. The ipsilateral ureter is completely absent in slightly more than half of the patients (Fortune, 1927; Collins, 1932; Ashley and Mostofi, 1960). Many of the remaining individuals have only a partially developed ureter. In no instance is the ureter totally normal. Partial ureteral development is associated with either complete luminal atresia or patency of a variable degree. A hemitrigone (in association with complete ureteral agenesis) or an asymmetrical trigone (in the presence of a partially developed ureter) is recognizable at cystoscopy. Segmental ureteral atresia on one side has been associated with contralateral ureteral or renal ectopia (Limkakeng and Retik, 1972). Except for ectopia or malrotation, anomalies of the contralateral kidney are very infrequently encountered (Longo and Thompson, 1952). However, abnormalities of the contralateral collecting system are

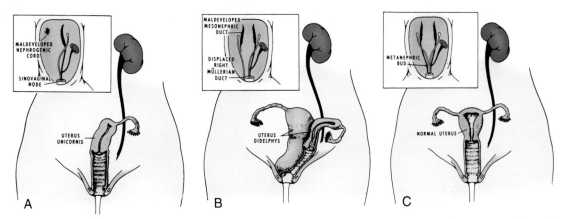

Figure 113–2. A to **C,** A proposed categorization of genital and renal anomalies in females. See text for details. (From Magee MC, Lucey DT, Fried FA: A new embryologic classification for uro-gynecologic malformations: The syndromes of mesonephric duct induced müllerian deformities. J Urol 1979;121:265.)

not uncommon, including ureteropelvic and ureterovesical junction obstruction in 11% and 7%, respectively (Cascio et al, 1999) and vesicoureteral reflux in 30% (Atiyeh et al, 1993; Cascio et al, 1999). Overall, as many as 65% may have another urologic abnormality (Kaneyama et al, 2004).

Ipsilateral adrenal agenesis is rarely encountered with URA: it is noted in fewer than 10% of autopsy reports (Fortune, 1927; Collins, 1932; Ashley and Mostofi, 1960) and in 17% of affected individuals evaluated by computed tomography (Kenney et al, 1985). This is not surprising in view of the different embryologic derivations of the adrenal cortex and medulla, which arise separately from the metanephros.

Genital anomalies are much more frequently observed. Despite the predominance of male infants with URA, reproductive organ abnormalities seem to occur with more regularity in females, occurring in at least 25% to 50% of cases, compared with 10% to 15% in males. Although a genital anomaly is easier to detect in the female, which may account for the difference in incidence between the two sexes, a more plausible explanation is related to the difference in timing and interaction of the male and female genital ducts in relation to the developing mesonephric duct and ureteral bud. The incidence of a genital organ malformation for both sexes varies from 20% to 40% (Smith and Orkin, 1945; Doroshow and Abeshouse, 1961; Thompson and Lynn, 1966). Regardless of the sex, both the ipsilaterally and contralaterally positioned testes are normal and the gonad is usually normal. But structures derived from the müllerian or wolffian duct are most often anomalous. In the male, the testis and globus major, which contains the efferent ductules and which arises from mesonephric tubules, are invariably present; all structures proximal to that point that develop from the mesonephric duct (the globus minor, vas deferens, seminal vesicle, ampulla, and ejaculatory duct) are frequently absent, with an incidence approaching 50% (Radasch, 1908; Collins, 1932; Charny and Gillenwater, 1965; Ochsner et al, 1972). In a review of the literature (Donohue and Fauver, 1989) of adult males with absence of the vas deferens, 79% were found to have an absent kidney on the ipsilateral side; left-sided lesions predominated in a ratio of 3.5:1. However, bilateral absence of the vas has been noted with URA (McCallum et al, 2001). Occasionally, the mesonephric duct structures are rudimentary or ectopic rather than absent (Holt and Peterson, 1974). Seminal vesicle cysts are being diagnosed with increasing frequency as pelvic ultrasound examinations are performed more often (Lopez-Garcia et al, 1998; Kaneyama et al, 2004): 6 cases (5%) were noted among 119 boys who were found to have URA during ultrasonic screening of schoolchildren (Shieh et al, 1990). Rarely has ipsilateral cryptorchidism been noted.

In the female, a variety of anomalies may result from incomplete or altered müllerian development caused by mesonephric duct maldevelopment. **Approximately one fourth to one third of women with URA have an abnormality of the internal genitalia** (Thompson and Lynn, 1966; Heinonen, 2004). Conversely, 43% of women with genital anomalies have URA (Semmens, 1962; Heinonen, 1997). Most common of these is a true unicornuate uterus with complete absence of the ipsilateral horn and fallopian tube or a bicornuate uterus with rudimentary development of the horn on the affected side (Candiani et al, 1997). The fimbriated end

of the fallopian tube, however, is usually fully formed and corresponds in its development to the globus major in the male (Shumacker, 1938).

Partial or complete midline fusion of the müllerian ducts may result in a double (didelphys) or septate uterus with either a single or a duplicated cervix (Radasch, 1908; Fortune, 1927). Complete duplication or separation of the vagina, proximal vaginal atresia associated with a small introital dimple, and even complete absence of the vagina have been reported (Woolf and Allen, 1953; D'Alberton et al, 1981). **Obstruction of one side of a duplicated system is not uncommon, and unilateral hematocolpos or hydrocolpos** associated with a pelvic mass and/or pain has been described in the pubertal girl (Weiss and Dykhuizen, 1967; Vinstein and Franken, 1972; Gilliland and Dick, 1976; Wiersma et al, 1976; Yoder and Pfister, 1976) (Fig. 113–3). In rare instances, this anomalous condition has been mistaken for a large or infected Gartner's duct cyst. Sometimes a true Gartner's duct cyst has been found in a prepubertal girl in association with an ectopic ureter that is blind ending at its proximal end or one that is connected to a rudimentary kidney (Currarino, 1982). Six percent of girls with URA were found to have a Gartner cyst on mass screening of schoolchildren (Shieh et al, 1990). Infertility occurs in as many as 33% of affected women with renal agenesis and unicornuate uterus (Heinonen, 1997).

Radiologic investigation of the upper urinary tract in individuals with anomalies of the internal genitalia often leads to the discovery of an absent kidney on the affected side (Bryan et al, 1949; Phelan et al, 1953; Heinonen, 1997).

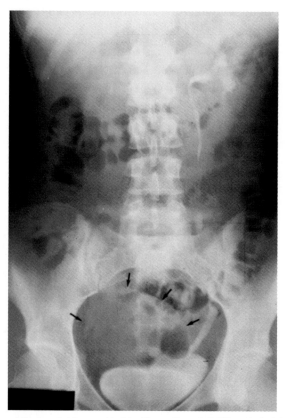

Figure 113–3. A 16-year-old girl with a solitary left kidney had abdominal pain and a pelvic mass that proved to be an obstructed duplicate vagina with hematocolpos. *Arrows* outline the obstructed vaginal segment.

In fact, because URA is so frequently associated with anomalies of the internal female genitalia, the clinician should evaluate the entire genitourinary system in any girl with one or more of the above-mentioned abnormalities (Heinonen, 2004). It is just as reasonable to investigate the pelvic area with ultrasound in boys diagnosed with URA because of its association with seminal vesicle abnormalities (Van den Ouden et al, 1998).

In addition, anomalies of other organ systems are found frequently in affected individuals. The more common sites involve the cardiovascular (30%), gastrointestinal (25%), and musculoskeletal (14%) systems (Emanuel et al, 1974) (Fig. 113–4). They include septal and valvular cardiac defects; imperforate anus and anal or esophageal strictures or atresia; and vertebral or phalangeal abnormalities (Jancu et al, 1976; Wheeler and Weaver, 2001; Rai et al, 2002). Several syndromes are associated with URA: Turner's syndrome, Poland's syndrome (Mace et al, 1972), Frazer's syndrome (Fryns et al, 1997), BOR (brachio-oto-renal) syndrome (Pierides et al, 2002), DiGeorge anomaly when associated with insulin-dependent diabetes mellitus in the mother (Wilson et al, 1993; Novak and Robinson, 1994), dysmorphogenesis, and, more recently, Kallmann's syndrome. Abnormalities of the *KAL1* locus at Xp22 in the X-linked autosomal dominant disorder have a high frequency of URA, 40% (Say and Gerald, 1968; Colquhoun-Kerr et al, 1999; Zenteno et al, 1999; Quinton et al, 2001), as does Townes-Brock syndrome with *SALL1* deletions (Salerno et al, 2000; Nishinakamura et al, 2001; Sato et al, 2003, 2004). Twenty to 30 percent of children with the

VACTERL association (*v*ertebral, imperforate *a*nus, *c*ardiac, *t*racheo-*e*sophageal atresia, *r*enal, and *l*imb anomalies) have URA (Barry and Auldist, 1974; Kolon et al, 2000). Children with supernumerary nipples (Urbani and Betti, 1996) and disorders of the ears with hearing loss (especially if it is a congenital abnormality) (Huang et al, 2001) and preauricular pits (Pierides et al, 2002) have a substantial incidence of URA. Therefore, a comprehensive review of all organ systems should be undertaken when more than one anomaly is discovered or when specific complexes of anomalies associated with renal agenesis are present. In a small number of children the constellation of defects is incompatible with life and gestational or neonatal death ensues.

KEY POINTS: UNILATERAL RENAL AGENESIS

- Unilateral agenesis occurs once in 1100 births.

- Males predominate in a ratio of 1.8:1.

- Absence of one kidney occurs somewhat more frequently on the left side.

- The ipsilateral ureter is completely absent in about half of the patients.

- Genital anomalies are much more frequently observed. Despite the predominance of male infants with URA, reproductive organ abnormalities occur with more frequency in females, occurring in 25% to 50% of cases, compared with 10% to 15% in males.

- Structures derived from the müllerian or wolffian duct are most often anomalous.

- Approximately one fourth to one third of women with URA have an abnormality of the internal genitalia.

- Anomalies of other organ systems are found frequently in affected individuals. The more common sites involve the cardiovascular (30%), gastrointestinal (25%), and musculoskeletal (14%) systems.

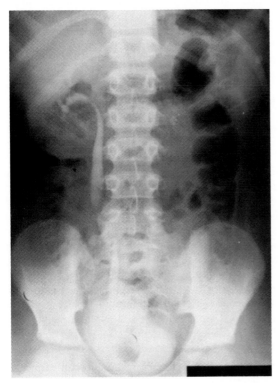

Figure 113–4. A 4-year-old girl had an excretory urogram because of imperforate anus and duplicate vagina. Note absence of left kidney and medial placement of the splenic flexure. At cystoscopy, a hemitrigone was noted.

Diagnosis. In general, **there are no specific symptoms heralding an absent kidney.** Previously, most reports were composed of surveys from autopsy series but now prenatal screening is detecting an absent kidney. The contralateral kidney does not appear to be more prone to disease from being solitary unless the absent kidney is truly secondary to a multicystic dysplastic organ that went unrecognized at birth, in which case there may be a mild UPJ obstruction in the remaining functioning kidney. The demands placed on the solitary kidney lead to compensatory enlargement even prenatally (Hill et al, 2000), which can then raise the possibility of contralateral agenesis.

The diagnosis should be suspected during a physical examination when the vas deferens or body and tail of the epididymis is missing or when an absent, septate, or hypoplastic vagina is associated with a unicornuate or

bicornuate uterus (Bryan et al, 1949). Bilateral absence of the vas (McCallum et al, 2001) and seminal vesical cysts have been associated as well (Calahorra Fernandez et al, 2002). Radiologically, an absent left kidney can be surmised when a plain film of the abdomen demonstrates the gas pattern of the splenic flexure of the colon in a medial position because the colon now occupies the area normally reserved for the left kidney (Mascatello and Lebowitz, 1976) (see Fig. 113–4). When this characteristic gas pattern is present, it is a very reliable sign. A similar finding showing the hepatic flexure positioned in the right renal fossa suggests congenital absence of the right kidney (Curtis et al, 1977). The diagnosis of agenesis usually can be confirmed by renal ultrasonography or excretory urography, which reveals an absent kidney or nephrogram on that side and compensatory hypertrophy of the contralateral kidney (Hynes and Watkin, 1970; Cope and Trickey, 1982). However, a multicystic kidney can easily be mistaken for true agenesis in an older individual, because the cysts involute as the fluid gets absorbed during the first several months of life. The colonic gas pattern will not occupy a position closer to the midline if a multicystic kidney was present during gestation, so this provides an excellent clue to the diagnosis when no kidney can be detected by ultrasonography later on in life. Prenatal and perinatal ultrasonography examinations are being performed more routinely today, and URA is being detected with increased frequency (Sipek et al, 1997). In addition, the ipsilateral adrenal gland may have a characteristic appearance—flattened or lying down—when the kidney never formed, alerting the clinician to URA (Hoffman et al, 1992).

Failure of one kidney to "light up" during the total body image phase of a radionuclide technetium scan is compatible with the diagnosis of an absent kidney, but this may not be infallible. **Radionuclide imaging of the kidney** using an isotope that traces renal blood flow will clearly differentiate URA from other conditions in which the renal function may be severely impaired (e.g., severe obstruction, high-grade reflux). Isotope scanning and ultrasonography have largely replaced arteriography in defining agenesis. When a fetus with suspected anomalies undergoes MRI, an absent kidney can be readily detected (Dell'Acqua et al, 2002). Fluoroscopic monitoring of the renal fossa at the end of a cardiac catheterization or renal ultrasonography at the end of echocardiography has demonstrated an absent kidney on occasion. The 28% incidence of contralateral reflux (Cascio et al, 1999) warrants cystography, either conventional or nuclear, in these individuals.

Cystoscopy, if performed, usually reveals an asymmetrical trigone or hemitrigone, suggesting either partial or complete ureteral atresia and renal agenesis. Cystoscopy has been relegated to a minor diagnostic tool since the development of other, more sophisticated, noninvasive radiographic studies (Kroovand, 1985).

Prognosis. **There is no clear-cut evidence that patients with a solitary kidney have an increased susceptibility to other diseases.** Most reviews dealing with this subject were conducted in the preantibiotic era, and they reported a high incidence of "pyelitis," nephrolithiasis and ureterolithiasis, tuberculosis, and glomerulonephritis. The increased ability to prevent infection and its sequelae has reduced the incidence of morbidity and mortality among patients with a solitary kidney. In Ashley and Mostofi's series (1960), only 15% of the patients died as a result of renal disease, the nature of which in almost every case would have been bilateral had two kidneys been present initially. Renal trauma resulted in death for 5%; some patients in this group might have lived had there been two kidneys (however, because the source of the autopsy material included many military personnel, the potential risk of injury was accentuated). In other words, URA with an otherwise normal contralateral kidney is not incompatible with normal longevity and does not predispose the remaining contralateral kidney to greater than normal risks (Gutierrez, 1933; Dees, 1960). One should be prudent, however, in advising individuals to participate in contact sports or strenuous physical exertion.

Rugui and associates (1986) found an increased occurrence of hypertension, hyperuricemia, and decreased renal function but no proteinuria in a small group of patients with congenital absence of one kidney. Only one patient had a renal biopsy, and this showed focal glomerular sclerosis, similar to what has been found in the remaining kidney in patients with the hyperfiltration syndrome noted after unilateral nephrectomy. The authors concluded that URA may carry the same potential factor. Focal glomerulosclerosis has been confirmed in six other individuals with URA (Nomura and Osawa, 1990). **Argueso and colleagues** (1992) **assessed 157 middle-aged patients with congenital URA and noted hypertension and proteinuria in 47% and in 19%, respectively, as well as mild renal insufficiency in 13%.** Despite these findings, survival was not impaired in this group of people. In addition, the ability of the kidney to excrete increased loads of protein was not impaired, even in patients with renal insufficiency or proteinuria (DeSanto et al, 1997). In another study of 206 women with uterine abnormalities, 33 (16%) had an absent kidney. The risk of hypertension in these affected women was 42% versus 18% of controls with no uterine defects and bilaterally present kidneys (Heinonen, 2004).

Supernumerary Kidney

Parenchymal development is controlled, in part, by an unidentified substance that acts to limit the amount of functioning renal tissue. It is, therefore, interesting to find that nature has created, albeit rarely, a condition in which the individual has three separate kidneys and an excessive amount of functioning renal parenchyma. In such instances, the two main kidneys are usually normal and equal in size, whereas the third is small. **The supernumerary kidney is truly an accessory organ with its own collecting system, blood supply, and distinct encapsulated parenchymal mass.** It may be either totally separate from the normal kidney on the same side or connected to it by loose areolar tissue (Geisinger, 1937). The ipsilateral ureters may be bifid or completely duplicated. The condition is not analogous to a single kidney with ureteral duplication, in which each collecting system drains portions of one parenchymatous mass surrounded by a single capsule.

Incidence. The true incidence of this anomaly cannot be calculated because of its very infrequent occurrence. **Approximately 100 cases have been reported since it was first described in 1656;** it represents a very rare anomaly of the urinary system (Sasidharan et al, 1976; McPherson, 1987). It affects males and females equally but has a higher predilection for the left side (N'Guessan and Stephens, 1983). Four cases of bilateral supernumerary kidneys have been reported (Campbell, 1970; Otto et al, 2002).

Embryology. The sequence of interdependent events involved in ureteral bud formation and metanephric blastema development, which is required for the maturation of the normal kidney, probably also allows for the occurrence of a supernumerary kidney. **It is postulated that a deviation involving both of these processes must take place to create the anomaly. A second ureteral outpouching off the wolffian duct or a branching from the initial ureteral bud appears as a necessary first step. Next, the nephrogenic anlage may divide into two metanephric tails, which separate entirely** when induced to differentiate by the separate or bifid ureteral buds (N'Guessan and Stephens, 1983). The twin metanephroi develop only when the bifid or separate ureteral buds enter them. N'Guessan and Stephens do not accept that this condition is the result of widely divergent bifid or separate ureteral buds. Geisinger (1937) proposed that the separate kidneys may have been caused either by fragmentation of a single metanephros or by linear infarction producing separate viable fragments that develop only when a second ureteral bud is present.

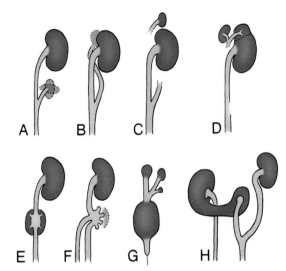

Figure 113–5. **A** to **H,** Various patterns of urinary drainage when ureters form a common stem. All kidney positions are relative only and are depicted on the left side for ease of interpretation. *Dashed lines* indicate that detail was not defined. (From N'Guessan G, Stephens FD: Supernumerary kidney. J Urol 1983;130:649.)

KEY POINTS: SUPERNUMERARY KIDNEY

■ The supernumerary kidney is truly an accessory organ with its own collecting system, blood supply, and distinct encapsulated parenchymal mass.

■ The supernumerary kidney is a distinct parenchymatous mass that may be either completely separate or only loosely attached to the major kidney on the ipsilateral side.

■ The ureteral interrelationships on the side of the supernumerary kidney are quite variable.

Description. The supernumerary kidney is a distinct parenchymatous mass that may be either completely separate or only loosely attached to the major kidney on the ipsilateral side. In general, it is located somewhat caudad to the dominant kidney, which is in its correct position in the renal fossa. Occasionally, the supernumerary kidney lies either posterior or craniad to the main kidney, or it may even be a midline structure anterior to the great vessels and loosely attached to each of the other two kidneys (Fig. 113–5). A pelvic supernumerary kidney has also been cited (Eberle et al, 2002).

The supernumerary kidney is reniform but generally smaller than the main ipsilateral organ. In about one third of cases, the kidney or its collecting system is abnormal. In almost half of the reported cases, the collecting system is severely dilated with thinned parenchyma, indicating an obstructed ureter.

The ureteral interrelationships on the side of the supernumerary kidney are quite variable (Kretschmer, 1929). Convergence of the ipsilateral ureters distally to form a

common stem and a single ureteral orifice occurs in 50% of the cases (Exley and Hotchkiss, 1944; N'Guessan and Stephens, 1983). Two completely independent ureters, each with its own entrance into the bladder, are seen in the other 50% of cases. The Weigert-Meyer principle (see Chapter 116) usually is obeyed, but in 10% the caudal kidney has a ureter that does not follow the rule and enters the trigone below the ipsilateral ureter (Tada et al, 1981) (Fig. 113–6). Rarely, the supernumerary kidney has a completely ectopic ureter opening into the vagina or introitus (Rubin, 1948; Carlson, 1950). Individual case reports have described calyceal communications between the supernumerary and the dominant kidney, or fusion of the dominant kidney's ureter with the pelvis of the supernumerary kidney (Kretschmer, 1929) to create a single distal ureter, which then enters the bladder (see Fig. 113–5). The vascular supply to the supernumerary kidney is, as might be expected, anomalous and depends on its position in relation to the major ipsilateral kidney. Although some investigators believe that the blood supply to the individual parenchymal masses should be separate to consider this a true supernumerary kidney (Kaneoya et al, 1989), this view is not held universally.

Associated Anomalies. Usually the ipsilateral and contralateral kidneys are normal. Except for an occasional ectopic orifice from the ureter draining the supernumerary kidney, no genitourinary abnormalities are present in any consistent pattern. Few of the case reports describe anomalies of other organ systems.

Symptoms. Although this anomaly is obviously present at birth, **it is rarely discovered in childhood. It may not produce symptoms until early adulthood, if at all.** The average age at diagnosis in all reported cases was 36 years. Pain, fever, hypertension, and a palpable abdominal mass are the usual presenting complaints. Urinary infection or obstruction, or both, are the major conditions that lead to an evaluation. Ureteral ectopia from the supernumerary kidney may produce urinary

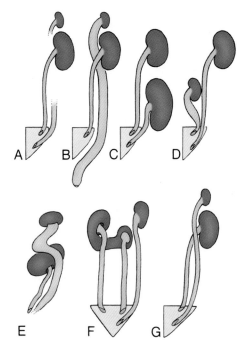

Figure 113-6. **A** to **G,** Various patterns of urinary drainage of supernumerary and ipsilateral kidneys when ureters are completely separated. All kidney positions are relative only and are depicted on the left side for ease of interpretation. *Dashed lines* indicate that detail was not defined. (From N'Guessan G, Stephens FD: Supernumerary kidney. J Urol 1983;130:649.)

incontinence, but this is extremely rare because of the hypoplastic nature of the involved renal element (Shane, 1942; Hoffman and McMillan, 1948).

A palpable abdominal mass secondary to development of carcinoma in the supernumerary kidney has been noted in two patients. In 25% of all reported cases, however, the supernumerary kidney remains completely asymptomatic and is discovered only at autopsy (Carlson, 1950).

Diagnosis. If the supernumerary kidney is normal and not symptomatic, it is usually diagnosed when excretory urography or abdominal ultrasonography is performed for other reasons. The kidney may be inferior and distant enough from the ipsilateral kidney that it does not disturb the latter's architecture (Conrad and Loes, 1987). If it is in close proximity, its mere presence may displace the predominant kidney or its ureter very slightly.

A supernumerary kidney may become symptomatic from hydronephrosis or even stone formation (Koureas et al, 2000). When it does it may distort the normal ipsilateral kidney and ureter, a condition that is detectable by ultrasonography. If the collecting system is bifid, the dominant kidney on that side is usually involved in the same disease process. If the ureters are separate, the ipsilateral kidney may show the effects of an abnormal supernumerary kidney. Voiding cystourethrography, ultrasonography, computed tomography (CT) with contrast medium enhancement, and even retrograde pyelography may be needed to help delineate the pathologic process. Radionuclide imaging provides information about relative function in the supernumerary as well as normal kidneys (Conrad and Loes, 1987). Cystoscopy reveals one or two ureteral orifices on the ipsilateral side, depending on whether

the ureters are completely duplicated and, if so, to what extent ureteral ectopia exists in or outside of the bladder. Occasionally a supernumerary kidney is not accurately diagnosed until the time of surgery or at autopsy.

ANOMALIES OF ASCENT
Simple Renal Ectopia

When the mature kidney fails to reach its normal location in the "renal" fossa, the condition is known as *renal ectopia*. The term is derived from the Greek words *ek* ("out") and *topos* ("place") and literally means "out of place." It is to be differentiated from renal ptosis, in which the kidney initially is located in its proper place (and has normal vascularity) but moves downward in relation to body position. The ectopic kidney has never resided in the appropriate location.

An ectopic kidney can be found in one of the following positions: pelvic, iliac, abdominal, thoracic, and contralateral or crossed (Fig. 113–7). Only the ipsilateral retroperitoneal location of the ectopic kidney is discussed here. Thoracic kidney and crossed renal ectopia (with and without fusion) are described later.

Incidence. Renal ectopia has been known to exist since it was described by 16th century anatomists, but it did not achieve clinical interest until the mid-19th century. In recent times, with greater emphasis on diagnostic acumen and uroradiologic visualization, including prenatal imaging, this condition has been noted with increasing frequency.

The actual incidence among autopsy series varies from 1 in 500 (Campbell, 1930) to 1 in 1200 (Stevens, 1937; Thompson and Pace, 1937; Anson and Riba, 1939; Bell, 1946), but the average occurrence is about 1 in 900 (Abeshouse and Bhisitkul, 1959). With increasing clinical detection, the incidence among hospitalized patients has approached the autopsy rate (Abeshouse and Bhisitkul, 1959). Autopsy studies reveal no significant difference in incidence between the sexes.

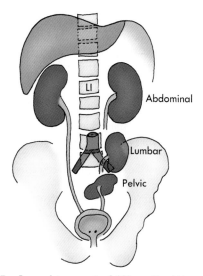

Figure 113-7. Incomplete ascent of kidney: The kidney may halt at any level of its ascent from the pelvis. (From Gray SW, Skandalakis JE: The kidney and ureter. In Gray SW, Skandalakis JE: Embryology for Surgeons. Philadelphia, WB Saunders, 1972.)

A recent review of prenatal ultrasounds detected an incidence of 0.003% in India, but even this may under-represent its true occurrence (Sanghvi et al, 1998). Clinically, renal ectopia is more readily recognized in females because they undergo uroradiologic evaluation more frequently than males as a result of their higher rate of urinary tract infection and/or associated genital anomalies (Thompson and Pace, 1937).

The left side is favored slightly over the right. Pelvic ectopia has been estimated to occur in 1 of 2100 to 3000 autopsies (Stevens, 1937). A solitary ectopic kidney occurs in 1 of 22,000 autopsies (Stevens, 1937; Hawes, 1950; Delson, 1975); by 1973, only 165 cases of a solitary pelvic kidney had been recorded (Downs et al, 1973). Bilateral ectopic kidneys are even more rarely observed and account for only 10% of all patients with renal ectopia (Malek et al, 1971).

Embryology. The ureteral bud, arising from the wolffian duct at the end of the 4th week, **grows craniad toward the urogenital ridge,** acquiring a cap of metanephric blastema by the 5th week. The developing metanephric tissue and ureteral bud **migrate cephalad, rotating medially on its long axis** as it does so. **The entire process is completed by the 8th week of gestation.** Factors that may prevent the orderly movement of kidneys include ureteral bud maldevelopment (Campbell, 1930), defective metanephric tissue that by itself fails to induce ascent (Ward et al, 1965), genetic abnormalities, and maternal illnesses or teratogenic causes, because genital anomalies are common (Malek et al, 1971). A vascular barrier that prevents upward migration secondary to persistence of the fetal blood supply has also been postulated (Baggenstoss, 1951), but the existence of an "early" renal blood supply does not prevent the affected kidney's movement to its ultimate position. More probably it is the end result, not the cause, of renal ectopia.

Description. The classification of ectopia is based on the position of the kidney within the retroperitoneum: the pelvic kidney is opposite the sacrum and below the aortic bifurcation; the lumbar kidney rests near the sacral promontory in the iliac fossa and anterior to the iliac vessels; and the abdominal kidney is so named when it is above the iliac crest and adjacent to the second lumbar vertebra (see Fig. 113–7). No single location is more common for the ectopic kidney (Dretler et al, 1971).

The ectopic kidney is usually smaller than normal, and it may not conform to the usual reniform shape, owing to the presence of fetal lobulations. The axis of the kidney is slightly medial or vertical, but it may be tilted as much as 90 degrees laterally, so that it lies in a true horizontal plane. **The renal pelvis is usually anterior (instead of medial) to the parenchyma because the kidney has incompletely rotated. As a result, 56% of ectopic kidneys have a hydronephrotic collecting system. Half of these cases result from obstruction at either the ureteropelvic or the ureterovesical junction (70% and 30%, respectively); 25% from reflux grade 3 or greater, and 25% from the malrotation alone** (Gleason et al, 1994). With the increased use of screening ultrasonography detecting more asymptomatic renal anomalies, these numbers for symptomatic abnormalities may be higher than is actually the case.

Overall, **vesicoureteral reflux has been found in 30% of children with ectopic kidneys** (Guarino et al, 2004). The length of the ureter usually conforms to the position of the kidney, but occasionally it is slightly tortuous. It is rarely redundant, in contrast to the ptotic kidney, in which the ureter has achieved its full length before the kidney drops (Fig. 113–8). **The ureter usually enters the bladder on the ipsilateral side with its orifice situated normally.** Therefore, cystoscopy will not distinguish renal ectopia from a normal kidney. The arterial and venous network is predictable only by the fact that it is anomalous; its vascular pattern depends on the ultimate resting place of the kidney (Anson and Riba, 1939). There may be one or two main renal arteries arising from the distal aorta or from the aortic bifurcation, with one or more aberrant arteries coming off the common or external iliac or even the inferior mesenteric artery. The kidney may be supplied entirely by multiple anomalous branches, none of which arises from the aorta. In no instance has the main renal artery arisen from that level of the aorta that would be its proper origin if the kidney were positioned normally.

KEY POINTS: SIMPLE RENAL ECTOPIA

- The left side is affected slightly more than the right.
- Pelvic ectopia has been estimated to occur in 1 of 2100 to 3000 autopsies.
- Fifty-six percent of ectopic kidneys have a hydronephrotic collecting system. Half of these cases result from obstruction at either the ureteropelvic or the ureterovesical junction (70% and 30%, respectively); 25% from reflux grade 3 or greater, and 25% from the malrotation alone.
- Vesicoureteral reflux has been found in 30% of children with ectopic kidneys.
- The incidence of genital anomalies in the patient with ectopia is about 15%.
- Most ectopic kidneys are clinically asymptomatic.
- The ectopic kidney is no more susceptible to disease than the normally positioned kidney.

Associated Anomalies. Although the contralateral kidney is usually normal, it is associated with a number of congenital defects. Malek and colleagues (1971) and Thompson and Pace (1937) found **the incidence of contralateral agenesis to be rather high,** suggesting that a teratogenic factor affecting both ureteral buds and/or metanephric blastemas may be responsible for the two anomalies (see Fig. 113–8). Bilateral ectopia is seen in a very small number of patients (Fig. 113–9). Hydronephrosis secondary to obstruction or reflux may be seen in as many as 25% of nonectopic contralateral kidneys (Gleason et al, 1994).

The most striking feature is the association of genital anomalies in the patient with ectopia. The incidence varies from 15% (Thompson and Pace, 1937) **to 45%** (Downs et al, 1973), depending on how carefully the patient is evaluated. Twenty to 66 percent of females have one or more of the following abnormalities of the reproductive organs: bicornuate

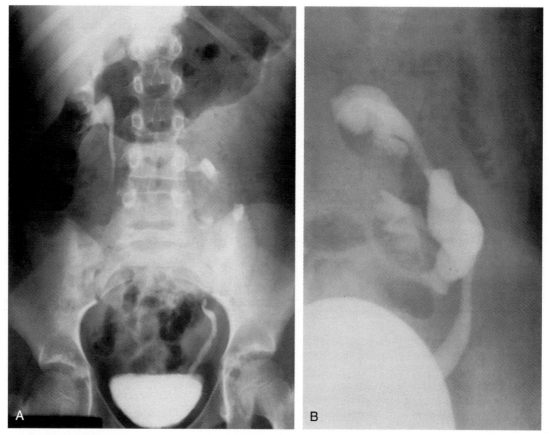

Figure 113–8. **A,** Excretory urography in a 9-year-old girl investigated for recurrent urinary tract infection shows a left lumbar kidney. **B,** Voiding cystourethrography demonstrates reflux to the ectopic kidney. At cystoscopy, the ureteral orifice was found to be located at the bladder neck.

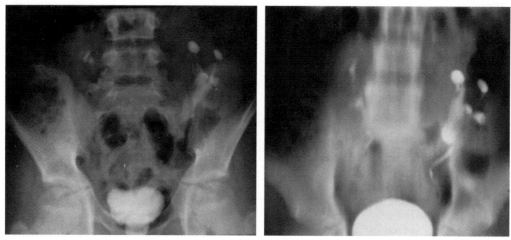

Figure 113–9. A palpable abdominal mass in an 8-year-old girl proved to be bilateral pelvic kidneys.

or unicornuate uterus with atresia of one horn (McCrea, 1942); rudimentary or absent uterus and proximal and/or distal vagina (Tabisky and Bhisitkul, 1965; D'Alberton et al, 1981); and duplication of the vagina. Among male patients, 10% to 20% have a recognizable associated genital defect; undescended testes, duplication of the urethra, and hypospadias are the most common (Thompson and Pace, 1937). Fourteen percent of patients with a cloacal malformation have an ectopic kidney (Warne et al, 2002).

Rarely, the adrenal gland is absent or abnormally positioned. Twenty-one percent of patients have anomalies of other organ systems (Downs et al, 1973); most of these involve the skeletal or cardiac systems.

Diagnosis. With the increasing use of radiography, ultrasonography, and radionuclide scanning to visualize the urinary tract, the incidence of incidental discovery of an asymptomatic ectopic kidney is also increasing.

Most ectopic kidneys are clinically asymptomatic. Vague abdominal complaints or frank ureteral colic secondary to an obstructing stone are still the most frequent symptoms leading to discovery of the misplaced kidney. The abnormal position of the kidney results in a pattern of direct and referred pain that is atypical for colic and may be misdiagnosed as acute appendicitis or as pelvic organ inflammatory disease in female patients. It is rare to find symptoms of compression from organs adjacent to the ectopic kidney. Patients with renal ectopia may also present initially with a urinary tract infection or a palpable abdominal mass. Several cases of a rare association of renal and ureteral ectopia causing urinary incontinence have been reported (Borer et al, 1993, 1998; Pattaras et al, 1999). The difficulty in diagnosing this condition is related to the poor function of the ectopic kidney. Dimercaptosuccinic acid (DMSA) scintigraphy or enhanced CT will delineate these unusual cases (Borer et al, 1998; Leitha, 1998; Pattaras et al, 1999).

Malposition of the colon (as discussed earlier in regard to renal agenesis) may be a clue to the ectopic position of a lumbar or pelvic kidney. The diagnosis is easily made when the excretory urogram or renal ultrasound study fails to reveal a kidney in its proper location. The fact that many of these kidneys overlie the bony pelvis, which obscures the collecting system, can lead to a misdiagnosis with failure to recognize the true position of the kidney.

Nephrotomography during an excretory urogram has been replaced by ultrasonography, radionuclide scanning, and MRI as diagnostic tools (Pattaras et al, 1999; Maher et al, 2000). Cystoscopy alone is rarely useful, because the trigone and ureteral orifices are invariably normal unless the ureteral orifice is also ectopic—a rare event. Arteriography may be helpful in delineating the renal vascular supply in anticipation of surgery on the ectopic kidney. This is especially important in cases of solitary ectopia.

Prognosis. The ectopic kidney is no more susceptible to disease than the normally positioned kidney except for the development of hydronephrosis or urinary calculus formation (Gleason et al, 1994; Benchekroun et al, 2002). This is in part a result of the anteriorly placed pelvis and malrotation of the kidney, which may lead to impaired drainage of urine from a high insertion of the ureter to the pelvis or an anomalous vasculature that partially blocks one of the major calyces or the upper ureter. In addition, there may be an increased risk of injury from blunt abdominal trauma because the low-lying kidney is not protected by the rib cage.

Renovascular hypertension secondary to an anomalous blood supply has been reported, but a higher than normal incidence is yet to be proved. Anderson and Harrison (1965), in a review of pregnant women with renal ectopia, could find no increased occurrence of difficult deliveries or maternal or fetal complications related to the ectopic kidney (Anderson and Harrison, 1965; Delson, 1975). Dystocia from a pelvic kidney is a very rare finding, but when it does occur, early recognition is mandatory and cesarean section is indicated. Although three cases of cancer in an ectopic kidney have been reported, **there does not appear to be an increased risk for malignant transformation.** No deaths have been directly attributable to the ectopic kidney, but in at least five instances a solitary ectopic kidney has been mistakenly removed because

the kidney was thought to represent a pelvic malignancy (Downs et al, 1973). This should not happen today, with the multiplicity of imaging techniques available to accurately diagnose the condition.

Cephalad Renal Ectopia

The mature kidney may be positioned more craniad than normal in patients who have had a history of omphalocele (Pinckney et al, 1978). When the liver herniates into the omphalocele sac with the intestines, the kidneys continue to ascend until they are stopped by the diaphragm. In all reported cases, both kidneys were affected and lay immediately beneath the diaphragm at the level of the 10th thoracic vertebra. The ureters are excessively long but otherwise normal. An angiogram in these patients demonstrates that the origin of each renal artery is more cephalad than normal, but no other abnormality of the vascular network is present. Patients with this anomaly usually have no symptoms referable to the malposition, and urinary drainage is not impaired.

Thoracic Kidney

The rarest form of renal ectopia exists when the kidney is positioned considerably higher than normal. **Intrathoracic ectopia denotes either a partial or a complete protrusion of the kidney above the level of the diaphragm into the posterior mediastinum. Fewer than 5% of all patients with renal ectopia have an intrathoracic kidney** (Campbell, 1930). This condition is to be differentiated from a congenital or traumatic diaphragmatic hernia, in which other abdominal organs as well as the kidney have advanced into the chest cavity.

Incidence. Before 1940, all reports of this condition were noted as part of autopsy series (DeCastro and Shumacher, 1969). Since that time, however, **at least 200 patients have been reported** in the literature (Donat and Donat, 1988; Lacasta Garcia et al, 1999), 4 of whom had bilateral thoracic kidneys (Berlin et al, 1957; Hertz and Shahin, 1969; Lundius, 1975; N'Guessan and Stephens, 1984; Liddell et al, 1989). There appears to be a slight left-sided predominance of 1.5:1, and the sex ratio favors males by 2:1 (Lozano and Rodriguez, 1975). This entity has been discovered in all age groups, from a neonate (Shapira et al, 1965) to a 75-year-old man evaluated for prostatic hypertrophy (Burke et al, 1967), but is most commonly detected in adults undergoing chest radiography for other reasons (Drop et al, 2003).

Embryology. The kidney reaches its adult location by the end of the 8th week of gestation. At this time, the diaphragmatic leaflets are formed as the pleuroperitoneal membrane separates the pleural from the peritoneal cavity. Mesenchymal tissues associated with this membrane eventually form the muscular component of the diaphragm. It is uncertain whether delayed closure of the diaphragmatic anlage allows for protracted renal ascent above the level of the future diaphragm or whether the kidney overshoots its usual position because of accelerated ascent before normal diaphragmatic closure (Spillane and Prather, 1952; Burke et al, 1967; N'Guessan and Stephens, 1984). Delayed involution of mesonephric tissue has been proposed as a causative factor (Angulo et al, 1992), because intrathoracic kidneys occur in only 0.25% of patients with a diaphragmatic hernia (Donat and Donat, 1988). Renal angiography has demonstrated either a normal site (Lundius, 1975) or a more cranial origin (Franciskovic and Martincic, 1959) for the renal artery takeoff from the aorta supplying the thoracic kidney.

Description. **The kidney is situated in the posterior mediastinum and usually has completed the normal rotation process** (Fig. 113–10). The renal contour and collecting system are normal. The kidney usually lies in the posterolateral aspect of the diaphragm in the foramen of Bochdalek. The diaphragm at this point thins out, and a flimsy membrane surrounds the protruding portion of kidney. Therefore, the kidney is not within the pleural space (N'Guessan and Stephens, 1984). The lower lobe of the adjacent lung may be hypoplastic secondary to compression by the kidney mass. The renal vasculature and the ureter enter and exit from the pleural cavity through the foramen of Bochdalek.

Associated Anomalies. **The ureter is elongated** to accommodate the excessive distance to the bladder, but it never enters ectopically into the bladder or other pelvic sites. The adrenal gland has been mentioned in only two reports; in one it accompanied the kidney into the chest (Barloon and Goodwin, 1957), and in the other it did not (Paul et al, 1960). However, N'Guessan and Stephens (1984) analyzed 10 cases and determined that the adrenal gland is below the kidney in its normal location in most of the patients. In unilateral cases the contralateral kidney is usually normal. No consistent anomalies have been described in other organ systems;

however, one child did have trisomy 18 (Shapira et al, 1965) and another patient had multiple pulmonary and cardiac anomalies in addition to the thoracic kidney (Fusonie and Molnar, 1966).

Symptoms. **The vast majority of affected individuals have remained asymptomatic.** Pulmonary symptoms are exceedingly rare, and urinary ones are even more infrequent. Most cases are discovered on routine chest radiography or at the time of thoracotomy for a suspected mediastinal tumor (DeNoronha et al, 1974). The first case of a ureteropelvic junction obstruction in a thoracic kidney causing flank pain was only recently reported (Hampton and Borden, 2002).

Diagnosis. **The diagnosis is most commonly made after a routine chest radiograph in which the affected hemidiaphragm is found to be elevated slightly.** A smooth, rounded mass is seen extending into the chest near the midline on an anteroposterior film and along the posterior aspect of the diaphragmatic leaflet on a lateral view. Excretory urography or renal scintigraphy (Williams et al, 1983) usually suffices to clarify the diagnosis. In some instances, retrograde pyelography may be needed. Rarely, when arteriography has been employed to delineate a cardiac or pulmonary anomaly, it has revealed a thoracic kidney at the same time (Fusonie and Molnar, 1966).

Prognosis. Neither autopsy series nor clinical reports suggest that a thoracic kidney can cause serious urinary or pulmonary complications. Because most patients are discovered fortuitously and have no specific symptoms referable to the

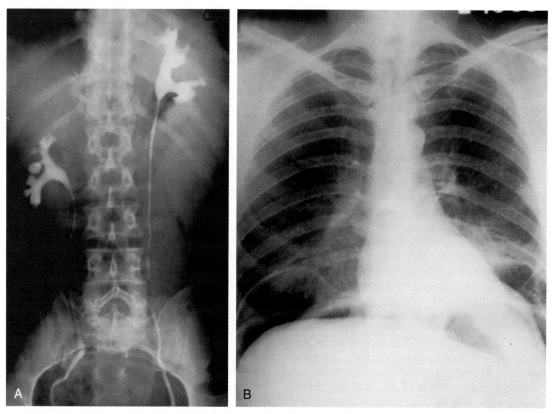

Figure 113–10. Radiograph of a thoracic kidney. The left kidney lies above the diaphragm. **A,** Diagnostic urogram. **B,** Diagnostic pneumoperitoneum. (From Hill JE, Bunts RC: Thoracic kidney: Case reports. J Urol 1960;84:460.)

misplaced kidney, no treatment is necessary once the diagnosis has been confirmed.

ANOMALIES OF FORM AND FUSION
Crossed Renal Ectopia with and without Fusion

When a kidney is located on the side opposite from which its ureter inserts into the bladder, the condition is known as *crossed ectopia.* Ninety percent of crossed ectopic kidneys are fused to their ipsilateral mate. Except for the horseshoe anomaly, they account for the majority of fusion defects. The various renal fusion anomalies associated with ectopia are discussed in this section; horseshoe kidney, the most common form of renal fusion, is described later.

Fusion anomalies of the kidney were first logically categorized by Wilmer (1938), but McDonald and McClellan (1957) refined and expanded that classification to include crossed ectopia with fusion, crossed ectopia without fusion, solitary crossed ectopia, and bilaterally crossed ectopia (Fig. 113–11). The fusion anomalies have been designated as (1) unilateral fused kidney with inferior ectopia; (2) sigmoid or S-shaped; (3) lump or cake; (4) L-shaped or tandem; (5) disc, shield, or doughnut; and (6) unilateral fused kidneys with superior ectopia (Fig. 113–12). Although this classification has little clinical significance, it does lend some order to understanding the embryology of renal ascent and rotation.

Incidence. The first reported case of crossed ectopia was described by Pamarolus in 1654. Abeshouse and Bhisitkul, in 1959, conducted the last significant review of the subject and collected exactly 500 cases of crossed ectopia with and without fusion. Subsequently, numerous case reports have been published.

Sixty-two patients with crossed ectopia without fusion have been reported (Diaz, 1953; Winram and Ward-McQuaid, 1959). This represents approximately 10% of all crossed ectopic kidneys (Lee, 1949). The anomaly occurs more commonly in males in a ratio of 2:1, and left-to-right ectopia is seen three times more frequently than right-to-left ectopia (Lee, 1949).

Solitary crossed ectopia has been reported in 34 patients (Miles et al, 1985; Gu and Alton, 1991). Males predominate in a ratio of 2:1. The crossed ectopia involves migration of the left kidney to the right side with absence of the right kidney, rather than the reverse, in a ratio of almost 2:1 (Kakei et al, 1976). In most cases the kidney fails to ascend and rotate completely. Bilateral crossed renal ectopia has been described in five patients (McDonald and McClellan, 1957; Abeshouse and Bhisitkul, 1959) and is considered the rarest form.

Abeshouse and Bhisitkul (1959) compiled 443 reports of crossed ectopia with fusion and estimated its occurrence at 1 in 1000 live births. This figure varies with the type of fusion anomaly; **the unilaterally fused kidney with inferior ectopia is the most common variety, whereas fusion with superior ectopia is the least common.** The autopsy incidence has been calculated at 1 in 2000 (Baggenstoss, 1951). There is a slight male predominance (3:2), and a left-to-right crossover occurs somewhat more frequently than its counterpart.

Embryology. The ureteral bud enters the metanephric blastema while the latter is situated adjacent to the anlage of the lumbosacral spine. During the next 4 weeks the developing kidney comes to lie at the level of the L1-L3 vertebrae. Because the factors responsible for the change in kidney position during gestation are still undetermined, **the reasons for crossed ectopia are similarly uncertain.** Wilmer (1938) suggested that crossover occurs as a result of pressure from abnormally placed umbilical arteries that prevent cephalad migration of the renal unit, which then follows the path of least resistance to the opposite side.

Potter (1952) and Alexander and coworkers (1950) theorized that crossed ectopia is strictly a ureteral phenomenon, with the developing ureteral bud wandering to the opposite side and inducing differentiation of the contralateral nephrogenic anlage. Ashley and Mostofi (1960) deduced that strong but undetermined forces are responsible for renal ascent and that these forces attract one or both kidneys to their final place on the opposite side of the midline.

Cook and Stephens (1977) postulated that crossover is the result of malalignment and abnormal rotation of the caudal end of the developing fetus, with the distal curled end of the vertebral column being displaced to one side or the other. As a result, either the cloaca and wolffian duct structures lie to one side of the vertebral column, allowing one ureter to cross the midline and enter the opposite nephrogenic blastema, or the kidney and ureter are transplanted to the opposite side of the midline during "normal" renal ascent (Hertz et al, 1977; Maizels and Stephens, 1979).

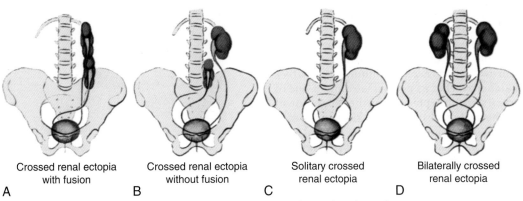

| Crossed renal ectopia with fusion | Crossed renal ectopia without fusion | Solitary crossed renal ectopia | Bilaterally crossed renal ectopia |
| A | B | C | D |

Figure 113–11. **A** to **D,** Four types of crossed renal ectopia.

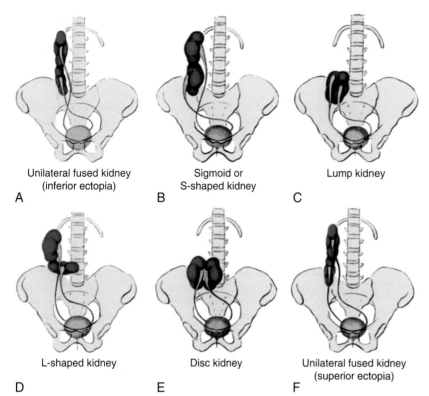

A Unilateral fused kidney (inferior ectopia)

B Sigmoid or S-shaped kidney

C Lump kidney

D L-shaped kidney

E Disc kidney

F Unilateral fused kidney (superior ectopia)

Figure 113–12. **A** to **F,** Six forms of crossed renal ectopia with fusion.

Kelalis and coworkers (1973) implicated teratogenic factors after they noted an increased incidence of associated genitourinary and other organ system anomalies. Finally, genetic influences may play a role, because similar anomalies have occurred within a single family (Greenberg and Nelsen, 1971; Hildreth and Cass, 1978).

Fusion of the metanephric masses may occur when the renal anlagen are still in the true pelvis before or at the start of cephalad migration, or it may occur during the latter stages of ascent. The extent of fusion is determined by the proximity of the developing renal anlagen to one another. After fusion, advancement of the kidneys toward their normal location is impeded by midline retroperitoneal structures—the aortic bifurcation, the inferior mesenteric artery, and the base of the small bowel mesentery (Joly, 1940).

Description. Fusion of a crossed ectopic kidney is related to the time at which it comes in contact with its mate. The crossed kidney usually lies caudad to its normal counterpart on that side. It is likely that migration of each kidney begins simultaneously but ascent of the ectopic renal unit lags behind because of crossover time. Therefore, **it is the superior pole of the ectopic kidney that usually joins with the inferior aspect of the normal kidney. Ascent continues until either the uncrossed kidney reaches its normal location or one of the retroperitoneal structures prevents further migration of the fused mass. The final shape of the fused kidneys depends on the time and extent of fusion and the degree of renal rotation that has occurred.** No further rotation is likely once the two kidneys have joined (Fig. 113–13). Therefore, the position of each renal pelvis may provide a clue as to the chronology of the congenital defect. An anteriorly placed pelvis suggests early fusion, whereas a medially positioned renal pelvis

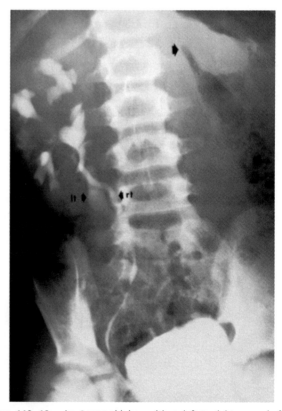

Figure 113–13. An 8-year-old boy with a left-to-right crossed, fused ectopia, in which the two kidneys lie abreast of one another (*arrows* marked Lt and Rt refer to both kidneys and their collecting systems on the right side of the abdomen). Splenic flexure lies in empty right renal fossa (*larger black arrow* accentuates gas pattern of splenic flexure in empty left renal fossa).

indicates that fusion probably occurred after rotation was completed.

Ninety percent of crossed ectopic kidneys are fused with their mate. When they are not fused, the uncrossed kidney usually resides in its normal dorsolumbar location and with proper orientation, while the ectopic kidney is inferior and in either a diagonal or a horizontal position with an anteriorly placed renal pelvis. The two kidneys are usually separated by a variable but definite distance, and each is surrounded by its own capsule of Gerota's fascia. In every case of crossed ectopia without fusion, the ureter from the normal kidney enters the bladder on the same side and that of the ectopic kidney crosses the midline at the pelvic brim and enters the bladder on the contralateral side.

In cases of solitary crossed ectopia, the kidney is usually located somewhat low but in the opposite renal fossa at the level of L1-L3 and is oriented anteriorly, having incompletely rotated on its vertical axis (Alexander et al, 1950; Purpon, 1963). When the kidney remains in the pelvis or ascends only to the lower lumbar region, it may assume a horizontal lie with an anteriorly placed pelvis because it has failed to rotate fully (Tabrisky and Bhisitkul, 1965). Here, too, the ureter crosses the midline above the S2 vertebra and enters the bladder on the opposite side (Gu and Alton, 1991). The contralateral ureter, if present, is often rudimentary (Caine, 1956). The patient with bilateral crossed ectopia may have perfectly normal-appearing kidneys and renal pelves, but the ureters cross the midline at the level of the lower lumbar vertebrae (Abeshouse and Bhisitkul, 1959). Arteriography has demonstrated anomalous vasculature to ectopic and crossed ectopic kidneys, which may account for stone formation from delayed drainage associated with the hydronephrosis and UPJ obstruction that is seen in a proportion of cases (Collura et al, 2004).

KEY POINTS: CROSSED RENAL ECTOPIA WITH AND WITHOUT FUSION

- When a kidney is located on the side opposite from which its ureter inserts into the bladder, the condition is known as crossed ectopia.

- The superior pole of the ectopic kidney usually joins with the inferior aspect of the normal kidney.

- Ninety percent of crossed ectopic kidneys are fused with their mate.

- In all the types of fusion anomalies, the ureter from each kidney is usually orthotopic.

- The highest incidence of associated anomalies occurs in children with solitary renal ectopia and involves both the skeletal system and genital organs.

Inferior Ectopic Kidney. Two thirds of all unilaterally fused kidneys involve inferior ectopia. The upper pole of the crossed kidney is attached to the inferior aspect of the normally positioned mate. Both renal pelves are anterior, so fusion probably occurs relatively early.

Sigmoid or S-Shaped Kidney. The sigmoid or S-shaped kidney is the second most common anomaly of fusion. The crossed kidney is again inferior, with the two kidneys fused at their adjacent poles. Fusion of the two kidneys occurs relatively late, after complete rotation on the vertical axis has taken place. Therefore, each renal pelvis is oriented correctly, and they face in opposite directions from one another. The lower convex border of one kidney is directly opposite the outer border of its counterpart, and there is an S-shaped appearance to the entire renal outline. The ureter from the normal kidney courses downward anterior to the outer border of the inferior kidney, and the ectopic kidney's ureter crosses the midline before entering the bladder.

Lump Kidney. The lump or cake kidney is a relatively rare form of fusion (Fig. 113–14). Extensive joining has taken place over a wide margin of maturing renal anlage. The total kidney mass is irregular and lobulated. Usually ascent progresses only as far as the sacral promontory, but in many instances the kidney remains within the true pelvis. Both renal pelves are anterior, and they drain separate areas of parenchyma. The ureters do not cross.

L-Shaped Kidney. The L-shaped or tandem kidney occurs when the crossed kidney assumes a transverse position at the time of its attachment to the inferior pole of the normal kidney (Fig. 113–15). The crossed kidney lies in the midline or in the contralateral paramedian space anterior to the L4 vertebra. Rotation about the long axis of the kidney may produce either an inverted or a reversed pelvic position. The ureter from each kidney enters the bladder on its respective side.

Disc Kidney. Disc, shield, doughnut, or pancake kidneys are kidneys that have joined at the medial borders of each pole to produce a doughnut- or ring-shaped mass; when there is more extensive fusion along the entire medial aspect of each kidney, a disc or shield shape is created. The lateral aspect of each kidney retains its normal contour. This type of fusion differs from the lump or cake kidney in that the reniform shape is

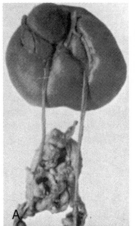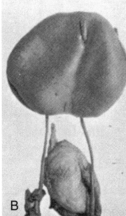

Figure 113–14. **A,** Lump kidney showing the unusual anatomy, with the anterior blood supply coming from above and the ureters leaving from below. **B,** Posterior view of **A,** with the blood supply entering from above and a deep grooving of the parenchyma indicating where the kidney pressed against the spine. (Courtesy of Dr. H. S. Altman.)

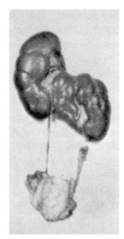

Figure 113–15. Renal fusion. L-shaped kidney in a 1-year-old child in whom a considerable portion of the left renal segment lies across the lower lumbar spine. On each side, the pelvic outlet faces anteriorly. (From Campbell MF: Anomalies of the kidney. In Campbell MF, Harrison JH [eds]: Urology, 3rd ed. Philadelphia, WB Saunders, 1970, vol 2.)

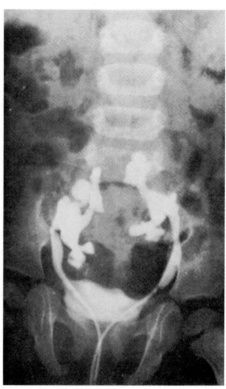

Figure 113–16. Pelvic fused kidney in a 2-year-old girl examined because of the low abdominal mass thought to be an ovarian cyst. (From Campbell MF: Anomalies of the kidney. In Campbell MF, Harrison JH [eds]: Urology, 3rd ed. Philadelphia, WB Saunders Company, 1970, vol 2.)

better preserved owing to the somewhat less extensive degree of fusion. The pelves are anteriorly placed, and the ureters remain uncrossed. Each collecting system drains its respective half of the kidney and does not communicate with the opposite side (Fig. 113–16).

Superior Ectopic Kidney. The least common variety of renal fusion is the crossed ectopic kidney that lies superior to the normal kidney. The lower pole of the crossed kidney is fused to the upper pole of the normal kidney. Each renal unit retains its fetal orientation, with both pelves lying anteriorly, suggesting that fusion occurred very early.

Regardless of the type of fusion encountered, the vascular supply to each kidney is variable and unpredictable. The crossed ectopic kidney is supplied by one or more branches from the aorta or common iliac artery (Rubinstein et al, 1976). The normal kidney frequently has an anomalous blood supply, with multiple renal arteries originating from various levels along the aorta. In one rare instance, Rubinstein and coworkers (1976) discovered that one renal artery had crossed the midline to supply the tandem ectopic kidney. The solitary crossed ectopic kidney is found to receive its blood supply generally from that side of the aorta or iliac artery on which it is positioned (Tanenbaum et al, 1970).

Associated Anomalies. **In all the types of fusion anomalies, the ureter from each kidney usually is not ectopic.** Except for solitary crossed ectopia, in which there may be a hemitrigone or a poorly developed trigone with a rudimentary or absent ureter on the side of the ectopic kidney, most patients with crossed ectopia have a normal trigone with no indication that an anomaly of the upper urinary tract is present (Magri, 1961; Tanenbaum et al, 1970; Yates-Bell and Packham, 1972). An ectopic ureteral orifice from the crossed renal unit has been observed about 3% of the time (Abeshouse and Bhisitkul, 1959; Magri, 1961; Hendren et al, 1976). Occasionally, the ureter from the uncrossed renal segment of a fusion anomaly has an ectopic orifice (Hendren et al, 1976). In one instance, Malek and Utz (1970) discovered an ectopic ureterocele associated with the uncrossed kidney. Vesicoureteral reflux is

noted in 20% of crossed ectopia and in 71% of bilateral crossed ectopia (Kelalis et al, 1973; Guarino et al, 2004). Currarino and Weisbruch (1989) collected 10 cases of midline renal fusion in which a single ureter divided into two pelves that stretched across the midline to drain one respective half of the total parenchymatous mass. In 4 of the 10 cases, a second ureter was present that drained a separate duplex system on either the right or left side. Most of the affected individuals had an imperforate anus or abnormal vertebrae, or both.

Most orthotopic renal units are normal. If an abnormality exists, it usually involves the ectopic kidney and consists of cystic dysplasia, UPJ obstruction (29%), reflux (15%), or carcinoma (Abeshouse and Bhisitkul, 1959; Gerber et al, 1980; Caldamone and Rabinowitz, 1981; Macksood and James, 1983; Nussbaum et al, 1987; Gleason et al, 1994).

The highest incidence of associated anomalies occurs in children with solitary renal ectopia and involves both the skeletal system and genital organs (Miles et al, 1985; Gleason et al, 1994). This seems to be related more to renal agenesis than to the ectopic anomaly per se. Fifty percent of patients with solitary crossed renal ectopia have a skeletal anomaly, and 40% have a genital abnormality (Gu and Alton, 1991). The most common of the latter in the male is either cryptorchidism or absence of the vas deferens; in the female, it is vaginal atresia or a unilateral uterine abnormality (Yates-Bell and Packham, 1972; Kakei et al, 1976). Imperforate anus has also been observed in 20% of the patients with solitary crossed ectopia.

In general, the occurrence of an associated anomaly in crossed renal ectopia, excluding solitary crossed ectopia, is low; the most frequent such conditions are imperforate anus (4%), orthopedic anomalies (4%), skeletal abnormalities, and septal cardiovascular defects.

Symptoms. Most individuals with crossed ectopic anomalies have no symptoms. The defects are often discovered incidentally at autopsy, during routine perinatal ultrasound screening, or after bone scanning. If manifestations do occur, signs and symptoms usually develop in the third or fourth decades of life and include vague lower abdominal pain, pyuria, hematuria, and urinary tract infection (Gleason et al, 1994). Hydronephrosis and renal calculi have been discovered in conjunction with some of these symptoms. It is believed that the abnormal kidney position and the anomalous blood supply may impede drainage from the collecting system, creating a predisposition to urinary tract infection and calculus formation (Collura et al, 2004).

In one third of patients, an asymptomatic abdominal mass is the presenting sign (Abeshouse and Bhisitkul, 1959; Nussbaum et al, 1987). In a few individuals, hypertension has led to the discovery of an ectopic fusion anomaly (Abeshouse and Bhisitkul, 1959), and in one case this was attributable to a vascular lesion in one of the anomalous vessels (Mininberg et al, 1971).

Diagnosis. In the past, the usual method of detection was by excretory urography, but ultrasonography and radionuclide scanning have revealed more asymptomatic cases recently (for unrelated reasons). Cystoscopy and retrograde pyelography were useful in mapping out the collecting system and pattern of drainage. Renal angiography was required before performing extensive surgery on the ectopic or normal kidney due to the anomalous blood supply to both kidneys. Ultrasound evaluation of the pelvic kidney demonstrated absence of renal sinus echoes, a normal finding associated with the extrarenal position of the pelvis and calyces (Barnewolt and Lebowitz, 1996). MRI, with its exquisite detail of soft tissues, has replaced most of these imaging modalities for defining the anatomy of an ectopic kidney.

Prognosis. Most individuals with crossed renal ectopia have a normal longevity and prognosis. However, some patients with an obstructive-appearing collecting system are at risk for development of urinary tract infection or renal calculi, or both (Kron and Meranze, 1949). Boatman and associates (1972) noted that one third of their symptomatic patients required a pyelolithotomy for an obstructing stone. More recently, extracorporeal shock wave lithotripsy therapy and percutaneous nephrolithotomy have rendered most of these unusual patients stone free (Semerci et al, 1997; Desai and Jasani, 2000).

Horseshoe Kidney

The horseshoe kidney is probably the most common of all renal fusion anomalies. It should not be confused with asymmetrical or off-center fused kidneys, which may give the impression of being horseshoe shaped. The anomaly consists of two distinct renal masses lying vertically on either side of the midline and connected at their respective lower poles by a parenchymatous or fibrous isthmus that crosses the mid-

plane of the body. It was first recognized during an autopsy by DeCarpi in 1521, but Botallo in 1564 presented the first extensive description and illustration of a horseshoe kidney (Benjamin and Schullian, 1950). Morgagni described the first diseased horseshoe kidney, and since then more has been written about this condition than about any other renal anomaly. Almost every renal disease has been described in the horseshoe kidney.

Incidence. Horseshoe kidney occurs in 0.25% of the population, or about 1 in 400 persons (Dees, 1941; Nation, 1945; Bell, 1946; Glenn, 1959; Campbell, 1970). A recent review of over 15,000 radiologic imaging studies revealed an incidence of 1 in 666 people (Weizer et al, 2003). As with other fusion anomalies, it is found more commonly in males by a slightly greater than a 2:1 margin (Basar et al, 1999; Weizer et al, 2003). The abnormality has been discovered clinically in all age groups ranging from fetal life to 80 years, but in autopsy series it is more prevalent in children (Segura et al, 1972). This early age prevalence is related to the high incidence of multiple congenital anomalies associated with the horseshoe kidney, some of which are incompatible with long-term survival (Scott, 2002).

Horseshoe kidneys have been reported in identical twins (Bridge, 1960) and among several siblings within the same family (David, 1974). From the rarity of these reports and the relative frequency of the anomaly, it is doubtful that these observations represent a particular genetic predisposition, but they might be the result of a genetic expression with a low degree of penetrance (Leiter, 1972).

Embryology. The abnormality occurs between the 4th and 6th week of gestation, after the ureteral bud has entered the renal blastema. In view of the ultimate spatial configuration of the horseshoe kidney, the entrance of the ureteral bud had to have taken place before rotation and considerably before renal ascent ensued. Boyden (1931) described a 6-week-old embryo with a horseshoe kidney, the youngest fetus ever discovered with this anomaly. He postulated that at the 14-mm stage (4.5 weeks), the developing metanephric masses lie close to one another; any disturbance in this relationship might result in joining at their inferior poles. A slight alteration in the position of the umbilical or common iliac artery could change the orientation of the migrating kidneys, leading to contact and fusion (Fig. 113–17). It has been postulated that an abnormality in the formation of the tail of the embryo or another pelvic organ could account for the fusion process (Cook and Stephens, 1977). Domenech-Mateu and Gonzales-Compta (1988), after studying a 16-mm human embryo, suggested that posterior nephrogenic cells migrate abnormally to form an isthmus or connection between the two developing kidneys to create the horseshoe shape.

Whatever the actual mechanism responsible for horseshoe kidney formation, the joining occurs before the kidneys have rotated on their long axis. In its mature form, the pelves and ureters of the horseshoe kidney are usually anteriorly placed, crossing ventrally to the isthmus (Fig. 113–18). Very rarely, the pelves are anteromedial, suggesting that fusion occurred somewhat later, after some rotation had taken place. In addition, migration is usually incomplete, with the kidneys lying lower in the abdomen than normal. It is

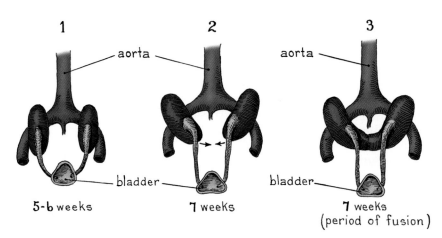

Figure 113–17. Embryogenesis of horseshoe kidney. The lower poles of the two kidneys touch and fuse as they cross the iliac arteries. Ascent is stopped when the fused kidneys reach the junction of the aorta and inferior mesenteric artery. (From Benjamin JA, Schullian DM: Observation on fused kidneys with horseshoe configuration: The contribution of Leonardo Botallo [1564]. J Hist Med Allied Sci 1950;5:315, after Gutierrez, 1931.)

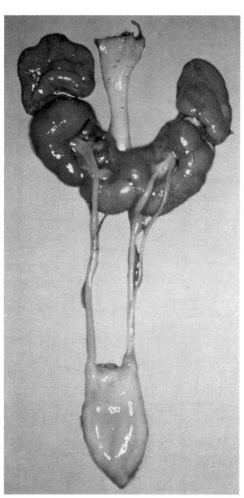

Figure 113–18. Specimen of a horseshoe kidney in a neonate who had multiple anomalies, including congenital heart disease. Note the thick parenchymatous isthmus.

presumed that the inferior mesenteric artery prevents full ascent by obstructing the movement of the isthmus.

Description. There are several variations in the basic shape of the horseshoe kidney. **In 95% of patients, the kidneys join at the lower pole; in a small number, an isthmus connects both upper poles instead** (Love and Wasserman, 1975).

Generally, the isthmus is bulky and consists of parenchymatous tissue with its own blood supply (Glenn, 1959; Love and Wasserman, 1975). Occasionally it is just a flimsy midline structure composed of fibrous tissue that tends to draw the renal masses close together. It is located adjacent to the L3 or L4 vertebra just below the origin of the inferior mesenteric artery from the aorta. As a result, the paired kidneys tend to be somewhat lower than normal in the retroperitoneum. In some instances, the anomalous kidneys are very low, anterior to the sacral promontory or even in the true pelvis behind the bladder (Campbell, 1970). The isthmus most often lies anterior to the aorta and vena cava, but it is not unheard of for it to pass between the inferior vena cava and the aorta or even behind both great vessels (Jarmin, 1938; Meek and Wadsworth, 1940; Dajani, 1966).

The calyces, normal in number, are atypical in orientation. Because the kidney fails to rotate, the calyces point posteriorly, and the axis of each pelvis remains in the vertical or obliquely lateral plane (on a line drawn from lower to upper poles). The lowermost calyces extend caudally or even medially to drain the isthmus and may overlie the vertebral column.

The ureter may insert high on the renal pelvis and lie laterally, probably as the result of incomplete renal rotation. It courses downward and has a characteristic bend as it crosses over and anterior to the isthmus, a deviation that is proportionate to the thickness of the midline structure. Despite upper ureteral angulation, the lower ureter usually enters the bladder normally and rarely is ectopic.

The blood supply to the horseshoe kidney can be quite variable (Fig. 113–19). In 30% of cases, it consists of one renal artery to each kidney (Glenn, 1959), but it may be atypical with duplicate or even triplicate renal arteries supplying one or both kidneys. The blood supply to the isthmus and lower poles is also variable. The isthmus and adjacent parenchymal masses may receive a branch from each main renal artery, or they may have their own arterial supply from the aorta originating either above or below the level of the isthmus. Not infrequently this area is supplied by branches from the inferior mesenteric, common or external iliac, or sacral arteries (Boatman et al, 1971; Kolln et al, 1972). Three cases of retrocaval ureter and isthmus have been reported (Eidelman et al, 1978; Hefferman et al, 1978).

KEY POINTS: HORSESHOE KIDNEY

- Horseshoe kidney occurs in 0.25% of the population, or about 1 in 400 persons.

- The isthmus is bulky and consists of parenchymatous tissue.

- The calyces, normal in number, are atypical in orientation. Because the kidney fails to rotate, the calyces point posteriorly, and the axis of each pelvis remains in the vertical or obliquely lateral plane.

- The blood supply can be quite variable.

- Horseshoe kidney is frequently found in association with other congenital anomalies.

- UPJ obstruction, causing significant hydronephrosis, occurs in as many as one third of individuals.

- Sixty percent of patients with horseshoe kidneys remained asymptomatic for an average of 10 years after discovery.

Table 113–1. Genitourinary Anomalies Associated with Horseshoe Kidneys

Genital Anomalies	
Hypospadias	4%
Undescended testes	4%
Bicornuate uterus	7%
Septate vagina	7%
Urinary Collecting System	
Ureteral duplication	10%
Ureteropelvic junction obstruction	20%
Vesicoureteral reflux	50%
Renal Parenchymal Abnormalities	
Multicystic dysplasia	1%
Autosomal recessive polycystic kidney	1%
Metabolic Derangements in Patients with Stones	
Hypercalciuria, hyperoxaluria, hypocitraturia, hypouricuria	50%

Associated Anomalies. The horseshoe kidney, even though it produces no symptoms, **is frequently found in association with other congenital anomalies** (Table 113–1). Boatman and coworkers (1972) discovered that almost one third of the 96 patients they studied had at least one other abnormality. Many newborns and young infants with multiple congenital anomalies have a horseshoe kidney. Judging from autopsy reports, the incidence of other anomalies is certainly greater in patients who die at birth or in early infancy than in those

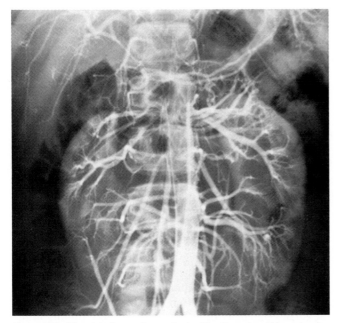

Figure 113–19. Arteriogram in a patient with a horseshoe kidney showing a multiplicity of arteries supplying kidney arising from aorta and common iliac arteries. (From Kelalis PP: Anomalies of the urinary tract: The kidney. In Kelalis PP, King LR [eds]: Clinical Pediatric Urology. Philadelphia, WB Saunders, 1976, p 492.)

who reach adulthood (Zondek and Zondek, 1964; Scott, 2002). This implies that a horseshoe kidney may occur more often in patients with other serious congenital anomalies. The organ systems most commonly affected include the skeletal, cardiovascular (primarily ventriculoseptal defects [Voisin et al, 1988]), and central nervous systems. Horseshoe kidney is found in 3% of children with neural tube defects (Whitaker and Hunt, 1987). Anorectal malformations are frequently encountered in these patients. Horseshoe kidney may also be seen in 20% of patients with trisomy 18 and as many as 60% of females with Turner's syndrome (Smith, 1970; Lippe et al, 1988) and in patients with Townes-Brock syndrome who have a *SALL1* transcription factor defect (Salerno et al, 2000).

Boatman and his colleagues (1972) **also discovered an increased occurrence of other genitourinary anomalies in patients with a horseshoe kidney.** Hypospadias and undescended testes each occurred in 4% of males, and a bicornuate uterus or septate vagina or both were noted in 7% of the females.

Duplication of the ureter occurs in 10% of patients (Zondek and Zondek, 1964; Boatman et al, 1972); in some cases this has been associated with an ectopic ureterocele. Vesicoureteral reflux has been noted in more than half of affected individuals (Segura et al, 1972; Pitts and Muecke, 1975; Cascio et al, 2002). UPJ dilation has been seen in over 20%, but on diuretic nuclear scanning less than 20% have an obstructive pattern (Cascio et al, 2002; Kao et al, 2003). Cystic disease, including multicystic dysplasia in one half (the upper pole) of one side (Novak et al, 1977; Boullier et al, 1992) and adult polycystic kidney disease, has been reported in patients with horseshoe kidney (Gutierrez, 1934; Campbell, 1970; Pitts and Muecke, 1975; Correa and Paton, 1976). DMSA scanning in 22 patients revealed asymmetrical function in 63% (Kao et al, 2003). Because stone formation has been seen commonly in these patients, evaluation in 37 revealed altered calcium, oxalate, uric acid, and citrate excretion in 50%, suggesting an underlying *metabolic* etiology (Raj et al, 2004). Thus, stone formation may not be due to just delayed drainage from the anatomic abnormality and other causes should be considered.

Symptoms. With increased ultrasound screening for renal anomalies it is likely that at least 50% of patients with horseshoe kidneys are asymptomatic rather than the 33% incidence reported in the past (Glenn, 1959; Kölln et al, 1972). In most instances, the anomaly is an incidental finding at autopsy (Pitts and Muecke, 1975). When symptoms are present, however, they are related to hydronephrosis, infection, or calculus formation. The most common symptom that reflects these conditions is vague abdominal pain that may radiate to the lower lumbar region. Gastrointestinal complaints may be present as well. The so-called Rovsing sign—abdominal pain, nausea, and vomiting on hyperextension of the spine—has been infrequently observed. Signs and symptoms of urinary tract infection occur in 30% of patients, and calculi have been noted in 20% to 80% (Glenn, 1959; Kölln et al, 1972; Pitts and Muecke, 1975; Evans and Resnick, 1981; Sharma and Bapna, 1986; Benchekroun et al, 1998). Five to 10 percent of horseshoe kidneys are detected after palpation of an abdominal mass (Glenn, 1959; Kölln et al, 1972). Horseshoe kidneys have been detected after angiography for evaluation of an abdominal aortic aneurysm (Huber et al, 1990; deBrito et al, 1991).

UPJ obstruction causing significant hydronephrosis occurs in as many as one third of individuals (Whitehouse, 1975; Das and Amar, 1984). The high insertion of the ureter into the renal pelvis, its abnormal course anterior to the isthmus, and the anomalous blood supply to the kidney may individually or collectively contribute to this obstruction.

Diagnosis. Except for the possibility of a palpable midline abdominal mass (Grandone et al, 1985), the horseshoe kidney does not by itself produce symptoms. The clinical features from a diseased kidney, however, are often vague and nonspecific. The anomalies, therefore, may not be suspected until a renal ultrasound or an excretory urogram is obtained. Prenatal ultrasonography is detecting horseshoe kidneys before birth (Sherer and Woods, 1992; Van Every, 1992). The classic radiologic features are easily recognized and a diagnosis is readily made (Fig. 113–20). Findings that suggest a horseshoe kidney singly or collectively include the following: kidneys that are somewhat low lying and close to the vertebral column; a vertical or outward axis, so that a line drawn through the midplane of each kidney bisects the midline inferiorly; a continuation of the outer border of the lower pole of each kidney toward and across the midline; the characteristic orientation of the collecting system, which is directly posterior to each renal pelvis, with the lowermost calyx pointing caudally or even medially; and the high insertion of the ureter into the pelvis as well as the anteriorly displaced upper ureter that appears to drape over a midline mass (Strauss et al, 2000). However, obstruction from either a calculus or a UPJ stricture may obscure the radiologic picture (Love and Wasserman, 1975; Christoffersen and Iversen, 1976). Other studies, such as retrograde pyelography or CT, may be necessary to confirm the diagnosis.

Prognosis. Although Smith and Orkin (1945) believed that horseshoe kidneys are almost always associated with disease, subsequent investigators have not found this to be so. **Glenn (1959) observed patients with horseshoe kidneys for an average of 10 years after discovery and found that almost 60% of these remained asymptomatic.** Only 13% had persistent urinary infection or pain, and 17% developed recurrent calculi. When stone disease is present, extracorporeal

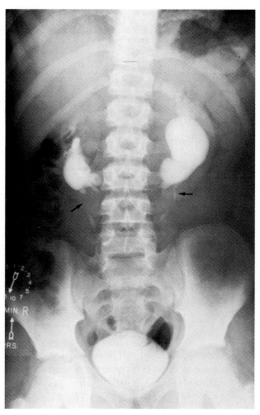

Figure 113–20. Excretory urogram in an 11-year-old boy evaluated for nocturnal incontinence reveals a horseshoe kidney. Note vertical renal axes and medial orientation of the collecting systems. The ureters *(arrows)* are laterally displaced and bow over the isthmus, causing a degree of hydronephrosis.

shock wave lithotripsy can render 68% of patients stone free, but percutaneous stone removal has achieved an 87.5% stone free rate (Kupeli et al, 1999; Raj et al, 2003). In Glenn's series, no patients benefited from division of the isthmus for relief of pain; as a result, this idea has now been largely repudiated (Glenn, 1959; Pitts and Muecke, 1975).

Many patients with a horseshoe kidney have other congenital anomalies, some of which are incompatible with life beyond the neonatal period or early infancy. Excluding that group, survival is not reduced merely by the presence of this anomaly. Often a horseshoe kidney is found incidentally, and it is rarely a cause for mortality (Dajani, 1966; Boatman et al, 1972).

Many disease processes have been described with a horseshoe kidney, but this only reflects the relative frequency of the congenital defect. **Renal carcinoma has been reported within a horseshoe kidney in 123 patients** (Buntley, 1976; Hohenfellner et al, 1992; Schubert et al, 1998); more than half of these cancers were renal cell carcinoma and included two cases of bilateral tumors (Romics et al, 2002). However, renal pelvic tumors and Wilms' tumor each accounted for 25% of the total. Overall, 41 of 8617 (0.48%) Wilms' tumors in the National Wilms' Tumor study occurred in horseshoe kidneys, mostly on the left side, rarely in the isthmus, and practically all with favorable histology (Neville et al, 2002). This incidence of Wilms' tumor in horseshoe kidneys is more than twice that expected in the general population (Mesrobian et al, 1985). Thirty-seven percent of these tumors were inoperable initially because the diagnosis is often missed until later when a palpable mass is detected. However, with reoperative chemotherapy most patients can be salvaged with a 75% preservation rate of renal parenchyma (Neville et al, 2002). Except for renal pelvic tumors, a surprisingly high number of these cancers appear to have arisen in the isthmus (Blackard and Mellinger, 1968). For this reason, it has been suggested that teratogenic factors are responsible for abnormal migration of nephrogenic cells to form an isthmus, which then leads to the horseshoe shape and the increased potential of carcinoma development in this portion of the kidney (Domenech-Mateu and Gonzales-Compta, 1988; Hohenfellner et al, 1992).

It has been suggested that the increased occurrence of chronic infection, obstruction, and stone formation may be instrumental in producing a higher than expected incidence of renal pelvic tumors in this group (Shoup et al, 1962; Castor and Green, 1975). Wilms' tumor may originate in the isthmus (Beck and Hlivko, 1960), creating a very bizarre radiologic picture (Walker, 1977). The incidence of tumors within horseshoe kidneys seems to be increasing when compared with the occurrence of tumors in the general population (Dische and Johnston, 1979). Survival from these tumors is related to the pathology and stage of the tumor at diagnosis and not to the renal anomaly (Murphy and Zincke, 1982). This may warrant surveillance for tumors in patients with symptomatic horseshoe kidneys.

Because it is located above the pelvic inlet, a horseshoe kidney should not adversely affect pregnancy or delivery (Bell, 1946). Glomerulocystic disease has been reported in children before 1 year of age but does not appear to be related specifically to the horseshoe anomaly (Craver et al, 1993). The development of renal failure associated with adult polycystic kidney disease is not any greater in the presence of a horseshoe kidney (Correa and Paton, 1976). The North American Pediatric Renal Transplant Cooperative Study (NAPRTCS, McDonald et al, 2000) and the Department of Health and Human Services 2000 Annual Report (U.S. Department of Health and Human Services, U.S. Scientific Registry of Transplant Recipients and the Organ Procurement and Transplantation Network, 2000) each failed to reveal any patient with a horseshoe kidney receiving a renal transplant. A worldwide review from the Netherlands noted that 23 whole and 57 split horseshoe kidneys have been transplanted into 120 patients with only a 7% initial failure rate (4.3%) for en bloc and a 13.4% failure rate for split transplants and an overall graft survival rate of 80% at 5 years (Strousma et al, 2001).

ANOMALIES OF ROTATION

The adult kidney, as it assumes its final position in the "renal" fossa, orients itself so that the calyces point laterally and the pelvis faces medially. When this alignment is not exact, the condition is known as _malrotation._ Most often, this inappropriate orientation is found in conjunction with another renal anomaly, such as ectopia with or without fusion or horseshoe kidney. This discussion centers on malrotation as an isolated renal entity. It must be differentiated from other conditions that mimic it and are caused by extraneous forces such as an abnormal retroperitoneal mass.

Incidence. The true incidence of this developmental anomaly cannot be accurately calculated because minor degrees of malrotation are never reported and generally do not cause much concern. Campbell (1963) found renal malrotation in 1 of 939 autopsies, and Smith and Orkin (1945) noted 1 case per 390 admissions. **It is frequently observed in patients with Turner's syndrome** (Gray and Skandalakis, 1972). Males are affected twice as often as females, but there does not appear to be any predilection for one side or the other.

Embryology. It is thought that **medial rotation of the collecting system occurs simultaneously with renal migration.** The kidney starts to turn during the 6th week, just when it is leaving the true pelvis, and it completes this process, having rotated 90 degrees toward the midline, by the time ascent is complete, at the end of the 9th week of gestation.

It has been postulated (Felix, 1912) that rotation is actually the result of unequal branching of successive orders of the budding ureteral tree, with two branches extending ventrally and one dorsally during each generation or division. Each ureteral branch then induces differentiation of the metanephrogenic tissue surrounding it to encase it as a cap. More parenchyma develops ventrally than dorsally, and the pelvis seems to rotate medially. Weyrauch (1939) accepted this theory of renal rotation as the result of excessive ventral versus dorsal branching of the ureteral tree and concluded that the fault of malrotation lies entirely with the ureter. A late-appearing ureteral bud may insert into an atypical portion of the renal blastema, leading to a lessened propensity for the developing nephric tissue to shift. Late appearance of the ureteral bud is almost always associated with an aberrant origin from the wolffian duct; this translates into ureteral ectopia at the level of the lower urinary tract. Mackie and colleagues (1975), however, did not describe any malrotation anomalies in their study of renal ectopia. The renal blood supply does not appear to be the cause or a limiting factor in malrotation but rather follows the course of renal hyporotation, hyper-rotation, or reverse rotation.

> ### KEY POINTS: ANOMALIES OF ROTATION
>
> - The adult kidney, as it assumes its final position in the "renal" fossa, orients itself so that the calyces point laterally and the pelvis faces medially. When this alignment is not exact, the condition is known as malrotation.
>
> - It is frequently observed in patients with Turner's syndrome.

Description. The kidney and renal pelvis normally rotate 90 degrees ventromedially during ascent. Weyrauch (1939), in an exhaustive and detailed study, outlined the various abnormal phases of medial and reverse rotation and labeled each according to the position of the renal pelvis (Fig. 113–21).

Ventral Position. The pelvis is ventral and in the same anteroposterior plane as the calyces, which point dorsally, since they have undergone no rotation at all. This is the most

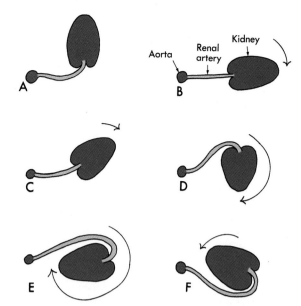

Figure 113–21. Rotation of the kidney during its ascent from the pelvis. The left kidney with its renal artery and the aorta are viewed in transverse section to show normal and abnormal rotation during its ascent to the adult site. **A,** Primitive embryonic position; hilus faces ventrad (anterior). **B,** Normal adult position; hilus faces mediad. **C,** Incomplete rotation. **D,** Hyper-rotation; hilus faces dorsad (posterior). **E,** Hyper-rotation; hilus faces laterad. **F,** Reverse rotation; hilus faces laterad. (From Gray SW, Skandalakis JE: Embryology for Surgeons. Philadelphia, WB Saunders, 1972.)

common form of malrotation. Very rarely, this position may represent excessive medial rotation, in which a complete 360-degree turn has occurred. In one such presumed case reported by Weyrauch (1939), the vasculature had rotated with the kidney and passed around dorsally and laterally to it before entering the anteriorly placed hilus.

Ventromedial Position. The pelvis faces ventromedially because of an incompletely rotated kidney. Excursion probably stops during the 7th week of gestation, when the kidney and pelvis normally reach this position. The calyces thus point dorsolaterally.

Dorsal Position. Renal excursion of 180 degrees occurs to produce this position. The pelvis is dorsal to the parenchyma, and the vessels pass behind the kidney to reach the hilum. This is the rarest form of malrotation.

Lateral Position. When the kidney and pelvis rotate more than 180 degrees but less than 360 degrees, or when reverse rotation of up to 180 degrees takes place, the pelvis faces laterally and the kidney parenchyma resides medially. The renal vascular supply provides the only clue to the actual direction of excursion. Vessels that course ventral to the kidney to enter a laterally or dorsolaterally placed hilum suggest reverse rotation, whereas a path dorsal to the kidney implies excessive ventral rotation. Both types of anomalous turning were cited in Weyrauch's series (1939).

In cases of isolated malrotation, certain other characteristic features may be present. The kidney shape may be discoid, elongated, oval, or triangular, with flattened anterior and posterior surfaces. Fetal lobulations are invariably present and accentuated beyond normal limits. A dense amount of fibrous tissue encases the hilar area, possibly even distorting

and fixing the pelvis. The UPJ may be distorted as well. The upper ureter initially courses laterally, and it, too, may be encased in this fibrous matting. The pelvis is elongated and narrow, and calyces, especially the superior calyx, may be stretched. The blood supply, as previously described, may vary widely, depending on the direction and degree of rotation. The vasculature may consist of a single vessel with or without multiple additional branches entering the parenchyma along the course of the renal artery. In addition, there may be a polar vessel in conjunction with the main renal artery. The vascular orientation around the kidney provides the only clue to the type and extent of renal rotation (i.e., whether medial or lateral rotation has occurred).

Symptoms. Rotation anomalies per se do not produce any specific symptoms. The excessive amount of fibrous tissue encasing the pelvis, UPJ, and upper ureter, however, may lead to a relative or actual obstruction of the upper collecting system. Vascular compression from an accessory or main renal artery or distortion of the upper ureter or UPJ may contribute to impaired drainage. Symptoms of hydronephrosis (namely, dull, aching flank pain) may be experienced during periods of increased urine production. This is the most frequent cause of symptoms. Hematuria, which occurs occasionally within a hydronephrotic collecting system, may be noted as well. Infection and calculus formation, each with its attendant symptoms, may also occur secondary to poor urinary drainage.

Diagnosis. The diagnosis may be surmised when a renal calculus is detected in an abnormal location, but confirmation should be obtained only from a renal ultrasound, excretory urogram, or retrograde pyelogram (Fig. 113–22). These studies should reveal the abnormal orientation of the renal pelvis and calyces, a flattened and elongated pelvis, a stretched superior calyx with blunting of the remaining calyces, and a laterally displaced upper third of the ureter. Bilateral malrotation is not uncommon and may lead to the diagnosis of a horseshoe kidney. However, careful inspection for an isthmus and observation of the lower pole renal outline should help to distinguish the two entities.

Prognosis. No abnormality of function of the kidney has been detected secondary to malrotation, and this anomaly is therefore compatible with normal longevity. Hydronephrosis resulting from impaired urinary drainage may lead to infection and calculus formation with their sequelae.

ANOMALIES OF RENAL VASCULATURE
Aberrant, Accessory, or Multiple Vessels

Knowledge of the anatomy of the renal blood supply is important to every urologic surgeon, and fortunately this subject lends itself to easy investigation. Anatomists were keenly interested in renal vascular patterns before the end of the 19th century, but the advent of aortography in the 1940s and 1950s spearheaded a systematic clinical approach to this topic. Most of the classic work was performed by investigators in the middle to late 1950s and early 1960s (Graves, 1954, 1956; Anson and Kurth, 1955; Merklin and Michele, 1958; Anson and Daseler, 1961; Geyer and Poutasse, 1962).

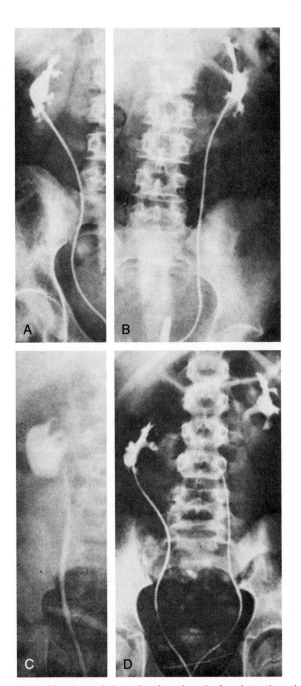

Figure 113–22. Congenital renal malrotation. **A,** Complete; the pelvis faces median. **B,** Pelvis faces posteriorly. **C,** Complete renal rotation in a 20-month-old girl with abnormally high insertion of the ureter into the pelvis. **D,** Diminutive malrotated pelvis in a 5-year-old girl. Urinary infection was the indication for urologic examination in all four cases. (From Campbell MF: Anomalies of the kidney. In Campbell MF, Harrison JH [eds]: Urology, 3rd ed. Philadelphia, WB Saunders, 1970, vol 2.)

The kidney is divided into various segments, each supplied by a single "end" arterial branch that usually courses from one main renal artery. *Multiple renal arteries* is the correct term to describe any kidney supplied by more than one vessel. The term *anomalous vessels* or *aberrant vessels* should be reserved for those arteries that originate from vessels other than the aorta or main renal artery. The term

accessory vessels denotes two or more arterial branches supplying the same renal segment.

Incidence. **Between 71%** (Merklin and Michele, 1958) **and 85%** (Geyer and Poutasse, 1962) **of kidneys have one artery that supplies the entire renal parenchyma.** A slightly higher percentage of right-sided kidneys (87%) have a single renal artery compared with left-sided organs (Geyer and Poutasse, 1962). This figure does not seem to be influenced significantly by either sex or race. True aberrant vessels are rare except in patients with renal ectopia, with or without fusion, and in individuals with a horseshoe kidney.

Embryology. **The renal arterial tree is derived from three groups of primitive vascular channels that coalesce to form the mature vascular pattern for all retroperitoneal structures.** The cranial group consists of two pairs of arteries dorsal to the suprarenal gland that shift dorsally to form the phrenic artery. The middle group is made up of three pairs of vessels that pass through the suprarenal area. They retain the same lateral position and become the adrenal artery. Finally, the caudal group has four pairs of arteries that cross ventral to the suprarenal area and become the main renal artery. Sometimes they are joined by the most inferior pair from the middle group (Guggemos, 1962). It is believed that during renal migration this network of vessels selectively degenerates and the remaining adjacent arteries assume a progressively more important function. By a process of elimination, one primitive renal arterial pair eventually becomes the dominant vessel, the completed process being dependent on the final position of the kidney (Graves, 1956). Polar arteries or multiple renal arteries to the normally positioned kidney represent a failure of complete degeneration of all primitive vascular channels. The multiple vessel pattern that has been described for renal ectopia should be considered as an arrested embryonic state for that particular renal position (Gray and Skandalakis, 1972).

Description. **On the basis of vascular supply, the renal parenchyma is divided into five segments: apical, upper, middle, lower, and posterior** (Fig. 113–23). The main renal artery divides initially into an anterior and posterior branch. The anterior branch almost always supplies the upper, middle, and lower segments of the kidney. The posterior branch invariably nourishes the posterior and lower segments (Sampaio and Aragao, 1990a). The vessel to the apical segment has the greatest variation in origin; it arises from (1) the anterior division (43%), (2) the junction of the anterior and posterior divisions (23%), (3) the main stem renal artery or aorta (23%), or (4) the posterior division of the main renal artery (10%) (Graves, 1954). Rarely, the upper segment is supplied from a branch totally separate from the main renal artery (Merklin and Michele, 1958). The arterial and venous tree of the kidney and its relationship to the collecting system was beautifully depicted in endocasts by Sampaio and Aragao (1990a, 1990b). These investigations showed that the least likely areas to encounter vessels when entering the collecting system, either endourologically or with open surgery, is directly end-on through a fornix or inferiorly on the posterior aspect of the pelvis.

The lower renal segment, however, is often fed by an accessory vessel. This vessel is usually the most proximal branch when it arises from the main renal artery or its anterior division (Graves, 1954). However, it may originate directly from the aorta near the main renal artery, or it may be aberrant, arising from the gonadal vessel. A summary of findings from Merklin and Michele (1958), who analyzed reports from almost 11,000 kidneys, is depicted in Table 113–2. The rela-

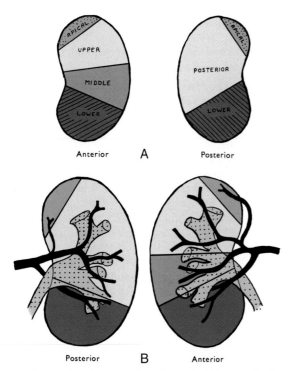

Figure 113–23. Usual pattern of arteries to the kidney. **A,** The five vascular lobes of Graves. **B,** Relationships of renal artery branch and renal pelvis to the five lobes. (From Graves FT: The anatomy of the intrarenal arteries and its application to segmental resection of the kidney. Br J Surg 1954;42:132.)

tionship of the main renal artery and its proximal branches to the renal vein can be seen in Figure 113–24. The venous drainage of the kidney has been carefully restudied by Sampaio and Aragao (1990b), who noted a close association between the inferior branch to the main renal vein and the anterior inferior aspect of the renal pelvis in 40% of kidneys. They cautioned that an endourologic incision of an obstructed UPJ should be done laterally and posteriorly instead of anteriorly to avoid injury to this vessel.

Symptoms. Symptoms attributable to renal vascular anomalies are those that might result from inadequate urinary drainage. Multiple, aberrant, or accessory vessels may constrict an infundibulum (Fig. 113–25A), a major calyx, or the UPJ (Yen et al, 2004) (Fig. 113–26). Pain, hematuria secondary to hydronephrosis, signs and symptoms of urinary tract infection, or calculus formation may result.

Diagnosis. Excretory urography may reveal multiple renal vessels or an aberrant artery (1) when a filling defect in the renal pelvis is consistent with an anomalous vascular pattern; (2) when hydronephrosis is noted along with a sharp cutoff in the superior infundibulum (see Fig. 113–25B) (Fraley, 1966, 1969); (3) when UPJ obstruction is seen in association with an angulated ureter near the renal pelvis and a kidney whose pole-to-pole axis is more vertical than normal; or (4) when differences are noted in the timing and concentration of one renal segment or in the entire kidney when compared with the opposite side (especially when hypertension is present). Renal angiography has been the gold standard for defining the vascular tree of the kidney, but less invasive imaging studies such as CT and MRI have been developed that are as accurate in delineating the precise anatomy with its variants and any disease states (Textor and Canzanello, 1996; Salcarga et al, 1999; Park et al, 2003).

Prognosis. None of these variations in the vascular tree increases the kidney's susceptibility to disease. Hydronephro-

Table 113–2.	**Variations in the Arterial Supply to the Kidney**		
		Condition	Percentage
		1 Hilar artery	71.1
		1 Hilar artery and 1 upper pole branch	12.6
		2 Hilar arteries	10.8
		1 Hilar artery and 1 upper pole aortic artery	6.2
		1 Hilar artery and 1 lower pole aortic artery	6.9
		1 Hilar artery and 1 lower pole branch	3.1
		3 Hilar arteries	1.7
		2 Hilar arteries, one with upper pole branch	2.7
		Other variations	—

From Gray SW, Skandalakis JE (eds): Embryology for Surgeons. Philadelphia, WB Saunders, 1972.

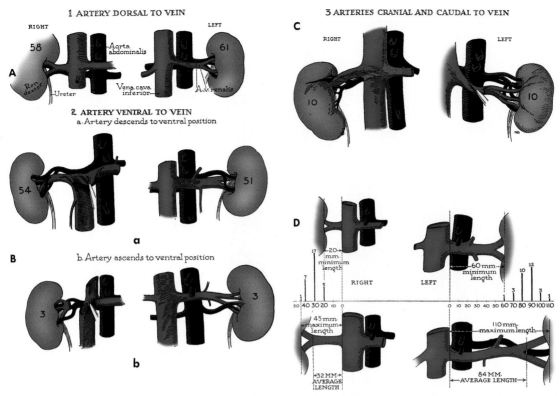

Figure 113–24. Relationships of renal arteries and veins. **A,** Artery dorsal to vein (47.6%). **B,** Artery ventral to vein (a, 42%; b, 2.4%). **C,** Artery cranial and caudal to vein (8.0%). **D,** Maximum, minimum, and average lengths of the renal pedicle in 30 successive specimens. (From Anson BJ, Daseler EH: Common variations in renal anatomy, affecting the blood supply, form and topography. Surg Gynecol Obstet 1961;112:439.)

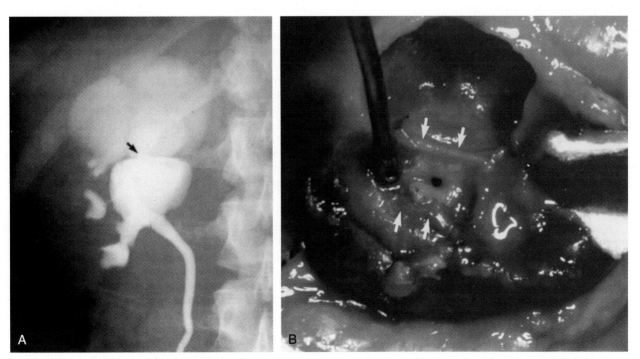

Figure 113–25. **A,** A 14-year-old girl with right flank pain underwent an excretory urogram, and this retrograde pyelogram revealed dilated upper calyces and a narrow upper infundibulum *(arrow)*. **B,** At surgery, the infundibular channel was found sandwiched between two segmental arteries *(arrows)*.

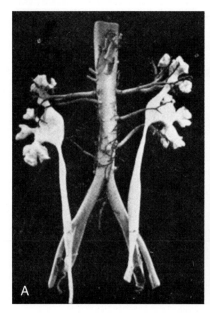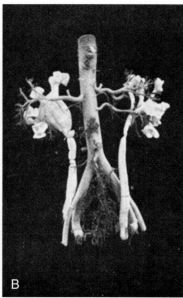

Figure 113–26. Accessory renal vessels demonstrated by celluloid corrosion preparation. **A,** In a full-term fetus, the renal pelves and ureters are shown in relationship to the main arterial distribution. On each side there are two accessory renal vessels above and one below, the lower one on the left being in proximity to the ureterovesical junction. **B,** In an 8-month-old fetus, the kidney on the right had one renal artery but the organ on the left had an accessory branch to the lower renal pole. Yet, the location of the lower accessory vessel on the left does not suggest that it might cause ureteral obstruction. On the right, there are early hydronephrosis, secondary kinking, and narrowing at the ureterovesical junction. (Courtesy of Dr. Duncan Morison.)

sis secondary to a vascular anomaly is a very rare finding, especially when one considers the relative frequency of all renal vascular variations. Hypertension is no more frequent in patients with multiple renal arteries than in those with a single vessel (Geyer and Poutasse, 1962). Nathan (1958) did report the development of orthostatic proteinuria in seven patients with a lower pole renal artery that wrapped around and compressed the main renal vein. He thought there might have been a causal relationship but did not prove it.

Renal Artery Aneurysm

Aneurysmal dilation was the first disease process of the renal artery to be recognized (Poutasse, 1957); it was considered a rare occurrence until selective renal angiography became widely available. Since then, **the overall incidence has been calculated to be between 0.1% and 0.3%.** Abeshouse (1951), in a comprehensive review, classified renal artery aneurysms as follows: saccular, fusiform, dissecting, and arteriovenous. The saccular aneurysm, a localized outpouching that communicates with the arterial lumen by a narrow or wide opening, is the most common type, accounting for 93% of all aneurysms (McKeil et al, 1966; Stanley et al, 1975; Hageman et al, 1978; Zinman and Libertino, 1982). Renal artery aneurysms have been associated with autosomal dominant polycystic kidney disease (Schievink, 1998). When the aneurysm is located at the bifurcation of the main renal artery and its anterior and posterior divisions or at one of the more distal branchings, it is considered to be congenital in origin and is called the fusiform type (Poutasse, 1957). The presence of similar aneurysms at branching points in the vasculature of other organ systems attests to this possible origin (Lorentz et al, 1984). Acquired aneurysms may be located anywhere and may result from inflammatory, traumatic, or degenerative factors. A localized defect in the internal elastic tissue and the media allows the vessel to dilate at that point. It is a true aneurysm because its walls are composed of most of the layers that make up the normal artery (Poutasse, 1957). The

outpouchings may vary in size from 1 to 2 cm up to 10 cm (Garritano, 1957) but 90% are smaller than 2 cm. There is no predilection for side but the right is favored and bilateral aneurysms are seen in 15% (Pfeiffer et al, 2003).

Most renal artery aneurysms are silent, especially in children (48%) (Sarker et al, 1991). Some produce symptoms at a later age in relation to their size because there is a tendency for them to enlarge with time. Pain (15%), hematuria (microscopic and macroscopic) (30%), and hypertension (55%) secondary to compression of adjacent parenchyma or to altered blood flow within the vascular tree can occur (Glass and Uson, 1967; Bulbul and Farrow, 1992). The hypertension is renin mediated, secondary to relative parenchymal ischemia (Lorentz et al, 1984). In a recent review, 13 cases of hydronephrosis secondary to an adjacent renal vessel aneurysm was noted (Miyagawa et al, 2001).

The diagnosis may be suspected when a pulsatile mass is palpated in the region of the renal hilum or when a bruit is heard on abdominal auscultation. A wreathlike calcification in the area of the renal artery or its branches (30%) is highly suggestive (Silvis et al, 1956), but this finding is often missed on a plain abdominal radiograph (Bulbul and Farrow, 1992). Excretory urography may suggest a vascular lesion in 60% of cases, and color Doppler imaging (Bunchman et al, 1991) will demonstrate decreased flow, but selective renal angiography (Cerny et al, 1968), digital subtraction angiography, or, more recently, color Doppler ultrasound (Okamoto et al, 1992) or magnetic resonance angiography (Takebayashi et al, 1994) is needed to confirm the diagnosis.

Many asymptomatic renal artery aneurysms come to light after the discovery and workup of hypertension. Fifty percent are diagnosed when a renal arteriogram is performed for other reasons (Zinman and Libertino, 1982), but CT is also readily detecting the lesion (Miyagawa et al, 2001; Nishimura et al, 2002). Generally, excision is recommended if (1) the hypertension cannot be easily controlled; (2) incomplete ring-like calcification is present; (3) the aneurysm is larger than 2.5 cm (Poutasse, 1975; Pfeiffer et al, 2003); (4) the patient is female and of child-bearing age, because rupture during pregnancy is a likely possibility (Cohen and Shamash, 1987); (5) the aneurysm increases in size on serial angiograms; or (6) an arteriovenous fistula is present. Over 30 cases of a ruptured aneurysm during pregnancy have been reported (Lacroix et al, 2001) so any aneurysm larger than 1.0 cm in younger women with the potential for child bearing should be repaired (Henke and Stanley, 2003). The likelihood of spontaneous rupture (about 10%), with its dire consequences, dictates attentive treatment in the foregoing situations. Recent improvements in endovascular techniques dictate early prophylactic treatment (Yamamoto et al, 1998).

KEY POINTS: RENAL ARTERY ANEURYSM

- The overall incidence has been calculated to be between 0.1% and 0.3%.

- Most renal artery aneurysms are silent, especially in children.

- The diagnosis may be suspected with a pulsatile mass in the region of the renal hilum or when an abdominal bruit is heard. A wreathlike calcification in the area of the renal artery or its branches (30%) is highly suggestive.

- Many asymptomatic renal artery aneurysms come to light after the discovery and workup of hypertension.

Renal Arteriovenous Fistula

Although rare, renal arteriovenous fistulas have been discovered with increasing frequency since they were first described by Varela in 1928. **Two types exist, congenital and acquired** (Maldonado et al, 1964), with the latter (secondary to trauma, inflammation, renal surgery, or percutaneous needle biopsy) accounting for the recent increased incidence. Only the congenital variant is discussed here.

Fewer than 25% of all arteriovenous fistulas are of the congenital type. They are easily identifiable by their cirsoid configuration and multiple communications between the main or segmental renal arteries and venous channels (Crummy et al, 1965; Cho and Stanley, 1978). Although they are considered congenital (because similar arteriovenous malformations can be found elsewhere in the body), they rarely present clinically before the third or fourth decade. Women are affected three times as often as men, and the right kidney is involved slightly more often than the left (Cho and Stanley, 1978; Ishikawa et al, 2004). The lesion is usually located in the upper pole (45% of cases), but not infrequently it may be found in the midportion (30%) or in the lower pole (25%) of the kidney (Yazaki et al, 1976). A total of 91 cases had been reported (Takaha et al, 1980) when the last review was conducted.

The exact cause remains an enigma, but the condition is thought to be either present at birth or the result of a congenital aneurysm that erodes into an adjacent vein and slowly enlarges (Thomason et al, 1972). The pathophysiology involved in the shunting of blood, which bypasses the renal parenchyma and rapidly joins the venous circulation and returns to the heart, results in a varied clinical picture. The myriad of symptoms are based on the size of the arteriovenous malformation and how long it has existed (Messing et al, 1976).

The hemodynamic derangement often produces a loud bruit (in 75% of cases). Diminished perfusion of renal parenchyma distal to the fistulous site leads to relative ischemia and renin-mediated hypertension (40% to 50%) (McAlhany et al, 1971). The increased venous return and high cardiac output with concomitant diminution in peripheral resistance may result in left ventricular hypertrophy and eventually in high-output cardiac failure (50%) (Maldonado et al, 1964). In addition, the arteriovenous fistula usually is located close to the collecting system. As a result, macroscopic and microscopic hematuria occurs in more than 75% of affected individuals (Messing et al, 1976; Cho and Stanley, 1978; Montoya et al, 2004). Although flank or abdominal pain may be present, a mass is rarely felt (10%).

Excretory urography may reveal diminished or absent function either in one segment or in the entire portion of the involved kidney (DeSai and DeSautels, 1973), an irregular filling defect in the renal pelvis or calyces (secondary to either clot or encroachment by the fistula), or calyceal distortion or obstruction distal to the site of the lesion (Gunterberg, 1968). Despite these specific radiographic features, an abnormality may be noted in only 50% of excretory urograms. **Three-dimensional Doppler ultrasound and MR angiography are more accurate and noninvasive tests** (Mohaupt et al, 1999; Ishikawa et al, 2004), but selective renal arteriography or digital subtraction angiography is the most definitive method for diagnosing the lesion. A cirsoid appearance with multiple small, tortuous channels; prompt venous filling; and an enlarged renal and possibly gonadal vein are pathognomonic for a renal arteriovenous fistula (DeSai and DeSautels, 1973).

The symptomatic nature of this lesion, which causes progressive alterations in the cardiovascular system, often dictates surgical intervention. The congenital variant rarely behaves like its acquired counterpart, which may disappear spontaneously after several months. Nephrectomy, partial nephrectomy, vascular ligation (Boijsen and Kohler, 1962), selective embolization (Bookstein and Goldstein, 1973), and balloon catheter occlusion (Bentson and Crandalls, 1972) have been employed to obliterate the fistula.

ANOMALIES OF THE COLLECTING SYSTEM
Calyx and Infundibulum

Calyceal Diverticulum

A calyceal diverticulum is a cystic cavity lined by transitional epithelium, encased within the renal substance, and situated peripheral to a minor calyx, to which it is connected by a narrow channel. This abnormality, first described by Rayer in 1841, may be multiple, with the upper calyx being most frequently affected.

An incidence of 4.5 per 1000 excretory urograms has been reported (Timmons et al, 1975). A similar incidence was noted in both children and adults, with no predilection for either side or sex. Most diverticula, labeled type I, occur adjacent to an upper- or occasionally a lower-pole calyx. Type II diverticula are larger and communicate with the renal pelvis directly; they tend to be the symptomatic ones (Wulfsohn, 1980).

Congenital and acquired factors have been suggested to explain the formation of calyceal diverticula. The similarity in incidence in children and adults is consistent with an embryologic etiology (Abeshouse, 1950; Mathieson, 1953; Devine et al, 1969; Middleton and Pfister, 1974). At the 5-mm stage of the embryo, some of the ureteral branches of the third and fourth generation, which ordinarily degenerate, may persist as isolated branches, resulting in the formation of a calyceal diverticulum (Lister and Singh, 1973).

A localized cortical abscess draining into a calyx has also been postulated as an etiologic factor. Other proposed causes include obstruction secondary to stone formation or infection within a calyx, progressive fibrosis of an infundibular stenosis, renal injury, achalasia, and spasm or dysfunction of one of the supposed sphincters surrounding a minor calyx. Small diverticula are usually asymptomatic and are found incidentally at excretory urography or renal ultrasonography. Over time these diverticula tend to progressively distend with trapped urine (Schneck et al, 1994). Infection, milk of calcium (crystallization of calcium salts without actual stone formation) (Patriquin et al, 1985), or true stone formation are complications of stasis or obstruction that can produce symptoms (Lister and Singh, 1973; Siegel and McAlister, 1979). Hematuria, pain, and urinary tract infection may be seen in the presence of stones. In the Mayo Clinic series (Timmons et al, 1975), 39% of patients with calyceal diverticula had calculi.

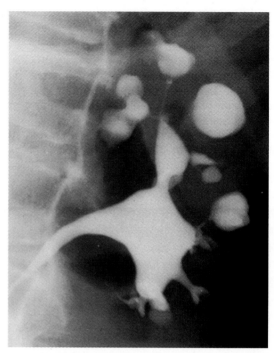

Figure 113-27. A 13-year-old girl with hematuria had a retrograde pyelogram demonstrating multiple calyceal diverticula.

> ## KEY POINTS: CALYCEAL DIVERTICULUM
>
> - A calyceal diverticulum is a cystic cavity lined by transitional epithelium, encased within the renal substance, and situated peripheral to a minor calyx, to which it is connected by a narrow channel.
>
> - The incidence is about 4.5 per 1000 excretory urograms.
>
> - The diagnosis is best made by excretory urography or CT.
>
> - Percutaneous removal of the stones and ablation of the mucosal surface is the modern treatment of choice.

The diagnosis is made by excretory urography or CT; one child in our series developed an abscess in her infected diverticulum that required percutaneous drainage (Ellis et al, 1990; Schneck et al, 1994). Delayed films are helpful in demonstrating pooling of contrast material in the diverticulum. Retrograde pyelography (Fig. 113–27) and, more recently, delayed imaging CT with contrast medium enhancement and MRI are sometimes useful in making the diagnosis and defining the

precise anatomy. Ultrasonography delineates a fluid-filled area more centrally located near the collecting system than a simple renal cyst. When it is filled with microcalculi, ultrasound characteristically demonstrates a layering effect within the diverticulum between clear fluid above and echo-dense debris without shadowing below (Patriquin et al, 1985). In fact, ultrasonography may be more definitive because it is easier to image the milk of calcium within the diverticulum as the patient changes position. Milk of calcium appears on excretory urography as a crescent-shaped density that changes as the patient assumes different positions. Reflux is found in as many as two thirds of the children, which may explain why some children present with urinary tract infection (Amar, 1975).

In general, patients who are asymptomatic do not require treatment. Persistent pain, resistant urinary tract infections, hematuria, and milk of calcium or true calculus formation are indications for surgery (Siegel and McAlister, 1979). **Partial nephrectomy was the treatment of choice in the past, but now percutaneous removal of the stones and ablation of the mucosal surface** and communication with the collecting system (Goldfischer et al, 1998), ureteroscopic enlargement of the diverticular communication with removal of the stones (Baldwin et al, 1998), and extracorporeal laparoscopic stone removal with marsupialization of the diverticulum (Hoznek et al, 1998) have been reported as successful kidney-sparing alternatives.

Hydrocalycosis

Hydrocalycosis is a very rare cystic dilation of a major calyx with a demonstrable connection to the renal pelvis; it is lined by transitional epithelium. It may be caused by a congenital or acquired intrinsic obstruction such as a parapelvic cyst (Fig. 113–28).

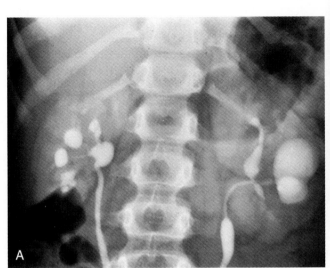

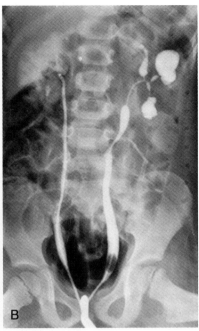

Figure 113–28. Hydrocalycosis of infundibulopelvic stenosis in a 3-year-old boy with bilaterally ectopic ureteral orifices (at the vesical neck) and other congenital anomalies, who presented with urinary infection. Reflux was not demonstrable, and the patient has remained uninfected on suppressive antibiotics. There has been no urographic change for 5 years. **A,** Long-term excretory urogram. Right infundibular and left infundibulopelvic stenosis. **B,** Retrograde ureteropyelogram (bilateral). Mildly dilated left ureter. Note diffuse tubular backflow on right. (From Malek RS: Obstructive uropathy: Calyx. In Kelalis PP, King LR [eds]: Clinical Pediatric Urology. Philadelphia, WB Saunders, 1976, p 235.)

Dilation of the upper calyx due to obstruction of the upper infundibulum by vessels or stenosis has been described (see Fig. 113–25) (Fraley, 1966; Johnston and Sandomirsky, 1972). Cicatrization of an infundibulum may result from infection or trauma. Conversely, hydrocalycosis has been reported to occur without an obvious cause (Williams and Mininberg, 1968). It has been postulated that achalasia of a ring of muscle at the entrance of the infundibulum into the renal pelvis causes a functional obstruction (Moore, 1950; Williams and Mininberg, 1968).

Mild upper calyceal dilation caused by partial infundibular obstruction is relatively common but usually asymptomatic. The most frequent presenting symptom is upper abdominal or flank pain. On occasion a mass may be palpated. Stasis can lead to hematuria or urinary infection, or both.

Hydrocalycosis must be differentiated from multiple dilated calyces secondary to ureteral obstruction, calyceal clubbing as a result of recurrent pyelonephritis or medullary necrosis, renal tuberculosis, a large calyceal diverticulum, and megacalycosis. These entities can be differentiated by a combination of excretory urography, findings at surgery, histopathology of removed tissue, and bacteriology.

Hydrocalycosis due to vascular obstruction is usually treated by dismembered infundibulopyelostomy, which changes the relationship of the infundibulum to the vessel. If the cystic dilation is caused by an intrinsic stenosis of the infundibulum, an intubated infundibulotomy or partial nephrectomy may be performed. Percutaneous treatment of these narrowed areas has also been successful and is probably the approach of choice today (Lang, 1991). Although clinical improvement is apparent in most instances, the radiologic appearance often is not altered significantly.

Megacalycosis

Megacalycosis is best defined as nonobstructive enlargement of calyces resulting from malformation of the renal papillae (Fig. 113–29). It was first described by Puigvert in 1963. The calyces are generally dilated and malformed and may be increased in number. The renal pelvis is not dilated, nor is its wall thickened, and the UPJ is normally funneled without evidence of obstruction. The cortical tissue around the abnormal calyx is normal in thickness and shows no signs of scarring or chronic inflammation. The medulla, however, is underdeveloped and assumes a falciform crescent appearance instead of its normal pyramidal shape. The collecting tubules are not dilated but are definitely shorter than normal, and they are oriented transversely rather than vertically from the corticomedullary junction (Puigvert, 1963). A mild disorder of maximal concentrating ability has been reported (Gittes and Talner, 1972), but acid excretion is normal after an acid load (Vela-Navarrete and Garcia Robledo, 1983). Other functions of the kidney—glomerular filtration, renal plasma flow, and isotope uptake—also are not altered (Gittes, 1984).

Megacalycosis is most likely congenital and has been diagnosed prenatally (Vidal Company et al, 2001). **It occurs predominantly in males in a ratio of 6:1 and has been found only in white patients. Bilateral disease has been seen almost exclusively in males, whereas segmental unilateral involvement occurs only in females** (Cacciaguerra et al, 1996). This suggests an X-linked partially recessive gene with reduced penetrance in females (Gittes, 1984). Except for one report of two affected brothers, the entity has not been thought to be familial (Briner and Thiel, 1988).

It was theorized by Puigvert (1964) and endorsed by Johnston and Sandomirsky (1972) that there is transient delay

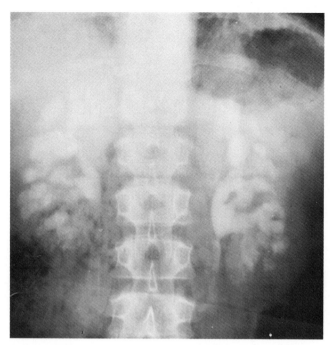

Figure 113–29. Bilateral megacalyces discovered in an 11-year-old boy with abdominal pain and hematuria. He had no history of urinary infection, and voiding cystography did not demonstrate vesicoureteral reflux.

in the recanalization of the upper ureter after the branches of the ureteral bud hook up with the metanephric blastema. This produces a short-lived episode of obstruction when the embryonic glomeruli start producing urine. The fetal calyces may dilate and then retain their obstructed appearance despite the lack of evidence of obstruction in postnatal life (Gittes and Talner, 1972). **The increased number of calyces frequently seen in this condition may be an aborted response by the branching ureteral bud to the obstruction.**

Primary hypoplasia of juxtamedullary glomeruli was suggested as an etiology by Galian and associates (1970); this theory nicely explains the reason for the lack of concentrating ability, but it has not been corroborated by others.

The abnormality is noticed in children, usually when x-ray studies are obtained after a urinary tract infection or as part of an evaluation when other congenital anomalies are present (Arambasic et al, 2003). Adults frequently present with hematuria secondary to renal calculi, which leads to excretory urographic investigation.

The calyces are dilated and usually increased in number, but the infundibuli and pelvis may not be enlarged. Although the UPJ does not appear obstructed, there may be segmental dilation of the distal third of the ureter (Kozakewich and Lebowitz, 1974). Megacalycosis associated with an ipsilateral segmental megaureter was described in 12 children (Mandell et al, 1987), mostly boys, and predominantly left-sided. A normal-caliber ureter was interposed between the two entities (Fig. 113–30). Not infrequently this anatomic picture has been

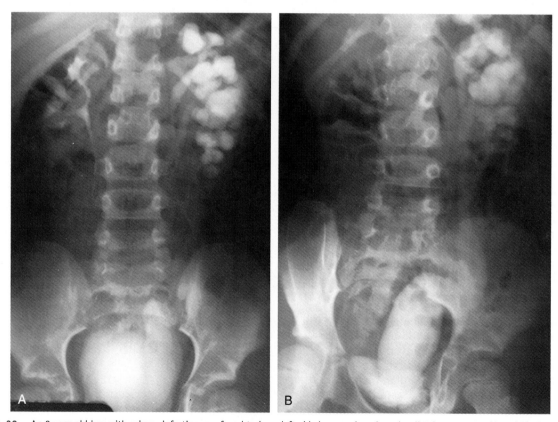

Figure 113–30. An 8-year-old boy with urinary infection was found to have left-sided megacalycosis and a distal megaureter (**A** and **B**). Note the normal-caliber upper ureter. A voiding cystogram revealed no reflux, and a diuretic renogram did not demonstrate any obstruction.

mistaken for congenital ureteropelvic or ureterovesical junction obstruction, with surgery being performed to correct the suspected defect. Postoperatively, the calyceal pattern remains unchanged.

Diuretic renography reveals a normal pattern for uptake and washout of the isotope, whether or not the Whitaker test generates high pressure in the collecting system (Gomes Tellado et al, 1997). Therefore, an obstructive picture cannot be proven. **Long-term follow-up of patients with this anomaly does not reveal any progression of the anatomic derangement or functional impairment of the kidney** (Gittes, 1984).

KEY POINTS: MEGACALYCOSIS

- Megacalycosis is best defined as nonobstructive enlargement of calyces resulting from malformation of the renal papillae.

- It occurs predominantly in males in a ratio of 6:1.

- Bilateral disease has been seen almost exclusively in males, whereas segmental unilateral involvement occurs only in females.

- Long-term follow-up of patients with this anomaly does not usually reveal any progression of the anatomic derangement or functional impairment of the kidney.

Unipapillary Kidney

The unipapillary kidney is an exceptionally rare anomaly in humans. Only 18 cases have been reported (Neal and Murphy, 1960; Sakatoku and Kitayama, 1964; Harrison et al, 1976; Morimoto et al, 1979; Toppercer, 1980; Kaneto et al, 1997). This anomaly is present not uncommonly in monkeys, rabbits, dogs, marsupials, insectivores, and monotremes. The cause is thought to be a failure of progressive branching after the first three to five generations (which create the pelvis) of the ureteral bud (Potter, cited by Harrison et al, 1976). The solitary calyx drains a ridgelike papilla. Nephrons attach to fewer collecting tubules, which then drain directly into the pelvis. Biopsies of these kidneys reveal glomerulosclerosis, tubular atrophy, and increased fibrosis (Bischel et al, 1978).

The kidney is smaller than normal but usually is in its correct location. Its function is often reduced (Smith et al, 1984; Kaneto et al, 1997). The arterial tree, although sparse, has a normal configuration. **The opposite kidney is frequently absent.** Genital anomalies are often present. The condition is frequently asymptomatic, being discovered fortuitously in most instances. More often than not there are abnormalities of the proximal ureter (i.e., megaureter, reflux, or ectopic insertion), suggesting an underlying ureteral bud defect as the cause (Smith et al, 1984; Kaneto et al, 1997). The anomaly has also come to light during a workup for urinary infection (Kaneto et al, 1997).

Extrarenal Calyces

Extrarenal calyces are an uncommon congenital anomaly in which the major calyces as well as the renal pelvis are outside the parenchyma of the kidney (Fig. 113–31). This entity was originally reviewed by Eisendrath in 1925 and then more extensively by Malament and coworkers in 1961. The kidney is usually discoid, with the pelvis and the major and minor calyces located outside the renal parenchyma. The renal vessels have an anomalous distribution into the kidney, usually at the circumferential edge of the flat, widened hilus. Malament considered this condition to be the result of abnormal nephrogenic anlage or a too early and rapidly developing ureteral bud.

Extrarenal calyces usually do not produce symptoms, although failure of normal drainage may lead to stasis, infection, and calculi. Sometimes, the calyces are blunted, mimicking the radiographic changes usually seen with pyelonephritis or obstruction, from which this condition should be distinguished. Surgery is reserved for those cases in which infection or obstruction is demonstrated.

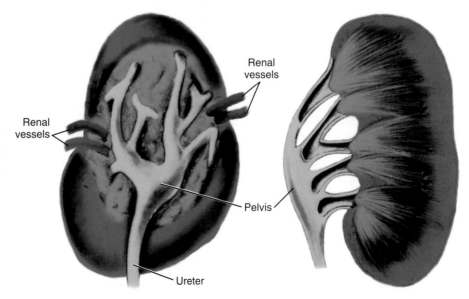

Figure 113–31. Extrarenal calyces. These represent delayed rather than insufficient ureteral growth. (From Malament M, Schwartz B, Nagamatsu GR: Extrarenal calyces: Their relationship to renal disease. AJR Am J Roentgenol 1961;86:823.)

Renal vessels

Renal vessels

Pelvis

Ureter

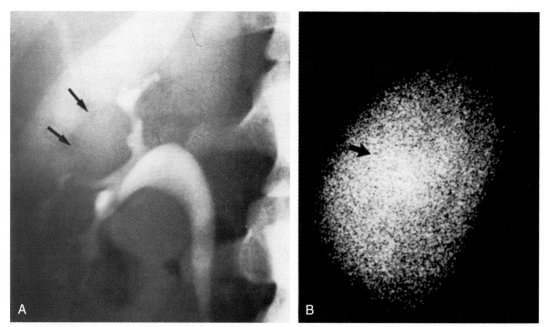

Figure 113–32. **A,** This child has a mass effect with splaying of the middle calyces. **B,** A renal scan demonstrates normal uptake in the area *(arrow)*, suggesting the pseudotumor is really a hypertrophied column of Bertin.

Anomalous Calyx (Pseudotumor of the Kidney)

A number of normal variants of the pyelocalyceal system in the kidney have been described. One such entity manifests as **a localized mass, usually situated between the infundibula of the upper and middle calyceal groups, and is called a hypertrophied column of Bertin** (Fig. 113–32). The column may be sufficiently large to compress and deform the adjacent pelvis and calyces, suggesting a mass on excretory urography; this is the so-called pseudotumor. The individual calyces, however, are normally shaped and developed.

It is important to differentiate this calyceal anomaly from true disease of the calyx and from a parenchymal tumor. **A renal scan shows normal uptake of the radioisotope in this area** (Parker et al, 1976), and a renal ultrasound study shows a normal echogenic pattern of parenchyma to the area in question.

Infundibulopelvic Dysgenesis

Infundibulopelvic stenosis most likely forms a link between cystic dysplasia of the kidney and the grossly hydronephrotic organ (Kelalis and Malek, 1981; Uhlenhuth et al, 1990). This condition includes a variety of radiographically dysmorphic kidneys with varying degrees of infundibular or infundibulopelvic stenosis that may be associated with renal dysplasia (Fig. 113–33). Although not called as such, the first case involving the entire pelvis and all the infundibuli of both kidneys was reported by Boyce and Whitehurst in 1976. Rayer had described a focal form of the disease in 1841, and several reports noting narrowing of one or two infundibuli appeared between 1949 and 1976 (Uhlenhuth et al, 1990). These authors tried to link the focal form to cystic dysplasia secondary to obstruction, in which multicystic kidney disease

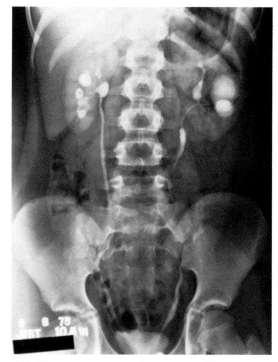

Figure 113–33. Excretory urogram in an 18-year-old male with a urinary tract infection shows severe stenosis of the infundibula and left ureteropelvic junction and a milder form of infundibulopelvic dysgenesis in the right kidney. Vesicoureteral reflux was absent on voiding cystourethrography. (Courtesy of Dr. Panos Kelalis.)

is the severest form in the spectrum. Uhlenhuth and coworkers (1990) believed that this phenomenon is the result of extensive dysgenesis of the pyelocalyceal system but with preservation of renal function. Reflux is not commonly observed in these patients.

KEY POINTS: INFUNDIBULOPELVIC DYSGENESIS

- Infundibulopelvic stenosis most likely forms a link between cystic dysplasia of the kidney and the grossly hydronephrotic kidney.

- Infundibulopelvic stenosis is usually bilateral and is commonly associated with vesicoureteral reflux, suggesting an abnormality of the entire ureteral bud.

Infundibulopelvic stenosis is usually bilateral and is commonly associated with vesicoureteral reflux, suggesting an abnormality of the entire ureteral bud (Kelalis and Malek, 1981). Patients usually present with urinary infection, hypertension, or flank pain. Sometimes, an asymptomatic child with multiple anomalies is evaluated and found to have this condition. Despite extensively dysmorphic kidney features, the function is either normal or only slightly affected (Kelalis and Malek, 1981). Long-term follow-up, however, reveals that progressive renal deterioration is common, leading to severe renal insufficiency or end-stage renal disease in all patients with bilateral involvement (Husmann et al, 1994). Biopsies in patients with renal failure demonstrate lesions consistent with hyperfiltration injury. Progressive hydronephrosis is not thought to be responsible for the deterioration in renal function, based on histologic assessment of renal tissue adjacent to dilated calyces. Therefore, infundibulotomy may be needed if there is a specific need (i.e., calyceal stones or loss of function) (Husmann et al, 1994).

Pelvis

Extrarenal Pelvis

An extrarenal pelvis is of clinical importance only when drainage is impaired. This is sometimes associated with a variety of kidney abnormalities, including malposition and malrotation, that predispose to urinary stasis, infection, and calculous disease. UPJ obstruction causing dilation of only the renal pelvis and not the calyces has been reported (Johnson, 1999).

Bifid Pelvis

Approximately 10% of normal renal pelves are bifid, the pelvis dividing first at or just within its entrance to the kidney to form two major calyces. A bifid pelvis should be considered a variant of normal. No increased incidence of disease has been reported in patients with this entity, although some who exhibit flank pain will have a bifid pelvis on radiographic imaging. A renal scan may show the yo-yo effect of urine ascending one limb after descending from another, which is thought but not proven, to be the cause of the symptoms (Chu et al, 2003). If further division of the renal pelvis occurs, triplication of the pelvis may result, but this is extremely rare.

SUGGESTED READINGS

Abeshouse BS, Bhisitkul I: Crossed renal ectopia with and without fusion. Urol Int 1959;9:63.

Anson BJ, Daseler EH: Common variations in renal anatomy, affecting the blood supply, form and topography. Surg Gynecol Obstet 1961;112:439.

Argueso LR, Ritchey ML, Boyle ET Jr, et al: Prognosis of patients with unilateral renal agenesis. Pediatr Nephrol 1992;6:412.

Ashley DJB, Mostofi FK: Renal agenesis and dysgenesis. J Urol 1960;83:211.

Atiyeh B, Husmann D, Baum M: Contralateral renal anomalies in patients with renal agenesis and noncystic renal dysplasia. Pediatrics 1993;91:812.

Baldwin DD, Beaghler MA, Ruckle HC, et al: Ureteroscopic treatment of symptomatic caliceal diverticular calculi. Tech Urol 1998;4:92.

Biedel CW, Pagon RA, Zapata JO: Müllerian anomalies and renal agenesis: Autosomal dominant urogenital adysplasia. J Pediatr 1984;104:861.

Bischel MD, Blustein WC, Kinnas NC, et al: Solitary renal calix. JAMA 1978;240:2467-2468.

Boatman DL, Culp DA Jr, Culp DA, Flocks RH: Crossed renal ectopia. J Urol 1972;108:30.

Boatman DL, Cornell SH, Kolln CP: The arterial supply of horseshoe kidney. AJR Am J Roentgenol 1971;113:447.

Boijsen E, Kohler R: Renal arteriovenous fistulae. Acta Radiol 1962;57:433.

Borer JG, Bauer SB, Peters CA, et al: Single system ectopic ureter draining an ectopic dysplastic kidney: Delayed diagnosis in the young female with continuous urinary incontinence. Br J Urol 1998;81:474-478.

Bulbul MA, Farrow GA: Renal artery aneurysms. Urology 1992;40;124.

Caldamone AA, Rabinowitz R: Crossed fused renal ectopia, orthotopic multicystic dysplasia and vaginal agenesis. J Urol 1981;126:105.

Candiani GB, Fedele L, Candiani M: Double uterus, blind hemivagina, and ipsilateral renal agenesis: 36 cases and long-term followup. Obstet Gynecol 1997;90:26.

Carlson HE: Supernumerary kidney: A summary of fifty-one reported cases. J Urol 1950;64:221.

Cascio S, Sweeney B, Granata C, et al: Vesicoureteral reflux and ureteropelvic junction obstruction in children with horseshoe kidney: Treatment and outcome. J Urol 2002;167:2566-2568.

Cascio S, Paran S, Puri P: Associated urological anomalies in children with unilateral renal agenesis. J Urol 1999;162:1081-1083.

Cho KJ, Stanley JC: Non-neoplastic congenital and acquired renal arteriovenous malformations and fistula. Radiology 1978;129:333.

Colquhoun-Kerr JS, Gu W-X, Jameson JL, et al: X-Linked Kallmann syndrome and renal agenesis occurring together and independently in a large Australian family. Am J Med Genet 1999;83:22-27.

Crummy AB Jr, Atkinson RJ, Caruthers SB: Congenital renal arteriovenous fistulas. J Urol 1965;93:24.

Curtis JA, Sadhu V, Steiner RM: Malposition of the colon in right renal agenesis, ectopia and anterior nephrectomy. AJR Am J Roentgenol 1977;129:845.

DeSai SG, DeSautels RE: Congenital arteriovenous malformation of the kidney. J Urol 1973;110:17.

Devine CJ Jr, Guzman JA, Devine PC, Poutasse EF: Calyceal diverticulum. J Urol 1969;101:8.

Donat SM, Donat PE: Intrathoracic kidney: A case report with a review of the world's literature. J Urol 1988;140:131.

Ellis JH, Patterson SK, Sonda LP, et al: Stones and infection in renal caliceal diverticula: Treatment with percutaneous procedures. AJR Am J Roentgenol 1990;156:995.

Evans WP, Resnick MI: Horseshoe kidney and urolithiasis. J Urol 1981;125:620.

Fitch N, Lachance RC: The pathogenesis of Potter's syndrome of renal agenesis. Can Med Assoc J 1972;107:653.

Fraley EE: Vascular obstruction of superior infundibulum causing nephralgia: A new syndrome. N Engl J Med 1966;275:1403.

Fraley EE: Vascular obstruction of superior infundibulum causing nephralgia: New syndrome. N Engl J Med 1966;275:1403.

Gittes RF: Congenital megacalices. Monogr Urol 1984;5:1.

Gittes RF, Talner LB: Congenital megacalyces vs. obstructive hydronephrosis. J Urol 1972;108:833.

Glass PM, Uson AC: Aneurysms of the renal artery: A study of 20 cases. J Urol 1967;98:285.

Glenn JF: Analysis of 51 patients with horseshoe kidney. N Engl J Med 1959;261:684.

Graves FT: The anatomy of the intrarenal arteries and its application to segmental resection of the kidney. Br J Surg 1954;42:132.

Gu L, Alton DJ: Crossed solitary renal ectopia. Urology 1991;38:556.

Guarino N, Tadini B, Camardi P, et al: The incidence of associated urological abnormalities in children with renal ectopia. J Urol 2004;172:1757-1759.

Guarino N, Tadini B, Camardi P, et al: The incidence of associated urological abnormalities in children with renal ectopia. J Urol 2004;172:1757-1759.

Harrison RB, Wood JL, Gillenwater JY: A solitary calyx in a human kidney. Radiology 1976;121:310.

Hendren WH, Donahoe PK, Pfister RC: Crossed renal ectopia in children. Urology 1976;7:135.

Hertz M, Rabenstein ZJ, Shairin N, Melzer M: Crossed renal ectopia: Clinical and radiologic findings in 22 cases. Clin Radioli 1977;28:339.

Hill LM, Nowak A, Hartle R, Tush B: Fetal compensatory renal hypertrophy with a unilateral functioning kidney. Ultrasound Obstet Gynecol 2000;15:191-193.

Hiraoka M, Tsukahara H, Ohshima Y, et al: Renal aplasia is the predominant cause of congenital solitary kidneys. Kidney Int 2002;61:1840-1844.

Hoffman CK, Filly RA, Callen PW: The "lying down" adrenal sign: A sonographic indicator of renal agenesis or ectopia in fetuses and neonates. J Ultrasound Med 1992;11:533.

Hohenfellner M, Schultz-Lampel D, Lampel A, et al: Tumor in the horseshoe kidney: Clinical implications and review of embryogenesis. J Urol 1992;147:1098.

Hoznek A, Herard A, Ogiez N, et al: Symptomatic caliceal diverticula treated with extraperitoneal laparoscopic marsupialization, fulguration and gelatin resorcinol formalin glue obliteration. J Urol 1998;160:352.

Husmann DA, Kramer SA, Malek RS, Allen TD: Infundibulopelvic stenosis: A long-term follow-up. J Urol 1994;152:837.

Jancu J, Zuckerman H, Sudarsky M: Unilateral renal agenesis associated with multiple abnormalities. South Med J 1976;69:94.

Kamba T, Higashi S, Kamoto T, et al: Failure of ureteric bud invasion: A new model of renal agenesis in mice. Am J Pathol 2001;159:2347-2353.

Kaneto H, Metoki R, Fukuzaki A, et al: Unicalyceal kidney associated with ureteral anomalies. Eur Urol 1997;32:328.

Kaneyama K, Yamataka A, Satake S, et al: Associated urologic anomalies in children with solitary kidney. J Pediatr Surg 2004;39:85-87.

Kolln CP, Boatman DL, Schmidt JD, Flocks RH: Horseshoe kidney: A review of 105 patients. J Urol 1972;107:203.

Koureas AP, Panourgias EC, Gouliamos AD, et al: Imaging of a supernumerary kidney. Eur Radiol 2000;10:1722-1723.

Kozakewich HPW, Lebowitz FL: Congenital megacalices. Pediatr Radiol 1974;2:251.

Lang EK: Percutaneous infundibuloplasty: Management of calyceal diverticula and infundibular stenosis. Radiology 1991;181:871.

Leitha T: The usefulness of Tc99m-DMSA SPECT and three-dimensional surface rendering in an asymptomatic patient with a single kidney in the pelvis. Clin Nucl Med 1998;23:414-416.

Lippe B, Geffner ME, Dietrich RB, et al: Renal malformations in patients with Turner syndrome: Imaging in 141 patients. Pediatrics 1988;82:852.

Lorentz WB Jr, Browning MC, D'Souza VJ, et al: Intrarenal aneurysm of the renal artery in children. Am J Dis Child 1984;138:751.

Magee MC, Lucey DT, Fried FA: A new embryologic classification for urogynecologic malformations: The syndromes of mesonephric duct induced müllerian deformities. J Urol 1979;121:265.

Mandell GA, Snyder HM 3rd, Haymen SK, et al: Association of congenital megacalycosis and ipsilateral segmental megaureter. Pediatr Radiol 1987;17:28.

Mascatello V, Lebowitz RL: Malposition of the colon in left renal agenesis and ectopia. Radiology 1976;120:371.

McKeil CF Jr, Graf EC, Callahan DH: Renal artery aneurysms: A report of 16 cases. J Urol 1966;96:593.

McPherson RI: Supernumerary kidney: Typical and atypical features. Can Assoc Radiol J 1987;38:116.

Merklin RJ, Michele NA: The variant renal and suprarenal blood supply with data on the inferior phrenic, ureteral and gonadal arteries: A statistical analysis based on 185 dissections and review of the literature. J Int Coll Surg 1958;29:41.

Mesrobian H-GJ, Kelalis PP, Hrabovsky E, et al: Wilms' tumor in horseshoe kidneys: A report from the National Wilms' Tumor Study. J Urol 1985;133:1002.

Mesrobian HG, Rushton HG, Bulas D: Unilateral renal agenesis may result from in utero regression of multicystic renal dysplasia. J Urol 1993;150:793.

Miles BJ, Moon MR, Bellville WD, Keesling VJ: Solitary crossed renal ectopia. J Urol 1985;133:1022.

Mohaupt MG, Perrig M, Vogt B: 3D ultrasound imaging: A useful noninvasive tool to detect A-V fistulas in transplanted kidneys. Nephrol Dial Transplant 1999;14:943.

Moore T: Hydrocalycosis. Br J Urol 1950;22:304.

Nathan J: Observation on aberrant renal arteries curving around and compressing the renal vein: Possible relationship to orthostatic proteinuria and to orthostatic hypertension. Circulation 1958;18:1131.

N'Guessan G, Stephens FD: Supernumerary kidney. J Urol 1983;130:649.

N'Guessan G, Stephens FD: Congenital superior ectopic (thoracic) kidney. Urology 1984;24:219.

Parker JA, Lebowitz R, Mascatello V, Treves S: Magnification renal scintigraphy in differential diagnosis of septa of Bertin. Pediatr Radiol 1976;4:157.

Patriquin H, Lafortune M, Filiatrault D: Urinary milk of calcium in children and adults: Use of gravity-dependent sonography. AJR Am J Roentgenol 1985;144:407.

Pitts WR, Muecke EC: Horseshoe kidneys: A 40 year experience. J Urol 1975;113:743.

Potter EL: Bilateral renal agenesis. J Pediatr 1946a;29:68.

Potter EL: Facial characteristics in infants with bilateral renal agenesis. Am J Obstet Gynecol 1946b;51:885.

Potter EL: Bilateral absence of ureters and kidneys: A report of 50 cases. Obstet Gynecol 1965;25:3.

Poutasse EF: Renal artery aneurysms. J Urol 1975;113:443.

Raj GV, Auge BK, Assimos D, Preminger GM: Metabolic abnormalities associated with renal calculi in patients with horseshoe kidneys. J Endourol 2004;18:157-161.

Roodhooft AM, Birnholz JC, Holmes LD: Familial nature of congenital absence and severe dysgenesis of both kidneys. N Engl J Med 1984;310:1341.

Rugui C, Oldrizzi L, Lupo A, et al: Clinical features of patients with solitary kidneys. Nephron 1986;43:10.

Salcarga ME, Arslan H, Unal O: The role of power Doppler sonography in the renal evaluation of fetal renal vasculature. Clin Imaging 1999;23:32.

Sampaio FJB, Aragao AHM: Anatomical relationship between the intrarenal arteries and the kidney collecting system. J Urol 1990a;143:679.

Sampaio FJB, Aragao AHM: Anatomical relationship between the renal venous arrangement and the kidney collecting system. J Urol 1990b;143:679.

Segura JW, Kelalis PP, Burke EG: Horseshoe kidney in children. J Urol 1972;108:333.

Siegel MJ, McAlister WH: Calyceal diverticula in children: Unusual features and complications. Radiology 1979;131:79.

Sipek A, Gregor V, Horacek J, et al: Incidence of renal agenesis in the Czech Republic from 1961-1995. Ceska Gynekol 1997;62:340-343.

Stewart TL, Irons MB, Cowan JM, Bianchi DW: Increased incidence of renal anomalies in patients with chromosome 22q11 microdeletion. Teratology 1999;59:20-22.

Stroup NE, Edmonds L, O'Brien TR: Renal agenesis and dysgenesis: Are they increasing? Teratology 1990;42:383-395.

Takaha M, Matsumoto A, Ochi K, et al: Intrarenal arteriovenous malformation. J Urol 1980;124:315.

Thompson DP, Lynn HB: Genital anomalies associated with solitary kidney. Mayo Clin Proc 1966;41:538.

Thompson GJ, Pace JM: Ectopic kidney: A review of 97 cases. Surg Gynecol Obstet 1937;64:935.

Timmons JW Jr, Malek RS, Hattery RR, DeWeerd J: Caliceal diverticulum. J Urol 1975;114:6.

Toppercer A: Unipapillary human kidney associated with urinary and genital abnormalities. Urology 1980;16:194.

Uhlenhuth E, Amin M, Harty JI, Howerton LW: Infundibular dysgenesis: A spectrum of obstructive renal disease. Urology 1990;35:334.

Weizer AZ, Silverstein AD, Auge BK, et al: Determining the incidence of horseshoe kidney from radiographic data at a single institution. J Urol 2003;170:1722-1726.

Weyrauch HM Jr: Anomalies of renal rotation. Surg Gynecol Obstet 1939;69:183.

Williams AG, Christie JH, Mettler SA: Intrathoracic kidney on radionuclide renography. Clin Nucl Med 1983;8:408.

Yoder IC, Pfister RC: Unilateral hematocolpos and ipsilateral renal agenesis: Report of two cases and review of the literature. AJR Am J Roentgenol 1976;127:303.

Zenteno JC, Mendez JP, Maya-Nunez G, et al: Renal anomalies in patients with Kallmann syndrome. Br J Urol Int 1999;83:383-386.

114 Renal Dysgenesis and Cystic Disease of the Kidney

KENNETH I. GLASSBERG, MD

Not so long ago the student of urology thought of normal kidney development simply in terms of a ureteric bud developing from the wolffian duct at 4 weeks of gestation and growing toward a cluster of mesenchymal cells, where it would induce metanephric development. Today, a basic knowledge of molecular genetics is required to better understand normal renal development, absence of renal development, and the effects of genetic mutations and abnormal signaling proteins on renal maldevelopment and cystic diseases. This chapter begins with a simplified interpretation of the molecular genetics of renal development. The remainder of the chapter is devoted to renal maldevelopment in terms of dysgenesis and cystic disease. Understanding the molecular genetics of renal development will help the reader to understand the genetic and molecular defects of many of the conditions discussed.

MOLECULAR GENETICS

If a mutant gene is responsible for maldevelopment of an organ in utero, then that gene in its normal form is likely to play an integral role in normal organogenesis. Likewise, if a mutant gene is responsible for the development of a tumor in an organ later in life, then that gene in its normal state most likely acts as a tumor suppressor gene postnatally and may play a role in regulating the growth of cells in utero. A number of the gene defects that are responsible for renal disease or maldevelopment are discussed in this section, including how some of these same genes, when normal, play a part in normal renal development. Further discussion on the specific genes involved with renal development appears in Chapter 106, "Normal Development of the Urogenital System," and in an article by Glassberg in 2002.

Classic Genetics

Typically, geneticists follow a sequence to identify a gene that causes a specific disease. The sequence starts with mapping the area of a chromosome where a gene is located. This is facilitated by finding common flanking genetic markers in a specific chromosomal area in multiple affected family members.

The genetic markers will be the same in all affected members within a family but will be different from the markers in unaffected family members. An effort is made to find closer flanking genetic markers that are "linked" to the disease gene, progressively leading to a very small area. Once the gene site is identified, the gene can be cloned. Geneticists then create defects in that gene in animal models and observe whether a similar malfunction, disease, or tumor results. When sporadic cases exist, the geneticist must determine whether the same gene defect is involved. For example, **von Hippel-Lindau (VHL) disease is inherited in 70% of patients but in 30% the disease is sporadic and is not present in other family members. That percentage will start to fall since some VHL disease patients without a family history are being found to have a parent who is mosaic for a** *VHL* **mutation, presumably a de novo one** (Murgia et al, 2000; Sgambat et al, 2000). **However, whether inherited or sporadic, the same gene is defective in both, although the defect may differ from patient to patient** (Zbar et al, 1996; Neumann and Zbar, 1997).

Genes and Their Products

The protein product of a gene often has the same name as the gene. Human genes usually appear in the literature capitalized and italicized. The protein product of a gene is in capitals but not italicized. For example, the *WNT4* gene produces the glycoprotein WNT4. Whether the *WNT4* gene is normal or abnormal, it is still called *WNT4*. In general, when a gene is normal its protein product is normal as well. When a gene is abnormal, it produces an abnormal protein that can lead to maldevelopment or disease. When a defective gene is responsible for a disease, that gene, when normal or even when abnormal, often is named after the disease. For example, the gene responsible for the entity von Hippel-Lindau (VHL) disease is called the *VHL* gene either in its normal state performing its normal activities or in its mutant state causing the disease to manifest. When normal, *VHL* is a tumor suppressor gene; when abnormal, it can play a role in mitogenesis.

Sometimes more than one gene is responsible for a specific disease. **For example, an abnormality of one of two genes is responsible for the entity tuberous sclerosis. One tuberous sclerosis gene,** *TSC1,* **is located on chromosome 2 and the second,** *TSC2,* **on chromosome 16. In autosomal dominant polycystic kidney disease (ADPKD), an abnormality in any one of three genes is responsible for manifestation of the disease. The** *PKD1* **gene is located on chromosome 16, and the** *PKD2* **gene is on chromosome 4; a** *PKD3* **gene is believed to exist, but its location has not yet been identified.** *PKD1* **and** *TSC2* **are located side by side on chromosome 16 and are referred to as contiguous gene syndromes. When cystic disease is manifest in neonates, then either condition's mutations can extend into the adjacent gene (see later).**

Polycystin-1 is a long-chain glycoprotein produced by the ADPKD gene *PKD1* on chromosome 16. Polycystin-2 is produced by the *PKD2* gene on chromosome 4. These two genes seem to play a role, along with the signaling gene *WNT4,* in normal tubulogenesis in the developing metanephrenic kidney. When either the *PKD1* or the *PKD2*

gene is abnormal, cystic kidneys can develop. Because defects of *PKD1* and *PKD2* manifest similarly, Qian and associates (1996) suggested that the gene product of each is involved in the same pathway and that an abnormality of either product results in similar manifestations of the disease.

KEY POINTS: MOLECULAR GENETICS

- Knudson's "two-hit theory" accounts for most heritable cystic disease conditions.

- The "two-hit theory" involves a first hit, that is, one allele of a gene already mutated at the germ cell level (germ cell mutation), and a second hit, that is, a mutation that develops in the second allele, the wild-type allele, in cells in one or more organs later in life (somatic cell mutation).

Two-Hit Theory

Each gene within a cell is one of a set of two; each is called an allele. One defective allele may be the carrier for the defect. Its normal allele is referred to as the "wild type." In Knudson's (1991) two-hit theory, the first hit in an inherited mutation is found in all cells of an individual (i.e., a germline mutation). The second hit occurs when the wild-type allele spontaneously mutates within a specific organ, although it may be a different mutation than in the primarily affected allele (Knudson, 1993).

For example, the typical somatic cells in the kidney and all other cells of a patient with VHL disease typically are heterozygous for the *VHL* gene located on chromosome 3; that is, the mutant *VHL* allele is inherited and its mate is the normal wild-type allele. However, the configuration of wild-type *VHL* makes it prone to spontaneous mutation. If the wild-type allele develops a defect within the cells of a specific organ, those cells no longer are able to produce normal pVHL with its suppressor properties. That organ then has the propensity to develop a tumor. In kidney cells of individuals with VHL disease, for example, heterozygosity is lost when the wild-type allele mutates, and there is a propensity to develop a clear cell renal cell carcinoma. To determine whether cysts lined with epithelial cells are predisposed to renal cell carcinoma (RCC), Lubensky and coworkers (1996) studied partial nephrectomy specimens of two patients with familial VHL disease with RCC who underwent renal-sparing surgery. The makeup of 26 cysts was studied with microdissection techniques. Each cyst was found to be lined with a single layer of clear epithelial cells. Twenty-five of the 26 cysts had a mutation of the wild-type allele; in only one case was the usual heterozygosity of the disease maintained. This finding supports the two-hit theory. Once the heterozygosity for *VHL* is lost in a specific organ, in this case the kidney, the cyst can progress into a tumor. However, the progression to RCC in VHL disease typically is slow.

The variability in manifestations of ADPKD may be related to a two-hit phenomenon as well. For example, ADPKD is a heterozygous condition in which one allele of the *PKD1* **or** *PKD2* **set is responsible for the genetic trans-**

mission of the disease but may not be enough for cystogenesis. A spontaneous mutation of the wild-type allele may be responsible for cystogenesis or for other manifestations of the disease. Qian and associates (1996) suggested that the *PKD1* gene has an unusual genomic structure that makes it readily mutable for a second hit, and the timing of this second hit may account for the phenotypic variability within one family. The second hit itself may occur only in a few cells, possibly accounting for the fact that fewer than 1% of nephrons in ADPKD eventually develop cysts (Qian et al, 1996). Within a cyst, many but not all of the lining cells have lost their heterozygosity (Brazier and Henske, 1997; Qian et al, 1999).

RENAL AGENESIS

Renal agenesis, or absent kidney development, can occur secondary to a defect of the wolffian duct, ureteric bud, or metanephric blastema. Bilateral agenesis occurs in 1 of every 4000 births and has a male predominance (Potter, 1965). Because the placenta filters the fetus's blood, it is not the lack of kidney tissue that causes early death but rather the lack of urine production and oligohydramnios. Affected infants are born with immature lungs and pneumothorax, Potter's facies (hypertelorism, prominent inner canthal folds, and recessive chin), and orthopedic defects secondary to intrauterine compression. The actual incidence of agenesis cannot be determined by imaging studies because aplastic kidneys can be misinterpreted as agenesis because they lack function and are too small to be visualized on any study. Most cases of bilateral agenesis are sporadic, and many are associated with other congenital anomalies, including urogenital sinus defects.

Unilateral agenesis is more common, with an incidence of 1 in 450 to 1000 births (Kass and Bloom, 1992). Because it may be secondary to a wolffian duct abnormality and the wolffian duct lies adjacent to the müllerian duct, renal agenesis may be associated with malformation of the ipsilateral uterine horn or fallopian tube or absence of the ipsilateral ovary in the female, or with absence of the ipsilateral testis, vas deferens, or seminiferous tubules in the male. The eponym Mayer-Rokitansky-Küster-Hauser syndrome refers to a group of associated findings that include unilateral renal agenesis or renal ectopia, ipsilateral müllerian defects, and vaginal agenesis.

Cascio and associates (1999) **found unilateral renal agenesis to be associated with other urologic abnormalities in 48% of patients, including primary vesicoureteral reflux (28%), obstructive megaureter (11%), and ureteropelvic junction obstruction (3%). These findings are similar to those associated with unilateral multicystic kidney disease, suggesting the possibility that some of these "agenetic" kidneys represent involuted multicystic dysplastic kidneys.** Furthermore, it implies that unilateral renal agenesis and unilateral multicystic kidney may have similar causes.

On rare occasions, when either unilateral or bilateral agenesis is associated with a group of other renal abnormalities within a family, the term *familial renal adysplasia* is used. Additional reading on renal agenesis may be found in Chapter 113, "Anomalies of the Upper Urinary Tract."

KEY POINTS: RENAL AGENESIS

- Bilateral renal agenesis is associated with oligohydramnios and Potter's facies (hypertelorism, prominent inner canthal folds, and recessive chin).

- Unilateral agenesis diagnosed at birth or thereafter may represent an in utero involuted multicystic kidney.

DYSPLASIA

Precise definitions as adopted in 1987 by the American Academy of Pediatrics (AAP) Section on Urology (Glassberg et al, 1987) are employed in this chapter. **Renal dysgenesis** is maldevelopment of the kidney that affects its size, shape, or structure. Dysgenesis is of three principal types: dysplastic, hypoplastic, and cystic. Although dysplasia is always accompanied by a decreased number of nephrons (i.e., hypoplasia), the converse is not true; hypoplasia may occur in isolation. When both conditions are present, the term *hypodysplasia* is preferred (Schwarz et al, 1981a). Aplastic dysplasia is represented by a nubbin of nonfunctioning tissue, not necessarily of reniform shape, that meets the histologic criteria for dysplasia. In-utero and postnatal follow-up by ultrasound has shown that some multicystic kidneys shrink with time into such nubbins. Therefore, some instances of aplasia may represent the involuted stage of a multicystic kidney.

Definition

Whereas dysplasia is the leading cause of renal failure in children, it still has no universal definition. First, it must be understood that dysplasia is a histologic diagnosis made by the presence of embryonic mesenchyme and primitive renal components. Metanephric development begins to take place, but formation into normal nephrons and collecting ducts may come to a halt at a time when a particular gene or genetic pathway malfunctions. Common histologic features include distortion of renal architecture, immature or primitive glomeruli, nephron precursors such as comma and S-shaped bodies, and cartilage and tubules encircled by collars of fibromuscular cells (referred to as primitive ducts) (Fig. 114–1). Cysts may or may not be present. There seems to be two types of dysplasia—one in which alterations in a genetic pathway important for nephron or collecting duct formation lead to abnormal development, sometimes with cyst formation, and the second caused by obstruction.

Primitive Duct

Ericsson and Ivemark (1958) considered primitive ducts to be the sine qua non finding of all dysplasia. However, the embryologic derivation of primitive ducts is still not clear. Possibilities include remnants of ureteric bud branches that have never connected with the nephron system and persistent nephron precursors that fail to develop further in the

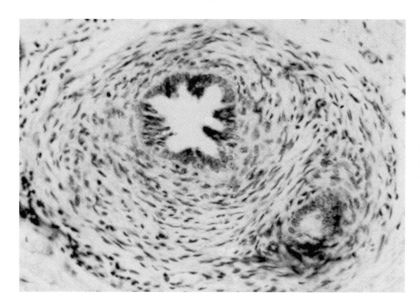

Figure 114–1. Primitive duct lined with columnar epithelial cells. Note concentric arrangement of spindle mesenchymal cells around the duct. Special staining is required to demonstrate smooth muscle cells.

face of early gestational obstruction. The latter is less likely because nephron differentiation appears to be independent of obstruction. The limited effect of obstruction on nephrogenesis is probably related to low filtration pressures during nephrogenesis.

KEY POINTS: DYSPLASIA

■ The hallmark of dysplasia is the "primitive duct," a duct encircled by a collar of fibromuscular cells.

■ Cartilage often accompanies dysplasia.

■ Dysplasia often is associated with ectopically located ureteral orifices.

Cystic and Other Forms of Dysplasia

Potter (1972) described four types of renal cystic disease, with type II and IV representing two distinct forms of cystic dysplasia. Type II is the typical multicystic dysplastic kidney, and type IV is dysplasia associated with obstruction. The latter form is often seen at the periphery of the kidney, at the nephrogenic zone, and frequently with subcapsular cysts. This type usually develops later on in gestation such as in the case of posterior urethral valves (PUV). Dysplasia may also be associated with ureteral ectopia, where it is not clear if it is the obstruction, aberrant ureteric bud formation, or some other factor that leads to the dysplasia. Dysplasia that is sometimes associated with vesicoureteral reflux would be included in this category. Lastly, dysplasia is associated with various dysmorphic clinical conditions (e.g., Fraser syndrome, brachiooto-renal (BOR) syndrome, renal-coloboma syndrome, Kallman syndrome, Simpson-Golabi-Behmel syndrome, Townes-Brocks syndrome). The kidney in association with these conditions may be composed mostly of normal functioning parenchyma with areas of dysplasia, or alternatively the entire kidney may be dysplastic.

When a cyst is identified, it is not always clear if that particular cyst resulted from abnormal development or some obstruction distal to it. Therefore, there is confusion as to when cysts are truly dysplastic or just examples of nephron stretching. We must be able to differentiate cysts that lend evidence to maldevelopment or dedifferentiation from those that develop secondary to stretching. Too often authors cite the development of cysts in animal models with obstruction as evidence of dysplasia, although other findings that are frequently associated with dysplasia are not mentioned. The multicystic form of dysplasia is discussed later in the chapter.

Obstruction

Fetal obstruction or obstruction in animal models created soon after birth can lead to dilatation at various segments of the nephron and collecting duct, inhibition of nephron development in the nephrogenic zone, increased transforming growth factor-β (TGF-β), architectural disorganization, the appearance of primitive glomeruli, and S-shaped bodies and cysts and, at times, can even lead to dedifferentiation, that is, conversion of epithelial cells back into mesenchymal cells and even of mesenchymal cells into myofibroblast (Peters et al, 1992; Nguyen et al, 1999; Matsell and Tarantal, 2002).

A number of questions regarding obstruction and dysplasia need to be answered. For example, why is dysplasia seen more often in association with PUV as compared with ureteropelvic junction obstruction? Why do some valve patients with apparently equally obstructive PUV have dysplastic kidneys (with the dysplasia usually at the periphery) while others do not? Why is the prognosis much worse for fetuses with PUV in which hydronephrosis appears before 24 weeks, and much more optimistic if the hydronephrosis first appears after 24 weeks? (Glassberg, 2002). Does this have to do with timing of urachal closure? Is there a way of prolonging patency of the urachus and thus avoid the need to create a vesicoamniotic shunt? Is there an age of gestation when in-utero shunting is too late? (Figs. 114–2 and 114–3).

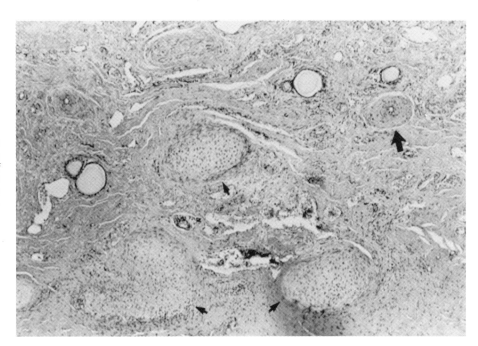

Figure 114–2. Histologic specimen of a nonfunctioning reflux kidney in a patient with posterior urethral valves. Note presence of nests of cartilage *(small arrows)*. Primitive ducts are scattered throughout the specimen *(large arrow)* (×100). The findings are compatible with dysplasia.

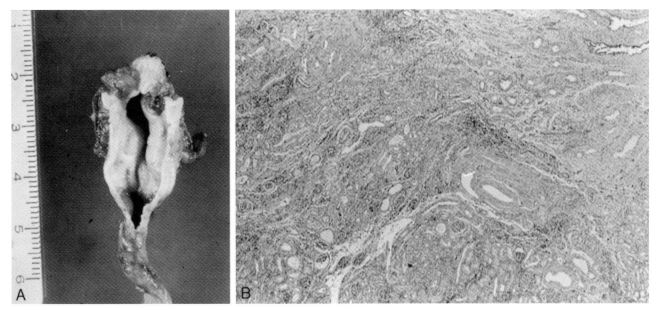

Figure 114–3. Upper pole of a duplex kidney associated with an ectopic ureterocele. **A,** Gross specimen has visible tiny cysts. **B,** On histology, primitive glomeruli are seen on left side and primitive ducts are seen in upper right corner (×40).

Bud Defects

The Mackie-Stephens (1975) bud theory suggests that ectopic (cephalad or caudal) ureteric bud formation leads to abnormal ureteric orifice location and penetration of the ureteric bud into a peripheral area of the metanephric blastema. The result is a marginal (i.e., hypoplastic or dysplastic) kidney. As of now, there is no direct experimental evidence to prove that an abnormal ureteric bud site leads to ureteric bud penetration at a peripheral area of the blastema. However, there is a plethora of findings supporting the idea that defects in genetic pathways can affect ureteric bud formation, branching morphogenesis within the metanephric blastema, and normal nephrogenesis (e.g., RET, RAR, BMP4, SLIT2-ROBO2, AT2) (Mendelsohn et al, 1994; Pope et al, 2001; Grieshammer et al, 2004). The genetic defect at each point may be the same, but the downstream pathway associated with the defect may vary for each process.

Familial Adysplasia

Renal agenesis, renal dysplasia, multicystic dysplasia, and renal aplasia usually appear as isolated, sporadic occurrences. On rare occasions, this group of anomalies may appear in many family members but heterogeneously. In other words, one family member may have renal agenesis while another has renal dysplasia and still another has a multicystic dysplastic or aplastic kidney. When all or part of this group of anomalies is seen in one family, an encompassing term for these four entities is used: *familial renal adysplasia.*

HYPOPLASIA AND HYPODYSPLASIA

Hypoplasia and hypodysplasia are subclassified in Table 114–1. The subdivision according to the nature of the ureteral orifice acknowledges the bud theory but is not necessarily intended to be an endorsement of that theory. **Hypodysplastic kidneys most often occur in conjunction with ectopic ureteral orifices, with the extent of dysplasia correlating with the degree of ectopia** (Schwarz et al, 1981a, 1981b, 1981c). However, hypodysplastic kidneys are seen in a few patients with normal ureteral orifices. In such cases, obstruction may or may not be present.

Renal Hypoplasia

To avoid perpetuating the confusion that has attended the use of the term *hypoplasia,* its use should be restricted to kidneys that have less than the normal number of calyces and nephrons but are not dysplastic or embryonic. The truly hypoplastic kidney may have a normal nephron density despite its small size.

Hypoplasia may be bilateral or unilateral. In unilateral cases, the other kidney usually shows greater compensatory growth than is characteristic in patients with renal atrophy caused by acquired disease. Hypoplasia can be associated with reflux, and the term *reflux nephropathy* is now applied to all types of abnormality associated with reflux. Segmental hypoplasia (Ask-Upmark kidney) probably is a type of reflux nephropathy.

Because of the similarity of the word *oligonephronia* (literally translated as a decreased number of nephrons) to oligomeganephronia, which is a specific clinical entity (see following discussion), the former term should not be used.

Oligomeganephronia

The combination of a marked reduction in the number of nephrons and hypertrophy of each nephron was described in 1962 (Habib et al, 1962; Royer et al, 1962) **and termed *oligomeganephronia.*** It is usually a bilateral condition, although a few instances of unilateral oligomeganephronia associated with contralateral renal agenesis have been reported (Griffel et al, 1972; Lam et al, 1982; Forster and Hawkins, 1994).

Clinical Features

While oligomeganephronia is a congenital disorder, it also is a nonfamilial one that affects boys more often than girls (3:1). It frequently is associated with low birth weight (2500 g). The condition usually is discovered soon after the child's birth or, if not, then usually by age 2 years. Infants most frequently are brought to medical attention because of vomiting, dehydration, intense thirst, and polyuria. The creatinine clearance is abnormal (10 to 50 mL/min/1.73 m^2), and the maximum specific gravity of the urine is 1.007 to 1.012. Moderate proteinuria may be present, but this is more likely to be a later finding.

Renal function remains below normal (although stable) for many years, but polydipsia and polyuria can worsen, and growth is severely retarded in many cases. As the patient enters his or her teens, the creatinine clearance begins to drop rapidly. Marked proteinuria (2 g/24 hr) is common.

Histopathology

The kidneys are smaller than normal (average weight at autopsy, 20 to 25 g) and are not always the same size. Van Acker and colleagues (1971) suggested that because of the reduced number of nephrons, those that do exist increase in size to compensate for the deficiency in number. The kidneys are pale and firm with a granular cortical surface and no clear distinction between the cortex and the medulla. The number of renal segments is reduced, usually to five or six, although unirenicular and birenicular kidneys have been described (Bernstein, 1968). The renal artery is small. There is a reduced normal of nephrons, which are all elongated, sometimes fourfold, and widened particularly at the proximal end (Fig. 114–4).

Evaluation

The kidneys may concentrate contrast medium adequately for an intravenous urogram, producing a picture of small kidneys, usually with normally formed calyces, although Morita and associates (1973) described a patient with dysmorphic calyces. The small kidneys also can be identified by sonography (Scheinman and Abelson, 1970).

Treatment

High fluid intake and correction of salt loss and acidosis are the initial steps. Daily dietary protein should be limited to 1.5 g/kg during the stable phase (Royer et al, 1962). Frank renal failure is managed by dialysis and transplantation. The allograft may come from a living related donor because the disease is not familial.

Table 114–1.   Classification of Hypoplasia and Hypodysplasia

Hypoplasia

True ("oligonephronia")
With normal ureteral orifice
With abnormal ureteral orifice
Oligomeganephronia
Segmental (Ask-Upmark kidney)

Hypodysplasia

With normal ureteral orifice
   With obstruction
   Without obstruction
With abnormal ureteral orifice
   Lateral ectopia
   Medial or caudal ectopia with ureterocele
With urethral obstruction
Prune-belly syndrome

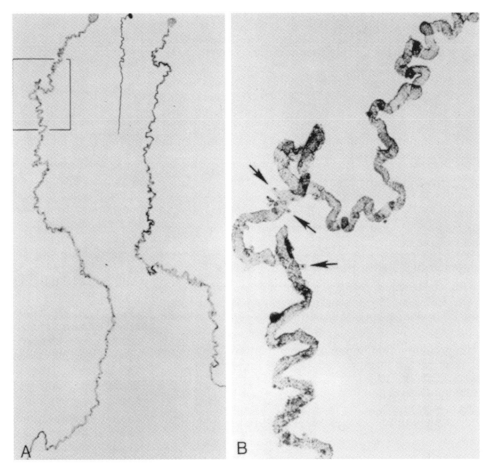

Figure 114-4. A, Mosaic photograph of two typical proximal tubules dissected from the kidney of a patient with oligomeganephronia. The silhouette in the top center is a diagrammatic representation to scale of an average proximal tubule from a kidney of an age-matched control. **B,** Enlargement of the *inset* in **A** showing the diverticula along the course of the nephron *(arrows)*. (From Fetterman GH, Habib R: Congenital bilateral oligonephronic renal hypoplasia with hypertrophy of nephrons [oligomeganephronia]. Am J Clin Pathol 1969;52: 199-207.)

KEY POINTS: HYPOPLASIA AND HYPODYSPLASIA

- Hypoplasia and hypodysplasia often are associated with ectopic orifices and sometimes with obstruction.

- Hypoplasia applies to kidneys with a decreased number of nephrons and calyces.

- Oligomegonephronia is a condition with small kidneys and elongated, widened nephrons.

- Ask-Upmark kidneys have segmented dysplasia, are seen most frequently in association with reflux, and are often accompanied by hypertension.

Ask-Upmark Kidney (Segmental Hypoplasia)

In 1929, Ask-Upmark described distinctive small kidneys in eight patients, seven of whom had malignant hypertension; six of these patients were adolescents.

Etiology

Although the Ask-Upmark kidney was originally thought to be a developmental lesion because of the youth of the first

patients, it more likely represents histologic changes secondary to infection even though areas of dysplasia sometimes can be seen.

Clinical Features

Most patients are 10 years of age or older at diagnosis. The disease is associated with severe hypertension, sometimes with headaches, either alone or together with hypertensive encephalopathy (Rosenfeld et al, 1973) and with retinopathy in half of the patients (Royer et al, 1971).

Proteinuria and some degree of renal insufficiency may be present if the disease is bilateral. Approximately half of the patients in the series described by Royer and associates (1971) had these signs at diagnosis.

Histopathology

The Ask-Upmark kidney is smaller than normal—12 to 35 g (Royer et al, 1971). Its distinctive feature is one or more deep grooves on the lateral convexity, underneath which the parenchyma consists of tubules resembling those in the thyroid gland. Usually, the hypoplastic segments are easily distinguished from adjacent areas. The medulla consists of a thin band, and remnants of the corticomedullary junction and arcuate arteries are seen. Arteriosclerosis is common, and juxtaglomerular hyperplasia may be seen (Bernstein, 1968; Meares and Gross, 1972; Kaufman and Fay, 1974; Arant et al, 1979).

Treatment

In patients with unilateral disease, partial or total nephrectomy may control the hypertension (Royer et al, 1971; Meares and Gross, 1972). Failure of this measure suggests an unrecognized scar or generalized arteriosclerosis in the remaining kidney (Arant et al, 1979). Bilateral disease with renal insufficiency usually is managed medically, although dialysis and transplantation may be needed. Correction of reflux may prevent further renal damage but probably will have no effect on the hypertension.

Renal Hypodysplasia

Hypodysplasia may be associated with a normal or abnormal ureteral orifice, ureterocele, urethral obstruction, or prune-belly syndrome.

Hypodysplasia with Normal Ureteral Orifice

With Obstruction. Primary obstructive megaureter and ureteropelvic junction obstruction usually are associated with small but normal-appearing and normally situated ureteral orifices. In general, this kidney has suffered diffuse damage because of hydronephrosis, although in a few cases small areas or even the entire kidney is hypodysplastic or shows multicystic dysplasia (Fig. 114–5).

Without Obstruction. The "dwarf" kidney, although usually described as hypoplastic, is in fact usually hypodysplastic. The calyces are normally cupped but generally fewer in number

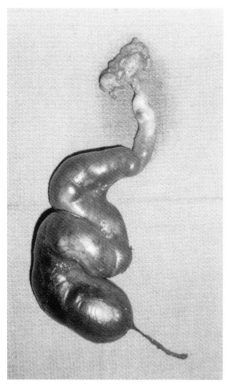

Figure 114–5. Small hypodysplastic kidney found in association with a severely obstructed primary megaureter. (From Glassberg KI, Filmer RB: Renal dysplasia, renal hypoplasia and cystic disease of the kidney. In Kelalis P, King LR, Belman AB [eds]: Clinical Pediatric Urology. Philadelphia, WB Saunders, 1985, pp 922-971.)

than would be expected from the size of the kidney. According to the bud theory, the dwarf kidney is the result of deficient metanephric blastema rather than a budding abnormality (Stephens, 1983).

Hypodysplasia with Abnormal Ureteral Orifice

The small kidney associated with an abnormally positioned orifice usually is thin with ectatic calyces. The thin parenchyma is thought to reflect insufficient divisions of the ureteral bud, with a consequent reduction in the number of nephrons induced (Stephens, 1983). The calyces generally are rounded, a picture characteristic of an earlier stage of development, before proliferating nephrons and papillary bulging indent the calyces to create the mature cup shape (Sommer and Stephens, 1981).

The radiographic appearance of rounded calyces should not be mistaken for the clubbing associated with reflux nephropathy, which is caused by parenchymal scars overlying the calyces rather than by the premature termination of calyceal development. On the basis of the view that abnormal budding leads to an ectopic ureteral orifice with thin renal parenchyma and ectatic calyces, Sommer and Stephens (1981) designated the condition the "pan-bud anomaly." Their theory seems particularly applicable in duplex systems in which the thin renal segment with ectatic calyces is associated with a ureter draining ectopically into either a medial (often obstructed) or a lateral ureteric orifice.

Lateral Ectopia. **Lateral ectopia usually is associated with reflux.** If the pan-bud theory is correct, the rounded calyces found in the newborn with no history of infection are the result of premature termination of calyceal development rather than of ballooning under the constant high-pressure assault by refluxing urine. Of course, infection leading to scarring and clubbing can confuse the picture, although pyelonephritic scars often create a characteristic indentation of the renal outline over the clubbed calyx (Hodson, 1981).

Medial or Caudal Ectopia and Ureteroceles. When the ureterovesical junction is displaced medially, the ureter and renal pelvis usually are dilated. The renal cortex may be thin, as in hydronephrosis, or severely dysplastic, perhaps with numerous small cysts (see Fig. 114–3). When obstruction is complete, as in blind ureterocele, the upper pole segment may mimic the multicystic kidney histologically (Stephens, 1983).

Hypodysplasia with Urethral Obstruction

According to Osathanondh and Potter (1964), **posterior urethral valves may be associated with two types of renal hypodysplasia.** In the less severe form, there are small, usually subcapsular cysts and nearly normal renal function, a picture that could be caused by increased pressure secondary to urinary outflow obstruction. In the second form, the cysts are larger and more widely distributed, and numerous islands of cartilage are present. This form usually is associated with earlier onset and more severe obstruction and reflux (see Fig. 114–2). Osathanondh and Potter (1964) believed that this highly abnormal condition has etiologic factors beyond urethral obstruction, and here again abnormal budding appears to be involved.

In patients with posterior urethral valves, the position of the ureteral orifice correlates well with the extent of hypodysplasia, as shown by Henneberry and Stephens (1980) and by Schwarz and colleagues (1981b). When the orifice is normally positioned, the kidney is histologically good but hydronephrotic, whereas a laterally placed orifice is associated with hypoplasia and an extremely lateral orifice is associated with hypodysplasia. This correlation is present regardless of the presence or absence of reflux or the degree of urethral obstruction, suggesting that obstruction is not the only factor involved in creating the histologic picture. Further evidence of the role of factors beyond obstruction comes from cases of congenital ureteropelvic junction obstruction or primary obstructive megaureter, in which the ureteral orifices are almost always normally positioned and the kidneys are rarely dysplastic.

Hypodysplasia Associated with Prune-Belly Syndrome

The features of the prune-belly syndrome (absent abdominal musculature, triad syndrome) include grossly deformed kidneys, which may have various degrees of dysplasia. The ureters are wide and tortuous, often with large and laterally placed orifices. The dysplasia in the kidneys of these patients is explainable by the abnormal budding theory of Mackie and Stephens (1975). Urethral obstruction or atresia may be present in the most severe cases, but usually there is no lower urinary tract obstruction.

CYSTIC DISEASE

The kidney is one of the most common sites in the body for cysts. Although the lesions themselves in the various cystic conditions are histologically similar (i.e., microscopic or macroscopic sacs lined with epithelium), their number, location, and clinical features are different. Some renal cysts are actually ectatic tubules or collecting ducts that are continuous with the nephron. Because any dilated duct or tubule within the kidney can be potentially referred to as a renal cyst, criteria have been suggested for specifying when a dilatation is appropriately called a cyst. Gardner (1988) suggested that ducts dilated to four times their normal diameter (i.e., 200 μm) be called cysts. Some cysts are saccular or fusiform structures that resemble diverticula and are located at various sites along the nephron. Other cysts may or may not communicate with a glomerulus, tubule, collecting duct, or calyx, or they may initially have communicated only to become isolated later on. Cysts may be located diffusely throughout the kidney or in one segment only. They may appear unilaterally or bilaterally. In some entities cysts may represent a form of dysplasia and may be accompanied by other findings of dysplasia.

When cysts are part of an inherited disorder, they may be present at birth or may develop sometime thereafter, perhaps even in adulthood. Some very different entities have similar features. For example, in ADPKD, tuberous sclerosis, VHL disease, and acquired renal cystic disease (ARCD), the cysts have a hyperplastic lining, sometimes with nodules of hyperplasia or polyps that project into the cyst lumen. However, these hyperplastic conditions are very different from each other. Another example of such similarities is the ectatic collecting ducts seen in two very different clinical entities,

autosomal recessive polycystic kidney disease (ARPKD) and medullary sponge kidney.

Most renal cystic conditions—congenital, sporadic, and acquired—arise from the nephrons and collecting ducts after they have formed, whether normally or abnormally. Multicystic dysplasia is an exception in that it arises before formation of the nephron, from abnormal induction of metanephric development, a primary abnormality of the nephrogenic blastema, or obstruction occurring early in renal development. Another exception, benign multilocular cyst, represents a neoplastic growth. The origin of simple cysts is not clear because they develop in kidneys that have apparently been normal throughout life.

Classification

Several classifications have been proposed. In this chapter, the system used is based on one proposed in 1987 by the Committee on Classification, Nomenclature and Terminology of the AAP Section on Urology, in which the primary distinction is between genetic and nongenetic disease and the various disorders are further classified according to their clinical, radiologic, and pathologic features (Table 114–2). A similar classification was offered by Stephens and Cussen (1983) and by Glassberg and Filmer (1985). Two discrete glomerulocystic entities have been added to the AAP classification; these are included in Table 114–2. In addition, because specific genes will soon be identified as the cause of most of the entities included in the nongenetic category, I have chosen to use the terms *heritable* and *nonheritable* for these two broad categories (Table 114–3).

The terms *multicystic* and *polycystic* should not be confused, even though both terms literally mean "many cysts." *Multicystic* refers to a dysplastic entity, and *polycystic* refers to a number of separate entities, most inherited, all without dysplasia and all with nephrons throughout the kidney. The term *polycystic kidney disease* traditionally leads the student to think predominantly of two conditions: ARPKD and ADPKD. Many of the polycystic kidney disease entities progress to renal

---

Table 114–2. Cystic Diseases of the Kidney

Genetic

Autosomal recessive (infantile) polycystic kidney disease
Autosomal dominant (adult) polycystic kidney disease
Juvenile nephronophthisis/medullary cystic disease complex
 Juvenile nephronophthisis (autosomal recessive)
 Medullary cystic disease (autosomal dominant)
Congenital nephrosis (familial nephrotic syndrome) (autosomal recessive)
Familial hypoplastic glomerulocystic disease (autosomal dominant)
Multiple malformation syndromes with renal cysts (e.g., tuberous sclerosis, von Hippel-Lindau disease)

Nongenetic

Multicystic kidney (multicystic dysplastic kidney)
Benign multilocular cyst (cystic nephroma)
Simple cysts
Medullary sponge kidney
Sporadic glomerulocystic kidney disease
Acquired renal cystic disease
Calyceal diverticulum (pyelogenic cyst)

Table 114–3. Characteristics of Various Forms of Cystic Kidneys

Entity	Site of Chromosomal Defect	Characteristic Renal Findings	Associated Anomalies	Incidence
Genetic Cystic Disease				
Autosomal recessive polycystic kidney disease (ARPKD)	6	In newborn usually large, homogeneous, echogenic kidneys; predominantly cysts of collecting ducts	Congenital hepatic fibrosis biliary dysgenesis	1:5,000 to 40,000
Autosomal dominant polycystic kidney disease (ADPKD)		Scattered renal cysts throughout parenchyma; if presenting in infancy may have glomerular cysts; large kidneys	Diverticulitis; liver, spleen and pancreatic cysts; mitral valve regurgitation; intracranial aneurysms; rare association with congenital hepatic fibrosis in neonatal cases	1:500 to 1,000
PKD1	16			~90% of cases
PKD2	4			~10% of cases
PKD3	Not mapped			<1% of cases
Juvenile nephronophthisis/medullary cystic disease complex				
Juvenile nephronophthisis (autosomal recessive)	2	Cysts at corticomedullary junction; develop after onset of renal failure; always thickened tubular basement membrane	80% of families have no extrarenal lesions	1:50,000
Senior-Loken syndrome (autosomal recessive)	Not mapped	Cyst at corticomedullary junction	Retinitis pigmentosa	1:200,000
Medullary cystic disease (autosomal dominant)	Not mapped	Cysts at corticomedullary junction; develop before onset of renal failure; tubular basement membrane may not be thickened	None	1:100,000
Congenital nephrosis Finnish type	19	Dilatation of proximal convoluted tubules; diffuse hypertrophy of podocytes; interstitial fibrosis	Enormously enlarged and edematous placenta; high amniotic α-fetoprotein	1:8200 in Finland; very rare elsewhere; reported in Minnesota
Diffuse mesangial sclerosis	Occasionally inherited	Dilatation of proximal convoluted tubules; diffuse hypertrophy of podocytes; interstitial fibrosis	Drash syndrome: nephrotic syndrome, Wilms' tumor, and male pseudohermaphroditism	Rare; more common worldwide than Finnish type
Familial glomerulocystic kidney disease	Not mapped	Small or normal size kidneys with glomerular cysts	None	Very rare
Tuberous sclerosis (autosomal dominant)		Cysts and angiomyolipomas throughout kidney; cysts even present in utero; 3% incidence of renal cell carcinoma	Adenoma sebaceum; epilepsy; mental retardation; cranial tumors	1:6,000 to 14,500
TSC1	9			
TSC2	16			
von Hippel-Lindau disease (autosomal dominant)	3	Cysts, adenomas, and clear cell renal carcinoma (35%–38% of cases)	Cerebellar hemangioblastoma; retinal angiomas; pheochromocytoma; cysts of pancreas and epididymis	1:30,000 to 50,000
Nongenetic Cystic Disease				
Multicystic dysplastic kidney	No genetic predisposition	Renal maldevelopment with diffuse cysts and remnants of early metanephric development; minimal if any nephron development	Not usual	Most frequent cystic disease in newborn
Benign multilocular cyst	No genetic predisposition	Benign cystic tumor of the kidney; remainder of kidney has normal nephrons that may become crushed by the expanding tumor	None	Present more often in males when younger than age 4 and females when older than age 30
Simple cysts	Rare genetic predisposition	Single or multiple cysts; normal nephrons throughout kidney	None	Very common in normal kidneys with increasing age
Medullary sponge kidney	Rare genetic predisposition	Ectactic collecting ducts; nephrons fairly normal	None	1:5,000 to 20,000
Sporadic glomerulocystic kidney disease	No genetic predisposition	Large kidneys, predominantly glomerular cysts; when seen in infancy, indistinguishable from ADPKD with glomerular cystic kidney disease	10% biliary dysgenesis; hepatic cysts	Very rare
Acquired renal cystic disease	No genetic predisposition (seen with end-stage renal disease)	Diffuse cysts; adenomas; occasionally renal cell carcinoma	None	Incidence increases with duration of end-stage renal disease

failure as the nephrons become more diseased. Other polycystic conditions include a number of diseases with "glomerulocystic" pathology. In tuberous sclerosis and VHL disease, there are hyperplastic cysts and the individual nephrons are normal. Only occasionally do the nephrons become compressed by the cysts or by associated tumors, and only in such situations does renal failure ensue.

Among the nongenetic cystic diseases, benign multilocular cysts and other variants are considered neoplasms. Medullary sponge kidney is a disease principally of dilated ectatic collecting ducts, with cysts playing a lesser role, although the size of the ducts by definition makes them cysts. The nephrons initially are normal.

It will be helpful to the reader to refer back to the genetic and nongenetic entities listed in Tables 114-2 and 114-3, which summarize many of the entities encountered later in the chapter.

KEY POINTS: CYSTIC DISEASE

■ A cyst can be a widened area of the nephron, a diverticulum of the nephron, or an isolated sac.

■ The terms *multicystic* and *polycystic* semantically mean the same but are used to label different conditions.

Bilateral Renal Cystic Disease

Bilateral renal cystic disease creates a dilemma in diagnosis at any age. The differential diagnosis includes ARPKD, ADPKD, tuberous sclerosis, VHL disease, bilateral simple cysts, and ARCD (Table 114–4). The cysts in ARPKD can manifest at any time from in utero to the age of 20 years, those in ADPKD from in utero to autopsy, those in tuberous sclerosis from in utero to any time in life but usually before the age of 30, and those in VHL disease infrequently in the first few years of life but almost always by the age of 30. Bilateral simple cysts can manifest at any age but particularly after age 35 years, and ARCD may become evident after end-stage renal disease (ESRD) develops.

Table 114–4. Sonographic Differential Diagnosis of a Newborn with Bilateral, Large, Cystic Kidneys

Homogenous, Hyperechogenic Kidneys Without Macrocysts	With Diffuse Macrocysts
Autosomal recessive polycystic kidney disease (characteristic appearance)	Autosomal recessive polycystic kidney disease (atypical appearance)
Autosomal dominant polycystic kidney disease (atypical appearance)	Autosomal dominant polycystic kidney disease (characteristic appearance)
Sporadic glomerulocystic kidney disease	Sporadic glomerulocystic kidney disease
Contrast nephropathy	Tuberous sclerosis
Renal vein thrombosis	

Heritable Cystic Disease

Genetic cystic diseases can be broadly classified as autosomal dominant and autosomal recessive forms of polycystic kidneys, autosomal dominant and autosomal recessive forms of medullary cystic kidneys, the autosomal recessive disorder congenital nephrosis, the autosomal dominant disorder familial hypoplastic glomerulocystic disease, and a group of rare disorders that have multiple systemic anomalies.

The genetically determined renal cystic diseases range from the very common to the very rare. Some of these disorders are caused by a single gene defect, some by an X-linked gene defect, and others by chromosomal defects. The specific gene or gene locus has been identified for almost every single-gene (mendelian) disorder (see Table 114–3).

AUTOSOMAL RECESSIVE ("INFANTILE") POLYCYSTIC KIDNEY DISEASE

When polycystic kidney disease is diagnosed in the neonate, it is most often of the recessive type (Cole et al, 1987). The autosomal recessive type in the past has been referred to as the "infantile" form. This confusing and inaccurate age designation should be discarded, because the disease can become manifest initially in adolescents and young adults, although significantly less frequently.

ARPKD has been reported as a rare disease, affecting about 1 of every 40,000 live births (Zerres et al, 1988), as a not so rare disease occurring in 1 of 10,000 births in Finland (Kääriäiren, 1987), and even occurring as frequently as 1 in 5,000 to 10,000 live births (Bernstein and Slovis, 1992). However, as many as 50% of affected newborns die in the first few hours or days of life, making for a significantly lower incidence among children who live for at least 1 year. Of those infants who survive the neonatal period, approximately 50% are alive at 10 years of age (Kaplan et al, 1989b).

ARPKD has a spectrum of severity, the most severe forms appearing earliest in life. If it is not apparent at birth, the disease will become apparent later in childhood (up to age 13 years or, rarely, up to age 20 years) and is bilateral. All patients have varying degrees of congenital hepatic fibrosis as well.

Genetics

Once the diagnosis of ARPKD is strongly suspected, referral for genetic evaluation and counseling is appropriate. A detailed history should be taken of at least three generations. **Because the disease is transmitted as an autosomal recessive trait, siblings of either sex have a 1 in 4 chance of being affected, and neither parent should show evidence of the disease.**

Despite the clinical variability of ARPKD, it appears that only mutations of a single gene named *PKHD1*, located on chromosome 6, is responsible for the disease. The gene produces a protein called fibrocystin (also known as polyductin) (Onuchic et al, 2002; Ward et al, 2002). Fibrocystin is abundant in fetal kidney collecting ducts but absent in the kidneys of some fetuses with ARPKD (Wilson, 2004).

Clinical Features

The earlier the age at which the disease is identified, the more severe the disease. No matter what the severity of the renal disease, all patients with ARPKD have liver involvement in the form of congenital hepatic fibrosis and vary in the degree of biliary ectasia and periportal fibrosis (CHF) (Habib, 1974; Kissane and Smith, 1975). Those with severe ARPKD have mild CHF and those with severe CHF have ARPKD. **Also, the younger the patient at presentation with ARPKD, the milder the liver disease; and, conversely, the younger the patient who presents with congenital hepatic fibrosis, the milder the renal cystic disease.** There also is a mild group of patients who present as teenagers or young adults.

The affected newborn usually has enormous, kidney-shaped, nonbosselated flank masses that are hard and do not transilluminate. In some cases, the kidneys are large enough to impede delivery. Oligohydramnios is common because of the lack of normal urine production by the fetus. The infant often displays Potter's facies and deformities of the limbs and may have respiratory distress as a consequence of pulmonary hypoplasia. Oliguria is to be expected. Because of in-utero "dialysis" by the placenta, the infant's serum creatinine and blood urea nitrogen (BUN) concentrations are those of the mothers' at birth but soon begin to rise.

Years ago those diagnosed as neonates had a very poor prognosis; however, since the routine use of in-utero ultrasound, the spectrum of ARPKD presenting in neonates is much greater and as a result prognosis overall is better. Those with the most severe disease usually die of respiratory failure. Those who survive the first month of life have a milder form of the disease and are likely to survive beyond 1 year. Some diagnosed as neonates can live beyond age 3 or 4 before going into renal failure (Cole et al, 1987; Avni, 2002).

For infants in whom ARPKD is evident at birth, the usual clinical course is death within the first 2 months as a result of uremia or respiratory failure. However, infants who survive their first 31 days have a good chance of living at least 1 year if they receive proper supportive therapy. Cole and associates (1987) monitored 17 such children for a mean of 6.1 years and found that 8 were doing well with glomerular filtration rates greater than 40 mL/min/1.73 m^2, although most were hypertensive. Moreover, three of the five patients who required hemodialysis had needed it before 7 years of age. In such survivors, the kidneys atrophy and shrink (Lieberman et al, 1971).

Children whose disease appears later in life develop renal failure and hypertension more slowly than those in whom ARPKD is manifest at birth. In general, their clinical problems are the consequence of liver disease rather than the renal condition, with hepatic fibrosis leading to portal hypertension, esophageal varices, and hepatosplenomegaly.

Histopathology

The kidneys retain their fetal lobulation. Small subcapsular cysts, representing generalized fusiform dilations of the collecting tubules, are grossly visible when the capsule is removed. In the sectioned kidney, the dilated tubules can be seen in a radial arrangement from the calyx outward to the capsule. The cortex is crowded with minute cysts. The renal pedicle is normal, as are the renal pelvis and ureter. In older children whose disease has been evident since birth, the cysts are large and spherical, similar to those seen in the dominantly inherited disease (see later discussion). The nephron configuration is normal except for small dilatations, leading Potter (1972) to suggest that the abnormality appears late in gestation, with the dilatations of the collecting ducts and nephrons resulting from hyperplasia. Guay-Woodford and colleagues (1998) made similar observations and believed that medullary duct dilatation occurs first and then is followed by cortical collecting duct dilatation. Among patients who survive into childhood, cortical cysts may be the principal finding (Guay-Woodford et al, 1998).

All children with ARPKD have lesions in the periportal areas of the liver (Habib, 1974; Kissane and Smith, 1975). Proliferation, dilatation, and branching of well-differentiated bile ducts and ductules accompany some degree of periportal fibrosis. Gross cysts are not found. Some have suggested that, just as all children with ARPKD have liver disease, all children with congenital hepatic fibrosis have ARPKD; however, it is not certain that this is the case. Darmis and associates (1970) found a 100% incidence of ARPKD in children with congenital hepatic fibrosis; however, there are reports of children with hepatic but not renal disease. Kerr and colleagues (1962) found evidence of ARPKD in 60% of children with congenital hepatic fibrosis using excretory urography. The kidneys were not studied histologically, however, so the true incidence of ARPKD in this series is unknown. Confusing the issue further is the fact that a small number of infants with ADPKD have been found to have congenital hepatic fibrosis (Cobben et al, 1990).

KEY POINTS: ARPKD

- ARPKD was previously called "infantile" polycystic kidney disease.

- ARPKD is secondary to a mutation of the *PKHD1* gene on chromosome 6.

- The severe form presents in utero or in infancy; milder cases can present later in childhood and rarely into the early 20s.

- All affected individuals have some degree of congenital hepatic fibrosis.

- When it manifests early, it is associated most often with very large kidneys that are homogeneously hyperechogenic.

- Discrete cysts appear more often as the child gets older.

- Affected newborns have dilated collecting ducts that radiate to the outer margins of the kidney.

Evaluation

The diagnosis may be suspected from in utero ultrasound examination and may be associated with oligohydramnios, a finding secondary to low urinary output. **In both fetus and newborn, sonography identifies very enlarged, homoge-**

neously hyperechogenic kidneys, especially when compared with the echogenicity of the liver. The increased echogenicity is a result of the return of sound waves from the enormous number of interfaces created by tightly compacted, dilated collecting ducts. In the normal newborn, the kidneys have an equal or slightly increased echogenicity compared with the liver. Within the normal newborn kidney, hypoechogenic areas are seen circumferentially and are very typical of newborn renal pyramids. In comparison, in ARPKD the pyramids are hyperechogenic because they blend in with the rest of the kidney and the kidneys typically have a homogeneous appearance (Fig. 114–6A). In ADPKD in newborns, the cysts if apparent are usually diffuse and large (see Fig. 114–6B). This appearance differs from that of severe bilateral hydronephrosis, in which the kidneys are enlarged with hypoechogenic calyces, or of multicystic kidney, in which hypoechogenic cysts lie within a nonreniform mass that has very little parenchyma. Bilateral mesoblastic nephroma, Wilms' tumor, does not appear as homogeneous masses, and the infant has functioning kidneys. Bilateral renal vein thrombosis produces renal enlargement but hypoechogenic medullary areas. If the diagnosis remains in doubt, computed tomography (CT) is valuable because it is more sensitive to inhomogeneity (and therefore to tumor) within abdominal masses. Macrocysts are rare in newborns but increase in frequency as the child gets older.

Occasionally a newborn with severe ADPKD can also have enlarged, homogeneously hyperechogenic kidneys. Typically, when ADPKD manifests at birth, cysts are apparent on the sonographic image. Macrocysts are rare in newborns with ARPKD but do increase in frequency as the child gets older, sometimes producing an appearance similar to that of the dominant disease. Cysts less than 1 cm appear more often than large cysts (Avni et al, 2002) (Fig. 114–7). However, with time and the development of renal failure, diffuse hyperechoic foci (i.e., white dots) that do not shadow appear. These may be composed of calcium oxalate or citrate (Lucaya et al, 1983; Avni et al, 2002) (Fig. 114–8). **Fetuses with sporadic glomerulocystic kidney disease also can have enlarged, hyperechogenic kidneys** (see Table 114–4).

Intravenous urography with delayed films may show functioning kidneys with characteristic radial or medullary streaking (sunburst pattern) caused by dilated collecting tubules filled with contrast medium. This picture can persist

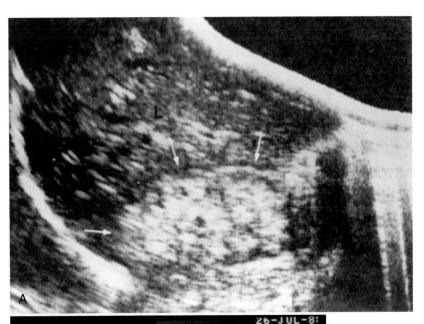

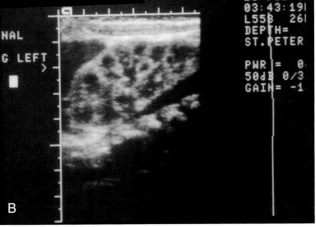

Figure 114–6. **A,** Sonogram of left kidney *(arrows)* in a newborn with autosomal recessive polycystic kidney disease (ARPKD). Note homogeneously hyperechogenic kidneys, especially in comparison with the less echogenic liver (L). Increased echogenicity is caused by the multiple interphases created by the dilated medullary ducts. **B,** In comparison, sonogram of kidney in a newborn with ADPKD. Note the nonhomogeneous appearance with multiple large cysts. (**A** from Grossman H, Rosenberg ER, Bowie JD, et al: Sonographic diagnosis of renal cystic diseases. AJR Am J Roentgenol 1983;140:81; **B** courtesy of Walter Berdon, MD.)

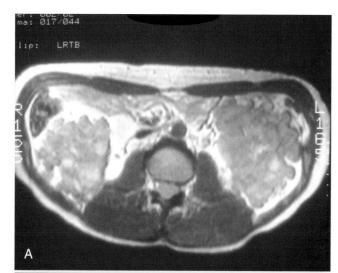

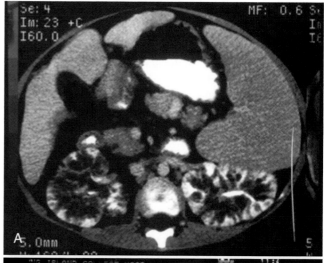

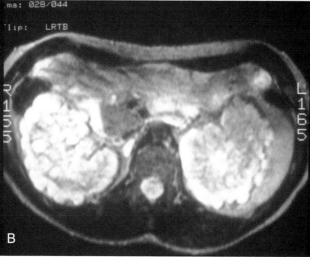

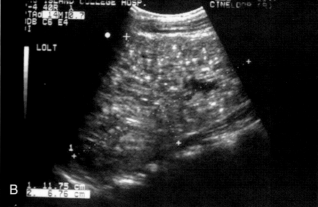

Figure 114–8. **A,** CT scan of a 4-year-old child with ARPKD. Note contrast puddling in collecting ducts. **B,** Sonogram demonstrates typical echogenic stippling seen in association with renal failure.

Figure 114–7. MR images of an 8-month-old child with ARPKD demonstrating multiple renal cysts. **A,** On T1-weighted image fluid content of cysts appears dark. **B,** On T2-weighted image the fluid content appears white. (Courtesy of Walter Berdon, MD.)

for as long as 48 hours after the study (Fig. 114–9). The calyces, renal pelvis, and ureter usually are not visible. In a few cases, the kidneys are already so dysfunctional that no opacification or only an increasingly dense nephrogram is apparent.

Some investigators have reported cases of transient neonatal nephromegaly that mimicked ARPKD after excretory urography and normalizing soon thereafter (Berdon et al, 1969; Stapleton et al, 1981; Avner et al, 1982).

A detailed family history covering at least three generations is needed when ARPKD is suspected. Once the diagnosis is confirmed, referral for genetic counseling is appropriate. Because this condition is transmitted in an autosomal recessive fashion, siblings of either sex have a 1 in 4 chance of being affected.

Treatment

No cure has been found for ARPKD. Respiratory care can ease or extend the child's life. Patients who survive may require treatment for hypertension, congestive heart failure, and renal and hepatic failure. Portal hypertension may be dealt with by decompressive procedures such as splenorenal shunt. Esophageal varices may be managed at least temporarily, by gastric section and reanastomosis. Endoscopic sclerotherapy is widely employed in pediatric and adults with bleeding varices. Hemodialysis and renal transplantation must eventually be considered in many patients.

AUTOSOMAL DOMINANT ("ADULT") POLYCYSTIC KIDNEY DISEASE

The autosomal dominant form of polycystic kidney disease is an important cause of renal failure, accounting for 7% to 15% of patients who receive hemodialysis (Hildenbrandt, 1995; Wilson, 2004). Its incidence is approximately 1 in 500 to 1,000 live births, and approximately 500,000 Americans have been diagnosed with the disease (Gabow, 1993). The protein products of these two genes, polycystin-1 and polycystin-2, are located in the renal tubular epithelia. The trait theoretically has a 100% penetrance; and, on average, because it is transmitted in an autosomal dominant fashion, 50% of an affected individual's offspring will likewise be affected. According to

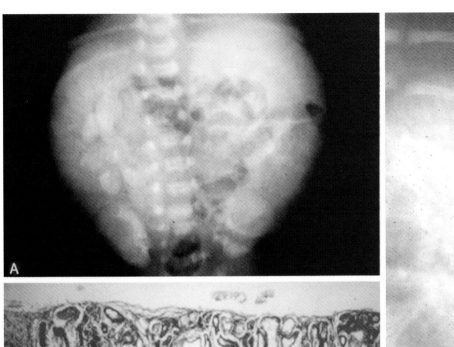

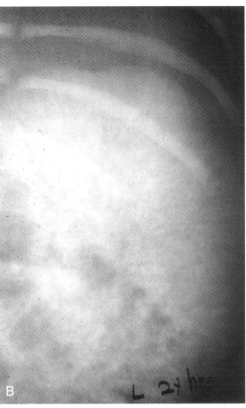

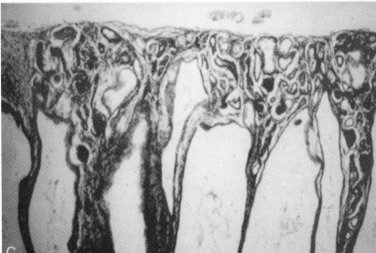

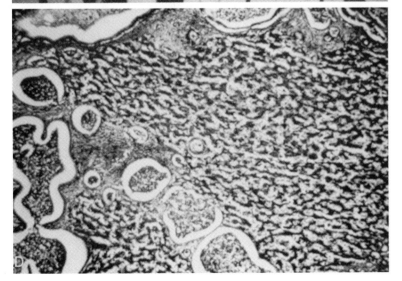

Figure 114–9. Newborn with abdominal mass and pulmonary hypoplasia. Neither parent had a history of renal cysts. **A,** On intravenous urography, 4 hours after injection of contrast medium, bilateral renomegaly is seen filling almost the entire abdomen with full and splayed out calyceal systems. Contrast medium can also be seen in the right kidney as rays stretching from the calyces to the periphery of the kidney. **B,** Twenty-four hours later, contrast medium still is seen within the left kidney in radially oriented dilated ducts. **C,** Renal histology also demonstrates dilated ducts radiating out to the periphery of the kidney. **D,** On liver histology, ectatic biliary ducts are seen in the left half of the figure and periportal fibrosis is seen at the upper edge. The final diagnosis was autosomal recessive polycystic disease.

Gabow (1991), 96% of affected persons will manifest the disease clinically by age 90 years.

The traditional descriptor of "adult" polycystic disease is inaccurate. Although most cases are identified when the patients are between 30 and 50 years of age, the condition has been recognized in newborns. Presumably, the typical age at diagnosis will decline as more members of families at risk for the trait are screened by genetic testing and by ultrasound examination. All affected individuals manifest the disease (although not necessarily symptomatically) if they live long enough, but renal failure is seldom seen before the age of 40 years, unless the disease manifests during infancy, in which case it is much more aggressive.

A number of associated anomalies are common, including cysts of the liver, pancreas, spleen, and lungs; aneurysms of the circle of Willis (berry aneurysms); colonic diverticula; aortic aneurysms; and mitral valve prolapse (Table 114–5).

Genetics

Two genes have been identified as the culprits for ADPKD: (1) the polycystic kidney disease (PKD1) gene localized on the short arm of chromosome 16 (Reeders et al, 1985; Breuning et al, 1987; Ryynanen et al, 1987; Pieke et al, 1989), **which accounts for 85% to 90% of cases, and (2) the PKD2 gene localized to chromosome 4** (Peters et al, 1993), **which accounts for 5% to 10% of cases.** The presence of a third locus (PKD3) is now accepted as the cause of disease in a very small percentage of patients who have been found to have neither a PKD1 nor a PKD2 gene defect (Dauost et al, 1993).

In general, although families with PKD1 and PKD2 gene defects share the same major manifestations, those with the PKD2 defect usually (but not uniformly) have a later onset of clinical symptoms and a slower progression of disease (Dauost et al, 1993). Median age of death or onset of renal failure (whichever comes first) is lower in PKD1 (53.0 years) versus PKD2 (69.1 years). In addition, the incidence of urinary tract infections and hypertension is higher for the PKD1 as compared with the PKD2 defect (Hataboer et al, 1999). Bear and associates (1992) suggested that the disease in general is more severe and manifests earlier when it is inherited from the mother rather than from the father. This phenomenon is referred to as *genetic imprinting*. The phenomenon of genetic anticipation is seen as well; it is manifested by progressively earlier presentation and increased severity in subsequent generations of patients with ADPKD (Fick et al, 1994; Zerres and Rudnick-Schöeheborn, 1995). (Additional information on the genetics of ADPKD was presented earlier, in the section on molecular genetics.)

Clinical Features

When the disease presents in utero with large cystic kidneys it may result in stillbirth or significant respiratory distress. In children who present after 1 year of age, the principal signs and symptoms are related to hypertension and enlarged and impaired kidneys (e.g., proteinuria, hematuria). Now that the families of ADPKD patients are being screened by sonography, large numbers of asymptomatic children with renal cysts are being identified before full-blown disease develops.

Typically, symptoms or signs first occur between the ages of 30 and 50 years (Glassberg et al, 1981). These include microscopic and gross hematuria, flank pain, gastrointestinal symptoms (perhaps secondary to renomegaly or associated colonic diverticula), and renal colic secondary either to clots or stone and hypertension. Microscopic or gross hematuria is seen in 50% of patients, and in 19% to 35% it is the presenting symptom (Milutinovic, 1984; Delaney et al, 1985; Zeier et al, 1988; Gabow et al, 1992). In the series of Gabow and associates (1992), 42% of patients had at least one episode of gross hematuria, the mean age at first episode being 30 ± 1 year. Only in 10% of patients did the first episode occur before the age of 16 years. In general, they found that increased episodes of gross hematuria were associated with higher serum creatinine levels. Because these patients with ADPKD have increased renal mass, erythropoietin levels are increased, making anemia unusual even when ESRD is present (Gabow, 1993).

Twenty to 30 percent of patients with ADPKD develop stones (Fick and Gabow, 1994), and these are treated by conservative means (i.e., urine alkalinization and extracorporal shock wave lithotripsy). However, the finding of hydronephrosis, which helps make the diagnosis of stones, may not be as useful in ADPKD patients because of the number of cysts camouflaging the findings (Choyke, 1996).

As blood pressure screening has become more widespread, hypertension more than hematuria has become the principal form of presentation (Zeier et al, 1988). The hypertension seems to be renin mediated and secondary to

Table 114–5.	**Comparison of Autosomal Recessive and Autosomal Dominant Polycystic Kidney Disease**	
Item	*Autosomal Recessive Polycystic Kidney Disease (ARPKD)*	*Autosomal Dominant Polycystic Kidney Disease (ADPKD)*
Gene defect	Chromosome 6	Chromosomes 4 and 16
Incidence	1:5,000 to 1:40,000	1:500 to 1:1,000
Usual age at clinical presentation	Perinatal	Third to fifth decades
Typical sonographic appearance of kidneys	Symmetrically enlarged, homogeneous, hyperechogenic kidneys	Large cystic kidneys, sometimes asymmetrical
Histology	Collecting duct ectasia; cysts derived principally from collecting duct	Microcysts and macrocysts derived from entire nephron
Liver	Always congenital hepatic fibrosis but of varying severity	Cysts, mostly in adults (on very rare occasions a newborn may have congenital hepatic fibrosis)
Other system involvement	None	Intracranial aneurysms; colonic diverticuli; mitral valve regurgitation; cysts of other organs

stretching of the intrarenal vessels around cysts, causing distal ischemia (Gabow, 1993).

As noted earlier, the polycystic condition in ADPKD is not confined to the kidneys. **Hepatic cysts, usually identified incidentally by sonography, help in making the diagnosis of ADPKD and usually appear later than renal cysts. These cysts are more likely to be found in adults than in children and more frequently in females** (Fick and Gabow, 1994). Such cysts were found by CT in almost 60% of one series of adults (mean age, 49 years) (Thomsen and Thaysen, 1988). Hepatic cysts often grow, but they seldom produce any clinically important effects. New ones may appear as the patient grows older (Thomsen and Thaysen, 1988). In rare instances, enlargement of hepatic cysts leads to portal hypertension and bleeding esophageal varices (Campbell et al, 1958). When secondary portal hypertension appears, differentiating ADPKD from ARPKD can be difficult. In ARPKD, portal hypertension is seen much more frequently and is always secondary to congenital hepatic fibrosis. However, congenital hepatic fibrosis on very rare occasions may accompany ADPKD as well, particularly when the diagnosis is made perinatally. When congenital hepatic fibrosis accompanies ADPKD, the clinical course is quite variable, just as it is in ARPKD. In three ADPKD families in which at least one family member had congenital hepatic fibrosis, the genetic defect was localized to *PKD1* on chromosome 16, clearly supporting a diagnosis of ADPKD rather than ARPKD (Cobben et al, 1990). In these three families, congenital hepatic fibrosis was not transmitted vertically with ADPKD but instead was found only in siblings.

Ten to 40 percent of patients have berry aneurysms, and approximately 9% of these patients die because of subarachnoid hemorrhages (Hartnett and Bennett, 1976; Grantham, 1979; Wakabayashi et al, 1983; Sedmon and Gabow, 1984; Ryu, 1990). Now with magnetic resonance imaging (MRI), even small berry aneurysms can be detected. Using MRI, Huston and associates (1993) found that families with a previous history of intracranial aneurysms had a higher incidence of berry aneurysms than families without a positive history. In their series, 6 (27%) of 27 patients with a family history and 3 (5%) of 56 patients without a family history were found to have aneurysms. The problem is what to do with these aneurysms when they are diagnosed, because they average only 6.1 mm. Although small aneurysms (1 cm) have a lower risk of rupture, patients with small aneurysms have a greater risk of rupture when there is a positive family history of ruptured intracranial aneurysms or the presence of ADPKD (Huston et al, 1993).

However, not all intracranial hemorrhages in patients with ADPKD represent subarachnoid bleeding secondary to berry aneurysms; in some patients, hemorrhage follows the rupture of intracerebral arteries, which is the usual type of intracranial hemorrhage seen in patients with hypertension who do not have ADPKD. Now, with earlier detection and treatment of hypertension, one can expect fewer deaths from intracranial hemorrhage.

Intracerebral bleeding has been reported in at least one child with ADPKD. This child also had hypertrophic pyloric stenosis (Proesmans et al, 1982), a condition that was reported in association with ADPKD in a set of identical twins and their father (Loh et al, 1977). Hypertrophic pyloric stenosis also has

accompanied ARPKD (Gaisford and Bloor, 1968; Lieberman et al, 1971; McGonigle et al, 1981). **Other abnormalities associated with ADPKD are mitral valve prolapse and colonic diverticulosis** (Scheff et al, 1980; Hossack et al, 1986; Kupin et al, 1987). Patients who have diverticulosis are more likely to have hepatic cysts and symptomatic berry aneurysms (Kupin et al, 1987).

When patients with ADPKD present clinically, they usually are found to have bilateral cysts. However, the disease can manifest asymmetrically, with cysts on only one side at first or with a unilateral renal mass (Fig. 114–10).

A variant form of ADPKD probably exists in which the renal cysts are located primarily in Bowman's space. The cytogenetic study of Reeders and associates (1985) provided evidence that such a condition is a form of ADPKD. They found that a fetus with cystic disease predominantly of the glomeruli had the same genetic linkages on chromosome 16 as did its ADPKD-affected mother. Bernstein and Landing (1989) suggested that glomerulocystic kidneys in members of families with ADPKD are variants; the glomerular cysts may be an early stage of ADPKD gene expression (Fig. 114–11). One caution: this condition should not be referred to as "glomerulocystic kidney disease," to avoid confusing it with sporadic glomerulocystic kidney disease, a condition that seems to be histologically identical to ADPKD in infants except for the absence of affected family members (Bernstein, 1993), or with other disorders associated with glomerular cysts, which are discussed later in this chapter. Both of these forms of glomerulocystic kidneys, sporadic glomerulocystic kidney disease and ADPKD with glomerular cysts, when diagnosed in neonates, are associated with about a 10% incidence of biliary dysgenesis (Bernstein, 1993).

KEY POINTS: ADPKD

- ADPKD was previously called "adult" polycystic disease.

- ADPKD is the most common cause of ESRD.

- It most often becomes clinically apparent after age 30 but may present in utero.

- Ninety-nine percent of affected individuals have a mutation either of the *PKD1* gene on chromosome 16 and less often of the *PKD2* gene on chromosome 4.

- The protein products of *PKD1* and *PKD2* are polycystin-1 and polycystin-2, which are important in normal cell polarity and structure.

- Cysts can be identified sonographically before age 20 in almost all affected individuals.

- ADPKD is associated with a high incidence of liver cysts that increases with age.

- Some patients may never clinically present or not present until their 60s, even though cysts already are present.

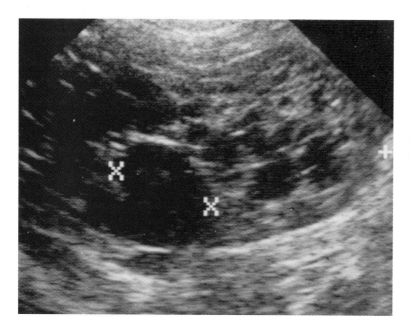

Figure 114–10. Asymmetrical presentation of ADPKD in a 9-year-old boy with hematuria. Sonogram demonstrates right kidney with multiple cysts. No cysts were identified in the left kidney. Subsequently, the diagnosis was made in the patient's brother and mother. Cysts can be expected to develop in the right kidney with time.

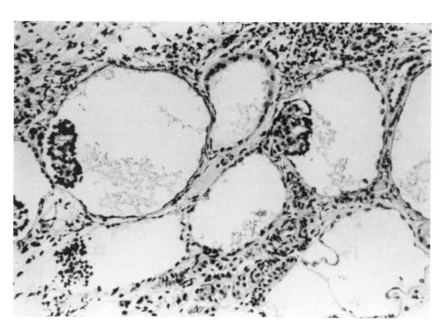

Figure 114–11. Glomerular cysts with a pattern compatible with that of ADPKD in early childhood (×190). (From Bernstein J, Gardner KD: Cystic disease and dysplasia of the kidneys. In Murphy WM [ed]: Urological Pathology. Philadelphia, WB Saunders, 1989, pp 483-524.)

Etiology

Epithelial cells have their own unique polarity, that is, certain proteins and protein receptors appear at one side of the cell as opposed to another. In the case of normal tubular epithelial cells, Na^+-K^+ ATPase (the sodium pump) and epithelial growth factor receptors (EGFRs) are located on the basal and lateral cell membranes. The base of the cell is the side lying above the basement membrane and extracellular matrix. When Na^+-K^+ ATPase is located at the apical side (i.e., luminal side) in addition to the basolateral sides, as occurs in ADPKD and ARPKD, sodium is pumped out of the cell and water follows, filling the tubular lumen. In ADPKD, the loss of polarity can occur in epithelial cells anywhere along the nephron or collecting duct, whereas in ARPKD the loss is only in those cells lining the collecting duct. In both conditions, in addition to EGFRs being located on the apical membrane, there is an increased level of epithelial growth factor (EGF) in the tubular fluid. As a result, cells proliferate and tubular walls fold inward or bulge outward, leading to tubular dilatation and outpouching and thus cyst formation. An outpouching can become pinched off and separate from the continuity of the tubule. Infoldings can cause tubular obstruction, leading to further dilatation proximally. The products of *PKD1* and *PKD2*, polycystin-1 and polycystin-2, and of *PKHD1*, fibrocystin, are proteins normally located at the cell membrane and likely play a role in cell polarity. When any of these genes are mutated, the associated protein will be lacking or abnormal and normal cell polarity will become affected (Grantham et al, 1987a, 1989; Avner et al, 1989; Wilson et al, 1991; Gabow, 1993; Wilson, 2004). For example, in normal kidney epithelium, polycystin-1 is located at the cell membrane but in ADPKD this protein is intracellular (Wilson, 1997). Fibrocystin is located abundantly in normal fetal collecting ducts, but in some patients with ARPKD it is absent (Gabow, 2004). A number of investigators believe that defects of the basement membrane and extracellular matrix also occur in ADPKD and account in part not only for the cystic disease of the kidney and liver but also for some associated anomalies such as mitral valve prolapse and colonic diverticula (Dalgaard and Norby, 1989; Gabow and Schrier, 1989).

Histopathology

The renal cysts range from a few millimeters to a few centimeters in diameter and appear diffusely throughout the cortex and medulla with communications at various points along the nephron (Kissane, 1974). Frequently, the epithelial lining resembles the segment of the nephron from which the cyst is derived, and it often is active in secretion and reabsorption (Gardner, 1988).

In affected fetuses the renal abnormality may develop earlier in ARPKD because the cortical cysts develop simultaneously with abnormal medullary differentiation, rather than as a subsequent event as in ADPKD, in which the kidneys are more normally differentiated (Guay-Woodford, 1998). The first pathologic finding in fetuses is focal tubular dilatation, which may occur anywhere along the nephron (Choyke, 1996).

Epithelial hyperplasia or even adenoma formation in the cyst wall is common, and the basement membrane of the wall is thickened. Arteriosclerosis is present in more than 70% of patients with preterminal or terminal renal failure; and interstitial fibrosis, with or without infiltrates, is common (Zeier et al, 1988). This fibrosis may be secondary to infection or to an inflammatory reaction set off by spontaneously rupturing cysts.

Apoptosis may play a role in the development of renal failure. It appears in the epithelial lining of the cysts and to a lesser degree in the cells lining nondilated nephrons (Winyard et al, 1996).

Gregoire and coworkers (1987) found a 91% incidence of hyperplastic polyps in kidneys removed from ADPKD patients either at autopsy or before transplantation. Some of the autopsies were performed on patients with normal renal function, yet polyps were still found. However, there was a greater predominance of polyps in patients with renal failure and in those receiving dialysis therapy. Because hyperplastic epithelium is seen in both chronic renal failure and ADPKD, a uremic toxin not removed by dialysis may be involved.

Association with Renal Cell Carcinoma

The incidence of renal adenomas is almost as high in ADPKD as in ESRD associated with ARCD (i.e., one in four to five patients). However, whereas ESRD is associated with an increased incidence of RCC, especially when associated with ARCD (three to six times the incidence seen in the general population), the incidence of RCC in patients with ADPKD is no higher than that in the general population. That the incidence of RCC is not increased in ADPKD is also surprising in view of the frequent finding of epithelial hyperplasia. For example, two other conditions, tuberous sclerosis and VHL disease, are associated with epithelial hyperplasia (and adenomas as well) and are associated with an increased incidence of RCC (tuberous sclerosis, 2%; VHL disease, 35% to 38%). Although it is recognized that there is no increased incidence of RCC in ADPKD patients, it is hard to account for certain findings considered typical of a predisposition to RCC that are seen more frequently in patients with ADPKD than in the general population. For example, RCC in ADPKD is more often concurrently bilateral (12% vs. 1% to 5% in the general population), multicentric (28% vs. 6%), and sarcomatoid in type (33% vs. 1% to 5%) (Keith et al, 1994).

Three factors may have contributed to the impression of a higher incidence of RCC in ADPKD. First, the chance association of these two rather common lesions is expected to be frequent. Second, some cases of simultaneous ADPKD and RCC may actually represent cancers in patients with VHL disease or tuberous sclerosis. Third, the epithelial hyperplasia of ADPKD, which is a precancerous lesion in other conditions, may have been considered precancerous in ADPKD as well, although available data do not at present justify this view (Jacobs et al, 1979; Zeier et al, 1988).

Evaluation

To make the diagnosis, it is important to have a history of the patient's family spanning at least three generations. Questions should be asked about renal disease, hypertension, and strokes. Abdominal sonography may reveal renal cysts as well as cysts in other organs. When there is no family history to support a diagnosis of ADPKD, a presumptive diagnosis can be made if bilateral renal cysts are present and two or more of the following symptoms are present as well: bilateral renal enlargement; three or more hepatic cysts; cerebral artery aneurysm; and a solitary cyst of the arachnoid, pineal gland, pancreas, or spleen (Grantham, 1993).

When ADPKD is manifested in utero or in infancy, 50% of affected kidneys are large with identifiable macrocysts (Pretorius et al, 1987). However, the kidneys may appear identical to those seen in ARPKD, having no apparent macrocysts and showing only enlargement and homogeneous hyperechoic features. In such situations, one must look for a parent with ADPKD to confirm the diagnosis. With time, cysts often larger than 1 cm will develop in most children (Avni et al, 2002).

On intravenous urography, the calyces may be stretched by cysts. However, the picture may simulate that of ARPKD, with medullary streaking of contrast medium. In adults, intravenous urography usually reveals bilateral renal enlargement, calyceal distortion, and a bubble or Swiss cheese appearance in the nephrogram phase. CT or MRI (or both) may be helpful in some cases and often is superior to sonography for detecting cysts in organs other than the kidney (Fig. 114–12; see Fig. 114–10). CT is helpful in making the diagnosis of hemorrhage within a cyst. More acute hemorrhage has a higher density (50 to 90 Hounsfield units [HU]) than old hemorrhage (Choyke, 1996). **MRI also may be helpful, particularly in patients with compromised renal function, because no contrast agent is needed** (Fig. 114–13).

According to Gabow and associates (1989b), patients with ADPKD have a reduced maximal urine osmolality (680 ± 14 mOsm) after overnight water deprivation and

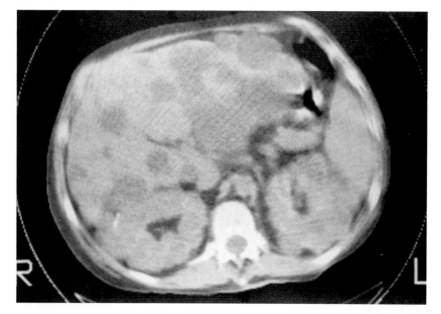

Figure 114–12. CT scan of an adult male patient with ADPKD. Bilateral renal cysts are seen in enlarged kidneys with calcification. Large asymptomatic cysts are seen throughout the liver as well.

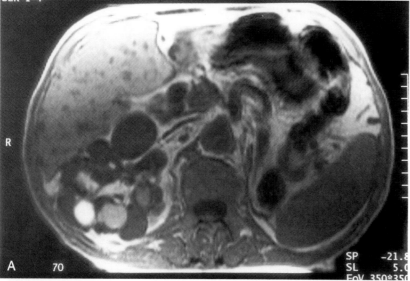

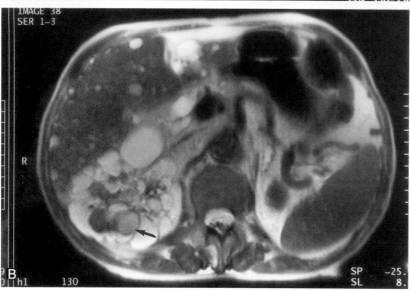

Figure 114–13. MR cholangiogram in a 55-year-old woman with ADKPD done for evaluation of biliary distention. Patient has had a left nephrectomy for pain. Right renal and hepatic cysts are seen on both T1- and T2-weighted coronal images. **A,** T1-weighted image demonstrates renal cysts with low and high (white) signals. High-signal cysts correlate with intracystic hemorrhage. **B,** On T2 weighting, hemorrhagic cysts are dark and cysts without hemorrhage are white. On T2 weighting with the patient in the supine position, cysts with blood tend to get darker more posteriorly *(arrow)*. (Courtesy of H. Zinn, MD.)

administration of vasopressin, a finding that may be helpful in identifying other family members with the disease. However, within the next few years cytogenetic screening should be readily available to identify the gene defects on chromosomes 4 and 16.

Examination of Family Members and Genetic Counseling

Because ADPKD is an autosomal dominant condition, 50% of the children of affected adults will also be affected. Therefore, when the disease is diagnosed, the patient's children should be examined by ultrasound. Before 1970, diagnosis of ADPKD before the age of 25 years was rare. With ultrasound, the possibility of making the diagnosis in affected individuals before this age is at least 85%. When genetic studies are used, the diagnostic accuracy approaches 100%.

When patients with a known *PKD1* defect were selected for renal sonographic screening, 40 (83%) of 48 individuals were found to have cysts before the age of 30 years, and all 48 had them after age 30 (Parfrey et al, 1990). Because the number of simple cysts increases with age, criteria to make the diagnosis need to change with increasing patient age.

At present, family members of an individual with ADPKD cannot obtain insurance before the age of 25 years because of the possibility of the disease (Dalgaard and Norby, 1989). Between the ages of 25 and 35 years, insurance is available but at higher rates; and after the age of 35 years, insurance can be obtained at normal rates if a sonogram has been negative. Now, with definitive cytogenetic diagnosis available, it may be time for insurance companies to revise their criteria of insurability.

Treatment and Prognosis

Men tend to have more renal involvement than women, manifesting with hypertension and renal insufficiency earlier than in women (Grantham, 1993). However, women seem to have more severe cystic involvement of the liver, which causes pain and requires treatment more often than that in men (Grantham, 1993).

More than 60% of patients with ADPKD who do not yet have renal impairment have hypertension (Gabow et al, 1984), which can worsen renal function, cause cardiac disease, and predispose the patient to intracranial hemorrhage. The complications of ADPKD can be reduced significantly by controlling the blood pressure.

The rate of renal deterioration seems to correlate with the rate of cyst growth, supposedly because the enlarging cysts cause pressure atrophy. **However, histologic studies by Zeier and coworkers** (1988) **revealed no evidence of pressure atrophy,** nor did these investigators find evidence of glomerular hyperperfusion, which had been thought to damage the remaining glomeruli after some had been destroyed.

Fifty to 70 percent of patients with ADPKD at some time have loin or back pain (Grantham, 1992). The pain can be colicky, acute, or chronic. Colicky pain occurs secondary to the passage of either stones or clots. Acute pain may be secondary to infection or hemorrhage into a cyst or to subcapsular bleeding. Chronic loin pain requiring narcotics is probably related to distention of cysts and the renal capsule. Rovsing, in 1911, described an operation that involved unroofing the cysts to relieve the pain. The procedure fell into some dispute because of reports that renal function could deteriorate after such a procedure. More recent reports, however, are repopularizing the procedure. Ye and associates (1986) reported that the incidence of relief of pain after Rovsing's operation was 90.6% after 6 months and 77.1% after 5 years, whereas Elzinga and colleagues (1992) found that 80% of patients were pain free at 1 year and 62% at 2 years. Of significance was the finding that renal function did not deteriorate after the procedure in either series; in fact, in the former study there was a significant improvement in renal function in some patients. When pain did return after an unroofing procedure, it often was less severe than it was preoperatively and required narcotics infrequently (Elzinga et al, 1992). Percutaneous cyst aspiration with or without instillation of a sclerosing agent such as alcohol (Bennett et al, 1987; Everson et al, 1990) also can play a therapeutic role. However, aspiration alone is more likely to be associated with reaccumulation of cyst fluid.

In 1993, Elzinga and associates suggested laparoscopic unroofing of cysts as an alternative to an open procedure in order to reduce the incidence of morbidity. More recently, Dunn and colleagues (2001) reported on 15 patients, 6 with bilateral cysts, who had undergone laparoscopic unroofing of cysts for the management of pain. With time, these authors have become more aggressive in their treatment, extending the number of cysts unroofed in some patients to more than 300 and the time of procedure to more than 5 hours. At a mean follow-up of 2.2 years, subjective pain was reduced by 62% in 11 of the 15 patients and those with bilateral unroofing faired better. The remaining 4 patients had less impressive results. The effect of laparoscopic unroofing in those patients with hypertension was quite variable.

Because only 1% of nephrons develop cysts in ADPKD, it is not clear why renal failure develops. Possible causes include compression of nondilated nephrons by the cysts; prominence of apoptosis in epithelial cells—not only in the cells lining the cysts but also in the nondilated nephrons (Winyard et al, 1996); and secondary effects of hypertension. The fact that unroofing of cysts does not dramatically improve renal function makes one question the role that compression plays.

Upper urinary tract infections are common in patients with ADPKD, especially women. Schwab and coworkers (1987) divided these cases into parenchymal and cyst infections. In their series, **87% of cyst infections and 91% of parenchymal infections occurred in women.** When a gram-negative enteric organism was the cause, 100% of the infections were seen in women. Presumably, in women the infection is an ascending one. The only dependable antibiotics are those that are lipid soluble, namely, trimethoprim-sulfamethoxazole, chloramphenicol, and fluoroquinolones (Schwab et al, 1987; Bennett et al, 1990). If a patient with suspected pyelonephritis does not respond to an antibiotic and if the antibiotic used is not lipid soluble, one must consider whether the infection may be present in a noncommunicating cyst (Gabow, 1993).

Symptomatic children usually are in the terminal stages of the disease, but their survival may be extended by supportive care for complications. As in affected adults, dialysis and transplantation may be appropriate. In the past, allografts from siblings were ruled out because of the frequency of ADPKD in such donors. However, now that siblings can be screened, this ban may no longer be appropriate.

Presymptomatic patients with ADPKD should be monitored with blood pressure measurements and tests of renal function. The advantages of such monitoring include the abilities to prevent or control infection and hypertension, to identify potential kidney donors from among the family, to offer advice on marriage and childbearing, and to provide prenatal diagnosis. The question of abortion of an affected fetus is an issue that the parents and the physician must consider in view of the improved prognosis for such patients.

PKD1 and *PKD2* testing is readily available, and mutation of one or the other can be identified by commercial laboratories 50% to 70% of the time. Research laboratories results exceed 90%. Amniocentesis can be used for genetic studies to differentiate whether in utero renal cystic disease is ADPKD, ARPKD, or tuberous sclerosis.

Churchill and associates (1984) calculated that patients with sonographically identifiable ADPKD have a 2% chance of developing end-stage renal failure by age 40 years, a 23% chance by age 50, and a 48% chance by age 73. Because of enhanced ability to deal with problems such as urinary infection, calculi, hypertension, and renal failure, the outlook for patients with ADPKD appears to be improving.

Emerging Therapeutics

Because polycystic kidney disease entities represent hyperplastic cystic conditions, Grantham (2000) suggested that it is time to treat polycystic kidney diseases like the neoplastic disorders they are. One such method would be to block the action of growth factors or their receptors. For example, EGF and its receptor (see previous discussion) are thought to play an important role in the genesis of ADPKD. Sweeney and coworkers (2000) have taken this information and developed an EGFR-tyrosine kinase inhibitor, EKI-785, which competes with EGF for its receptor site and used it to treat postnatal mice with polycystic kidney disease between days 7 and 14. Untreated mice died by day 24 with collecting duct cysts, renal failure, and severe biliary abnormalities. Those treated until day 48 were alive and well, with normal renal function, much less cyst formation, and significantly fewer biliary abnormalities. If the EGFR of these mice is the same or similar to that in humans with ARPKD and ADPKD, EKI-785 or a similar agent may be useful in the treatment of these diseases.

JUVENILE NEPHRONOPHTHISIS/ MEDULLARY CYSTIC DISEASE COMPLEX

Juvenile nephronophthisis was first described by Fanconi and colleagues in 1951. Medullary cystic disease was first reported by Smith and Graham in 1945. Although the two conditions are similar anatomically and clinically, they have a different mode of transmission and a different clinical onset.

Although juvenile nephronophthisis is the more common condition and is responsible for 10% to 20% of cases of renal failure occurring in children (Cantani et al, 1986), this relatively high incidence does not appear to correlate with the low incidence (1 in 50,000 births) reported by Lirenman and associates (1974). A frequency of less than 1 in 100,000 was reported for medullary cystic disease by Reeders (1990).

Genetics

Although either condition can occur sporadically, juvenile nephronophthisis usually is inherited as an autosomal recessive trait. There are three distinct types—juvenile, adolescent, and infertile—caused by mutations to the following corresponding genes: *NPH1*, *NPH2*, **and** *NPH3* (Antignac et al, 1993; Hildebrandt et al, 2000; Omran et al, 2001). **Renal failure develops at a mean age of 13 years and almost always before 25 years** (Neumann et al, 1997). Medullary cystic disease usually is inherited in an autosomal dominant fashion caused by mutations in either the *MCKD1* or *MCKD2* genes. When it manifests in early adulthood it is a milder disease. ESRD most often develops in the third or fourth decade. Because it is transmitted in an autosomal dominant fashion, 50% of all offspring will have the disease. It will manifest in all by 50 years of age (Bernstein and Gardner, 1979b). Because patients with either condition theoretically can be fertile in their early childbearing years, the risk of transmitting the condition to offspring must be acknowledged: 1% for juvenile nephronophthisis and 50% for medullary cystic disease (Neumann et al, 1997) (Table 114–6).

Clinical Features

Juvenile nephronophthisis and medullary cystic disease both cause polydipsia and polyuria in more than 80% of

Table 114–6. Juvenile Nephronophthisis/Medullary Cystic Disease Complex*

Item	Juvenile Nephronophthisis	Medullary Cystic Disease
Inheritance	Autosomal recessive (chromosome 2)	Autosomal dominant (chromosome ?)
Incidence	1 : 50,000	1 : 100,000
End-stage renal disease	By age 13 yr	20–40 yr
Medullary cysts	Develop after renal failure	May develop before onset of renal failure
Tubular basement membrane	Thickened	May not be thickened
Symptoms	Polyuria, polydipsia, anemia, growth retardation (usually after age 2)	Polyuria, polydipsia, anemia; may have hematuria and proteinuria (symptoms usually appear after patient is fully grown)

*Both have tubulointestinal nephritis and small kidneys with granular surface; medullary cysts are not essential for diagnosis and are not present in all cases.

cases, but not to the extent observed in patients with diabetes insipidus (Gardner, 1984a; Cantani et al, 1986). The polyuria is attributable to a severe renal tubular defect associated with an inability to conserve sodium. The polyuria is resistant to vasopressin, and a large dietary salt intake frequently is necessary. Hypertension is not associated with juvenile nephronophthisis, because these patients have a salt-losing nephropathy. On the other hand, medullary cystic disease nephropathy is associated with hypertension because these patients do not have a salt-losing problem. Proteinuria and hematuria usually are absent. In children, growth gradually slows and malaise and pallor may appear in advanced disease. These latter findings are secondary to anemia, which may be attributable to a deficiency of erythropoietin production by the failing kidneys (Gruskin, 1977). Renal failure usually ensues 5 to 10 years after initial presentation (Cantani et al, 1986).

Juvenile nephronophthisis often is associated with disorders of the retina (particularly retinitis pigmentosa), skeletal abnormalities, hepatic fibrosis, and Bardet-Biedl syndrome, which is a combination of obesity, mental retardation, polydactyly, retinitis pigmentosa, and hypogenitalism. **Sixteen percent of patients with juvenile nephronophthisis have associated retinitis pigmentosa** (Hildebrandt et al, 1993). When the two entities coexist, the condition is referred to as renal-retinal or Senior-Løken syndrome. However, if one member in a family with juvenile nephronophthisis has retinal disease, that does not mean that others in the family with nephronophthisis necessarily also have retinal disease. Alström's syndrome, a nephropathy accompanied by blindness, obesity, diabetes mellitus, and nerve deafness, may be a form of juvenile nephronophthisis (Bernstein, 1976). Eighty percent of families have no extrarenal lesions (Neumann et al, 1997). Extrarenal abnormalities classically have been associated only with juvenile nephronophthisis.

Histopathology

Early in the disease course, the kidneys may be of normal size (Cantani et al, 1986). In clinically manifest cases, the kidneys almost always demonstrate interstitial nephritis, with round cell infiltrates and tubular dilatation with atrophy. The corticomedullary junction is poorly defined. Atrophy begins in the cortex, but later the entire organ becomes very small and has a granular surface.

Cysts are present in the kidneys of many patients, particularly those with medullary cystic disease (incidence: 85% vs. 40% for patients with juvenile nephronophthisis) (Mongeau and Worthen, 1967). These cysts, which range in diameter from 1 mm to 1 cm, appear usually at the corticomedullary junction and less often in the medulla, generally within the distal convolutions and the collecting ducts (Fig. 114–14) (Cantani et al, 1986). Biopsies do not always reveal cysts, however, both because affected areas may be missed and because cysts tend to appear only with renal failure in the recessive disease. In the dominant disorder, medullary cysts are sometimes seen before the development of renal failure (Lirenman et al, 1974; Steele et al, 1980; Garel et al, 1984; Cantani et al, 1986; Kleinknecht and Habib, 1992).

Evaluation

In the early stages of the disease, intravenous urography may show a normal or slightly shrunken kidney (Habib, 1974; Chamberlin et al, 1977). Homogeneous streaking of the medulla may be found, presumably secondary to retention of contrast medium within dilated tubules, or ring-shaped densities at the bases of papillae may be seen, again perhaps representing contrast-filled tubules (Olsen et al, 1988). In the late stages of the disease, intravenous urography is of little value. Calcifications are not seen.

Sonography may show smaller than normal kidneys in juvenile nephronophthisis. Cysts may be seen on imaging studies if they are large enough (Rosenfeld et al, 1977), but early in the disease cysts are rarely visible. For example, Garel and associates (1984) demonstrated medullary cysts in 17 of 19 patients with ESRD but not in twins who had only mild uremia. The parenchyma may appear hyperechogenic

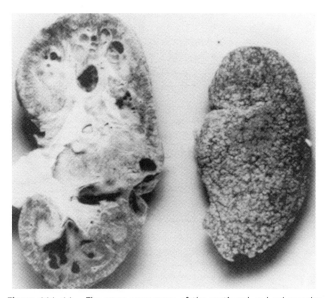

Figure 114–14. The gross appearance of the sectioned and subcapsular surface of a kidney from a patient with medullary cystic disease. Note that the cysts are concentrated at the corticomedullary junction, not at the papillae as in medullary sponge kidney. (From Kissane JM: Pathology of Infancy and Childhood, 2nd ed. St. Louis, CV Mosby, 1975.)

secondary to tubulointerstitial fibrosis (Resnick and Hartman, 1990) (Fig. 114–15).

McGregor and Bailey (1989) described the CT appearance of juvenile nephronophthisis in a 19-year-old patient. In this case, cysts approximately 0.5 cm in diameter were apparent throughout the medulla, although no cysts were visible by sonography. These investigators recommended CT rather than sonography for examining relatives of known cases. Even though the cysts may be prominent and may help in diagnosis, renal failure probably results not from the cysts but from the tubulointerstitial changes. However, as Wise and colleagues (1998) pointed out, CT may require the use of a contrast agent, which often is contraindicated in renal failure. They see a future for MRI in the diagnosis of this entity, especially with such new advances as fast spin-echo and breath-hold sequences, which overcome breathing and motion artifact.

Treatment

Sodium replacement is indicated early in the course of the disease. Later, dialysis and transplantation must be considered. Allografts apparently are not susceptible to the same process that destroyed the native kidney, because there is no evidence of serum antibodies to the basement membrane or other renal structural proteins (Cantani et al, 1986; Cohen and Hoyer, 1986).

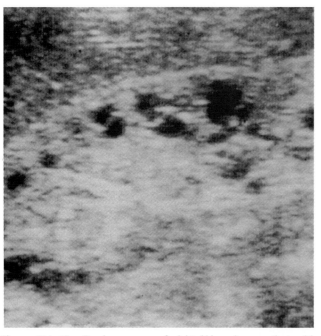

Figure 114–15. Renal sonogram of right kidney in a patient with medullary cystic disease. Note small to medium-size cysts located predominantly at outer edge of medulla and a few well within the medulla. The hyperechogenicity is secondary to the tubulointerstitial fibrosis. (From Resnick JS, Hartman DS: Medullary cystic disease. In Pollack HM [ed]: Clinical Urography. Philadelphia, WB Saunders, 1990, pp 1178-1184.)

CONGENITAL NEPHROSIS

Congenital nephrosis is predominantly of two types. The more common variety, referred to as the Finnish type (CNF), has, as the name suggests, been reported principally in Finland, where the incidence is 1 in 8200 (Norio, 1966; Lanning et al, 1989). It has also been reported in other areas, including Minnesota (Kestilä et al, 1994). The other type, described by Habib and Bois in 1973, is referred to as diffuse mesangial sclerosis (DMS). The Finnish type is recessive (Norio, 1966) and has been localized to chromosome 19 (Kestilä et al, 1994), but only 10 of the 30 reported cases of DMS were familial (Habib et al, 1989). More recently, Kestilä (1998) cloned the gene *(NPHSI)*, which encodes a protein called nephrin that plays a significant role in functional renal development (Ruotsalainen et al, 1999). Both conditions are associated with dilatation of the proximal convoluted tubules. The term *microcystic disease* is now rarely used.

Clinical Features

CNF usually is discovered because of an enormously enlarged and edematous placenta, which accounts for more than 25% of the birth weight (Norio and Rapola, 1989). In DMS, the placenta usually is not enlarged.

In infants with CNF, proteinuria is present in the first urinalysis. Edema usually develops within the first few days and always by the age of 3 months. Essentially, these infants starve because of their severe loss of protein in the urine; without treatment, they probably would die of sepsis before renal failure killed them. Without dialysis half of the patients die by the age of 6 months, and the rest die before their fourth birthday (Huttunen, 1976).

In DMS, the onset of symptoms is variable and the diagnosis is usually made by the age of 1 year. All children have terminal renal failure by the age of 3 years.

Habib and colleagues (1985) demonstrated that the nephropathy of Drash syndrome (nephrotic syndrome and Wilms' tumor with or without male pseudohermaphroditism) is, in fact, DMS. Of the 35 cases of DMS diagnosed by Habib and coworkers (1989), 13 were associated with Drash syndrome.

Histopathology

CNF and DMS are both characterized by normal-sized kidneys, initially with pronounced proximal tubular dilatation. DMS is distinctive in that the glomeruli have an accumulation of periodic acid–Schiff–positive and silver phosphate–staining mesangial fibrils. With advanced disease, the glomerular tufts sclerose and contract (Norio and Rapola, 1989; Habib et al, 1989). Diffuse hypertrophy of the podocytes is also found.

CNF is characterized by a proliferation of the glomerular mesangial cells. In both DMS and CNF, as in all types of nephrosis, there is fusion of the glomerular podocytes. Interstitial fibrosis is present in both conditions but is more pronounced in DMS (Norio and Rapola, 1989).

Evaluation

The diagnosis of CNF can be made at about 6 weeks of gestation because of the greatly elevated concentrations of amniotic α-fetoprotein secondary to fetal proteinuria. The use of α-fetoprotein to diagnose DMS in utero has not been demonstrated.

In the later stages of disease postnatally, ultrasonography reveals enlarged kidneys with cortices that are more echogenic than those of the liver or spleen. The pyramids are small and hazy, and the corticomedullary junction is indistinct or absent. In one study, the kidneys continued to enlarge and the corticomedullary junction became more effaced as the disease become worse (Lanning et al, 1989).

Treatment

After the kidneys have failed, transplantation is curative. Neither type of disease responds to corticosteroids.

FAMILIAL HYPOPLASTIC GLOMERULOCYSTIC KIDNEY DISEASE (CORTICAL MICROCYSTIC DISEASE)

In 1982, Rizzoni and coworkers described two families in which a mother and two daughters were affected by what these investigators called hypoplastic glomerulocystic disease. Melnick and associates (1984) described the same condition under the name cortical microcystic disease, and Kaplan and colleagues (1989a) reported it in a mother and son. This condition is autosomal dominant.

The diagnosis of familial hypoplastic glomerulocystic disease requires four features. First, stable or progressive chronic renal failure must be present. Second, the kidneys must be small or of normal size with irregular calyceal outlines and abnormal papillae. Third, the condition must be present in two generations of a family. Last, histologic evidence of glomerular cysts must be found. These cysts are thin walled and tend to be subcapsular. Tubular atrophy with some normal glomeruli and tubules in the deeper cortex is also observed. Marked prognathism is present in some patients (Kaplan et al, 1989a; Rizzoni et al, 1982).

MULTIPLE MALFORMATION SYNDROMES WITH RENAL CYSTS

Renal cysts are a feature of several syndromes characterized by multiple malformations (Table 114–7). Tuberous sclerosis and VHL disease are autosomal dominant disorders and are the ones most likely to be encountered by urologists. Meckel's syndrome, Jeune's asphyxiating thoracic dystrophy, and Zellweger's cerebrohepatorenal syndrome are some of the more common autosomal recessive syndromes. Many of these conditions involve glomerular cysts, and some have cystic dysplasia as a feature.

Tuberous Sclerosis Complex

Bourneville described tuberous sclerosis in 1880. The incidence seems to be rising with each report, now ranging between 1 in 6,000 and 1 in 14,500 (Webb et al, 1991; O'Hagan et al, 1996). The rise is the result not of an increased incidence but rather of an increased awareness of the disease and its manifestations.

Classically, tuberous sclerosis is described as part of a triad of epilepsy (80% of cases), mental retardation (60% of cases), and adenoma sebaceum (75% of cases) (Lagos and Gomez, 1967; Pampigliana and Moynahan, 1976). The lesions of adenoma sebaceum are flesh-colored papules of angiofibroma and are especially prevalent in the malar area. An earlier skin lesion that is a white papule in the shape of an "ash leaf" is sometimes identified (Shepherd et al, 1991). An examination of the skin with ultraviolet light may reveal cutaneous lesions earlier and should be part of a diagnostic evaluation.

The hallmark lesion of the central nervous system is a superficial cortical hamartoma of the cerebrum, which sometimes looks like hardened gyri, creating the appearance of a tuber (root). Hamartomas often affect other organs as well, especially the kidneys and eyes. Periventricular subependymal nodules also occur frequently.

The kidneys of these patients may be free of lesions (Stillwell et al, 1987) or may display cysts, angiomyolipomas, or both (Figs. 114–16 and 114–17).

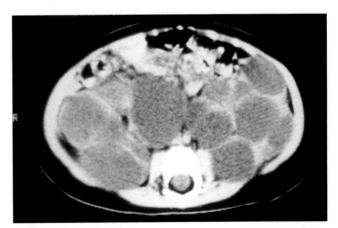

Figure 114–16. CT of 4-month-old with tuberous sclerosis and diffuse renal cysts. (Courtesy of Walter Berdon, MD.)

Table 114–7. Multiple Malformation Syndromes Associated with Renal Cysts

Genetics	Syndrome	Features	Cyst Characteristics	Other Renal Lesions	Renal Sequelae
Mendelian (single gene disorders)					
Autosomal dominant	Tuberous sclerosis	Adenoma sebaceum, epilepsy, mental retardation, cranial calcifications	Variable size, eosinophilic hyperplastic lining*	Angiomyolipomas (more common than cysts), renal cell carcinoma (2% incidence)	Occasionally masses compress or obstruct kidney, leading to renal failure.
	von Hippel-Lindau disease	Cerebellar hemangioblastomas, retinal angiomatosis, pheochromocytoma, cysts of pancreas and epididymis	Variable size; hyperplastic lining	Clear cell carcinoma (35%–38% incidence)	Rarely, masses compress or obstruct kidney, leading to renal failure
Autosomal recessive	Meckel's syndrome	Microcephaly, polydactyly, posterior encephalocele	Large with fibromuscular collars that probably arise from collecting ducts	Dysplasia, hypoplasia	Possible renal failure
	Jeune's asphyxiating thoracic dystrophy	Small chest, respiratory failure	From subcapsular cortical microcysts to dysplasia with cystic component; generalized dilatation of various segments of nephron (similar to ADPKD)	Dysplasia	Possible renal failure or chronic nephritis
	Zellweger's cerebrohepatorenal syndrome	Hypotonia, high forehead, hepatomegaly	From glomerular microcysts to 1-cm cortical cysts	—	Rarely, mild azotemia; usually no manifestations
	Ivemark's syndrome (renal-hepatic-pancreatic dysplasia)	Biliary dysgenesis, dilated intrahepatic ducts, pancreatic dysplasia	Diffuse, microscopic to large	Dysplasia	Possible renal failure
X-linked dominant disorders	Orofaciodigital syndrome I	Hypertrophic lingular and buccal frenula; cleft lip, palate, and tongue; hypoplasia of alinasal cartilage, brachydactyly, syndactyly, alopecia	Develop with age	—	Hypertension, renal failure
Chromosomal disorders	Trisomy 13 (Patau's syndrome) Trisomy 18 (Edwards' syndrome) Trisomy 21 (Down syndrome)		Any cystic changes usually are not clinically significant. Findings are variable, but cysts generally are microscopic (dysplastic cysts, subcortical cysts, glomerular cysts)		

ADPKD, autosomal dominant polycystic kidney disease.
*May resemble ADPKD in imaging studies.
Adapted from Glassberg KI: Cystic disease of the kidney. Curr Probl Urol 1988;2:157; and Glassberg KI: Renal cystic diseases. Curr Probl Urol 1991;1:137.

Genetics

Although it is transmitted as an autosomal dominant trait in 25% to 40% of cases, in the remainder tuberous sclerosis occurs either sporadically or as an example of the genetic condition with variable or incomplete penetrance.

Because it is a heterogeneous genetic disorder with variable manifestations, it usually is referred to as tuberous sclerosis complex (TSC). **Two genes, *TSC1* on chromosome 9 and *TSC2* on chromosome 16, have been identified as being responsible for the autosomal dominant transmission of tuberous sclerosis** (Kandt et al, 1992; Brook-Carter et al, 1994). However, in a review of 10 previously reported cases (in addition to 1 new patient in whom severe bilateral cystic

disease was diagnosed by the age of 4 months), 6 of the infants had no family history of tuberous sclerosis, in 3 no family history was available, and in only 1 was the disease found to be familial (Campos et al, 1993). In another study (Brook-Carter et al, 1994) of 6 patients with tuberous sclerosis and a known history of diffuse bilateral cystic disease in early infancy, all were found to have deletions not only at the *TSC2* gene site on chromosome 16 but also in the adjacent *PKD1* gene, the gene responsible for ADPKD. There were no signs of tuberous sclerosis in parents or other family members, suggesting that in these 6 patients the disease probably represented a new mutation. It is interesting that of the 11 cases reviewed by Campos and colleagues (1993) and the 6 studied by Brook-Carter and associates (1994) with diffuse bilateral

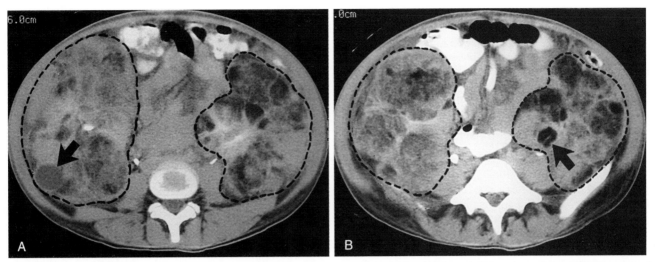

Figure 114-17. A 24-year-old woman was known to have tuberous sclerosis since early childhood. Enhanced CT scan demonstrates bilateral renomegaly with multiple renal cysts and angiomyolipomas. **A,** Arrow points to a cyst with a CT value of +10 HU. **B,** The *arrow* points to an angiomyolipoma with a negative CT value (−50 HU) secondary to its high fat content.

cystic disease in early infancy, the disease was identified as familial in only 1 child.

In summary, **when severe polycystic kidneys are present in patients, particularly infants, with tuberous sclerosis, the condition represents a contiguous gene syndrome (i.e., defects in both *TSC2* and *PKD1*).** Such contiguous gene syndromes are relatively rare phenomena. In an infant with polycystic kidney disease, other findings associated with tuberous sclerosis should be investigated to exclude the diagnosis of tuberous sclerosis (Gillis et al, 1997).

TSC1 encodes the protein hamartin, whereas *TSC2* incodes tuberin. Both proteins work together as a complex playing a role in several cell-signaling events. Therefore, a mutation of either gene will lead to similar clinical manifestations.

Histopathology

The renal cysts are of a unique histologic type in that they have a lining of hypertrophic, hyperplastic eosinophilic cells (Bernstein and Meyer, 1967; Stapleton et al, 1980). These cells have large, hyperchromatic nuclei; and mitoses are seen occasionally. The cells often aggregate into masses or tumorlets (Bernstein and Gardner, 1986, 1989). Later in the disease, the cyst walls may atrophy into a thickened, unidentifiable lining (Mitnick et al, 1983). In a few patients, predominantly glomerular cells have been seen (Bernstein and Gardner, 1989). The cystic disease can lead to renal failure with or without the presence of angiomyolipomas. The probable mechanism is compression of the parenchyma by the expanding cysts. Hypertension may also be present.

Angiomyolipomas occur in 40% to 80% of patients (Chonko et al, 1974; Gomez, 1979). They are rarely identified before the age of 6 years but are common after age 10 (Bernstein et al, 1986). By themselves, these lesions probably do not cause renal failure (Okada et al, 1982; Bernstein et al, 1986). Also, belying their aggressive histologic appearance, which is characterized by pleomorphism and mitoses, no evidence of metastases has been presented.

Evaluation

The rising incidence of identified tuberous sclerosis is in part the result of full investigation of patients with seizure disorders, of children with hypomelanotic macules, and of some infants and young children misdiagnosed as having ADPKD who actually have tuberous sclerosis. The most significant primary diagnostic finding is multiple calcified subepididymal nodules penetrating into the ventricle by CT or MRI (Roach et al, 1992).

Sometimes both renal cysts and angiomyolipomas can be identified by sonography in tuberous sclerosis, the former lesions being sonolucent and the latter having a fluffy, white appearance. When renal cysts are present without angiomyolipomas, the sonographic appearance of the kidneys in tuberous sclerosis is very similar to that in ADPKD. Therefore, it is not that unusual for a patient in whom cysts typical of ADPKD are identified to be diagnosed as having ADPKD, only to develop the stigmata of tuberous sclerosis a few years later. To help make the diagnosis, abdominal CT can be useful in demonstrating angiomyolipomas that may be present in the kidney or other organs (findings that are compatible with tuberous sclerosis) and in revealing cysts in other organs (compatible with ADPKD). MRI or CT of the head may demonstrate the classic cranial calcifications associated with tubers or gliosis (Okada et al, 1982). Ultraviolet light examination of the skin may reveal cutaneous lesions before they become manifest grossly and should be part of the differential diagnosis.

Clinical Features and Prognosis

Renal cysts develop in approximately 20% of patients and most often manifest before 3 years of age; one third of children are younger than 1 year of age at presentation. Patients with large cysts or polycystic kidney disease may be identified by in-utero ultrasound or may present with an abdominal mass and distended abdomen in the first year of life. Most patients with renal cysts do not develop any serious renal compromise, but when the disease is more widespread within the kidney and large cysts are present, renal failure may develop in the milder form with polycystic kidney disease. If any renal failure develops, it is uncommon before the fourth decade (Glazier et al, 1996). The cysts probably originate from nephrons lined with hyperplastic cells that may be present even at birth (Bernstein, 1993).

Because more patients with tuberous sclerosis now survive their central nervous system lesions than in the past, the urologist is more likely to be called on for management of the renal problems (Stillwell et al, 1987). Shepherd and associates (1991) found that renal disease was the leading cause of death (11 of 40 deaths). Of 355 patients they observed at the Mayo Clinic, 49 had died, 9 from disease not related to tuberous sclerosis, 10 from brain tumors, 4 from lymphangiomatosis of the lung, 13 from causes secondary to status epilepticus or bronchopneumonia, and 11 from renal disease. Of these 11 patients, 2 died of metastatic RCC, 2 of massive hemorrhage associated with renal angiomyolipomas, and 6 of renal failure secondary to the cysts, angiomyolipomas, or both.

Large angiomyolipomas are more likely to bleed. Van Baal and coworkers (1994) have recommended careful monitoring of the size of angiomyolipomas and prophylactic embolization or surgical excision if they enlarge to greater than 4 cm.

Association with Renal Cell Carcinoma

The numerous reports of RCC in patients with tuberous sclerosis make it clear that this association is more than coincidental and may be as frequent as 2% (Bernstein et al, 1986; Bernstein, 1993). However, the incidence of RCC is considerably less than that seen in other conditions involving hyperplastic epithelial cells, specifically VHL disease and ARCD of chronic renal failure (although it is more frequent than that seen in another condition with hyperplastic cells, ADPKD, which may not even have an increased incidence).

These cancers appear in patients who are younger than would be expected (7 to 39 years); they may be single or multiple and unilateral or bilateral (Bernstein and Gardner, 1989). The karyotype of the cells near the tumor is similar to that of the tumor itself, and it is reasonable to suspect that the lining of the cysts evolves into the cancer (Ibrahim et al, 1989).

Von Hippel-Lindau Disease

von Hippel, a German ophthalmologist, published two articles describing retinal angiomatosis in 1904 and 1911. One of his patients developed renal cancer and was reported on in 1921. Four years later, Lindau published a series of patients with retinal and cerebellar tumors, with four of his patients also having renal cysts and renal cancer.

VHL disease is an autosomal dominant condition manifested by cerebellar and retinal hemangioblastomas; cysts of the pancreas, kidney, and epididymis; epididymal cystadenoma; pheochromocytoma; and clear cell RCC. It has an incidence of approximately 1 in 35,000 (Neumann and Wiestler, 1991).

KEY POINTS: MULTIPLE MALFORMATION SYNDROMES

- Tuberous sclerosis complex is an autosomal dominant condition that includes the triad of epilepsy, mental retardation, and adenoma sebaceum. It is associated with renal cysts (20% of patients), renal angiomyolipoma (40% to 80%), and RCC (2%).

- There are two different gene mutations associated with tuberous sclerosis: *TSC1* on chromosome 9 and *TSC2* on chromosome 16.

- *TSC2* is a gene located adjacent to *PKD1* on chromosome 16, and together they are referred to as a contiguous gene syndrome. In tuberous sclerosis a mutation of *TSC2* may involve part of *PKD1* and, vice versa, a mutation of *PKD1* in *ADPKD* may involve a part of *TSC2*.

- von Hippel-Lindau (VHL) disease is an autosomal recessive condition associated with cerebellar and retinal hemangioblastomas; cysts of the pancreas, kidney (76%), and epididymis; pheochromocytoma (10% to 12%); and clear cell RCC (50% incidence and 30% to 40% of death).

- VHL disease is associated with a recessively inherited mutation of the *VHL* gene on chromosome 3.

- *VHL* is a tumor suppressor gene, involved in regulation of hypoxia-inducible factor (HIF) target genes including *VEGF*; abnormal or absent VHL leads to increased tissue levels of specific growth factors and, in particular, VEGF, the most prominent growth factor in RCC.

Genetics

The gene associated with the transmission of VHL disease is located on chromosome 3 (Latif et al, 1993). Seventy percent of patients will have a mutation of one *VHL* allele (i.e., *VHL+/−*). For the disease to manifest, the second allele must develop a spontaneous mutation as well (i.e., *VHL +/+*) at some time later in life.

The *VHL* gene is characterized as a recessive tumor-suppressor gene, and its gene product is referred to as VHL. Many different mutations of the *VHL* gene have been identified, five of which are seen most frequently (Zbar et al, 1996). The disease can be divided into type 1 with a low risk of pheochromocytoma and type 2 with a high risk for pheochromocytoma. Type 2 has a high risk both for pheochromocytoma and renal cell carcinoma, and type 2B has a high risk only for pheochromocytoma (Kaelin, 2003). A different mutation of the *VHL* gene often is associated with familial RCC and some sporadic RCC cases.

The genetic nature of VHL disease mandates careful screening. However, because of molecular genetic advances, the screening process for the disease in family members can now be more selective. Previously, asymptomatic relatives

required routine ophthalmoscopic examination to rule out retinal angiomas, as well as frequent abdominal CT scans. Now only genetically affected family members require screening.

The recommendations of Levine and colleagues (1990) for all asymptomatic relatives now applies only to those with genetic evidence of the disease. For example, ophthalmoscopic examination for retinal angiomas is useful, and an abdominal CT scan should be obtained when an asymptomatic genetically affected relative is between the ages of 18 and 20 years. If no disease is found, reevaluation is recommended at 4-year intervals (Levine et al, 1990). If cysts or small indeterminate lesions are identified, CT examination should be repeated every 2 years, perhaps with narrow-screen collimation (Levine et al, 1990). The goal is to diagnose the disease early so that malignancies can be identified before they metastasize.

The diagnosis can be made without a family history if a patient has two cardinal manifestations. In such families, germline mutations may be present without clinical manifestations and should be screened for.

VHL acts as a tumor suppressor protein via at least two routes: it destabilizes β-catenin strengthening GSK-3 and APC bonds to β-catenin, and it binds to and inactivates hypoxia-inducible factor (HIF), a protein when not suppressed that can stimulate the formation of hemangioblastomas and RCC. When these bonds are weaked by the absence of VHL, β-catenin is overproduced and cellular proliferation as in RCC can follow. HIF targets specific genes that encode growth factors that seem to play a role in tumorigenesis, including platelet-derived growth factor (PDGF), transforming growth factor-α (TGF-α), and VEGF, the last of which is particularly prominent in RCC. Attempts at producing drugs that will inactivate HIF, VEGF, PDGF, and TGF-α are being made to curb the effect of the absence of VHL (Kaelin 2003). (Additional discussion of the genetics of von Hippel-Lindau disease is included in the discussion of molecular genetics earlier in this chapter.)

Histopathology

When present, renal cysts and tumors often are multiple and bilateral. The cysts usually simulate simple benign cysts, with flattened epithelium that some investigators consider precancerous. When Poston and associates (1993) studied cysts that were surgically removed along with specimens of RCC, they found that cysts larger than 2 cm were more likely than smaller cysts to have components of RCC. Frank cancer usually appears between the ages of 20 and 50 years (Jennings and Gaines, 1988). Loughlin and Gittes (1986) found that the hyperplastic lining cells frequently resembled the clear cell type of RCC, the most common type in these patients. Ibrahim and coworkers (1989) studied the cysts adjacent to carcinomas and found, much as in tuberous sclerosis, that the karyotype resembled that of the tumors. This similarity is evidence that the hyperplastic cells of the cyst lining are precursors of the carcinomas.

Solomon and Schwartz (1988) believed that a spectrum of pathology is found within the kidneys of patients with VHL disease. At one extreme is a simple cyst with a single layer of bland epithelium. The next step is a typical proliferative cyst with layers of epithelial cells. In the ensuing step, there are complex neoplastic projections into the cyst lumen. If one agrees with the arbitrary distinction between adenoma and carcinoma on the basis of size, the next stage would be adenoma. Finally, there is the full-blown RCC. In some cases, one might stretch the spectrum two steps further: sclerosing RCC with residual foci of malignant epithelium and completely hyalinized fibrotic nodules lacking epithelial foci. The latter condition may represent the endpoint of evolution of the RCC. All of these stages may be found within a single kidney (Solomon and Schwartz, 1988). Lubensky and associates (1996) presented molecular evidence supporting the concept that benign-appearing cysts are indeed representative precursors to RCC in individuals with VHL disease.

Evaluation

Sonography is useful in diagnosing the typical benign cystic features of VHL disease: absence of internal echoes, well-defined margins, and acoustic enhancement. On CT, sharp, thin walls are seen around homogeneous contents without enhancement after contrast medium injection. Because multiple lesions (cysts, tumors, or both) are often present, CT frequently is more useful than sonography. CT often is useful in examining the adrenal glands for pheochromocytomas.

When the lesions are small, it is impossible to distinguish tumors from cysts. In such cases, patients should have regular CT scans with narrow-screen collimation (Levine et al, 1982). With larger lesions, and whenever RCC is suspected, renal angiography with magnification or subtraction is advisable (Kadir et al, 1981; Loughlin and Gittes, 1986). This type of study helps to reveal any additional tumors and indicates the appropriateness of conservative surgery (Kadir et al, 1981; Loughlin and Gittes, 1986). Intra-arterial administration of epinephrine is sometimes helpful because it causes vasoconstriction of the normal vessels but has no effect on tumor neovascularity.

MRI has not been very useful for small tumors of the kidney unless the shape of the kidney is altered. The lesions on MRI have a signal intensity that is similar to that of normal renal parenchyma on T1- and T2-weighted images. However, gadolinium is useful because it enhances RCC. The heterogeneous nature of the larger tumors makes them more readily diagnosed (Rominger et al, 1992).

Clinical Features: Association with Renal Cell Carcinoma

The mean age at presentation is 35 to 40 years (Neumann and Zbar, 1997). There is no sex preference for the disease or for RCC development. (Sporadic RCC in individuals without VHL disease occurs more often in males and usually after age 50.)

Renal cysts, the most common and often earliest manifestation, are seen in 76% of patients (Levine et al, 1982). The cysts are bilateral 75% of the time and multifocal in 87% (Reichard et al, 1998). Diagnosis of RCC usually occurs in the fourth or fifth decade of life, whereas in the general population it more often manifests in the sixth decade (Reichard et al, 1998). RCC occurs in approximately 50% of affected individuals. The renal cysts as well as the tumors usually are asymptomatic, although large tumors may cause pain or a mass. Hematuria may occur after rupture of the tumor into the pelvicalyceal system. When cysts are present, typically they are large. Only rarely do images typify ADPKD and even less often do cysts cause renal failure.

Pheochromocytoma occurs in 10% to 17% of affected individuals and appears to be confined to specific families (Horton et al, 1976; Levine et al, 1982). Patients may present with seizures or dizziness secondary to hemangioblastomas of the central nervous system. Cerebellar hemangioblastomas usually become symptomatic between 15 and 40 years of age (Jennings and Gaines, 1988). Retinal angiomas (hemangiomas) frequently manifest early. Bleeding may cause blurred vision, retinal detachment, and blindness. Early diagnosis is important because these tumors respond to laser therapy or cryotherapy.

Because of the high incidence of RCC in patients with VHL disease, the urologist's primary role is careful surveillance so that small tumors can be identified and treated before they metastasize. Annual or perhaps biannual CT examinations are advised. Although central nervous system hemangioblastomas account for more than half of the deaths, RCC causes its own share, approximately 30% (Reichard et al, 1998).

Treatment

Frydenberg and associates (1993) recommended conservative surgery, that is, excision or partial nephrectomy, for small low-grade tumors but more aggressive surgery for tumors that are larger than 5 cm. The outlook is poorer with bilateral tumors. Low-grade bilateral tumors can be treated cautiously like unilateral tumors with close monitoring. Patients with bilateral high-grade tumors are probably served best with bilateral nephrectomy (Frydenberg et al, 1993). Between 1977 and 1997, approximately 20 patients with VHL disease received a kidney transplant. However, it is not known whether the immunosuppressive drugs required for transplantation increase the growth rate of other lesions associated with VHL disease (Neumann and Zbar, 1997). The most important need in improving survival is careful surveillance to identify tumors early and even more careful surveillance after surgery because of the multicentric characteristics of the tumor.

Classically, the survival rate after nephrectomy has been only 50%. However, in the closely monitored series of seven patients treated by Loughlin and Gittes (1986), six patients were monitored for 4 months to 8 years and only one death from metastatic disease was reported. With renal-sparing surgery, there is a 75% incidence of recurrence in the same or opposite kidney (Malek et al, 1987).

MULTICYSTIC DYSPLASTIC KIDNEY

Historically, the terms *multicystic* and *polycystic* were used interchangeably in discussing the kidney. However, in 1955, Spence stressed that these terms designated completely different entities. He included them separately in his classification, and subsequent investigators have done likewise.

The multicystic kidney represents a severe form of nongenetic dysplasia that is sometimes described as multicystic dysplasia. The kidney does not have a reniform configuration, and no calyceal drainage system is present. Typically, the

kidney has the appearance of "a bunch of grapes," with little stroma between the cysts (Fig. 114–18A). Renal size is highly variable, from slightly less than normal to enormous, filling most of the abdomen. When the cysts are small, even microscopic, and stroma predominates, the condition is referred to as solid cystic dysplasia (see Fig. 114–18B). And when an identifiable renal pelvis is associated with what appears to be a multicystic dysplastic kidney, the condition is referred to as the hydronephrotic form of multicystic kidney (see Fig. 114–18C) (Felson and Cussen, 1975).

The multicystic dysplastic kidney represents an active process, not an end result. Some areas of the kidney have increased expression of genes active in nephrogenesis and anti-apoptosis (e.g., *IGF2, WT1, PAX2, WNT4, BCL2*), whereas in other areas a lack of expression of these genes might be associated with increased cell death. The size of a multicystic dysplastic kidney and its cysts results from a balance (or imbalance) between the two. Whether a multicystic dysplastic kidney grows and dilates, shrinks, or stays the same size is dependent on this balance. It is of interest that Matsell and colleagues (1996) had the opportunity to study two human fetal multicystic dysplastic kidney specimens (14 and 19 weeks of age) and identified normal zones of nephrogenesis dispersed throughout the kidneys. The authors suggest that these scattered areas found early in development are part of this balance and disappear with gestational age. Because it is recognized that there is an increased expression of growth and transcription factors in multicystic dysplastic kidney, it might be worthwhile to consider whether some of the anecdotal cases of Wilms' tumors that have developed in multicystic kidneys might be secondary to overexpression of these genes. In addition, the fact that the contralateral kidney often has a dilated nonobstructed renal pelvis, and sometimes even a ureteropelvic junction obstruction, makes one wonder if multicystic dysplastic kidney is the result of obstruction. However, no one has succeeded in producing multicystic dysplastic kidney in animal models by creating obstruction. One must also consider why there is a 15% association of vesicoureteral reflux on the contralateral side. Is there a common molecular genetic defect? The observation that these kidneys usually are associated with ipsilateral ureteral atresia may have nothing to do with obstruction (although it might). Perhaps a similar damaged pathway leads to both deficient ureteric bud branching and ureteral atresia.

Although it is often stated that the large cysts of multicystic dysplastic kidney do not connect with each other, it must be realized that this is an impression made from imaging studies. In fact, when contrast agent is injected into one cyst, invariably it passes to others through a network of ducts. A single ostium is located in each calyx and usually is easily seen opening into a set of channels. The fact that this ostium is visible to the naked eye makes one consider that the large cysts are derived from the ureteric bud rather than the blastema.

Etiology

In the view of Felson and Cussen (1975), the multicystic kidney is an extreme form of hydronephrosis that occurs secondary to atresia of the ureter or renal pelvis, which is a frequent concomitant condition. The fact that the left kidney is the one more often affected supports this view, because this is

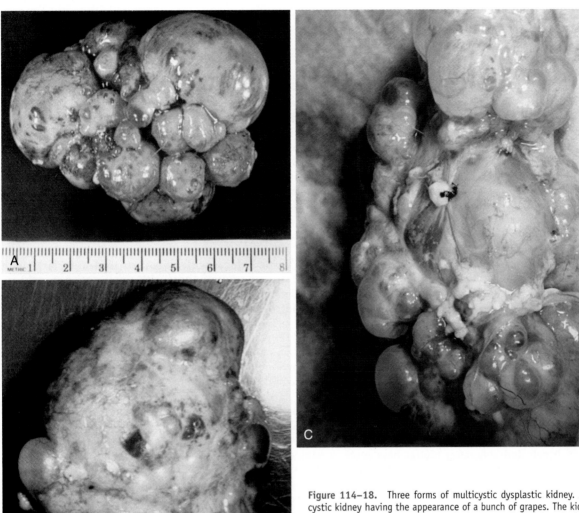

Figure 114–18. Three forms of multicystic dysplastic kidney. **A,** A typical multicystic kidney having the appearance of a bunch of grapes. The kidney was composed almost entirely of cysts with very little stroma. **B,** Nonfunctioning solid cystic dysplastic kidney, which differs from classic multicystic kidney in that it has smaller and fewer cysts and is composed predominantly of stroma. **C,** Hydronephrotic form of multicystic kidney, which has a medial pelvis that typically is larger than any of the cysts in its associated kidney.

the kidney more often associated with primary obstructive megaureter (Glassberg, 1977) and ureteropelvic junction obstruction (Johnston et al, 1977). In testing this hypothesis, several investigators have attempted to establish an animal model by ligating the ureter at various points in gestation (Beck, 1971; Tanagho, 1972; Fetterman et al, 1974). This approach is not effective in middle or late gestation; early ligation of the fetal lamb ureter produces renal dysplasia but not multicystic dysplasia (Beck, 1971). However, Berman and Maizel (1982) were unable to obtain similar results in the chick. Similarly, other investigators have been able to induce dysplasia, but no one as yet has been able to induce a multicystic dysplastic kidney.

Other theories have been offered by Hildebrandt (1894) and by Osathanondh and Potter (1964). Hildebrandt (1894) suggested that failure of the union between the ureteric bud and the metanephric blastema leads to cystic dilatation in the latter; this hypothesis, like the obstructive view, is supported by the high incidence of concomitant ureteral atresia. Osathanondh and Potter (1964) postulated that Potter type IIA kidneys, the type with large cysts, result from an ampullary abnormality in which the ampullae stop dividing early and therefore produce fewer generations of tubules. In this view, the last generation of tubules produced is cystic and does not induce metanephric differentiation, and the occasional normal or near-normal nephron is the result of a rare normal ampulla and collecting tubules.

Clinical Features

Multicystic dysplasia is the most common type of renal cystic disease, and it is one of the most common causes of an abdominal mass in infants (Longino and Martin, 1958; Melicow and Uson, 1959; Griscom et al, 1975). Widespread prenatal ultrasound evaluation has greatly increased the frequency with which the condition is identified. Although the pathogenetic process leading to a multicystic kidney probably is operative by the 8th week in utero, the mean age at the time of antenatal diagnosis is about 28 weeks, with a range of 21 to 35 weeks (Avni et al, 1987). The reason is not apparent. In less severely affected patients, the condition may be an incidental finding during evaluation of an adult for abdominal pain, hematuria, hypertension, or an unrelated condition. At any age, the condition is more likely to be found on the left (Friedman and Abeshouse, 1957; Fine and Burns, 1959; Parkkulainen et al, 1959; Pathak and Williams, 1964; Griscom et al, 1975). Males are more likely to have unilateral multicystic dysplastic kidneys (2.4:1), whereas bilateral multicystic kidneys appear twice as often in females (Lazebnick et al, 1999). Unilateral multicystic kidneys, when not associated with other renal or nonrenal anomalies, rarely involve a chromosomal disorder. Bilateral disease, however, is associated with other anomalies as well as chromosomal anomalies. Such information may be important for genetic counseling (Lazebnick et al, 1999).

The contralateral system frequently is abnormal as well. For example, contralateral ureteropelvic junction obstruction is found in 3% to 12% of infants with multicystic kidney and contralateral vesicoureteral reflux is seen even more often, in 18% to 43% of infants (Heikkinen et al, 1980; Atiyeh et al, 1992; Flack and Bellinger, 1993; Wacksman and Phipps, 1993; Al-Khaldi et al, 1994). Because the high incidence of reflux, voiding cystourethrography usually has been considered advisable in all newborns with a multicystic kidney. However, Ismali and colleagues (2004) have more recently questioned the routine need for a voiding cystourethrogram. Instead they believe that if a normal contralateral kidney is seen on ultrasound in the first week of life and again on a repeat ultrasound within a few weeks, it is unlikely that reflux is present on the contralateral side and, if it is, it is very mild and likely will disappear.

When a diagnosis of multicystic kidney is made in utero by ultrasound, the disease is found to be bilateral in 19% to 34% of cases (Kleiner et al, 1986; Al-Khaldi et al, 1994). Those with bilateral disease often have other severe deformities or polysystemic malformation syndromes (Al-Khaldi et al, 1994). In bilateral cases, the newborn has the classic abnormal facies and oligohydramnios characteristic of Potter's syndrome. The bilateral condition is incompatible with survival, although one infant reportedly survived for 69 days (Kishikawa et al, 1981). Another association, between multicystic kidney and contralateral renal agenesis, likewise is incompatible with life. The association of any of several entities—renal agenesis, renal dysplasia, multicystic dysplastic kidney, and renal aplasia—within one family has been referred to as *familial renal adysplasia* (see earlier discussion).

Involution sometimes occurs in the multicystic kidney, either antenatally or postnatally (Hashimoto et al, 1986; Avni et al, 1987). This involution may be so severe that the affected kidney disappears from subsequent sonograms. In such cases, the kidney may be only a "nubbin," and the condition is referred to as "renal aplasia" or "aplastic dysplasia" (Bernstein and Gardner, 1989; Glassberg and Filmer, 1992). Previously, aplastic kidneys, which often are associated with atretic ureters, were thought to be a separate entity. Now, with the

experience of monitoring multicystic kidneys sonographically, it is apparent that most aplastic kidneys represent involuted multicystic organs.

Multicystic dysplasia can involve one segment of a horseshoe kidney (Greene et al, 1971; Walker et al, 1978; Borer et al, 1994) or one pole of a duplex kidney.

Cystic dysplasia of the testes, a benign rare lesion of the rete testis, may be associated with an ipsilateral multicystic dysplastic kidney, although more often with renal agenesis. Some of the cases of unilateral agenesis probably represent involuted multicystic dysplastic kidney. The common etiology in such cases would seem to be abnormalities of the ipsilateral wolffian duct that cause anomalies in both the testis and kidney (Wojcik et al, 1997; Lane et al, 1998).

Histopathology

Multicystic kidneys with large cysts tend to be large with little stroma, whereas those with small cysts generally are smaller and more solid. The blood supply likewise is variable, ranging from a pedicle with small vessels to no pedicle at all (Parkkulainen et al, 1959). Usually the ureter is partly or totally atretic, and the renal pelvis may be absent. Griscom and associates (1975) referred to the form without a renal pelvis as "pyeloinfundibular atresia" and reported finding no evidence of communication between the cysts. However, others have shown distribution of contrast medium among the cysts by means of connecting tubules (Saxton et al, 1981). I have found these tubules by probing gross specimens and by injecting contrast medium into one of the cysts and visualizing the connections between the cysts radiographically (Fig. 114–19). Felson and Cussen (1975) referred to the variety with a renal pelvis as the "hydronephrotic type" and demonstrated connections between the cysts and the renal pelvis. Thirty-three multicystic kidneys, including 7 of our own cases and 11 of

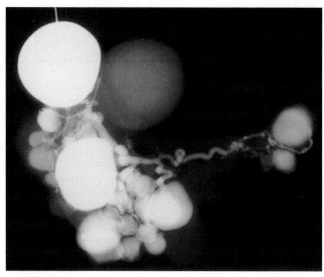

Figure 114–19. Contrast study of a multicystic kidney representing one component of a horseshoe kidney removed at surgery. Contrast medium injected into one cyst demonstrates communication between the cysts by tubular structures. (From Borer JG, Glassberg KI, Kassner G, et al: Unilateral multicystic dysplasia in one component of a horseshoe kidney: Case report and review of the literature. J Urol 1994;152:1568.)

Dewan and Goh's cases, were injected with contrast agent intracystically. Seven of the 33 kidneys were of the hydronephrotic type (Dewan and Goh, 1994; Glassberg and Kassner, 1998). Connections between cysts were identified in 30 of the 33 kidneys injected. In other words, the vast majority of multicystic dysplastic kidneys, including both the hydronephrotic and nonhydronephrotic variants, had communication between cysts. We found, as did Griscom and coworkers (1975) previously, the presence of one or more pits or orifices at the hilum side of each cyst. These pits were found to communicate with the tubular structures that are seen on radiographic examination between the cysts.

Microscopically, the cysts are lined by low cuboidal epithelium. They are separated by thin septa of fibrous tissue and primitive dysplastic elements, especially primitive ducts. Frequently, immature glomeruli are present, and on occasion a few mature glomeruli are seen.

KEY POINTS: MULTICYSTIC DYSPLASTIC KIDNEY

- Multicystic dysplastic kidney is a dysplastic kidney with cysts, is associated with active expression of genes involved with nephrogenesis, and has a changing morphology.

- Kidneys usually get smaller or disappear from view on imaging studies (i.e., renal aplasia), very occasionally increase in size, and very rarely are associated with Wilms' tumor.

- The patient needs to be monitored for tumor and hypertension, at least in the first 5 years of life.

- There is no clear indication for removal of the kidney unless an increased amount of solid tissue is identified.

- Fifteen percent of patients have associated contralateral reflux, and debate exists regarding whether or not to obtain a voiding cystourethrogram in all or only in those with some degree of fullness in the contralateral collecting system.

Evaluation

Renal masses in infants most often represent either multicystic kidney disease or hydronephrosis, and it is important to distinguish between the two, especially if the surgeon wishes to remove a nonfunctioning hydronephrotic kidney or repair a ureteropelvic junction obstruction while leaving a multicystic organ in situ. In newborns, ultrasonography usually is the first study performed. In a few cases, it is difficult to differentiate multicystic kidney disease from severe hydronephrosis (Gates, 1980; Hadlock et al, 1981). **In general, however, the multicystic kidney has a haphazard distribution of cysts of various sizes without a larger central or medial cyst and without visible communications between the cysts. Frequently, very small cysts appear between the large cysts. In comparison, in ureteropelvic junction**

obstruction the cysts or calyces are organized around the periphery of the kidney, connections usually can be demonstrated between the peripheral cysts and a central or medial cyst that represents the renal pelvis, and there is absence of small cysts between the larger cysts (Fig. 114–20). When there is an identifiable renal sinus, the diagnosis is more likely to be hydronephrosis than multicystic kidney.

In these difficult cases, radioisotope studies may be helpful. **Hydronephrotic kidneys usually show some function on a dimercaptosuccinic acid (DMSA) scan, whereas renal uptake is seldom seen in multicystic kidneys.** Angiography reveals an absent or small renal artery in the multicystic kidney, but this study is rarely indicated. Cystoscopy may reveal a hemitrigone and absent ureteral orifice on the affected side; more often, however, an orifice is present but retrograde urography demonstrates ureteral atresia. Again, this study is seldom performed.

In a few cases, diagnostic studies are not performed until the patient is older. In these instances, the plain abdominal film often reveals renal calcifications. These deposits usually appear as annular or arcuate shadows (Felson and Cussen, 1975).

As mentioned previously, voiding cystourethrography is indicated in the workup because of the high incidence of reflux into the single functioning kidney.

Treatment and Prognosis

It has often been stated that the multicystic kidney can be ignored unless its bulk is inconvenient (Pathak and Williams, 1964; Griscom et al, 1975) and that attention should be directed instead to identifying any abnormalities of the contralateral urinary tract. Certainly, the need in the past to explore some multicystic kidneys to rule out malignancy (e.g., cystic Wilms' tumor, congenital mesoblastic nephroma) has largely been erased by new diagnostic tools. Kidneys that do contain malignancies are likely to be explored because of the retention of some function as seen by excretory urography or nuclear medicine studies (Walker et al, 1984); therefore, routine exploration solely to rule out malignancy is inappropriate.

A nonfunctioning hydronephrotic kidney could be mistaken for a multicystic kidney, although complete nonfunction on a nuclear medicine study is unusual in kidneys affected by ureteropelvic junction obstruction. Even if the correct diagnosis is missed in such a case, however, there are unlikely to be significant consequences, because a totally nonfunctioning hydronephrotic kidney is rarely salvageable and probably will cause no problems other than a predisposition to infection or hyperkalemia.

Of greater concern is the potential for malignant degeneration in a multicystic kidney. In very few reports has the diagnosis of multicystic kidney been made before the diagnosis of an associated cancer (Oddone et al, 1994).

Most case reports have been of Wilms' tumor and less often RCC that developed in a previously "unrecognized" multicystic dysplastic kidney. Because many tumors have cystic components (e.g., cystic partially differentiated nephroblastoma), one cannot absolutely conclude that such a kidney was a multicystic dysplastic one at birth. Beckwith (1997) cited examples of reports in the literature of Wilms' tumor in a

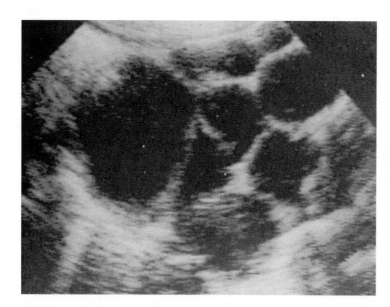

Figure 114–20. Female neonate with left multicystic kidney. Note large cysts arranged in a haphazard manner without any evidence of connections to or the presence of a large central or medial cyst. (Gross specimen appears in Figure 114–18A.)

multicystic dysplastic kidney that, on his review of the photomicrographs, were not Wilms' tumor but nephrogenic rests.

Two reports in the literature might be interpreted as reinforcing the arguments in favor of prophylactic surgical removal. Dimmick and coworkers (1989) and Noe and coworkers (1989) described a total of 120 patients, of whom 5 had nephrogenic rests of nodular renal blastema. In addition, one of the patients in the series of Dimmick and coworkers (1989) had Wilms' tumorlets in the hilar region. Although these findings suggest a hazard in leaving a multicystic kidney in situ, it is unusual for nodular renal blastema or even Wilms' tumorlets to develop into frank Wilms' tumor. For example, nodular renal blastema has been reported in 0.25% to 0.5% of normal kidneys (Bennington and Beckwith, 1975; Bove and McAdams, 1976; Beckwith, 1986), yet the incidence of Wilms' tumor in the general population is much lower. Therefore, although nodular renal blastema and Wilms' tumorlets may be part of a nephroblastomatosis/Wilms' tumor spectrum, the majority of these lesions involute in time without ever becoming malignant.

Trying to predict what percentage of multicystic kidneys will develop Wilms' tumors, Noe and associates (1989) used Beckwith's estimated 1% incidence of Wilms' tumor development in nodular renal blastema. They then calculated, using a 5% incidence of nodular renal blastema in multicystic kidneys, that 2000 nephrectomies for multicystic kidney disease would have to be performed to prevent one Wilms' tumor. Accordingly, the risk of surgery must be weighed against that of Wilms' tumor. If one elects to monitor without surgery, the cost-benefit ratio or even the effectiveness of long-term follow-up must be considered. Because nodular renal blastema occurs most often in the hilum (Dimmick et al, 1989), and because most kidneys that shrink lose only cyst fluid, leaving the dysplastic tissue, follow-up by sonography may not be helpful (Colodny, 1989).

In an effort to determine whether there is a relationship between multicystic dysplasia and neoplasia, Jung and coworkers (1990) performed flow cytometric analyses on specimens from 30 patients. No evidence of tetraploidy or aneuploidy, as would be expected in a preneoplastic condition,

was found. This report is comforting to the surgeon who does not routinely remove multicystic kidneys. Still, one must be aware that some malignant cells retain a diploid karyotype. In a more recent study, Perez and colleagues (1998) identified only five reported cases in the United States of Wilms' tumor developing in a multicystic dysplastic kidney over the preceding 14 years. They estimated the incidence of this progression to be 3 to 10 times greater than in the general population. This number corresponds with Beckwith's report of a fivefold incidence of nephrogenic rests in persons with multicystic kidney compared with the general population.

Of the 7500 Wilms' tumor specimens reviewed by Beckwith (1997) over 18.75 years, only 5 cases had occurred in a multicystic dysplastic kidney. Beckwith thought it unlikely that the incidence of Wilms' tumor developing in multicystic dysplastic kidneys is greater than fourfold, citing an incidence of 1 in 8000 in the general population and 1 in 2000 in the multicystic dysplastic population. He concluded that this fourfold increase does not make a case for prophylactic nephrectomy. He further pointed out that if Wilms' tumor does develop, the condition is not as severe as in the past, because the survival rate is now greater than 90%.

Homsy and associates (1997) reported perhaps the two best documented cases of previously diagnosed multicystic dysplastic kidneys that went on to develop Wilms' tumor.

Another management question in multicystic kidney disease is the frequency of hypertension. Gordon and associates (1988) reviewed this topic in a thoughtful article. They noted that since 1966 only nine well-documented cases of hypertension in association with multicystic kidneys in situ had been published. In three of these cases, the hypertension resolved after nephrectomy (Javadpour et al, 1970; Burgler and Hauri, 1983; Chen et al, 1985).

In more recent reports, hypertension resolved after nephrectomy in two of three hypertensive patients studied by Webb and colleagues (1997) and in two of four children studied by Snodgrass (2000). Of 887 patients in the AAP Multicystic Kidney Disease Registry, only 6 (0.7%) had hypertension, and the etiology of the hypertension was questionable in most.

In a series of 20 patients older than 11 years who had multicystic kidney disease, Ambrose (1976) found that 2 had hypertension, and in neither of these patients was the blood pressure controlled by nephrectomy. **In summary, hypertension occurs infrequently with multicystic dysplastic kidney and it may or may not normalize after nephrectomy. The role of peripheral vein renin is not clear** (Snodgrass, 2000). Nevertheless, the incidence of hypertension is not high enough to warrant nephrectomy, although it certainly is a finding warranting routine blood pressure monitoring. Other reports suggest that the incidence of hypertension may actually be greater than that reported in the literature (Emmert and King, 1994; Hanna, 1995; Webb et al, 1997).

A large number of patients have now been monitored for longer than 5 years by the National Multicystic Kidney Registry (Table 114–8). When the status of neonatal multicystic kidneys is monitored over a period of time, the vast majority either become smaller or stay the same size, and only a very small percentage become larger. If the kidney becomes larger, depending on the surgeon's inclinations, consideration can be given to removal. When the kidney stays the same size, it actually becomes smaller in proportion to the size of the child as he or she gets older. Most kidneys that become smaller do so during the first year of follow-up, and an increasing number of those that become smaller disappear from view with time on ultrasound examination. None of the multicystic kidneys in the registry has developed a tumor during follow-up. However, a number of kidneys were removed at the time of entry into the study by decision of the individual surgeon and a smaller number were removed later because of increasing size during follow-up. As a result, it cannot be determined whether the kidneys that were selected for nephrectomy had a greater potential for malignancy or hypertension. Hypertension has developed in only five of the patients in the registry, and it is not clear from the data how many of these cases of hypertension were thought to be secondary to the multicystic kidney. Occasional urinary tract infections have been seen, but it is unclear whether the multicystic kidney had anything to do with them, particularly because many of these patients also have contralateral reflux.

Questions still must be answered. Does the disappearance of a multicystic kidney on imaging studies mean that there is no longer a potential risk? When these kidneys disappear from view, it means only that the fluid within the cysts has disappeared; the cells still remain. How necessary is it to follow those patients who are not operated on, because many inevitably will be lost to follow-up? Perez and coworkers (1998) recommended renal ultrasound every 3 months until

8 years of age, when the incidence of Wilms' tumor is almost nil. From the experience of Ambrose (1976), it appears that flank pain as an adult is the chief risk of a multicystic kidney that is left in situ, and in such cases the pain usually responds to nephrectomy.

Elder and coworkers (1995) reported on 30 multicystic kidneys that were removed in an ambulatory setting within an operative time of 20 to 70 minutes, making the case for an alternative approach to nonsurgical management. In the clinical setting, however, parents will respond differently to the suggestion that surgery provides less risk than long-term follow-up of a disease that has a low association with development of malignancy. Certainly the prejudices of the individual surgeon presenting the choice of surgery or conservative follow-up play a significant role in a parent's decision.

If we use the recommendations of Perez and colleagues (1997) for conservative management including a renal ultrasound study every 3 months until 8 years of age, the cost ($2,000 to $5,000) is still not more than for a simple nephrectomy ($5,000 to $7,000). In summary, although the incidence of Wilms' tumor developing in a multicystic dysplastic kidney may be higher than in a normal kidney (3- to 10-fold), the numbers do not make a strong case for either prophylactic nephrectomy or conservative nonsurgical follow-up.

BENIGN MULTILOCULAR CYST (CYSTIC NEPHROMA)

A multilocular cystic lesion in a child's kidney may be a benign multilocular cyst, a multilocular cyst with partially differentiated Wilms' tumor, a multilocular cyst with nodules of Wilms' tumor, or cystic Wilms' tumor (Fig. 114–21). These four lesions form a spectrum, with benign multilocular cyst at one extreme and cystic Wilms' tumor at the other. There has been some debate as to whether these represent a spectrum of one disease with one etiology lying between a benign multilocular cyst and a cystic adenocarcinoma or some other cystic renal tumor.

A multilocular cyst is not a renal segment affected by multicystic kidney disease; these conditions differ clinically, histologically, and radiographically. However, controversy continues about whether the multilocular cyst is a segmental form of renal dysplasia (Powell et al, 1951; Osathanondh and Potter, 1964; Johnson et al, 1973); a hamartomatous malformation (Arey, 1959); or a neoplastic disease (Boggs and Kimmelstiel, 1956; Christ, 1968; Fowler, 1971; Gallo and

Table 114–8. National Multicystic Kidney Registry: Sonographic Follow-up

Follow-up	No. of Children	Not Identifiable	Smaller	Larger	Unchanged
1–3 mo	140	7 (5.0%)	64 (45.7%)	16 (11.4%)	53 (37.9%)
4–66 mo	181	13 (7.2%)	119 (65.7%)	9 (5.0%)	40 (22.1%)
7–9 mo	134	13 (9.7%)	73 (54.5%)	4 (3.0%)	44 (32.0%)
10–12 mo	96	14 (14.6%)	41 (42.7%)	5 (5.2%)	36 (37.5%)
1–3 yr	622	99 (15.9%)	286 (46.0%)	26 (4.2%)	211 (33.4%)
3–5 yr	183	42 (22.9%)	63 (34.4%)	10 (5.5%)	68 (37.2%)
>5 yr	159	38 (23.9%)	60 (37.7%)	2 (1.3%)	59 (37.1%)

Data supplied by J. Wacksman and L. Phipps, National Multicystic Kidney Registry, American Academy of Pediatrics, October, 2000.

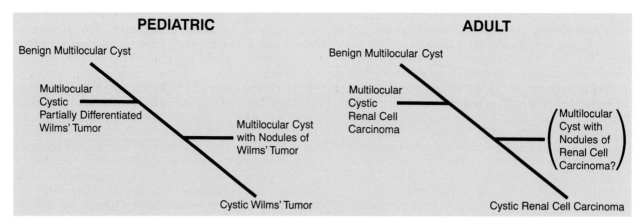

Figure 114–21. The spectrum of multilocular cystic lesions in children and adults. There is no evidence that one lesion can convert into the other. Benign cystic partially differentiated Wilms' tumor and multilocular cystic renal cell carcinoma act as benign lesions. When nodules of tumor are present the lesion should be considered malignant, although the prognosis of this lesion as well as cystic Wilms' tumor and cystic renal cell carcinoma seems to be better than that of the corresponding solid lesions. It is not clear whether clinical examples of "multilocular cyst with nodules of renal cell carcinoma" actually exist, but this entity is placed in the spectrum for consideration. For simplicity, the multilocular-appearing lesions of other cystic tumors (e.g., cystic oncocytoma, cystic hamartoma of the renal pelvis) are not included in the figure.

Penchansky, 1977). The confusion arises in part from the variability of the histologic picture: the appearance of the primitive stroma, the maturity of tubular and even on occasion of muscle elements, and the degree of epithelial atypia that differs not only from patient to patient but also within the same lesion.

Past use of many nonspecific terms—such as lymphangioma, partial or focal polycystic kidney, multicystic kidney, and cystic adenoma—makes it difficult to identify relevant published cases for review (Aterman et al, 1973). Edmunds used the term *cystic adenoma* in 1892 in what was probably the first published description of this lesion. I favor the term *benign multilocular cyst* because the descriptor "benign" separates this lesion from other multilocular cystic lesions and the words "multilocular cyst" clearly describe the gross appearance of the lesion. Joshi and Beckwith (1989) prefer the term *cystic nephroma* because it implies a benign but neoplastic lesion. Some refer to the spaces within the lesion as *loculi*, and others use the term *cysts*.

Clinical Features

The great majority of patients present before the age of 4 years or after 30 years. Five percent present between 4 and 30 years. The patient is twice as likely to be male if younger than 4 years and eight times as likely to be female if older than 30 years of age (Eble and Bonsib, 1998).

The signs and symptoms differ according to the age at presentation. In children, an asymptomatic flank mass is the most common finding, whereas most adults present with either a flank mass, abdominal pain, or hematuria. The bleeding is secondary to herniation of the cyst through the transitional epithelium into the renal pelvis (Uson and Melicow, 1963; Aterman et al, 1973; Madewell et al, 1983).

Seven cases of bilateral benign multilocular cysts of the kidney have been described (Castillo et al, 1991); in one of these patients, the lesion recurred after excision (Geller et al, 1979). Also, at least two instances are known in which multi-locular cysts arose in kidneys known to have been normal previously (Uson and Melicow, 1963; Chatten and Bishop, 1977). Such cases support a neoplastic theory of the origin of this lesion.

Histopathology

These lesions are bulky and are circumscribed by a thick capsule. Normal renal parenchyma adjacent to the lesion frequently is compressed by it. The lesion may extend beyond the renal capsule into the perinephric space or renal pelvis. The loculi, which range from a few millimeters to centimeters in diameter, do not intercommunicate. They contain clear, straw-colored or yellow fluid and are lined by cuboidal or low columnar epithelial cells. In some cases, eosinophilic cuboidal cells project into the cyst lumen, creating a hobnail appearance (Madewell et al, 1983). The definitions of multilocular cystic kidney given by Powell and coworkers (1951) and by Boggs and Kimmelstiel (1956) require a normal epithelial lining for the diagnosis. **Joshi and Beckwith (1989) also defined the septa of a benign multilocular cyst as being composed of fibrous tissue in which well-differentiated tubules may be present but poorly differentiated tissues and blastemal cells are not present.**

When Castillo and associates (1991) reviewed the literature on multilocular cysts, they included lesions that had interlocular septa containing tissue of two different types: (1) fibrous tissue only or (2) embryonic-type tissue. Adults in general have only the first type, whereas children, principally those younger than 3 years of age, have either type. Joshi and Beckwith (1989) referred to the embryonic type as an immature form. They prefer the term *cystic partially differentiated nephroblastoma* (Joshi, 1980), because histologically this form is different from the first group, which they believe is the typical benign multilocular cyst. To make the diagnosis of a cystic partially differentiated nephroblastoma, blastemal cells must be present. Often varying amounts of poorly differentiated tissues such as tubules, glomeruli, mesenchyme, skeletal muscle, and, rarely, cartilage are admixed with the blastemal cells (Joshi and Beckwith, 1989). These elements are not present in benign multilocular cysts. Supportive evidence that the second variety should not be called a benign multilocular cyst lies in the histories of Joshi and Beckwith's (1989) 18 patients with cystic partially differentiated nephroblastoma: 1 patient had a contralateral anaplastic Wilms' tumor, and another had two local recurrences after nephrectomy.

Eble and Bonsib (1998) believe that cystic nephroma in children is a different entity than in adults. They believe that benign multilocular cyst and cystic partially differentiated Wilms' tumor are the same disease in childhood. Because neither metastasizes, they prefer to call both conditions in childhood *cystic partially differentiated nephroblastoma* and to leave the term *cystic nephroma* to the adult variety.

As noted earlier, benign multilocular cysts **can be considered as part of a spectrum. Within that spectrum lies cystic partially differentiated nephroblastoma** (see Fig. 114–21). I prefer the term *multilocular cystic partially differentiated Wilms' tumor* to *cystic partially differentiated nephroblastoma*, because two of the other entities within the spectrum are described with the category Wilms' tumor. For example, when nodules of Wilms' tumor are present, Joshi (1980) designates the lesion as a *multilocular cyst with nodules of Wilms' tumor*. The term *cystic Wilms' tumor* is reserved for the rare cases of tumor in which cysts are lined by epithelial cells. This entity should not be confused with Wilms' tumors that have sonolucent or radiolucent cyst-like spaces attributable to tumor necrosis.

Although in children there may be a continuum from benign multilocular cyst to cystic Wilms' tumor, and although all of these lesions may be derived from similar cells or tissues, no evidence suggests that one entity transforms into another. Furthermore, **none of the genetically determined conditions associated with Wilms' tumor (e.g., hemihypertrophy, aniridia) has accompanied a benign multilocular cyst** (Banner et al, 1981).

In adults there also is a spectrum of multilocular cystic lesions. For example, **if an adult is identified with a multilocular cystic lesion, it can be either a multilocular cystic RCC, a cystic RCC, a cystic oncocytoma, or some rare tumor such as cystic hamartoma of the renal pelvis.** Eble and Bonsib (1998) found 44 reported adult cases of "multilocular cystic RCC." One year later, Kirsh and coworkers (1999) added four of their own cases, but they preferred the term *benign adenomatous multicystic kidney tumor* because of the lesion's benign nature. This tumor has also been referred to as Perlmann's tumor, because Perlmann (1928) was the first to describe the lesion. Perlmann, however, interpreted his findings as representing a cystic lymphangioma (Perlmann, 1928; Kirsh et al, 1999). Just as cystic partially differentiated Wilms' tumor in children falls in the spectrum between benign multilocular cyst and cystic Wilms' tumor, so does multilocular cystic RCC in adults fall in the spectrum between a benign multilocular cyst and a cystic RCC. Also, just as in partially differentiated Wilms' tumor there are blastema cells lying in the septa between loculi and sometimes lining the loculi, so, too, in multilocular cystic RCC, clear cells and clear epithelial cells lie between the loculi and line the loculi. Neither condition has expansile nodules, and neither condition metastasizes

(Eble and Bonsib, 1998). It is not clear whether there is a condition in adults that resembles the next lesion in the pediatric spectrum—multilocular cyst with nodules of Wilms' tumor. The cystic component of the tumor at the carcinomatosis end of the spectrum in both children and adults (i.e., cystic Wilms' tumor and cystic RCC) improves the prognosis of the malignant lesion (Kirsh et al, 1999). In adults, as in children, there is no evidence that one lesion can convert into another. As an education tool, the spectrum of multilocular cystic lesions in children and adults may be considered in a parallel fashion. I therefore suggest use of the parallel terms *multilocular cystic partially differentiated Wilms' tumor* and *multilocular cystic RCC* (Fig. 114–22).

An even rarer tumor in adults, cystic hamartoma of the renal pelvis, also cannot be differentiated from other multilocular cystic tumors on imaging studies. Although the tumor arises centrally within the kidney, its proximity to the pelvis and often herniation into the pelvis give it its name. The benign tumors are composed of microcysts and tubules. The stroma consists of spindle cells. Mitotic figures do not appear (Eble and Bonsib, 1998).

KEY POINTS: BENIGN MULTILOCULAR CYST

- A benign multilocular cyst is a benign, nondysplastic, neoplastic lesion that occurs most commonly either before the age of 4 years, when it appears most frequently in males, or after 30 years, when it is seen predominantly in females.

- The only way to determine the diagnosis of a multilocular cystic lesion identified on imaging studies, in either a child or adult, is by surgical excision.

- The diagnosis in an adult will either be a benign multilocular cyst, a multilocular cyst with partially differentiated Wilms' tumor, a multilocular cyst with nodules of Wilms' tumor, or cystic Wilms' tumor.

Evaluation

A number of tests may be useful, including intravenous urography, sonography, CT, MRI, cyst puncture with aspiration and double-contrast cystography, and arteriography. **Ultrasound and CT can distinguish multicystic kidney and multilocular cyst, but neither study is sufficiently reliable to distinguish multilocular cyst, multilocular cyst with foci of Wilms' tumor or adenocarcinoma, mesoblastic nephroma, cystic Wilms' tumor, and clear cell sarcoma.** Typically, the septa are highly echogenic with sonolucent loculi, although if there is debris in a loculus, it may appear more solid. On CT, the septa are less dense than normal parenchyma; when myxomatous material is present, the density is equal to that of solid structures (Wood et al, 1982). Calcification is rarely visible in such lesions in children (Madewell et al, 1983).

In the few cases in which angiography was performed, vascular, hypovascular, and hypervascular patterns were seen (Davides, 1976; Madewell et al, 1983; DeWall et al, 1986). A

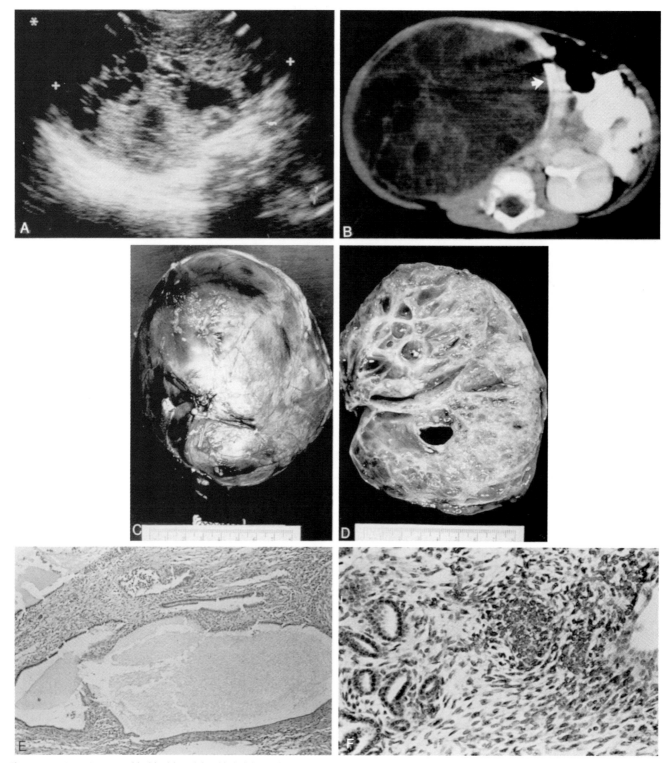

Figure 114–22. A 4-year-old girl with a right-sided abdominal mass. **A,** Renal sonogram shows multiple cysts throughout the left kidney. **B,** On contrast medium–enhanced CT scan, a large, smoothly outlined left renal mass is seen with fine septa throughout the mass. Residual preserved parenchyma and the pelvicalyceal system are compressed medially and pushed to the contralateral side *(arrow).* **C,** Uncut gross specimen reveals a smooth-walled, encapsulated renal mass. **D,** Cross section of mass reveals multiple noncommunicating loculations. **E,** On histology, a hypocellular cystic area is seen with monotonous stroma (×100). **F,** Between loculi, nests of blastemal cells are visualized along with tubular elements *(left),* making the diagnosis of multilocular cyst with partially differentiated Wilms' tumor (×200).

tumor blush and neovascularity that sometimes was extensive were apparent in some cases (Madewell et al, 1983).

Clear to yellow fluid is recovered by cyst puncture. Contrast agents opacify only those loculi through which the needle has passed, because the loculi do not communicate (Madewell et al, 1983).

Treatment

The treatment for benign multilocular cyst, multilocular cystic partially differentiated Wilms' tumor, and multilocular cystic RCC is nephrectomy. If the lesion is localized enough and there is well-preserved normal tissue, excision of the lesion or partial nephrectomy is feasible. Children who have a multilocular cyst with nodules of Wilms' tumor or a cystic Wilms' tumor should be treated as for Wilms' tumor, recognizing the generally favorable outlook. Similarly, cystic RCC in adults should be managed as a malignant lesion, again, however, recognizing its better prognosis. In adults, benign multilocular cysts more often are associated with larger amounts of normal renal tissue, making partial nephrectomy more often feasible. In a report by Castillo and associates (1991), 24 of 29 patients underwent renal-sparing surgery, including 2 who were children. The treatment for multilocular cystic lesions in most children is nephrectomy, because the lesion usually is associated with little preserved tissue. In children, two questions must be answered in selecting the treatment for a multilocular cystic lesion: (1) Is the contralateral urinary tract normal? and (2) Is the abnormal kidney involved with Wilms' tumor? At least four of the cystic tumors in the National Wilms' Tumor Study (NWTS) metastasized (Beckwith and Palmer, 1978); therefore, these lesions clearly have malignant potential, although they appear to be less aggressive than classic Wilms' tumor.

The treatment of a multilocular cyst in most children is nephrectomy. If pathologic review shows cystic Wilms' tumor, further treatment should be given according to the NWTS recommendations for the appropriate stage of disease. However, if the focus of tumor does not exceed 2 cm, nephrectomy alone may be sufficient. If enucleation or partial nephrectomy is chosen, recurrence is possible. However, with more Wilms' tumors being treated by local excision, the case for enucleation or partial nephrectomy combined with close follow-up by sonography and CT is stronger, even if malignancy is found within the lesion. In comparison, if a clear cell sarcoma is found after enucleation, the remaining ipsilateral renal tissue should be removed because of the aggressiveness of this cancer. The recurrence of a multilocular cyst not containing malignancy probably reflects inadequate excision of the initial lesion.

SIMPLE CYSTS

A simple cyst is a discrete finding that may occur well within a kidney or on its surface. It is usually oval to round, has a smooth outline bordered by a single layer of flattened cuboidal epithelium, and is filled with transudate-like clear or straw-colored fluid. It is not connected to any part of the nephron, although it may originate initially from a portion of the nephron. Simple cysts may be singular or multiple and unilateral or bilateral.

Simple cysts may manifest at any time in utero and have been diagnosed as early as 14 weeks of gestation. **Sonography done on 29,984 fetuses in succession revealed 0.09% of 11,000 pregnancies to have renal cysts** (Blazer et al, 1999). In 25 fetuses the cysts resolved before birth. Of two cysts that remained after birth, one was the first sign of a multicystic kidney. All 28 children were healthy without genitourinary system anomalies and with no chromosomal anomalies (Blazer et al, 1999). Between birth and 18 years of age, the incidence of simple renal cysts is fairly stable, ranging from 0.1% to 0.45%, with an average incidence of 0.22% (McHugh et al, 1991). However, in adults the frequency rises with age. Using CT, Laucks and McLachlan (1981) demonstrated that the incidence of cysts was 20% by age 40 years and approximately 33% after age 60. On autopsy, Kissane and Smith (1975) identified a 50% incidence of simple renal cysts after age 50. Most reports show no gender predilection; however, in at least two studies, men were affected more frequently than women (Bearth and Steg, 1977; Tada et al, 1983).

Clinical Features

In both children and adults, cysts rarely call attention to themselves. Instead, they are discovered incidentally on sonography, CT, or urography performed for a urinary tract or other pelvic or abdominal problem. However, cysts can produce an abdominal mass or pain, hematuria secondary to rupture into the pyelocalyceal system, and hypertension secondary to segmental ischemia (Rockson et al, 1974; Lüscher et al, 1986; Papanicolaou et al, 1986). Cysts can cause calyceal or renal pelvic obstruction as well (Wahlqvist and Grumstedt, 1966; Evans and Coughlin, 1970; Hinman, 1978; Barloon and Vince, 1987). They may or may not increase in size with time. Of 23 cysts in 22 children who underwent sonographic follow-up for up to 5 years, McHugh and associates (1991) found that 17 cysts (74%) remained unchanged in size.

Cysts can rupture into the pelvicalyceal system, maintain a communication, and become a pseudocalyceal diverticulum. The reverse is also possible: closure of the communication of a diverticulum can create a simple cyst (Mosli et al, 1986; Papanicolaou et al, 1986). These two sequences of events can be distinguished only by histologic examination. **Theoretically, diverticula should have linings of transitional epithelium, whereas simple cysts should be lined by a single layer of flattened or cuboidal epithelium.**

Histopathology

Simple cysts vary considerably in size, ranging from less than 1 cm to greater than 10 cm. The majority are less than 2 cm in diameter, however (Tada et al, 1983). The wall is fibrous and of varying thickness and has no renal elements. The cyst lining is a single layer of flattened or cuboidal epithelium.

Because cysts are increasingly common with age, they have been considered an acquired lesion. Bearth and Steg (1977) found greater ectasia and cystic dilatation of the distal tubules and collecting ducts in patients older than 60 years of age and considered these changes to be precursors of macroscopic cysts.

KEY POINTS: SIMPLE CYSTS

- Simple cysts are seldom seen in children; in adults, simple cysts are seen increasingly more frequently with age.

- To make the diagnosis of a benign simple cyst on sonography, it should have a sharply defined, thin distinct smooth wall, be spherical or oval with no internal echoes, and have good transmission of sound waves with acoustic enhancement behind the cyst. When these criteria are not met, CT with contrast medium enhancement needs to be made.

- Relevant CT guidelines for determining when and not to explore or remove a complex cyst are often based on the Bosniak CT classification (see Table 114–9).

Evaluation

One can safely make the diagnosis of a classic benign simple cyst by sonography when the following criteria are met: (1) absence of internal echoes; (2) sharply defined, thin, distinct wall with a smooth and distinct margin; (3) good transmission of sound waves through the cyst with consequent acoustic enhancement behind the cyst; and (4) spherical or slightly ovoid shape (Goldman and Hartman, 1990). If all of these criteria are satisfied, the chance that malignancy is present is negligible (Fig. 114–23) (Lingard and Lawson, 1979; Livingston et al, 1981).

When some of these criteria are not met (e.g., when there are septations, irregular margins, calcifications, or suspect areas), further evaluation by CT or perhaps needle aspiration or MRI is indicated (Bosniak, 1986). A cluster of cysts is another indication for further study, because they may be hiding a small carcinoma. CT is better than sonography in

defining such a camouflaged lesion (Bosniak, 1986). Peripelvic cysts often require CT confirmation because they frequently are interspersed between structures of the collecting system and hilum, which can create artificial echoes (Bosniak, 1986).

The CT criteria for a simple cyst are similar to those used in sonography: (1) sharp, thin, distinct, smooth walls and margins; (2) spherical or ovoid shape; and (3) homogeneous content. The density ranges from −10 to +20 HU, similar to the density of water, and no enhancement should occur after the intravenous injection of contrast medium. Bosniak (1986) stated that he had not seen a tumor with a density of less than 20 HU on a contrast medium–enhanced scan, but a truly benign cyst can have fluid with a density greater than 20 HU. In these cases, intravenous contrast medium injection is particularly helpful.

When the cyst fluid is hyperdense (i.e., between 20 and 90 HU), it still is likely to be a simple cyst if no enhancement occurs when intravenous contrast agent is injected and if the other criteria of CT and sonography are met. Hyperdense cysts must be evaluated with narrow window settings to make sure that they are homogeneous. Other criteria that must be met to avoid further evaluation of hyperdense cysts (e.g., cyst puncture or exploration) include size (the lesion should be 3 cm or smaller) and location (at least one fourth of the cyst's circumference should extend beyond the renal contour so that the smoothness of a good portion of the cyst can be evaluated) (Bosniak, 1991a, 1991b; Hartman et al, 1992). When reviewing the CT study of a hyperdense cyst with the radiologist, the urologist must be reassured that the Hounsfield units were calibrated by using fluid in the gallbladder or unopacified urine. Still, on rare occasions, although all criteria for a benign hyperdense cyst are carefully met, a cystic RCC may be missed (Hartman et al, 1992). Technical factors can affect the results, for example, injecting too little contrast agent or waiting too long to scan after injection (Macari and Bosniak, 1999).

Because cysts have no blood vessels and do not communicate directly with nephrons, they should not enhance;

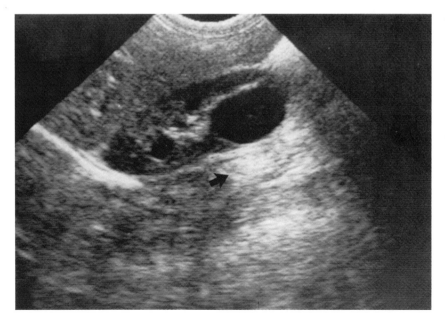

Figure 114–23. Two renal cysts in an 8-year-old boy. Note evidence of enhancement of sound wave transmission through the larger oval cyst by the hyperechogenicity (whiteness) of the image behind the cyst. Family history or even sonographic evaluation of family should be considered to rule out ADPKD, especially when more than one cyst is present. In children, it is not unusual for ADPKD to first manifest with one or two cysts.

enhancement therefore implies vascular tissue or contrast medium mixing with fluid. However, for several days after the injection of contrast medium, the fluid in a benign cyst may enhance (Hartman, 1990). Despite the diagnostic utility of contrast enhancement, the first scan should always be performed without enhancement because contrast medium may obscure calcification, small amounts of fat, or recent hemorrhage (Bosniak, 1986). When the aforementioned criteria are respected, the accuracy of diagnosis of a simple cyst by CT approaches 100% (Figs. 114–24 and 114–25) (McClennan et al, 1979). Occasionally, a high-density (>30 HU), well-marginated lesion may be noticed on a postcontrast CT when no record of density of the previously unrecognized lesion was obtained (Macari and Bosniak, 1999). In such situations one can look for "de-enhancement," a finding that occurs after the initial flow of contrast agent to an organ and that offers proof of vascularity (i.e., neoplasm). Macari and Bosniak

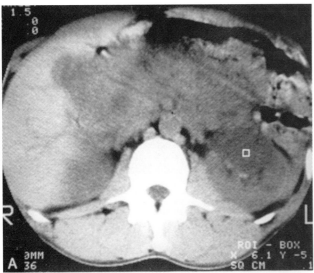

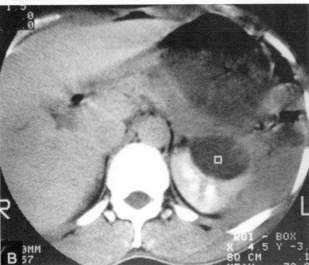

Figure 114–24. **A,** Hyperdense renal cysts on precontrast CT scan measuring +33 HU. **B,** After contrast agent administration, CT scan values were +30 HU. Absence of enhancement, spherical shape, and fine outline are findings compatible with the diagnosis of a simple cyst despite CT values greater than +20 HU.

(1999) found 15 minutes to be a sufficient period of delay to detect de-enhancement. If there is still a question of de-enhancement, the patient can be taken off the table and returned 30 or more minutes later.

When sonographic or CT criteria are not met, such as when there is a thick wall, calcification, septation, nonhomogeneous or hyperdense fluid, or fluid with internal echoes, conditions other than simple cyst must be considered. Other possibilities are complicated cysts (i.e., those containing blood, pus, or calcification) and cystic neoplasms. One of the more common sources of confusion is the parenchymal beak classically seen on intravenous urography when the tissue partially engulfs the cyst margin. When seen in cross section on sonography or CT, this beak can create the appearance of a thick wall (Segal and Spitzer, 1979). Cyst puncture and aspiration with or without contrast medium injection was popular in the 1960s and 1970s. Fluid from cystic RCC may be hemorrhagic or may contain elevated levels of protein, lactic dehydrogenase, or fat (Marotti et al, 1987). Today, with the improvements in sonography and CT, cyst puncture is less likely to be needed. The remaining indications for cyst puncture are (1) suspected infection, in which case puncture may be therapeutic as well as diagnostic; (2) the presence of low-level echoes on sonography but a classic cyst on CT; and (3) a borderline lesion in a poor surgical candidate.

Bosniak (1986) believed that hyperdense cysts larger than 3 cm in diameter require further evaluation or close follow-up because there are few data on the nature of hyperdense lesions of this size. In such cases, the following options might be considered, depending on the patient's age and general health: (1) cyst puncture with aspiration for cytologic study, (2) puncture and injection of contrast medium, or (3) follow-up by sonography or CT at progressively longer intervals.

When evaluating a possibly infected cyst, one must be aware that the wall may be thickened and sometimes calcified. Debris is often present (Hartman, 1990). Calcification may also be present in the absence of infection or malignancy; 1% to 3% of renal cysts are calcified (Daniel et al, 1972; Bree et al, 1984). Such calcification is dystrophic and usually occurs secondary to hemorrhage, infection, or ischemia (Hartman, 1990). Also, 6% of simple cysts can hemorrhage (Jackman and Stevens, 1974; Pollack et al, 1979). In 1971, 31% of hemorrhagic cysts were reported to be malignant (Gross and Breach, 1971), but it was deemed necessary at that time to explore the majority of such cysts. Today, even if blood is present, the decision to operate usually can be made on the basis of sonographic or CT findings.

MRI offers little information beyond that available from sonography and CT, although it is more specific in identifying the nature of the cyst fluid. Marotti and coworkers (1987) found that if the fluid has low signal intensity (similar to that of urine) on T1-weighted images, the cyst is benign even if the wall is thick or septa are present. If this report is substantiated by additional studies, MRI may prove valuable in deciding which indeterminate cysts are benign and which should be considered for exploration. **The T2-weighted images identify bloody fluid with an extremely bright image.**

Technical points need to be made about the evaluation of simple cysts by each of these imaging methods. First, when poor acoustic enhancement or low-level internal echoes are identified by real-time sonography, the findings may be an

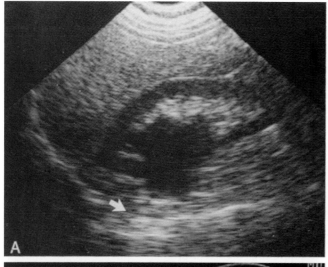

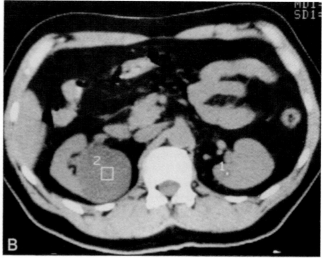

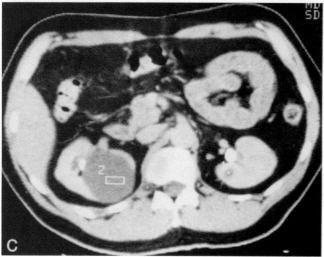

Figure 114–25. A 56-year-old man with an indeterminate, left renal cyst on renal sonography. **A,** Note the nonspherical, non–smoothly outlined sonolucent mass in the left kidney. However, there is good sound wave transmission through the cysts (acoustic enhancement), which is illustrated by the intensity (whiteness) of the sonogram image behind the cyst *(arrow)*. **B,** On precontrast CT scan, a very small cyst (1) is seen in the left kidney. The right renal cyst (2) that was identified on sonography measures 17 HU. **C,** After contrast agent administration, the CT value (2) was 16 HU, signifying no enhancement. CT values between −10 and +20 HU are characteristic of cysts. No enhancement with contrast agent confirms the diagnosis of a simple renal cyst. The small cyst (1) was not large enough for determining accurate CT values. (Courtesy of G. Laungani, MD.)

artifact of the method. Weinreb and coworkers (1986) suggested that, in these cases, a static ultrasound scan should be obtained to see whether the findings are reproducible before performing CT. If no internal echoes are seen or if acoustic enhancement is clearly demonstrable, the contrary findings on the real-time scan can be considered artifactual and CT can be avoided. Second, problems may occur in judging the density of cyst fluid by CT if the scanner is not regularly calibrated against gallbladder fluid or urine without contrast medium in the renal pelvis or bladder. These fluids should have densities near that of water (−10 to +20 HU). Third, it must be remembered with MRI that ventilatory and bowel motions can degrade the signal intensity of cyst fluid as well as lesion definition (Marotti et al, 1987).

To summarize, in most cases of simple cysts, the diagnosis is readily made. **When the cyst is indeterminate, the most important diagnostic question is whether the cyst is a manifestation of malignancy. When the cysts are diffuse, multiple, or bilateral, the possibility of ADPKD must be considered. The sonographic and CT appearance of these two types of lesions can be identical. Diagnosis then depends on identifying other family members with ADPKD or finding reduced renal function or other signs of ADPKD, such as hepatic cysts. In its early stages, ADPKD is not always represented by multiple bilateral cysts; it may initially appear sonographically as a single renal cyst, multiple unilateral cysts, or cysts localized to one portion of the kidney.**

Treatment and Prognosis

The propensity of simple cysts to enlarge is not clear. Laucks and McLachlan (1981) found that cyst diameter increases with age. Contrary data were reported by Richter and associates (1983), who found an increase in cyst size in only 2 of 31 patients who were observed for as long as 10 years. Also, Dalton and coworkers (1986) monitored 59 patients by sonography and found no significant changes in cyst size, although they did see an increase in the number of cysts in 20% of cases.

Before 1970, most simple cysts in children were treated surgically. However, a number of large series published in the 1970s indicated that cysts could be managed much like those in adults because they are the same type of lesion. Once malignancy has been ruled out, unroofing or removal of an asymptomatic cyst is not indicated (Gordon et al, 1979; Bartholomew et al, 1980; Ravden et al, 1980; Siegel and McAlister, 1980).

When a benign simple cyst causes pyelocalyceal obstruction or hypertension, the problem may be corrected either surgically, by unroofing the cyst, or percutaneously, by aspirating the fluid and perhaps injecting a sclerosing agent, particularly if fluid has reaccumulated after an earlier aspiration. Several sclerosing agents have been used, including glucose, phenol, iophendylate (Pantopaque), and absolute ethanol, but none has been sufficiently impressive for its use to become dominant (Holmberg and Hietala, 1989).

Holmberg and Hietala (1989) managed simple cysts in 156 patients in one of three ways. In one group, no treatment was given; in 25% of these patients, the cysts grew during a mean follow-up period of 3 years. In a second group, cyst aspiration was performed. In this group, the cysts disappeared in 10% of patients and the mean size of the cysts in the remainder declined to 90% of the original volume after 24 months. In the third group, cyst aspiration was followed by sclerotherapy with bismuth phosphate. In this group, the cysts disappeared in 44% of patients and the mean size of the cysts in the remainder was only 21% of the original size after 3 to 4 years.

On the basis of this study and another study by Westberg and Zachrisson (1975), in which all bismuth-treated cysts shrank, it appears that, when treatment is needed for a simple cyst because of pain or compression effects, sclerosis of the cyst lining with instilled bismuth phosphate is a method worthy of consideration. Newer approaches to recalcitrant cysts are percutaneous resection and intrarenal marsupialization (Hubner et al, 1990; Hulbert and Hunter, 1990; Meyer and Jonas, 1990) and laparoscopic unroofing, either transperitoneally (Morgan and Rader, 1992) or retroperitoneally (Raboy et al, 1994).

Simple Cyst Variations

Two variations of simple cysts must be considered: unilateral renal cystic disease and autosomal dominant simple cyst disease.

Unilateral Renal Cystic Disease

Large renal cysts of varying size appearing side by side, often more numerous at one pole, have been referred to as *unilateral renal cystic disease.* Evidence from Levine and Huntrakoon (1989) strongly supports the view that this condition is a discrete, unilateral, nongenetic entity. On sonography the appearance is that of multiple simple cysts lying side by side; on CT, normal parenchyma separates the cysts (Levine and Huntrakoon, 1989). These cysts do not seem to be separated into one encapsulated mass lesion. Because the entity seems to represent nothing more than multiple simple cysts lying side by side within a kidney, it seems reasonable to consider it as a variation of the presentation of simple cysts.

It is important not to overdiagnose unilateral simple cyst disease, because the entity itself is rare and when first identi-

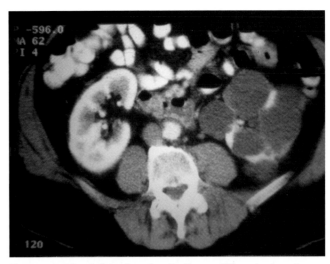

Figure 114-26. Unilateral renal cystic disease. Diffuse simple cysts were evident in one kidney. There was no discrete mass nor evidence of multiple malformation syndrome. (Courtesy of Jeffrey Newhouse, MD.)

fied in an individual it is more likely to represent a unilateral asymmetrical presentation of ADPKD (Glassberg, 1991). **Such a diagnosis therefore requires long-term follow-up demonstrating absence of cyst development in the contralateral kidney and no family members with cystic disease** (Glassberg, 1999). In previous reports, cysts have not been identified in other organs. The term *unilateral polycystic kidney disease* (Lee et al, 1978; Kossow and Meek, 1982) should not be employed because it confuses the diagnosis with ADPKD. If warranted, studies to rule out VHL disease and tuberous sclerosis should be considered. Now that genetic studies are becoming available for ADPKD, tuberous sclerosis, and VHL disease, the diagnosis of unilateral renal cystic disease can more readily be confirmed (Fig. 114–26).

Autosomal Dominant Simple Cyst Disease

Our group studied the families of five children with simple cysts sonographically to determine whether simple cysts in children might in some cases be inherited. In two of the five families, several members were found to have simple cysts (Schulsinger et al, 1994). In one of the families four siblings, the father, and the paternal grandmother also had renal cysts. In the second affected family the mother, but not the father or siblings, had simple cysts. Genetic linkage studies were unable to identify ADPKD in these two families. In addition, neither family had findings associated with tuberous sclerosis or VHL disease. The evidence so far leads us to conjecture that we might be identifying a new entity, *autosomal dominant simple cyst disease*. Until there is further genetic proof that it is a new entity, I prefer not to include autosomal simple cyst disease as a formal separate entity in this classification.

Plas and Hübner (1993) investigated the long-term results (median follow-up, 45.7 months) in 10 patients who underwent percutaneous resection of a renal cyst. There was no evidence of renal cyst in 50% of the patients at follow-up, a recurrence in 30%, and a 45% decrease in size in 20%. In all 10 patients the symptoms that made the cyst resection

Table 114–9. Bosniak's Classification of Simple and Complex Cysts

Category I	Simple benign cyst with (1) good through-transmission (i.e., acoustic enhancement), (2) no echoes within the cyst, (3) sharply, marginated smooth wall; requires no surgery.
Category II	Looks benign with some radiologic concerns including septation, minimal calcification, and high density; requires no surgery.
Category II F	Although calcification in wall of cyst may even be thicker and more nodular than in category II, the septa have minimal enhancement, especially those with calcium; requires no surgery.
Category III	More complicated lesion that cannot confidently be distinguished from malignancy, having more calcification, more prominent septation of a thicker wall than a category II lesion; more likely to be benign than malignant; requires surgical exploration and/or removal.
Category IV	Clearly a malignant lesion with large cystic components, irregular margins; solid vascular elements; requires surgical removal.

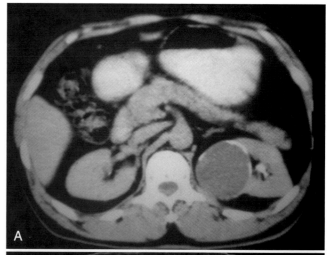

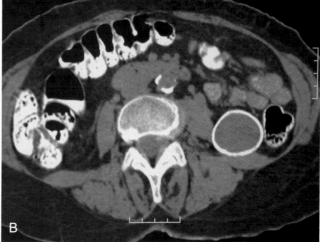

Figure 114–27. **A** and **B**, Two examples of Bosniak category II F cysts with diffuse calcification but no enhancement of septa on CT. (Courtesy of Jeffrey Newhouse, MD.)

necessary disappeared, and in none of the patients were there any late complications.

In an attempt to sort out the difficult cases into surgical and nonsurgical ones, Bosniak suggested a classification in 1986 that was clarified further in 1997 and modified by Israel and Bosniak in 2003 (Table 114–9).

Category I cyst is the typical benign cyst. Category II cysts are benign cystic lesions that are minimally complicated, such as by septations, small calcifications, infection, or high density, and do not require surgery. For example, when all the criteria for a simple cyst are met except that a fine line of calcification or a short segment of slightly thickened calcification is seen in the wall or septa, the lesion should be considered a benign cyst, and exploration is not required. Another example is the cyst with fine traversing strands, perhaps containing calcium. In this case, exploration is not required unless the septa are numerous, irregular, or thick.

Category II F was described by Israel and Bosniak (2003) for complex cysts that cannot be classified either as category II or III. These lesions may contain increased calcification. The calcification may even be thicker and nodular, but although the septa may have minimal enhancement those septa with calcium do not enhance. Calcification seems to represent a less significant finding in making a lesion suspicious as a malignancy than previously thought. More focus is placed on tissue enhancement. There is little concern if calcification increases with time but much concern if the wall or septa becomes thicker or irregular. **Category II F does not require surgical exploration** (Israel and Bosniak, 2003) (Fig. 114–27).

Category III cysts are more complicated lesions with radiologic features that are also seen in malignancy. One example is the lesion with more extensive calcification, especially if the wall is not pencil-point thin or is irregular. Other type III cysts are those with septations, suggesting a multilocular cystic lesion, or chronic infection with a thickened wall. **These lesions are more problematic and require a surgical approach that is individualized.** In some cases, one

might consider violating Gerota's fascia to expose the kidney for examination of the lesion or partial nephrectomy.

Bosniak category IV lesions are cystic malignant tumors and are dealt with as such, namely, by radical nephrectomy.

MEDULLARY SPONGE KIDNEY

The condition known as medullary sponge kidney was recognized by Beitzke in 1908, and its radiographic features were described by Lenarduzzi in 1939. The name of this disorder dates from a 1949 publication by Cacchi and Ricci. **The characteristic features of medullary sponge kidney are dilatation of the distal portion of the collecting ducts with numerous associated cysts and diverticula. The dilated ducts can be counted individually on an intravenous pyelogram and have the appearance of the bristles on a brush. At times the collecting ducts are more ectatic and are filled with calcifications, giving an appearance suggestive of a "bouquet of flowers."** The term *precalyceal canalicular ectasia* sometimes is used for this entity, especially in Europe, because it describes a condition in which dilatation is predominantly of the papillary portion of the collecting ducts (Fig. 114–28).

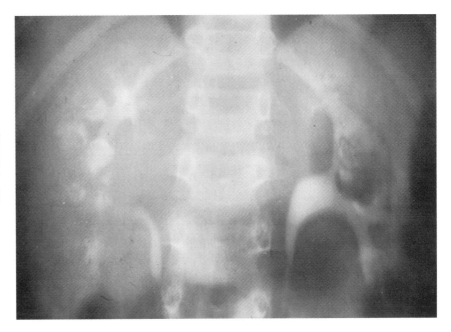

Figure 114–28. Intravenous urogram in a 9-year-old girl with hematuria. Characteristic puddling of contrast medium in the ectatic papillary collecting ducts makes the diagnosis of medullary sponge kidney. (From Glassberg KI, et al: Congenital anomalies of kidney, ureter, and bladder. In Kendall AR, Karafin L [eds]: Goldsmith's Practice of Surgery: Urology. New York, Harper & Row, 1981, pp 1-82.)

A significant number of patients with medullary sponge kidney are asymptomatic, and their condition is never diagnosed. As a result, the true incidence of the condition is unknown. Among patients undergoing intravenous urography for various indications, 1 in 200 were found to have medullary sponge kidney (Palubinskas, 1961; Myall, 1970). Bernstein and Gardner (1986), on the basis of a literature review, estimated the incidence in the general population to be between 1 in 5000 and 1 in 20,000 persons.

KEY POINTS: MEDULLARY SPONGE KIDNEY

- Usually a nonheritable condition associated with dilated collecting ducts that appear as bristles on a brush on intravenous pyelography and sometimes filled with calcifications.

- High incidence of renal colic (50% to 60%), urinary tract infections (20% to 33%), gross hematuria (10% to 18%), and hypercalciuria (33%).

Clinical Features

Any clinical presentation usually occurs after age 20, although Hamberger and colleagues (1968) found, in more than 100 cases, that the first symptoms appeared at ages ranging from 3 weeks to 71 years. **The most common presentation is renal colic (50% to 60%), followed by urinary tract infection (20% to 33%) and gross hematuria (10% to 18%)** (Kuiper, 1976b). In many cases, the diagnosis is made when a patient is evaluated by intravenous urography for some unrelated problem, such as a renal mass, benign prostatic hyperplasia, or hypertension. Rarely is such hypertension attributable to the medullary sponge kidney unless there is pyelonephritis.

The incidence of medullary sponge kidney in stone formers differs widely in the reported series, ranging from 2.6% to 21%. The incidence appears to be higher in female than in male stone formers (Palubinskas, 1961; Lavan et al, 1971; Parks et al, 1982; Sage et al, 1982; Wikstrom et al, 1983; Vagelli et al, 1988; Yendt, 1990). Urinary tract infections likewise seem to be more common in female patients with medullary sponge kidney (Parks et al, 1982).

One third to one half of the patients with medullary sponge kidney have hypercalcemia (Ekstrom et al, 1959; Harrison and Rose, 1979; Parks et al, 1982; Yendt, 1990). The etiology does not appear to be the same in all cases. Maschio and coworkers (1982) found a renal calcium leak in eight patients and increased calcium absorption in two. Yendt (1990) found increased parathyroid hormone levels in 2 of 11 patients with medullary sponge kidney. In the absence of infection, the stones passed by patients with medullary sponge kidney are composed of calcium oxalate either alone or in combination with calcium phosphate.

Although medullary sponge kidney is not considered a genetic disease, there are a small number of isolated reports of autosomal dominant and autosomal recessive inheritance. In addition, medullary sponge kidney has been reported in association with rare congenital anomalies such as hemihypertrophy, Beckwith-Wiedemann syndrome (macroglossia, omphalocele, and gigantism), Ehler-Danlos syndrome, anodontia, and Caroli's disease. Beetz and associates (1991) reported on a case of bilateral medullary sponge kidney in a 14-year-old girl with Beckwith-Wiedemann syndrome, hemihypertrophy, and Wilms' tumor. Twenty other patients have been reported with congenital hemihypertrophy and fewer with Beckwith-Wiedemann syndrome (Gardner, 1992).

Histopathology

The principal finding is dilated intrapapillary collecting ducts and small medullary cysts, which range in diameter from 1 to 8 mm and give the cross-sectioned kidney the appearance of a sponge. The cysts are lined by collecting duct epithelium (Bernstein, 1990) and usually communicate with the collecting tubules. The cysts and the dilated collecting ducts may have concretions mostly made of pure apatite (calcium phosphate) and less frequently apatite and calcium oxalate (Ekstron et al, 1959) in the remaining three. The cysts contain a yellow-brown fluid and desquamated cells or calcified material.

Diagnosis

In general, intravenous urography is more sensitive than CT in detecting mild cases of medullary sponge kidney. In 75% of patients the disease is bilateral (Kuiper, 1976a), but in some only one pyramid is affected. **The urographic features of the disorder are as follows: (1) enlarged kidneys, sometimes with calcification, particularly in the papillae; (2) elongated papillary tubules or cavities that fill with contrast medium; and (3) papillary contrast blush and persistent medullary opacification** (Gedroyc and Saxton, 1988). In some cases the papillae resemble bunches of grapes or bouquets of flowers, and in others discrete linear stripes appear that can be counted readily.

On occasion, the intravenous urogram of an older child or young adult with one of the milder forms of ARPKD mimics the appearance of medullary sponge kidney (Yendt, 1990). In these instances, the liver should be evaluated before a diagnosis is made.

When nephrocalcinosis is found, other hypercalciuric states, such as hyperparathyroidism, sarcoidosis, vitamin D intoxication, multiple myeloma, tuberculosis, and milk alkali syndrome, must be ruled out. In these conditions the calcium deposits are in collecting ducts of normal caliber, whereas in medullary sponge kidney the calcifications occur in dilated ducts (Levine and Grantham, 1990).

Given that the cysts are small, sonography is not expected to be helpful. However, because children have less renal sinus fat and overlying muscle than adults, sonographic resolution is better, and hyperechoic papillae are seen on occasion (Patriquin and O'Regan, 1985). The hyperechogenicity is secondary to the multiple interfaces created by the dilated ducts and small cysts and to any intraductal calcification.

Treatment and Prognosis

It is the complications of medullary sponge kidney—calculus formation and infection—that require management. As noted earlier, many of these patients have hypercalciuria. **Thiazides are effective for lowering hypercalciuria and limiting stone formation. If thiazides cannot be used, inorganic phosphates may be appropriate. For those patients with renal lithiasis, thiazides should be administered even if hypercalciuria is not present.** Yendt (1990) reported that these drugs prevent calcium stones and arrest the growth of stones already present. If thiazides are ineffective or not tolerated, inorganic phosphates should be tried. However, they should not be used in patients with urinary tract infections caused by urease-producing organisms because of the risk of struvite stones.

Because infections are not unusual in patients with medullary sponge kidney, especially if stones are present, cultures should be obtained frequently, and long-term prophylaxis should be considered in some cases. Infections by coagulase-positive staphylococci are common in patients with

stones and should be treated even when the colony count in the cultures is less than 100,000/mL (Yendt, 1990).

Stones can now be removed by extracorporeal lithotripsy and percutaneous nephrolithotomy. Therefore, open surgery is rarely necessary.

SPORADIC GLOMERULOCYSTIC KIDNEY DISEASE

Glomerulocystic disease is a specific entity, but the term has often been applied as a catchall to include all conditions in which there are glomerular cysts. The term *glomerulocystic* means that cysts of the glomeruli or Bowman's space are present diffusely and bilaterally. However, cysts of the glomeruli are present in many forms of renal cystic disease, and they may or may not be the predominant pathology. Therefore, the presence of glomerular cysts does not prove that the patient has glomerulocystic disease.

Table 114–10 shows the Bernstein and Landing classification of conditions with glomerular cysts, as modified by Glassberg and Filmer (1992) to make it compatible with the AAP classification. The diagnosis of sporadic glomerulocystic disease should be made only when the disorder conforms to the 1941 definition of Roos and the 1976 definition of Taxy and Filmer. That is, glomerulocystic disease is a noninheritable condition producing bilaterally enlarged kidneys containing small cysts, predominantly of Bowman's space. Characteristically, no other family members are affected, and no associated anomalies are present, although in the case described by Taxy and Filmer (1976) subcapsular hepatic cysts were present. Sporadic glomerulocystic disease clearly is different from familial hypoplastic glomerulocystic disease. It is not an inherited disorder, and the kidneys are larger.

The patients evaluated by Bernstein and Landing (1989) after referral and those they found described in the literature differed in age of presentation, clinical course, and renal morphology. These investigators suggested that, in some of the published cases, features of other syndromes were overlooked or family members were inadequately screened for ADPKD. They recommended the use of the term *sporadic glomerulocystic disease* to show that the condition is not genetic.

Bernstein (1993) believed that sporadic glomerulocystic kidney disease in young infants is indistinguishable from ADPKD when the latter is seen in infants and glomerular

---

Table 114–10. Conditions Associated with Glomerular Cysts

Sporadic glomerulocystic kidney disease
Familial hypoplastic glomerulocystic disease
Autosomal dominant polycystic disease
Juvenile nephronophthisis in association with hepatic fibrosis
Multiple malformation syndromes
  Zellweger's syndrome
  Trisomy 13
  Meckel's syndrome
  Short-rib polydactyly (Majewski type)
  Tuberous sclerosis
  Orofaciodigital syndrome type I
  Brachymesomelia renal syndrome
  Renal-hepatic-pancreatic dysplasia

cysts are a major histologic finding. The only difference clinically or histologically between the two is that no family history can be identified in the sporadic entity. Bernstein went so far as to question whether sporadic glomerulocystic kidney disease represented a new mutation of classic ADPKD rather than a different disease. He concluded that the question was at that time unanswerable.

ACQUIRED RENAL CYSTIC DISEASE

In 1977, Dunhill and coworkers described ARCD in patients in renal failure. **At first, ARCD was thought to be confined to patients receiving hemodialysis. However, it shortly became apparent that the disorder is almost as common in patients receiving peritoneal dialysis** (Thompson et al, 1986) and that it may develop in patients with chronic renal failure who are being managed medically without any type of dialysis (Fisher and Horvath, 1972; Ishikawa et al, 1980; Kutcher et al, 1983; Miller et al, 1989). Therefore, ARCD appears to be a feature of end-stage kidneys rather than a response to dialysis. Ishikawa (1985) suggested that the term *uremic acquired cystic disease* be applied to this entity (Fig. 114–29).

The incidence of ARCD differs among institutions, perhaps as a result of population differences or diagnostic criteria. To make the diagnosis one should see at least three to five cysts on ultrasound, CT, or MRI, recognizing that ultrasound is the least sensitive of these modalities.

The significance of ARCD lies in two areas: (1) the symptoms it may produce (pain and hematuria) and (2) the high incidence of benign and malignant renal tumors that accompany the condition. The incidence of renal tumors warrants special consideration.

Incidence: Association with Renal Cell Carcinoma

In 1984, Gardner identified 160 patients with ARCD among 430 patients receiving long-term hemodialysis, an incidence of 34% (Gardner, 1984b). This incidence represents an overall figure, because the incidence of ARCD rises with time on dialysis and perhaps also with the duration of chronic renal failure and the age of the patient. For example, Ishikawa and coworkers (1980) found ARCD in 44% of patients who had been receiving hemodialysis for less than 3 years but in 79% of those who had been receiving hemodialysis for a longer time. Hughson and coworkers (1986) found a 2.9:1 male-to-female ratio for ARCD, which is striking when one considers that the number of male patients undergoing dialysis only slightly exceeds the number of female patients.

When ARCD is present in men, it usually is more advanced. African Americans, and perhaps Japanese, are more prone than Americans of European descent to develop ARCD (Reichard et al, 1998). **ARCD can occur in children as well.** Hakim and associates (1994) found a 23% incidence of ARCD in a group of 22 children with ESRD who had been receiving dialysis for a period of 7 to 49 months. Because simple cysts in children are rare, they thought that the presence of ARCD should be considered even when there are only one or two cysts. A Japanese study group investigated the incidence of ARCD in 56 children undergoing continuous ambulatory peritoneal dialysis. The patients were grouped according to length of time on dialysis: 0 to 4 years (n = 33), 5 to 9 years (n = 16), and longer than 10 years (n = 5). The corresponding incidences of ARCD were 9.1%, 50%, and 80%. In general, the number and size of cysts increased with the duration of dialysis (Kyushu Pediatric Nephrology Study Group, 1999).

The incidence of ARCD appears to be higher in patients with ESRD secondary to nephrosclerosis than in those in whom renal failure was the result of diabetes (Fallon and Williams, 1989; Miller et al, 1989). However, the lower incidence of ARCD in diabetic patients may well be a result of their shorter survival time on dialysis (Fallon and Williams, 1989).

Renal neoplasms, principally adenomas, occur in 10% of patients receiving chronic hemodialysis, and when ARCD is present the incidence of neoplasms is even higher, ranging from 20% to 25% (Gardner and Evan, 1984). **When RCC**

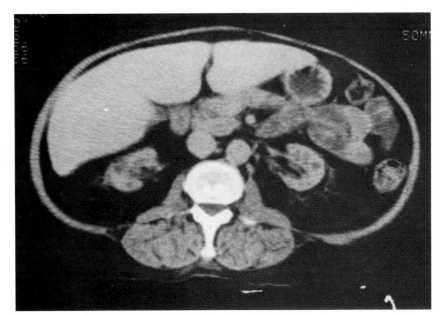

Figure 114–29. Small kidneys with multiple small cysts in a hemodialysis patient with acquired renal cystic disease.

develops in ESRD, 80% of the time it is associated with ARCD; and when RCC is associated with ARCD, it frequently occurs at an earlier age than in the general population, often in the third or fourth decade. In these cases, the cysts are pronounced. When RCC appears after the age of 60 years in a patient with ARCD there usually are fewer cysts (Hughson et al, 1986).

In Japan, the incidence of RCC among dialysis patients is several times to 20 times higher than it is in the general population (Ishikawa, 1993), whereas in the United States it is three to six times higher based on an annual incidence of 8 per 100,000 among the general population (Resseguie et al, 1978; Levine et al, 1991). In Michigan, a fivefold increase of RCC among dialysis patients was reported, correlating well with the overall U.S. statistic (Port et al, 1989). Perhaps the difference in incidence of RCC in Japan and the United States is a result of the stronger push in Japan toward routine screening of the kidneys by CT after 3 years of dialysis. According to Levine and associates (1991), CT screening at approximately $600 per study would amount to a cost of $36 million a year, making the cost of such mass screening almost prohibitive.

RCC occurring in ESRD is different biologically in a number of ways from classic RCC: (1) the age at occurrence averages 5 years younger in patients with ESRD; (2) the male-to-female ratio is significantly greater in ESRD patients with RCC than in the general population with RCC (7:1 and 2:1, respectively); and (3) the incidence of RCC in ESRD is 3 to 6 times that of the general population and may be as high as 10 times the incidence in blacks (Matson and Cohen, 1990; Cohen, 1993). These differences probably reflect the high incidence of epithelial hyperplasia, renal cysts, and adenomas seen in patients with ESRD.

A 15-year follow-up report on 39 ARCD patients found that if no RCC had developed before 10 years of chronic dialysis, development after 10 to 15 years was unusual. The study also found that kidney size tended to plateau in males after 13 years of dialysis but that significant enlargement of cysts occurred in females after 18 years of dialysis (Ishikawa et al, 1997).

Etiology

As noted earlier, the initial view that ARCD is a consequence of hemodialysis per se has been shown to be incorrect. However, if uremic toxins are the principal risk factor, why are there different incidences of ARCD at various institutions? It is possible that different durations of predialysis medical therapy or different dialysis regimens are important, but no data have been collected on this point.

A number of findings suggest a role for toxins. First, the cysts, adenomas, and carcinomas usually are multiple and bilateral, as are the carcinomas induced experimentally in rats by toxins. Second, there is a regression of the cysts after successful transplantation (Ishikawa et al, 1983), suggesting that some cystogenic or carcinogenic toxin of uremia is being eliminated by the allograft. Third, if transplantation fails and dialysis is resumed, the cysts return.

Another theory suggests that loss of functioning renal tissue leads to the production of renotrophic agents that induce hyperplasia of remaining glomeruli, cyst development, and, in

---

> ## KEY POINTS: ACQUIRED RENAL CYSTIC DISEASE
>
> - Acquired renal cystic disease is associated with chronic renal failure and most often seen in patients on long-term hemodialysis.
>
> - It consists of hyperplastic renal cysts and frequently adenomas; either can progress to RCC.
>
> - If RCC develops, it mostly does so before 10 years of dialysis.
>
> - The cysts usually regress with transplantation, and even when this occurs there still is some suggestion that the risk of developing RCC still persists but at a much lower incidence.

extreme cases, renal tumors (Harris et al, 1983; Yamamoto et al, 1983).

Clinical Features

The most common presentation of ARCD is loin pain, hematuria, or both. Bleeding occurs in as many as 50% of patients (Levine, 1996). When it occurs, whether into the kidney or into the retroperitoneum, it may be secondary to renal cysts or to RCC. Feiner and coworkers (1981) suggested that cystic bleeding is secondary to rupture of unsupported sclerotic vessels in the wall. If the cyst communicates with the nephron, hematuria may result. In some patients, bleeding occurs after heparinization during dialysis. Also, in some cases, the serum hemoglobin concentration is elevated secondary to increased renal production of erythropoietin (Shalhoub et al, 1982; Ratcliffe et al, 1983; Mickisch et al, 1984).

Histopathology

The cysts develop predominantly in the cortex, although the medulla may be affected, and usually they are bilateral (Fig. 114–30). They average 0.5 to 1.0 cm in diameter, but some have been reported to reach 5.0 cm (Miller et al, 1989). The cysts are filled with clear, straw-colored or hemorrhagic fluid and often contain calcium oxalate crystals (Miller et al, 1989). Some resemble simple retention cysts, with a flat epithelial lining.

The nuclei of the epithelial cells in these cases are round and regular, without prominent nucleoli (Hughson et al, 1980). However, some cysts (atypical or hyperplastic) are lined by epithelial cells with larger, irregular nuclei that contain prominent nucleoli and may show mitotic activity. This hyperplastic lining is thought by some to be a precursor of renal tumors. Moreover, some hyperplastic cysts have papillary projections, and to some observers the distinction between cyst and neoplasm becomes blurred when papillary hyperplasia predominates.

The renal adenomas usually are multiple and often are bilateral. Miller and colleagues (1989) performed autopsies on 155 patients with ESRD and found 25 to have small renal cor-

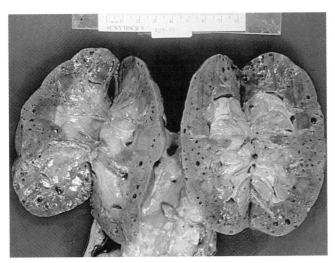

Figure 114–30. Kidneys on autopsy from a 55-year-old man who was receiving chronic hemodialysis demonstrate acquired renal cystic disease with numerous small, diffuse renal cysts.

tical nodules (adenomas). These nodules were multiple, and all were smaller than 2.5 cm in diameter. They usually arose from the walls of the atypical (hyperplastic) cysts.

Differentiating renal tumors into adenomas and carcinomas is arbitrary at times. In Bell's classic 1935 article, renal tumors larger than 3 cm in diameter were considered carcinomas, whereas the smaller ones were considered adenomas. However, even in Bell's work, tumors as small as 1 cm were associated with metastases in a few cases. Also, although the majority of RCCs in patients with ARCD are larger than 2.0 to 3.0 cm, some have measured only 1.0 to 1.5 cm (Feiner et al, 1981; Chung-Park et al, 1983; Hughson et al, 1986). The smallest RCC associated with known metastases was 1.2 cm in diameter (Ishikawa, 1988a, 1988b). In sum, most renal nodules that are smaller than 1 cm in diameter are adenomas and most that are larger than 3 cm in diameter are carcinomas. Tumors between 1 and 3 cm in diameter must be considered a gray zone.

It is not clear whether renal adenomas undergo malignant transformation. The large incidence of renal adenomas in the general population and the even larger incidence in uremic patients, combined with the low incidence of RCC in both populations, suggest that the frequency of malignant transformation is low if it occurs at all. However, because of the higher incidence of both RCC and adenomas in patients with ARCD, one cannot rule out malignant transformation.

Bretan and associates (1986) postulated a continuum ranging from simple cysts to epithelial hyperplasia to carcinoma. In support of their hypothesis, they offered the finding of renal tumors in the hyperplastic epithelial lining of some cysts. However, no study to my knowledge has demonstrated such a continuum. A curiosity is the morphologic similarity of the nuclei in the hyperplastic cells to those of RCC and the lack of similarity of the nuclei of the adenoma cells to those seen in either of the other lesions.

Hughson and coworkers (1986) believed that atypical hyperplastic epithelium occurs even without cyst formation and that it is these cells that are the precursors of both atypical cysts and adenomas. This theory accounts for the finding

of end-stage kidneys containing multiple adenomas without cysts. These investigators also believed that either hyperplastic cysts or adenomas can become RCCs. Therefore, one must not ignore the native kidney left in situ during a renal transplantation. Whereas the cysts as precursors of RCC may disappear, the cells lining the cysts and the small adenomas probably persist, and these, too, may be premalignant lesions. Hyperplastic cyst epithelium has been considered a possible precursor of RCC in other cystic diseases, in particular, VHL disease and tuberous sclerosis (Fayemi and Ali, 1980).

Evaluation

In uremic patients with fever, one should consider the diagnosis of ARCD and the possibility of an infected cyst (Bonal et al, 1987). Sonography usually shows small, hyperechoic kidneys with cysts of various sizes. Cyst wall calcification may be visible, but it is more readily seen on CT. Infection should be suspected if sonographic examination shows internal echoes or a thickened wall. Cyst puncture can be used to confirm the diagnosis and to identify the infecting microorganism.

Ultrasound has been the most common modality used to diagnose and monitor patients with ARCD. CT and MRI identify more cysts, and MRI is probably better at demonstrating and characterizing small lesions in particular (Heinz-Peer et al, 1998).

CT examination may identify cyst wall thickening in cases with infection. If the patient is receiving dialysis, contrast medium can be given safely to see whether it causes enhancement (Levine et al, 1984). In some cases, one can identify a metastatic retroperitoneal RCC but cannot identify the primary lesion in the kidney.

In the differential diagnosis of ARCD, the etiology of the renal failure must be considered and, in particular, the possibility of ADPKD. Usually, patients with ARCD have smaller kidneys and smaller cysts and are free of the extrarenal manifestations of ADPKD. In patients receiving hemodialysis, kidneys affected by ARCD usually are less than 300 g; ADPKD kidneys usually are larger than 800 g (Feiner et al, 1981) (Fig. 114–31).

The chief presentations of both cysts and tumors in patients receiving hemodialysis are abdominal or flank pain and gross hematuria. Gehrig and coworkers (1985) found that 11 of 24 patients with ARCD and symptomatic bleeding had renal tumors; 8 of these 11 proved to have RCCs. The tumors themselves may be asymptomatic, revealing their presence only by metastases. The most common manifestation is loin pain, sometimes secondary to a retroperitoneal mass rather than to the primary tumor.

Treatment

If heparinization is associated with hematuria during hemodialysis, peritoneal dialysis may be substituted. Other options are embolization and nephrectomy.

For an infected cyst, percutaneous drainage may be effective. When it is not, surgical drainage or nephrectomy should be considered.

Neumann and associates (1988) recommended that patients who have been receiving hemodialysis for longer than

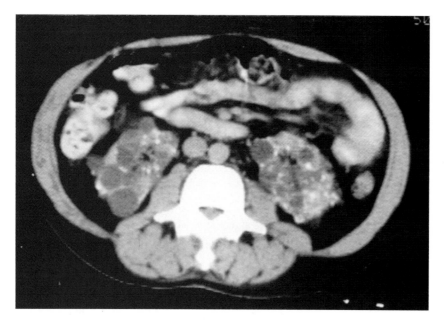

Figure 114-31. Bilateral multiple renal cysts and diffuse calcification in enlarged kidneys in a patient undergoing chronic hemodialysis. The findings simulate those of ADPKD. However, cystic disease was not the cause of the uremia, and the diagnosis of acquired renal cystic disease was made. (Courtesy of D. Gordon, MD.)

3 years be screened by ultrasound and CT and then monitored by ultrasonography every 6 months if the kidneys are without cysts and tumors or by both ultrasonography and CT on the same schedule if cysts or tumors smaller than 2 cm are identified. However, more recently a less aggressive approach has been taken in the United States toward routine CT screening because of the high cost attached to such a program.

Reichard and associates (1998) **suggested that screening of patients should be considered when known risk factors exist, such as prolonged dialysis, presence of ARCD, and male gender.**

A number of investigators have found that the cysts of ARCD regress after renal transplantation (Fig. 114–32) (Ishikawa et al, 1983; Kutcher et al, 1983; Thompson et al, 1986). Tajima and colleagues (1998) found improvement in regard to number and size of cysts in 16 (64%) of 25 ARCD patients 1 year after transplantation. Therefore, it was considered that the incidence of RCC might fall after transplantation as well. However, Ishikawa and associates (1991) found that although the majority of cysts either disappeared or became smaller, 18% of patients developed new cysts after transplantation. And more recently, Levine and Gburek (1994) reported four cases of renal carcinoma occurring in the native kidney 3 to 8 years after transplantation and suggested that the risk of carcinoma does not lessen after transplantation. In a series of 96 transplantation patients, Heinz-Peer and coworkers (1995) found that RCC had developed in 6 patients and that 5 of the 6 had associated ARCD. They suggested that the malignant potential of ARCD persists for many years after transplantation. They also found a higher incidence of RCC in older transplantation patients and in men. It must be kept in mind that, although the native kidneys may become smaller after transplantation and although the cysts may disappear from view on ultrasound follow-up, it does not necessarily mean that the cells that previously surrounded these cysts have disappeared.

The immunosuppression received by these patients in itself makes them vulnerable to carcinoma. Native kidneys account for 4.5% of all malignancies in renal transplantation recipients (Penn, 1979).

CALYCEAL DIVERTICULUM (PYELOGENIC CYST)

A calyceal diverticulum is a smoothly outlined, intrarenal sac that communicates with the pelvicalyceal system by means of a narrow neck. Diverticula usually arise from the fornix of a calyx and most often affect upper pole calyces. Some investigators reserve the term *calyceal diverticulum* for those lesions that communicate with a calyx or infundibulum and use the term *pyelogenic cyst* to designate lesions that communicate with the renal pelvis. Other workers employ the term *pyelocal calyceal diverticulum* to encompass both entities (Friedland et al, 1990). This entity is discussed in Chapter 113, "Anomalies of the Upper Urinary Tract."

PARAPELVIC AND RENAL SINUS CYSTS
Definitions

A number of terms have been used for cysts adjacent to the renal pelvis or within the hilum: peripelvic cysts, parapelvic cysts, renal sinus cysts, parapelvic lymphatic cysts, hilus cysts, cysts of the renal hilum, and peripelvic lymphangiectasis. Some peripelvic cysts are, in fact, simple cysts that arise from the renal parenchyma but happen to abut the renal pelvis, with or without obstruction. Clearly, these are not cysts of the renal sinus. **The terms *peripelvic* and *parapelvic* generally describe cysts around the renal pelvis or renal sinus. Cysts derived from the renal sinus have no parenchymal etiology.**

To avoid confusion, the terms *peripelvic* and *parapelvic* should be used only to describe location. I prefer to use these terms only as adjectives to describe simple parenchymal cysts adjacent to the renal pelvis or hilum, that is, a peripelvic simple parenchymal cyst (Fig. 114–33). The term *renal sinus cyst* should be reserved for all other cysts in the hilum, that is,

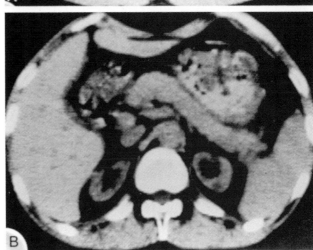

Figure 114–32. Effect of renal transplantation on acquired cystic kidney disease. **A,** CT scan obtained 1 month before renal transplantation in a patient who had been receiving dialysis for 7.5 years. Numerous bilateral renal cysts are present. **B,** Ten months after successful renal transplantation, almost all cysts, except one in the left kidney, have regressed. The kidney size has decreased considerably. (From Ishikawa I, et al: Regression of acquired cystic disease of the kidney after successful renal transplantation. Am J Nephrol 1983;3:310.)

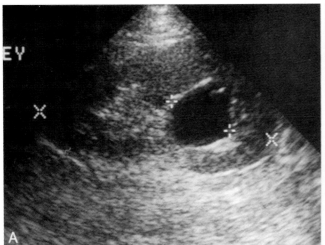

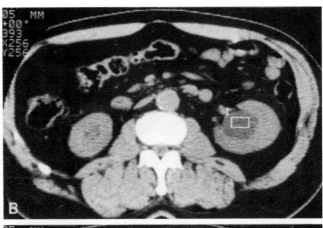

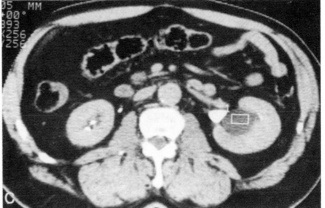

Figure 114–33. Simple cyst with peripelvic location. **A,** Renal sonogram reveals a centrally located left renal cyst. **B,** On precontrast CT scan, the cyst measures 3 HU. **C,** After contrast agent administration the cyst is calibrated to 2 HU. Note how the cyst is situated between a calyx and the renal pelvis. This is a simple parenchymal cyst in a peripelvic location and should not be confused with a renal sinus cyst.

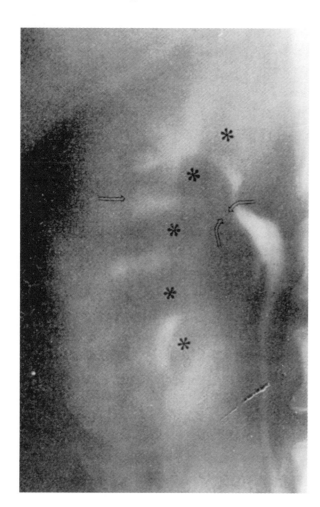

Figure 114–34. "Polycystic disease of the renal sinus" simulating renal pelvic lipomatosis. Nephrotomography demonstrates multiple renal lucencies in the renal sinus *(asterisks)* with medial displacement of the renal pelvis and elongation and stretching of infundibula *(arrows)*. (From Vela-Navarrete R, Robledo AG: Polycystic disease of the renal sinus: Structural characteristics. J Urol 1983;129:700.)

those that are not derived from the renal parenchyma but rather from the other structures of the sinus, such as arteries, lymphatics, and fat.

Renal Sinus Cysts

The predominant type of renal sinus cyst appears to be one derived from the lymphatics. Most often these cysts are multiple, and often they are bilateral. The majority appear after the fifth decade, and they may be associated with inflammation, obstruction, or a calculus (Jordan, 1962; Kutcher et al, 1982).

A condition previously described in the Spanish literature (Paramo and Segura, 1972; Vela-Navarrete et al, 1974; Paramo, 1975) but only recently described in the English literature has been called *polycystic disease of the renal sinus* (Vela-Navarrete and Robledo, 1983), a problematic term because of the possible confusion with polycystic disease of the kidney. Vela-Navarrete and Robledo (1983) described 32 patients with this condition, some in multiple generations of a family (Vela-Navarrete, personal communication, 1990).

Vela-Navarrete and Robledo (1983) found nephrotomography and CT to be particularly useful in defining the lesions.

Sonography was less helpful, perhaps because of the limitations of the equipment then available. On nephrotomography, radiolucencies are identifiable in the renal sinus, along with stretching of the infundibula. Therefore, the appearance is similar to that of renal sinus lipomatosis, a fact that led Vela-Navarrete and Robledo (1983) to suggest that many cases of lipomatosis would be identified as polycystic disease of the renal sinus if CT were used (Fig. 114–34). On CT, the cysts can be seen within the renal sinus as they displace the calyces peripherally (Fig. 114–35). The columns of Bertin may appear attenuated. In the Spanish series, 9 of the 32 patients had small renal calculi visible on plain film.

In 5 patients in the Spanish series, the lesions were explored. Multiple cysts were found, ranging from 2 to 4 cm in diameter and intertwined with stretched infundibula. The fluid was clear, with a plasma-like chemical composition. Histologically, the cyst walls were suggestive of a lymphatic vessel.

This entity has a benign natural history except for the small calculi. These concretions may be secondary to stasis.

Most multiple cystic structures in the area of the renal sinus will turn out to be lymphatic cysts, whereas most singular cysts will be found to be derived from the renal parenchyma. Continued study of cases by CT should clarify the nature of parapelvic and renal sinus cysts.

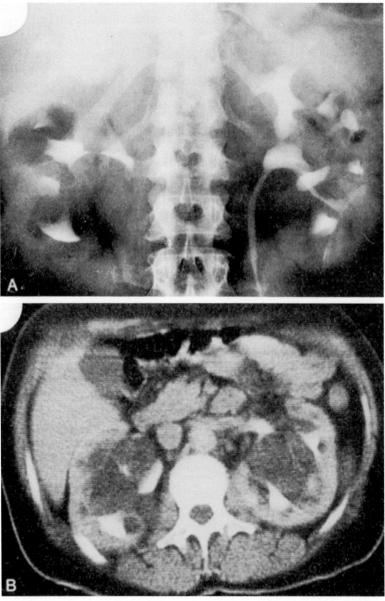

Figure 114–35.   "Polycystic disease of the renal sinus," a form of renal sinus cysts. **A,** Intravenous urogram with enlargement of both kidneys, stretching of infundibula, and trumpet-shaped calyces. **B,** CT scan in midportion of kidneys demonstrates multiple sinus cysts with peripheral displacement of renal pelvis and calyces. (From Vela-Navarrete R, Robledo AG: Polycystic disease of the renal sinus: Structural characteristics. J Urol 1983;129:700.)

SUGGESTED READINGS

Beck AD: The effect of intra-uterine urinary obstruction upon the development of the fetal kidney. J Urol 1971;105:784.

Bernstein J: Developmental abnormalities of the renal parenchyma: Renal hypoplasia and dysplasia. Pathol Annu 1968;3:213.

Bosniak MA: The current radiological approach to renal cysts. Radiology 1986;158:1.

Feiner HD, Katz LA, Gallo GR: Acquired renal cystic disease of kidney in chronic hemodialysis patients. Urology 1981;17:260.

Felson B, Cussen LJ: The hydronephrotic type of congenital multicystic disease of the kidney. Semin Roentgenol 1975;10:113.

Gardner KD Jr: Pathogenesis of human cystic renal disease. Annu Rev Med 1988;39:185.

Glassberg KI: Normal and abnormal development of the kidney: A clinician's interpretation of current development. J Urol 2002;167:2339-2351.

Glassberg KI, Stephens FD, Lebowitz RL, et al: Renal dysgenesis and cystic disease of the kidney: A report of the Committee on Terminology, Nomenclature and Classification, Section on Urology, American Academy of Pediatrics. J Urol 1987;138:1085.

Grantham JJ: Polycystic kidney disease: Hereditary and acquired. Adv Intern Med 1993;38:409.

Kandt RS, Haines JL, Smith M, et al: Linkage of an important gene locus for tuberous sclerosis to a chromosome 16 member for polycystic kidney disease. Nat Genet 1992;2:37.

Kim E, Arnould T, Sellin LK, et al: The polycystic kidney disease 1 gene product modulates Wnt signaling. J Biol Chem 1999;274:4947.

Levine E, Collins DL, Horton WA, et al: CT screening of the abdomen in von Hippel-Lindau disease. AJR Am J Roentgenol 1982;139:505.

Mackie GG, Stephens FD: Duplex kidneys: A correlation of renal dysplasia with position of the ureteral orifice. J Urol 1975;114:274.

Madewell JE, Goldman SM, Davis CJ Jr: Multilocular cystic nephroma: A radiographic pathologic correlation of 58 patients. Radiology 1983;146:309.

Mendelsohn C, Lohnes D, Decimo D, et al: Function of retinoic acid receptors (RARs) during development: II. Multiple abnormalities at various stages of organ genesis in RAR double mutants. Development 1994;120:2749.

O'Hagan AR, Ellsworth R, Secic M, et al: Renal manifestations of tuberous sclerosis complex. Clin Pediatr 1996;183.

Osathanondh V, Potter EL: Pathogenesis of polycystic kidneys: Historical survey. Arch Pathol 1964;77:459.

Pope JC 4th, Brock JW 3rd, Adams MC, et al: Congenital anomalies of the kidney and urinary tract: Role of the loss of function mutation in the pluripotent angiotension type 2 receptor gene. J Urol 2001;165:196.

Roach ES, Smith M, Huttenlocker P, et al: Diagnostic criteria: Tuberous sclerosis complex. Report of the Diagnostic Criteria Committee of the National Tuberous Sclerosis Association. J Child Neurol 1992;7:221.

Sedman A, Bell P, Manco-Johnson M, et al: Autosomal dominant polycystic kidney disease in childhood: A longitudinal study. Kidney Int 1987;31:1000.

Spence HM: Congenital unilateral multicystic kidney: An entity to be distinguished from polycystic kidney disease and other cystic disorders. J Urol 1955;74:893.

Winyard PJD, Nauta J, Lirenman DS, et al: Deregulation of cell survival in cystic and dysplastic renal development. Kidney Int 1996;49:135.

115 Anomalies and Surgery of the Ureteropelvic Junction in Children

MICHAEL C. CARR, MD, PhD • ALAA EL-GHONEIMI, MD

EVIDENCE

ETIOLOGY

SYMPTOMS/PRESENTATION

DIAGNOSIS

SURGICAL REPAIR

OUTCOME

SUMMARY

There is ongoing debate as to whether a hydronephrotic kidney is obstructed, primarily because the tools we use to measure or define obstruction are less than precise. A ureteropelvic junction (UPJ) obstruction can be thought of as a restriction to flow of urine, from the renal pelvis to the ureter, which, if left uncorrected, leads to progressive renal deterioration (Whitaker, 1975; Koff et al, 1986; Koff, 1990). The response to obstruction is the development of renal pelvic hypertrophy, in which the kidney compensates to maintain adequate urinary flow. Eventually, there are further changes to the renal pelvis and pressure-induced injury that leads to irreversible renal damage.

This chapter considers only congenital UPJ obstruction. Other conditions that delay drainage of the proximal urinary tract and secondarily affect the UPJ are discussed elsewhere in this text.

EVIDENCE

UPJ obstruction occurs in all pediatric age groups, but there tends to be a clustering in the neonatal period because of the detection of antenatal hydronephrosis and again later in life because of symptomatic occurrence. At one point, about 25% of cases were discovered within the first year of life (Williams

and Kenawi, 1976), but today the majority of cases are identified and diagnosed in the perinatal period (Brown et al, 1987). **UPJ obstruction is the most common cause of significant dilation of the collecting system in the fetal kidney**, accounting for 48% of all dilation of the collecting system and far exceeding the incidence of multicystic dysplastic kidney (Colodny et al, 1980; Brown et al, 1987). Kidneys with an anterior-posterior diameter greater than 20 mm seen prenatally are certainly at greater risk for requiring surgery postnatally (Dhillon, 1998). The problem that exists today is that the diagnosis of UPJ is "made" at the time of prenatal ultrasonography, so that expectant parents are often informed that their fetus will most likely require surgical intervention as a neonate. This has contributed to ongoing anxiety and altered parental enjoyment during pregnancy (Harding et al, 1999).

Beyond the neonatal period, UPJ obstruction is seen during childhood and adolescence but to a lesser degree. Often, the cause is an aberrant lower pole parenchymal vessel that crosses over the UPJ (Lowe and Marshall, 1984). **Obstruction occurs more commonly in boys than in girls** (Williams and Karlaftis, 1966, Kelalis et al, 1971; Johnston et al, 1977), especially in the newborn period, when the ratio exceeds 2:1 (Robson et al, 1976; Williams and Kenawi, 1976; Johnston et al, 1977). Left-sided lesions predominate, particularly in the neonate (approximately 67%). Bilateral UPJ obstruction is present in 10% to 40% of cases (Nixon, 1953; Uson et al, 1968; Robson et al, 1976; Williams and Kenawi, 1976; Johnston et al, 1977; Lebowitz and Griscom, 1977), with both synchronous and asynchronous occurrences. This tends to occur in infants younger than 6 months of age (Perlmutter et al, 1980; Snyder et al, 1980), and it has been known to affect members of more than one generation (Cohen et al, 1978).

ETIOLOGY

The precise cause of UPJ obstruction remains elusive despite investigation along a number of lines: embryologic (Osathanondh and Potter, 1963; Allen, 1973; Ruano-Gil et al, 1975), anatomic (Nixon, 1953; Johnston, 1969), functional (Whitaker, 1975), and histologic (Murnaghan, 1958; Notley, 1968; Hanna et al, 1976). A narrowing of the UPJ is often found (Allen, 1973; Lebowitz and Griscom, 1977), but whether this is a result of developmental arrest (Osathanondh and Potter, 1963; Allen, 1973) or of incomplete recanalization of the ureter (Ruano-Gil et al, 1975) is not yet known.

Intrinsic

The typical finding at the time of pyeloplasty is a narrowed segment of the ureter at the UPJ that is probe patent (Fig. 115–1). This finding may be the result of an interruption in the development of the circular musculature of the UPJ (Murnaghan, 1958) or an alteration of the collagen fibers and composition between and around the muscle cells (Notley, 1968; Hanna et al, 1976; Hanna, 2000). The muscle fibers become widely separated and attenuated, leading to a functional discontinuity of the muscular contractions and ultimately to insufficient emptying. Further characterization of the UPJ by Starr and colleagues (1992) noted a significant increase in the lamina muscularis and in the number of inner longitudinal muscular bundles of the UPJ complex of obstructed kidneys in infants younger than 1 year compared with age-matched healthy infants. These findings suggest a dramatic response by the muscular layers to obstruction. Further work has shown that the expression of transforming growth factor β (TGF-β) is increased in the pelvis of partially obstructed kidneys (Seremetis and Maizels, 1996), which may help explain some of the histologic and electron microscopic findings that were described by Notley and Hanna and their colleagues.

Other causes of intrinsic UPJ obstruction include valvular mucosal folds (Maizels and Stephens, 1980), persistent fetal convolutions (Leiter, 1979), and upper ureteral polyps (Colgan et al, 1973; Gup, 1975; Williams and Kenawi, 1976; Williams et al, 1980; Thorup et al, 1981).

Congenital folds are a common finding in the upper ureter of fetuses after the fourth month of development and may persist until the newborn period. Such folds are mucosal infolds with an axial offshoot and adventitia that does not flatten out when the ureter is distended or stretched. The epithelial folds are secondary to differential growth rates of the ureter and the body of the child, with excessive ureteral length occurring early in gestation. This provides a "length reserve" for the ureter, which traverses a shorter distance in the newborn than in the adult (Östling, 1942). Östling thought that these folds were a precursor of UPJ obstruction because they frequently were discovered in babies who had a contralateral UPJ obstruction. This concept has evolved, and "Ostling's folds" are now considered folds that are not obstructive and disappear with a person's linear growth (Leiter, 1979) (Fig. 115–2). They are rarely seen in an older child or adult. On the other hand, persistent fetal folds containing muscle and high insertion of a valvular leaflet at the UPJ may become obstructive (Maizels and Stephens, 1980). This type of obstruction sometimes can be relieved by dissection of the folds and elimination of the kinking (Johnston, 1969), but more commonly the ureteral portion containing the valve must be excised.

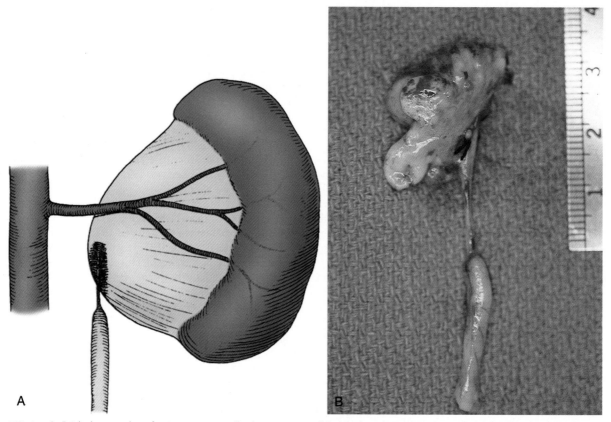

Figure 115–1. **A,** Intrinsic narrowing of upper ureter contributing to ureteropelvic junction obstruction. **B,** Surgical specimen of nonfunctioning kidney with significant proximal ureteral narrowing.

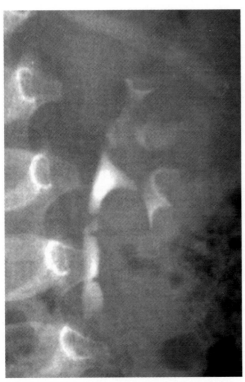

Figure 115–2. Early image of left kidney from intravenous urogram of 4-month-old girl with prenatal hydronephrosis, depicting Östling's folds.

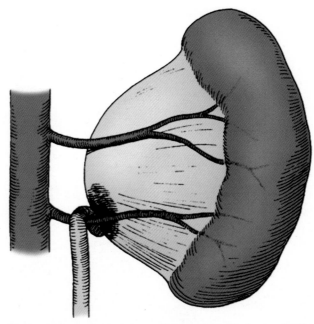

Figure 115–3. A lower pole–crossing vessel contributes to significant kinking at the ureteropelvic junction and resultant intermittent obstruction. Often, when the ureter is mobilized, no evidence of intrinsic narrowing is found. Insertional anomaly and peripelvic fibrosis may also be present as secondary obstructive factors.

Extrinsic

An aberrant, accessory, or early-branching lower pole vessel is the most common cause of extrinsic UPJ obstruction (Fig. 115–3). These vessels pass anteriorly to the UPJ or proximal ureter and contribute to mechanical obstruction. Nixon (1953) reported that 25 of 78 cases of UPJ obstruction were secondary to vascular compression; other reported incidences have varied between 15% and 52% (Ericsson et al, 1961; Williams and Kenawi, 1976, Johnston et al, 1977; Stephens, 1982; Lowe and Marshall, 1984). This is a major cause of UPJ obstruction in adults.

Whether the aberrant vessel causes obstruction or is a covariable that exists along with an intrinsic narrowing is unclear. Stephens (1982) theorized that when an aberrant or accessory renal artery to the lower pole of the kidney is present and the ureter courses behind it, the ureter may angulate at both the UPJ and the point at which it traverses over the vessel as the pelvis fills and bulges anteriorly. Further angulation of the ureter occurs as it becomes adherent to the UPJ secondary to an inflammatory process. A two-point obstruction ensues, with kinking of the ureter at the UPJ and at the point where the ureter drapes over the vessel. Stephens (1982) could find no evidence of stricture or fibrosis at these points when the ureter was freed of its adhesions and lifted off the vessel. However, he suggested that, over time, these areas may become ischemic, fibrotic, and finally stenotic.

Secondary Ureteral Pelvic Junction Obstruction

UPJ obstruction may also be seen with severe vesicoureteral reflux (VUR); these conditions coexist in 10% of cases. The ureter elongates and develops a tortuous course in response to the obstructive element of reflux. A kink may develop in the UPJ area, a point of relative fixation, and may cause obstruction secondarily (Lebowitz and Blickman, 1983). In such a situation the obstructive lesion needs to be corrected initially, even though the VUR contributed to the initial problem (Fig. 115–4). With the advent of injectable biomaterials such as Deflux (Q-Med, Uppsala, Sweden) and Macroplastique (Uroplasty, Minneapolis, MN), consideration should be given to correcting the proximal obstruction as well as the distal reflux by an endoscopic approach.

Lower Pole Ureteral Pelvic Junction Obstruction

Lower pole UPJ obstruction can occur in kidneys with an associated incomplete renal duplication. Hydronephrosis of the lower pole moiety can be delineated with a well-performed sonogram. Such a finding can suggest the presence of a lower pole UPJ obstruction, which is an unusual finding. The incidence of renal duplication is predicted to be 0.3% to 6%. Incomplete duplications are found approximately 70% of the time in comparison with complete duplications (Privett et al, 1976). The anatomy of lower pole UPJ obstruction is either a short bifurcating ureteral segment distal to the UPJ or a longer bifurcating ureteral segment. Such a long ureteral segment lends itself to a typical dismembered pyeloplasty, whereas the

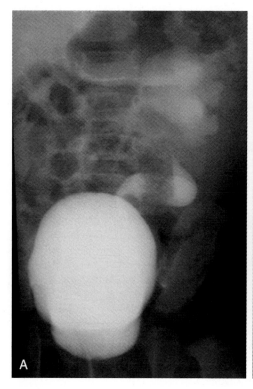
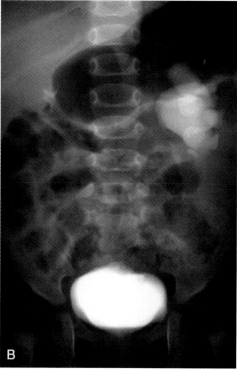

Figure 115–4. **A,** Voiding cystourethrogram demonstrating left vesicoureteral reflux. Note dilutional effect of contrast in renal pelvis. **B,** Postvoid view demonstrating right grade II vesicoureteral reflux and significant retained contrast in left renal pelvis. Patient developed worsening left hydronephrosis, which was observed on subsequent ultrasound imaging, and underwent a left dismembered pyeloplasty. There was evidence of a lower pole–crossing vessel contributing to intermittent kinking of the ureter.

short ureteral segment is better handled by opening the renal pelvis, excising the stenotic ureteral bifurcation, and performing an end-to-side pyeloureterostomy (Fig. 115–5) (Joseph et al, 1989).

Associated Anomalies

Congenital renal malformations are commonly seen in association with UPJ obstruction. Other urologic abnormalities may be found in 50% of affected infants (Uson et al, 1968; Robson et al, 1976; Lebowitz and Griscom, 1977). **UPJ obstruction is the most common anomaly** encountered in the opposite kidney; it occurs in 10% to 40% of cases. Renal dysplasia and multicystic dysplastic kidney are the next most frequently observed contralateral lesions (Williams and Karlaftis, 1966). In addition, unilateral renal agenesis has been noted in almost 5% of children (Robson et al, 1976; Williams and Kenawi, 1976; Johnston et al, 1977). UPJ obstruction may also occur in either the upper or the lower half (usually the latter) of a duplicated collecting system (Amar, 1976; Joseph et al, 1989) (see Fig. 115–5) or of a horseshoe or ectopic kidney (Fig. 115–6).

UPJ obstruction was noted in 21% of children with the VATER (vertebral defects, imperforate anus, tracheoesophageal fistula, and radial and renal dysplasia) association (Uehling et al, 1983), whereas a more recent review showed a 9% incidence of UPJ obstruction, along with the majority of patients having some degree of hydronephrosis but no obstruction or reflux, solitary renal kidneys, or a small percentage with multicystic dysplastic kidneys (Kolon et al, 2000).

VUR has been found in as many as 40% of affected children (Williams and Kenawi, 1976; Juskiewenski et al, 1983; Lebowitz and Blickman, 1983). This degree of reflux is often low grade, not contributing to upper urinary tract obstruc-

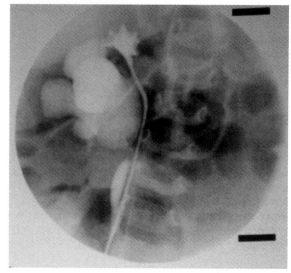

Figure 115–5. Retrograde pyelogram demonstrating anatomy of right incomplete renal duplication with lower pole ureteropelvic junction obstruction.

tion, and with a high likelihood of spontaneous resolution. In certain situations, high-grade VUR can have a profound effect on the UPJ, as previously noted. Anomalies of other organ systems are frequently observed but without any consistent pattern of inheritance.

SYMPTOMS/PRESENTATION

The dichotomy of presentation of infants and children with UPJ obstruction is that **most infants are asymptomatic and most anomalies in children are discovered because of their**

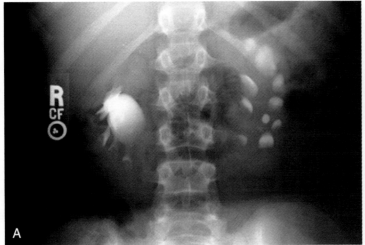

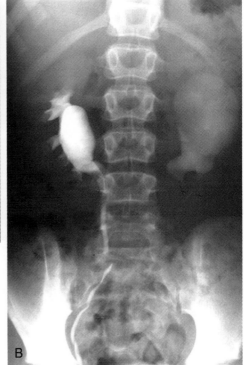

Figure 115–6. **A,** Intravenous urogram (10-minute image) showing delayed uptake and excretion of contrast from left kidney. **B,** Thirty-minute image demonstrating horseshoe kidney and wisp of contrast in proximal left ureter. Patient was found to have high insertion and intermittent kinking of the ureter, which was contributing to periodic abdominal pain. He presented with gross hematuria after being struck by a soccer ball.

symptoms. Previously, infants were discovered to have UPJ obstruction because of a palpable mass (Williams and Karlaftis, 1966; Robson et al, 1976; Johnston et al, 1977). Now, the almost universal use of prenatal sonography has made discovery of UPJ obstruction a common occurrence. It has changed our approach to evaluation because now we are attempting to prove that a problem exists in an otherwise asymptomatic infant. There are still occasionally infants who present with failure to thrive, feeding difficulties, sepsis secondary to urinary tract infection, or pain or hematuria related to nephrolithiasis. Urinary tract infection is the presenting sign in 30% of affected children beyond the neonatal period (Snyder et al, 1980).

In the older child, episodic flank or upper abdominal pain, sometimes associated with nausea and vomiting related to intermittent UPJ obstruction, is a prominent symptom (Kelalis et al, 1971; Williams and Kenawi, 1976) (Fig. 115–7). At other times, cyclic vomiting alone is caused by intermittent UPJ obstruction. The pathology may be manifested only during the episode of cyclic vomiting or abdominal pain, or both. Hematuria, which is seen in 25% of children, may occur after minor abdominal trauma (Kelalis et al, 1971; Williams and Kenawi, 1976). This hematuria is believed to be caused by disruption and rupture of mucosal vessels in the dilated collecting system (Kelalis et al, 1971). In the young adult, episodic flank or abdominal pain, particularly during diuresis, is a common manifestation. Occasionally, a patient with the UPJ obstruction presents with hypertension (Squitieri et al, 1974; Johnston et al, 1977; Munoz et al, 1977; Grossman et al, 1981). The pathophysiology is thought to be a functional ischemia with reduced blood flow caused by the enlarged collecting system that produces a renin-mediated hypertension (Belman et al, 1968).

DIAGNOSIS

In the evaluation of prenatal hydronephrosis, a number of different recommendations and algorithms have been devised (Homsey et al, 1990; Blyth et al, 1993; Cendron et al, 1994). Postnatal ultrasound imaging has traditionally been deferred until day 2 or 3 of life to allow improvement in the relative oliguria, which could lead to underestimation of the degree of hydronephrosis. A comparison of the initial postnatal ultrasound study performed in the first 48 hours of life and 7 to 10 days of life yielded a difference in the degree of hydronephrosis between the first and second sonograms. The authors argued that the initial postnatal ultrasound study should be performed at age 7 to 10 days in newborns with a history of unilateral or mild bilateral hydronephrosis but early scans should be reliable if significant obstruction or potential loss to follow-up is suspected (Wiener and O'Hara, 2002). Docimo (2003), on the basis of his prior evaluation and a review of Weiner's data, argued that there is no reason to delay the first neonatal ultrasound examination beyond 48 hours. The fetal and neonatal kidney may appear to be hydronephrotic on ultrasonography secondary to the sonolucent appearance of the medullary area and pyramids. This appearance tends to resolve after parenchymal maturation, which occurs at 3 months of age. Further evaluation includes a voiding cystourethrogram or nuclear voiding cystourethrogram study to rule out the presence of VUR, which is reported to occur in 13% to 42% of infants studied (Zerin et al, 1993; Anderson et al, 1997). Some investigations have reported a predominance of boys detected with VUR (Bouachrine et al, 1996), whereas results of others are evenly divided between boys and girls (Anderson et al, 1997). Each instance underscores the need for postnatal investigation of infants with a

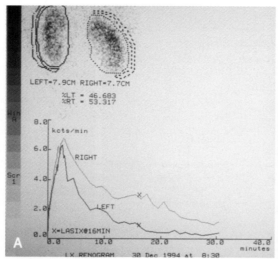

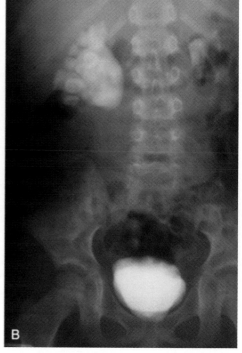

Figure 115–7. **A,** Mercaptoacetyltriglycine (MAG3) Lasix renogram of patient with mild to moderate right hydronephrosis and a history of intermittent abdominal pain. **B,** Intravenous urogram obtained after the patient developed right flank pain and hematuria following a fall from bicycle, consistent with ureteropelvic junction obstruction.

renal pelvic measurement of 5 mm or greater and reinforces the notion that a normal postnatal ultrasound scan does not preclude the presence of VUR (Jaswon et al, 1999).

A number of diagnostic studies have been and are still used to define whether a kidney is obstructed. They have generally been used in adult patients and then applied to the pediatric or neonatal population. The neonatal kidney is undergoing considerable growth and development. Ongoing obstruction may lead not only to functional deterioration but also to impairment of the functional potential of the kidney (Peters, 1995). Some of the diagnostic tests that have been used and some of the newer methods that complement these studies are presented here.

Ultrasonography

Ultrasonography is the standard method for identifying hydronephrosis in infancy. The size of the renal pelvis (anteroposterior diameter) can correlate with the likelihood of obstruction, but this does not diagnose obstruction, nor can it answer whether the hydronephrosis will improve or worsen. This is particularly true in the newborn, in whom hydronephrosis may transiently disappear after birth or fluctuate significantly with time, hydration, and bladder fullness. Sequential studies become meaningful because they define a trend with regard to the hydronephrosis. Worsening hydronephrosis usually indicates obstruction, and improved hydronephrosis suggests the opposite.

To improve further the diagnostic accuracy of ultrasonography, the renal parenchyma-pelvicaliceal area has been measured and compared with the result of conventional diuretic renography. A ratio of less than 1.6 correlates well with an obstructive process and need for pyeloplasty, whereas patients with a ratio greater than 1.6 can be safely observed (Cost et al, 1996). These measurements are more stringent than measurements of anteroposterior diameter but are certainly more operator dependent. On the other hand, they reflect the amount of pelvocaliectasis that exists, which is more meaningful than pelvic diameter alone.

Serial ultrasound measurements can provide another useful parameter in helping to confirm the presence or absence of obstruction by monitoring changes in the growth rate of the normal kidney opposite the hydronephrosis (Koff et al, 1994; Koff and Peller, 1995). Obstruction of one kidney can lead to functional changes in its contralateral mate, affecting its rate of growth. A renal growth–renal function chart was generated with four reproducible, clinically relevant diagnostic patterns derived. Obstruction of one kidney manifests as a decrease of overall function as well as an increase in the growth rate of its contralateral mate. Application of this technique at other institutions did not reveal a significant correlation between unilateral hydronephrosis and contralateral renal length (Brandell et al, 1996).

Renal duplex Doppler ultrasonography has also shown promise as a means of identifying obstruction. A resistive index (RI) is defined as the peak systolic velocity minus the lowest diastolic velocity divided by the peak systolic velocity. Infants younger than 1 year of age had a greater RI (0.66) than children older than 1 year of age (0.57). In hydronephrotic kidneys, the **RI values were much higher in the kidneys that had an obstructive pattern on diuretic renography** (RI ≥ 0.75) (Gilbert et al, 1993). When these Doppler studies were modified by the addition of furosemide, the differences between obstructed and nonobstructed kidneys were further accentuated. In addition, follow-up of these patients demonstrated that the RI normalized after successful pyeloplasty (average preoperative RI, 0.87; average postoperative RI, 0.63) (Ordorica et al, 1993).

Radionuclide Renography

Intravenous urography was in the past the primary radiographic study used to define UPJ obstruction. In most institutions, this has been supplanted by radionuclide renography, which provides differential renal function data and an assessment of washout from the individual kidney. On the other hand, in situations where an intermittent UPJ obstruction is believed to occur, an intravenous pyelogram at the time that the patient presents with pain is an ideal study to define the anatomy, is readily available at most hospitals, and can generally be done on short notice when a patient presents to an emergency department. In addition, some pediatric urologists still prefer radiographic visualization of the UPJ to assure families that the cause of hydronephrosis is a UPJ variant that will not lead to a problem in the future.

Radionuclide renography lends itself to a more objective interpretation. Despite guidelines and consensus protocols, renographic procedures differ among centers, causing difficulties in comparison and controversy in the interpretation of results (Eskild-Jensen, 2004). Early attempts at standardization of the technique were due to the increasing detection of asymptomatic neonates with hydronephrosis. The concept of the "well-tempered" diuretic renogram was advanced as a result of a dialogue between the Society for Fetal Urology and the Pediatric Nuclear Medicine Council (Conway and Maizels, 1992).

The well-tempered renogram stipulated that infants would be prehydrated with 10 to 15 mL/kg of saline and that a catheter would be placed at the time the study was being performed. Early studies used ^{99m}Tc-diethylenetriaminepentaacetic acid (DTPA) as the radionuclide, which has since been supplanted by ^{99m}Tc-mercaptoacetyltriglycine (MAG3) at many institutions. DTPA is a small molecule that is exclusively filtered by glomeruli with an extraction coefficient of 20% in the mature kidney (Rehling, 2003). Because it is excreted only by glomerular filtration, this agent provides an indirect means of measuring the glomerular filtration rate (GFR). Differential GFR can be determined by comparing the amount of uptake in each kidney during the first 1 to 3 minutes after intravenous injection (Rowell et al, 1986).

MAG3 is cleared by the kidneys by secretion in the proximal tubules (Eshima, 1992) with a higher extraction fraction than DTPA (about 50% in mature kidneys) and MAG3 remains essentially within the intravascular space. This provides a high target-to-background ratio, good image quality, and more accurate numerical values, particularly when the kidney function is low or immature.

As experience was gained in applying the well-tempered renogram, there was an increased realization that a number of factors need to be taken into consideration, including renal maturation, body proportions, differential renal function, pelvic capacity, tubular reabsorption, the timing and effect of the diuretic, as well as the influences of gravity and the bladder on drainage (Gordon, 2004).

There is no correct time to give a diuretic. Some institutions prefer the diuretic prior to tracer (usually 15 minutes, F −15), some with the tracer (times 0 or 2 to 3 minutes, F 0), and other institutions give the diuretic when the renal pelvis is full of tracer (15 to 20 minutes, F +20). The effect of the diuretic on the tracer is different, which adds another physiologic variable to the drainage curve. With F −15, the tracer enters a renal pelvis that is full of nonisotopic urine; with F 0, the high urine flow rate and tracer occur simultaneously, suggesting that the urine and the tracer are well mixed in the dilated pelvis; and with F +20, the pelvis is full of tracer so that the diuresis is of urine with little tracer and the degree of pelvic filling at the start of the diuresis is variable. There is no wrong or right technique, and every institution should adopt a standard protocol for these infants and children (Fig. 115–8).

It is well known that a full bladder can inhibit drainage from the pelvis (Amarante et al, 2003). This is the rationale for either placing a catheter in the bladder prior to the initiation of the study or acquiring a postmicturition image at the end of the dynamic diuretic renogram (Gordon and Riccabona, 2003). For most infants and toddlers who have been given a diuretic, there is little difficulty in facilitating micturition. Such simple maneuvers as changing the baby's position and putting the infant on the mother's shoulder can facilitate this. Furthermore, this change in posture also allows gravity to have its full effect because the renogram is normally done in a supine position. The timing of this postmicturition image is another variable factor that should be standardized in each institution. **If a kidney with antenatal unilateral hydronephrosis is shown to maintain a stable differential renal function and pelvic diameter, this kidney is by definition not obstructed** (Koff, 2003). Furthermore, this kidney may be said to be in equilibrium inasmuch as the filtration at the glomerulus is constant (allowing maturation and growth), and the urine production has not resulted in progressive enlargement in the renal pelvis.

Such a kidney would then have a renogram with the normal three phases: uptake, a peak, and a falling third phase. However, the slope of the uptake phase depends on the differential renal function. The peak of the renogram varies depending on the combination of pelvic volume and timing of the diuretic challenge. Thus, the lower the differential renal function and the bigger the renal pelvis, the longer it takes to achieve a renogram with all three phases. For historical and convenience reasons, diuretic renograms usually have data acquisition for approximately 40 minutes; clearly, with some kidneys this is too short. With such variables, it may not be possible to undertake the postmicturition image at different delayed times for each child, and thus it would make sense to adopt a standard time for this delayed postmicturition data acquisition. Clearly, this should be at least 20 minutes after the diuretic with F +20 or F −15. With F 0 it could be 40 minutes or longer (Gordon, 2004).

The analysis of the drainage curve should then take into account the function of the kidney, allow gravity to have its full effect, and ensure that the bladder is empty. Employing different analysis techniques, poor drainage has been recorded in kidneys that were not operated upon and had stable function and stable size of the renal pelvis on follow-up studies. Given the complexity of such a study, it is clear that **only looking at the slope of the drainage curve is a simplistic approach to a complex parameter.** Impaired drainage can be explained on a pathophysiologic basis so that dilation with impaired drainage is not by definition a sign of obstruction.

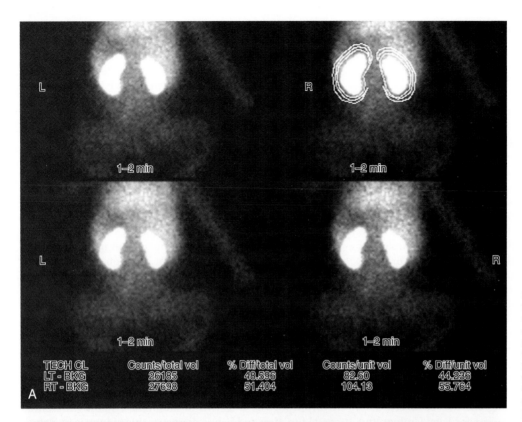

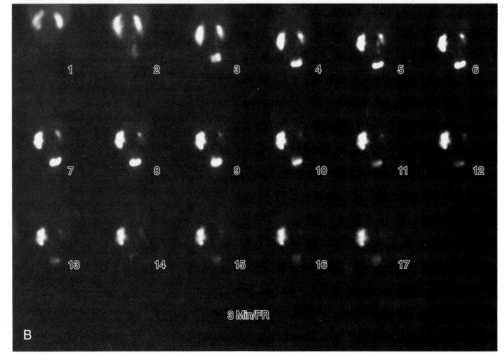

Figure 115–8. A, Mercaptoacetyl-triglycine (MAG3) Lasix renogram with differential renal function obtained between 1 and 2 minutes showing relatively symmetric function. **B,** Images obtained every 3 minutes showing adequate blood flow to both kidneys; cortical transit in both kidneys is 3 to 4 minutes, which is within normal limits. Historically, it was shown that the normal transit of a radiotracer through the kidney is 3 to 5 minutes, so that the renal pelvis can be identified on the second frame (3- to 6-minute image). Lasix (1 mg/kg) was administered intravenously at 27 minutes (frame 7).

Impaired drainage in infants with a prenatal ultrasound diagnosis of hydronephrosis who are asymptomatic may not then be used as a definition of obstruction (Gordon, 2004).

The nuclear renogram is one test that can help define whether obstruction exists. A kidney that shows symmetric uptake and good washout is by definition not obstructed. In many situations with hydronephrotic kidneys, there is a small difference in the differential function of the affected kidney compared with its contralateral mate and the Lasix renogram shows some impairment of drainage. Depending upon the patient's age and the concern about an indolent obstruction, a repeated renal scan after several months may help determine the trend because an ongoing partial obstruction would be

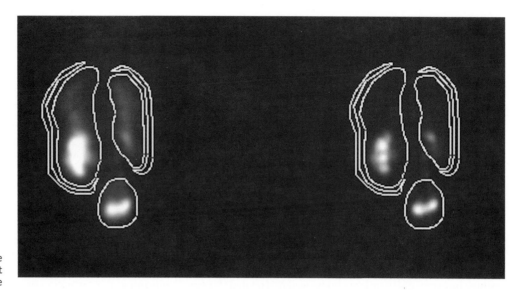

Figure 115–8, cont'd. C, Time activity curve showing good washout from right kidney and moderate retention of radiotracer in left kidney with some response to Lasix administration.

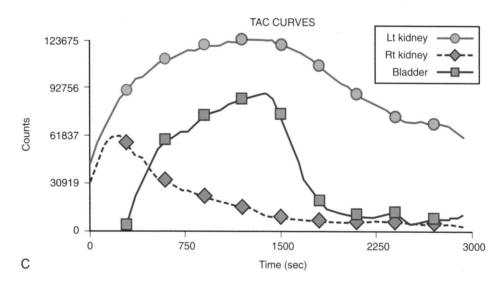

C

expected to cause a further decline in the overall renal function and potentially a worsening in the washout curve. A snapshot of the kidney's function over time can be helpful in deciding whether surgery is necessary or not. In addition, following successful surgery a postoperative renal scan can provide an assessment of the overall residual function in the kidney, particularly if this function was diminished prior to surgery. In such a situation, it is reasonable to perform such a study 6 to 12 months following a successful pyeloplasty to obtain an accurate assessment of the residual renal function.

Magnetic Resonance Imaging

New, ultrafast magnetic resonance imaging (MRI) offers unique advantages for evaluating renal blood flow, anatomy, and urinary excretion. Anatomic analysis of MRI noncontrast studies showed precise dilatation of the hydronephrotic pelvis and corticomedullary junction in a rat model with unilateral congenital hydronephrosis (Fichtner et al, 1994). This technology is now routinely being utilized in pediatric patients, with much of the work originating from Emory University and Children's Health Care of Atlanta. Much like the work that was done to define the utility of nuclear renography in the evaluation of children with hydronephrosis, MRI urography is being investigated to define urinary tract anatomy, calculate differential renal function, and assess urinary tract obstruction (Grattan-Smith et al, 2003). In comparison with ultrasonography and nuclear renography, dynamic contrast enhanced MRI is superior (Fig. 115–9). The differential renal function, as determined by calculating the volume of enhancing renal parenchyma, is comparable to that determined by nuclear renography. When assessing the utility of each modality, as determined by the decision to proceed with surgery or not, MR urography has been shown to be as sensitive, more specific, and of greater diagnostic efficiency than renal scintigraphy. Because there is no absolute test that exists to define obstruction precisely, the surgery itself becomes the endpoint (Grattan-Smith et al, 2003).

Further refinements in dynamic contrast material enhanced MR urography include the calculation of renal transit time

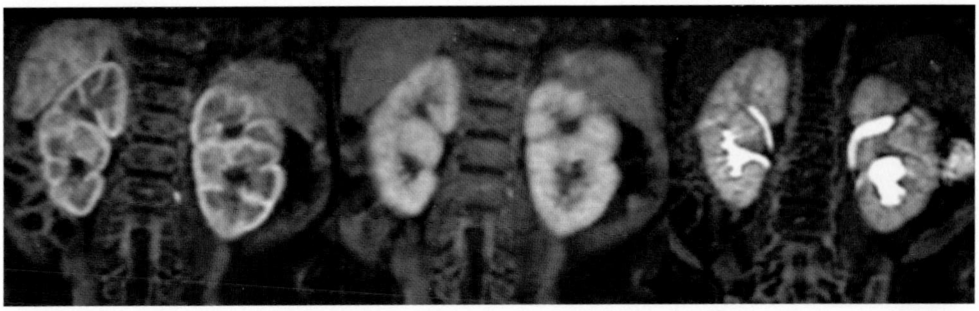

Perfusion　　　　　　Uptake　　　　　　Excretion

Figure 115–9. Post–gadolinium-diethylenetriaminepentaacetic acid (DTPA) infusion sequential images reveal perfusion, uptake, and excretion phases. (From Perez-Brayfield MR, Kirsch AJ, Jones RA, Grattan-Smith JD: A prospective study comparing ultrasound, nuclear scintigraphy and dynamic contrast enhanced magnetic resonance imaging in the evaluation of hydronephrosis. J Urol 2003; 170:1331.)

(Jones et al, 2004). This calculation complements the determination of differential renal function. The procedure involves prehydrating the patient for 30 minutes with an intravenous infusion of 10 mL/kg body weight lactated Ringer solution and catheterizing the patient to ensure constant bladder drainage. Sedation involves a standard protocol in which chloral hydrate was used in children younger than 1 year and intravenous pentobarbital plus fentanyl in children between 1 and 7. Sedation was administered and monitored by a trained pediatric sedation nurse using continuous pulse oximetry. Patients were placed in a supine position on an imaging bed of a 1.5 T unit filled with 30 MT/m gradient coils. Scout images were acquired to determine kidney and bladder positions in order to optimize the signal-to-noise ratio. Furosemide, 1 mg/kg with a maximum dose of 20 mg, was administered intravenously. Images were acquired using various parameters that optimize the anatomic reference images. The images obtained with the heavily T2-weighted sequence provided the basis for a precontrast maximum intensity projection of the collecting systems, ureters, and bladder (Rohrschneider et al, 2002).

The acquisition of three-dimensional dynamic gradient-echo images was initiated and a bolus of 0.1 mmol/kg gadopentetate dimeglumine (Magnevist; Berlex Laboratories, Wayne, NJ) was hand injected 15 minutes after the injection of furosemide to coincide with the maximal diuretic effect. Volume acquisitions require 15 seconds, so that continuous acquisitions occur during the first 5 minutes of the dynamic study, with subsequent imaging at 1-minute intervals. If both ureters were clearly visualized 10 minutes after the injection of contrast medium, no more dynamic images were acquired. The renal transit time (RTT) was then calculated following archiving of all the images. The first volume that showed clear enhancement of the cortex and the first volume that clearly showed contrast material in the ureter at or below the level of the lower pole of the kidney were determined, with the difference in the time of acquisition between these two volumes representing the RTT. In kidneys with poor drainage, in which no contrast was seen in the ureter at the end of 15 minutes of dynamic imaging, the RTT was 900 seconds (15 minutes) (Jones et al, 2004). Analogous to the half-life ($t_{1/2}$) that is calculated for nuclear scintigraphy studies, RTT defined normal kidneys (less than or equal to 245 seconds), equivocal (RTT between 245 and 490 seconds), or obstructive (RTT greater than 490 seconds). This was based upon the evaluation of 126 patients with hydronephrosis (Fig. 115–10).

The authors found there to be an excellent correlation between the $t_{1/2}$ of renal signal decay following furosemide administration and the RTT, showing that both tests yield meaningful information on response of the diuretic challenge. These observations hold true when defining a UPJ obstruction but not necessarily in the case of the ureterovesical junction obstruction. Furthermore, the quality of functioning renal tissue can affect the interpretation of obstructive uropathy with MR urography. In the presence of both poor function and hydroureteronephrosis, the signal increases only gradually, making the calculation of RTT somewhat more subjective.

MRI and nuclear medicine studies were equally sensitive in detecting obstruction, but the definition of obstruction becomes somewhat arbitrary because there is no reference test to define obstruction. MRI does not involve ionizing radiation so that multiple follow-up studies can be performed to monitor hydronephrosis. This must be balanced with the higher expense, need for sedation, and higher frequency of adverse reactions to the contrast agent. Further refinements in the technique and more widespread application to other centers will be forthcoming. Data acquisition from MR urography is being evaluated to calculate an index of glomerular filtration. Research is ongoing with diffusion (Jones and Grattan-Smith, 2003; Pedersen et al, 2003) and blood oxygenation level–dependent imaging (Prasad et al, 1996; Ries et al, 2003) of the kidney being explored. The diversity of information promises to make MR urography an attractive method for assessment of obstructive uropathy.

Pressure-Flow Studies

Whitaker (1978) defined obstruction in the kidney as impedance to flow such that proximal pressure must be raised to transmit the usual flow rate through it. His study involved placing catheters into the renal pelvis and bladder, infusing fluid at a rate of 10 mL/sec into the kidney, and measuring the intrapelvic pressure of the kidney. A differential pressure between kidney and bladder could then be indicative of obstruction to the kidney. Whitaker studies are usually not performed in pediatric patients, but the concept of measuring intrapelvic pressure to help delineate whether obstruction exists remains. For example, infusion of the renal pelvis of hydronephrotic kidneys is performed, and the decrease in pressure with time is determined as a pressure decay curve (Fung et al, 1996). As might be expected, renal units without

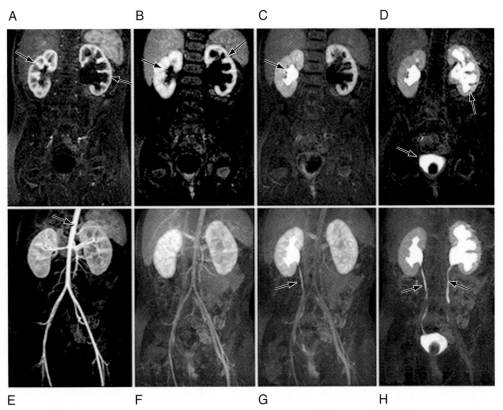

Figure 115–10. **A** to **D,** T1-weighted images of a coronal section obtained through anterior region of the kidneys in a 3-year-old girl with obstruction of ureteropelvic junction of left kidney. Each image is a single section from dynamic volumes acquired at four time points. **E** to **H,** Maximum intensity projections (MIPs) derived from full volumes (30 sections) at same time points. Arrows in A and E correspond to intense cortical and vascular enhancement, respectively. B and F were acquired approximately 1 minute after cortical phase of enhancement and arrows in B indicate that signal from both cortex and medulla was enhanced; this phase was used for calculation of differential renal function. C and G were obtained approximately $2^1/_2$ minutes after cortical phase. Arrows in C highlight enhancement of right collection system, and in G, the corresponding right ureter *(arrow)* is also seen. D was obtained approximately 12 minutes after cortical phase. In D, the left collecting system *(top arrow)* and bladder *(bottom arrow)* are also seen. In corresponding MIP in H, both ureters *(arrows)* are visible. (From Jones RA, Perez-Brayfield MR, Kirsch AJ, et al: Renal transit time with MR urography in children. Radiology 2004;233:44.)

elevated pelvic pressure during infusion at a high physiologic flow rate have relatively rapid pressure decay, whereas those with elevated renal pelvic pressure during infusion are associated with much slower pressure decay. The diuretic nuclear renography half-lives have no correlation with collecting system pressure dynamics. **The pressure decay half-life reflects both efficient urine transport and the relative compliance and volume of the collecting system.** Further refinements with this technique of antegrade nephrostomy have included measurement of the ureteral opening pressure, which is defined as the pressure at which contrast material is first seen beyond the suspected site of obstruction (Fung et al, 1998). In all patients with a renal pelvic pressure greater than 14 cm H_2O, the pressure-flow study also demonstrated evidence of obstruction. In contrast, negative ureteral opening pressure had a much lower specificity or negative predictive value.

Pressure-flow measurements that define outflow resistance have also been used to help define obstruction. Servoregulating the infused flow to preset pressure levels was used to assess patients with hydronephrotic kidneys so that steady-state flow was achieved at pressures of 5, 10, 15, 20, 25, and 30 mm Hg greater than the intra-abdominal pressure. This was compared with the standard Whitaker procedure at an infusion rate of

10 mL/min following the percutaneous puncturing of the renal pelvis. The Whitaker test proved to be of no value for calculating outflow resistance in UPJ obstruction. A pressure-flow study was found to be superior to the Whitaker test and allowed categorization of the patients requiring surgery or observation (Wahlin et al, 2001).

Biochemical Parameters

Various biochemical markers have been used as indicators of renal tubular injury in the setting of obstructive uropathy. Such markers could be assessed to determine the need for intervention, based on a detrimental change. *N*-Acetyl-β-D-glucosaminidase (NAG) was measured in patients who were thought to have a UPJ obstruction (Carr et al, 1994). Urinary NAG levels were consistently elevated in urine obtained directly from the kidney, although bladder urines did not provide a significant discriminator when compared with control urinary NAG levels. A similar observation was made when urinary TGF-β1 was measured in children with UPJ obstruction (Palmer et al, 1997). The presence of TGF-β messenger RNA was noted in the renal pelvis after both clinical and experimental UPJ obstruction and may be related to the adaptive molecular responses that increase muscle and collagen in the renal pelvis (Seremetis and Maizels, 1996). Urinary TGF-β1 was found to be fourfold higher in bladder urine in patients with upper tract obstruction compared with control subjects. Voided urine then could be assayed for TGF-β1 on a repetitive basis to assist in the diagnosis of upper urinary tract obstruction (Furness et al, 1999). Furthermore, postoperative urines could be assayed for TGF-β1 in order to confirm that there is no longer upper tract obstruction. In a small series of patients using a bladder urine concentration of 29 pg/mg creatinine as a cutoff between obstruction and no obstruction, TGF-β1 was 80% sensitive, 82% specific, and 81% accurate for the diagnosis of obstruction (El-Sherbiny et al, 2002). A biochemical or molecular marker that is found in the urine and is easily assayed would hold the greatest promise of improving diagnostic ability in obstructive uropathy.

SURGICAL REPAIR

Evolution in the surgical correction of UPJ obstruction has occurred on a number of fronts, with open surgical techniques yielding way to endoscopic and laparoscopic approaches. The open techniques that have had the greatest applicability can be classified into three main groups: the flap type, the incisional-intubated type, and the dismembered type. The Anderson-Hynes pyeloplasty (1949) has become the most commonly employed "open" surgical procedure for the repair of UPJ. This repair had as its underpinnings both the Foley Y-V plasty (1937) and the Davis intubated ureterotomy (1943).

The Foley operation was designed for the correction of UPJ with a high ureteral insertion (Fig. 115–11). As such, this technique cannot be used in conjunction with transposition of a lower pole vessel, nor does it allow any significant reduction of the renal pelvic size. The Davis intubated ureterotomy depends on secondary epithelialization from the incised ureter. It is applicable when multiple or extensive strictures of the proximal ureter are present but cannot be bridged by a pelvic flap (Fig. 115–12). Its use requires maintenance of ureteral continuity on at least one side and the presence of an indwelling ureteral stent for 6 weeks, the time needed for full circumferential regeneration of all layers of the ureter.

Culp and DeWeerd's (1951) spiral flap is created from the renal pelvis, which is used to repair the defect at the UPJ. Such a flap is able to bridge the gap between the pelvis and healthy ureter over a distance of several centimeters (Fig. 115–13). Scardino and Prince (1953) described a vertical flap that can be used in the situation of a dependent UPJ with a large, square-shaped extrarenal pelvis (Fig. 115–14). The rare cases of giant hydronephrosis that may be associated with a completely atretic ureter can be corrected by reconstructing the entire ureter using redundant pelvic tissue (Kheradpir, 1983).

Dismembered Pyeloplasty

The technique of dismembering the ureter was born out of necessity in the repair of a retrocaval ureter (Anderson and Hynes, 1949) (Fig. 115–15). This technique was embraced by English surgeons in the repair of UPJ obstruction, but there was reluctance on the part of surgeons elsewhere because of concerns about severing the neural continuity between pelvis and ureter. Later work, however, demonstrated that the bolus of urine is the peristaltic stimulus. Furthermore, injection studies (Douville and Hollingshead, 1955) demonstrated that

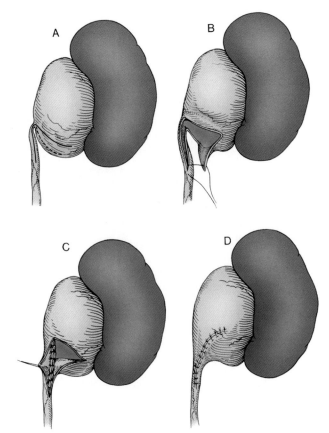

Figure 115–11. **A,** A Foley Y-V plasty is best applied to a ureteropelvic junction obstruction associated with a high insertion of the ureter. The flap is outlined with tissue marker or stay sutures. The base of the V is positioned on the dependent, medial aspect of the renal pelvis and the apex at the ureteropelvic junction. The incision from the apex of the flap, which represents the stem of the Y, is then carried along the lateral aspect of the proximal ureter well into an area of normal caliber. **B,** The flap is developed with fine scissors. The apex of the pelvic flap is brought to the inferiormost aspect of the ureterotomy incision. **C,** The posterior walls are approximated utilizing interrupted or running fine absorbable sutures. **D,** The anastomosis is completed with approximation of the anterior walls of the pelvic flap and ureterotomy.

the arborization of blood vessels in the renal pelvis would ensure appropriate healing even with dismembering.

The principal reasons for the universal acceptance of the dismembered pyeloplasty are (1) broad applicability, including preservation of anomalous vessels; (2) excision of the pathologic UPJ and appropriate repositioning; and (3) successful reduction pyeloplasty. This operation is generally easy to perform and can be accomplished by a number of surgical approaches, including anterior subcostal, flank, and posterior lumbotomy.

A dismembered pyeloplasty may be problematic if there is inadequate ureteral length. A spiral flap from the renal pelvis can overcome this problem. Alternatively, excision of all scar tissue along with a dismembered technique is often possible when the kidney is completely mobilized and brought down as a "reverse" nephropexy. This can provide an additional 5 cm of length, avoiding such maneuvers as bowel interposition, ureterocalicostomy, or autotransplantation.

The age and size of the patient and the position of UPJ are factors that must be considered when choosing a surgical

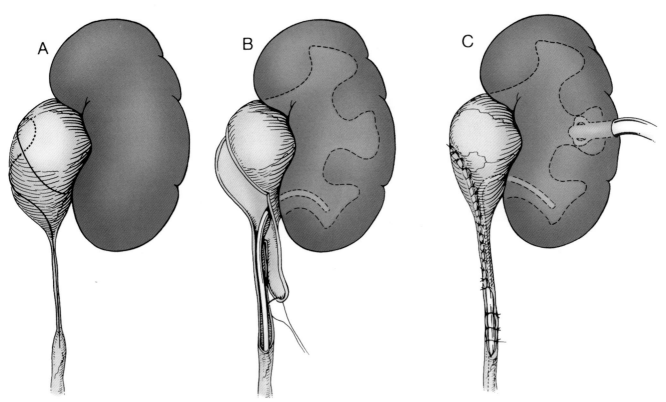

Figure 115–12. **A,** The intubated ureterotomy may be of value when a ureteropelvic junction obstruction is associated with extremely long or multiple ureteral strictures. A spiral flap is outlined and developed as described in Figure 115–13. The ureterotomy incision will be carried completely through the long strictured area or through each of the multiple areas of stricture. **B,** The flap is developed, taking care to use minimal dissection of the ureter in order to preserve its blood supply. In contrast to uncomplicated repairs, nephrostomy tube drainage is utilized routinely. A self-retaining, soft, inert internal ureteral stent is placed and positioned proximally in the renal pelvis or lower infundibulum and distally in the bladder. The apex of the flap is brought as far down as possible over the stent on the ureterotomy. The flap is closed with interrupted or running absorbable sutures. **C,** The distal aspect of the ureterotomy is left open to heal secondarily by ureteral regeneration. A few fine absorbable sutures may be placed loosely to keep the sides of the ureter in apposition to the stent.

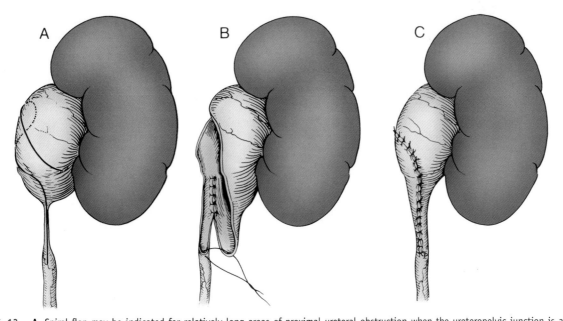

Figure 115–13. **A,** Spiral flap may be indicated for relatively long areas of proximal ureteral obstruction when the ureteropelvic junction is already in a dependent position. The spiral flap is outlined with the base situated obliquely on the dependent aspect of the renal pelvis. The base of the flap is positioned anatomically lateral to the ureteropelvic junction, between the ureteral insertion and the renal parenchyma. The flap is spiraled posteriorly to anteriorly or vice versa. The anatomically medial line of incision is carried down completely through the obstructed proximal ureteral segment into normal caliber ureter. The site of the apex for the flap is determined by length of the flap required to bridge the obstruction. The longer the segment of proximal ureteral obstruction, the farther away is the apex, as this makes the flap longer. To preserve vascular integrity to the flap, however, the ratio of flap length to width should not exceed 3:1. **B,** Once the flap is developed, the apex is rotated down to the most inferior aspect of the ureterotomy. **C,** The anastomosis is completed, usually over an internal stent, utilizing fine absorbable sutures.

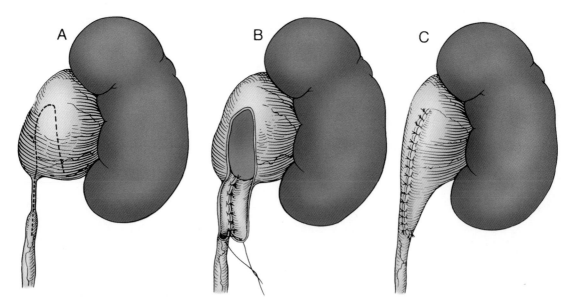

Figure 115–14. **A,** Vertical flap technique may be utilized when a dependent ureteropelvic junction is situated at the medial margin of a large, box-shaped extrarenal pelvis. In contrast to the spiral flap, the base of the vertical flap is situated more horizontally on the dependent aspect of the renal pelvis, between the ureteropelvic junction and the renal parenchyma. The flap itself is formed by two straight incisions converging from the base vertically up to the apex on either the anterior or posterior aspects of the renal pelvis. As for the spiral flap, the position of the apex determines the length of the flap, which should be a function of the length of the proximal ureter to be bridged. The medial incision of the flap is carried down the proximal ureter completely through the strictured area into normal caliber ureter. **B,** The apex of the flap is rotated down to the inferiormost aspect of the ureterotomy. **C,** The flap is closed by approximating the edges with interrupted or running fine absorbable sutures.

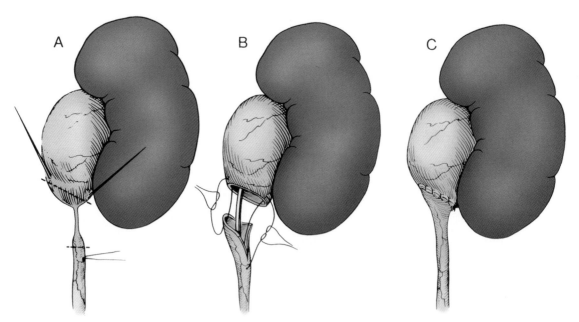

Figure 115–15. **A,** Traction sutures are placed on the medial and lateral aspects of the dependent portion of the renal pelvis in preparation for dismembered pyeloplasty. A traction suture is also placed on the lateral aspect of the proximal ureter, below the level of the obstruction. This suture will help maintain proper orientation for the subsequent repair. **B,** The ureteropelvic junction is excised. The proximal ureter is spatulated on its lateral aspect. The apex of this lateral, spatulated aspect of the ureter is then brought to the inferior border of the pelvis while the medial side of the ureter is brought to the superior edge of the pelvis. **C,** The anastomosis is performed with fine interrupted or running absorbable sutures placed full thickness through the ureteral and renal pelvic walls in a watertight fashion. In general, we prefer to leave an indwelling internal stent in adult patients. The stent is removed 4 to 6 weeks later.

approach. A posterior lumbotomy affords good exposure in the neonate but may not be a good choice in a muscular adolescent. The position of the UPJ can be determined from an intravenous urogram, but most surgeons now perform renal scans instead. Therefore, retrograde pyelography can be used for making this determination. Cockrell and Hendren (1990) noted the benefits of performing retrograde pyelography at the time of pyeloplasty. Findings included a discrete area of narrowing, a long segment of narrowing, tortuosity of the upper ureter, more than one area of narrowing, high insertion of the ureter on the renal pelvis, and compression of the ureter by the lower pole of the kidney. Rushton and colleagues (1994) noted that their surgical findings confirmed obstruction at the UPJ in all patients. Undiagnosed distal ureteral obstruction was not seen, and therefore routine retrograde pyelography is not necessary.

The actual repair for the modified Anderson-Hynes dismembered pyeloplasty, as performed through an anterior subcostal incision, is as follows:

1. The anterior subcostal incision is a muscle-splitting incision that is made with the patient supine and a roll placed transversely beneath the patient to elevate the flank (Fig. 115–16).

2. Each muscle layer encountered is split in the direction of the muscle fibers until Gerota's fascia is identified by sweeping the peritoneum medially. The fascia is then incised posteriorly over the lateral aspect of the kidney.

3. The renal pelvis is identified by medial retraction of the peritoneum and lateral traction of the kidney. If the renal pelvis is significantly dilated, an Angiocath can be inserted to decompress the pelvis and facilitate identification of the UPJ.

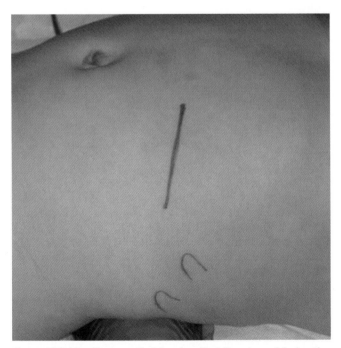

Figure 115–16. Three-month-old male with left ureteropelvic junction obstruction positioned for anterior subcostal approach to dismembered pyeloplasty. The tips of the 11th and 12th ribs are marked and the patient is placed on a gel roll for elevation of flank.

4. Anterior exposure is usually better when a dismembered pyeloplasty is being performed. **Once the ureter and UPJ are identified, a traction suture is displaced anteriorly through the proximal ureter** to minimize subsequent handling.

5. The area of UPJ is dissected free to allow a clear area in which to perform the anastomosis. Traction sutures of 6-0 Prolene may be placed in the renal pelvis superiorly, medially, laterally, and inferiorly to the UPJ. When adequate ureteral length is confirmed and the pathology of UPJ identified, the ureter can be transected at the UPJ. If the ureter is short, the kidney is completely mobilized to determine whether it can be brought down sufficiently to allow a primary tension-free anastomosis.

6. After transection of the UPJ, the renal pelvis may not spontaneously drain until it is incised. This should be done after the site for anastomosis is chosen.

7. The **ureter is spatulated on the side opposite to the traction suture** using Potts tenotomy scissors. The distance over which the ureter is opened is variable, until healthy ureter is encountered, which springs open when forceps are placed into it.

8. The **portion of pelvis is excised**, usually a diamond-shaped segment that is present within the traction sutures that were placed in the renal pelvis. It is better to leave too much renal pelvis than too little, especially when resecting along the medial aspect of the renal pelvis. Infundibula can be encountered if one is not careful (Fig. 115–17).

9. The ureter and renal pelvis are aligned to ensure that the anastomosis can be accomplished without tension. If a nephrostomy tube is to be used, it is placed at this time. An inferior calix is chosen, preferably where the overlying parenchyma is not too thick. A Malecot catheter works well and is positioned away from the repair to minimize the chance of the catheter's causing urinary blockage through the reconstructed UPJ.

10. The anastomosis is started by placing the first 7-0 Maxon (Davis and Geck) suture at the apex of the "V" in the ureter and into the tip of the inferior pelvic flap. As the suture is tied down, the ureter and renal pelvis are brought together to minimize tension on the repair. A small feeding tube is placed into the ureter; it can be used to stabilize the ureter during the anastomosis. A **"no-touch" technique is employed with the ureter to minimize trauma** and edema to the ureteral tissue. Either interrupted sutures or a running closure may be used, depending on the surgeon's preference. The area of the initial anastomosis is critical to ensuring a water-tight closure.

11. Before the repair is completed, the renal pelvis is irrigated to remove any blood clots or debris that could obstruct the UPJ. If an indwelling JJ ureteral stent is employed, it should be placed now, with care taken to place the stent into the bladder and renal pelvis without kinking it.

12. A Penrose drain is placed adjacent to the repair and brought out through a separate stab wound.

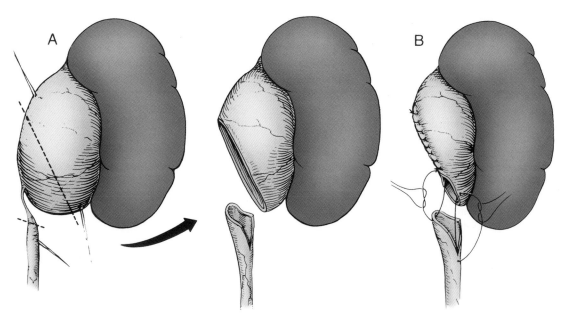

Figure 115–17. A, For a large or redundant pelvis, a reduction pyeloplasty is performed by excising the redundant portion between traction sutures. **B,** The cephalad aspect of the pelvis is then closed with running absorbable sutures down to the dependent portion. The dependent aspect of the pelvis is anastomosed to the proximal ureter as described in Figure 115–15.

13. The kidney is returned to its native position, and perinephric fat, if available, is placed over the anastomosis.

14. Closure of the three fascia is readily accomplished, followed by closure of Scarpa's fascia and subcuticular skin.

15. A Foley catheter, which was placed at the beginning of the procedure, may be left in place for 24 to 48 hours postoperatively. The Penrose drain usually can be removed before discharge or, if left in place, it can easily be removed in the office 7 to 10 days postoperatively.

Posterior Lumbotomy

The patient is placed in a prone position with a roll under the chest, pelvis, and knees. After the skin incision, Scarpa's fascia is sharply incised and a vertical incision is made through the lumbodorsal fascia (posterior lamella). The lateral edge of the lumbodorsal fascia is elevated, and the sacrospinalis muscle is medially retracted. An incision is made through the middle and anterior lamella of the lumbodorsal fascia, taking care not to injure the iliohypogastric nerve. The quadratus lumborum muscle is retracted, exposing Gerota's fascia beneath the paranephric fat, and then this fascia is opened. The renal pelvis is identified, and several holding stitches are placed in the pelvis. The ureter is identified, a holding stitch is placed in the ureter, and the surgeon proceeds with the dismembered pyeloplasty.

Flank Approach

The patient is placed over the kidney rest in a flank position; the kidney rest is elevated and the operating room table is flexed. The skin incision is made off the tip of the 12th rib, or, if necessary, a supracostal 12th rib incision is made. The external oblique and latissimus dorsi muscles are divided. Next the internal oblique and serratus posterior inferior muscles are divided. The transversalis muscle is often thin and can be divided with digital dissection. The peritoneum is identified and retracted medially. Gerota's fascia is then encountered and opened longitudinally to gain exposure to the perinephric space. After identification of the renal pelvis and the ureter, a dismembered pyeloplasty can be performed as described earlier.

Minimally Invasive Techniques

Minimally invasive approaches in the repair of UPJ obstruction include endoscopic approaches and pyeloplasties performed laparoscopically (Schuessler et al, 1993; Chen et al, 1998; Tan, 1999).

Endoscopic Approaches

The endoscopic approach to the UPJ has been successful in both an anterograde and retrograde fashion. The initial attempts at balloon dilatation (Tan et al, 1995) have been superseded by the use of an Acucise device (Applied Medical, ureteral cutting balloon catheter, No. 5 Fr) (Bolton et al, 1994). Postoperative stenting is required for 6 weeks, with a 100% success rate being reported in a small series of patients. In a much larger series of adult patients, Kim and colleagues (1998) reported an overall success rate of 78%. Two patients required angiographic studies and embolization of lower pole branching arteries because they developed gross hematuria after Acucise endopyelotomy.

Antegrade endopyelotomy can readily be accomplished in both adults and preadolescent or adolescent patients. Figenshau and Clayman (1998) recommended this procedure for any patient with a reasonably functioning kidney, mild to moderate hydronephrosis, and no evidence of a crossing vessel. Computed tomography or MRI can be used for preoperative assessment of a crossing vessel, or endoluminal ultrasonography can be performed before the procedure. The antegrade endopyelotomy requires access to the kidney through a midpole posterior calix. Direct visualization of UPJ obstruction allows use of a cold knife, electrocautery, and even contact laser fiber to achieve the endopyelotomy (Renner et al, 1998). After fluoroscopic documentation of successful incision or dilation of the UPJ, or both, a double-pigtail ureteral stent is placed under direct vision in the renal collecting system and fluoroscopically positioned into the bladder.

The need for fluoroscopy for urologic intervention along with two and sometimes three anesthetics for preoperative stent placement (nephrostomy tube placement), endopyelotomy, and subsequent stent removal must be weighed against the more invasive open dismembered pyeloplasty. Older pediatric patients may be managed with the less invasive procedures, with the expectation of good results (80% to 85% success) and improved postoperative convalescence. In one of the largest pediatric experiences to date, endopyelotomy in children ranging in age from 4.5 to 17 years was successful 89% of the time (Tallaiet et al, 2004). The ideal situation exists in the case of a failed pyeloplasty because the UPJ should be in a dependent location (Fig. 115–18). A nephrostomy tube may already be in place and a stricture or stenosis is most likely to be encountered at the UPJ. After a successful endopyelotomy, a double-pigtail ureteral stent is maintained for 6 weeks. Unlike the adult endopyelotomy stent (No. 14 Fr/7 Fr), a pediatric endopyelotomy stent does not exist. The ideal stent would be a biodegradable stent that would not require removal (Lumiaho et al, 2000).

Laparoscopic Pyeloplasty

Laparoscopic pyeloplasty was introduced in adults in 1993 (Kavoussi and Peters, 1993; Schuessler et al, 1993). In the initial report of five cases, the operative time ranged from 3 to 7 hours. The procedure has gained in popularity, and more recent series have reported a success rate of over 95% (Ben Slama et al, 2000). Laparoscopic pyeloplasty in children has followed the same evolution as nephrectomy. The procedure was first described through a transperitoneal approach. Tan (1999) reported the first pediatric series of transperitoneal laparoscopic dismembered pyeloplasty in 18 children aged 3 months to 15 years. Mean operative time was 89 minutes. Two patients with persistent obstruction underwent repeated laparoscopic pyeloplasty.

Yeung and coworkers (2001) have reported their initial experience with retroperitoneal dismembered pyeloplasty in 13 patients, 1 of whom required open conversion. The mean operative duration was 143 (range 103 to 235) minutes. The longer time needed for the retroperitoneal approach is probably related to the limit of the working space that renders suturing more difficult.

In our experience with 52 retroperitoneal laparoscopic pyeloplasties in children (Fig. 115–19), aged between 22 months and 15 years, open conversion has been necessary in 4 cases because of technical difficulties during suturing (El-Ghoneimi et al, 2003; Bonnard et al, 2005). With a mean follow-up of 18 months (range 6 months to 5 years), one redo case was necessary for early persistent postoperative obstruction. The learning curve is significant, with mean operative time decreasing from 4 to 3 hours without a need for open conversion in our last 35 cases. More recently, the average time

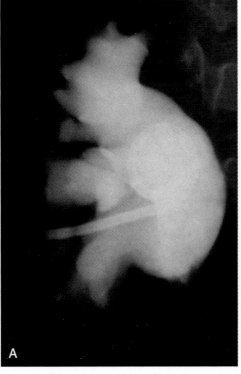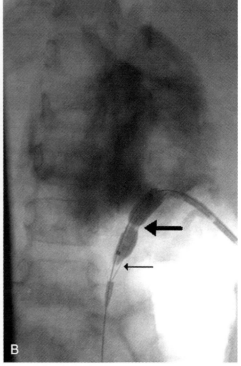

Figure 115–18. **A,** Right antegrade nephrostogram performed 2 months after dismembered pyeloplasty, demonstrating persistent obstruction at the ureteropelvic junction. A nephrostomy tube was placed 2 weeks after surgery, after the patient developed flank pain, fever, and *S. aureus* urinary tract infection. **B,** Acucise balloon being inflated across the ureteropelvic junction narrowing. Note waist present in balloon *(upper arrow)* and cutting wire positioned laterally *(lower arrow)*.

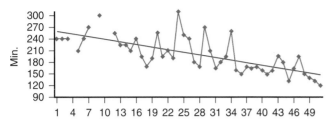

Figure 115–19. The learning curve of retroperitoneal laparoscopic pyeloplasty. The figure represents the global experience in retroperitoneal laparoscopic experience. Each point corresponds to one child; 52 cases are consecutive from 1999 to 2004. Cases that needed conversion to open surgery (four cases, 8%) are not presented with points on the operative time curve. The trend line of the learning curve is also shown.

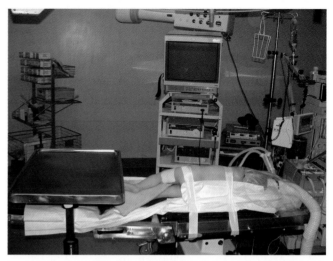

Figure 115–20. Positioning of patient for left retroperitoneal laparoscopic renal surgery. The patient is placed lateral, with sufficient flexion of the operating table to expose the area of trocar placement, between the last rib and the iliac crest; for younger children as shown, a lumbar support is sufficient for the exposure. The child is wrapped by two adhesive bands, one on the greater trochanter level and a second on the chest to keep the child on a perpendicular angle with the table. The surgeon, assistant, and scrub nurse are all on the back side of the child. The front side of the child is left free for the monitor.

to complete a case was less than 150 minutes. An aberrant crossing vessel was found in 24 cases, and dismembered pyeloplasty enabled ureteral transposition in all of them.

In our current practice, children younger than 2 years undergo a posterior lumbotomy to avoid the technical difficulties of suturing in young children through the retroperitoneal approach. It has been our observation that the open pyeloplasty through a posterior lumbotomy incision is well tolerated and the benefits of a laparoscopic procedure for the child would not be significant.

Robotically assisted surgery may be ideally suited for a pyeloplasty, allowing one to overcome the difficulties encountered with laparoscopic suturing. Peters has presented the first preliminary results of robotically assisted laparoscopic transperitoneal pyeloplasty in children (Peters et al, 2002; Peters, 2004a, 2004b). Olsen and Jorgensen (2003, 2004) have reported their unique experience of retroperitoneal robot-assisted pyeloplasty. They compared a group of 8 children operated by the robot-assisted procedures with a previous group of 15 children operated by the standard laparoscopic procedure. The median operative time with the robot was lower than with standard equipment (172 versus 210 minutes); the shortest operative time with the robot was 110 minutes. The first impression is that the robot-assisted technique makes suturing easier and may expand advanced laparoscopic reconstructive surgery to a larger number of surgeons without expertise in advanced laparoscopic surgery. Teaching laparoscopic pyeloplasty was not feasible when the surgeon did not have advanced experience in laparoscopy (Farhat et al, 2003).

Soulie and associates (2001) have compared retroperitoneal laparoscopic versus open pyeloplasty with a minimal incision in 53 consecutive nonrandomized adults. The mean operating time (165 versus 145 minutes) was similar in both groups. Incidence of complications, hospital stay, and functional results were equivalent for both groups, but the return to painless activity was more rapid with laparoscopy in younger patients. Bauer and coauthors (1999) did a similar study, with no difference in the postoperative outcome between laparoscopic and open pyeloplasty. We have compared retroperitoneal laparoscopic versus open pyeloplasty in 37 consecutive children (Bonnard et al, 2005). Mean operative time was 96 minutes (50 to 150) versus 219 minutes (140 to 310) for the open surgery and the laparoscopy groups, respectively (P < .0001). Mean hospital stay was 2.4 days (1 to 5) and 5 days (3

to 7) for the laparoscopy and the open surgery groups, respectively (P < .0001). The use of analgesics was less in the laparoscopic group, but further confirmation by a randomized prospective study is needed.

Midterm results confirm that dismembered retroperitoneal laparoscopic pyeloplasty is a safe and feasible approach in children. Although the technique is highly demanding, it has the advantage of duplicating principles of the gold standard open approach. Transperitoneal approach may be better adapted in young infants. Long operative time may be reduced with experience and with the new robot-assisted equipment.

Renal Access

Access to the kidney can be achieved by a retroperitoneal or transperitoneal approach.

Retroperitoneal Access

Lateral Approach

The patient is placed laterally, with sufficient flexion of the operating table to expose the area of trocar placement, between the last rib and the iliac crest (Fig. 115–20). In infants and younger children (under 6 years), our preference is to use lumbar padding to flex the patient laterally without flexing the operating table. Yeung and colleagues (2001) used different positioning based upon the kidney requiring surgery; semiprone for the right side and semilateral for the left side. Retroperitoneal access is achieved through the first incision, 15 to 20 mm in length, and one finger width from the lower border of the tip of the 12th rib (Fig. 115–21). The use of narrow retractors with long blades allows a deep dissection with short incision. Gerota's fascia is approached by a muscle splitting blunt dissection, opening under direct vision and

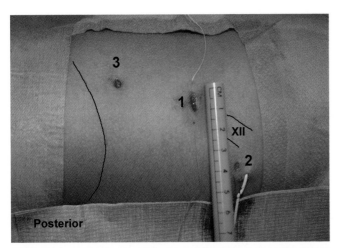

Figure 115–21. Ports placement and landmarks for left retroperitoneal laparoscopic pyeloplasty. Retroperitoneal access is achieved by the first incision (1), at the tip of the 12th rib, and is used for the laparoscope. Second port (2), placed in the costovertebral angle, is used for the needle holder, scissors, and to place the double J stent. Third port (3) is placed near the iliac crest at the anterior axillary line and is used for the grasping forceps. The first port is 3 or 5 mm in diameter and the other ports are 3 mm. In this case, a transanastomotic pyelostomy stent was used.

placing the first blunt trocar (3 or 5 mm) directly inside Gerota's fascia. A working space is created by gas insufflation dissection, and the first trocar is fixed with a purse-string suture that is applied around the deep fascia to ensure an airtight seal and yet allow traction on the main trocar if needed to increase the working space. This type of fixation is preferable to the single-use self-retaining trocars, which are larger and interfere with the mobility of instruments. A second trocar (3 mm) is inserted posteriorly in the costovertebral angle, in front of the lumbosacral muscle. A third trocar (3 mm) is inserted in the anterior axillary line, a finger width from the top of the iliac crest. To avoid transperitoneal insertion of this trocar, the working space is fully developed and the deep surface of the anterior wall muscles is identified before the trocar is inserted. Insufflation pressure does not exceed 12 mm Hg, and the CO_2 flow rate is progressively increased from 1 to 3 L/min. Access to the retroperitoneum and creation of the working space are the keys to success in retroperitoneal renal surgery. Age is not a limiting factor for this approach. Young children have less fat and the access is easier. This approach has been used for a nephrectomy in a neonate as young as 3 weeks of age (El-Ghoneimi, 2005).

Prone Posterior Approach

The access begins with an incision in the costovertebral angle at the edge of the paraspinous muscles. The secondary trocars are placed just above the iliac crest, one medially at the edge of the paraspinous muscles and one laterally at the posterior clavicular line (Peters, 2000).

Another Technique for Access to the Retroperitoneal Space

Since the description by Gaur (1992), balloon dissection has been the method applied by most urologists. Disadvantages of

balloon dissection are the cost of disposable materials and the possible complications with rupture of the balloon (Adams et al, 1996). On the other hand, balloon dissection creates a working space without opening Gerota's fascia, which is important for performing a radical nephrectomy.

Capolicchio and coauthors (2003) described a modification of lateral access by inserting the first trocar through the costovertebral angle. This modification helped the authors to avoid an accidental peritoneal tear during access through the first lateral incision and allowed a smaller incision for the laparoscope. Micali and colleagues (2001) reported the use of the Visiport visual trocar for direct access to the retroperitoneal space. The advantage of this method is the use of a small incision for the first trocar, which may benefit reconstructive surgery.

Transperitoneal Access

Several options exist for positioning the patient. The most frequently described is the flank position (Peters, 2000). The pneumoperitoneum is created through an open umbilical approach. The child is positioned with the surgeon standing in front of the abdomen (opposite side of pyeloplasty) (Fig. 115–22A). The most frequent configuration has been an umbilical port and two ipsilateral ports in the midclavicular line above and below the umbilicus. A fourth trocar may be placed in the midaxillary line to allow liver or spleen retraction, if needed. The kidney is exposed by medial mobilization of the colon. Ideally, the laparoscope is placed through the umbilicus, and the operating trocars are inserted midway between the umbilicus and the symphysis pubis and between the umbilicus and the xiphoid process (Fig. 115–22B). This configuration is available for both sides and has been used successfully in cases of horseshoe kidney.

Technique of Laparoscopic Retroperitoneal Pyeloplasty

A three-trocar technique is currently employed (El-Ghoneimi et al, 2003) (see Fig. 115–21). First, a 3- or 5-mm trocar for the laparoscope is placed (at the tip of the 12th rib), the second 3-mm trocar is inserted in the costovertebral angle (used for the needle driver on the left side pyeloplasty), and the third trocar is inserted at the top of the iliac crest (used for the needle driver on the right side pyeloplasty). The kidney is approached posteriorly and the renal pelvis is first identified. The pyeloureteral junction is identified and minimal dissection is done to free the junction from connective tissue. Small vessels are divided using bipolar electrocoagulation. Care is taken not to section ureteral blood vessels. A stay stitch is placed at the junction (Fig. 115–23). Aberrant crossing vessels are identified. The renal pelvis is partially divided using scissors at the most dependent part, and gentle traction on the stay suture helps to define this point. Keeping the traction, the ureter is partially divided and incised vertically for spatulation. The traction suture helps to mobilize the ureter so that the scissors can be in the axis of the ureter, usually introduced through the last trocar. The anterior surface of the kidney is left adherent to the peritoneum so that the kidney is retracted medially without the need for individual kidney retraction.

The ureteropelvic anastomosis begins using a 6-0 absorbable suture with a tapered 3/8 circle needle, placed from

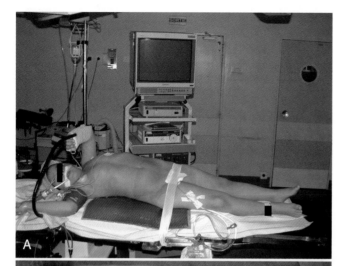

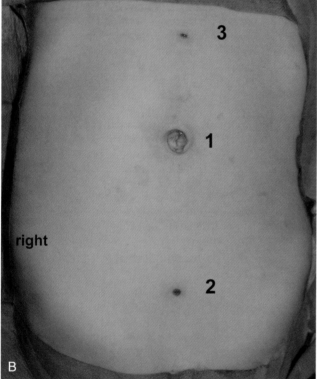

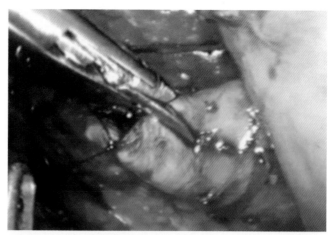

Figure 115–23. The traction suture, the "key point" for laparoscopic pyeloplasty by a retroperitoneal approach. A stay suture is placed at the pyeloureteral junction (PUJ) for traction and the renal pelvis partly divided by scissors at the most dependent part; gentle traction on the stay suture helps to define this point. The traction suture also helps to mobilize the ureter so that the scissors can be in the axis of the ureter. Note that the PUJ and the trimmed part of the pelvis remain undismembered for traction and stabilization of the suture line and are removed only after the last suture is placed.

Figure 115–22. Positioning of patient and trocars for left transperitoneal laparoscopic renal surgery. The child is positioned on semiflank position with the surgeon standing in front of the abdomen (opposite side of pyeloplasty) (**A**). First port (1) is inserted under vision through a midline transumbilical incision and is used for the laparoscope (**B**). Second port (2) is inserted midway between the umbilicus and the symphysis pubis and is used for the needle holder and scissors. Third port (3) is placed midway between the umbilicus and xiphoid and is used for the grasping forceps. The same configuration can be used for the opposite side after modification of the child's position.

the most dependent portion of the pelvis to the most inferior point or vertex of the ureteral spatulation. The suture is tied using the intracorporeal technique with the knots placed outside the lumen. The same stitch is used to run the anterior wall of the anastomosis. The UPJ is kept intact for traction and stabilization of the suture line and removed just before tying the last suture on the pelvis. This stay suture may be fixed

to the psoas muscle to give stability and to facilitate the suturing. A double-pigtail stent is inserted through the costovertebral angle trocar, and, if there is doubt, its position in the bladder is ensured under fluoroscopy. The posterior ureteropelvic anastomosis is then done. To avoid a second general anesthesia to remove the stent, a transanastomotic pyelostomy stent is used. The stent is closed on the first postoperative day and removed at 1 week in the outpatient clinic. A double-pigtail stent is used with an intrarenal pelvis because of the technical difficulties of inserting the pyelostomy stent. The pelvis is trimmed if needed. In case of aberrant crossing vessels (Fig. 115–24), the technique is slightly different. After placement of the stay suture, the ureter is completely divided and the UPJ and the pelvis are delivered anterior to the vessels with the help of the stay suture. Then the anastomosis is performed as described. If a double J stent is used, a Foley catheter is left in the bladder for 24 hours postoperatively.

Technique of Laparoscopic Transperitoneal Pyeloplasty

The surgical steps are identical to those in the retroperitoneal approach. A traction suture may be inserted through the anterior abdominal wall to stabilize the suture line.

In our experience, we have used the transperitoneal approach only in five cases of UPJ obstruction in a horseshoe kidney. The anterior position of the UPJ in this specific anatomic variant makes it easier by the anterior transperitoneal approach (Fig. 115–25).

Special Situations

Special situations include hydronephrosis secondary to low UPJ, retrocaval ureter, horseshoe kidney, ectopic kidney, ureterocaliceal anastomosis, and redo surgery.

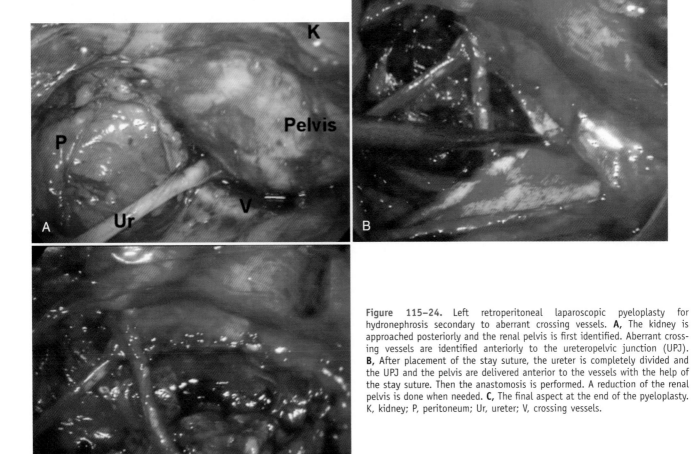

Figure 115-24. Left retroperitoneal laparoscopic pyeloplasty for hydronephrosis secondary to aberrant crossing vessels. **A,** The kidney is approached posteriorly and the renal pelvis is first identified. Aberrant crossing vessels are identified anteriorly to the ureteropelvic junction (UPJ). **B,** After placement of the stay suture, the ureter is completely divided and the UPJ and the pelvis are delivered anterior to the vessels with the help of the stay suture. Then the anastomosis is performed. A reduction of the renal pelvis is done when needed. **C,** The final aspect at the end of the pyeloplasty. K, kidney; P, peritoneum; Ur, ureter; V, crossing vessels.

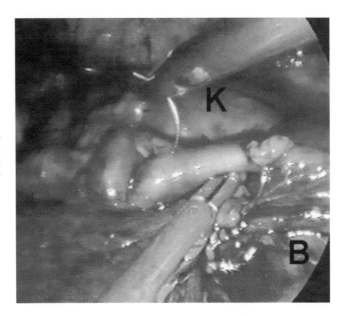

Figure 115-25.   Left transperitoneal laparoscopic pyeloplasty for horseshoe kidney. A stay suture is placed at the ureteropelvic junction (UPJ). Crossing vessels are anterior to the UPJ. In this case a double J stent was inserted preoperatively. B, bridge of parenchyma between the two parts of the horseshoe kidney; K, kidney.

The retroperitoneal lateral approach provides the advantage of dealing with most situations requiring a pyeloplasty. Thus far, the only indications for performing a transperitoneal approach are the horseshoe kidney and the ectopic kidney. Even the presence of a retrocaval ureter was easily diagnosed, allowing transposition of the ureter without difficulty. A case of severe hydronephrosis with significant calyceal dilation and minimal pelvic dilation lent itself to a ureterocalyceal anastomosis. This was readily accomplished with a lateral retroperitoneal approach as well.

Thus far, only two children have required redo surgery. The first was stenosis after retroperitoneal laparoscopic pyeloplasty. A transperitoneal approach was used, but open conversion was needed to dissect the UPJ. The second case was a child who had renal transplantation and extensive stenosis of the donor ureter. A transperitoneal approach allowed laparoscopic anastomosis between the native ureter and the renal pelvis of the graft.

OUTCOME

Adherence to sound surgical principles, minimal handling of the ureter at the time of repair, and judicious use of internal stenting or nephrostomy tube drainage ensure a successful outcome. Success is defined as improvement in hydronephrosis and stabilization or improvement in function on renal scan along with a decrease in washout time. In situations in which symptomatic presentation occurred, resolution of flank or abdominal pain or vomiting should also occur.

Imaging of the kidneys postoperatively depends on whether a nephrostomy tube has been used. A nephrostogram performed 10 to 14 days after surgery allows visualization of the anastomosis. Others have simply clamped the nephrostomy tube for 24 hours and checked the residual in the renal pelvis. If the residual is less than 15 mL, the nephrostomy tube is removed (Flint et al, 1998). If a double-pigtail ureteral stent is left indwelling, it is removed 2 to 6 weeks after the initial procedure. A renal ultrasound scan is obtained 6 weeks after pyeloplasty or after stent removal to ensure that the hydronephrosis (pelvocaliectasis) is improving. A renal scan may be obtained 1 year after the pyeloplasty to provide a relative assessment of the overall renal function. This is particularly helpful if the initial renal scan showed diminished renal function to the affected kidney. A new baseline is then established, which may be helpful for long-term outcome. On the other hand, if the renal function was not significantly affected at the time that surgery was performed, an overall decrease in the degree of pelvicaliectasis over time is a good indication that the obstruction has been relieved. Long-term imaging at 3 years may be obtained to look for the rare situation of delayed cicatrization and restenosis of the UPJ. Table 115–1 lists the results from a number of contemporary series of pyeloplasties.

Early complications of pyeloplasty are uncommon and usually involve prolonged urinary leakage from the Penrose drain. Depending on the amount of drainage, observation is generally the best approach. If it persists beyond 10 to 14 days, placement of a retrograde ureteral stent can often rectify the situation. Spontaneously delayed opening of the anastomosis has occurred as late as several months after the repair. If a patient presents postoperatively with fever, flank pain, and

Table 115–1. Results from Contemporary Series of Pyeloplasties		
Author and Year	*Patients/Kidneys*	*Success (%)*
Poulsen et al, 1987	35	100
O'Reilly, 1989	30	83-93
MacNeily et al, 1993	75	85
Shaul et al, 1994	32/33 (2 mo old)	97
	30/33 (>2 mo old)	93
Salem et al, 1995	100	98
McAleer and Kaplan, 1999	79	90
Austin et al, 2000	135/137	91
Houben et al, 2000	186/203	93
Casale et al, 2004*	19	94
Bonnard et al, 2005†	20	96

*Transperitoneal laparoscopic.
†Retroperitoneal laparoscopic.

significant hydronephrosis, a nephrostomy tube may be necessary to decompress the kidney. Lack of drainage for a prolonged period would necessitate further intervention, including an endopyelotomy, redo pyeloplasty, or even ureterocalicostomy (Fig. 115–26). The majority of times, repeated dismembered pyeloplasty was successful in correcting the problem. An anteriorly elongated flank incision facilitated exposure, a transperitoneal approach avoided some of the dense scarring that often occurs, and a nephrostomy tube was left postoperatively (Rohrmann et al, 1997). Ureterocalicostomy was performed when there was evidence of extensive proximal ureteral strictures, an intrarenal pelvis, or diminished pelvis that prevented the performance of a tension-free anastomosis. Experience with the laparoscopic redo pyeloplasty is thus far rare.

Careful preoperative planning is mandatory before embarking upon redo surgery. The location and the extent of the diseased segment are assessed with preoperative imaging including antegrade, retrograde, or intravenous urography and nuclear renography to assess renal function. In performing a ureterocalicostomy, key points include amputating the lower pole of the kidney, preserving all periureteral tissue and blood supply, creating a widely spatulated tension-free, mucosa-to-mucosa anastomosis, and adequate internal stenting. Perioperative fat can be placed around the anastomosis, but closing the lower pole capsule over the renal parenchyma should be avoided (Matlaga et al, 2005).

SUMMARY

Future surgical progress will be made in understanding the underlying factors that contribute to the formation of UPJ obstruction, along with continuing improvements in successful surgical approaches. There will continue to be debate about what constitutes surgical obstruction. Our tools that are used to define and measure the problem are imprecise. Newer modalities such as magnetic resonance urography may shed light on the problem and help surgeons in their decision-making process. In the end, though, it is an assimilation of radiographic studies, the patient's history, and the surgeon's experience that collectively guide the therapy.

Laparoscopic pyeloplasty is still a challenging procedure and its expansion is limited by the technical difficulties. More

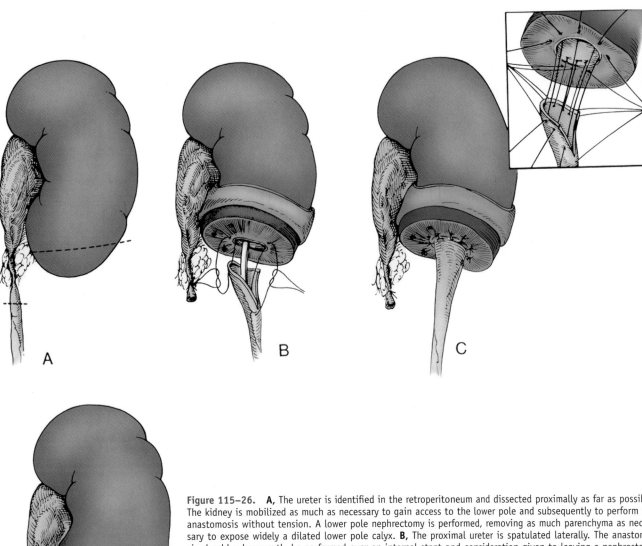

Figure 115–26. **A,** The ureter is identified in the retroperitoneum and dissected proximally as far as possible. The kidney is mobilized as much as necessary to gain access to the lower pole and subsequently to perform the anastomosis without tension. A lower pole nephrectomy is performed, removing as much parenchyma as necessary to expose widely a dilated lower pole calyx. **B,** The proximal ureter is spatulated laterally. The anastomosis should subsequently be performed over an internal stent and consideration given to leaving a nephrostomy tube. The initial suture is placed at the apex of the ureteral spatulation and the lateral wall of the calyx, with another suture placed 180 degrees from that. **C,** The anastomosis is completed in an open fashion, placing each suture circumferentially but not securing them down until the anastomosis has been completed. **D,** The renal capsule is closed over the cut surface of the parenchyma whenever possible. However, the capsule should not be closed close to the anastomosis itself as that may compromise the lumen by extrinsic compression. Instead, the anastomosis should be protected with a graft of perinephric fat or with a peritoneal or an omental flap.

KEY POINTS

- Ureteropelvic junction obstruction is typically due to either an intrinsic narrowing in which the ureteral segment has an interruption in the development of the circular musculature of the ureteropelvic junction, an alteration in collagen fibers in and around the muscular cells, or an extrinsic obstruction that is seen in association with aberrant, accessory, or an early branching lower pole vessel that passes anteriorly to the UPJ or proximal ureter and contributes to mechanical obstruction.

- Congenital renal malformations can be commonly seen in association with a ureteropelvic junction, with a contralateral UPJ obstruction being the most common anomaly followed by renal dysplasia and multicystic dysplastic kidneys.

- Nuclear renography is considered the radiographic study that best defines the presence of a ureteropelvic junction obstruction. Differential renal function is quantitated along with the kidney's response to diuretic challenge. A number of variables have been shown to affect the washout curve following Lasix administration, which must be accounted for in the interpretation of the study.

- Pressure-flow studies that require a nephrostomy tube or percutaneous access to the renal pelvis may be used in situations in which other radiographic modalities are ambiguous. These studies underscore the importance of the compliance of the renal pelvis and its effect upon ultimate renal function.

- The surgical approach favored in the repair of a ureteropelvic junction obstruction is the dismembered pyeloplasty, which has been shown to be effective because of its broad applicability, means of allowing excision of the pathologic segment in question, and facilitation of a reduction pyeloplasty when necessary.

- Laparoscopic pyeloplasties provide excellent visualization of the anatomy, enhance cosmesis, and duplicate the results of open pyeloplasties with short-term follow-up. The technical challenges of this approach have been facilitated by the use of a robot-assisted procedure that improves the anastomotic repair.

- Complications from a pyeloplasty include prolonged urinary drainage postoperatively, lack of improvement in renal function or improvement in washout, and occasionally worsening hydronephrosis and diminished renal function postoperatively. Such a situation may lend itself to a repair using ureterocalicostomy or a redo dismembered pyeloplasty.

than 5 years of experience with the technique was needed to standardize the procedure and to achieve a "reasonable" operative time. The limitation of the number of centers routinely performing this technique is an indication that more efforts are needed to facilitate the suturing technique. The retroperitoneal approach procedure is safe; it gives functional results as good as those of open surgery but with better cosmetic appearance and a more comfortable postoperative course. The emerging generation of young surgeons already experienced in advanced laparoscopic surgery should optimize the expansion of the technique in the near future.

SUGGESTED READINGS

Bonnard A, Fouquet V, Carricaburu E, et al: Retroperitoneal laparoscopic versus open pyeloplasty in children. J Urol 2005;173:1710-1713.

Eskild-Jensen A, Gordon I, Piepsz A, et al: Interpretation of the renogram: Problems and pitfalls in hydronephrosis in children. BJU Int 2004;94:887-892.

Grattan-Smith JD, Perez-Brayfield MR, Jones RA, et al: MR imaging of kidneys: Functional evaluation using F-15 perfusion imaging. Pediatr Radiol 2003;33:293-304.

Koff SA: Pathophysiology of ureteropelvic junction obstructions. Urol Clin North Am 1990;17:263-272.

Peters C: Laparoscopic and robotic approach to genitourinary anomalies in children. Urol Clin North Am 2004;31:595-605.

Rohrmann D, Snyder HM III, Duckett JW Jr, et al: The operative management of recurrent ureteropelvic junction obstruction. J Urol 1997;158:1257-1259.

Salem YH, Majd M, Rushton HG, Belman AB: Outcome analysis of pediatric pyeloplasty as a function of patient age, presentation and differential renal function. J Urol 1995;154:1889-1893.

116 Ectopic Ureter, Ureterocele, and Other Anomalies of the Ureter

RICHARD N. SCHLUSSEL, MD • ALAN B. RETIK, MD

TERMINOLOGY

EMBRYOLOGY

ANOMALIES OF TERMINATION

ANOMALIES OF STRUCTURE

ANOMALIES OF NUMBER

ANOMALIES OF POSITION

TERMINOLOGY

Ureteral anomalies are some of the most significant anomalies in all of pediatric urology because they directly affect overall renal function. These congenital problems may manifest acutely or insidiously. Similarly, if they are incorrectly treated, the adverse outcome may not be appreciated for years. Appropriate management is predicated on knowledge of the relevant embryology, anatomy, and physiology, as well as of all the variants thereof. Finally, the urologist entrusted with the care of these children must be familiar with the many reconstructive techniques available so that an optimal outcome can be achieved.

The study of ureteral anomalies has yielded a rich array of terms and descriptions. Many of these terms and categories were put forth by some of the founders of pediatric urology. Because all of medicine is based on effective communication, this chapter summarizes classifications used in the past, defines current common usages, and proposes a standard rational nomenclature that, it is hoped, will allow accurate communication.

Because ureteral anomalies are at times associated with duplications of the kidney, it is prudent to review renal terminology. A *duplex kidney* is one that has two separate pelvicalyceal systems. A duplex kidney has an upper pole and a lower pole. The ureters may join at any point. If they join at the level of the ureteropelvic junction, the configuration is termed a *bifid system*. If the ureters join more distally but are still proximal to the bladder level, the configuration is termed *bifid ureters* (Fig. 116–1A). Double ureters are ureters that drain their respective poles and empty separately into the genitourinary tract. This represents a complete duplication (see Fig. 116–1B). A ureter that drains the upper or lower pole should be referred to respectively as the "upper pole ureter" and the "lower pole ureter."

The word *ectopia* is derived from the Greek ex ("out") and topos ("place"); any ureter whose orifice terminates anywhere other than the normal trigonal position is considered ectopic. Lateral ectopia implies an orifice more cranial and lateral than normal. Caudal ectopia implies that the orifice is more medial and distal than the normal position. Such an orifice may theoretically be found between the normal orifice position and the bladder neck. However, in general practice, **the term ectopic ureter is meant to imply a ureter whose orifice terminates even more caudally, such as in the urethra or outside the urinary tract.**

Ericsson (1954) characterized ureteroceles as either simple or ectopic. A "simple ureterocele" was defined as one that lies completely within the bladder, whereas those that extended to the bladder neck or distally to the urethra were considered to be "ectopic." Stephens (1958, 1964, 1971, 1983) described ureteroceles as either stenotic, sphincteric, or sphincterostenotic or as a cecoureterocele. A stenotic ureterocele is one whose narrowed or pinpoint opening is found inside the bladder (Fig. 116–2). **If a ureterocele has an orifice distal to the bladder neck, it is termed *sphincteric* (Fig. 116–3). If a ureterocele has an orifice that was both stenotic and distal to the bladder neck, it is considered a sphincterostenotic ureterocele (Fig. 116–4A). A cecoureterocele has an intravesical orifice and a submucosal extension that dips into the urethra.** This type of ureterocele can distend with urine and obstruct the urethra (see Fig. 116–4B).

Several terms for ureteroceles in common use are confusing. They are listed here not to encourage their use but to clarify their intended meaning. A "simple ureterocele" is frequently used to mean a single-system ureterocele. The "adult ureterocele" has the same implication. An "orthotopic ureterocele" is a ureterocele contained within the bladder. Often, the phrase "ectopic ureterocele" is used to explain a ureterocele associated with a duplicated system.

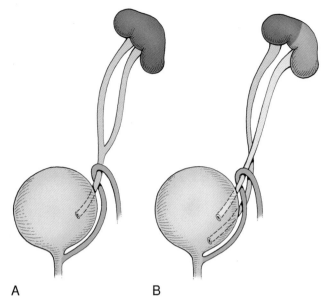

Figure 116–1. **A,** A bifid ureter is depicted; the upper pole and lower pole ureters join proximal to the bladder. **B,** Double ureters are seen when the upper pole ureter and lower pole ureter empty separately into the bladder.

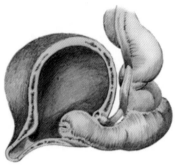

Figure 116–2. The orifice of a stenotic ectopic ureterocele may be located at the tip or at the superior or inferior surface of the ureterocele.

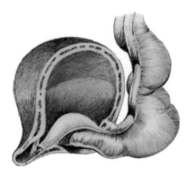

Figure 116–3. Sphincteric ectopic ureteroceles.

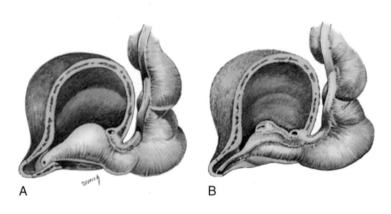

Figure 116–4. A, Sphincterostenotic ectopic ureterocele. **B,** Cecoureterocele lumen extends distal to the orifice as a long tongue beneath the ureteral submucosa. The orifice communicates with the lumen of the bladder and is large and incompetent.

Obviously, these terms are not completely clear because they are nondescriptive and sometimes inaccurate. In an effort to eliminate this ambiguity and confusion, the Committee on Terminology, Nomenclature and Classification of the Section of Urology of the American Academy of Pediatrics proposed standardized terms that are both descriptive and accurate (Glassberg et al, 1984). According to this classification, **a ureterocele is *intravesical* if the ureterocele is contained in the bladder in its entirety, and it is ectopic if any portion of the ureterocele extends to the bladder neck or the urethra** (Fig. 116–5). Ureteroceles are classified further according to the number of systems (single or duplex) and the type of orifice involved (e.g., stenotic, sphincteric, sphincterostenotic or as a cecoureterocele). Therefore, by way of example, the ureterocele seen in Figure 116–6 would be categorized as an intravesical ureterocele of a left single system with a stenotic orifice, and the ureterocele shown in Figure 116–4A would be categorized as an ectopic ureterocele of a duplicated left

system. Such classifications lead to little doubt, and their use should be encouraged.

EMBRYOLOGY

An understanding of normal renal development is critical to an appreciation of how ureteral anomalies evolve and whether they are clinically significant. At 4 weeks' gestation, an outpouching arises from the distal mesonephric duct. This outpouching is the ureteric bud, and it interacts with a mass of mesenchyme that is the metanephric blastema. This interaction results in the ureteric bud's branching and developing into the calyces, renal pelvis, and ureter. The metanephric blastema is induced to form all elements of the nephron, including the collecting duct, distal convoluted tube, loop of Henle, proximal convoluted tubule, and glomerulus. **The segment of mesonephric duct distal to the ureteric bud is the common excretory duct** (Fig. 116–7). The point of origin of

Figure 116-5. A, An intravesical ureterocele located entirely within the bladder. **B,** The distal portion of an ectopic ureterocele extends outside the bladder and into the urethra.

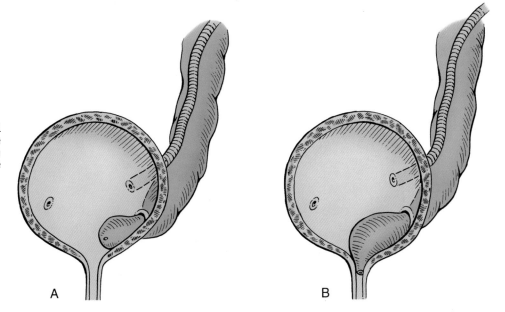

A

B

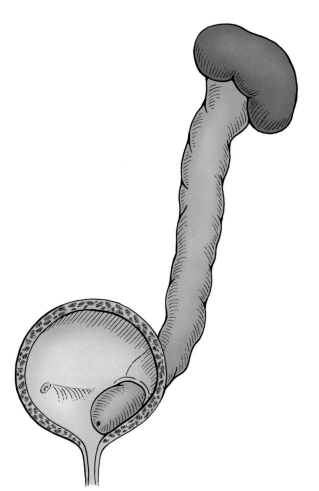

Figure 116-6. A single-system intravesical ureterocele.

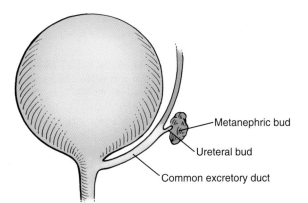

—Metanephric bud

—Ureteral bud

—Common excretory duct

Figure 116-7. The structures of the urinary tract originate from the primitive metanephric blastema and the ureteral bud, which arises from the mesonephric duct. The common excretory duct is the portion of the mesonephric duct that is distal to the ureteral bud.

the ureteric bud is the ureteral orifice. When the ureteral orifice enters the bladder it begins to migrate in the bladder in a cranial and lateral direction (Moore, 1988).

If the ureteric bud arises off the mesonephric duct more distally than normally, the ureteral orifice enters the bladder earlier than usual and hence has a greater period for cranial and lateral migration (Mackie and Stephens, 1975; Tanagho, 1976; Schwartz et al, 1981). This results in lateral ectopia. **If the ureteric bud arises more proximally on the mesonephric duct than normally, the ureteral orifice has less time in the bladder to undergo its normal migration and results in a ureteral orifice more medial and caudal than is usual** (Fig. 116-8). An even further proximal ureteric bud position on the mesonephric duct may result in the ureteral orifice's remaining on the mesonephric duct, with the end result being that

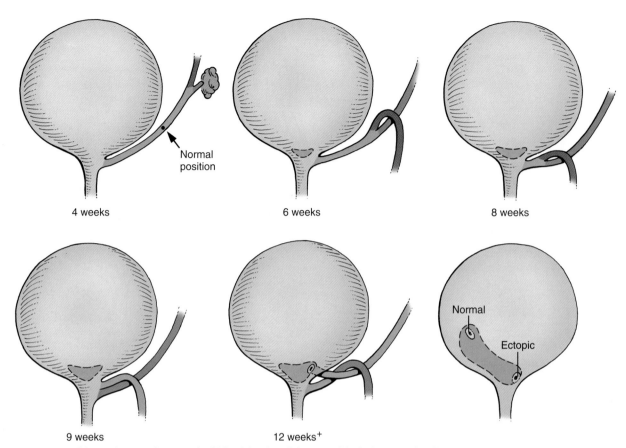

4 weeks   6 weeks   8 weeks

9 weeks   12 weeks+

Figure 116–8. Caudal ectopia occurs because of a high origination of the ureteral bud. The ureteral orifice has less time to be absorbed into the bladder and has a caudal, medial trigone location or is extravesically located along the path of the mesonephric duct remnants.

the orifice terminates outside the bladder altogether. In the male, the embryologic equivalents of the mesonephric duct are the epididymis, vas deferens, seminal vesicles, and prostate. In the female, the mesonephric duct proximal to the ureteric bud becomes the epoöphoron, oophoron, and Gartner's duct. An ectopic ureter draining into any of these female structures can rupture into the adjoining fallopian tube, uterus, upper vagina, or vestibule.

The conventional model of ureteral bud integration into the bladder and formation of the trigone indicates a mesonephric duct origin, yet recent evidence has suggested this may not be correct. Trigonal tissues appear to originate in the urogenital sinus. The implications of these observations on the etiology of ectopic ureters and ureteroceles remain to be determined (Batourino et al, 2005).

The interaction of the ureteric bud with the metanephric blastema is critical to the correct ontogeny of the ureter and collecting system and the future kidney. Examination of the developing kidney reveals close cell-to-cell interactions between the ureteric bud and the metanephric blastema (Saxen, 1987). Experimental models have shown that if these interactions are altered or disrupted, the blastema fails to differentiate into normal nephrons (Grobstein, 1956; Kirrilova et al, 1982; Sariola et al, 1988).

In clinical practice, it appears that renal units drained by ureters that terminate in positions other than the trigone do, in fact, have problems with proper development. Recalling the embryology of the trigone and ureteral orifice, it is likely that an abnormal ureteral orifice position reflects an abnormal

point of origin of the ureteric bud from the mesonephric duct. This ureteric bud would be poorly positioned for the necessary interactions with the metanephric blastema. Therefore, these clinical and experimental observations combine to support the commonly held notion that dysplasia is the product of inadequate ureteric bud-to-blastema interaction (Mackie and Stephens, 1975).

After its emergence from the mesonephric duct, the ureteric bud can become a split or bifid structure. The splitting creates two separate collecting systems that join eventually in a common ureter (Fig. 116–9). As mentioned previously, this anatomic arrangement is termed a *duplex kidney with a bifid ureter*. The ureter distal to the bifurcation has arisen from a normal position on the mesonephric duct, and therefore its single ureteral orifice is in the normal trigonal location.

If two separate ureteric buds originate from the mesonephric duct, two complete and separate interactions will develop between the ureter and the metanephric blastema. The result is two separate renal units and collecting systems, ureters, and ureteral orifices. Using our earlier terminology, this complete duplication is synonymous with a duplex system drained by double ureters (Fig. 116–10). The final position of the ureteral orifices has important clinical implications. Both Weigert (1877) and Meyer (1946) noted that there is a constant trigonal relationship between the upper and lower pole orifices. When performing a cystoscopic examination, it is important to remember this counterintuitive concept: the so-called lower or distally placed orifice is in fact the orifice of the upper pole, and the so-called higher or

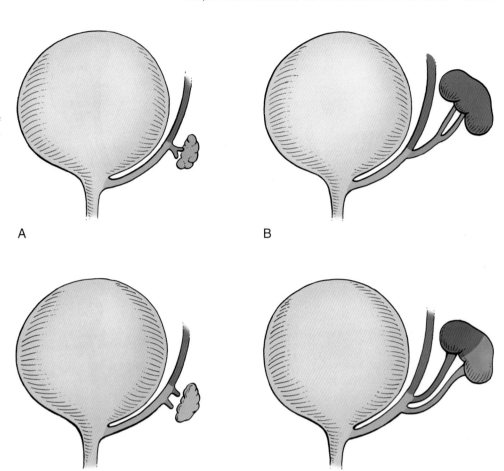

Figure 116–9. **A** and **B,** Branching of the ureteral bud after it arises from the mesonephric duct creates a bifid ureter.

Figure 116–10. When two separate ureteral buds come off the mesonephric duct, they develop into an upper pole and its ureter and a lower pole and its ureter, each having distinct ureteral orifices in the bladder.

A   B

A   B

cranial orifice is the lower pole orifice. The lower pole orifice is more cranial and lateral to the caudad, medial upper pole orifice. To achieve these positions, the two ureters and orifices rotate 180 degrees clockwise on their longitudinal axes (Fig. 116–11). The Weigert-Meyer rule of complete duplicated systems yields a fairly constant anatomy that is important for radiologic, cystoscopic, and reconstructive considerations.

All congenital anomalies of the ureter can be considered as falling into one of the categories in which we have organized this chapter: anomalies of termination, anomalies of structure, anomalies of number, and anomalies of position.

ANOMALIES OF TERMINATION
Ectopic Ureters

As mentioned previously, in the strictest sense, a ureter whose orifice is laterally and cranially located in the bladder could be considered ectopic. However, the term "ectopic ureter" has universally been used to describe a ureter that terminates at the bladder neck or distally into one of the aforementioned mesonephric duct structures. We employ this general terminology in the following discussion.

The true incidence of an ectopic ureter is uncertain, because many cause no symptoms. Campbell (1970) noted 10 examples in 19,046 autopsies in children (an incidence of 1 in 1900) but thought that some had been overlooked. **Of all ectopic orifices, 80% are associated with a duplicated col-** lecting system. **In females, more than 80% are duplicated, but in males, most ectopic ureters drain single systems** (Schulman, 1976; Ahmed and Barker, 1992). This is particularly true when ectopic ureteroceles are excluded from consideration.

Ectopic ureters appear more commonly in females clinically, from 2 to 12 times more frequently, with the lesser frequency probably reflecting the incidence more accurately (Eisendrath, 1938; Mills, 1939; Burford et al, 1949; Lowsley and Kerwin, 1956). Ellerker (1958) noted 366 females and 128 males in his review of 494 ectopic ureters, including autopsies, for a female-to-male ratio of 2.9:1. Between 5% and 17% of ectopic ureters appear bilaterally (Eisendrath, 1938; Ellerker, 1958; Malek et al, 1972; Mandell et al, 1981; Ahmed and Barker, 1992). A small percentage involve a solitary kidney. With unilateral ectopic ureter, a contralateral ureteral duplication is not uncommon. Various other abnormalities, including imperforate anus and tracheoesophageal fistula, may be found in association with the ectopic ureter (Ahmed and Barker, 1992). **The internal genitalia may be disordered, with duplicated vaginas, hemivaginas, and bicornuate uteruses described** (Krishnan et al, 2003; Acien et al, 2004; Sameshima et al, 2005).

The distribution of ectopic ureters is itemized by location in Table 116–1. **In the male, the posterior urethra is the most common site of termination of an ectopic ureter. Drainage into the genital tract involves the seminal vesicle three times more often than the ejaculatory duct and vas deferens com-**

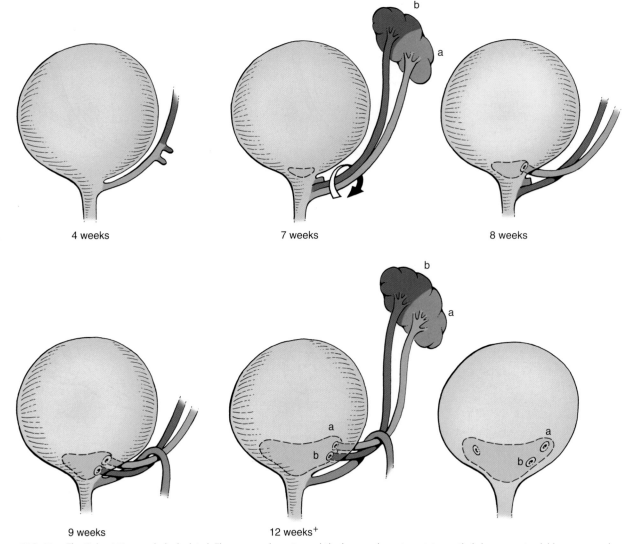

Figure 116–11. The Weigert-Meyer rule is depicted. The upper pole ureter and the lower pole ureter rotate on their long axes to yield an upper pole orifice (b) that is medial and caudal to the lower pole orifice (a).

Table 116–1. **Location of 494 Ectopic Ureters (Including Autopsies)**

Type	No.	%
128 Male Subjects		
Posterior urethra	60	47
Prostatic utricle	13	10
Seminal vesicle	42	33
Ejaculatory duct	7	5
Vas deferens	6	5
366 Female Subjects		
Urethra	129	35
Vestibule	124	34
Vagina	90	25
Cervix or uterus	18	5
Gartner's duct	3	<1
Urethral diverticulum	2	<1

From Ellerker AG: The extravesical ectopic ureter. Br J Surg 1958;45:344.

bined (Riba et al, 1946; Ellerker, 1958; Lucius, 1963; Sullivan et al, 1978; Squadrito et al, 1987). **In the female, the urethra and vestibule are the most common sites.** The age at diagnosis ranges widely, with many examples not detected during life (Ellerker, 1958).

The earlier reports failed to provide adequate descriptions of the upper tracts, but later reports emphasized that **the more remote the ureteral opening, the greater the degree of renal maldevelopment** (Schulman, 1976). With duplicated systems, this means hypoplasia or dysplasia of the upper pole segment. Of 10 cases involving an ectopic ureter that drained a single system and opened into the male seminal tracts, the kidney was not visualized radiographically in any (Rognon et al, 1973). Of 16 single renal ducts drained by an ectopic ureter, renal dysplasia was present in 7 (Prewitt and Lebowitz, 1976). The kidney drained by an ectopic ureter may be in an abnormal position as well (Utsunomiya et al, 1984; Borer et al, 1993, 1998; Bozorgi et al, 1998; Moores et al, 1997). This kidney is often quite small and difficult to localize on imaging studies.

Ectopic ureters draining single systems appear to be seen more frequently in Japan (Gotoh et al, 1983; Suzuki et al, 1993; Moores et al, 1997; Wakhlu et al, 1998). In Borer's report of single-system ectopic ureters, each child was initially believed to have a solitary hypertrophied kidney and all had received erroneous diagnoses and undergone multiple diagnostic investigations (average 10) before the correct diagnosis was made. In seven of their eight patients, the single-system ectopic ureter terminated in the vagina.

The ectopic ureter itself is also abnormal, usually to a greater degree in the single system than in the duplicated system. Usually, the ureter is variably dilated and drainage is impaired (Williams and Royle, 1969). Muscle cells may show severe alterations on ultrastructure studies. Whether these changes are developmental or acquired is not yet known (Hanna et al, 1977).

Clinical presentation of an ectopic ureter usually differs in males and females, reflecting the differing termination of the ectopic ureters in the two genders. Recalling the embryology of ureteral ectopia, when the ureteric bud arises more proximally on the mesonephric duct than it normally should, the ureteral orifice remains on the mesonephric duct caudally and is not absorbed in the bladder. **In the female, these parts of the mesonephric duct become the epoöphoron, oophoron, and Gartner's duct. If an ectopic ureter drains into any of these respective female structures, they can rupture or be incorporated into any of the nearby müllerian duct structures, such as the vagina, uterus, cervix, or fallopian tubes** (Fig. 116–12). Therefore, in the female patient, an ectopic ureteral orifice may be within (e.g., bladder neck, proximal urethra) or outside the realm of the urinary sphincter, making ectopic ureters one of the more important causes of urinary incontinence in girls (Freedman and Rickwood, 1994). **Continuous incontinence in a girl with an otherwise normal voiding pattern after toilet training is the classic symptom of an ectopic ureteral orifice.**

On occasion, incontinence becomes apparent at a later age and may be confused with stress incontinence, incontinence associated with neurogenic bladder dysfunction, or psychogenic incontinence. A persistent vaginal discharge from an ectopic orifice located in the vagina is another clinical sign (Acien et al, 1990; See and Mayo, 1991; Gharagozloo and Lebowitz, 1995). Most ectopic ureters are associated with acute or recurrent urinary tract infection. A patient may also present with abdominal pain, failure to thrive, and chronic infection (Fig. 116–13). Patients with ectopic ureters draining into the proximal urethra often experience reflux, and urge incontinence is common. An ectopic ureter may be severely obstructed, causing massive hydronephrosis and hydroureter, and it may manifest as an abdominal mass (Uson et al, 1972) or be detected on prenatal ultrasonographic evaluation.

In males, the mesonephric duct structures eventually form the epididymis, vas deferens, and seminal vesicles. Therefore, an ectopic ureter in the male patient can drain into the bladder neck, the prostatic urethra, or the previously mentioned wolffian duct structures (see Fig. 116–12). All of these locations are proximal to the external sphincter. Therefore, males with ectopic ureters do not suffer from urinary incontinence as females do.

Because their ectopic ureters drain most commonly into the prostatic urethra and bladder neck, males most often

Female

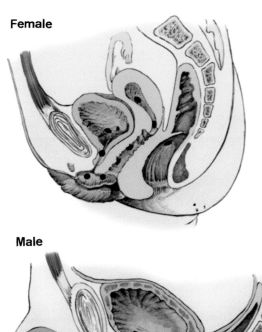

Male

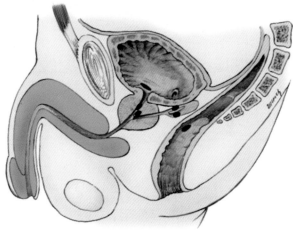

Figure 116–12. Sites of ectopic ureteral orifices in the male and female.

present with urinary tract infection. They may also experience urgency and frequency. In some instances, the ureter ends in the wolffian duct remnants (seminal vesicles, vas deferens, or epididymis), predisposing the individual to epididymitis (Williams and Sago, 1983; Umeyama et al, 1985). Therefore, epididymitis in a prepubertal boy should prompt the physician to consider the presence of an ectopic ureter. In males, the symptoms may not be as obvious as incontinence in females; males may complain of constipation, abdominal pain, pelvic pain, or discomfort during ejaculation, and they may even be infertile (Squadrito et al, 1987). A stone may form in the ectopic ureter. It is most important to remember that boys will be continent because the ectopic ureter always drains proximal to the external sphincter. Urgency and frequency in a male patient, caused by the ectopic ureter's draining into the prostatic fossa, should not be mistaken for incontinence.

Diagnosis

Prenatal sonographic diagnosis of ectopic ureters has become common. The condition is identifiable by virtue of the hydronephrosis produced by the obstruction. If this is isolated to the upper pole of a duplex system and the bladder is normal, the diagnosis is relatively straightforward. In other situations, prenatal findings serve to initiate a postnatal evaluation that will specifically identify the condition.

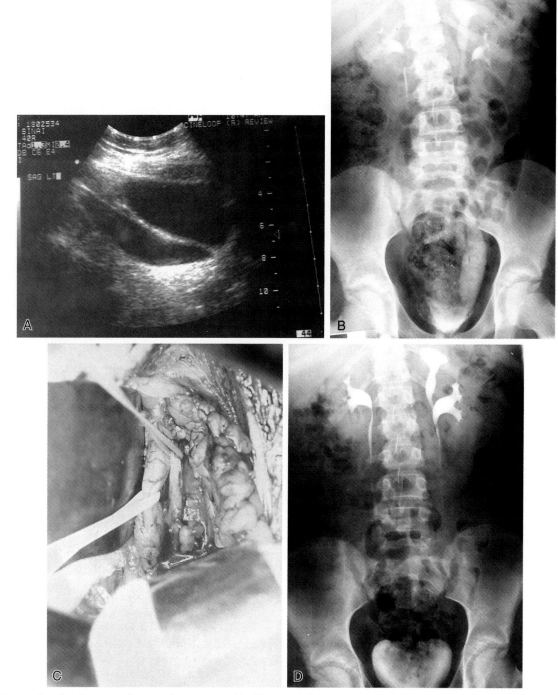

Figure 116–13. Ectopic left upper pole ureter in a teenage girl with chronic abdominal pain. **A,** Sonogram of dilated ureter entering bladder neck. **B,** Intravenous pyelogram demonstrating severe upper pole hydroureteronephrosis with dilated ureter entering the bladder neck. **C,** Intraoperative photograph of dilated medial upper pole ureter and normal-caliber lateral lower pole ureter. **D,** Intravenous pyelogram after upper pole to lower pole ureteroureterostomy. The patient was free of symptoms immediately after the procedure.

In a girl, sometimes the diagnosis of an ectopic ureter can be made by physical examination. Direct visualization of the vulva may reveal continuous urinary dribbling or wetness. In the absence of neurogenic vesical dysfunction or a urethral sphincter defect, an ectopic ureter is likely. Often, a punctum or orifice is apparent in the urethrovaginal septum (Fig. 116–14). Perineal and genital skin erythema or maceration may reflect the irritating effect of the urine that continually bathes this area.

The ultrasonographic findings of an ectopic ureter include the dilated pelvis and collecting system of the upper pole and a dilated ureter behind an otherwise normal bladder (Fig. 116–15). A large ectopic ureter may press against the bladder and create an indentation that appears much like

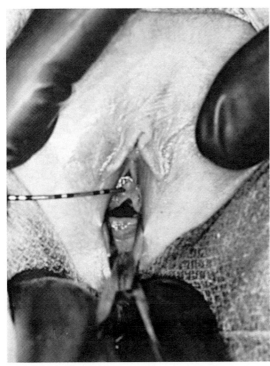

Figure 116–14. Photograph at the time of cystoscopy of an ectopic ureteral orifice in the urethrovaginal septum. A ureteral catheter is in the orifice.

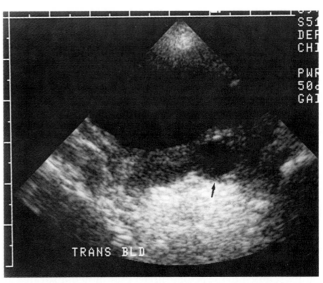

Figure 116–15. Distal ureteral dilatation is seen sonographically as a round, hypoechoic area behind the bladder *(arrow)*.

a ureterocele and is termed a *pseudoureterocele* (Diard et al, 1987; Sumfest et al, 1995). The difference is that an ectopic ureter is clearly extravesical, with a thick septum of bladder muscle between the ureteral lumen and bladder lumen. In contrast, in a ureterocele the septum is thin and delicate and the ureteral lumen is partially intravesical. Sumfest and associates (1995) noted that their patients had ectopic ureteral drainage into mesonephric duct cysts; these mesonephric duct cysts can rupture into the vagina or bladder. The renal parenchyma associated with a ectopic ureter is often thinner than that of a normally draining lower pole (Nussbaum et al, 1986).

The diagnosis of an ectopic ureter can be confirmed by excretory urography (Fig. 116–16). The usual radiographic feature is a nonvisualizing or poorly visualizing upper pole of a duplex system that may be massively hydronephrotic. **The upper pole displaces the lower pole downward and outward, creating the so-called drooping lily appearance.** When the upper pole does not excrete contrast medium and make the duplicated system readily apparent, there are several other clues to suggest that a duplicated system is present. First, the calyces of a lower pole are fewer than in the normal kidney. Second, the axis of the lowest to uppermost calyx does not point toward the midline. Third, the uppermost calyx of the lower pole unit is usually farther from the upper pole border than is the lowest calyx from the corresponding lower pole limit. In addition, the lower pole pelvis and the upper portion of its ureter may be farther from the spine than on the contralateral side, and the lower pole ureter may also be scalloped and tortuous secondary to its wrapping around a markedly dilated upper pole ureter (similar to the findings of upper pole

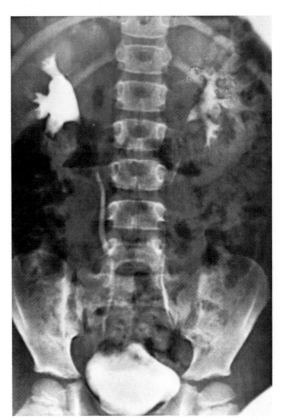

Figure 116–16. Excretory urogram in a 5-year-old girl with urinary incontinence shows a nonvisualizing upper pole on the right side that is displacing the lower pole downward and outward. Also, note that the right renal pelvis and upper ureter are farther from the spine than are the structures on the left.

hydroureteronephrosis in the child with a ureterocele in Figure 116–30). When an ectopic ureter drains a nonvisualizing, diminutive, dysplastic renal unit, these typical radiologic features may not be demonstrated. Care must be taken to identify exactly which kidney is responsible for the ectopic ureter and the incontinence, because there may be bilateral duplicated systems. Failure to make the correct identification may result in removing the wrong upper pole and the patient's experiencing the same symptoms postoperatively! Particular attention should be paid to the contralateral kidney on excretory urography to avoid missing bilateral ureteral ectopia. This is reported to occur in 5% to 17% of cases but was noted in 25% of cases in one series (Campbell, 1951).

The functional status of the upper pole renal segment of duplex systems may be evident on excretory urography, but more precise assessment may become important if upper pole salvage is considered. Isotopic renal scanning using technetium 99m-labeled dimercaptosuccinic acid (^{99m}Tc-DMSA) has proved to be the most adequate, although differentiating between the function of the upper and lower poles may be difficult.

Voiding cystourethrography demonstrates reflux into the lower pole ureter in at least half of the cases. More importantly, reflux into the ectopic ureter may be demonstrated at different phases of voiding, providing evidence of the location of the orifice (Fig. 116–17). If the reflux into the ectopic ureter is seen before voiding, the orifice is proximal to the bladder neck; reflux only with voiding suggests an orifice in the urethra. The latter finding may be evident only with several cycles of voiding monitored fluoroscopically (Wyly and Lebowitz, 1984). Sphincteric orifices may not produce reflux at all.

Occasionally, the renal parenchyma is difficult to locate and may be identified only by alternative imaging studies (Giles

et al, 1982; Gharagozloo and Lebowitz, 1995). In such cases, in which an ectopic ureter is strongly suspected because of incontinence yet no definite evidence of the upper pole renal segment is found (Simms and Higgins, 1975), computed tomography (CT) or magnetic resonance imaging (MRI) has demonstrated the small, poorly functioning upper pole segment (Braverman and Lebowitz, 1991) (Fig. 116–18).

MRI offers several advantages in regard to localizing otherwise hard to find small, dysplastic upper poles and their ureters terminating in ectopic positions. MRI does not require intravenous contrast media and does not use ionizing radiation. Most importantly, the T2-weighted images are particularly suited for finding and defining fluid-filled structures such as the ectopic ureter. The MRI in the sagit-

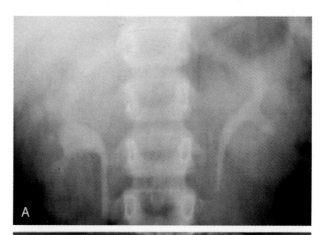

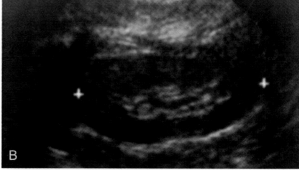

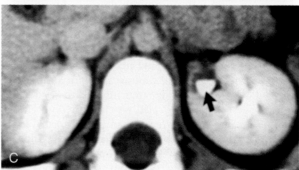

Figure 116–18. **A,** Excretory urogram in 10-year-old girl with constant wetting. No definite evidence for an upper pole segment is present. **B,** Left renal ultrasound in the same patient, also without a clear indication of the presence of an upper pole segment. **C,** Contrast medium–enhanced CT scan in the same girl specifically demonstrates the small upper pole segment *(arrow)* associated with the ectopic ureter. Upper pole nephrectomy cured the wetting.

Figure 116–17. A cystogram demonstrates reflux into an ectopic ureter that enters the urethra immediately distal to the bladder neck.

tal plane can even demonstrate the exact point of termination of the ectopic ureter (Gylys-Morin et al, 2000; Krishnan and Baskin, 2005). **The MRI may also add information regarding abnormalities of the internal reproductive structures.**

If ^{99m}Tc-DMSA scanning and CT are done in a delayed fashion, small, poorly functioning kidneys that are unapparent on other studies or renal upper poles may be visualized for the first time (Utsunomiya et al, 1984; Pantuck et al, 1996; Moores et al, 1997; Borer et al, 1998; Bozorgi et al, 1998; Komatsu et al, 1999). The position of the ectopic kidney on a nuclear scan can direct the radiologist to order thin cuts of the CT scan through the suspected ectopic renal location.

Ectopic ureteral orifices may be identified at the time of cystourethroscopy and vaginoscopy. Careful inspection of the vestibule, urethra, and vagina sometimes reveals the ectopic orifice. Often, the orifice is difficult to identify amid the various mucosal folds of these structures. If an orifice is identifiable, a ureteral catheter can be passed into it and a retrograde pyelogram can be performed to better delineate the anatomy. If there is a single-system ectopic ureter, the characteristic features are a hypertrophied contralateral kidney and the cystoscopic findings of an absent ureteral orifice and absent ipsilateral hemitrigone.

We have not found the intravenous injection of indigo carmine to be particularly helpful because of the delayed function of the segment drained by the ectopic ureter. It has been suggested that two oral doses of phenazopyridine (Pyridium) given the night before and the morning of cystoscopy improve visualization of the ectopic ureter (Weiss et al, 1984). Filling the bladder with a dye solution, such as methylene blue or indigo carmine, is sometimes helpful in detecting the elusive ectopic orifice. If a clear fluid continues to drain into the vulva, one can be certain that an ectopic orifice is present. Deep flank palpation at the time of the examination may result in expression of urine and thereby reveal the orifice location.

Sometimes, the diagnosis must be made by exclusion, that is, the vestibule is damp, no orifice is found, the excretory urogram shows subtle changes suggesting a tiny dysplastic upper segment of a duplex system, and the patient is cured by an upper pole nephrectomy. With current imaging techniques and an appropriate degree of suspicion, the diagnosis is invariably made before surgery.

Treatment

Most ectopic ureters drain renal moieties (either an upper pole or a single-system kidney) that have minimal function. Therefore, upper pole nephrectomy (or nephrectomy in a single system) is often recommended (Sullivan et al, 1978; Plaire et al, 1997). In some cases, particularly with single-system ectopic ureters, renal function is worth salvaging. This may become more commonplace as antenatal sonography brings such patients to medical attention at an earlier stage and possibly before the damaging long-term effects of obstruction. Either ureteropyelostomy or common sheath ureteral reimplantation for a duplicated system, or solitary reimplantation for a single system, will achieve the goal of relief of obstruction. In our experience, many of these reconstructive procedures have resulted in decreased dilatation of the upper urinary tract and improved function (Fig. 116–19).

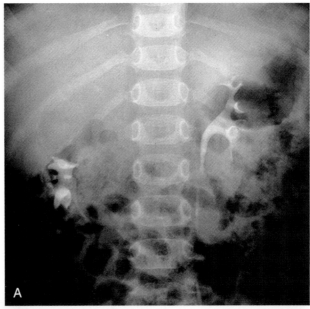

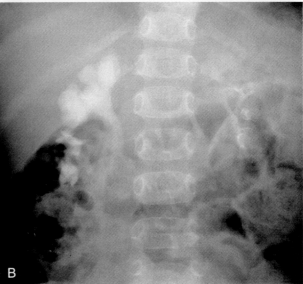

Figure 116–19. Preoperative (**A**) and postoperative (**B**) intravenous pyelograms demonstrate relief of the right upper pole obstruction after ureteroureterostomy between the upper and lower pole ureters.

Heminephrectomy and ureteropyelostomy are well described elsewhere (Mor et al, 1994), but several technical points deserve emphasis (Fig. 116–20). A flank approach for heminephrectomy usually offers better exposure to the upper pole vessels. Of primary concern is the need to avoid damaging the viable lower pole. The kidney should be retracted gently so as not to cause any vascular embarrassment. **Transecting the upper pole ureter and placing a traction stitch on the proximal portion of this ureter affords the surgeon a good method of retraction and manipulation of the upper pole.** The ureter is passed behind the main renal vessels. The dissection around the renal vessels should be done carefully to avoid damage to the lower pole. The upper pole vessels (most often two to three in number) are sequentially ligated. Demarcation of the upper pole parenchyma becomes apparent after

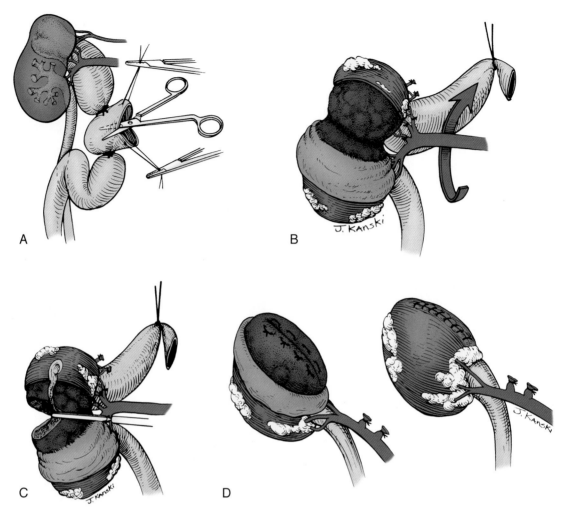

Figure 116–20. Technique of upper pole nephrectomy. **A,** The upper pole ureter is usually very dilated and tortuous and can be identified readily at the lower pole of the kidney. It is separated carefully from the lower pole ureter, divided, and used to improve access to the upper pole moiety. **B,** The upper pole ureter is passed beneath the hilar renal vessels and retracted upward. Small feeding vessels to the upper pole are individually ligated and divided. Any larger vessels that may be supplying the upper pole can be temporarily clamped to determine the extent of their distribution. The capsule of the upper pole is bluntly stripped away, exposing the often coarse and cystic parenchyma of the upper pole. This can usually be distinguished from the smooth texture of the normal lower pole. Often, an indented demarcation is seen between the two poles. **C,** While traction is applied to the lower pole ureter, the upper pole is excised with the use of electrocautery. Vascular control is achieved by temporary clamping of the lower pole vessels. This may also be accomplished by gentle finger compression of the lower pole. Individual vessels are identified and ligated during this part of the procedure. **D,** The parenchyma of the lower pole is approximated at the site of removal of the upper pole with the use of broad mattress sutures. The redundant capsule is then brought over the site of repair and sewn together with a running suture.

the upper pole vessels are ligated. Stripping the capsule off the upper pole in continuity allows it to be used in the closure. During upper pole nephrectomy, we have favored atraumatic clamping of the renal pedicle. This approach enables us to work in a bloodless field. Administration of an intravenous osmotic diuretic (e.g., mannitol) moments before and after clamping of the pedicle helps avert acute tubular necrosis. Topical vasodilating agents (e.g., papaverine) should be available in case vasospasm occurs. When performing the upper pole ureterectomy, it is of utmost importance to maintain the dissection immediately on the wall of the upper pole ureter as much as possible to preserve the blood supply to the remaining lower pole ureter.

If, in addition to obstruction, there is concomitant reflux into the ectopic ureter, a second incision is necessary (i.e., a Gibson incision) to resect the ureter in its entirety. Care must be taken to avoid injury to the vas deferens in male patients.

As mentioned previously, dissection should be performed strictly along the wall of the upper pole ureter. To prevent complications that may arise from dissection within a common sheath of two ureters (especially distally), the back wall of the upper pole ureter should be left attached to the lower pole ureter. The remainder of the upper pole ureter should be removed (Fig. 116–21). Such a maneuver prevents damage to the lower pole ureteral blood supply, which courses between both ureters. Resection is carried out to the level of the bladder, where several vesicle sutures are placed to close the upper pole ureteral hiatus.

A Penrose drain (brought through a separate stab wound) is placed in such a fashion as to drain the renal fossa and the area of the ureteral dissection. Postoperative evaluation includes an upper urinary tract study (intravenous pyelogram or nuclear renal scan) to demonstrate the anatomy and function in the lower pole.

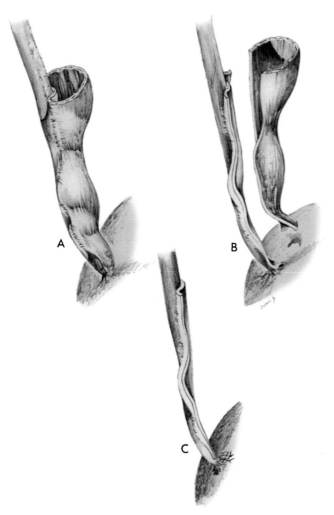

Figure 116–21. Surgical management of the refluxing ureteral stump. **A,** It is difficult to completely separate the distal 2 to 3 cm of the upper pole ureter from the lower pole ureter. The ectopic ureter is excised to this point. **B,** The outer wall of the ectopic ureter is excised to the bladder level. **C,** A transfixing suture obliterates its lumen, with care being taken not to injure the orthotopic ureter.

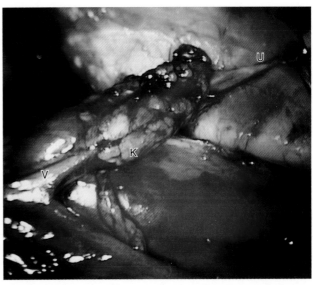

Figure 116–22. Laparoscopic view of a minimally functioning left kidney that was drained by an ectopic ureter in a 16-year-old incontinent girl. Laparoscopic nephrectomy resulted in immediate continence. U, ureter; K, kidney; V, vessels.

The procedure of ureteropyelostomy can be done either through a flank incision or via a dorsal lumbotomy approach, which is both effective and less morbid than a muscle-dividing flank incision.

Another surgical option is laparoscopic nephrectomy or heminephrectomy (Fig. 116–22). This can be done by either a transabdominal or a retroperitoneal approach. Laparoscopic procedures putatively offer reduced morbidity in regard to less postoperative pain, earlier return of gastrointestinal function, sooner discharge home, and presumably a quicker return to work for the parents (Jordan and Winslow, 1993; Rassweiler et al, 1993; Suzuki et al, 1993; Figenshau et al, 1994; Janetschek et al, 1997; El-Ghoneimi et al, 1998; Kobashi et al, 1998; Prabhakaran and Lingaraj, 1999; Yao and Poppas, 2000; Lee et al, 2004). Other advantages include direct lighting and increased magnification of the operative field, improved cosmesis, and avoidance of a second incision that is often needed for the distal ureterectomy of a nephroureterectomy.

Laparoscopic heminephrectomy can be performed in very small infants, and the operative time has decreased as expe-

rience and skill have increased (El-Ghoneimi, 2003; Wang et al, 2004). **Newer equipment such as the LigaSure device** (Valleylab, Boulder, CO) **and the Harmonic Scalpel** (Ethicon EndoSurgery, Cincinnati, OH) **allow for resection of the upper pole in a bloodless field.**

Some authors believe that cystoscopic placement of a ureteral catheter allows for easier identification of the ureter at the time of laparoscopy (Prabhakaran and Linaraj, 1999; Yao and Poppas, 2000). Laparoscopic heminephrouretectomy begins similarly to the open procedure in that the pathologic ureter is grasped as a handle and dissected closely to its wall to avoid compromise of the blood supply to the normal ureter. The polar renal vessels are then ligated with clips or divided with electrocautery; this allows for a more discernible demarcation of the affected upper pole. After the polar element is removed with electrocautery, one can check for collecting system leakage with intravenous injection of methylene blue (Yao and Poppas, 2000). Janetschek and colleagues (1997) place fibrin glue and hemostatic agents on the cut surface and then cover it with Gerota's fascia to aid in hemostasis.

When performing a partial nephrectomy, robotic-assisted laparoscopy offers significant advantages over standard laparoscopy. The magnification is augmented and the dexterity of the robotic instruments allows for greater precision when working around the renal pedicle and controlling the upper pole vessels.

Laparoscopic complications are inversely related to surgeon experience (Peters, 1996). In the above-cited reports, complications were uncommon but included inferior vena cava laceration; duodenal perforation and total nephrectomy; and peritoneal tears (if done via the retroperitoneum).

Alternative treatments have been described in special situations. If the ectopic ureter terminates proximal to the urinary sphincter, endoscopic dilation of the insertion site can relieve obstruction (Akbal et al, 2004; Lee et al, 2004). **When the offending ectopic ureter is from a single-system**

kidney that has scant function, embolization of that kidney will cause cessation of function and hence an end to urine production and incontinence (Kudoh et al, 2003; Solinas et al, 2004).

Bilateral Single-System Ectopic Ureters

Bilateral single-system ectopic ureters are fortunately rare, because they present a complex therapeutic problem (Koyanagi et al, 1977; Ahmed and Barker, 1992). In this condition, the ureters usually drain into the prostatic urethra in the male and into the distal urethra in the female. Embryologically, the portion of the urogenital sinus between the orifices of the wolf-fian duct and the ureter develops into the bladder neck musculature. This development does not occur if both ureters remain in the position of the wolffian duct orifice. Because there is no formation of the trigone and base plate, a very wide, poorly defined, incompetent vesical neck results. In rare instances, bilateral single ectopic ureters are associated with agenesis of the bladder and urethra. This condition is usually, but not always, incompatible with life (Glenn, 1959).

Commonly, the involved kidneys are dysplastic or display varying degrees of hydronephrosis (Fig. 116–23). The ureters are usually dilated, and reflux is often present. The bladder neck is incompetent, so the child dribbles continuously. Because there is poor resistance, the bladder does not have the opportunity to distend with urine and has a small capacity (Fig. 116–24). In the male, incontinence is not as severe as in the female and bladder capacity may be greater because the external sphincter provides a variable degree of control.

At cystoscopy, the ureteral orifices can be identified in the male, usually just distal to the bladder neck. The lax bladder neck and small bladder are clearly evident. In the female, it can be difficult to find both ureteral orifices, which usually are located in the distal urethra but occasionally enter the genital tract.

The abnormality is akin to epispadias, with the basic defect being a short urethra and incompetent bladder neck. However, in contrast to epispadias, there is a high incidence of renal and urethral abnormalities in addition to the small bladder capacity.

Treatment usually consists of ureteral reimplantation and reconstruction of the bladder neck for continence by one of the tubularization procedures, such as the Young-Dees-Leadbetter (Leadbetter, 1985), Kropp (Kropp and Angwafo, 1986), or Salle (Rink et al, 1994) procedures. It is often helpful to employ vesicourethral suspension at the same time. Increased exposure through symphyseal splitting has been helpful during these reconstructions (Peters and Hendren, 1989). The success rate is higher in boys than in girls. Bladder capacity often increases in the child who gains satisfactory control. Enterocystoplasty to increase bladder capacity may be necessary in selected cases.

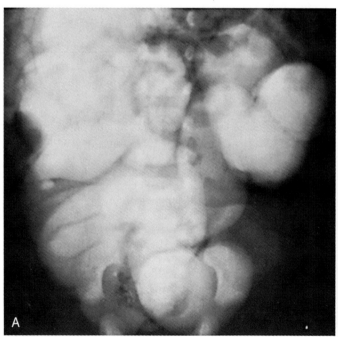

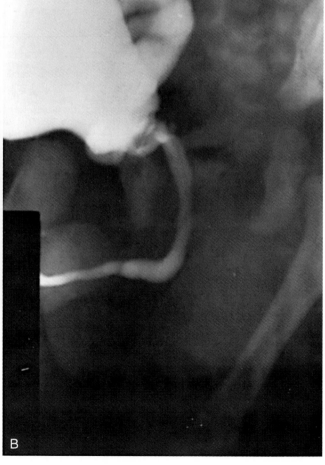

Figure 116–23. **A,** Excretory urogram in a 6-day-old boy shows severe bilateral hydronephrosis and hydroureter. **B,** A voiding cystourethrogram demonstrates refluxing ectopic ureters draining into the prostatic urethra.

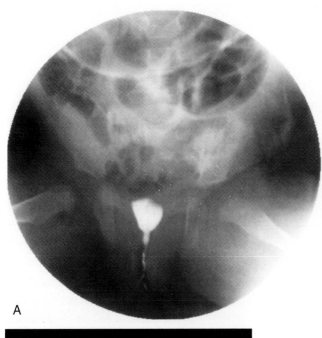

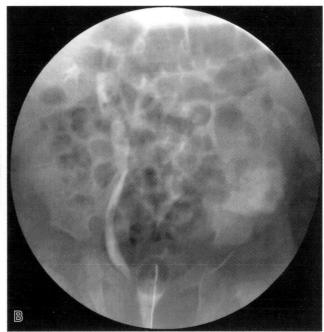

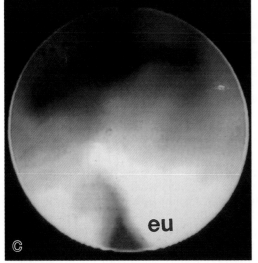

Figure 116–24. A 6-month-old girl was diagnosed with a solitary right kidney drained by an ectopic ureter entering the urethra. **A,** Diminutive bladder was seen on voiding cystourethrogram (VCUG). **B,** Reflux seen on VCUG. **C,** Cystoscopic image of wide bladder neck anteriorly and ectopic ureter (eu) entering just below it into the urethra.

ANOMALIES OF STRUCTURE
Ureteroceles

Few entities in pediatric urology present as great a clinical challenge as ureteroceles. Ureteroceles have varied effects in regard to obstruction, reflux, continence, and renal function; hence, each ureterocele must be managed on an individual basis and not by a simple algorithm. It is imperative for the treating physician to be acquainted with the multiple presentations, radiologic appearances, and treatment options of ureteroceles, as well as the complications to avoid. Such knowledge yields the best possible clinical results.

Embryology

A ureterocele is a cystic dilatation of the terminal ureter. How this develops has been the subject of several discussions. At 37 days' gestation, Chwalle's membrane, a two-layered cell structure, transiently divides the early ureteric bud from the urogenital sinus (Chwalle, 1927). The stenotic orifice commonly seen in the ureterocele has led several researchers to postulate that this dilatation results from incomplete dissolution of Chwalle's membrane. Others have theorized that the affected intravesical ureter suffers from abnormal muscular development; without the appropriate muscular backing, the distal ureter assumes a balloon morphology (Tokunaka et al, 1981). A third theory implicates a developmental stimulus responsible for bladder expansion acting simultaneously on the intravesical ureter (Stephens, 1971). Incontrovertible evidence does not exist to uphold any of these theories, which, in fact, have very little effect on clinical practice.

Diagnosis

As with ectopic ureters, ureteroceles are increasingly diagnosed by prenatal ultrasound studies. Prenatal ultrasonography is capable of demonstrating both the hydronephrosis and the intravesical cystic dilatation. Shekarriz and associates (1999) reported that 30% of their ureteroceles were diagnosed prenatally; however, this series began in 1979, when obstetric sonography was performed less commonly than today. More recent series reveal a high proportion of prenatally diagnosed ureteroceles. Pfister and colleagues (1998) reported that 31 of their 35 patients with ureteroceles were diagnosed prenatally. In the latter half of their study, Husmann and coworkers (1995) reported a median age at diagnosis of ureterocele of 3 months, with the implication that many of these cases were diagnosed prenatally. Di Benedetto and Monfort (1997) reported that all 25 of their patients with ureteroceles presenting between 1980 and 1994 were diagnosed in utero. **Fetal diagnosis of a ureterocele can be accomplished with MRI. Although this is not the primary modality for ureterocele diagnosis in utero, MRI can overcome issues of suboptimal fetal position, maternal obesity, and oligohydramnios, which may hinder obstetrical ultrasounds** (Sozubir et al, 2003).

If ureteroceles are diagnosed prenatally, the physician is alerted to perform a more comprehensive postnatal evaluation and to administer prophylactic antibiotics at birth.

Ureteroceles have a particular predilection for race and gender (Brock and Kaplan, 1978; Mandell et al, 1980; Cobb et al, 1982; Caldamone and Duckett, 1984; Scherz et al, 1989; Monfort et al, 1992; Rickwood et al, 1992). **They occur most frequently in females (4:1 ratio) and almost exclusively in whites. Approximately 10% are bilateral. Eighty percent of all ureteroceles arise from the upper poles of duplicated systems.** Single-system ureteroceles are sometimes called simple ureteroceles and are usually found in adults. These single-system ureteroceles are less prone to the severe obstruction and dysplasia associated with duplicated systems.

However, many ureteroceles are still diagnosed clinically (Upadhyay et al, 2002; Chertin et al, 2003; DeFoor et al, 2003). The most common presentation is that of an infant who has a urinary tract infection or urosepsis (Gonzales, 1992; Monfort et al, 1992; Retik and Peters, 1992; Coplen and Duckett, 1995). We have seen patients whose ultrasound and intraoperative findings revealed frank pus in the obstructed upper pole collecting system, and this has also been noted by others (Glazier and Packer, 1997). For this reason, all children with a ureterocele (or, less specifically, any significant hydronephrosis) should be given prophylactic antibiotics. Of 33 patients prescribed prophylactic antibiotics after their prenatal diagnosis, only 1 developed a urinary tract infection (Husmann et al, 1995). Stasis of urine in this obstructed system can lead not only to infection but also to calculus formation (Thornbury et al, 1977; Rodriguez, 1984; Moskovitz et al, 1987). Some children present with a palpable mass in their abdomen, which is a hydronephrotic kidney. The ureterocele, if ectopic, can prolapse out of the urethra as a vaginal mass (Fig. 116–25).

If the ureterocele is large enough, it can obstruct the bladder neck or even the contralateral ureteral orifice and result in hydronephrosis of that collecting system (Diard et al, 1981). The bladder outlet obstruction causing bilateral hydronephrosis can even be diagnosed prenatally (Gloor et al, 1996; Austin et al, 1998). **Ectopic ureteroceles can cause incontinence by hindering the normal sphincteric function at or distal to the**

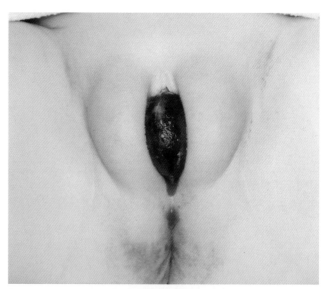

Figure 116–25. A prolapsed ureterocele presented as an interlabial mass in a 3-week-old girl.

bladder neck. Patients with ureteroceles may have a varied pattern of voiding dysfunction, including urgency and incontinence. Sherman and associates (2003) found that patients with bilateral ectopic ureteroceles had poor bladder emptying and recurrent urinary tract infection after surgical treatment of the ureteroceles.

Infrequently, a child with a ureterocele can present with hematuria. Ureteroceles may have an insidious clinical course, resulting in no specific urologic symptoms but manifesting only as a failure to thrive or as abdominal or pelvic pain. Usually, lengthy evaluation of other organ systems ensues before the problem is correctly localized to the urinary tract.

Imaging studies that are now available afford a great deal of insight into the effects of the ureterocele on normal anatomy and physiology. **The first study obtained in these evaluations is usually an ultrasound** (Geringer et al, 1983b; Cremin, 1986; Teele and Share, 1991). Most commonly, the ureterocele is associated with a duplicated collecting system. Sonographically, two separate renal pelves surrounded by their echogenic hila can be seen. This duplex kidney is larger than a kidney associated with a single collecting system. A dilated ureter emanates from a hydronephrotic upper pole (Fig. 116–26). This finding should signal the examiner to image the bladder to determine whether a ureterocele is present. If the lower pole is associated with reflux, or if the ureterocele has caused delayed emptying from the ipsilateral lower pole, this lower pole may likewise be hydronephrotic. Similarly, the ureterocele may impinge on the contralateral ureteral orifice or obstruct the bladder neck and cause hydronephrosis in the opposite kidney. The upper pole parenchyma drained by the ureterocele will exhibit varying degrees of thickness and echogenicity. Increased echogenicity correlates with dysplastic changes. The bladder frequently displays a thin-walled cyst that is the ureterocele (Fig. 116–27).

There are several pitfalls in ultrasound diagnosis. If the bladder is overdistended, the ureterocele may be effaced and go unnoticed. At times the bladder may be empty, in which

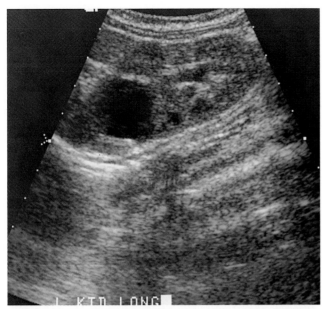

Figure 116–26. Sonographic appearance of upper pole hydronephrosis caused by a ureterocele.

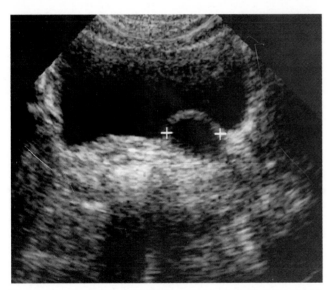

Figure 116–27. An intravesical ureterocele in a 2-month-old girl is outlined by the cursors on an ultrasound image.

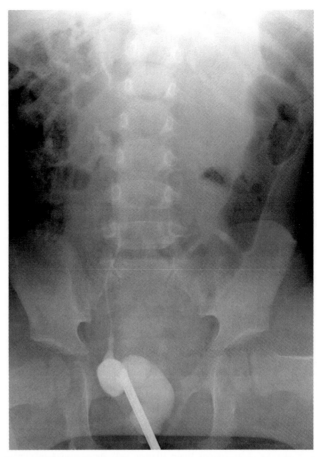

Figure 116–28. Ureterocele disproportion demonstrated via retrograde pyelography. Note the disparity between the large ureterocele and the thin ureter and nondilated collecting system.

case it is difficult to discriminate between the wall of the ureterocele and the wall of the bladder. In such instances, the empty bladder with a ureterocele may be interpreted as simply a partially filled bladder. The dilated ureter should be seen posterior to the bladder. On occasion, a large ureterocele is associated with a diminutive ureter and collecting system. The corresponding upper pole parenchyma can be so small as to be nonvisualized. The diagnosis of ureterocele may be overlooked because the duplicated collecting system cannot be identified. This entity has been termed both *nonobstructive ectopic ureterocele* (Bauer and Retik, 1978) and *ureterocele disproportion* (Share and Lebowitz, 1989) (Fig. 116–28).

On occasion, a dilated *ectopic* ureter may be seen immediately posterior to the bladder and may impinge on the **bladder wall, giving the appearance that the dilated ureter is intravesical.** This may give the false impression of a ureterocele, the pseudoureterocele referred to previously (Diard et al, 1987; Sumfest et al, 1995). The difference between the two entities is that a ureterocele is separated from the bladder space by its thin wall, whereas an ectopic ureter has the thicker bladder wall separating it from the intravesical space. A mesonephric duct cyst that communicates with an ectopic ureter can open into the bladder and mimic a ureterocele on radiographic studies (Sumfest et al, 1995).

Intravenous pyelography is a valuable imaging study in the evaluation of a ureterocele. There are several hallmarks of a urogram in a patient with a ureterocele (Geringer et al, 1983a; Muller et al, 1988), and these findings are similar to those mentioned in the discussion on ectopic ureters. **In the great majority of cases, the upper pole functions poorly and excretes contrast agent in a delayed fashion or not at all. This upper pole is deviated laterally from the spine because of its hydronephrosis.** This same upper pole hydronephrosis is responsible for pushing the lower pole laterally and inferiorly (Fig. 116–29). Because only the lower pole calyces are seen, the number of calyces is less than the complement of a normal kidney.

Whereas the upper pole ureter is infrequently seen on the intravenous pyelogram because of the lack of contrast excretion, its presence may be inferred from its effect on the lower

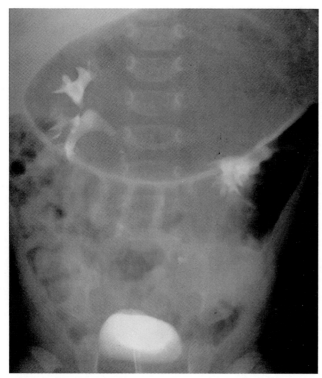

Figure 116–29. Left upper pole hydronephrosis causes lower pole displacement inferiorly and laterally, which is referred to as the drooping lily sign.

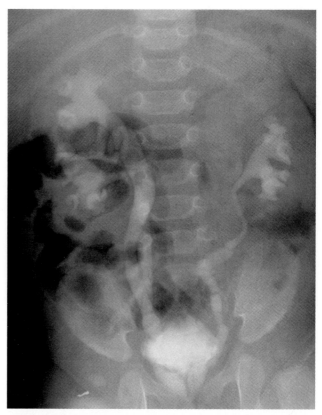

Figure 116–30. An intravenous pyelogram reveals the effects of left upper pole hydronephrosis caused by its obstructing ureterocele. The left upper pole is not visualized, the left lower pole ureter takes a serpiginous course around the dilated upper pole ureter, and there is contralateral hydronephrosis owing to obstruction of the bladder neck by the ureterocele.

pole ureter. **The lower pole ureter can be seen as laterally deviated, taking a serpiginous course, and notched. These characteristics all result from its association with the dilated, tortuous upper pole ureter** (Fig. 116–30). As mentioned earlier in the section on ultrasonography, hydronephrosis may be seen in the contralateral kidney as a result of obstruction by the ureterocele.

Voiding cystourethrography can demonstrate the size and location of the ureterocele as well as the presence or absence of vesicoureteral reflux. Assessing the severity of such reflux is critical to future management. Reflux into the ipsilateral lower pole is common (Feldman and Lome, 1981; Caldamone, 1984) (Fig. 116–31). Pfister and colleagues (1998) noted an incidence of reflux of 49%. Shekarriz and coworkers (1999) reported an overall incidence of reflux of 59% (intravesical ureteroceles, 44%, and extravesical ureteroceles, 63%). In Husmann and colleagues' series (1999), the incidence of reflux was 67%. Sen and associates (1992) reported reflux in 80 (54%) of 148 ipsilateral lower pole ureters. Rickwood and coworkers (1992) noted that 15 (65%) of 23 patients had ipsilateral lower pole reflux. Forty percent of patients with ureteroceles in Monfort and coworkers' series had reflux (1992). Reflux may also be seen in the contralateral system if the ureterocele is large enough to distort the trigone and the opposite ureteral submucosal tunnel. Pfister and colleagues (1998) noted that 9% of their patients had reflux into the contralateral kidney. In Sen's series, 35 (28%) of 127 patients had reflux in the contralateral unit. Reflux into the ureterocele and its ureter may be present but is uncommon and should alert the physician to the possibility of an ectopic ureterocele whose open mouth in the urethra is allowing reflux.

Images should be obtained from early in the filling phase, because some ureteroceles may efface later in filling and may not be seen. The ureterocele may evert into the ureter and appear to be a diverticulum (Fig. 116–32). Bellah and coworkers (1995) reported on 12 children who were noted to have vesicoureteral reflux and an ipsilateral bladder diverticulum. At surgery, each of these children had a ureterocele associated with a duplex system, and in 5 the ureterocele was not correctly identified preoperatively. These authors made the point that the lower pole ureter actually enters into a bladder diverticulum that is present because of attenuation of the bladder musculature by the ureterocele. They believed that in these cases the ureterocele is not everting into its own ureter but is rather everting through a weakened bladder wall and dragging the lower pole ureteral orifice along with this segment of herniated bladder mucosa. This description may explain the clinical finding of infrequent resolution of reflux associated with a ureterocele.

When it is performed diligently, cystography demonstrates the ureterocele in the bladder. It **appears as a smooth, broad-based filling defect located near the trigone.** It is frequently eccentrically located, and the superior portion of the ureterocele may be angled to one side, thereby giving a clue as to which side the ureterocele is associated with (Fig. 116–33). However, on cystography, the ureterocele is often centrally placed, and it may not be helpful in this regard. In such instances, cystoscopy may shed light on the issue. If the

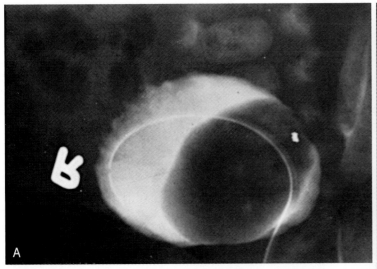

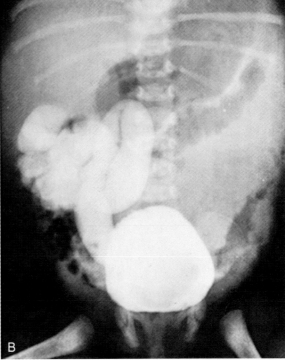

Figure 116–31. **A,** Cystogram outlines a left ureterocele. **B,** Postvoiding film shows reflux to the right lower pole. This girl had bilateral ureteroceles, with the right one being a small ureterocele that was not demonstrated on the cystogram.

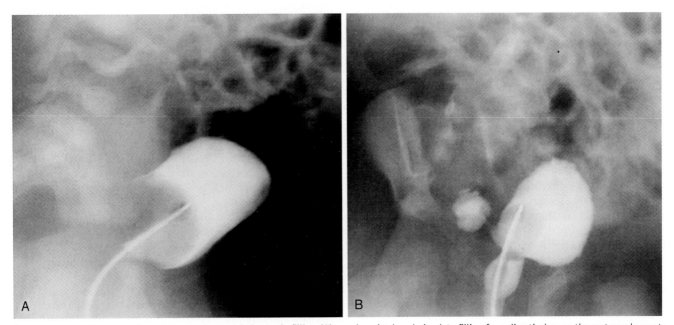

Figure 116–32. A ureterocele seen on a cystogram during early filling (**A**) may be mistaken during late filling for a diverticulum as the ureterocele everts into its own ureter (**B**).

cystoscopic findings are inconclusive, the answer can be obtained by injecting contrast material into the ureterocele; this method should define the side from which the ureterocele originated (Fig. 116–34). Injection of contrast medium into the ureterocele can verify the diagnosis of ureterocele disproportion when the upper tract findings are difficult to interpret. Such information is obviously necessary in planning the surgical approach.

Nuclear scans with agents such as DMSA and diethylene-triaminepentaacetic acid (DTPA) or mercaptoacetyltriglycine (MAG3) can give valuable estimates of upper pole contribution to overall renal function as well as degrees of obstruction (Arap et al, 1984). It is important to trace the regions of interest correctly and consistently to obtain accurate information. This information is often helpful in determining whether the upper pole moiety is worth saving.

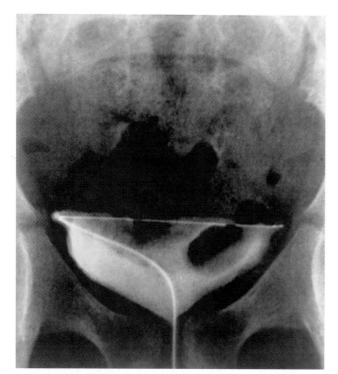

Figure 116–33. A smooth, lateral filling defect is the classic appearance of a ureterocele on a cystogram.

Treatment

It should once again be stressed that, before any surgical intervention, the surgeon must obtain as much information as possible regarding the patient's altered anatomy and physiology. Only then can a rational treatment plan be devised.

Because ureteroceles have a broad spectrum of presentation, anatomy, and pathophysiology, each child must be treated individually. No single method of surgical repair suffices for all cases. The goals of therapy should be clearly defined and factored into the clinical decisions. **These goals are preservation of renal function; elimination of infection, obstruction, and reflux; and maintenance of urinary continence. Minimizing surgical morbidity is a goal that must be included in this consideration.** The management of a ureterocele associated with an upper pole of a duplicated system has generated much debate. Although the goals of treatment could certainly generate a consensus, the means to achieving those goals have not necessarily been agreed on. **One area of agreement is that early institution of daily prophylactic antibiotics can result in a low rate of urinary tract infections.**

A primary concern is the preservation of renal parenchyma if at all possible. This goal is achieved by correcting obstruction and preventing reflux with its risks of renal parenchymal damage from infection. At times, it is necessary to balance one against the other, because relieving the obstruction of a ureterocele may induce reflux in either or both poles of the involved duplication. In other instances, the same action may cause existing lower pole reflux to resolve. Several means of achieving these goals of therapy are available. Because there are a sizable number of permutations when one considers all the possible combinations and degrees of ipsilateral and contralateral reflux, ipsilateral and contralateral obstruction,

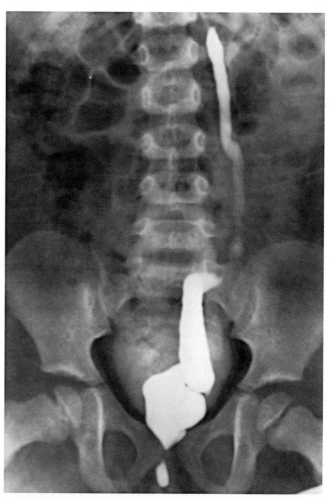

Figure 116–34. Endoscopic injection of a ureterocele outlines the upper pole and the distal extent of the ureterocele.

varying degrees of salvageable function, infection, and age, one can easily see why most people believe that when dealing with ureteroceles each case must be managed on an individual basis.

Ureteroceles can cause bladder outlet obstruction resulting in hydronephrosis and oligohydramnios. Prenatal decompression of the ureterocele (via laser incision or needle disruption) or vesicoamniotic shunting has been described in case reports as treatment for fetal bladder outlet obstruction (Hansen et al, 2002).

However, ureteroceles are overwhelmingly dealt with postnatally. Although one might reason that a prenatal diagnosis could lead to earlier relief of obstruction and presumably a greater chance of recovery of upper pole function, the evidence in the literature seems to show that loss of function of the upper pole occurs equally in those diagnosed prenatally and postnatally (Upadhyay et al, 2002). In most instances, the upper pole contributes little, if at all, to overall renal function.

Histologic lesions of the upper pole can take the form of interstitial fibrosis and inflammation, glomerular and tubular sclerosis, atrophy, and dysplasia (Bolduc et al, 2003). Approximately one third of their patients had preservation of function of the upper pole; that preservation rate was the same for intravesical versus ectopic ureteroceles and also for antenatal versus postnatal diagnosis. Severe thinning of the parenchyma seen on preoperative ultrasound and minimal function of the upper pole on renal scan (= 4% of overall function) were statistically reliable predictors of severe histologic lesions. Increased parenchymal echogenicity and degree of hydronephrosis also were associated with severe histologic lesions. Upadhyay and associates (2002) found that on nuclear renal imaging more than half of their patients had nonfunction of the upper pole draining into the ureteroceles.

The aim therefore is to deal with this affected renal moiety in a manner that is geared not only toward alleviating obstruction and its potential for recurrent infection but also toward the cessation of reflux that is present in about half of the cases. There is a diversity of opinion in this regard. One group of surgeons advocates the so-called upper tract approach; this approach consists of upper pole nephrectomy and partial ureterectomy, or, less commonly, when significant upper pole function is present, a ureteropyelostomy (Mandell et al, 1980; Cendron et al, 1981; Feldman and Lome, 1981; Caldamone et al, 1984; Reitelman and Perlmutter, 1990). With either of these procedures, the ureterocele should decompress and, with return of the trigone to a more normal configuration, resolution of the ipsilateral lower pole reflux may occur. The advantages of this approach are avoidance of the morbidity of a second surgical procedure and, it is hoped, elimination of a potentially difficult bladder neck and urethral dissection. If a second procedure is eventually required, it can be performed when the child is older on an elective basis (King et al, 1983). Mandell and associates (1980) treated 18 patients in this manner. In 14 of these patients, a one-stage procedure was planned; only 3 patients (21%) required reoperation (the indications being persistent lower pole reflux, reflux into the ureteral stump, and failure of ureterocele decompression). They are proponents of the upper pole approach because it meets the goals of a low reoperative rate and resolution of the problems described earlier. They do state, however, that if a patient has high-grade reflux into the ipsilateral lower pole ureter, a combination of upper pole nephroureterectomy, ureterocele excision, and lower pole ureteral reimplantation may be necessary. This combined approach would be recommended because these severe degrees of reflux are less likely to disappear spontaneously and would probably require a second procedure.

Another scenario that should prompt consideration for a single-stage repair at the kidney and bladder level is the case of lower pole reflux associated with a large everting ureterocele and a poorly functioning upper pole. This, too, is unlikely to result in reflux resolution, because the muscular backing necessary for ureteral compression is usually lacking in everting ureteroceles.

Caldamone and associates (1984) had a similar rate for secondary procedures using the upper tract approach. Of 36 patients managed in this way (including 4 who underwent ureteropyelostomy), only 7 (19%) needed secondary procedures. Four had bladder outlet obstruction, and 3 had persistent reflux associated with poor renal growth, renal scarring, or recurrent urinary tract infections. Ten of their patients had delayed reflux (i.e., reflux that appeared after an upper tract procedure in a patient with no preoperative reflux), and only 3 of these 10 patients had spontaneous

resolution of the reflux. The authors concluded that most patients can be managed with an upper urinary tract approach alone.

Similarly, Perlmutter and associates (Kroovand and Perlmutter, 1979; Reitelman and Perlmutter, 1990) directed their attention to removal of the upper pole of the kidney. They combined this procedure with a total ureterectomy to the level of the bladder to prevent possible problems from a retained stump (e.g., pyoureter, diverticulum). When the upper pole merited salvage, they performed either an ipsilateral ureteropyelostomy or a distal ureteroureterostomy. In most instances, there was a reasonable chance for resolution of the reflux after decompression of the ureterocele. Upper pole nephrectomy can be performed laparoscopically even in children younger than 12 months. Removal of the upper pole can be done with monopolar electrode or ultrasound scalpel (Valla et al, 2003).

One of the more extensive experiences in the literature is that of Scherz and colleagues (1989). They reported their clinical observations in 60 patients with ectopic ureteroceles (defined as either a ureterocele associated with an upper pole of a duplicated system or a ureterocele in an ectopic position). They also compared the need for further surgery in patients treated with the upper urinary tract approach alone and in those who had a combined upper and lower urinary tract approach. The combined approach uses two incisions to achieve upper pole heminephrectomy, partial ureterectomy, and intravesical excision and marsupialization of the ureterocele, along with correction of reflux when present. **Of 19 evaluable patients who had the upper urinary tract approach alone, 9 (47%) required reoperation for recurrent reflux or infection. In contrast, of 28 patients who were treated with the combined approach, only 4 (14%) required reoperation, all for reflux.** These authors believed that marsupialization of the ureterocele was less likely to cause sphincter damage than enucleation. They also emphasized the need for passing a large catheter antegrade through the bladder neck to ascertain that all mucosal lips that might act as obstructing valves had been removed. They believed that the combined approach is a superior one because of its lower reoperative rate. With the exception of the acutely ill child with urosepsis, Hendren and Mitchell (1979) also advocated a complete repair, namely, upper pole nephrectomy, ureterocele excision, and ureteral reimplantation.

Gotoh and colleagues (1988) reported use of the presence or absence of radiographic eversion of the ureterocele, the separation between the upper and lower orifices, and the upper pole function to determine the means of correction. In cases with eversion and separation of the orifices, upper pole function was always absent. When the orifices were adjacent, function was absent in one third of cases. Upper pole nephrectomy was performed with an extravesical resection of the ureterocele and repair of the bladder wall, without lower pole reimplantation.

The reports of Decter and associates (1989) and Gonzales (1992) reiterated the need to consider each case individually. They used an upper tract approach in infants who had low-grade or no reflux in the ipsilateral lower pole. In those infants who were likely to need a secondary procedure (e.g., those with high-grade reflux or a prolapsed ureterocele) and in septic patients not responding to antibiotic therapy, they advocated initial decompression of the ureterocele via endoscopic incision.

A body of evidence has begun to emerge from the literature delineating the difference in success of treatment based on whether the ureteroceles were intravesical versus ectopic and whether there was associated reflux. In regard to upper pole nephrectomy for the treatment of a ureterocele, Shekarriz and associates (1999) noted that of their 41 extravesical ureteroceles treated with an upper tract approach, 17 (41%) required reoperation. The reoperation rate varied based on the degree of preoperative reflux. If there was no reflux, only 20% required reoperation. Low-grade reflux required reoperation in 30% of cases, and high-grade reflux required reoperation in 53%. The same upper tract approach in intravesical ureteroceles resulted in two of six patients' requiring a second operation.

Husmann and colleagues (1999) similarly noted a high reoperative rate when upper pole nephrectomy was performed for an ectopic ureterocele associated with reflux. Their overall need for a second procedure after a partial nephrectomy for an ectopic ureterocele was 65%. A partial nephrectomy was the definitive procedure for 85% of patients if there was no reflux, but for only 16% of those with grade III or greater reflux.

Churchill and coworkers (1992) divided their 43 patients into three groups based on the number and severity of the renal units jeopardized by hydronephrosis and reflux. Group 1 was defined as those patients with an ectopic ureterocele whose only renal unit with significant hydronephrosis was the upper pole that drained into the ureterocele. This group was successfully treated with an upper tract approach 89% of the time. Group 2 (ipsilateral lower pole significant hydronephrosis and/or reflux) and group 3 (ipsilateral lower pole significant hydronephrosis and/or reflux and a contralateral kidney with significant hydronephrosis and/or reflux) required a second surgical procedure 71% and 60% of the time, respectively.

Defoor and coworkers (2003) found that by retrospectively categorizing their ureterocele patients using this system they could predict successful responses to various surgical interventions. When totaling success rates for endoscopic puncture, upper tract approach and lower tract approach, they noted success rates of 73%, 48%, and 20% for grades 1, 2, and 3 ureteroceles, respectively.

Prenatal versus postnatal diagnosis also seems to be a way to stratify success rates with ureterocele procedures. Those with prenatal diagnosis needed a secondary procedure 22% of the time as compared with 45% of those diagnosed after birth. For those patients undergoing endoscopic decompression of the ureteroceles, the need for secondary procedures for prenatally and postnatally diagnosed patients was 33% and 70%, respectively (Upadhyay et al, 2002).

The technique of upper pole nephrectomy for nonfunctioning upper poles due to ureteroceles is the same technique as upper pole nephrectomy described previously in this chapter for ectopic ureters (see Fig. 116–20).

Our intravesical approach to the ureterocele begins with a transverse incision of the ureterocele between two stay sutures (Fig. 116–35). Proximally, a plane is obtained between the ureterocele wall and the wall of the bladder. The ureterocele is dissected off the bladder to the point at which it joins the lower pole ureter. Then the ureters are dissected as a unit, the upper pole ureter is tapered as needed, and both ureters are reimplanted submucosally. Amar (1978) advocated submucosal saline injection to facilitate creation of the submucosal tunnel. The distal portion of the ureterocele is dissected in the same plane to the level of the bladder neck, where it is resected. **The detrusor muscle is plicated if it is attenuated and it appears that it may offer insufficient backing.** Bladder mucosal flaps are raised to cover the area of the removed ureterocele.

Once again, several technical points regarding ureterocele excision and common sheath reimplantation deserve mention. **Separation of the duplicated ureters during intravesical dissection should be discouraged, because it can lead to sacrifice of the common blood supply running longitudinally between the two ureters. Plication of the detrusor muscle underlying the ureterocele may be necessary to shore up any areas of muscle deficiency. Furthermore, the distal portion of the ureterocele may extend below the bladder neck. Extreme care must be taken in this part of the dissection to avoid injury to the sphincter mechanisms.**

Upper pole biopsy at the time of renal exploration may aid in assessing whether the tissue is dysplastic or viable (Coplen and Duckett, 1995). Before that procedure, radiographic imaging can provide information regarding the presence of function. An intravenous pyelogram that demonstrates an upper pole that excretes contrast agent, either *concurrently* with the lower pole or even in only a slightly delayed fashion, is suggestive of parenchyma with recoverability. A nuclear medicine renal scan with an agent such as ^{99m}Tc-DMSA, which binds to the functional nephron tubules, can demonstrate an upper pole that may have salvageable renal parenchyma despite obstruction. The goal in these cases is to create effective drainage of the upper pole collecting system.

One option used to achieve this goal is the upper urinary tract anastomotic techniques of ureteroureterostomy or ureteropyelostomy. This results in the upper pole system's draining into the lower pole system. Such high anastomoses are preferable to a distal ureteroureterostomy, because the latter is prone to the travel of urine boluses down one ureter and then, at the ureteral-ureteral junction, retrograde up the other ureter. This phenomenon is sometimes referred to as the yo-yo effect. It can detrimentally affect urinary drainage and lead to stasis, infection, and ureteral dilatation.

When performing the upper tract anastomoses, dissection should be limited to an absolute minimum, especially medially, to prevent disruption of either ureter's blood supply. The upper pole ureter may be considerably larger than the lower pole ureter. A generous longitudinal ureterotomy made in the lower pole ureter is performed to overcome such disproportion, and the anastomosis is performed in an end-to-side fashion. The distal portion of the upper pole ureter should be aspirated with a fine feeding tube to decompress the ureterocele. The distal upper pole ureter is resected as far inferiorly as possible, with care taken to stay directly on this ureter's wall and avoid the vasculature of the adjacent lower pole ureter. If the ureterocele does not reflux, the resection is taken as distally as the wound allows and the remnant lower portion of ureter may be left open.

Ureterocele excision with common sheath reimplantation also achieves the goal of upper tract drainage. The technical

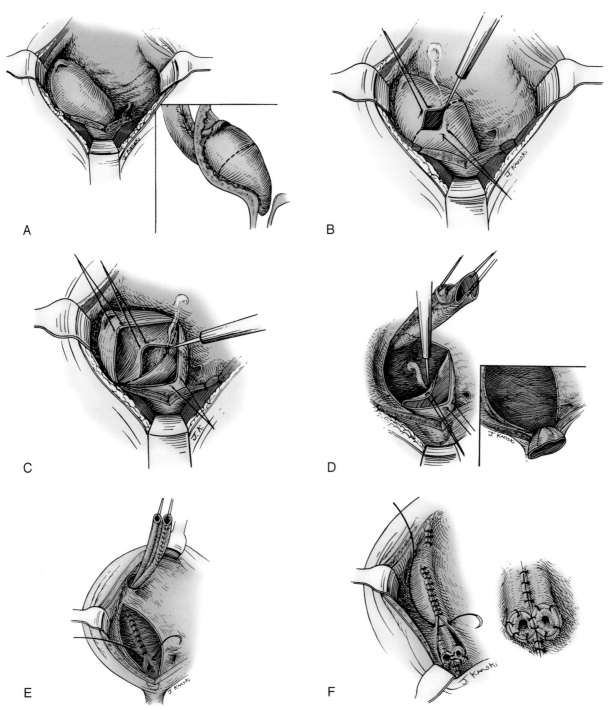

Figure 116–35.   Technique for excision of ectopic ureterocele and common sheath reimplantation of upper and lower pole ureters. **A,** Appearance of right-sided ureterocele with open bladder, viewed from below. Note proximity of the contralateral ureteral orifice. *Inset,* Cutaway side view demonstrating the close association of the two polar ureters with a common vascular supply. The *dotted line* indicates the planned initial incision of the ureterocele. **B,** After stay sutures are placed, the ureterocele is incised with electrocautery in a transverse direction, exposing the inner cavity of the ureterocele. **C,** The posterior mucosal wall of the ureterocele is incised transversely, revealing the often thinned posterior muscular wall of the bladder. This incision will then be continued around the bladder mucosal edge of the ureterocele, including the orifice of the lower pole ureter. Stay sutures are important to provide adequate exposure. **D,** The upper and lower pole ureters have been mobilized and are retracted into the bladder. The distal aspect of the ureterocele is being mobilized in a similar fashion. The bladder mucosal surface will also be incised around the edge of the ureterocele to permit complete removal of the ureterocele. *Inset,* The fully mobilized distal ureterocele is retracted caudally, revealing its narrowing attachment at the bladder neck. **E,** The dilated upper pole ureter associated with the ureterocele has been tapered and remains in continuity with the lower pole ureter. Both have been brought into the bladder through a newly formed muscular hiatus to provide adequate tunnel length for the ureteral reimplantation. The thinned-out posterior bladder wall has been repaired with multiple interrupted sutures to provide adequate muscular backing for the ureters. The bladder mucosa surrounding the ureterocele defect has been mobilized to permit covering of the ureters. **F** *left,* The ureters have been reimplanted into the new ureteral tunnel, have been sutured distally after spatulation, and are being covered with bladder mucosa. The lower pole orifice is medial. *Right,* Final appearance of the ureteral tunnel after completion of the reimplantation.

aspects of this approach were described earlier. The disadvantage of this approach compared with the flank upper pole to lower pole anastomoses just described is that the bladder approach has the added morbidity of hematuria, bladder spasm, and several days of bladder drainage with a catheter. In addition, the dissection of the ureterocele bed may be a more involved one and has the potential problems of bladder neck injury.

Descriptions of ureterocele incisions date back to Zielinski's technique of a low transverse incision (Zielinski, 1962) and a longitudinal ureterocele incision proposed by Hutch and Chisholm (1966). These so-called meatotomies were performed via open surgery.

There has been an increased interest in the endoscopic treatment of ureteroceles (Cobb et al, 1982; Monfort et al, 1992; Blythe et al, 1993; Coplen and Duckett, 1995; Hagg et al, 2000; Chertin et al, 2003; Ben Meir et al, 2004; Castagnetti et al, 2004). Although transurethral resection was satisfactory in achieving decompression (Wines and O'Flynn, 1972; Tank, 1986), it often led to massive reflux of the involved system. As a result, this procedure fell out of favor, except in cases of sepsis when urgent relief of obstruction was needed. However, improvements in equipment and refinements in technique have led to a reevaluation of the role of ureterocele incision. Blythe and coworkers (1993) described their technique of using a No. 3 Fr Bugbee electrode to puncture the ureterocele near its base and proximal to the bladder neck. The new opening should have an intravesical position while the bladder is empty, to avoid obstruction by the bladder neck. With the use of such a technique, obstruction is relieved and the roof of the ureterocele presumably should collapse onto the floor of the bladder and act as a flap valve mechanism to prevent reflux. With this technique, 73% of their patients needed no further procedures. However, when analyzing their data further, they concluded that intravesical ureteroceles fared better than ectopic ureteroceles with regard to decompression (93% vs. 75%), preservation of upper pole function (96% vs. 47%), newly created reflux (18% vs. 47%), and need for secondary procedures (7% vs. 50%). Based on these findings, they recommended ureterocele incision in all neonates as well as in older children with either an intravesical ureterocele, a ureterocele associated with a functioning upper pole, or a single-system ureterocele.

Hagg and associates (2000) presented a more recent compilation of patients from the same group; in this series, they used a slightly modified method of endoscopic ureterocele decompression. With endoscopic ureterocele puncture, rather than incision, 19 (37%) of 51 patients with a ureterocele associated with a duplicated system required a secondary open procedure. Twenty-two of these patients had an intravesical ureterocele, and 5 of them (23%) required a secondary open procedure. Of the 29 patients with an ectopic ureterocele, 14 (48%) required a secondary open procedure. For ectopic ureteroceles, these authors recommended puncture of the intravesical component just proximal to the bladder neck and omission of the puncture of the urethral component of the ureterocele. Of note, none of the nine intravesical single-system ureteroceles that were endoscopically punctured required a secondary open procedure. Nineteen of the 51 patients had iatrogenic reflux, and 7 went on to ureteral reimplantation. **Ben Meir and coworkers (2004) reviewed**

published data for incision and puncture of ureteroceles and found no significant difference in de novo reflux between the two decompression techniques.

Endoscopic puncture of the ureterocele is nearly uniformly successful at achieving decompression (91%) in the experience of Chertin and colleagues (2003). In regard to reflux, 59% of patients with reflux had spontaneous resolution after puncture of the ureterocele. However, 35 of 52 patients underwent a secondary procedure (9 nephrectomies, 10 upper pole nephrectomies, 15 endoscopic treatments of reflux, and 1 ureteral reimplantation).

Stated another way, 60% or more of children will need no further procedures after endoscopic decompression of a ureterocele, which is a 15-minute outpatient procedure with almost no morbidity. This argument sways many urologists to choose endoscopic decompression as the first line of surgical treatment in many cases of ureteroceles.

However, there is an opposing school of thought that perhaps ureterocele incision is not quite as effective and should not be employed as the initial approach in the majority of ureteroceles. This disaffection with transurethral incision appears to be directed more toward the ectopic ureterocele than the intravesical ureterocele. Husmann and associates (1999) treated 25 patients with intravesical ureteroceles with endoscopic decompression; only 3 required a second procedure (2 for failed decompression and 1 for reflux into the ureterocele). Two patients were treated with repeat endoscopy, and the patient with reflux was treated with ureteral reimplantation. There appeared to be no difference in the success rate whether the decompression was achieved via ureterocele puncture or via ureterocele incision. However, in regard to ectopic ureteroceles, the incision was markedly less successful. If the ectopic ureterocele was associated with no reflux, only 36% of the patients were spared a second procedure. If the ureterocele was associated with grade III reflux or greater, then only 16% required no further surgery. The upper pole nephrectomy had no better success in this group of patients with high-grade preoperative reflux.

Pfister and associates (1998) **also observed a difference in the success of ureterocele incision based on the type of ureterocele (i.e., intravesical vs. ectopic).** Of the 16 intravesical ureteroceles incised, only 1 required a second procedure. Of the 21 patients with ectopic ureteroceles, 4 required a second procedure for incomplete decompression, 7 required reoperative surgery for preoperative reflux that persisted in all 7 patients, and 8 patients required ureteral reimplantation for reflux into the ureterocele that did not resolve in follow-up ranging from 12 to 36 months. Therefore, although incision of the ectopic ureterocele appeared to be mostly successful in regard to decompression, it did not achieve the goal of correcting preexisting reflux, and it resulted in a significant incidence of reflux into the ureterocele itself (30%). The authors did note, however, that there were 14 patients whose upper pole was subtended by a ureterocele that was presumed to have no preoperative function. Of these, 10 had return of function to the upper pole (as seen by intravenous pyelogram) after ureterocele incision.

In contrast, in Castagnetti and associates' series (2004) **approximately half of patients required a secondary surgical procedure after endoscopic compression irrespective of their ureteroceles being intravesical or ectopic.**

Husmann and coworkers (1999) concluded that neither transurethral incision nor upper pole nephrectomy adequately addresses the needs of patients with an ectopic ureterocele and significant reflux, and lower tract complete reconstruction may be the optimal approach. Shekarriz and associates (1999) also expressed a lack of enthusiasm for the transurethral incision of ectopic ureteroceles. The intravesical ureteroceles that were incised in their series had an acceptable reoperative rate of only 23%. All 13 patients with ectopic ureteroceles that were cystoscopically incised needed secondary procedures. The reoperative rate in the literature for ectopic ureteroceles treated with upper pole nephrectomy varies but can be as high as 62% (Caldamone et al, 1984; Rickwood et al, 1992; Husmann et al, 1995). Their success rate with upper pole nephrectomy for the ectopic ureterocele associated with preoperative high-grade reflux was only 47%. They therefore concluded that endoscopic incision has a limited application and should be used only in cases of intravesical ureteroceles or ectopic ureteroceles causing bladder outlet obstruction and sepsis. However, for the ectopic ureterocele with significant preoperative reflux, they believed that patients are best served by complete lower tract reconstruction. This is defined as

ureterocelectomy and ureteral reimplantation. They treated 18 patients who had an ectopic ureterocele with this approach (of whom 83% had preoperative reflux), and none required secondary surgery. Approximately half of their patients were operated on before 1 year of age, and all of the patients were continent on follow-up. They believed that their experience refuted the commonly held notion that lower tract reconstruction for ureterocele in the young child is fraught with complications and should be avoided.

We have endoscopically incised ureteroceles in selected cases. In our experience, ureterocele incision resulted in partial or complete decompression of all ureteroceles (Fig. 116–36). More importantly, the radiographic appearance of the upper tract improved in 20 of 22 cases (Fig. 116–37). Five of 12 children who had reflux into the ipsilateral lower pole had their reflux resolve after ureterocele incision, and three others had their reflux decrease in grade. Transurethral incision of the ureterocele resulted in reflux into the ureterocele ureter in 44% of the cases; this induced reflux was equivalent for ectopic and intravesical ureteroceles as well as single and duplicated systems. One third of the patients underwent a second operative procedure, primarily for reflux. One could

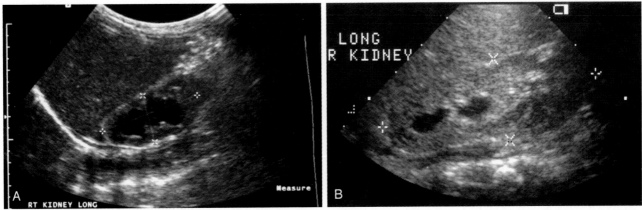

Figure 116–36. **A,** Sonographic appearance of right upper pole hydronephrosis secondary to a ureterocele. **B,** Same patient 3 months after cystoscopic incision of ureterocele; the upper pole has been significantly decompressed.

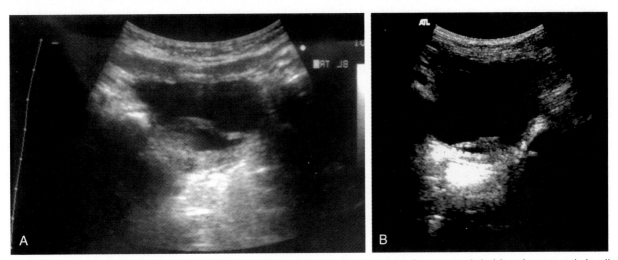

Figure 116–37. **A,** Sonogram of a ureterocele 3 months after cystoscopic incision. **B,** Ten months after cystoscopic incision, the ureterocele is collapsed. (Bladder volume is the same in both images.)

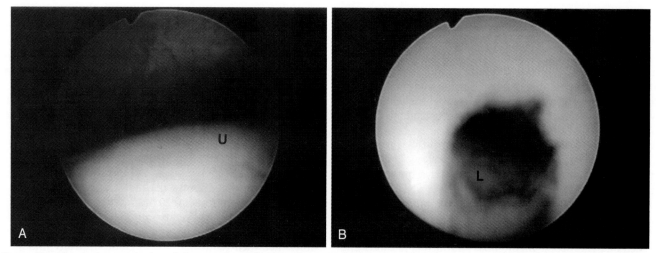

Figure 116–38. **A,** Cystoscopic view of the smooth-walled dome of a ureterocele (u) with the bladder cavity in the distance. **B,** Magnified cystoscopic view of the ureterocele and its lumen (L) after endoscopic puncture of the ureterocele.

argue that this minimally invasive outpatient procedure is of benefit to the remainder of the patients who require no further surgery. If future reimplantation surgery is performed, the ureter is less dilated and easier to manipulate.

We have made several observations based on our experience with transurethral incisions of ureteroceles. When performing routine cystoscopy in a female patient, it is acceptable to blindly pass the cystoscope sheath and obturator into the bladder via the urethra. However, blind passage of a cystoscope in a child with a ureterocele may result in a tearing of the ureterocele. Therefore, we pass the cystoscope under direct vision. In addition, we try to instill a minimum of irrigation so as not to collapse the ureterocele. The entire bladder is inspected to ascertain the position of the ipsilateral lower pole ureteral orifice and the contralateral ureteral orifice.

Our preferred method of incising the ureterocele is similar to the one described by Rich and colleagues (1990): a transverse incision through the full thickness of the ureterocele wall using the cutting current. Making the incision as distally on the ureterocele and as close to the bladder floor as possible lessens the chance of postoperative reflux into the ureterocele. One can either use a Bugbee electrode or the metal stylet of a ureteral catheter, which is extended just beyond the catheter. We favor the latter instrument because it has a finer tip and allows for more precision. The No. 3 Fr straight and angle-tipped wires are also acceptable for ureterocele incision.

The ureterocele should be incised deeply, because ureteroceles are often thick walled. Adequacy of ureterocele incision is confirmed either by the escape of a jet of urine from the ureterocele or by viewing the urothelium of the inside of the ureterocele (Fig. 116–38). For the ectopic ureterocele that extends into the urethra, several people advocate either a longitudinal incision that extends down from the intravesical portion into the urethral portion or two separate punctures, one in the intravesical portion of the ureterocele and one in the urethral portion of the ureterocele.

If reflux occurs in the upper pole or persists in the lower pole, the reflux can be managed with subureteric injections

(Diamond and Boston, 1987; Yachia, 1993), although the anticipated success is likely to be low.

Coplen and Austin (2004) described an interesting subset of patients with ureteroceles and multicystic dysplastic kidneys in the associated upper tract segment. This group had either low-grade or no reflux and no ureteral dilatation. These prenatally diagnosed patients were managed nonoperatively and had a benign clinical course.

Single-System Ureteroceles

Although the single-system ureterocele usually manifests in adults, it is sometimes seen in children. The ureterocele in these cases is almost always intravesical and occupies the proper trigonal position. Although most single-system ureteroceles have obstructing pinpoint orifices, unobstructed ureteroceles do exist. The degree of obstruction is probably not significant in most adult cases and likewise tends to be less severe than the obstruction seen in duplicated systems in children (Sen et al, 1992).

The ureterocele may vary from a tiny cystic dilatation of the submucosal ureter to a large balloon that fills the bladder. Histologically, the wall of the ureterocele contains varying degrees of attenuated smooth muscle bundles and fibrous tissue. The ureterocele is covered by vesical mucosa and lined with ureteral mucosa.

Most children with simple ureteroceles present with symptoms of urinary tract infection. Prenatal ultrasonography has detected other, asymptomatic cases. Stasis and infection predispose the patient to stone formation in the ureterocele and upper urinary tract. Rarely, large simple ureteroceles prolapse through the bladder neck, causing urinary obstruction.

Excretory urography often demonstrates the characteristic cobra-head (or spring-onion) deformity, an area of increased density similar to the head of a cobra with a halo or less dense shadow around it (Fig. 116–39). The halo represents a filling defect, which is the ureterocele wall, and the oval density is contrast medium excreted into the ureterocele from the functioning kidney. Larger ureteroceles often fail to fill early with contrast material, resulting in a sizable filling

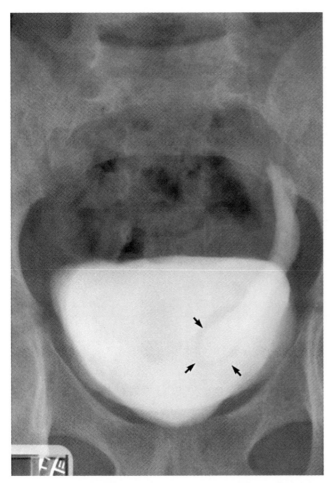

Figure 116–39. Contrast material in the ureterocele from a functioning renal unit looks like a cobra head on the intravenous pyelogram because of the filling defect of the ureterocele wall.

contrast to the grapelike cluster that typifies rhabdomyosarcoma (see Fig. 116–25). The color may vary from pink to bright red to the necrotic shades of blue, purple, or brown. The ureterocele usually slides down the posterior wall of the urethra, and therefore the urethra can be demonstrated anterior to the mass and can be catheterized. The vagina (and the corresponding masses that emanate from it, such as hydrometrocolpos) is posterior to the ureterocele.

The prolapse can be intermittent and may cause vesical obstruction and, consequently, bilateral renal obstruction. Alternatively, the child may be able to void around the ureterocele. In the former scenario, the patient may have varying degrees of hydronephrosis and azotemia and may be septic.

The short-term goal is to decompress the ureterocele. The prolapsing ureterocele may be manually reduced back into the bladder, but, even if this is successful, the prolapse is likely to recur. Upper pole nephrectomy (as previously described) combined with aspiration of the ureterocele from above is usually effective in achieving decompression. However, this decompression may not occur rapidly enough in the acutely ill child. In an effort to decompress the ureterocele rapidly, one can make a transverse incision in the ureterocele at the level of the vagina. Because the wall of the ureterocele may be thick, the incision should be appropriately deep. This maneuver is not uniformly successful because the bladder neck in its resting state is closed and this may keep the intravesical ureterocele, which is proximal to the point of incision and proximal to the bladder neck, distended.

Therefore, if interlabial incision is not effective, endoscopic incision of the ureterocele in its intravesical portion may be necessary. If all these measures fail and the child remains in extremis, open surgical unroofing or marsupialization of the ureterocele is indicated. Common sheath ureteral reimplantation to correct the ensuing reflux can be carried out on an elective basis when the child is older.

Ureteral Stenosis and Stricture

Congenital anatomic narrowing or narrowing of the ureteral lumen as detected by calibration is referred to as congenital ureteral stenosis or congenital ureteral stricture, but developmentally the term *stricture* should refer only to obstructions involving a histologic lesion in the ureter. Cussen (1971), in his series of 147 ureteral lesions, noted 81 (55%) with ureteral stenosis. His histologic studies of the stenotic zone revealed normal transitional epithelium, a diminished population of otherwise normal-appearing smooth muscle cells, and no increase in fibrous tissue in the wall of the stenotic zone. Ultrastructural studies were not conducted.

The cause of congenital ureteral stenosis is not certain, but ultrastructural studies such as those of Notley (1972) and Hanna and associates (1976, 1977) may provide the answer. Developmentally, simple narrowing probably results from a disturbance in embryogenesis around the 11th to 12th weeks, with disturbed development of the mesenchyme contributing to the ureteral musculature (Allen, 1977). A spectrum of histologic abnormalities, with or without demonstrable anatomic narrowing, may occur at the zone of obstruction (Hanna et al, 1976). **Three areas of the ureter are particularly liable to ureteral stenosis. In order of decreasing frequency, they are the ureteropelvic junction, the distal ureter just**

defect in the bladder. These findings are associated with varying degrees of hydronephrosis and hydroureter. The upper urinary tract changes associated with a simple ureterocele are usually not as severe as those associated with an ectopic ureterocele. At cystoscopy, the ureterocele usually expands rhythmically with each peristaltic wave that fills it and then shrinks as a thin jet of urine drains, usually continuously, through the small orifice.

Single-system ureteroceles more readily lend themselves to transvesical excision and reimplantation, with any muscular defect corrected as necessary. **These ureteroceles are also more amenable to endoscopic incision** (Rich et al, 1990) and are less likely to exhibit postoperative reflux into the incised ureterocele.

Prolapsing Ureteroceles

A ureterocele that extends through the bladder neck and the urethra and presents as a vaginal mass in girls is termed a *prolapsing ureterocele* (Orr and Glanton, 1953). This mass can be distinguished from other interlabial masses (e.g., rhabdomyosarcoma, urethral prolapse, hydrometrocolpos, periurethral cysts) by virtue of its appearance and location (Witherington and Smith, 1979; Nussbaum and Lebowitz, 1983). The prolapsed ureterocele has a smooth, round wall in

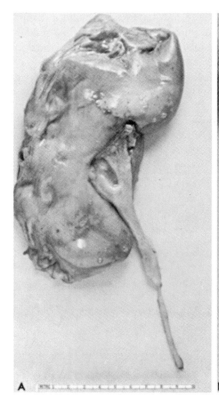 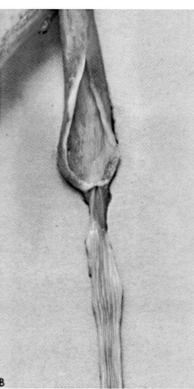

Figure 116–40. Congenital ureteral valve. **A,** Extended view. **B,** Long section showing greatly dilated ureter above the valve and normal size below. (From Simon HB, Culp OS, Parkhill EM, et al: Congenital ureteral valves: Report of two cases. J Urol 1955;74:336.)

above the extravesical junction, and, rarely, the mid ureter at the pelvic brim (Allen, 1970; Campbell, 1970). More than one area of segmental stenosis may be present in the same ureter, with a widened length of ureter between the segments, suggesting a developmental defect that affects the entire ureteric bud.

The clinical manifestations and treatment of ureteral stenosis and stricture involving the ureteropelvic junction are included in the section on ureteropelvic junction obstruction.

Ureteral Valves

Ureteral valves are uncommon causes of ureteral obstruction, consisting of transverse folds of redundant mucosa that contain smooth muscle (Wall and Wachter, 1952). These are single annular or diaphragmatic lesions with a pinpoint opening (Figs. 116–40 and 116–41). The ureter is dilated above the obstruction and normal below it. As determined in a review of 40 congenital ureteral valves, the valves are distributed throughout the length of the ureter, although least commonly in the middle third or the pelviureteral junction (Dajani et al, 1982). Presenting symptoms include flank pain, urinary tract infection, incontinence, hypertension, and hematuria. The valves appear to occur equally in boys and girls and equally on the right and left sides (Sant et al, 1985).

Transverse, nonobstructing mucosal folds are present in 5% of ureters in newborns and gradually disappear with growth (Wall and Wachter, 1952). They may be one of the normal findings described by Östling (1942) and by Kirks and associates (1978). Cussen (1971, 1977) identified what he termed ureteral valves in 46 of 328 abnormal ureters from infants and children at surgery or at autopsy. Unlike the

diaphragmatic valves described previously, these are cusps that can be demonstrated by perfusing the upper ureter with fixative, dilating the lumen, flattening the mucosa, and accentuating the valves. In a patient with valvular obstruction, Cussen noted that the long axis of the distal ureter was eccentric relative to the long axis of the dilated proximal segment, with the fold being an eccentric cusp (Fig. 116–42). He also noted that these flaps could be found in the presence of a normal or stenotic distal ureter. In Cussen's series of 328 intrinsic ureteral lesions, there were 24 primary valves with no distal obstruction. A total of 19 valves were reported to be associated with a more distal obstruction.

Others have observed ureteral obstructions from eccentric cusps, believed to be distinct from secondary folds and kinks associated with ureteral dilation and elongation (Maizels and Stephens, 1980; Gosalbez et al, 1983). The cusp need not contain smooth muscle (Gosalbez et al, 1983; Reinberg et al, 1987). However, Williams (1977) believed that eccentric obstructing valves may be more infrequent than Cussen reported. Many of the apparent valves may be artifacts of distention because the dilated ureter at its junction with the undilated segment assumes a kinked and eccentric position resulting from elongation and pull of the surrounding adventitia.

In summary, diaphragmatic annular valves are a rare, although definite, form of ureteral obstruction. Eccentric, cusplike flaps or folds can be obstructing, but they can also be secondary to the elongation and tortuosity that occurs with ureteral distention at the site of an underlying anatomic or functional obstruction. It has been postulated that several of these anomalies may appear transiently in utero and may be responsible for the milder forms of hydronephro-

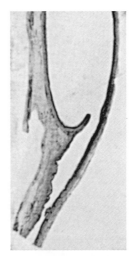

Figure 116–42. A 12-year-old girl with obstructing distal congenital ureteral valve in an ectopic, duplicated ureter. (Courtesy of Dr. Laurence R. Wharton.)

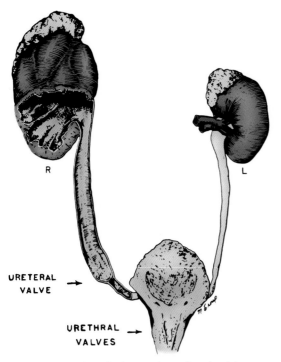

Figure 116–41. Complete diaphragm obstructing the right ureter, with hydroureter and hydronephrosis above. (From Roberts RR: Complete valve of the ureter: Congenital urethral valves. J Urol 1956;76:62.)

sis that are found postnatally to be nonobstructive. If the lesion is in fact obstructive, an intravenous pyelogram and a retrograde pyelogram should be obtained, because these studies deliver the most complete anatomic information about the ureter. Resection of this obstructing lesion with primary reanastomosis is then curative. The involved kidney may be devoid of significant function and require nephrectomy (Sant et al, 1985).

Spiral Twists and Folds of the Ureter

Campbell (1970) observed this anomaly only twice in 12,080 autopsies of children (Fig. 116–43). He ascribed it to failure of the ureter to rotate with the kidney. This explanation may be simplistic, because the illustration shows more than one twist. Obstruction and hydronephrosis may result from spiral twists. The condition may arise from one of a number of possible persistent manifestations of normal fetal upper ureteral development, as described by Östling (1942) (Fig. 116–44; see also Fig. 116–43). These manifestations include ureteral mucosal redundancy and apparent folds and convolutions that may have a spiral appearance. Occasionally, ureteral convolutions that are enclosed by investing fascia persist as a form of ureteropelvic obstruction (Gross, 1953).

Persistent fetal folds were described in a previous paragraph. An isolated single fold or kink demonstrated radiographically with an otherwise normal upper urinary tract may be acquired, nonobstructing, and reversible and represents acute or intermittent elongation of the ureter with distal obstruction or reflux. Campbell (1970) believed that isolated primary obstructing congenital kinks could occur as an uncommon disorder, but the example he presented did not

demonstrate convincing obstruction. Nevertheless, this sort of deformity is often one manifestation of ureteropelvic junction obstruction in association with ensheathment by dense fibrous bands (Gross, 1953).

Ureteral Diverticula

Diverticula of the ureter have been classified by Gray and Skandalakis (1972) into three categories: (1) abortive ureteral duplications (blind-ending bifid ureters), discussed later; (2) true congenital diverticula containing all tissue layers of the normal ureter; and (3) acquired diverticula representing mucosal herniations. Congenital diverticula are very uncommon and have been reported as arising from the distal ureter above the ureterovesical junction, mid ureter, and ureteropelvic junction (Culp, 1947; McGraw and Culp, 1952). These diverticula can become very large, and secondary hydronephrosis can ensue. The patient may present with abdominal pain or renal colic and a palpable cystic mass. McGraw and Culp's patient, a 64-year-old woman, had a cystic lesion at surgery, extending from under the right costal margin to the pelvic brim.

A typical diverticulum in a 20-year-old man is shown in Figure 116–45. Even small diverticula may be symptomatic. Sharma and coworkers (1980) reported on two patients with repeated infections and a girl with intermittent colic. Fluoroscopy in the second patient demonstrated stasis and peristaltic dysfunction with back-and-forth ureter-to-diverticulum reflux. She was cured by diverticulectomy.

As discussed in the section on blind-ending duplications, congenital diverticula below the level of the ureteropelvic junction arise from premature cleavage of the ureteric bud with abortive development of the accessory limb. Those from the ureteropelvic junction region arise from primitive calyceal formation that similarly failed to encounter metanephric tissue (Gray and Skandalakis, 1972).

Single acquired diverticula may be associated with strictures or calculi and may occur after trauma (Culp, 1947). Multiple diverticula that are small (5 mm) have been ascribed to the

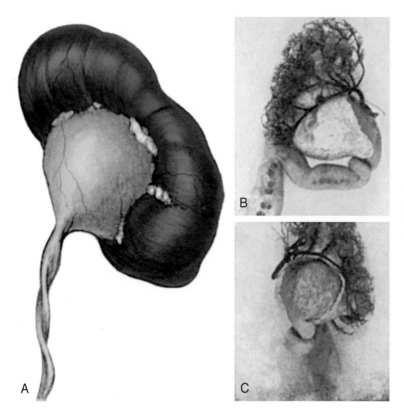

Figure 116–43. Torsion (spiral twists) of the ureter. **A,** Torsion observed in an infant at autopsy. There is secondary hydronephrosis. **B** and **C,** Corrosion specimens from late fetal life: anterior view and lateral view from pelvic aspect. (Courtesy of Dr. Karl Östling.)

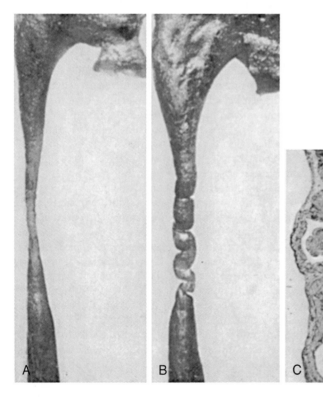

Figure 116–44. Embryologic considerations in the genesis of ureteral folds, kinks, and strictures. **A,** Cast of the ureter and the renal pelvis in a newborn. There is physiologic narrowing of the upper ureter, below which is the normal main spindle of the ureter. No ureteral folds are present. **B,** Cast of the ureter and the renal pelvis in the newborn. The ureteral folds proceed alternately from the opposite sides. **C,** Ureteral kinks that appear as muscular folds with axial offshoots of the loose adventitia. (Courtesy of Dr. Karl Östling; from Campbell MF: In Campbell MF, Harrison JH [eds]: Urology, 3rd ed. Philadelphia, WB Saunders, 1970, vol 2.)

effect of chronic infection (Holly and Sumcad, 1957; Rank et al, 1960). However, Norman and Dubowy (1966) reported two cases of multiple diverticula that were demonstrable by retrograde ureteropyelography. Such lesions, demonstrable only by supraphysiologic pressures, may be congenital variants with weaknesses of the ureteral wall rather than acquired conditions (Hansen and Frost, 1978). However, the published reports do not contain histologic observations to support either hypothesis. Large diverticula usually can be removed without sacrificing the kidney.

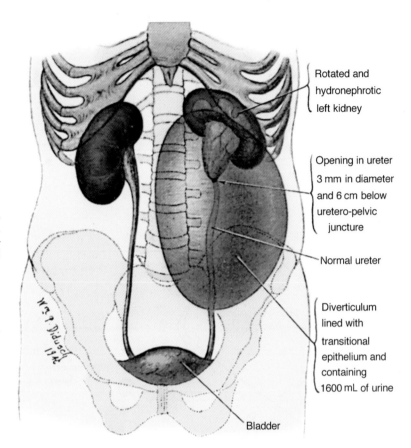

Figure 116–45. Congenital diverticulum of left ureter containing 1600 mL of urine. The kidney was hydronephrotic. (From Culp OS: Ureteral diverticulum: Classification of the literature and report of an authentic case. J Urol 1947;58:309.)

Labels on figure:
Rotated and hydronephrotic left kidney

Opening in ureter 3 mm in diameter and 6 cm below uretero-pelvic juncture

Normal ureter

Diverticulum lined with transitional epithelium and containing 1600 mL of urine

Bladder

ANOMALIES OF NUMBER

The reported incidence of ureteral duplication varies widely in different series, depending in part on whether the survey was based on autopsy or clinical data and on the composition of patient material and on whether bifid pelves were separately recorded (Fig. 116–46). Because it is generally recognized that clinical series usually contain a disproportionate number of duplication anomalies, unselected autopsy data are more accurate in predicting the true incidence. At least two large autopsy series have provided data not too dissimilar regarding partial and complete ureteral duplication (Nation, 1944; Campbell, 1970). **Combining Nation's autopsy series and Campbell's adult series, the projected incidence of duplication is 1 in 125, or 0.8%.**

Despite a wealth of information about gender differences in the incidence of duplication in clinical series (the anomaly is identified in women at least two times more frequently than in men), there are no reliable data on gender differences in unselected series. Campbell's autopsy data do not document such a difference. Of Nation's 109 autopsy cases, 56 were female and 53 male. However, only 40% of the 16,000 autopsies were performed in women. Calculating a correction for this difference, one could project a female-to-male ratio of 1.6:1. These statistics, however, may not be reliable in view of the small number of cases recorded.

Nevertheless, clinical and autopsy data are in substantial agreement about other aspects of duplication (Table 116–2). **Unilateral duplication occurs about six times more often than bilateral duplication, with the right and left sides being involved about equally.** Excluding bifid pelvis, there does not appear to be a difference in the literature in the incidence of bifid ureter versus double ureters. A small percentage of individuals with bilateral duplications have a mixed condition, such as bifid ureter on one side and double ureters on the other.

Genetics

Evidence exists that duplication may be genetically determined by an autosomal dominant trait with incomplete penetrance (Cohen and Berant, 1976). **In parents and siblings of probands with duplication, the incidence of duplication increases from the predicted 1 in 125 to 1 in 8** (Whitaker and Danks, 1966) **or 1 in 9** (Atwell et al, 1974). Two reports of geographic foci suggest that environmental factors can also play a role (Philips et al, 1987; Barnes and McGeorge, 1989).

Position of Orifices

In double ureters, the two orifices are characteristically inverted in relation to the collecting systems they drain. The orifice to the lower pole ureter occupies the more cranial and lateral position, and that of the upper pole ureter has a caudal and medial position (see Fig. 116–11). As mentioned previously, this relationship is so consistent that it has been termed the *Weigert-Meyer law*. When the two orifices are not immediately adjacent, the orifice from the upper pole can be found anywhere along a predictable pathway, which Stephens (1958, 1963) called the ectopic pathway.

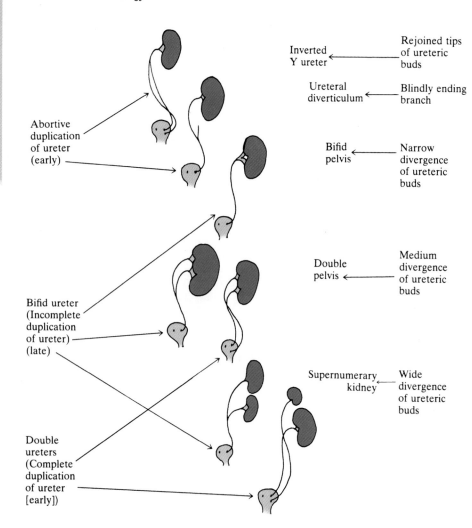

Inverted Y ureter ← Rejoined tips of ureteric buds

Ureteral diverticulum ← Blindly ending branch

Bifid pelvis ← Narrow divergence of ureteric buds

Double pelvis ← Medium divergence of ureteric buds

Supernumerary kidney ← Wide divergence of ureteric buds

Abortive duplication of ureter (early)

Bifid ureter (Incomplete duplication of ureter) (late)

Double ureters (Complete duplication of ureter [early])

Figure 116–46. Gradations in ureteral and kidney duplications. (From Gray SW, Skandalakis JE [eds]: Embryology for Surgeons. Philadelphia, WB Saunders, 1972.)

Rare exceptions to the Weigert-Meyer law have been observed, in which the upper pole orifice is cranial, although it is still medial to the orthotopic orifice. Stephens (1958) collected four examples from the literature and added seven more. Stephens studied the positional relationship between the lower portions of the ureters and noted that it, too, varies according to the terminal position of the upper pole orifice. With the rare cranially placed upper pole orifice, the ureter lies anterior to the lower pole ureter, with the ureters being uncrossed. With a medial orifice the upper pole ureter lies medially, and with a caudally placed orifice it spirals in an anterior-to-medial direction around the lower pole ureter as it descends, terminating posterior to the lower pole orifice. Ahmed and Pope (1986) documented a case of uncrossed complete ureteral duplication and reflux into the upper pole, which fits this pattern.

An embryonic hypothesis to explain the exception to the Weigert-Meyer law was proposed by Stephens (1958) and is based on the premise that an upper pole orifice located craniomedially arises from a junctional ureteric bud, one that bifurcated immediately, rather than from a second bud.

Associated Findings

The distribution of the renal mass drained by each ureter in duplication varies somewhat. On average, about one third of the renal parenchyma is served by the upper collecting system. In a detailed radiographic review, Privett and associates (1976) reported a number of observations about duplication. **The mean total number of calyces for single-system kidneys was 9.4, and for duplex units it was 11.3, with a mean of 3.7 calyces in the upper collecting system and 7.6 in the lower collecting system.** These investigators also observed that 97% of the single-system kidneys in their series were radiographically normal, whereas 29% of the duplex units had scarring or dilatation, or both. Reflux also was more common in the duplex units in patients who had voiding cystograms. Two (12%) of 17 nonduplex units generated reflux, compared with 13 (42%) of 31 duplex units.

Hydronephrosis of the lower pole segment is not infrequent and is generally associated with severe reflux into that unit. However, primary ureteropelvic junction obstruction can involve the lower pelvis (Dahl, 1975; Christofferson and Iversen, 1976; Privett et al, 1976).

Other anomalies are encountered with increased frequency. In Nation's (1944) series, 27 (12%) had other urinary tract anomalies, with just over half of these being on the same side. The anomalies included renal hypoplasia and aplasia (today these conditions would probably be termed *dysplasia*) and various ureteral anomalies, among them ectopic insertion of the upper pole ureter in four cases (3% of the complete duplications). Coexisting urologic anomalies were encountered in

116–2. Ureteral Duplication: Clinical, Radiographic, and Autopsy Studies

Study	Database	No. Duplications	F	M	Unilateral	Bilateral	Complete	Partial	Unilateral Complete/Partial	Bilateral Complete/Partial	Bilateral Mixed
Archangelskj, 1926	110	R 619 / A 3 (2.7%)			502 (80%)	117 (20%)					
Colosimo, 1938	1,500	X 50 (3.3%)	88 (6.8%)								
Nation, 1944	16,000	A 109 (0.68%) / C 121	*(63%) / 88 (73%)	* / 33	177 (77%)	53 (23%)	102 (44%)	118 (51%)	78 (44%)/99 (56%)	35 (45%)/19 (36%)	10 (4.3%)
Nordmark, 1948	4,744	X 138 (2.8%)			119 (86%)	19 (14%)	70 (51%)	65 (47%)	59/60	11/5	3 (2.1%)
Payne, 1959		C 141	87 (62%)	54	120 (85%)	21 (15%)	45	78 + 18 bifid pelvis			
Johnston, 1961	5,000	X 83 / C 73 / A 9	57 (70%)	25			63 (77%)	19 (33%)			
Kaplan and Elkin, 1968	(Partial duplications only)	X 51	33 (65%)	18	43 (84%)	8 (16%)					
Campbell, 1970	51,880 (19,046 children) (32,834 adults)	A 342 (0.65%) / 61 (0.32%) / 281 (0.85%)			293 (85%)	53 (15%)	101 (30%)			4	"1 in 5 cases"
Timothy et al, 1971		C 46	39 (85%)	7			24 (52%)	16 (35%)	13/15	11/1	
Privett et al, 1976	5,196 (1,716 children; 3,480 adults [2,896 male; 2,300 female])	X 91 (1.8%)	63 (66%)	32	79 (85%)	16 (15%)	33 (29%) (but 21 not known)	57 (52%)			6 (13%)

A, autopsy; C, clinical; R, review; X, X-ray.
*See text.

29 of Campbell's (1970) series of 342 duplications. Nonurologic anomalies were found in 63 cases. These were not recorded in detail, but most of the urologic anomalies were, as in Nation's series, a variety of ipsilateral renal and ureteral lesions; 22 were anomalies of the contralateral kidney. The nonurologic lesions mainly involved the gastrointestinal tract plus a few cardiopulmonary lesions. However, both of these were autopsy series. Rarely, the pelvicalyceal systems communicate, presumably from later fusion of the ureteric buds during pelvicalyceal expansion (Braasch, 1912; Beer and Mencher, 1938).

The increased incidence of duplications in investigations of childhood urinary tract infections is well established. Campbell (1970) reported a personal series of 1102 children with pyuria, 307 of whom proved to have ureteropelvic anomalies. Of these, 82 (27%) had duplications, or 7.5% of the total group. Kretschmer (1937) reviewed 101 cases of hydronephrosis in infancy and childhood and noted 24 nonureteral anomalies, more than half of which were duplications.

Based on three cases of duplication with some form of ureteral ectopy, coexistent renal dysplasia, and nodular renal blastema, Cromie and colleagues (1980) raised the possibility that this pattern of findings might be more than a coincidental association, accounting for an increased risk of neoplasm (Pendergrass, 1976). This concept deserves further investigation.

Bifid ureter is often clinically unimportant, but stasis and pyelonephritis do occur. When the Y junction is extravesical, free to-and-fro peristalsis of urine from one collecting system to the other may appear, with preferential retrograde waves passing into slightly dilated limbs instead of down the common stem. This results in stasis that is more marked when the Y junction is more distal, when the bifid limbs are wide, or when the Y junction is large. Increased urinary reprocessing from vesicoureteral reflux may enhance this phenomenon, and loin pain can result. About one fourth of the patients studied with nuclear renography by O'Reilly and coworkers (1984) had significant urodynamic abnormalities. Treatment by ureteroneocystostomy is effective when the junction is sufficiently close to the vesical wall that resection of the common sheath or common stem permits placement of both orifices within the bladder. Reimplantation of the common stem may be effective when vesicoureteral reflux is severe and the Y junction is higher up.

Blind-Ending Duplication of the Ureter

Rarely, a ureteral duplication does not drain a renal segment, hence the term *blind ending*. Most blind-ending ureteral duplications involve one limb of a bifid system; even more unusual is one involving complete duplication (Szokoly et al, 1974; Jablonski et al, 1978). Although the Y junction in the bifid type may be at any level, most are found in the mid or distal ureter. Blind-ending segments are diagnosed three times more frequently in women than in men and twice as often on the right side (Schultze, 1967; Albers et al, 1971). The condition has been reported in twins (Bergman et al, 1977) and in sisters (Aragona et al, 1987). Many of these blind segments

cause no problems. Symptomatic patients most often complain of vague abdominal or chronic flank pain, sometimes complicated by infection or calculi, or both (Marshall and McLoughlin, 1978). The majority of cases are not diagnosed until the third or fourth decade of life.

Because the blind segment does not always fill on excretory urography, retrograde pyelography may be required for diagnosis (Fig. 116–47). This may be the cause of the pain (van Helsdingen, 1975). Because the lesion is more common in women and on the right side, the propensity for dilation of the right urinary tract with pregnancy might explain the relatively late onset of symptoms.

The embryogenesis of blind-ending ureteral duplication is similar to that for duplications in general. It is postulated that the affected ureteric bud is abortive and fails to make contact with the metanephros. Histologically, the blind segment contains all normal ureteral layers. The blind end tends to have a bulbous dilation. Most of these blind segments

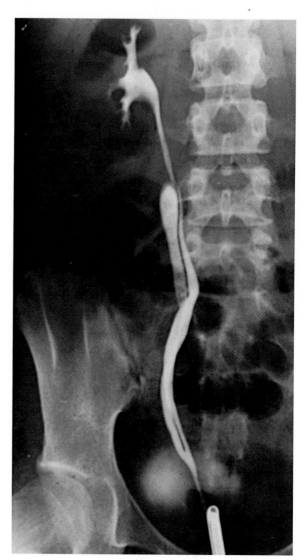

Figure 116–47. Retrograde pyelogram. Blind-ending duplication in an 18-year-old girl was noted in evaluation of transitory hematuria. Only the distal portion of this blind-ending duplication has been visualized on intravenous pyelogram.

are not surrounded by any abortive renal tissue, but in a few segments there is a fibrous stalk (ureteral atresia) extending into a dysplastic renal segment. The blind limb may vary from a short stump of a few centimeters to one extending all the way into the renal fossa.

The area of union between the two limbs is invested in a common sheath that may be attenuated proximally. The blind segment and the adjacent normal ureter share a common blood supply (Albers et al, 1968; Peterson et al, 1975). When surgery is necessary, excision of the blind segment is indicated. Because the ensheathment is less dense at the upper or proximal end, the dissection should start there. Care should be taken to denude only the blind segment and not to enter the normal ureter. Some investigators suggest leaving a short stump at the junction with the common stem (Peterson et al, 1975; Rao, 1975).

Diverticula of the ureter have also been described. Controversy exists in the literature about the distinction between some diverticula and blind-ending duplications. In most cases, it may simply be a matter of terminology. For example, Campbell (1936) described a case of a finger-like extension from the lower ureter that he called a ureteral diverticulum, but he ascribed it developmentally to an abortive duplication. Similarly, Youngen and Persky (1965) labeled as a diverticulum a tubular, finger-like appendage from the pelvis but also ascribed its origin to an abortive budding. Rank and coworkers (1960) and Gray and Skandalakis (1972) agreed that congenital ureteral diverticula have the same embryogenesis as blind duplications. Gray and Skandalakis specifically noted that a diverticulum from the ureteropelvic area represents a primitive calyx that has failed to meet nephrogenic mesenchyme. Sarajlic and colleagues (1989) believed that all of these lesions could be described as congenital diverticula.

For some investigators, the distinction between a diverticulum and a blind-ending ureter is one of morphology. The typical blind-ending ureteral segment of a Y ureter joins the normal ureter at an acute angle and extends upward parallel to the normal ureter. It is at least twice as long as it is wide (Culp, 1947). A congenital diverticulum, in comparison, has a ballooned appearance. Histologically, both are similar and both arise from disordered ureteric budding. Additional descriptions of ureteral diverticula were presented in a previous section.

Inverted-Y Ureteral Duplication

This is the rarest of the anomalies of ureteral branching. It consists of two ureteral limbs distally that fuse proximally to become a single channel draining the kidney. This condition is more common in females than in males. **One of the distal ureteral limbs not uncommonly ends in an ectopic ureter or ureterocele** (Klauber and Reid, 1972; Beasley and Kelly, 1986; Harrison and Williams, 1986; Mosli et al, 1986; Ecke and Klatte, 1989). In several cases, one distal segment was atretic (Britt et al, 1972; Suzuki et al, 1977). In one case of bilateral inverted-Y duplication in a 12-year-old girl, there was an atretic distal limb on each side, each with a calculus (Suzuki et al, 1977).

The embryology of inverted-Y ureteral duplication is ascribed to two separate ureteric buds whose tips coalesce and fuse into a single duct before joining the metanephros. The frequently ectopic position of one limb is caused by widely separated buds on the mesonephric duct, with the second bud relatively cephalad. To explain the distal atresia of the ectopic limb in their case, Britt and associates (1972) offered two possibilities. One was failure of Chwalle's membrane to rupture. The second, also postulated by Hawthorne (1936), was atresia of the wolffian duct's normal regression in the female before absorption of the too cephalad second ureteric bud into the urogenital sinus distally. Bingham (1986) reported on a woman with a single right ureter that divided into two segments and then rejoined, showing the features of a bifid ureter distally and an inverted-Y proximally. He postulated that the ureteric bud split after migration began and then re-fused before entering the metanephros. Treatment, usually resection of the accessory channel, is directed toward any problems that result from an ectopic limb.

Ureteral Triplication and Supernumerary Ureters

Just as two buds from the mesonephric duct or premature fission of a single bud can explain double and bifid ureters, so the presence of three buds from the mesonephric duct or two with early fission of one of them can explain the rarely encountered complete and partial triplications (Marc et al, 1977). Most investigators use the classification of Smith (1946), who distinguished four varieties of triplicate ureter:

Complete triplication: three ureters from the kidney, with three draining orifices to the bladder, urethra, or elsewhere.

Incomplete triplication: a bifid ureter plus a single ureter, with three ureters from the kidney and two orifices draining below.

***Trifid ureter:* all three ureters unite and drain through a single orifice; this appears to be the most common form encountered.**

Two ureters from the kidney, one becoming an inverse Y bifurcation, resulting in three draining orifices below.

In one apparently unique case, Fairchild and associates (1979) reported a typical bifid system with a third, lateral ureter that appeared to communicate with the lower pole calyx.

Triplication has been reported with renal fusion anomalies (Pode et al, 1983; Golomb and Ehrlich, 1989). Patients with triplication also may, of course, present with symptoms and signs of reflux and obstruction, ureterocele (Arap et al, 1982; Finkel et al, 1983; Rodo Salas et al, 1986; Juskiewinski et al, 1987), or ectopia, as in duplication anomalies. Treatment is based on the same principles as for duplication anomalies.

ANOMALIES OF POSITION
Vascular Anomalies Involving the Ureter

A variety of vascular lesions can cause ureteral obstruction. With these lesions, the vascular system rather than the urinary system is anomalous. With the exception of accessory renal blood vessels, all of these lesions are relatively uncommon, although all have clinical relevance.

Accessory Renal Blood Vessel

Accessory or aberrant vessels to the lower pole of the kidney can cross ventral to the ureteropelvic junction, causing obstruction.

Preureteral Vena Cava

Anatomy. This anomaly is commonly known to urologists as circumcaval or retrocaval ureter, terms that are anatomically descriptive but misleading in regard to development (Lerman et al, 1956; Dreyfuss, 1959; Peisojovich and Lutz, 1969). In the case reported by Dreyfuss, there was also a small branch vein between the vena cava and right iliopsoas muscle, over which (cephalad to it) the ureter coursed to enter the retrocaval area. **The term *preureteral vena cava* emphasizes that the circumcaval ureter results from altered vascular, rather than ureteral, development. This is the more accurate term.**

This disorder involves the right ureter, which typically deviates medially behind (dorsal to) the inferior vena cava, winding about and crossing in front of it from a medial to a lateral direction, to resume a normal course, distally, to the bladder. The renal pelvis and upper ureter are typically elongated and dilated in a J or fishhook shape before passing behind the vena cava (Fig. 116–48). However, the collecting system is not inevitably obstructed. Bateson and Atkinson (1969), Crosse and associates (1975), and Kenawi and Williams (1976) classified circumcaval ureters into two clinical types: (1) the more common type I has hydronephrosis and a typically obstructed pattern demonstrating some degree

of fishhook-shaped deformity of the ureter to the level of the obstruction, and (2) type II has a lesser degree of hydronephrosis or none at all. Here, the upper ureter is not kinked but passes behind the vena cava at a higher level, with the renal pelvis and upper ureter lying almost horizontal before encircling the vena cava in a smooth curve. In type I, the obstruction appears to occur at the edge of the iliopsoas muscle, at which point the ureter deviates cephalad before passing behind the vena cava. In type II, the obstruction, when present, appears to be at the lateral wall of the vena cava as the ureter is compressed against the perivertebral tissues.

Embryology. The definitive inferior vena cava develops on the right side from a plexus of fetal veins (Fig. 116–49). Initially, the venous retroperitoneal pathways consist of symmetrically placed vessels, both central and dorsal. The posterior cardinal and supracardinal veins lie dorsally, and the subcardinal veins lie ventrally. These channels, with their anastomoses, form a collar on each side through which the ascending kidneys pass. Normally, the left supracardinal veins and the lumbar portion of the right posterior cardinal vein atrophy. The subcardinal veins become the internal spermatic veins. The definitive right-sided inferior vena cava forms from the right supracardinal vein. **If the subcardinal vein in the lumbar portion fails to atrophy and becomes the primary right-sided vein, the ureter is trapped dorsal to it.**

When the definitive vena cava forms normally and the ventral portion of the primitive ring also persists, a double right vena cava is formed because of the persistence of both

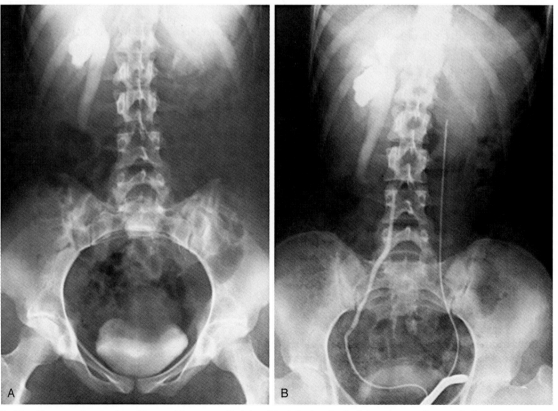

Figure 116–48. Circumcaval ureter in a 20-year-old woman with intermittent flank pain. **A,** Intravenous pyelogram. **B,** Retrograde ureteropyelogram.

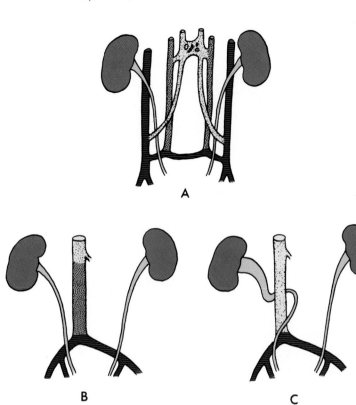

Figure 116–49. Fetal venous ring (**A**), normal vena cava (**B**), and preureteric vena cava (**C**). (Redrawn from Hollinshead WH: Anatomy for Surgeons. New York, Hoeber Medical Division of Harper & Row, 1956, vol 2.)

■ Posterior cardinal v.   ▨ Supracardinal v.   ▨ Subcardinal v.

the right subcardinal vein dorsally and the right subcardinal vein ventrally. This double vena cava traps the right ureter between its limbs (Fig. 116–50) (Gruenwald and Surks, 1943; Sasai et al, 1986).

Although bilateral vena cava or left-sided vena cava can occur (Clements et al, 1978; Mayo et al, 1983), a bilateral circumcaval ureter has been described in a case of situs inversus (Brooks, 1962). In cases of bilateral vena cava associated with a circumcaval ureter, the circumcaval ureter has been reported only on the right side, denoting that the right vena cava developed abnormally from a persistent subcardinal vein, whereas the left vena cava developed from the left supracardinal vein but otherwise normally (Pick and Anson, 1940).

Incidence. The incidence of preureteral vena cava at autopsy is about 1 in 1500 (Heslin and Mamonas, 1951), and the anomaly is three to four times more common in male than in female cadavers. Gray and Skandalakis (1972) considered this frequency to be too high because of the preponderance of male autopsies performed, but the 4:1 male-female ratio appears to be seen clinically as well (Xiaodong et al, 1990).

Kenawi and Williams (1976), in reviewing the literature, recorded 114 male and 41 female patients. The symptoms of preureteral vena cava are those of obstruction. **Although the lesion is congenital, most patients do not present until the third or fourth decade of life** (Kenawi and Williams, 1976).

Diagnosis. Clinically, patients may present with symptoms of flank or abdominal pain or infection or the disorder may be discovered incidentally during other radiologic tests. Excretory urography often fails to visualize the portion of

the ureter beyond the J hook (i.e., extending behind the vena cava), but retrograde ureteropyelography demonstrates an S curve to the point of obstruction (see Fig. 116–48), with the retrocaval segment lying at the level of L3 or L4 (Kenawi and Williams, 1976). Cavography is no longer a necessary diagnostic test.

Ultrasound (Schaffer et al, 1985; Murphy et al, 1987) and CT or MRI also have been useful in defining the vascular malformation. When necessary, CT may be the procedure of choice to confirm the diagnosis and avoid retrograde ureteropyelography (Hattori et al, 1986; Sasai et al, 1986; Murphy et al, 1987; Kellman et al, 1988). Helical CT (which is quite useful in visualizing ureteral stones) can demonstrate the course of the ureter. Nuclear renal furosemide scanning can categorize the anomaly as obstructed or nonobstructed (Pienkny et al, 1999). **MRI can nicely demonstrate the course of a preureteral vena cava and may be a more detailed and less invasive imaging modality when compared with CT and retrograde pyelography** (Uthappa et al, 2002).

Treatment. Briefly, surgical correction involves ureteral division, with relocation and ureteroureteral or ureteropelvic reanastomosis, usually with excision or bypass of the retrocaval segment, which can be aperistaltic. It is important to be mindful of the ureter's blood supply from the renal artery and aorta superiorly and the iliac vessels inferiorly (Hellsten et al, 1980). This blood supply must be preserved during the ureteral dissection. As stated earlier, the preferred approach for the obstructed ureter is ureteral division and relocation; however, in the case of a solitary kidney, division

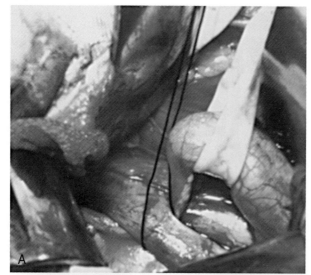

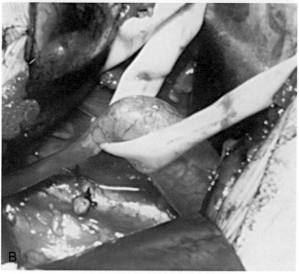

Figure 116–50. A 4-year-old boy presented with right ureteral obstruction from a double right vena cava. The site of obstruction is apparent distally, because the ureter lies between the ventral and dorsal limbs of the double cava. Intraoperative photographs were taken before (**A**) and after (**B**) division of the ventral limb.

of the anomalous inferior vena cava and its reposition behind the ureter may be contemplated. Laparoscopic reconstruction of the preureteral vena cava has been described both via the transperitoneal and retroperitoneal approaches (Bhandarkar et al, 2003; Ramalingam and Selvarajan, 2003; Tobias-Machado et al, 2005).

Other Anomalies of Position

Several instances of horseshoe kidney have been reported (Cukier et al, 1969; Cendron and Reis, 1972; Eidelman et al, 1978; Heffernan et al, 1978; Kumeda et al, 1982; Taguchi et al, 1986). Anomalies include a variety of left renal anomalies, such as agenesis, hydronephrosis, malrotation, and hypoplasia (Kenawi and Williams, 1976). There has been one case of left hydronephrosis with ensheathing of both ureters by a single fibrous membrane below the level of the venous anomaly

(Salem and Luck, 1976). An obstructing branch of the right spermatic vein has mimicked circumcaval ureteral obstruction (Psihramis, 1987), as has an anomalous tendon of the iliopsoas muscle (Guarise et al, 1989).

Preureteral Iliac Artery (Retroiliac Ureter). A ureter coursing behind the common iliac artery is rare (Dees, 1940; Corbus et al, 1960; Seitzman and Patton, 1960; Hanna, 1972; Iuchtman et al, 1980; Radhkrishnan et al, 1980). Either side can be involved; in two cases, the condition was bilateral (Hanna, 1972; Radhrishnan et al, 1980). Obstruction occurs at the level of L5 or S1 as the ureter is compressed behind the artery. Coexisting anomalies are common (Nguyen et al, 1989).

Gray and Skandalakis (1972) believed that this condition was vascular in origin. Normally, the primitive ventral root of the umbilical artery is replaced by development of a more dorsal branch between the aorta and the distal umbilical artery. Persistence of the ventral root as the dorsal root fails to form traps the ureter dorsally (Fig. 116–51). Dees (1940) also considered the possibility that aberrant upward migration of the kidney in the case he reported might have placed it dorsal to the iliac artery, which was redundant.

Ureteral or mesonephric duct ectopia is often present. In Dees' case, there was evidence, although not definite proof, that the ureteral orifice was ectopic in the vesical neck, supporting the concept of anomalous renoureteral development. The case of Seitzman and Patton (1960) involved an ectopic ureter that emptied, along with the ipsilateral vas deferens, via a persistent common mesonephric duct into the proximal posterior urethra. In the case of Radhrishnan and colleagues (1980), bilateral retroiliac ureters also involved bilateral ectopic termination of the vasa deferentia into the ureters. Iuchtman and associates (1980) described ectopic vaginal termination of the involved ureter, with urometrocolpos from an imperforate hymen.

Taibah and coworkers (1987) reported the unusual finding of left ureteral obstruction from a retrointernal iliac artery ureter in an otherwise normal young woman.

Vascular Obstruction of the Distal Ureter. Obstruction of the distal ureter from uterine, umbilical, obturator, and hypogastric vessels close to the bladder has been described (Hyams, 1929; Campbell, 1933, 1936, 1970; Greene et al, 1954; Young and Kiser, 1965; Scultety and Varga, 1975). However, it is not always clear that vascular impressions on a dilated ureter are the cause of the obstruction. At times, these findings may be an artifact, as when a dilated ureter from an intrinsic obstruction is secondarily compressed against the adjacent vessel (Campbell, 1970). Judging from the paucity of contemporary reports describing this lesion, it is likely that primary terminal ureteral obstruction by vascular lesions is a rare occurrence.

Herniation of the Ureter. Herniation of the ureter is another extremely rare condition. Dourmashkin (1937) searched the literature and tabulated a series of inguinal, scrotal, and femoral herniations of the ureter. Most of these were paraperitoneal, that is, a loop of herniated ureter extended alongside a peritoneal hernial sac. Only a minority were extraperitoneal (i.e., with no hernial sac present). In paraperitoneal ureteral hernias, the ureteral loop is always medial

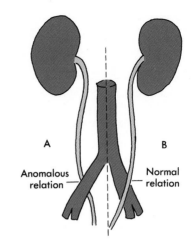

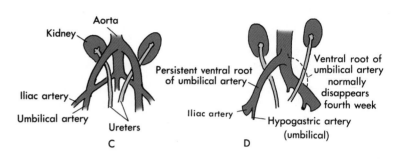

Figure 116–51. Preureteral iliac artery (postarterial ureter). **A,** Anomalous relationship of ureter and artery. **B,** Normal relationship of ureter and artery. **C,** Relationships between the ureter and the iliac and umbilical arteries in the embryo. **D,** Development of a normal iliac channel on the right and an anomalous iliac channel (persistence of proximal umbilical artery) on the left. (From Gray SW, Skandalakis JE [eds]: Embryology for Surgeons. Philadelphia, WB Saunders, 1972.)

to the peritoneal sac. Of six scrotal hernias, four did not have peritoneal sacs. When the ureter extended into the scrotum, it was more likely to be dilated, causing upper tract obstruction.

Watson (1948) collected 102 cases of inguinal or femoral hernia involving the ureter. Jewett and Harris (1953) described a case of left ureteral hernia into the scrotum in a 9-year-old boy with left hydronephrosis (Fig. 116–52). This hernia was of the extraperitoneal type: a mesentery-like blood source supplied two loops of ureter within the scrotum that were adherent to the cord structures. Powell and Kapila (1985) reported a unique case of a 1-week-old male infant with bilateral megaureters presenting as a left inguinal hernia. The loop of the dilated left ureter was lateral, in the inguinal canal, to an incomplete hernial sac.

Dourmashkin (1937) believed that herniation of the ureter could be acquired or congenital, with the acquired form being a so-called sliding hernia and the congenital form being present since birth. In the latter form, he proposed that the loop of ureter had been drawn down with the descent of the testis and the developing ureter had adhered to the migrating vas.

Internal hernias of the ureter are even more exceptional. Reports have been published of a sciatic hernia containing a ureter—one of which was diagnosed by CT in an elderly woman (Lindblom, 1947; Beck et al, 1952; Oyen et al, 1987)—and of herniation between the psoas muscle and iliac vessels (Page, 1955).

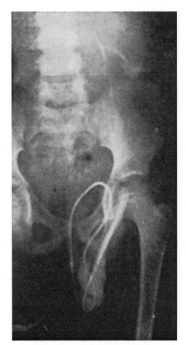

Figure 116–52. A 9-year-old boy with herniation of the left ureter into the scrotum. No hernial sac is present. The obstructed system was treated by ureteral resection and reanastomosis. (Courtesy of Dr. Hugh J. Jewett.)

KEY POINTS: ECTOPIC URETER, URETEROCELE, AND OTHER ANOMALIES OF THE URETER

- An intravesical ureterocele is one that sits entirely within the bladder. An ectopic ureterocele is one that extends to the bladder neck or urethra.

- Ureteral ectopy occurs when the ureteric bud arises more proximally than normal on the mesonephric duct.

- The Weigert-Meyer rule of complete ureteral duplication states that the lower pole orifice is more cranial and lateral to the caudad, medial upper pole orifice.

- In the male, the posterior urethra is the most common site of termination of an ectopic ureter. The symptoms of an ectopic ureter in a male are related to infection and obstruction.

- In the female, an ectopic ureter can drain into the vagina, uterus, cervix, or fallopian tubes. The urethra and vestibule are the most common sites of female ectopic ureter drainage.

- Continuous incontinence in a girl with an otherwise normal voiding pattern after toilet training is the classic symptom of an ectopic ureteral orifice.

SUGGESTED READINGS

Chertin B, de Caluwe D, Puri P: Is primary endoscopic puncture of ureterocele a long-term effective procedure? J Pediatr Surg 2003;38:116-119; discussion 116-119.

Glassberg KI, Braren V, Duckett JW, et al: Suggested terminology for duplex systems, ectopic ureters and ureteroceles. J Urol 1984;132:1153.

Malek RS, Kelalis PP, Stickler GB, et al: Observations on ureteral ectopy in children. J Urol 1972;107:308.

Mandell J, Bauer SB, Colodny AH, et al: Ureteral ectopia in infants and children. J Urol 1981;126:219-222.

Pfister C, Ravasse P, Barret E, et al: The value of endoscopic treatment for ureteroceles during the neonatal period. J Urol 1998;159:1006-1009.

Scherz HC, Kaplan GW, Packer MG, et al: Ectopic ureteroceles: Surgical management with preservation of continence: Review of 60 cases. J Urol 1989;142:538.

Shekarriz B, Upadhyay J, Fleming P, et al: Long-term outcome based on the initial surgical approach to ureterocele. J Urol 1999;162:1072-1076.

Stephens FD: Caecoureterocele and concepts on the embryology and aetiology of ureteroceles. Aust N Z J Surg 1971;40:239.

Upadhyay J, Bolduc S, Braga L, et al: Impact of prenatal diagnosis on the morbidity associated with ureterocele management. J Urol 2002;167:2560-2565.

Xiaodong Z, Shukun H, Jichuan Z, et al: Diagnosis and treatment of retrocaval ureter. Eur Urol 1990;18:207.

117 Reflux and Megaureter

ANTOINE KHOURY • DARIUS J. BÄGLI

INTRODUCTION

Vesicoureteral reflux (VUR) represents the retrograde flow of urine from the bladder to the upper urinary tract. VUR is a common clinical entity. Its clinical challenges arise from the fact that it is usually asymptomatic. When it is not, however, it is responsible for pyelonephritic scarring and can be associated with congenital renal dysmorphism. There are many unresolved issues regarding the etiology, diagnosis, and management of VUR. This chapter attempts to reconcile some of these areas by interpreting the best available information in the literature. Some areas, however, will continue to await more rigorous study. Some may remain unresolved for quite some time.

HISTORICAL PERSPECTIVE

VUR has a unique distinction of having evolved from an anatomic curiosity around the first century AD into one of the most contentious and complex areas of urology today. Galen and da Vinci made the first references to VUR by Western medicine when they alluded to the ureterovesical junction (UVJ) as a mediator of unidirectional flow of urine from the kidneys to the bladder. Even though VUR was first demonstrated to be a normal finding in dogs and rabbits (Semblinow, 1907), it was a gynecologic misadventure that revealed that VUR in human adults may not be a normal state (Pozzi, 1893). Sampson, in 1907, suggested that the oblique course of the ureter through the bladder wall created a locking mechanism at the UVJ, and he was also the first to imply that VUR might lead to renal infection. Although it was not possible to uniformly demonstrate VUR in all people in cadaveric studies (Young, 1898), it was not until the UVJ had been more clearly dissected that it was realized that the incidence of VUR varied with the length of the ureter's obliquity in the bladder and the formation of the trigone (Gruber, 1929).

Pivotal discoveries occurred in 1952, when Hutch reported on a relationship between VUR and chronic pyelonephritis in paraplegic patients (Hutch, 1952), and in 1959, with Hodson's observation that urinary tract infection (UTI) and renal scarring carried a high likelihood of VUR in children (Hodson, 1959).

Two seminal bodies of work defined the modern era of VUR. The first, the work of Ransley and Risdon (1979), defined the pathophysiology of reflux nephropathy by demonstrating the relationship between infection, reflux, and pyelonephritic scarring. Second, these observations complemented the clinical studies of Jean Smellie and coworkers, who galvanized the related concepts inherent in clinical UTI, bacterial pyelonephritis, renal scarring, and VUR. In 1985, a consensus system for the grading of reflux was published by Lebowitz and colleagues based on deliberations of the International Reflux Study Group.

Until recently, the virtues of medical therapy to avert infection and surgical therapy to correct reflux itself had been evenly debated for over 20 years. However, recent introduction of the biodegradable cross-linked polysaccharide dextranomer and stabilized hyaluronic acid for use in injectable endoscopic correction of reflux, as well as reexamination of the basis for medical therapy and the risks associated with reflux, has single-handedly triggered a reevaluation of virtually all aspects of reflux. From the age-related impact of reflux through the use of antibiotics for medical prophylaxis, the invasiveness of cystography, and the traditional indications for surgery, the impact of reflux and its management are being openly explored today. Although the fundamental biologic importance of reflux disease is not in question, many facets of how diagnosis and management of reflux are approached may take new shape in the coming decade.

DEMOGRAPHICS
Prevalence

The tendency for VUR to resolve spontaneously on the one hand or persist beyond its natural resolution rate because of abnormal bladder dynamics makes it difficult to confidently generalize the true prevalence of reflux from a given population. In one meta-analysis of studies of children undergoing cystography for various indications (Sargent, 2000), the prevalence of reflux was estimated to be approximately 30% in children with UTI and 17% in those without infection. **In contrast, reflux may be present in up to 70% of infants with UTI** (Baker et al, 1966). In a population of 157 adults investigated for incidental hypertension without any evidence of renal abnormality, the prevalence of VUR was estimated to be 19%, with high-grade reflux being present in more than half the refluxing group (Barai et al, 2004). Reflux is relatively uncommon in men (Chapple et al, 1990). In asymptomatic infants monitored for antenatal hydronephrosis, the prevalence of reflux ranged from 15% in infants with absent or mild hydronephrosis on postnatal ultrasound (Phan et al, 2003) to 38% in a group of neonates with various postnatal upper tract sonographic anomalies, including hydronephrosis, renal cysts, and renal agenesis (Zerin et al, 1993).

KEY POINTS: DEMOGRAPHICS

- The younger the child with UTI, the greater the likelihood of discovering reflux.
- VUR is relatively rare in children of African descent.

Gender

Differences in reflux rates between males and females may suggest a sexual dichotomy in the function of the lower urinary tract, bladder outlet, and urethra. In a study of 117 infants assessed for reflux after fetal upper tract dilation, 76% of refluxing infants were male (Ring et al, 1993). In later life, the likelihood of having reflux if a UTI is present is higher in males than females (Shopfner, 1970), even though the great majority (85%) of prevailing reflux in older children occurs in females. A confounding factor in understanding true gender differences in reflux between males and females is the gender-driven predisposition to UTI. Uncircumcised male infants have a 12-fold greater risk for UTI than circumcised infants, as well as a greater propensity for harboring periurethral uropathogenic flora (Wiswell et al, 1988; Wiswell and Hachey, 1993). The greater incidence of UTI will necessarily invite more frequent evaluation and therefore detection of VUR in this population. It is not known whether the incidence of reflux detection would rise in females if they were to be incidentally evaluated for reflux as often as male infants are. In a related finding, only 10% of patients entered in to the International Reflux Study in Children from the United States were boys as compared with 24% entered from Europe. The circumcision rate in the latter group was only 5%, versus 62% in the U.S. group ($P < .001$) (Weiss et al, 1992b).

Reflux in the Fetus

Most studies of fetal reflux do not in fact detect reflux per se in the fetus but relate fetal hydronephrosis parameters to reflux in the neonatal period. However, fetal hydronephrosis is common, often resolves, and has low specificity for postnatal VUR. Nevertheless, fetal hydronephrosis is commonly associated with postnatally detected reflux. Zerin et al (1993) reported a 38% detection rate of reflux in 130 neonates with prenatal hydronephrosis. In 19%, the reflux was bilateral. It is suggested that the lower the threshold for defining hydronephrosis (in millimeters of pelvic diameter) in the fetus, the more often reflux will be detected postnatally (Anderson et al, 1997). If this reasoning were pursued to the extreme and the hydronephrosis threshold were reduced to zero (i.e., no hydronephrosis), even more reflux would be expected postnatally. This leads to speculation regarding whether reflux is a normal variant in the population but becomes clinically relevant only in some because of a predisposition to UTI, a conclusion supported by the observation that reflux without infection is often of little clinical significance. Boys appear to harbor postnatal reflux more commonly, with a 6:1 male-to-female ratio being reported in one study of 27 cases (Marra et al, 1994). The highest grades of reflux are most commonly associated with renal scintigraphic abnormalities. In many cases, even in the absence of any history of infection from birth, the presence of a small kidney with globally reduced scintigraphic function my indicate that renal dysplasia is the developmental result of a ureteral bud abnormality associated with high-grade reflux or secondary to the reflux itself (Oliveira et al, 1998; Stock et al, 1998).

Age

As stated previously, because the natural history of reflux involves spontaneous resolution over time, it is self-evident that reflux would be less prevalent in older children than in infants (Table 117–1). Even in the presence of infection or asymptomatic bacteriuria, reflux is more common in younger patients (Smellie, 1991).

Race

Little is known about racial predisposition to reflux worldwide because reflux studies have generally been restricted to Western countries. **One difference established over several**

Table 117–1. Incidence of Reflux in Patients with Urinary Tract Infections	
Age (yr)	Incidence (%)
<1	70
4	25
12	15
Adults	5.2

From Baker R, Maxted W, Maylath J, et al: Relation of age, sex, and infection to reflux: Data indicating high spontaneous cure rate in pediatric patients. J Urol 1966;95:27.

studies is the relative 10-fold lower frequency of reflux in **female children of African descent** (Skoog and Belman, 1991; Chand et al, 2003). In addition, reflux resolved sooner in this population ($P < .005$). In a series of children of color with a 4:1 male-to-female ratio, 58% of whom were younger than 1 year and had UTI (72%), voiding difficulties (10%), or other malformations (14%), reflux was present in only 10% (West and Venugopal, 1993). Even in follow-up of antenatal hydronephrosis, reflux was found in 17.6% of 51 nonblack versus 0% of 58 black infants (Horowitz et al, 1999). Such differences may involve a delay in maturation of the antireflux mechanism in white patients inasmuch as the race-associated frequency of reflux becomes equal regardless of race after 10 years of age (Melhem and Harpen, 1997).

INHERITANCE AND GENETICS
Sibling Reflux

A recent meta-analysis of sibling reflux studies suggests the prevalence of VUR in siblings to be approximately 32% (Hollowell and Greenfield, 2002). However, the prevalence may be as low as 7% in older siblings (Connolly et al, 1996) or as high as 100% in identical twin siblings (Kaefer et al, 2000). **The latter finding undeniably supports the notion that VUR can be an inherited condition** and that the genetic mode of transmission may be autosomal dominant. Although a heightened prevalence of reflux exists in siblings of refluxing index patients, the natural history of reflux would suggest that siblings who are older harbor reflux less often than do relatively younger siblings because of spontaneous resolution of reflux (Connolly et al, 1996). However, none of the existing sibling studies rigorously state whether the prevalence of sibling reflux is dependent on whether the sibling is younger or older than the index patient. By virtue of its detection via screening, sibling reflux is usually asymptomatic at the time of diagnosis. Furthermore, the tendency for reflux to have resolved before any renal changes such as focal scarring detected by imaging can be reliably ascribed to the reflux itself further complicates the management of reflux in siblings. These clinical features underscore the difficulties inherent in formulating meaningful recommendations for the management of sibling reflux detected by screening.

Much of the concern for sibling reflux detected by screening stems from reports of renal abnormalities identified by ultrasound or nuclear scintigraphy in these patients. In a retrospective study of 123 screened siblings, 44 (36%) demonstrated VUR on voiding cystography (Houle et al, 2004).

Thirty-seven of these patients underwent renal imaging. Ultrasound findings were abnormal in 30%, and renal scintigraphy, when performed, was abnormal in 28%. However, in siblings older than 2 years, renal scintigraphic abnormalities were twice as common as in the entire group of siblings. The authors concluded that renal damage was therefore progressive in the older siblings and proposed earlier screening in siblings of refluxing index patients. However, this study fails to address the fact that renal damage or aberrant formation may have occurred very early and may appear progressive only when imaged beyond 2 years of age. Scintigraphic results may become exaggerated by normal cortical growth surrounding a scarred region that has failed to grow or by compensatory hypertrophy of a contralateral kidney. **The missing link is a prospective scintigraphic or sonographic follow-up of asymptomatic refluxing sibling children from birth onward.** Finally, the reporting of scintigraphic results by many sibling reflux studies is confounded by failure to differentiate between congenital dysplasia secondary to the aberrant renal development often associated with higher grades of reflux and true scarring secondary to infection and inflammation. Moreover, the ability to modulate the course of processes that mediate congenital dysplasia is not possible presently, as it is with scarring. In the absence of such data and faced with the invasive nature of the gold standard test for reflux—cystography—one is left with the following questions.

Is asymptomatic reflux in a sibling of clinical concern? If the propensity for UTI itself, with or without VUR, could be reliably determined to be genetically regulated, it would strengthen the case for screening for reflux in a sibling. Because the propensity for biologic infection cannot be reliably determined in either index patients or their siblings, the mere likelihood of development of a UTI cannot be used to support screening siblings for reflux. Therefore, one must rely on the aggregate clinical information available for the sibling in question. **Because it is the renal consequences of reflux that are at issue rather than reflux itself, siblings may be better served by noninvasive screening for cortical abnormalities first before screening for reflux itself.** The intensity of renal assessment, using ultrasound for general screening or a nuclear scan for highest accuracy, could then be tempered by clinical factors, including family history, patient and family compliance with follow-up, blood pressure, and a history of UTI, fever, and voiding dysfunction. The absence of renal structural abnormalities would allow the clinician to conclude that reflux, if present, has not yet been of any renal consequence.

Should screening depend on sibling age? Because the risk for new renal scarring after pyelonephritis is low in children older than 5 years, older siblings would probably suffer fewer consequences from recent reflux-induced pyelonephritis and therefore stand to benefit less from confirming a diagnosis of reflux and instituting antibiotic prophylaxis than would an infant or younger sibling. Nevertheless, a history of untreated febrile infections would support a decision to consider renal assessment or even obtain a cystogram in an older sibling.

Thus, by imaging the kidneys first, followed by assessing the integrity of the UVJs, a rational top-down approach to sibling reflux screening emerges. Such an approach helps strike a balance between avoiding the invasive nature of reflux detection and the classic commitment to prophylaxis versus failing to detect existing renal cortical abnormalities that might be the result of past or ongoing reflux. If consideration of age and renal integrity are combined, a possible graded approach to screening can be developed for siblings older or younger than 5 years, with or without renal structural abnormalities. The proximate urologic and voiding history must also play a deciding role in whether a sibling is ultimately screened by cystography for VUR. Thus, in siblings 5 years or older with normal kidneys, little would be gained from detecting reflux that could not be addressed by responding to a febrile UTI in the usual fashion as for the general pediatric population. Indeed, the knowledge that the index patient has VUR might heighten attention to family or self-reporting regarding urinary symptoms in older siblings. In siblings 5 years or older with renal abnormalities, the suggestion would be of past or continuing reflux. Ruling the diagnosis in or out by cystography could then depend on the prevailing voiding habits and proximate urologic history. Management of a sibling younger than 5 years with normal kidneys would be based on clinical judgment regarding the likelihood for infection rather than an immediate need to diagnose reflux. A sibling younger than 5 years with renal cortical defects would have the most to lose by a febrile infection in the face of reflux and the attendant risk for additional cortical loss after reflux-induced pyelonephritis triggered by an infection. In this case, knowledge of the potentially higher prevalence of reflux in siblings would logically support obtaining a screening cystogram. In any sibling, if reflux is diagnosed, the indications for correction of reflux remain the same as for the general refluxing pediatric population.

KEY POINTS: INHERITANCE AND GENETICS

- The prevalence of reflux is higher in siblings.

- There is a tendency for an autosomal dominant pattern of inheritance.

- Probably many genes are involved.

- It cannot be assumed that all cortical abnormalities in refluxing siblings are acquired. The lack of prospective studies should temper the notion of mass screening of siblings.

Genes Involved

In addition to sibling reflux, a prospective screen of the progeny of refluxing patients revealed a 66% rate of reflux in the offspring (Noe et al, 1992), which further strengthens the notion of an autosomal dominant component to the genetic mechanism of reflux. The substantially higher rate of reflux in the siblings and progeny of index patients than in the general population defines these patients as susceptible to renal morbidity. Segregation and linkage analysis has implicated a number of loci in the pathogenesis of VUR, although no specific gene product or functional role of these loci in reflux has yet been identified (Chapman et al, 1985; Feather et al, 2000). Several studies have used a morphogenetic approach to search for candidate genes that may underlie VUR. The original ureteral budding studies of Mackie and Stephens, in which the position of ureteral budding from the mesonephric (wolffian) duct was correlated with that of the final ureteral orifice, provide a modern basis for a genetic interpretation of VUR. Several genes have been observed to regulate these developmental processes and, by extension, are believed to serve as potential regulators of UVJ integrity. Indeed, genetic misregulation of ureteral budding is believed to underlie many congenital anomalies of the kidney and urinary tract (often referred to as CAKUT) (Miyazaki and Ichikawa, 2003). *PAX2* is a transcription factor regulating kidney, central nervous system, and ocular development in mice. It is necessary for ureteric budding in mice (Keller et al, 1994). *PAX2* is located on human chromosome 10q, and mutations have been reported in human syndromes involving colobomas and renal anomalies, including hypoplasia, dysplasia, glomerulonephritis, and VUR (Sanyanusin et al, 1995). However, *PAX2* has not been shown to be a major determinant of primary VUR (Choi et al, 1998; Cunliffe et al, 1998). Glial-derived neurotrophic factor (GDNF) and its receptor RET show strong involvement in UVJ formation in mice (Yu et al, 2004). Overexpression of RET in mice leads to abnormal placement of the ureteral bud and is associated with a 30% incidence of VUR at birth versus 4% in wild-type mice. Nevertheless, the GDNF-RET signaling complex has not been found to mediate VUR in humans (Shefelbine et al, 1998). Another fascinating animal model of VUR is observed after depletion of the uroplakin III gene (*UPK3*) (Hu et al, 2000). However, no structural *UPK3* gene alterations have been noted in human cohorts with VUR (Giltay et al, 2004; Jiang et al, 2004). One explanation for this current finding may be that major uroplakin mutations are developmentally lethal in humans. Finally, members of the renin-angiotensin family of proteins have been implicated in several renal and ureteral developmental anomalies, including ureteropelvic junction (UPJ) obstruction and megaureter (Hohenfellner et al, 1999). Although associations between angiotensin receptor 2 (*AGTR2*) (Yoneda et al, 2002) and angiotensin-converting enzyme (*ACE*) (Liu et al, 2004) genes with VUR have been sought, no definitive etiologic link with VUR has been found. Notwithstanding an observed pattern of autosomal dominant inheritance in some families, the failure to identify any strong genetic mechanism in primary VUR in humans despite the presence of convincing animal genetic models of reflux argues for a more complex polygenetic mechanism of disease in humans.

EMBRYOLOGY OF THE URETEROVESICAL JUNCTION

A full discussion of the embryology of the trigone and ureteric orifice is found elsewhere in this text. In brief, two events proceed simultaneously to govern the ultimate position and integrity of the UVJ. At one point, the embryonic ureter buds from the mesonephric or wolffian duct to define the metanephric duct or early fetal ureter. The wolffian duct (early vas deferens) and early ureter can be thought of as forming the two upper arms of a "Y," with the distal mesonephric duct being the stem of the "Y." While budding is occurring, the distal mesonephric duct is being drawn and incorporated into the region of the urogenital sinus (UGS), which later becomes the bladder. Incorporation continues until the entire stem is absorbed, with the two arms of the "Y" left to enter the bladder separately: one as the ureter and the other as the vas and ejaculatory duct in the male prostatic urethra or the vestigial Gartner duct in the female vagina. The two arms of the "Y" also rotate relative to each other once they contact the UGS/bladder wall such that the ureteral orifice is located proximal to the ejaculatory duct orifice. If the ureteral bud reaches the UGS too soon (believed to be due to early budding), overrotation draws it high and lateral in the bladder wall and leads to inadequate incorporation, insufficient intramural length in the bladder wall, and reflux (Mackie et al, 1975). If the ureteral bud reaches the UGS too late (because of budding late), insufficient rotation occurs and results in an ectopic ureter that is drawn distally and medially, often causing obstruction in the bladder neck region or elsewhere. Furthermore, early or late budding is also thought to mistarget the contact between bud epithelium and the metanephros and lead to renal malformations, dysplasia, hypoplasia, or even agenesis. Indeed, the association between vasal and renal agenesis would be explained by agenesis of the wolffian duct; with no source for the ureteral bud, no tissue can combine with the mesonephros to trigger kidney formation.

FUNCTIONAL ANATOMY OF THE ANTIREFLUX MECHANISM

The phenomenon of VUR represents a balance of several factors. Abnormality in any of these factors alone or in combination will allow or cause retrograde flow of urine from the bladder up the ureter and ultimately to the renal pelvis and

tubules. These factors include functional integrity of the ureter, anatomic composition of the UVJ, and functional compliance of the bladder.

First, for purposes of reflux prevention, the ureter represents a dynamic conduit that adequately propels the urine presented to it in a bolus fashion, antegrade, by neuromuscular propagation of peristaltic activity. In so doing, reflux is actively opposed. Moreover, if reflux were to occur, depending on its degree and timing, antegrade flow might be expected to keep refluxing urine from reaching the renal pelvis. The second component is the anatomic design of the UVJ. At the heart of this unique mechanism lies an intramural portion of ureter that travels within the detrusor muscle as it traverses the bladder wall (Fig. 117-1) (Elbadawi, 1972). At the extravesical bladder hiatus, the three muscle layers of the ureter separate. The outer ureteral muscle merges with the outer detrusor muscle to form Waldeyer's sheath. The latter contributes to formation of the deep trigone. The intramural ureter remains passively compressed by the bladder wall during bladder filling to prevent urine from entering the ureter. Adequate intramural length plus fixation of the ureter between its extravesical and intravesical points is required to create this antirefluxing compression valve. Paquin's early dissections of the UVJ in children revealed an approximate 5:1 ratio of tunnel length to ureteral diameter in nonrefluxing junctions versus a 1.4:1 ratio in refluxing UVJs (Paquin, 1959) (Table 117-2). Intravesically, the inner muscle of the ureter merges with the detrusor muscle to contribute to the superficial trigone. Some of these inner ureteral fibers pass medially to contribute to the intraureteric ridge (Mercier's bar). The cellular and molecular details that characterize normal and refluxing UVJs are still unknown. However, it is likely that in addition to architectural deficiencies in tunnel length,

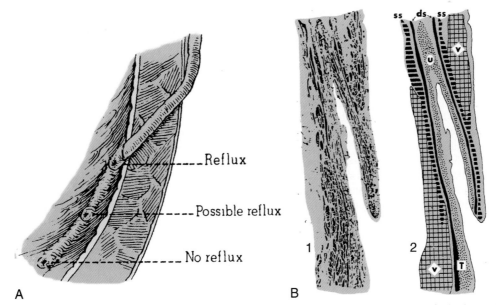

Figure 117-1. A, A refluxing ureterovesical junction has the same anatomic features as a nonrefluxing orifice, except for inadequate length of the intravesical submucosal ureter. Some orifices with marginal submucosal tunnels may reflux intermittently. **B,** Ureterovesical junction in longitudinal section. 1, Photomicrograph; 2, diagrammatic representation. The ureteral muscularis (u) is surrounded by superficial (ss) and deep (ds) periureteral sheaths that extend in the roof of the submucosal segment and continue beyond the orifice into the trigonal muscle (t). The relationship of the superficial sheath to the vesical muscularis (v) is clearly seen. Transverse fascicles in the superior lip of the ureteral orifice belong to the superficial and deep sheaths. No true space separates ureter from bladder. (**A,** From Glenn J [ed]: Urologic Surgery, 2nd ed. New York, Harper & Row, 1975; **B,** from Elbadawi A: Anatomy and function of the urethral sheath. J Urol 1972;107:224.)

SECTION XVII

Table 117–2. Mean Ureteral Tunnel Length and Diameter in Normal Children

Age (yr)	Intravesical Ureteral Length (mm)	Submucosal Ureteral Length (mm)	Ureteral Diameter at the Ureterovesical Junction (mm)
1-3	7	3	1.4
3-6	7	3	1.7
6-9	9	4	2.0
9-12	12	6	1.9

From Paquin AJ: Ureterovesical anastomosis: The description and evaluation of a technique. J Urol 1959;82:573.

abnormalities in ureterovesical smooth muscle and extracellular matrix composition, and neural function may contribute to reflux (Oswald et al, 2004).

Opening of the UVJ is achieved by active contraction of the longitudinal muscles within the tunnel. This draws the extravesical and intravesical points of the intramural ureter closer together, shortens and widens the tunnel, and allows passage of the urine bolus into the bladder. Indeed, when viewed cystoscopically, lateral displacement of the ureteral orifice accompanies the classic jet of urine into the bladder. Although such lateral displacement is functionally normal and necessary to permit urine to pass, permanent lateral displacement by virtue of a constitutively short tunnel characterizes the cystoscopic view of a refluxing ureteral orifice. Closure of the UVJ results from both compression of the intramural ureter and return to its full tunnel length as the ureteral muscle relaxes. Thus, active and passive mechanisms dynamically reconfigure the tunnel as needed to allow antegrade passage of urine while preventing retrograde flow. Finally, the existence of local efferent and afferent neuromuscular coordination between the UVJ and the periureteric bladder wall is suggested by neurophysiologic studies that induce an elevation or decrease in intraluminal UVJ pressure during bladder filling (Shafik, 1996).

ETIOLOGY OF VESICOURETERAL REFLUX

As mentioned previously, the occurrence of VUR represents a balance of several factors. The degree to which each contributes to the pathology largely defines whether the reflux is considered primary or secondary. In general, reflux is considered primary if the main reason for reflux is a fundamental deficiency in the function of the UVJ antireflux mechanism while the remaining factors (bladder and ureter) remain normal or relatively noncontributory. Secondary reflux, then, implies reflux as a result of the normal function of the UVJ being overwhelmed. Bladder dysfunction of a congenital, acquired, or behavioral nature is frequently the root cause of secondary reflux. It is also accepted that reflux is often considered secondary if its absence was documented at some point before its detection.

Primary Reflux

As just stated, primary reflux represents a congenital defect in the structure and therefore the function of the UVJ. Reflux occurs despite an adequately low-pressure urine storage profile in the bladder. The length-diameter ratio of the intramural ureteral tunnel is almost always less than that described by Paquin. Although inadequate tunnel length rather than excessive ureteral diameter usually underlies primary reflux, a dilated ureter often poses a challenge when a nonrefluxing ureterovesicostomy is required. This has traditionally prompted either long tunnels (>5 cm) or a reduction in ureteral diameter by tapering or plication, or both, to reconstruct a successful antireflux mechanism. On the other hand, construction of a new tunnel with a full 5:1 length-to-diameter ratio may not be absolutely required to correct reflux.

KEY POINTS: FUNCTIONAL ANATOMY

■ Integrity of the antireflux mechanism depends on balancing the anatomic and functional relationships between the ureter **and** the bladder.

■ Secondary reflux may be of anatomic or functional origin in the UVJ, bladder, or bladder outlet.

Secondary Reflux

Any number of obstructing bladder pathologies can create hostile and excessive storage and emptying pressures that eventually overwhelm a normal antirefluxing intramural flap-valve mechanism. Such abnormalities can be functional or anatomic.

The natural history of reflux to resolve suggests that the length-diameter ratio gradually evolves toward functional competency over time. Given that there is probably a range of tunnel lengths that can protect against reflux, as well as a spectrum of obstructional voiding etiologies in the refluxing population, it is reasonable to assume that some degree of secondary reflux may coexist with primary reflux.

The most common anatomic obstruction of the bladder in the pediatric population is posterior urethral valves (PUVs). Reflux is present in 48% to 70% of patients with PUVs (Reuter and Lebowitz, 1985; Puri and Kumar, 1996; Hassan et al, 2003; Priti et al, 2004). Relief of PUV obstruction appears to be responsible for resolution of reflux in about a third of patients. In one of these series, 78% of reflux resolved within 6 months of valve ablation (Priti et al, 2004). Such observations argue for the secondary nature of reflux caused by elevated voiding pressure in PUV bladders. Even prostatic enlargement and its relief are associated with VUR and its resolution, respectively (Morita, 1987). In females, anatomic bladder obstruction is rare. The most common structural obstruction is from a ureterocele that prolapses into the bladder neck (Merlini and Lelli Chiesa, 2004). In such cases, reflux in the contralateral ureter is probably due to the ensuing outlet obstruction and often resolves with decompression of the ureterocele. In general then, if relief of the obstruction results in rapid resolution of reflux, the reflux was probably secondary.

In contrast to anatomic obstruction, neurofunctional causes of elevated bladder pressure also predispose to VUR. In particular, a neurogenic bladder associated with spina bifida is at risk for reflux (Bauer et al, 1982). This fact must be borne in mind during evaluation of a child with UTI. Special attention to the potential for occult spinal dysraphism, including a sacral dimple or hairy patch, gluteal cleft abnormality, diminished rectal tone, or significant constipation or encopresis, should prompt consideration of investigation for coexistent spinal cord abnormalities.

Urodynamic extremes may also exist and predispose to reflux in the absence of overt neurologic pathology. Some studies suggest that a secondary aspect of neonatal reflux is a peculiarity of male infants. In a study by Yeung et al (1998), 22 of 24 refluxing infants with urodynamic evidence of instability (overactivity) or inadequate or obstructive voiding patterns were male. Normal or immature voiding patterns were observed in all infants in the nonrefluxing control group, of whom 16 of 21 were male. In infants, higher voiding pressure is associated with reflux, particularly in boys (Chandra et al, 1996), and may contribute to the male preponderance of reflux in infants. Urodynamic evaluation suggests that these elevated infant bladder pressures may be due to inadequate sphincter relaxation (Chandra and Maddix, 2000) during this stage of development. However, detrusor activity in such infants is largely normal during filling, with slightly diminished bladder capacities in some (Podesta et al, 2004), although uninhibited activity during filling has been observed, again predominantly in male infants (Yeung et al, 1998). In view of the fact that the high prevalence of reflux in infants coexists with urodynamic evidence of elevated voiding pressure, these observations suggest that infant voiding patterns may be a part of normal development. Thus, even though the UVJ matures with age, infant voiding patterns predispose to a form of secondary reflux that resolves with normalization of urodynamic parameters as these infants grow older.

In older children, acquired abnormalities in voiding parameters, commonly known as dysfunctional voiding or dysfunctional elimination, have been associated with reflux. The precise cause of voiding dysfunction is variable but may evolve from persistence of the expected early attempts to suppress bladder contractions during the toilet training months by volitional contraction of the external sphincter (Allen, 1985). If this behavior becomes prolonged or intensifies, often driven by the child's overwhelming desire for continence, bladder voiding pressure increases. Continence is gradually exchanged for incomplete emptying and thus results in a higher risk for UTI. Although investigation of UTI might necessarily lead to the diagnosis of persistence of primary reflux in some subjects, the elevated bladder pressure gradually distorts bladder and UVJ architecture and may create (secondary) reflux (Koff, 1992). Structural failure of the UVJ is probably a critical determinant because high voiding pressures of approximately 100 cm H_2O are common in normal bladders and structurally intact nonrefluxing UVJs. Indeed, with structural failure of the UVJ, reflux occurs very easily and at low voiding pressure or during early filling and is a poor prognostic factor for resolution of reflux (Koff, 1992; Hinman et al, 2002). Uninhibited bladder contraction is the most common urodynamic abnormality associated with reflux in neurologically normal children. In one study of 37 girls with "primary" reflux, 75% had uninhibited contractions (Taylor et al, 1982). However, the observation that treatment of such patients with oxybutynin can virtually eliminate reflux in up to 80% of refluxing ureters strongly argues that uninhibited contractions can

frequently be responsible for reflux, either by causing secondary reflux or by perpetuating primary reflux (Koff and Murtagh, 1983; Homsy et al, 1985). Thus, it is apparent that primary and secondary reflux may not always be mutually exclusive.

Clinical Correlates

The preceding discussion clearly suggests that multiple opportunities exist for modifying the course of reflux if secondary causes are appreciated, identified, and treated. Van Gool and colleagues (1992) reported that 18% of children enrolled in the European arm of the International Reflux Study in Children harbored voiding dysfunction associated with more frequent UTI and greater persistence of reflux than did subjects without voiding dysfunction. Failure to address voiding abnormalities can also adversely affect the outcome of antireflux surgery (Koff et al, 1998). Although voiding dysfunction is discussed in detail elsewhere in this text, a thorough evaluation of a toilet-trained child with reflux must recognize dribbling, urgency, or incontinence as signs of coexisting voiding disorders. Girls will also exhibit procrastination about voiding or demonstrate curtsying behavior, and boys may squeeze their penis in an attempt to suppress bladder contractions. The close proximity of the bladder and anal outlets often leads to sympathetic contraction of the anal sphincter as well, thereby resulting in the frequent association of constipation and encopresis with reflux and UTI (O'Regan and Yazbeck, 1985; O'Regan et al, 1986; Chase et al, 2004). Constipation must be recognized and eliminated as much as possible to establish optimal conditions for successful spontaneous or surgical resolution of reflux. The initial report of McGuire et al (1981) suggested that pressure in excess of 40 cm H_2O measured at full capacity is associated with reflux and upper tract deterioration. Treatments to maintain pressure below this value result in significant resolution of reflux (Flood et al, 1994).

LOWER URINARY TRACT INFECTION AND REFLUX

Reflux is not a general cause of UTI. In the absence of bladder symptoms or inflammation, reflux is most readily considered a clinical accelerant of bacteruria by mechanically delivering infected urine to the renal pelvis. Infection-related cystitis is expected to incite bladder irritability and dysuria, upset the voiding pattern, and lower the threshold for reflux in a given UVJ. However, animal studies differ on whether infection itself can perpetuate VUR. In primate studies, surgically created reflux followed by the introduction of pathogenic bacteria into the bladder was associated with persistence of reflux (Roberts et al, 1988), whereas spontaneously occurring primary reflux in the presence of chronic infection did not delay the resolution of reflux (Lewis and Roberts, 1986).

Significant hydroureter and hydronephrosis associated with high-grade reflux could, in theory, act as a reservoir for the repeat antegrade reintroduction of pathogenic organisms into the bladder. Colonized urine might then cyclically reflux retrograde to the upper tracts. Similarly, ureteral atony secondary to the effects of endotoxin could be associated with failure to expel infected urine from the upper tracts, but this does not appear to reduce the ultimate resolution of reflux (Roberts and Riopelle, 1978).

KEY POINTS: LOWER URINARY TRACT INFECTION AND REFLUX

- Reflux is not a general cause of UTI.
- Reflux facilitates pyelonephritis.

GRADING OF REFLUX

Grading systems generally exist to help prognosticate the behavior of the disease that they classify. In 1981, the International Reflux Study Committee proposed a system of five grades of reflux that remains in current use today in North America (Duckett and Bellinger, 1982; Lebowitz et al, 1985). Five grades of reflux that depict the appearance of the ureter, renal pelvis, and calyces as seen on radiographic contrast images generated by the voiding cystourethrogram (VCUG) are currently used (Table 117–3 and Fig. 117–2). The use of such a system serves several purposes. Grading standardizes the description of the degree of reflux for clinical management of individual patients, as well as for grouping research subjects in the design of clinical studies and trials. Grading facilitates documentation of the natural history of the reflux process in an individual patient. It also permits establishing quantitative

associations between reflux and other clinical parameters to determine whether such associations hold multivariate clinical relevance. Most importantly, description of the initial grade of primary reflux is the most significant parameter associated with prediction of reflux resolution (see later).

Despite widespread use of the five-point grading system, several shortcomings exist. For example, the expected concordance between ureteral and calyceal dilation does not always occur (Fig. 117–3). Either the ureter or the calyces may demonstrate dilation out of proportion to the calyces or ureter, respectively. Whether this reflects an anomaly in the biomechanical tissue properties or peristaltic activity of the excessively dilated structure as compared with the typical refluxing upper tract is unknown. Nevertheless, such anatomy is difficult to grade with the current system. Similarly, it is unknown whether the propensity for either scarring in the face of infection or resolution of reflux is altered in such systems.

Attempts have also been made to grade reflux with radionuclide cystography (RNC). Because RNC does not provide discrete images of the ureteral and calyceal architecture required to assign reflux grade, classifying reflux by RNC is difficult. Alternative RNC grading has been proposed (Zhang et al, 1987) and provides reasonable concordance to the objectives of the classic grading system by collapsing grades II and III and grades IV and V into low-grade and high-grade reflux, respectively (Fig. 117–4). The impact of the reduction in grading detail from five grades (I to V) to two (low and high) on understanding reflux pathophysiology and on the design of clinical studies has yet to be determined.

Table 117–3. **International Classification of Vesicoureteral Reflux**	
Grade	**Description**
I	Into a nondilated ureter
II	Into the pelvis and calyces without dilatation
III	Mild to moderate dilatation of the ureter, renal pelvis, and calyces with minimal blunting of the fornices
IV	Moderate ureteral tortuosity and dilatation of the pelvis and calyces
V	Gross dilatation of the ureter, pelvis, and calyces; loss of papillary impressions; and ureteral tortuosity

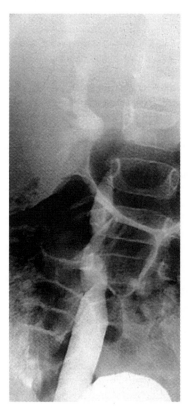

Figure 117–3. A refluxing ureter with significant dilatation of the lower segment but no distortion of the collecting system may be different from the typical system with grade II reflux.

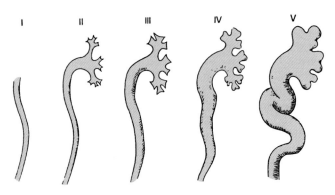

GRADES OF REFLUX

Figure 117–2. International classification of vesicoureteral reflux.

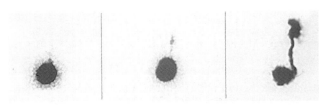

Figure 117–4. Nuclear voiding cystography showing right-sided reflux. Radionuclide tracer can be quantitated (from left to right) as grade 1 (grade I of the international grading system), grade 2 (grade II-III of the international grading system), and grade 3 (grade IV-V of the international grading system).

Grading is purely a classification of the appearance of contrast in the upper tract, and therefore ascribing an absolute value to the grade has the potential to cast the reflux in unequivocal terms to the exclusion of other factors that modulate reflux at the time that the images are acquired. Inherent bladder dynamics, the bladder outlet, and even ipsilateral UVJ obstruction all influence the degree of reflux at any given assessment (Lebowitz, 1992). Grade, reflux detection, and reflux resolution are all interrelated and influenced by the degree of bladder filling, the voiding cycle, the number of filling cycles during the contrast cystogram, and whether the reflux occurs during filling or only during voiding. None of these parameters are built into the grading system for reflux used currently. However, given that the principal role of a reflux grading system is to help prognosticate resolution of reflux, future incorporation of other parameters may provide additional clinical acumen. Finally, it must be remembered that reflux grade is still presently determined by an imaging study that requires invasion of a sensitive anatomic region. For a given reflux grading result, the aforementioned variables of bladder dynamics, filling, and voiding cannot necessarily be replicated with certainty in a given patient every time that they are studied. It is reasonable to speculate that reflux grade could easily vary up or down by at least one grade were sequential studies to be performed in a given patient. Thus, the entire reflux literature itself, which historically reports results in terms of five separate grades, must be considered with some circumspection because the veracity of grade at the time of the contrast study may, to some extent, be arbitrary.

DIAGNOSIS AND EVALUATION OF VESICOURETERAL REFLUX
Confirmation of Urinary Tract Infection

Because preventable reflux nephropathy is predicated on the combined effects of UTI and reflux, confirmation plus documentation of true UTI is paramount in the appropriate management of a patient with reflux. Many variables are responsible for accurate assessment and interpretation of UTI in the context of reflux, including the clinical history and presence of fever; age of the patient; circumcision status; method of collection, storage, and delivery of the urine specimen; and the results of urine dipstick and microscopic analysis. Although confirming true pyuria by dipstick or microscopic analysis, in addition to the presence of bacteriuria, will help

differentiate infection from colonization, colonization alone in the presence of reflux may still pose a threat to the upper tracts. Attention to these details cannot be overemphasized because major management decisions, including operative intervention for correction of reflux, often rest solely on a diagnosis of UTI. Conversely, confirming microbial growth in a urine specimen is of little value if the mode of collection is highly suspect and likely to harbor contamination. Confirmation of UTI begins with collection of the urine specimen. If storage is necessary, specimens should be maintained at 4°C until transfer to the laboratory.

In infants, specimen collection will often entail placement of an adhesive urine collection bag over the genitalia. Although topical cleansing of the area is reasonable to reduce contamination and false-positive culture results, care must be taken to avoid introducing the disinfection agent into the specimen. Unfortunately, routine practice is so variable that such guidelines are often difficult to follow or confirm, and **microbial contamination of bagged specimens is common. Conversely, this method is most useful if the resulting urine culture is negative.** Even though fever is common in infants, UTI is present in only 5% of children with fever (Hoberman and Wald, 1997). Thus, the ability to easily rule out UTI in a febrile infant with reflux facilitates management. If there is high clinical suspicion for UTI in an infant, the more accurate method is to obtain a catheterized specimen. Even this method may prove suspect in an uncircumcised male infant whose preputial skin is not yet retractable to easily reveal the urethral meatus. In this and other instances in which the urethral route is difficult or compromised in patients of any age, suprapubic needle aspiration of bladder urine provides the most accurate method of obtaining a urine sample. In a younger child, however, repeated catheterization for the acquisition of specimens, as well as radiographic assessment (see later), should be considered carefully. This hitherto routine practice is coming under greater scrutiny as the long-term sequelae of this invasive maneuver become appreciated (Stashinko and Goldberger 1998) and could in fact become a factor in patient compliance with follow-up and therefore management decisions for reflux.

In patients who can void spontaneously, a clean voided midstream catch specimen is preferred. The initial urine is discarded because it is rich in periurethral organisms.

The guidelines just presented pertain to patients with both unknown and known reflux status. In the former, the decision to look for reflux depends on the propensity for acquired reflux nephropathy in the individual patient. In a patient known to have reflux, the prevailing propensity for acquired reflux nephropathy, as well as compliance with proper voiding habits, antibiotic prophylaxis, and timely reporting, will influence further management (see later).

Evaluating Urinary Tract Infection

A number of factors support a search for reflux in a patient with UTI. The probability of finding VUR in children with UTI is 29% to 50% (Anonymous, 1981). Furthermore, in some patients, higher grades of reflux may be associated with various degrees of existing renal parenchymal maldevelopment (see the section "Embryology of the Uterovesical Junction") (Nakai et al, 2003). In addition, because reflux has a tendency to resolve over time, it is reasonable that UTI is more commonly associated with reflux in younger patients (Smellie et al, 1981), whose renal parenchyma is at more risk for scarring after a given incident of pyelonephritis than is the case in older children. Smellie and associates also suggest that the presence of reflux does not usually provide any unique clinical features in a patient with UTI. Thus, as with the search for sibling reflux, radiologic investigation of a patient with UTI is tailored to those who are placed at greatest renal functional risk from the presence of VUR. For this reason, **radiographic investigation for VUR has generally been directed to children younger than 5 years, all children with a febrile UTI, and any male with a UTI regardless of age or fever, unless sexually active.**

The high repeat UTI rate after a first UTI has prompted a recommendation for some form of VUR workup. However, the current state of the VUR debate makes it difficult to know which patients by such evaluations might harbor clinically significant reflux, given how common UTI is in children. Some reassurance can be provided if a voiding study is negative for VUR. However, parental concern over the invasiveness of a cystogram may first limit the evaluation only to ultrasonography to rule out any existing gross structural defects. As such, after taking the appropriate voiding, fever, and family histories into account, a sonographic study of the bladder and kidneys can be considered a reasonable minimum evaluation in an infant or child after a UTI if a cystogram is deemed overly aggressive by the family or treating physician. Even detection of reflux after the treatment of UTI could be of questionable significance if the child is older or no fever accompanied the UTI, or both. On the other hand, the presence of structural renal anomalies or significant asymmetry would support proceeding with a cystogram. More recent studies of racial predilection for reflux have supported a lower prevalence in children of African origin (Askari and Belman, 1982; Horowitz et al, 1999), but the prevalence in children of Hispanic origin (Pinto, 2004) is similar to that of white children.

The advent of prenatal ultrasound has probably augmented the detection of asymptomatic reflux in newborns as a result of mass surveillance for persistent postnatal hydronephrosis and the ensuing performance of cystography in these infants. It must be remembered that the sonographic finding of hydronephrosis is generally much more common than hydronephrosis caused by a renal moiety actively refluxing at the time of the sonogram. Indeed, there is little correlation between the degree of antenatal hydronephrosis and the existence of reflux (Farhat et al, 2000). A corollary study also demonstrated normal postnatal ultrasound findings in 25% of patients with VUR and antenatal hydronephrosis (Lebowitz, 1993).

ASSESSMENT OF THE LOWER URINARY TRACT
Cystographic Imaging

The basis of reflux detection lies in demonstrating the retrograde passage of an imaging contrast material from the bladder to the ureter and renal pelvicalyceal system. The

KEY POINTS: DIAGNOSIS AND EVALUATION OF VESICOURETERAL REFLUX

- The method of urine collection is of utmost importance in the diagnosis of UTI to avoid false-positive culture results.

- Radiologic studies should be tailored to age, gender, and mode of manifestation (i.e., fever).

- The gold standard study for the diagnosis of reflux requires bladder catheterization.

- Nuclear cystograms, though more sensitive, provide much less anatomic detail than a VCUG does.

- Parental perceptions of reflux management must be considered when treating a child with reflux.

- Routine cystoscopy is *contraindicated* in reflux management.

- Upper tract assessment is based on serial studies.

- The intensity of upper tract studies should be proportional to the propensity for renal damage.

- The challenge in imaging is to differentiate congenital reflux–associated renal dysmorphism from scarring acquired after infection.

currently available methodologies require a source of contrast agent in the bladder. Two approaches, the so-called indirect and direct cystograms, can be used, depending on whether the contrast enters the bladder indirectly after excretory urography or directly, usually by urethral catheterization. Indirect cystography, though avoiding the invasive nature of urethral catheterization, is prone to false-positive interpretation because contrast that does not originate from the bladder remains in the ureter or pelvis after filtration and antegrade passage (Conway et al, 1975), although it has been suggested that the value of indirect cystography may lie in ruling out the presence of VUR (Carlsen et al, 1986).

The VCUG and RNC are therefore the two common forms of direct cystography and constitute the present-day gold standard approaches to detection of reflux. More recently, to eliminate the need for ionizing radiation, some studies have demonstrated a growing interest in sonographic detection of reflux with either color Doppler imaging (Haberlik, 1997; Oak et al, 1999; Galia et al, 2004) or echo-enhancing contrast agents (Berrocal et al, 2001; Darge et al, 2001; Darge and Troeger, 2002; McEwing et al, 2002; Tasic and Todorovska, 2003; Valentini et al, 2004; Vassiou et al, 2004; Darge et al, 2005). Direct imaging of reflux is affected by several parameters, including bladder contraction during voiding, the fluid volume instilled into the bladder, and the presence of infection and therefore inflammation of the UVJ mucosa. Reflux may occur during filling or only during the active bladder contraction associated with voiding. Consequently, if a patient is unable to void in the artificial setting of the radiography suite, false-negative results may ensue. More importantly, even during voiding, reflux may not be demonstrated on a single filling-voiding cycle. Several studies have demonstrated a roughly 12% to 20% greater detection rate for VUR if a cyclic study is performed (Paltiel et al, 1992; Papadopoulou et al, 2002; Novljan et al, 2003). A cyclic VCUG involves a second or third cycle of bladder filling and emptying under fluoroscopic observation. A similar cyclic strategy is commonly used for RNC as well (Fettich and Kenda, 1992). Reflux may also be demonstrated during catheter filling of the bladder. Because filling assumes far lower intravesical pressure than voiding does, reflux during filling, or passive reflux, is generally considered a poor prognostic sign for resolution of reflux and suggests the presence of a fixed decompensation of the UVJ. This finding is common in patients with acquired or neurogenic voiding dysfunction, wherein high-resistance voiding gradually remodels the bladder wall and UVJ and leads to complete failure of the latter's antireflux mechanism and immediate reflux at virtually any volume of the filling phase (Koff, 1992). This situation is in contrast to reflux that occurs only during the higher-pressure milieu of bladder emptying and contraction. Thus, technical inconsistencies in the ratio of instilled volume to bladder capacity during the radiographic technique can lead to variations in rates of reflux detection: if the bladder is overfilled or underfilled for a given degree of progressive UVJ incompetency, reflux may be overdetected or underdetected, respectively.

One difficult dilemma in the performance of voiding studies involves cystography during active infection. On one hand, some UVJs maintain only borderline antireflux mechanisms that are competent in a sterile milieu but become incompetent from the edema and inflammation associated with mucosal inflammation during cystitis. Such patients will often have VCUG studies negative for reflux in the absence of infection, but they suffer from repeated pyelonephritic episodes. Cystograms in such patients may demonstrate reflux if obtained during active infection. On the other hand, evoking reflux during active cystitis, by definition, will transmit bacteria to the upper urinary tract and renal pelvis and risks iatrogenic pyelonephritis. Nevertheless, the general consensus has been to delay the voiding study for at least a week or longer to allow for adequate recovery from the acute infection episode (Craig et al, 1997). Only if it is imperative to make the diagnosis of reflux in children with a history of recurrent pyelonephritis and repeatedly negative voiding studies in the intercurrent periods should cystography during UTI be considered.

The VCUG is a fluoroscopic study that provides information on both the functional dynamics and the structural anatomy of the urinary tract. The detailed technique of a VCUG is discussed more fully elsewhere in the text. Bladder contrast is instilled by gravity after urethral catheterization. Bladder capacity is recorded when contrast influx ceases. Static images record bladder contour, the presence of diverticula or ureteroceles, the grade of reflux, the configuration and blunting of calyces, and intrarenal reflux. Passive or active reflux is demonstrated dynamically during fluoroscopy while filling and voiding, respectively. In addition, bladder neck anatomy, funneling or dilation, and urethral patency are additional parameters derived from the VCUG. **Delayed or postvoid films are crucial in documenting clearance of contrast from the upper tracts inasmuch as retained contrast, particularly with dilated pelvicalyceal systems, could signify the presence of a concomitant UPJ obstruction,** either primarily or secondarily as a result of distortion of the UPJ by massive retrograde filling of the pelvis by the reflux (Hollowell et al, 1989). **If both the UPJ and UVJ meet the criteria for operative repair, the UPJ should be repaired first to avoid the incipient obstruction that may ensue if resistance is added to the UVJ when the reflux is corrected** (Hollowell et al, 1989). With care, both processes may be repaired simultaneously when it is clear that they are independent significant problems.

RNC has historically enjoyed a reputation for requiring approximate 1% of the radiation exposure generated by a VCUG (Blaufox et al, 1971; Diamond et al, 1996a). Presently, the reduced radiation requirements of modern digital techniques have significantly narrowed the difference between fluoroscopy and RNC. Although little anatomic detail is afforded by RNC, it is ideal both as a screening modality and for monitoring the natural history or surgical follow-up of reflux. In contrast to the VCUG, the instilled bladder contrast material, usually technetium Tc 99 pertechnetate, is itself the radiation source. Reflux is detected by scintigraphic gamma camera images (Fig. 117–5). **Lack of the confounding imaging densities typical of fluoroscopy, as well as the ability to obtain prolonged exposures, allows for greater sensitivity of RNC in grades II to V reflux.** Ironically, **grade I reflux into the distal part of the ureter is often poorly detected because of the overlying exposure generated by contrast within the bladder itself.** Thus, RNC and VCUG imaging can be used complementarily to balance radiation exposure with the need for dynamic information and anatomic detail. Notwithstanding the forgoing discussion, modern digital fluoroscopic equipment has further reduced the radiation exposure of conventional fluoroscopy, thereby narrowing the difference in radiation exposure between the two modalities.

Another modality gaining popularity in some centers is ultrasonic cystography to detect reflux. Modern transducers coupled with the use of echo-enhancing contrast agents are able to image reflux quite well in older children (Novljan et al, 2003; Riccabona et al, 2003; Tasic and Todorovska, 2003; Galia et al, 2004), but the technique remains of limited use in neonates (McEwing et al, 2002). Furthermore, although radiation exposure is eliminated, bladder catheterization remains a necessary feature with this approach.

Challenging the Assessment of Reflux

The well-recognized distress of the family and patient associated with urethral catheterization, particularly in children, coupled with the advent of low-morbidity outpatient correction of reflux with endoscopic approaches, appears to be shaking the foundations of conventional reflux management and therapy. All aspects of VUR, including the modern incidence of renal scarring and failure, peak ages of renal susceptibility, and indications for correction of reflux, together with the assumption that permanent correction of reflux is an absolute necessity, are coming under scrutiny. This has given rise to added pressure to avoid bladder catheterization. Cystography can have traumatic aftereffects in young patients

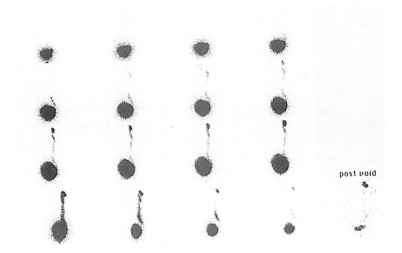

post void

Figure 117–5. Radionuclide cystogram showing right-sided reflux that worsens with bladder filling. The upper collecting system drains fully with voiding.

(Stashinko and Goldberger, 1998; Elder, 2005) and must be approached with sensitivity and awareness of the developmental stage of the patient. Sedation (Stokland et al, 2003), topical urethral anesthesia (Gerard et al, 2003), and more recently, hypnosis (Butler et al, 2005) have all been effective in mitigating the deleterious psychological effects of cystography. Nevertheless, it is clear that **parental perception of the nature of the medical modalities involved in reflux management will influence the choice of therapy** for their children (Ogan et al, 2001). **This should in no way be construed as license for the abandonment of conventional observational therapy, including antibiotic prophylaxis and periodic cystography, in favor of immediate correction of reflux in all patients** (Aaronson, 2005). Rather, the evolution of less invasive imaging modalities for the detection of reflux and reduced morbidity of reflux correction should be encouraged in parallel.

Uroflowmetry

Evaluation of the lower urinary tract during clinical assessment of VUR cannot rely solely on imaging. Because reflux is a dynamic phenomenon, the prevailing functional status of the bladder must also be considered. Although full pressure-volume urodynamic studies of the bladder are not required in all reflux patients, a minimal survey of bladder-emptying characteristics can be obtained by uroflowmetry. Details of the uroflowmetry technique are discussed elsewhere in this text. In refluxing patients, it is important to establish whether the bladder outlet is functioning relatively normally or harbors the more resistive characteristics that are highly prevalent in younger patients. Elements of uroflow such as lack of smoothness of the flow-velocity curve suggest incomplete relaxation of the bladder outlet during voiding. This implies the existence or development of relatively higher pressure during voiding that could delay the natural history of reflux resolution or even perpetuate reflux. An increased postvoid residual volume may be a risk factor for UTI. In the setting of passive reflux, carrying an infected postvoid residual urine can also lead to ascending infection and pyelonephritis.

Cystoscopy and the PIC Cystogram

Modern management of reflux does not include routine cystoscopy. It is rare for cystoscopy to add any information that will alter management of a patient with reflux, either at the time of initial diagnosis or during follow-up. Its routine use, especially in children with UTI or reflux, should be considered an anachronism. Similarly, the appearance and configuration of the ureteral orifices and intramural tunnel length that are afforded by cystoscopy and once considered useful parameters have over time provided little correlation with either the diagnosis or grade of reflux (Duckett, 1983). Cystoscopy can provide useful information immediately before open surgery, such as confirmation of orifice position and duplication and the proximity of diverticula to the orifice, and clarify urethral patency if indicated. Similarly, such cystoscopic parameters will become immediately available in all patients at the time of endoscopic reflux correction.

A recently developed, though still controversial (Elder, 2005) cystoscopic modality termed the PIC technique (positioning instillation of contrast at the ureteral orifice) purports to detect reflux under general anesthesia in patients with febrile UTIs but a normal VCUG. Contrast is instilled under low pressure through a ureteral catheter directly toward the ureteral orifice under direct cystoscopic vision and simultaneous fluoroscopy (Rubenstein et al, 2003). It is conceivable that antireflux mechanisms may be barely functional in some patients with recurrent UTI. The unique, but unphysiologic nature of the PIC technique may then reveal reflux in such cases. However, PIC cystography does not allow for age-adjusted instillation pressures; some pressures may be too high in younger patients and may be creating iatrogenic reflux rather than unmasking relevant, physiologically borderline reflux. In the study by Rubenstein et al (2003), 5 of 39 renal units from control patients without infection or bladder abnormalities and with normal VCUGs nevertheless showed reflux on PIC cystograms. It is also possible that the revealed reflux is clinically irrelevant to the recurrent febrile UTIs in some patients. The role of p-fimbriated organisms, which are responsible for many cases of febrile UTI without reflux, has not yet been accounted for in this approach. Finally, 26 of the 30 patients with recurrent febrile UTI and positive PIC cystograms with negative VCUGs were managed by instituting prophylactic antibiotics, a therapy that could be started on the basis of the infections alone, without PIC cystography. Although the remaining four patients were free of infection after surgical correction of reflux, this number is insufficient to validate this approach as an indication for surgery. Currently, PIC cystography provides seductive evidence and rationale for antireflux therapy in a new subset of patients, particularly since endoscopic correction could theoretically and easily follow the fluoroscopy at the same time. However, the urologist must exercise caution in this approach until more precise standardization of the technique is available. Prospective randomized controlled trials with sufficient numbers of patients that account for organism strain and the true rate of persistent recurrent infection after correction of reflux are required.

ASSESSMENT OF THE UPPER URINARY TRACT

Rationale for Serial Assessment of the Upper Tracts

The known effects of VUR on the upper tracts are largely what direct the need for diagnosis and correction of reflux. Pyelonephritis propagated by reflux causes renal scarring, impedes attainment of full renal growth potential, and increases the risk for renovascular hypertension. Therefore, imaging of the upper tracts is directed at assessing renal structure and function with attention to the aforementioned parameters. A fundamental goal in upper tract imaging in patients with VUR is to ascertain whether the abnormalities are due to ongoing or resolved reflux and differentiate them from intrinsic developmental disturbances, medical renal disease, or resistance to antegrade flow. Almost always, particularly in the youngest patients in whom VUR has the greatest potential to adversely affect renal function, these goals are best achieved through serial imaging of the kidneys over a period of months to years.

However, a meta-analysis of 63 studies in which the value of routine diagnostic imaging after initial UTI in children was assessed for the prevention of renal damage found no accurate evidence to support this practice (Dick and Feldman, 1996). Many observational studies raised concern for the sequelae of UTIs, as well as highlighted the potential for successful intervention. The reason to image the upper tracts after a UTI may be independent of knowledge of the reflux status of the lower tract. Reflux status may be known, suspected, or completely unknown. These three considerations, coupled with the age of the patient, gender, race, family history of reflux, and bladder functional status, serve as a guide to selective imaging that attempts to balance the intensity of imaging studies with the propensity for renal damage.

Renal Sonography

The mainstay of renal imaging in VUR management is ultrasonography. As a nonionizing, noninvasive imaging platform, coupled with its ability to assess the renal vasculature, it is ideally suited to serial follow-up of renal growth and development. Ultrasonography has supplanted routine excretory urography as the imaging modality of choice to monitor renal status over time.

Ultrasound lends itself well to quantitative assessment of renal dimensions (Rodriguez et al, 2001; Chen et al, 2002), which can then be used to monitor renal growth over time. Renal growth can be referenced to standard renal growth curves. In reflux diagnosed in the neonatal period, baseline renal dimensions are obtained and appropriate renal growth can be monitored over time. The impact of any intercurrent febrile UTI can be gauged by observing the effects on renal growth. Similarly, if the UTI history between follow-up visits for reflux is unclear, serial assessment of renal dimensions can help the urologist determine the need for further assessment of renal function by scintigraphy or the need for correction of reflux. Indeed, in the presence of reflux, modern postnatal renal sonography provides excellent correlation between renal length and scintigraphic hypoplasia (Farhat et al, 2002a).

Ultrasonography also images the degree of corticomedullary differentiation in the kidney. Loss of corticomedullary differentiation, or an increase in the overall echogenicity of the kidney, is associated with some degree of renal functional impairment. In neonates in particular, these parameters can be quite useful in assessing the overall status of a renal unit in the context of higher grades of reflux, even before any episode of UTI or pyelonephritis has occurred. Coupled with a relatively smaller ipsilateral kidney, loss of corticomedullary differentiation or increased echogenicity suggests a degree of intrinsic renal dysplasia that developmentally accompanies high-grade reflux. In a neonate with no infection history, such findings should not be confused with renal scarring, which is a direct sequela of inflammation and infectious pyelonephritis. In general, a routine sonogram is noninvasive, is performed relatively quickly, and does not require intravenous access for contrast agents. From a practical point of view, it is virtually an extension of the urologic physical examination and is still commonplace in urologists' offices. Accordingly, just as serial documentation of height, weight, and blood pressure is a basic component of most pediatric encounters, most urologists commonly perform serial sonography every 6 to 24 months during follow-up of reflux, if only to confirm that renal growth is proceeding normally.

Notwithstanding the value of renal sonography, it must be remembered that a single ultrasound study cannot reliably diagnose either VUR or renal obstruction. Although it is tempting to speculate on the presence of reflux when postnatal hydronephrosis is detected on sonography, particularly higher grades of hydronephrosis, there is no significant correlation between a normal ultrasound finding and the absence of reflux (Farhat et al, 2000a; Zamir et al, 2004).

Modern enhancements in ultrasound technology permit imaging of perfusion abnormalities in tissue. In reflux nephropathy imaged by color Doppler ultrasound, renal resistive index measurements derived from blood flow in the interlobar and arcuate arteries are significantly increased in the presence of higher grades of reflux and correlate positively with scintigraphic findings from the same renal unit (Radmayr et al, 1999). Resistive indices are likewise higher in patients with bona fide pyelonephritis confirmed by nuclear scintigraphy than in patients with lower tract infection alone (Ozcelik et al, 2004). Animal studies have also demonstrated that contrast-enhanced harmonic ultrasound can detect histologically confirmed regions of reflux-induced pyelonephritis with great sensitivity and positive and negative predictive values higher than 80% (Farhat et al, 2002b).

Renal Scintigraphy

The gold standard for imaging functioning renal parenchyma is scintigraphy with ^{99m}Tc-labeled dimercaptosuccinic acid (DMSA). The radiotracer is taken up only by functioning proximal tubular tissue mass, where it binds for several hours. Uptake of DMSA provides a good proportional representation of glomerular filtration (Taylor, 1982). Because pyelonephritis impairs tubular uptake of radiotracer, these areas will fail to radioemit photons and appear as unexposed or underexposed regions in the resultant renal cortical images (Fig. 117–6). Even though many such affected areas in the kidney resolve, especially if prompt medical treatment is possible (Fernández-Menéndez et al, 2003), when they persist, irreversible renal damage or scarring is said to have occurred (Rushton et al, 1992). In a study of 79 children monitored for 1 to 4 years, DMSA scanning provided 98% sensitivity and 92% specificity for scar detection (Merrick et al, 1980). Once pyelonephritis has occurred, any subsequent scarring is independent of the presence or absence of VUR (Rushton et al, 1992). Indeed, considering the overall incidence of pyelonephritis in children, VUR is present in 22% to 39% of such patients (Hoberman et al, 2003; Lin et al, 2003). Nonetheless, the importance of VUR lies in the realization that it remains a spontaneously resolving or surgically treatable cause of this ascending group of renal infections (Majd et al, 1991).

One advance in nuclear scintigraphy of the kidneys is single-photon emission computed tomography (SPECT). This approach reconstructs three-dimensional images of the renal cortical architecture, which can be viewed in any aspect in 360 degrees of rotation. Though providing slightly higher sensitivity for detection of cortical defects, SPECT images do not appreciably add to standard pinhole DMSA images in the clinical management of reflux (Majd et al, 1996).

Much has been written in the literature on the role of DMSA scanning in the management of VUR, as an indirect entrée to the diagnosis of reflux itself, for the detection of reflux-associated renal damage and acute pyelonephritic changes, and for follow-up of reflux. However, no consensus exists on the precise use of DMSA scanning in reflux management. For example, growing concern over the nature and frequency of voiding studies has prompted some to propose cystography after UTI only in children with persistent postinfection renal lesions on DMSA scan, citing that just a minority of post-UTI cystograms are positive for reflux (Hansson et al, 2004). DMSA and ultrasound are often used complementarily, particularly when knowledge of relative renal function is desired (Riccabona et al, 1993). As a general rule, the utility of scintigraphy can best be appreciated in the context of the data that it provides relevant to reflux: imaging cortical defects and relative renal function. The usefulness of this information will depend on which associated clinical and radiology data are at hand. If reflux and infection history are unclear or unknown in a new patient referred for evaluation after UTI, scintigraphy can provide the gold standard for demonstration of cortical defects for any reason and help with counseling on additional studies. If the significance or febrile nature of a potential pyelonephritis is unclear, particularly in a younger patient, a follow-up DMSA scan 4 to 6 months after UTI can rule out subsequent scarring, especially if a scan from a previous evaluation is normal. DMSA scanning can be particularly useful if the diagnosis of pyelonephritis is unclear during an acute infection. Confirmation of photopenic radioemission and acute pyelonephritis can help ensure that adequate antimicrobial therapy is provided. If surgical intervention is planned and significant renal asymmetry exists on ultrasound, quantification of relative function by scintigraphy can help decide between correction of reflux and nephrectomy.

DMSA scanning has also demonstrated that congenital cortical maldevelopment can exist, particularly in high-grade reflux, even in the absence of any history of UTI or outlet obstruction (Wallin and Bajc, 1994; Nguyen et al, 2000). This underscores the fact that cortical defects detected by DMSA scanning are not always the byproduct of infection and that all DMSA defects are not necessarily scars. The distinction is an important one in the design of clinical studies and interpretation of the reflux literature, where congenital cortical defects may be erroneously construed and evaluated as though they were due to postinfection scarring. One corollary to this observation is that scintigraphic renal defects detected for the first time in a child in whom the reflux history from birth cannot be confidently known could be secondary to reflux-associated pyelonephritic scarring, even though the reflux has resolved by the time of the study. Failure to appreciate that reflux often resolves in early childhood before scanning detects cortical defects for the first time makes it difficult to know whether these defects were or were not associated with reflux.

CORTICAL DEFECTS
Congenital Defects versus Acquired Scar

The term *scar* is defined as fibrous tissue replacing normal tissue destroyed by injury or disease. In a renal context, the

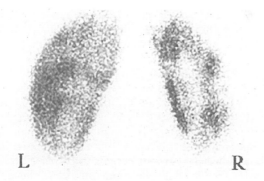

Figure 117–6. Dimercaptosuccinic acid renal scintigraphy. Pinhole images show a normal left kidney and a right kidney with multiple cortical defects.

term is most accurately used to describe the fibrous, contracted regions of the kidney that have been destroyed by infection. These areas of scar often appear smaller and photopenic by scintigraphy or hyperechoic and shrunken on sonographic images. The importance of such scars lies in the realization that they are a preventable complication of pyelonephritis, the latter being directly influenced by VUR in the presence of a bladder infection.

However, VUR, particularly of higher grades, may result in renal dysplasia, which often appears scintgraphically or sonographically identical to postinfection pyelonephritic scars. Thus, over time in the literature and in clinical practice, the terminology of scarring, which is ideally defined to describe an end product of infection, has become contaminated by the inclusion of reflux-associated congenital dysmorphism. However, until such time that primary reflux can be averted prenatally, dysmorphism will remain a nonpreventable developmental sequela of reflux. Failure to appreciate this important distinction has tainted and confused study design and interpretation in the reflux literature.

Reflux-Associated Renal Dysmorphism

The association of renal maldevelopment with the highest grades of reflux is expected by the theory of Mackie and Stephens, which suggests that an abnormal origin of the ureteral bud will interact suboptimally with the metanephric blastema (Fig. 117–7). The latter process is currently believed to be the probable cause of the renal dysmorphism associated with reflux. Several studies have confirmed the association between VUR and a smaller than normal ipsilateral kidney, an overall reduced relative renal function, and global or focal

areas of poor uptake by scintigraphy (Najmaldin et al, 1990; Burge et al, 1992). These infants tend to be male, and the preponderance of refluxing renal units are grade IV or V (Marra et al, 1994; Marra et al, 2004) (Fig. 117–8 and Table 117–4). Indeed, boys tend to be spared an infectious cause of reflux-associated scarring because they have a lower incidence of recurrent UTIs (Wennerstrom et al, 2000).

Renal dysplasia is not unique to primary isolated VUR but may also occur in a variety of urologic settings. Duplex renal moieties (Mackie and Stephens, 1975), prune-belly syndrome (Manivel et al, 1989), and PUVs may all exhibit reflux-associated renal dysmorphism, particularly when the grade of reflux has been high.

The Requirement for Urinary Microorganisms

It is now firmly established that nephropathy from VUR requires the colonization of urine with pathogenic bacteria. Indeed, the basis of current expectant medical management of reflux is to maintain urinary sterility while allowing the reflux to resolve naturally. In the absence of infection, sterile urinary reflux is insufficient to cause renal damage. This concept has been most definitively demonstrated by an elegant series of experiments by Ransley and Risden. Reflux was induced experimentally in a pig model by unroofing the intravesical ureteral tunnel. Only if the urine was subsequently infected could pyelonephritis and reflux nephropathy be induced. Without urine infection, no nephropathy could be created (Ransley and Risdon, 1981). Large clinical studies have also reiterated these experimental findings by demonstrating new reflux-associated scarring only in children with recurrent UTIs (Smellie et al, 1975; Huland and Busch, 1984). These observations conflict somewhat with earlier animal studies by Hodson in which reflux was induced with sterile urine (Hodson et al, 1975). However, bladder outflow obstruction was also included in this model and led to a finding of atrophic pyelonephritis similar to obstructive nephropathy. Scarring was nevertheless intensified by the presence of urinary microorganisms. Thus, abnormal hydrodynamic bladder characteristics may modulate even sterile reflux, but reflux is unlikely to be of any clinical significance in the absence of infection with relatively normal bladder function. These earlier observations of Hodson, however, underscore the importance of maintaining good lower tract emptying and minimizing any elements of bladder outlet obstruction while awaiting resolution of reflux.

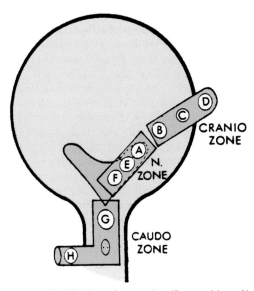

Figure 117–7. Classification of ureteral orifice position. Obstruction usually occurs in the caudo zone, and ureters positioned in the cranio zone are likely to result in reflux. Ureters positioned in the normal (N) zone are associated with normal kidneys. Because of ureteral bud abnormality, renal dysplasia occurs with ureters projecting from both abnormal positions. (From Mackie GC, Stephens FD: Duplex kidneys: A correlation of renal dysplasia with position of the ureteral orifice. J Urol 1975;114:274.)

KEY POINTS: CORTICAL DEFECTS

- Sterile reflux is considered benign.
- The youngest patients are at greatest risk for postpyelonephritic renal scarring.
- Most scarring probably follows the first episode of pyelonephritis.
- Somatic growth is an accurate reflection of renal cortical integrity.

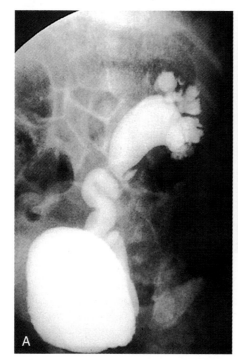

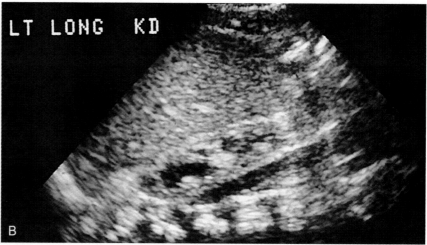

Figure 117–8. **A,** Massive reflux in a boy with antenatally diagnosed hydronephrosis. **B,** Ultrasound demonstrating a kidney with poor internal differentiation. No function was seen on scan.

Table 117–4. **Congenital Renal Scarring**			
Grade of Vesicoureteral Reflux	**No. of Patients**		
	Normal	*Slight Damage*	*Severe Damage*
I-III	13 (100%)	—	—
IV	8 (53%)	5 (34%)	2 (13%)
V	2 (15%)	5 (38%)	6 (46%)

Adapted from Marra G, Barbieri G, Dell'Agnola CA, et al: Congenital renal damage associated with primary vesicoureteric reflux. Arch Dis Child Fetal Neonatal Ed 1994;70:F147.

Pathophysiology of Acquired Scarring

Renal scarring is a sequela of infectious pyelonephritis. A full discussion of the pathophysiology of renal scarring is covered elsewhere in this text. However, VUR exploits several conditions that predispose to scarring. Most importantly, **reflux provides a mechanical hydrodynamic mechanism that facilitates the ascension of microorganisms from the bladder to the kidneys. As such, reflux may be considered an accelerant for renal tissue infection after bacterial colonization of the bladder.** This principle has been confirmed by studies showing a higher incidence of pyelonephritis in high- compared with low-grade reflux (Majd et al, 1991). Furthermore, the frequency of scarring itself appears to be directly proportional to the grade of reflux with which it is associated (Winter et al, 1983; Weiss et al, 1992b). This principle is also supported by observations after correction of reflux. In one study of 74 patients in whom preoperative and postoperative scintigraphic studies were available, more than 90% of the renal units corrected for reflux showed no new scars during a mean follow-up period of 19 months despite asymptomatic bacteriuria in 47% of the patients during follow-up (Choi et al, 1999).

Age. **The kidney's predilection for postpyelonephritic scarring is inversely proportional to age. This point is a guiding principle that must be considered in all decisions regarding the diagnosis of reflux, as well as the choice of therapy. The greatest risk for postinfectious renal scarring occurs within the first year of life** (Winberg, 1992). Similarly, patients younger than 4 years are more prone to scarring after a single UTI than older children are (Smellie and Normand, 1985), although scarring may still occur beyond 5 years of age (Smellie et al, 1985; Benador et al, 1997). Indeed, although younger patients are the most vulnerable to scarring, scarring in older children is frequently the result of late diagnosis, delayed or inadequate treatment of infection, and social factors that often interfere with patient management. Thus, in older children with reflux in whom a consideration to relinquish care from the urologist back to the family physician is being contemplated, it is vital that the fundamental principles of an adequate clinical index of suspicion for UTI and prompt UTI management be reiterated before transfer.

The seminal studies of **Ransley and Risdon proposed a "big bang" theory for the origin of scars after infant pyelonephritis. They observed that most of the scarring to which the kidney is ultimately susceptible occurs after the initial bout of pyelonephritis and that further scarring in the absence of repeated pyelonephritic episodes is unlikely to occur** (Ransley and Risdon, 1981). Consequently, little change in the initial scarring pattern is to be expected in follow-up scintigraphic imaging.

Papillary Anatomy. Another factor governing renal susceptibility to scarring is the configuration of the papillae as their ducts open to the calyces. Papillae with a concave architecture (compound papillae) have their ducts directed at right angles, whereas more convex papillae possess ducts that end obliquely and produce a valvular effect that guards against backflow of urine into the medullary collecting ducts (Fig. 117–9). The more polar calyces are composed preferentially of compound papillae as compared with the middle calyces. The former are more commonly the site of intrarenal reflux (reflux into the ducts) and are the prime regions of susceptibility to scarring. Furthermore, necropsy studies have determined that reflux into compound papillae occurs at lower pressure than does reflux into simple papillae (Funston and Cremin, 1978). Intrarenal reflux can occur with as little as 2 mm Hg pressure in a neonate (Fig. 117–10). By 1 year of age, the pressure required is 1 order of magnitude greater (Funston and Cremin, 1978) and helps explain the relative infrequency of intrarenal reflux in older children.

Bacterial Virulence. Bacteria possess phenotypes that provide an infective advantage when exposed to the lumen of the urinary tract. Chief among these is the ability to adhere to uroepithelium. Adherence is mediated by interaction between specific molecules or ligands located on bacterial fimbriae and specific receptors on host uroepithelial cells. A full discussion of the mechanism of action of uropathogenic bacteria is found elsewhere in this text. Once bacteria bind to host epithelium, specific biologic responses are activated in both the microorganism and host cell. Bacterial responses are designed to facilitate their survival and proliferation, as well as inhibit host defenses. Such responses include release of endotoxin and reduction of ureteral peristalsis, which may lead to urinary stasis and reduced antegrade flow of urine. The host inflammatory response perpetuates the classic symptoms of UTI. Although a more systematic understanding of bacterial-host interactions in the propensity for reflux-associated renal scarring is not yet available, it appears that the bacteria responsible for postpyelonephritic scars in the presence of reflux often express fewer than three virulence factors (Lomberg et al, 1984). Ironically then, less virulent bacteria are most often sufficient to produce scarring in the presence of reflux.

Host Susceptibility and Response. Nonhematogenous bacterial access to the urinary tract rests essentially with periurethral organisms. Thus, the type and number of vaginal and preputial organisms will determine individual propensity for bladder colonization. Local factors such as hygiene and bowel habits will also influence the bacterial load presented to the perineal surface from the intestinal tract, the latter being the principal repository for organisms that infect the urinary tract. The functional diversity of the host receptors for bacterial adherence also plays a role in the success or failure of bacteria to gain entry to the bladder. In one study, girls with recurrent UTI harbored far heavier periurethral colonization than did a control group of girls who were free of infection, thus suggesting a variation in the function of antibacterial defenses in susceptible females (Bollgren and Winberg, 1976b). Furthermore, such factors may exhibit both gender- and age-related dimorphism (Bollgren and Winberg, 1976b). The great majority of UTIs in both sexes younger than 6 months is confined to uncircumcised boys (Rushton and Majd, 1992) and is consistent with the observation that *Escherichia coli* colonization is dense in infant boys but sparse in girls (Bollgren and Winberg, 1976a).

Perhaps the greatest tangible factor in promoting susceptibility to UTI is urinary dwell time. Postvoid urine volume is traditionally singled out as being suspect in providing sanctuary for ascending urethral organisms. Perhaps more important, however, is the overall dwell time between voids, which provides the greatest advantage to bacterial proliferation. **When the average doubling time for *E. coli* is measured in minutes, it is self-evident that a quantity of microorganisms sufficient for clinical infection can easily incubate exponentially in a bladder that is not emptied for several hours.**

Recent advances have also been made in understanding the renal epithelial response to pathogens. The classic components of the innate immune response to infection include activation of the complement system, recruitment of neutrophils and macrophages with scavenging ability, and production of a variety of cytokines, chemokines, and defensins (antimicrobial peptides). One family of receptors, the toll-like receptors (TLRs), respond to highly constant antigens expressed in bacteria (Chowdhury et al, 2004). The best studied of these, TLR4, detects lipopolysacaraide (LPS). A breakthrough in

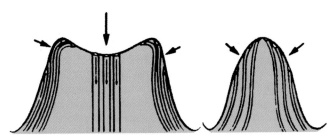

Figure 117–9. Papillary configuration in intrarenal reflux. A convex papilla (*right*) does not reflux because the crescentic or slitlike openings of its collecting ducts open obliquely onto the papilla. In contrast, a concave (*left*) or flat papilla refluxes because its collecting ducts open at right angles onto a flat papilla. (From Ransley PG, Risdon RA: Reflux and renal scarring. Br J Radiol 1978;14[Suppl]:1.)

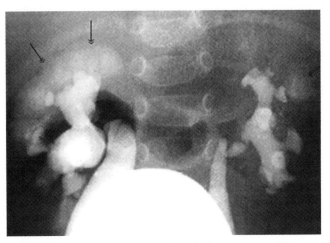

Figure 117–10. Intrarenal reflux (*arrows*) shown on a voiding cystourethrogram.

understanding renal infection came with the demonstration that mutations encoding the *TLR4* gene were responsible for LPS hyporesponsiveness (Hoshino et al, 1999). Nevertheless, molecules accessory to TLR4 are important to its response to LPS. Similarly, molecules such as CXCR1 and CXCR2 are receptors for interleukin-8, the principal renal epithelial secreted chemokine responsible for neutrophil migration (Godaly et al, 2000). Deficiencies in CXCR expression and function may underlie human susceptibility to pyelonephritis (Frendeus et al, 2000; Frendeus et al, 2001). Such advances placed into the context of VUR provide interesting and powerful opportunities to modify the natural history of the condition.

As well as orchestrating assembly of the phagosome for bacterial clearance, **the fallout of these renal epithelial processes that constitute the inflammatory response leads to local tissue damage and scarring.** Hallmarks of the response include capillary congestion, ischemia and reperfusion injury, and release of free oxygen radicals and inflammatory cytokines (Roberts, 1990; Roberts, 1992). Microabscess formation later coalesces into scar typical of the histologic changes of chronic pyelonephritis (Roberts, 1995). Although limiting the inflammatory response to reduce scarring may appear logical, no specific pyelonephritis anti-inflammatory pharmacotherapy is yet available. Traditional nonspecific anti-inflammatory agents, both steroidal and nonsteroidal, are not currently indicated for the treatment of pyelonephritis; in their current formulations the latter can pose a threat to renal function (Schaller and Kaplan, 1998). Nevertheless, the concept has been demonstrated experimentally in animals (Huang et al, 1999). A full understanding of the specific pathways involved in reflux-associated pyelonephritis could provide key strategies to limit specific renal inflammatory fallout without limiting bacterial clearance. Until then, antimicrobial prophylaxis instituted in a timely fashion, usually within 24 to 48 hours, is the single most effective pharmacologic strategy to date to limit the scarring consequences of pyelonephritis in both young and older children (Ransley and Risdon, 1981; Smellie et al, 1985).

Hypertension. VUR has long been held as the primary cause of significant hypertension in children. Arterial derangements in the renin-angiotensin system and sodium-potassium adenosine triphosphatase activity (Goonasekera and Dillon, 1998) may be involved, but the precise pathophysiology is not clear. Although methodologic flaws (Farnham et al, 2005) taint many studies of hypertension in the pediatric urology population, one recent study involving continuous ambulatory blood pressure monitoring revealed some correlation between progression to hypertension and more severe reflux nephropathy in children (Lama et al, 2003). A recent adult review of 157 patients with hypertension but no evidence of abnormal renal parameters discovered by cystography that latent VUR was present in 20% of the subjects, thus demonstrating that a significant association between reflux and hypertension exists in adulthood (Barai et al, 2004). The striking association between VUR diagnosed for the first time only in adulthood and arterial hypertension continues to underscore the importance of remaining vigilant about untreated infections in the reflux population (Kohler et al, 1997). Nevertheless, it remains unclear whether it is the nephropathy

associated with postinfection scarring, congenital dysmorphism and dysplasia associated with reflux, or some combination of both that predisposes to hypertension (Wolfish et al, 1993). This latter observation questions, then, whether prevention of postinfection scarring per se in the management of VUR will specifically help offset future hypertensive risk in patients in whom congenital renal dysmorphism is already present. There is obvious potential for the cause of reflux-related hypertension to rest with deranged renal microvascular mechanisms associated with parenchymal defects. This suggests that successful correction of reflux alone is unlikely to ameliorate blood pressure (Wallace et al, 1978). Indeed, removal of renal segments verified by selective renal vein sampling of arteriolar or segmental vessel renin levels has provided durable normalization of blood pressure in carefully selected patients (Tash et al, 2003). On occasion, complete removal of a small unilateral, congenitally dysmorphic, or globally scarred and shrunken kidney may also correct renovascular hypertension (Dillon and Smellie, 1984) because such kidneys are clearly not amenable to partial nephrectomy for any discrete segment.

Renal Growth. Several studies have attempted to demonstrate that correction of reflux will restore retarded renal growth associated with reflux, particularly when the growth defect is in a unilaterally affected kidney. However, reflux correction is a poor predictor of catch-up up growth in such kidneys (Hagberg et al, 1984; Shimada et al, 1988). A significant factor governing growth of an ipsilateral kidney is the function of its contralateral mate. Although forestalling infection in the presence of VUR will maintain the normal trajectory of renal growth in most cases (Smellie et al, 1981), it must be remembered that compensatory hypertrophy of the contralateral kidney will magnify the perceived impact of infection on renal growth because the contralateral developing kidney will assume the required renal function whenever the ipsilateral kidney is unable to contribute optimally to function. When correction of reflux has been associated with improved renal growth, it is likely that it is due to removal of the propensity for ascending infection rather than elimination of the reflux per se (Willscher et al, 1976a; Willscher et al, 1976b).

Renal Failure and Somatic Growth. In 2005, renal failure caused by primary VUR-associated infection should be an anachronism (although it is still seen) largely because of the virtual paradigm shift in reflux management championed by Smellie and coworkers during their pivotal studies of reflux and infection in children during the 1970s and 1980s. Over the past 30 years, the incidence of chronic pyelonephritis as a primary cause of end-stage renal disease has fallen from 15% to 25% (Human Renal Transplant Registry, 1975) to less than 2% (North American Pediatric Renal Transplant Committee, 2004). (Reflux nephropathy in all its forms, however, was the fourth most common primary diagnosis in nonblack pediatric transplant recipients [North American Pediatric Renal Transplant Committee, 2004].) The medical renal disease (Hinchliffe et al, 1994) that accompanies renal scarring can include hyperfiltration, concentrating defects, proteinuria, microalbuminuria (Lama et al, 1997), renal tubular acidosis (Guizar et al, 1996), and defects in fractional excretion of sodium and magnesium. Although all these parameters are probably the direct result of tubular and parenchymal damage or dysmorphism, concentrating defects have been reported in the presence of sterile reflux, independent of any history of infection (Walker et al, 1973). The concentrating defect is proportional to the grade of reflux and improves after cessation of reflux. These observations have suggested that a relative flow resistance may be created by the retrograde nature of reflux and raise the possibility of a functionally obstructive parameter in reflux pathogenesis. However, the precise relationship between antegrade flow, retrograde flow, and bladder dynamics in this theoretical mechanism has not been fully articulated.

One of the best global parameters of renal function in children is the somatic growth curve. Many children with VUR fall below the normal age-adjusted growth curve, particularly those with bilateral reflux and some degree of renal damage. Furthermore, successful suppression of pyelonephritis through either medical prevention of infection or surgical correction of reflux itself can result in catch-up growth, both in height and in weight (Polito et al, 1996; Polito et al, 1997). Although clear superiority has yet to be demonstrated between medical and surgical therapy to achieve improvement in growth or subsequent renal scarring after an initial pyelonephritic insult, surgical correction of reflux can benefit somatic growth when recurrent breakthrough infection indicates failure of antibiotic prophylaxis (Sutton and Atwell, 1989).

ASSOCIATED ANOMALIES AND CONDITIONS

Ureteropelvic Junction Obstruction

VUR and UPJ obstruction are two of the most common pathologic conditions in pediatric urology. Thus, it is not unusual that these two conditions coexist. Whether the concomitant presence of these two conditions is a random event or is causally related remains unclear. It has been speculated that a developmental ureteral bud anomaly may be responsible for the imperfect formation of both the UVJ and UPJ (Bomalaski et al, 1997a).

The incidence of VUR associated with UPJ obstruction ranges from 9% to 18% (Lebowitz and Blickman, 1983; Maizels et al, 1984; Hollowell et al, 1989; Bomalaski et al, 1997a; Kim et al, 2001). When the two conditions were primarily present, most of the patients in these studies had reflux that was coincidentally discovered, was of low grade, and resolved spontaneously with time. Such patients typically exhibited a significant discrepancy between the minimal degree of ureteral dilatation and the significantly dilated renal pelvis; thus, the apparent grade of reflux may be overestimated, and management decisions based on the grade of reflux would be inaccurate at best.

Conversely, the incidence of UPJ obstruction in patients with reflux ranges from 0.75% to 3.6% (Lebowitz and Blickman, 1983; Bomalaski et al, 1997a), with **high-grade reflux being five times more likely than lower grades of reflux to be associated with UPJ obstruction** (Lebowitz and Blickman, 1983; Bomalaski et al, 1997a). Indeed, in one study of children with reflux and hydronephrosis, 50% of patients with high-grade sonographic hydronephrosis, commonly associated with the highest grades of reflux, showed an obstructive pattern on furosemide (Lasix) scintigraphy (Stauss et al, 2003).

Three radiologic signs might suggest the existence of UPJ obstruction in the setting of reflux. First, if the pelvis shows little or no filling whereas the ureter is dilated by contrast, it may indicate a point of kinking secondary to reflux, or it may occur as a result of primary UPJ obstruction itself (Fig. 117–11). Second, contrast that does enter the pelvis may be poorly visualized because of dilution in a large pelvic volume, and the pelvis will exhibit markedly reduced radiodensity in comparison to the ureter or bladder. Finally, a large pelvis that fails to exhibit prompt drainage but retains contrast is also suggestive of UPJ obstruction.

Radiographic studies of UPJ obstruction associated with VUR may indicate true anatomic obstruction or simply dilation associated with pelviureteral dilation from higher grades of reflux. Hollowell and colleagues (1989) referred to three clinical categories of concomitant obstruction and reflux. Group 1 had primary UPJ obstruction and incidental low-grade reflux, and group 2 had secondary UPJ obstruction from high-grade reflux. These two groups represent true anatomic obstruction, for which pyeloplasty is recommended. Group 3 represents only significant dilation of the upper tracts, which is confirmed by documenting good drainage by cystography or renal scintigraphy.

The etiology of secondary UPJ obstruction is unclear. Several factors are thought to predispose to or even aggravate a potential narrowing at the level of the UPJ. High-grade reflux may result in kinking of the upper ureter and adjacent pelvic junction. The chronic effects of reflux may also stretch the renal pelvis so that atonicity and an inability to propel urine through the UPJ may occur (Whitaker, 1973). In the setting of UTI propagated to the upper tracts by reflux, inflammation and ureteritis can also contribute to transient or chronic obstruction at the UPJ.

The convergence of two seminal ureteral anomalies in the same patient raises additional management questions when treatment of one anomaly may affect the natural history of the other. Nevertheless, the guiding therapeutic principle is preservation of renal function. Although sterile reflux may be observed, obstruction, even in the absence of infection, may jeopardize renal function. Therefore, in the presence of reflux, if scintigraphy with catheter drainage confirms obstruction, pyeloplasty should be performed. The secondary insult to the UPJ from reflux is an evolving process that cannot be efficiently or adequately corrected by surgical repair of the reflux itself. Furthermore, reflux correction alone risks amplifying upper tract dilation during the phase of postoperative edema in the lower ureter, as well as risks introducing infection in a renal pelvis still harboring obstruction at the UPJ.

Simultaneous open correction of UPJ obstruction and reflux has always raised concern over surgical manipulation of both the upper and lower ureteral segments at the same time and its potential negative impact on ureteral vascularity. However, the advent of endoscopic injection raises the possibility of correcting reflux at the time of pyeloplasty for secondary or primary UPJ obstruction. The indications for correction of reflux are being reevaluated since the advent of endoscopic therapy and are discussed in the later section on endoscopic management.

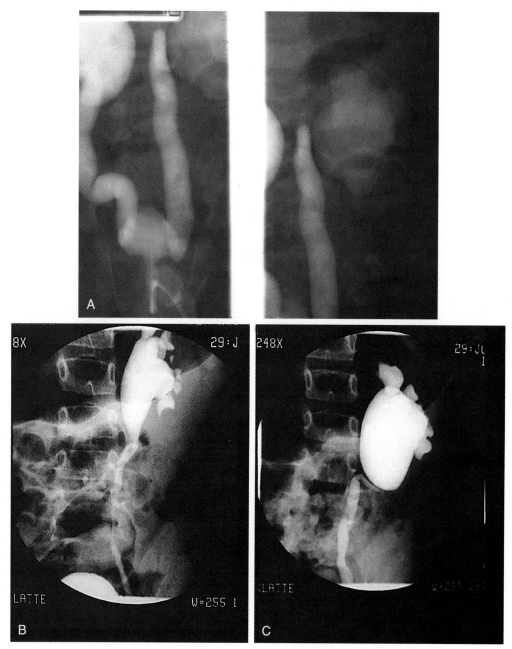

Figure 117–11. Reflux and ureteropelvic junction (UPJ) obstruction. **A,** Significant reflux fills the left ureter to the level of the UPJ. Minimal filling of the pelvis can be a sign of obstruction at this level. **B,** In a different patient, reflux is seen as the bladder fills. **C,** Significant kinking of the UPJ occurs with voiding.

Ureteral Duplication

VUR is the most common abnormality associated with complete ureteral duplication. The embryologic origin of the duplicated ureter supports the observation that reflux occurs most commonly into the lower pole. This relationship is based on the studies of Weigert (1877) and Meyer (1946), who documented a more lateral and proximal insertion of the lower pole ureter associated with a shorter intramural ureter at the UVJ (Fig. 117–12).

The incidence of reflux is increased in patients with complete ureteral duplication (Privett et al, 1976). Earlier studies provide a limited view of whether reflux in a duplex moiety carries increased patient risk because of lack of control groups, arbitrary patient selection, and short follow-up. There has been some tendency to correct reflux based on the existence of the duplication anomaly itself. Even in the absence of obstruction from a ureterocele or ureteral ectopia, duplication with low-grade reflux may take longer to resolve than in single-system reflux, although it carries no increased risk of increasing grade, breakthrough infection, or scarring (Ben-Ami et al, 1989; Husmann and Allen, 1991). The most recent series supports this finding in low-grade reflux but notes that high-grade reflux into lower pole ureters in females is more prone to breakthrough infection and scarring and may therefore warrant more aggressive management (Afshar et al, 2005).

Bladder Diverticula

A full discussion of bladder diverticula is found elsewhere in this text. The outpouching of mucosa between detrusor muscle bundles without any true muscle backing itself, commonly defining a bladder diverticulum, has the theoretical

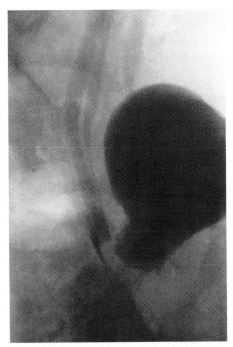

Figure 117–12. Reflux into both ureters of a complete duplication, as shown here, is less common than reflux into the lower pole ureter alone.

potential to affect the natural history of VUR in two ways. Most commonly, if the UVJ is distorted by a so-called paraureteral diverticulum that shares an anatomic point of origin at or near the UVJ, it is theoretically possible that the configuration of the diverticulum could compromise the antireflux configuration of the UVJ and cause reflux (Fig. 117–13). Second and more rarely, a large paraureteral diverticulum could expand within Waldeyer's fascia and cause ureteral obstruction, or it could project forward into the bladder and obstruct the bladder outlet, much as a ureterocele, and incite secondary reflux (Boechat and Lebowitz, 1978). Although the latter would require cystoscopic confirmation, neither cystoscopy nor imaging is predictive of whether paraureteral diverticula truly compromise the resolution of reflux, as has commonly been believed. Hutch (1952) was the first to recognize that bladder diverticula were congenital abnormalities that occurred primarily in smooth-walled normal bladders in children. A 40-year review of the literature from 1966 to 2004 failed to provide any objective case-control or cohort studies to support the routine repair of reflux when the sole indication was the presence of a paraureteral or Hutch diverticulum. However, a contemporary retrospective cohort analysis of 84 patients with paraureteral diverticula and reflux showed no significant difference in spontaneous resolution rates (60%, 39%, and 22% for grades I-II, III, and IV-V reflux with a paraureteral diverticulum versus 52%, 28%, and 33% in a matched control group of 95 refluxing patients without a diverticulum). Rates of UTI and scarring were similar in both groups. Multivariate analysis revealed reflux grade to be the only predictor of resolution in both groups (Afshar, 2005). Thus, **reflux associated with paraureteral diverticula resolves at rates similar to those of primary reflux and should be managed according to the prevailing indications**

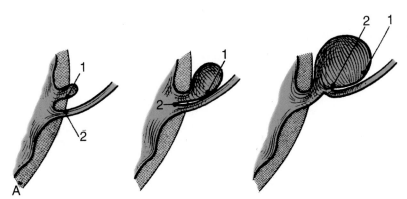

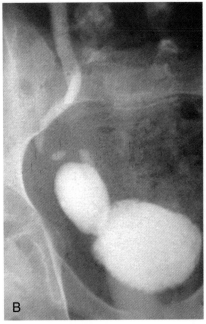

Figure 117–13. A, Schematic representation of a bladder diverticulum. A small amount of mucosa initially herniates through a congenital defect in the bladder musculature. The defect enlarges with voiding. Finally, the ureteral orifice is incorporated into the diverticulum. **B,** Reflux into a right-sided paraureteral diverticulum and ureter seen on voiding cystography. (**A,** From Hernanz-Schulman M, Lebowitz RL: The elusiveness and importance of bladder diverticula in children. Pediatr Radiol 1995;15:399-402.)

for the reflux itself, irrespective of the diverticulum. However, when a refluxing ureter enters a diverticulum, the latter is no longer paraureteral. With no muscular support for the UVJ, reflux is not expected to resolve. In a given patient, indications for repair require the combined consideration of the potential impact of unresolved reflux, if any, along with whether the diverticulum itself is of sufficient size or conformation to incite complications.

Renal Anomalies

By definition, reflux represents a dysfunction of the UVJ. Because development of both the UVJ and the kidney itself is linked to the origin and fate of the ureteral bud, it is reasonable to consider the existence of reflux whenever an anomaly in renal form or number is present. **The cardinal renal anomalies associated with reflux are multicystic dysplastic kidney (MCDK) and renal agenesis, and the presence of either condition mandates a VCUG.** In the largest series to date, 75 patients with MCDK had a 25% prevalence (19 patients) of contralateral reflux, and half of these were low grade (I to II) (Miller et al, 2004). Spontaneous resolution occurred in a mean of 4.4 years, regardless of grade. Only one patient had reflux corrected surgically. In a small series of ureteral ectopia, one patient with MCDK had the contralateral ureter enter into the ductus deferens (Wunsch et al, 2000), thus further underscoring the importance of documenting the contralateral kidney's ureteral conformation in patients with MCDK. Although contralateral renal growth often displays compensatory hypertrophy, one study observed somewhat less compensatory hypertrophy by 1 year of age (Zerin and Leiser, 1998) when contralateral reflux was also present (5.1 vs. 6.2 cm median renal length, $P < .001$).

Renal agenesis is associated with an even higher prevalence of contralateral VUR. In a retrospective study of 46 children with solitary renal agenesis, the rate of contralateral renal pathology was 46%. VUR was by far the most common contralateral defect (28%) (Cascio et al, 1999), with UVJ and UPJ obstruction seen in 11% and 7%, respectively. Both UPJ obstruction and reflux were present in one patient. In another study, 19 cases of contralateral reflux were observed in 51 patients with ipsilateral renal agenesis (Song et al, 1995). Reflux repair or persistence was documented in 9 and 7 patients, respectively, with spontaneous resolution observed in only 3 patients. Whether renal agenesis represents one extreme on a continuum that includes MCDK is unclear. Nevertheless, these data suggest that contralateral reflux associated with renal agenesis may show less tendency for spontaneous resolution than that associated with MCDK.

Megacystis-Megaureter Association

Massive bilateral VUR can cause a gradual remodeling of the entire upper urinary tract. The gross inefficiency of the bladder, which expels urine to both the exterior and the upper tracts, results in gradual bladder dilation as the refluxed urine returns to the bladder. This perpetuates marked ureteral dilation and leads to the radiographic appearance of massive hydroureter and a thin-walled enlarged bladder (Burbige et al, 1984). The phenomenon is referred to as the megacystis-megaureter association or syndrome. This configuration is even discernible in utero (Mandell et al, 1992). It is more frequent in males, and differentiation from PUV is crucial. Whereas the latter is due to an obstructive lesion, the megacystis-megaureter association is a nonobstructive condition akin to cardiac dilation that is caused by regurgitation from incompetent valves. Voiding studies will readily demonstrate an open posterior urethra and differentiate megacystis-megaureter from PUV or prune-belly syndrome. The persistent large residual urine volume is a significant risk factor for recurrent UTI. Vesicostomy can temporize by eliminating the residual urine volume and establishing safe drainage of the upper tracts until ureteral reimplantation can be performed. Given the propensity for reflux to exacerbate the effects of bacteriuria and the fact that UVJ dysfunction is the primary factor perpetuating the syndrome, surgical correction of the reflux is indicated. Treatments aimed at improving an already patent bladder outlet are contraindicated, risk infection, and will fail to correct the primary cause. A period of bladder rehabilitation by strict attention to emptying in the postoperative period (Koefoot et al, 1981) usually results in return to normal bladder volume and contractile behavior. This suggests that potentially normal underlying bladder physiology can be realized if the propensity for reflux is corrected.

Other Anomalies

VUR has also been described in association with a number of congenital conditions and syndromes. No precise common genetic insult has been determined to explain such associations. A complete survey of the Online Mendelian Inheritance in Man Database developed by Johns Hopkins University and maintained by the National Center of Biotechnology Information reveals over 40 different syndromes in which VUR has been described, including the VACTERL association (vertebral, anal, cardiac, tracheoesophageal, renal, and limb anomalies), CHARGE syndrome (coloboma, heart disease, atresia choanae, retarded development, genital hypoplasia, and ear anomalies), and imperforate anus. In cases in which VUR is anticipated, a VCUG is the initial study of choice to disclose both dysfunction at the UVJ and overall bladder and bladder outlet anatomy.

Pregnancy and Reflux

The morphology of the urinary tract is altered with the onset of pregnancy and increases throughout gestation (Beydoun, 1985). **Bladder tone decreases because of edema and hyperemia, changes that predispose the patient to bacteriuria. In addition, urine volume increases in the upper collecting system as the physiologic dilatation of pregnancy evolves.** The slower drainage that results can enhance the growth of organisms and increase the propensity for the development of pyelonephritis. It seems logical to assume that during pregnancy the presence of VUR in a system already prone to bacteriuria would lead to increased morbidity. A number of studies have been conducted to examine this relationship.

The presence of active reflux appears to present a risk factor for the affected mother. In 1958, Hutch described a higher incidence of pyelonephritis during pregnancy in 23 women with a history of reflux and recurrent bacteriuria. Heidrick and associates (1967) evaluated 321 women with cystography either during the last trimester or within 30 hours after delivery. The incidence of pyelonephritis was 33% in women with reflux versus less than 5% in women without reflux. Finally, cystograms performed 4 to 6 months postpartum in 100 women with a history of asymptomatic bacteriuria during pregnancy showed reflux in 21%. Bacteriuria was easier to clear in patients without reflux (67%) than in those with reflux (33%) (Williams et al, 1968).

Maternal history also becomes a factor if past reflux, renal scarring, or a tendency for UTIs is included. Martinell and colleagues (1990) compared the outcome of pregnancy in matched controls with that in 41 women with and without renal scarring after childhood UTI. They found that women with a history of previous infections had a high incidence of bacteriuria during pregnancy whereas those with renal scarring and persistent reflux were more prone to the development of acute pyelonephritis. In a similar study, the outcome of pregnancy was assessed in 88 women with previous bacteriuria. Women with known scars had a 3.3-fold increased incidence of hypertension, a 7.6-fold increased risk for preeclampsia, and a higher rate of obstetric interventions. Women with normal kidneys and reflux also had an increased risk for hypertension during the last trimester (McGladdery et al, 1992). Pregnant women with bilateral renal scars were shown to have a higher incidence of preeclampsia than those with unilateral scarring (24% vs. 7%, respectively) (El-Khatib et al, 1994), and those with elevated creatinine levels are also at risk (Jungers et al, 1987). In a large study of 158 women with reflux nephropathy, pregnancy was uneventful in patients with normal blood pressure and renal function, whereas the risk for fetal demise and accelerated maternal renal disease was increased in women with impaired renal function (Jungers et al, 1996).

The implications of reimplantation surgery were studied by Austenfeld and Snow (1988), who found an increased risk for UTI and fetal loss in 31 women who had undergone ureteral reimplantation as children, despite correction of the anomaly. In a follow-up study comparing these patients with a new cohort of historical controls, women with UTI and reflux who underwent reimplantation (suggesting an initially higher degree of reflux and increased renal scarring) were still at significant risk for UTI during pregnancy (Mansfield et al, 1995). However, they were not at higher risk for miscarriage than the general population. In a larger study of 77 pregnancies in 41 women whose ureters had been reimplanted, Bukowski and coworkers (1998) reported that the incidence of pyelonephritis during pregnancy was slightly higher than in the general population but that the fetus and mother were at significant risk when renal scarring or hypertension was present.

In summary, the majority of studies examining the effects of VUR on pregnancy suggest that women with a history of reflux have increased morbidity during pregnancy because of infection-related complications, regardless of whether the reflux has been corrected. **Women with hypertension and an element of renal failure are particularly at risk.** Those with uncorrected reflux appear to be especially at risk and should have their reflux corrected before pregnancy to minimize maternal and fetal morbidity. The morbidity during pregnancy in women with persistent reflux but no renal scarring remains poorly defined, but the tendency for UTI seems to be increased. Because of the difficulty in predicting an outcome

for this subset of patients, most clinicians recommend surgical correction for girls with reflux that persists beyond puberty. However, there has been a trend toward discontinuation of prophylactic antibiotics and expectant management in older girls with active reflux. Long-term follow-up studies of these patients through puberty are unavailable (see later discussion).

> **KEY POINTS: PREGNANCY AND REFLUX**
>
> ■ Physiologic changes in the ureter and bladder during pregnancy may influence the propensity for reflux-associated pyelonephritis in pregnant patients with reflux.
>
> ■ In the absence of definitive studies to the contrary, correction of reflux should be accomplished before pregnancy.

NATURAL HISTORY AND MANAGEMENT
Spontaneous Resolution

The one feature of VUR that provides the greatest relief to parents and caregivers while at the same time creating confusion in reflux study design and literature interpretation is spontaneous resolution. Indeed, the basis of contemporary medical therapy is predicated on an expected rate of spontaneous resolution. At birth, the probability of spontaneous resolution of primary reflux is roughly inversely proportional to the initial grade. If a patient is encountered at a later age, resolution from any point in time forward will depend on the initial grade of reflux, if it is known, and the age at initial evaluation. For example, unilateral grade III reflux at birth should resolve in 70% of cases by 5 years of age. However, if a 6-year-old with normal bladder function is found to have grade III reflux, it is much less likely to resolve. Given a growing tendency among some clinicians to reassess females for persistent reflux and possible endoscopic correction after a "holiday period" of non–follow-up (between 5 years and the teenage years), it is possible that new information remains to be learned about resolution of reflux. Reflux probably resolves spontaneously because of remodeling of the UVJ over time, with progressive elongation and consolidation of the intravesical ureter and antireflux mechanism, as well as stabilization of bladder dynamics. Conversely, failure of the latter probably accounts for persistence of reflux beyond the statistical norms in many patients. Indeed, an inability to strictly understand bladder dynamics may have skewed earlier determinations of absolute reflux resolution rates, but in doing so it provided a "real-world" picture of spontaneous resolution.

Resolution by Grade

Most cases of low-grade reflux (grade I and II) will resolve. Several studies have documented this high rate of spontaneous resolution. However, the variance in reported resolution rates for low-grade reflux (63% of grade II [Duckett,

1983], 80% of grade II [Arant, 1992], 85% of grade II [Edwards et al, 1977]) belies the fact that lower urinary tract dynamics may also play a role in mitigating spontaneous resolution.

Grade III reflux will resolve in approximately 50% of cases (Duckett, 1983; McLorie et al, 1990). Very few cases of higher-grade reflux (grades IV and V and bilateral grade III) will resolve spontaneously. Analyses from several sources, including the International Reflux Study in Children, support a uniformly low prevalence of resolved high-grade reflux, with no more than 25% (Weiss et al, 1992a) and as few as 9% (Skoog et al, 1987) of patients demonstrating spontaneous resolution. It is possible that no real difference exists in the resolution rates of high-grade reflux (Tamminen-Mobius et al, 1992). When one considers the fact that any given reflux grade is assigned on the basis of a dynamic voiding study, the possibility for variability by at least one grade, especially in assigning higher grades to reflux, is quite real. Thus, attempting to discriminate true differences in resolution rates for grade III and higher reflux may not be particularly clinically relevant.

Resolution by Age

The age at which reflux begins or is first encountered will play a more potent role in the management of a patient with reflux than will the grade itself. **It is self-evident that if reflux is a congenital disorder with an inherent tendency to resolve spontaneously over time, it will be most prevalent in neonates and young children and will demonstrate the greatest tendency to resolve in this group.** Conversely, in any analysis, if the reflux is truly primary and is encountered in an older child in whom it has been present since birth, it has already demonstrated a propensity to persist and is therefore self-selected for reflux that is unlikely to resolve (Skoog et al, 1987). The American Urological Association (AUA) guidelines data provide a synthesis of large numbers and reasonable statistical estimates of resolution rates segregated by age and grade (Fig. 117–14). Interpretation of more recent follow-up studies (Connolly et al, 2001) suggests that diagnosis at age 5, as well as in infancy, is associated with a similar resolution rate (20% per year), regardless of age. However, as stated at the outset, it must be remembered that resolution 5 years after age

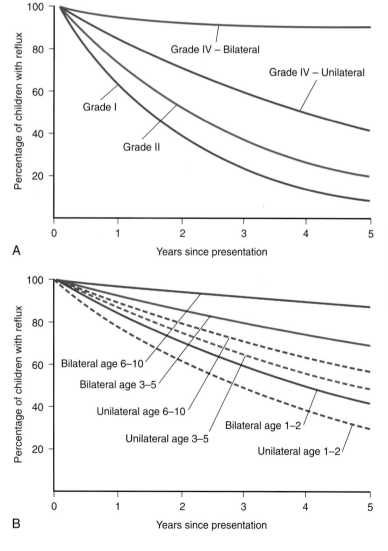

Figure 117–14. **A,** Percent chance of persistence of grades I, II, and IV reflux for 1 to 5 years after initial evaluation. **B,** Percent chance of persistence of grade III reflux by age for 1 to 5 years after initial evaluation. (From American Urological Association: Report on the Management of Vesicoureteral Reflux in Children. Baltimore, American Urological Association, Pediatric Vesicoureteral Reflux Clinical Guidelines Panel, 1997.)

5 implies that reflux has required 10 years to resolve versus resolution 5 years after birth. Moreover, the observation by McLorie and colleagues (1990) that high-grade reflux in patients evaluated after birth showed no difference in resolution rates between subjects younger and older than 1 year may reflect the generally poor resolution rate of high-grade reflux to begin with. Thus, persistence in early life will imply persistence when older. These principles probably underlie the observation that when reflux resolves, it often does so within the first few years of life. The study by Skoog and associates (1987) observed that reflux resolved in 30% to 35% of subjects each year. Reflux resolved in younger patients (<12 months old) more quickly (1.44 versus 1.85 years, $P < .02$), with grade III requiring slightly more time than grade II to resolve (1.56 versus 1.97 years, $P < .04$).

The traditional period of observation for resolution is 5 years, probably because the greatest proportion of growth and anatomic remodeling of the UVJ is complete. In the McLorie study, 92% of resolved grade III reflux occurred within 4 years. There is a tendency to ascribe a benefit to the observation of interval reduction in grade. Such a finding could herald progression to resolution, but in the end it still carries the same risk of escalating a UTI to pyelonephritis and thus should be interpreted with caution when counseling families. Resolution rates for VUR monitored into the teenage and adult years remain unknown. Clearly then, what constitutes resolution of reflux depends on the period over which resolution is sought.

KEY POINTS: NATURAL HISTORY AND MANAGEMENT

■ Reflux has a natural tendency to resolve spontaneously.

■ The likelihood of resolution is inversely proportional to grade.

■ Maintaining urine sterility (through both prophylactic antibiotics and frequent bladder emptying) is the cornerstone of "watchful waiting" medical management.

■ The success rate of surgical correction is very high.

Principles of Management

Medical and surgical therapy for reflux has purported to offer similar benefit to patients (Table 117–5). This has fueled the debate between fundamental choices of therapy for decades. The tension embedded in decision-making for reflux management stems from the almost perfect results attainable by surgical correction of reflux, now commonly successful in more than 98% of cases. However, traditional practice in management of reflux has held that the end does not justify the means: reflux correction is not indicated merely because it can be corrected easily and reliably. As stated earlier, almost 80% of low-grade and half of grade III reflux will resolve spontaneously. Walker (1994) has summarized the essential tenants of reflux management.

Table 117–5. Outcomes of Medical and Surgical Therapy for Children with Primary Vesicoureteral Reflux and Renal Scarring

Registrant	No. of Patients	New Scars	Thinning
Europe			
Medical	155	19 (12%)	11 (7%)
Surgical	151	20 (13%)	15 (10%)
United States			
Medical	66	14 (20%)	9 (13%)
Surgical	64	16 (25)%	2 (3%)

1. Spontaneous resolution of reflux is very common.
2. High-grade reflux is less likely to resolve spontaneously.
3. Sterile reflux is benign.
4. Extended use of prophylactic antibiotics is benign.
5. The success rate with surgical correction is very high.

Rather than providing strict guidelines for treatment, the foregoing principles provide ample room to individualize treatment based on the particular preferences and tolerances of physicians, families, and patients for the various burdens that each of the principles entails. **The classic approach has been to offer daily low-dose prophylactic antibiotic suppression of infections as the first line of treatment under the principle that every case of reflux should be offered time to resolve spontaneously, despite grade.** Clearly, age at initial encounter and grade will factor into predicting when and whether resolution is likely to occur. In addition, the diagnosis of reflux in patients after one or more episodes of pyelonephritis or the presence of scarring on renal scintigraphy may temper a decision for extended prophylaxis and observation, particularly if scarring is extensive, the reflux is high grade, renal function is already globally depressed, or congenital dysmorphism of one or both kidneys is present. In such cases, tolerance for yet another infection despite the presence of prophylaxis may be low, or simple disquiet with the notion of ongoing reflux may invite strong consideration for correction of reflux.

As stated previously, it is not clear how long to wait for resolution of reflux in an individual patient. In newborn patients, it is reasonable to wait until approximately 5 years of age, assuming that no intercurrent breakthrough infections occur. Beyond this age, the kidneys become less prone to scarring after pyelonephritis (Olbing et al, 2003). Thus, some practitioners are withdrawing prophylaxis as the child approaches the age of 5. After this age, boys with asymptomatic reflux will require little or no formal follow-up as long as lifelong attention to good bladder habits is reinforced and they are counseled to seek prompt medical attention, as well as reassessment of their reflux status, if pyelonephritis were to occur in the future. Nevertheless, there would still be disagreement regarding whether to correct asymptomatic bilateral high-grade reflux with normal renal parenchyma and function in an older boy despite the belief that sterile reflux is benign. Girls have traditionally undergone open surgical correction, even for asymptomatic reflux that fails to resolve by the age of 5, on the premise that it will reduce maternal and fetal morbidity during future pregnancy. Using the rationale of antibiotic withdrawal in an older child, one study demonstrated that recurrent febrile UTIs mandating surgical correction of reflux will subsequently develop in less than 10% of patients (Cooper et al, 2000), albeit with limited clinical follow-up and using only ultrasound imaging to assess renal health. Clinical guidelines for reflux management in children are presented in Table 117–6.

Adult patients who have nonobstructive flank pain, febrile UTI, or pyelonephritis and are found to have VUR have traditionally been offered antireflux surgery. Endoscopic correction of uncomplicated adult reflux should also be possible.

The Emerging Role for Endoscopic Correction of Reflux. Endoscopic management is discussed in greater detail later. In North America, the relative ease and low morbidity associated with endoscopic correction have begun to transform the indications for correction of unresolved reflux in females. Indeed, whereas open antireflux surgery is more technically demanding, as well as more taxing on older female patients, endoscopic correction can be easily performed well into the teenage years and beyond. Between the age of 5 and the mid to late teens, girls with asymptomatic reflux may be treated in the same fashion as boys and have their antibiotic prophylaxis withdrawn and follow-up imaging suspended for several years in the absence of any febrile UTI. Such management will also afford the opportunity for a new cohort of older patients to provide longer-term resolution rates on a systematic basis. Girls may then return for a final cystogram. If reflux is still present, endoscopic injection is performed, followed by a postinjection cystogram. Formal prospective trials of this proposition will be required to validate the principle.

Moreover, studies of parental preference in reflux management are revealing that endoscopic treatment may sometimes be preferred over either antibiotic prophylaxis or open surgery, depending on the perceived duration for resolution of the reflux (Ogan et al, 2001; Capozza et al, 2003). However, such studies must be interpreted with caution in that any therapy that combines low morbidity and technical ease can become a seductive choice, especially since endoscopic therapy was preferred despite an acknowledged lower success rate than with open surgery and the potential for more than one anesthetic. Alternatively, others may tolerate only definitive open surgical correction.

Notwithstanding the ethical considerations of proffering endoscopic treatment for correction of reflux, endoscopic indications have wider theoretical potential than is the case with open surgery. For example, even if the durability of endoscopic correction is not indefinite, by recognizing that the prime age for postpyelonephritic scarring is younger than 5 years, one could conceive of temporary reflux correction by endoscopy in the early years and thereby obviate the need for several years of prophylaxis in either males or females. Beyond 5 years, postinjection recurrence of asymptomatic reflux in males, were it to occur, would be of little clinical consequence. Males would require reevaluation only if pyelonephritis were to develop anytime after the age of 5 years. In females, a demonstration of the durability of injection therapy extending from infancy to at least the end of the child-bearing years would be required. One recent long-term study documented a 5- to 7-year durability rate of only 80% (Dodat et al, 2004); thus, in one fifth of patients, reflux recurs. Moreover, these results were achieved with Macroplastique. Similar

data are as yet unavailable for Deflux. Nevertheless, regardless of the substance injected and the uneven durability in comparison to open correction of reflux reported to date, the endoscopic approach to reflux management has gained favor over the last several years in many European centers (Puri et al, 2003).

Medical Management: Watchful Waiting

Although some reports have suggested the existence of "water hammer" renal damage from high-grade reflux of sterile urine against the renal papillae (Hodson et al, 1975; Hagen and Klevmark, 1991), no such clinical entity has been predictably demonstrated. Because it is not reflux per se that is actually being managed, **the hallmark of observational therapy in reflux disease can be more accurately termed "watchful waiting" while maintaining urinary sterility through the judicious use of single daily low-dose antimicrobial prophylaxis.** Often, antibiotics are given as oral suspensions once per day and preferably at night. **Nighttime dosing allows for concentration of antibiotic in the bladder urine over the longest period of expected physiologic retention, when infection is most likely to develop.** In children younger than 2 months, the most commonly used medications are trimethoprim and amoxicillin. **Children younger than 2 months possess relative hepatic immaturity and are unable to clear sulfamethoxazole efficiently; the drug displaces fetal bilirubin and leads to jaundice.** After 2 months of age, the antibiotic of choice becomes trimethoprim-sulfamethoxazole (TSX, Septra, Bactrim). Like virtually any drug, some mild side effects, including gastrointestinal upset and allergy, should be kept in mind. Although transient leukopenia has been reported with TSX, it is rare, resolves with discontinuation of the drug, and is not believed to be significant enough to warrant regular monitoring of white blood cell counts in all children taking the drug. The other drug most commonly used is nitrofurantoin (Macrodantin). Nitrofurantoin may minimize the development of resistance to fecal organisms, the latter being the largest reservoir for urine infectivity. This drug is known to cause pulmonary fibrosis and, rarely, interstitial pneumonia. However, oral tolerance is less than with TSX because of taste, and the gastrointestinal symptoms are subjectively worse. A recent comprehensive literature review of the use of these drugs by Karpman and Kurzrock (2004) in children revealed a very low incidence of significant hepatic (five patients) or pulmonary (nine patients) involvement, almost always associated with full-dose rather than once-a-day low-dose therapy. Finally, a growing literature on the use of probiotics (live microorganisms such as strains of *Lactobacillus*, which may displace and suppress the growth of uropathogenic bacteria) is beginning to address UTI prophylaxis in children (Bruce and Reid, 2003; Reid and Devillard, 2004; Salvini et al, 2004). The mechanisms that underlie the demonstrated benefit of probiotic use are now emerging (Reid, 2000). Further studies will be required to define the use of this attractive approach in the medical treatment of patients with reflux.

Breakthrough febrile UTIs or pyelonephritis during antibiotic prophylaxis are generally considered an indication for

Table 117-6. Treatment Recommendations for Boys and Girls with Primary Vesicoureteral Reflux*

Clinical Manifestation		Initial (Antibiotic Prophylaxis or Open Surgical Repair)			Follow-up† (Continued Antibiotic Prophylaxis, Cystography, or Open Surgical Repair)		
VUR Grade and Laterality	Age (yr)	Guideline	Preferred Option	Reasonable Option	Guideline	Preferred Option	No Consensus‡
For Children without Scarring at Diagnosis							
I-II, unilateral or bilateral	<1	Prophylaxis					Boys and girls
	1-5	Prophylaxis					Boys and girls
	6-10	Prophylaxis					Boys and girls
III-IV, unilateral or bilateral	<1	Unilateral: prophylaxis					
	1-5	Prophylaxis	Bilateral: prophylaxis		Bilateral: surgery if persistent§	Unilateral: surgery if persistent§	
	6-10		Unilateral: prophylaxis / Bilateral: surgery	Bilateral: prophylaxis	Surgery if persistent§	Surgery if persistent§	
V, unilateral or bilateral	<1		Prophylaxis				
	1-5		Bilateral: prophylaxis	Bilateral: prophylaxis / Unilateral: surgery	Surgery if persistent§	Surgery if persistent§	
	6-10	Surgery					
For Children with Scarring at Diagnosis							
I-II, unilateral or bilateral	<1	Prophylaxis					Boys and girls
	1-5	Prophylaxis					Boys and girls
	6-10	Prophylaxis					Boys and girls
III-IV, unilateral	<1	Prophylaxis			Girls: surgery if persistent§	Boys: surgery if persistent§	
	1-5	Prophylaxis			Girls: surgery if persistent§	Boys: surgery if persistent§	
	6-10	Prophylaxis					
III-IV, bilateral	<1		Prophylaxis				
	1-5		Prophylaxis	Surgery	Surgery if persistent§		
	6-10	Surgery			Surgery if persistent§		
V, unilateral or bilateral	<1		Prophylaxis				
	1-5	Bilateral: surgery	Unilateral: surgery	Surgery	Surgery if persistent§	Surgery if persistent§	
	6-10	Surgery					

*Recommendations were derived from a survey of preferred treatment options from 36 clinical categories of children with reflux. The recommendations are classified as follows:
Guidelines: treatments selected by 8 or 9 of 9 panel members, given the strongest recommendation language.
Preferred Options: treatments selected by 5 to 7 of 9 panel members.
Reasonable Alternatives: treatments selected by 3 to 4 of 9 panel members.
No Consensus: treatment selected by no more than 2 of 9 panel members.
†For patients with persistent uncomplicated reflux after extended treatment with continuous antibiotic therapy.
‡No consensus was reached regarding the role of continued antibiotic prophylaxis, cystography, or surgery.
§See the text regarding the length of time that clinicians should wait before recommending surgery.
From American Urological Association: Report on the Management of Vesicoureteral Reflux in Children. Baltimore, American Urological Association, Pediatric Vesicoureteral Reflux Clinical Guidelines Panel, 1997.

termination of watchful waiting and correcting the reflux. However, individual documentation and verification of true breakthrough infection vary widely. As such, it is likely that instances of premature reflux correction (false positive), as well as failure to proceed with reflux correction (false negative), are to be expected. This possibility underscores the importance of proper antibiotic dosing, patient and parental acceptance and compliance with the chosen therapy, and meticulous attention to proper collection and handling of urine culture specimens (see earlier). Although the interaction between host defenses and bacterial virulence factors is what ideally dictates breakthrough infection, **Smellie has provided useful interpretations surrounding practical causes of breakthrough infection: (1) if the organism is sensitive to the prescribed prophylactic antibiotic, the child or parent has probably not been compliant or the dose is too low, and (2) if the organism is resistant to the prescribed antibiotic, either the residual bladder volume is too high too often, or the dose is too high** (Smellie, 1991). Indeed, many referrals for definitive reflux correction result from breakthrough UTI after full-dose antibiotic prophylaxis for extended periods.

Once radiographic resolution of reflux has been documented, antibiotic prophylaxis is terminated, usually a few days after the cystogram. However, because resolution of reflux will probably herald a discharge from regular urologic follow-up, this is also the precise time for reinforcing lifelong adoption of good toileting and bladder behavior.

The Landmark Studies

The efficacy of medical management rests with a few key studies that came to define and establish watchful waiting as a cornerstone of therapy for reflux disease. Jean Smellie and coworkers led a series of studies that repeatedly demonstrated the ability of low-dose prophylactic antibiotics to prevent infection and renal scarring while reflux resolved in a significant majority of children (Edwards et al, 1977). Since then, two additional large-scale prospective studies have validated this approach and helped further define the natural history of VUR.

The International Reflux Study in Children. This North American (Weiss et al, 1992a) and European (Tamminen-Mobius et al, 1992) cooperative study randomized children younger than 9 years with high-grade reflux to watchful waiting with prophylaxis or corrective open surgery (see Table 117–5). **Although surgery was complicated by temporary postoperative obstruction in some patients, it was more effective than prophylaxis in reducing, but not eliminating the occurrence of pyelonephritis. Nevertheless, the incidence of UTI (38%) was the same with both modalities. Furthermore, both modalities were equally effective in reducing, but not eliminating new scar formation.** Only the European arm stratified data for the effect of dysfunctional voiding behavior (18%) (van Gool et al, 1992). **When untreated, voiding dysfunction was associated with more UTIs, more persistent cases of reflux, and greater grade variation during follow-up.**

The Birmingham Reflux Study. Medical and surgical management was prospectively compared in a randomized cohort of 104 patients with high-grade reflux (Birmingham Reflux Study Group, 1987) over a 5-year period. Again, the incidence of new scars was the same with either treatment modality. Although more than half the patients continued to reflux at 5 years, all cases of new scarring occurred within the first 2 years, consistent with the "big bang" concept of postinfectious renal injury mentioned previously.

Additional Prospective Studies. Medical management alone was assessed in 59 patients (84 refluxing ureters, grades I to III) by the Southwest Pediatric Nephrology Group (Arant, 1992). Resolution occurred in 67%, breakthrough infection in 33%, and new scarring in 10% of the low-grade and 28% of the grade III patients. Scholtmeijer (1993) demonstrated resolution in 57% of 47 cases of grade III to IV reflux, followed by watchful waiting and prophylaxis for 5 years. Interestingly, 15 patients underwent surgical correction after breakthrough infection, and new scars subsequently developed in 6 of them, whereas new scars developed in 2 of the patients managed medically.

Antibiotic prophylaxis is not a panacea—this approach is destined to fail without adequate teaching and periodic review of perineal hygiene techniques, timely bladder emptying habits, and anticonstipation measures. Similarly, family compliance with antibiotic administration and follow-up visits for imaging may vary widely (Wan et al, 1996). Careful discussion of obligations and expectations should take place to assess whether watchful waiting is appropriate in each case. Given the need for strict compliance with such an approach, alternative regimens, such as alternate-day dosing of prophylactic antibiotics, or no prophylaxis with early aggressive treatment of UTI using full-dose antibiotics, though conceptually attractive, will be at risk for decreasing compliance, especially when new opportunities for relaxing a daily routine and awareness are introduced into the management profile. If families or patients are willing but unable to maintain all the elements of a watchful waiting treatment regimen, consideration for open or endoscopic correction of VUR may be relatively indicated.

SURGICAL MANAGEMENT

Starting with Hutch's initial report on the successful correction of VUR in seven out of nine paraplegic patients (Hutch, 1952), multiple surgical techniques have been described to effectively correct VUR. Currently, the principles from these techniques have been incorporated into a handful of procedures with excellent results. The choice of procedure is individualized according to the surgeon's experience and the patient's condition.

Surgical Principles of Reflux Correction

The principles of surgical correction of reflux include the following:
- Exclusion of causes of secondary VUR
- Adequate mobilization of the distal ureter without tension or damage to its delicate blood supply

- Creation of a submucosal tunnel that is generous in caliber and satisfies the 5:1 ratio of length to width recommended by Paquin (1959)
- Attention to the entry point of the ureter into the bladder (hiatus), the direction of the submucosal tunnel, and the ureteromucosal anastomosis to prevent stenosis, angulation, or twisting of the ureter
- Attention to the muscular backing of the ureter to achieve an effective antireflux mechanism
- Gentle handling of the bladder to reduce postoperative hematuria and bladder spasms

The surgical procedures can be classified according to the approach to the ureter as *intravesical*, *extravesical*, or *combined*; furthermore, they can be classified according to the position of the submucosal tunnel in relation to the original hiatus as *suprahiatal* or *infrahiatal*.

The following components apply to all of the various surgical techniques. The surgeon is free to select the appropriate components tailored to the patient's anatomy to achieve successful ureteral reimplantation. Prophylactic antibiotics may be administered with induction of anesthesia. Patients are generally admitted the morning of the surgery unless specific reasons require preoperative admission. Enemas are reserved only for select cases because all issues related to dysfunctional elimination should be addressed when the diagnosis of VUR is made.

Cystoscopy

Historically, many centers performed cystoscopy after the diagnosis of VUR on the premise that it offers a predictive assessment of the likelihood of spontaneous resolution of VUR. Parameters such as shape (except for the golf hole orifice associated with high-grade reflux) and location of the ureteral orifice and submucosal tunnel length were subsequently found to not have predictive value (Duckett and Bellinger, 1982). Therefore, cystoscopy in the course of conservative management of VUR is indicated only to confirm or manage abnormalities found on other imaging modalities (Ferrer et al, 1998).

Some surgeons choose to perform cystoscopy at the time of ureteral reimplantation surgery after induction of anesthesia. This is helpful in identifying subtle anomalies not detected on preoperative imaging, particularly if an extravesical technique is used and the bladder is not opened. Preoperative cystoscopy may uncover inflammatory changes, trabeculation, duplication anomalies, or anatomic anomalies at the UVJ, such as small ureteroceles or diverticula.

The bladder should be examined as it is distending because a paraureteral diverticulum may not be apparent until the bladder is moderately to fully distended. PIC cystography (Rubenstein et al, 2003; Edmondson et al, 2006) has also been recommended for the detection of occult reflux in children who have had a febrile UTI and a negative VCUG. In both of these techniques the tip of the cystoscope is positioned at the ureteral orifice and flow of the irrigating fluid (with or without radiographic contrast) is directed at the ureter. Elevation of the anterior wall of the ureter to allow visualization of the ureteral lumen or retrograde flow of contrast detected by fluoroscopy is considered to be indicative of an incompetent UVJ that might reflux during a UTI or after contralateral surgery, but such signs remain to be validated.

At the completion of cystoscopy, the bladder is left half full if an intravesical technique is contemplated. If an extravesical technique will be used, a Foley catheter connected to a three-way adapter can be inserted to allow bladder distention to facilitate dissection of the detrusor flaps.

Positioning

The child is positioned supine, and to facilitate exposure of the bladder, especially in older children and adolescents, a rolled towel may be placed at the level of the upper sacrum, or a slight break in the table can be used to raise the lower pelvis and hips. All pressure points are appropriately padded and wide surgical preparation is performed. The hips are abducted slightly to allow access to the urethra in girls if required; in boys, the penis is prepared and draped in the field.

Incision

A Pfannenstiel skin incision is made along a skin crease, about 2 cm above the symphysis pubis to the lateral edges of the rectus muscles. If the child is exceptionally overweight, the classic Pfannenstiel incision can be extended. The anterior rectus fascia is opened in a transverse fashion and elevated superiorly to just below the umbilicus and inferiorly to the symphysis pubis. The pyramidis muscles attach between the pubic bone and the anterior rectus sheath and should not be separated from the rectus sheath. The bellies of the recti are then separated in the midline to expose the bladder. Alternatively, after the skin and Scarpa's fascia are incised, the skin can be mobilized off the anterior rectus sheath, and the linea alba can then be opened in the midline vertically.

KEY POINTS: SURGICAL CORRECTION

- Exclude secondary reflux.
- Adequate ureteral mobilization and protection of the ureteral blood supply are essential.
- A generous submucosal tunnel should be fashioned.
- Attention should be directed to angulation and twisting.
- Attention to muscular backing is important.
- Bladder tissues must be handled gently.
- Always consider bladder function preoperatively, as well as in all cases of persistent or recurrent reflux.
- Until appropriate prospective studies prove otherwise, indications for correction of reflux are the same regardless of whether the planned approach is open, endoscopic, or laparoscopic.

Intravesical Procedures

Approaching the Ureters

The peritoneum is gently swept off the dome of the bladder, which is easier with a moderately full bladder. The bladder is opened in the midline down to about 2 cm proximal to the bladder neck. Figure-of-eight stay sutures with 3-0 Prolene are placed at the junction of the lateral edges with the bladder dome and at the inferior apex of the incision to prevent extension of the incision into the bladder neck. A Dennis-Brown retractor provides excellent exposure. Saline-soaked sponges are folded and gently packed into the dome of the bladder and also placed along the lateral edges of the bladder incision. Three blades of the retractor are used to retract the lateral walls of the bladder and the dome. The retractor blades should be placed with utmost care, and minimal touching, suctioning, or rubbing of the bladder mucosa is recommended to prevent edema or inflammation of the mucosa, which can lead to bleeding and difficult mucosal dissection and may aggravate the bladder spasms in the postoperative period.

Intravesical Mobilization of the Ureter

The ureter or ureters are cannulated with a 3 or 5 French Silastic feeding tube that is sutured to the bladder mucosa at the inferior edge of the ureteral orifice with 5-0 Prolene. This serves to maintain orientation of the ureter during all phases of the procedure and is used to handle the ureter and apply gentle traction. Before ureteral mobilization, some surgeons inject 1:200,000 epinephrine submucosally to reduce the bleeding. With a needle-point cautery a circumscribing incision is made in the bladder mucosa about 1 to 2 mm away from the ureteral orifice. With gentle traction on the feeding tube, the ureter can now be mobilized into the bladder. Mobilization of the ureter is best started at the 6-o'clock position by spreading the blades of the tenotomy scissors gently in a posterior direction initially. Once the correct plane is entered, the dissection is carried out circumferentially. The adventitia of the ureter must not be violated to prevent ischemic injury to the ureter. The ureter is freed from its attachments to the bladder with a fine right-angle clamp and electrocautery, aided by gentle traction on the feeding tube. Dissection of the ureter is continued until it can reach the contralateral bladder wall without tension. At that point the surgeon is ready to develop the submucosal tunnel via the same ureteral hiatus or a suprahiatal technique, depending on experience and preference.

Suprahiatal Tunnels

Politano-Leadbetter Technique

The principle behind this technique, which was originally described in 1958 (Politano and Leadbetter, 1958), is to bring the ureter in through a new hiatus superior to the original insertion. A submucosal tunnel is created in the direction of the trigone, medial to the original orifice. The advantage of this technique is that a long tunnel can be created, which is valuable in the higher grades of reflux. This antireflux mechanism can also be further supported by a psoas hitch.

Technique. After completion of the ureteral mobilization intravesically, the location of the new hiatus is selected so that it lies in a **straight line superior to the original orifice** (Fig. 117–15). With the bladder open and the lateral walls retracted, an inexperienced surgeon might be inclined to position the new hiatus too laterally on the posterior wall. Once the bladder is closed and full, the ureter enters on the anterolateral wall and then hooks back posteriorly toward the trigone to create the classic "hooking," which is an important cause of postoperative ureteral obstruction. In the original description of the Politano-Leadbetter technique the new hiatus was created blindly by passing a right-angle clamp from the original hiatus behind the bladder to puncture through the posterior wall of the bladder at the new hiatal opening. This blind maneuver must be discouraged because it is the cause of significant complications that may be associated with this procedure, such as routing of the ureter intraperitoneally and injury to the bowel, vas deferens, vagina, or other nearby structures. The current approach is to retract the superior lip of the original hiatus with a stay suture or a vein retractor and clear the back wall of the bladder bluntly under direct vision. A right-angle clamp is then used to create a new hiatus through which the ureter enters the bladder. The submucosal tunnel is created in the direction of the trigone, medial to the original orifice. The length of the tunnel depends on the diameter of the ureter; a 5:1 ratio (length to width) as suggested by Paquin is a helpful guide. It is important to lift the mucosa off the detrusor at the point of entry of the ureter into the bladder so that the mucosa can be closed properly over the new hiatus. The tunnel should be capacious enough to prevent constriction of the ureter. The ureter is pulled through the tunnel and the feeding tube is removed.

Ureteral Anastomosis. The ureter is spatulated ventrally (at the 6-o'clock position), and the edges are freshened if necessary. Three interrupted sutures of 5-0 polyglactin placed relatively close to each other anchor the ureter to the trigone by suturing it to the bladder muscle and mucosa. The anchoring sutures should be placed very carefully because the apex of the spatulation is the narrowest point of the ureter. The remainder of the ureteral anastomosis is carried out with interrupted 5-0 polyglactin sutures at the 3-, 9-, and 12-o'clock positions. The 12-o'clock suture may be also used to evert the anterior wall of the ureter, thus creating a small cuff. Although a 5 French feeding tube passed up the ureter confirms patency and the absence of kinks, the most reassuring sign that the ureteral reimplant is not obstructed is to see a jet of urine emerging from the orifice. It is thus important to communicate to the anesthesiologist the importance of adequate fluid administration throughout the procedure. The mucosa overlying the new hiatus is closed with running 5-0 polyglactin suture. The bladder is closed in two layers with 3-0 polyglactin suture. A Foley catheter is used to drain the bladder for 48 hours; drains and stents are used only for more complex cases.

Paquin Technique

Paquin described a combined extravesical/intravesical technique in 1959. The new ureteral hiatus is created from outside the bladder, thus avoiding the difficulties associated with this maneuver in the Politano-Leadbetter technique. As with most of the other open techniques, a success rate of greater than 95% for primary VUR is achieved with this method (Woodard and Keats, 1973).

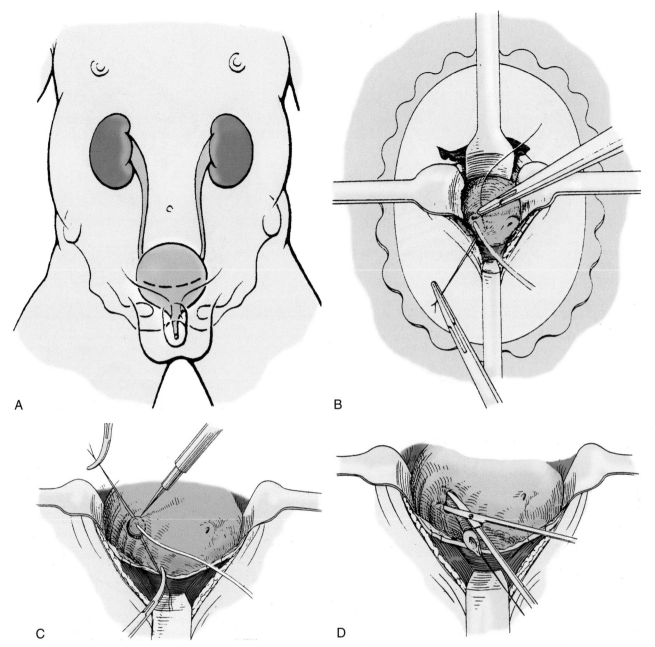

Figure 117–15. Politano-Leadbetter technique. **A,** Typical approach to the bladder for reimplantation. A transverse, lower abdominal incision is made along a skin crease one or two fingerbreadths above the symphysis pubis. **B,** Fine sutures are placed above and below the ureteral orifice for handling. A feeding tube in the ureter aids in the initial dissection. **C,** A needle-tip cautery outlines a circumferential incision around the orifice. **D,** Tenotomy scissors initially establish the plane of dissection inferiorly, where ureteral damage can be avoided. The plane is then carried around the ureter.   *Continued*

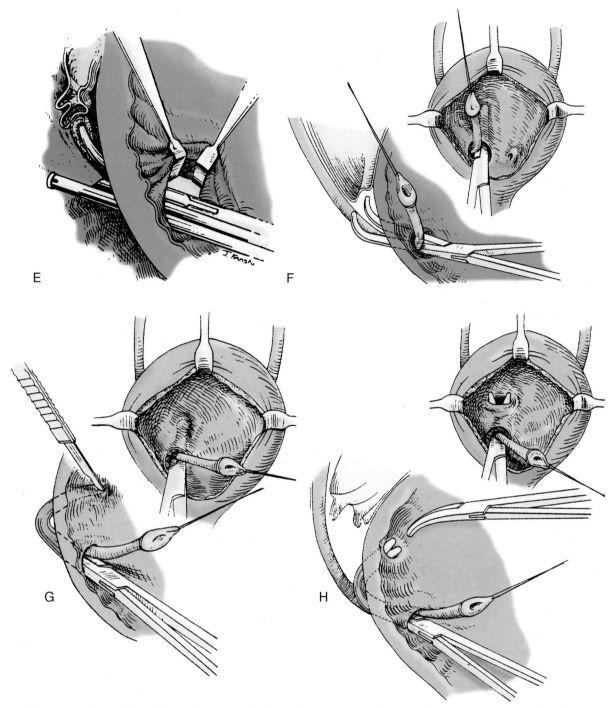

Figure 117–15, cont'd. **E,** With the aid of a lighted suction tip and two Senn retractors, a fine gauze dissector is used to sweep the peritoneum from the posterior bladder wall. **F,** After sweeping the peritoneum away, a blunt right-angle clamp indents the bladder from behind at a new hiatus approximately 2.5 cm superior and somewhat medial to the original hiatus. **G,** The clamp is incised upon from within and generously spread to make certain that the new hiatus is wide enough. **H,** A second right-angle clamp follows the first from within the bladder to the original hiatus. *Continued*

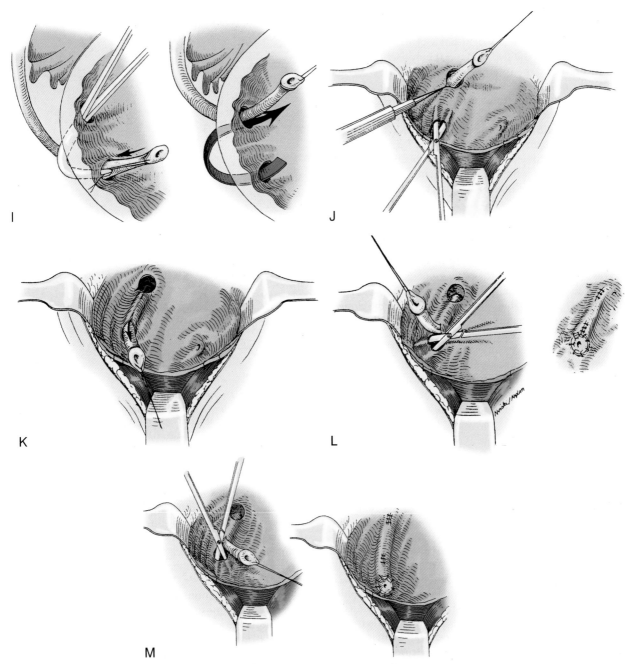

Figure 117–15, cont'd.   I, The right-angle clamp grasps the stay suture, and the ureter is pulled through the new hiatus. **J,** The inferior lip of muscle at the new hiatus is divided for a few millimeters to eliminate any ureteral angulation at its entrance to the submucosal tunnel that is created with scissors. **K,** The ureter is brought through the new tunnel to the original hiatus. **L,** The ureter is anastomosed to the original hiatus in the classic Politano-Leadbetter technique. Proximal mucosa can be closed over the ureter to give the tunnel additional length. **M,** Ureteral advancement is also helpful, especially if the original hiatus is laterally positioned. A second submucosal tunnel can be created toward the bladder neck to place the new orifice in a more inferior position and gain additional length for the reimplant. (**A** to **D** and **F** to **M,** From Retik AB, Colodny AH, Bauer SB: Pediatric urology. In Paulson DF [ed]: Genitourinary Surgery, vol 2. New York, Churchill Livingstone, 1984, pp 757-763; **E,** from Keating MA, Retik AB: Management of failures of ureteroneocystostomy. In McDougal WS [ed]: Difficult Problems in Urologic Surgery. Chicago, Year Book, 1989, p 121.)

The ureter in the Paquin technique can be approached extravesically (see the later section "Extravesical Procedures") before opening the bladder. A right-angle clamp is applied at the UVJ, the ureter is divided, and a 3-0 polyglactin suture is used to suture-ligate the original hiatus. The bladder is then opened in the midline, and a new hiatus located cephalad to the previous position is created. The peritoneum is carefully cleared off the back wall of the bladder at the site of the new hiatus. A right-angle clamp is passed from inside the bladder under direct vision, and one end of a 5-mm Penrose drain is pulled into the bladder. A mosquito snap applied to the Penrose drain acts as a holder and facilitates creation of the submucosal tunnel. The mucosa is dissected off the detrusor circumferentially at the new hiatus. The length of the submucosal tunnel is governed by the diameter of the ureter, and a 5:1 ratio is usually achievable. In more complex cases, a psoas hitch may be required to achieve longer tunnel length. The tunnel is developed by carefully lifting the mucosa off the detrusor with tenotomy scissors. Countertraction on the mucosa is helpful, especially in redo cases and when the bladder wall is trabeculated. Once the tunnel is developed, the remainder of the reimplant operation is similar to the Politano-Leadbetter procedure.

The modified Paquin technique is particularly well suited for dilated ureters and complex (El-Sherbiny et al, 2002) and failed (Mesrobian et al, 1985) reimplants because of the versatility offered by the combined extravesical/intravesical approach to the ureter and the ability to achieve longer submucosal tunnel length.

Infrahiatal Tunnels

Glenn-Anderson Technique

In 1967 Glenn and Anderson described their technique of ureteral reimplantation (Fig. 117–16). By using the same hiatus and advancing the ureter distally toward the bladder neck, the potential complications associated with the Politano-Leadbetter technique are avoided, specifically, kinking of the ureter. The ureter is mobilized as described earlier. A submucosal tunnel is created toward the bladder neck with tenotomy scissors. The distance from the hiatus to the bladder neck limits the length of the tunnel. Glenn and Anderson (1978) later described a modification that allows creation of a longer tunnel by incising the detrusor proximally at the original hiatus. The detrusor edges are then reapproximated distal to the ureter. With advancement of the ureter toward the bladder neck, the distal anastomosis of the ureter could be challenging with this technique. As with the other procedures, the results with this technique are excellent, with a 98% success rate (Gonzales et al, 1972).

Cohen Cross-Trigonal Technique

Cohen's technique, which was described in 1975, overcomes the limitation of tunnel length in the Glenn-Anderson technique by directing the tunnel across the trigone toward the contralateral bladder wall (Figs. 117–17 and 117–18). The difficulty with the distal anastomosis in the Glenn-Anderson technique is also eliminated.

Cohen's technique is particularly well suited for small bladders or thick-walled bladders (PUV or neuropathic) because

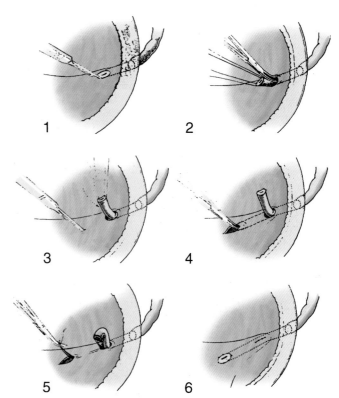

Figure 117–16. Glenn-Anderson technique. The ureter is mobilized and advanced beneath a new submucosal tunnel. (From Glenn JF, Anderson EE: Distal tunnel ureteral reimplantation. J Urol 1967;97:623.)

ureteral advancement across the back wall of the bladder rarely results in kinks or obstruction. Cross-trigonal reimplantation is also the procedure of choice in conjunction with bladder neck reconstructive procedures because the superior displacement of the ureters provides room for adequate elongation of the bladder neck.

As a result of its simplicity and reliable results (up to 99% [Glassberg et al, 1985; Kennelly et al, 1995; McCool and Joseph, 1995; El-Ghoneimi et al, 1999]), Cohen's procedure has become the most commonly used technique for intravesical reimplantation.

Critics of this technique cite the difficulty of retrograde catheterization of the superolaterally positioned ureteral orifice for radiographic studies, insertion of stents, or management of ureterolithiasis as a significant disadvantage. Suggested approaches to overcome this problem include suprapubic cystotomy by trocar (Lamesch, 1981) or a 14-gauge, 5-cm-long intravenous cannula in conjunction with cystoscopy to direct the ureteral catheter into the ureter, the use of a curved-tip vascular access catheter and an angle-tipped guide wire with a torque device (Wallis et al, 2003), or the use of a flexible ureteroscope.

Method

1. The technical methods of the Cohen and Glenn-Anderson procedures are similar in many aspects.
2. The ureter is approached and mobilized by the standard intravesical approach.
3. A hiatal groove may be created on the medial side of the ureter to reduce the angulation of the ureter as it crosses

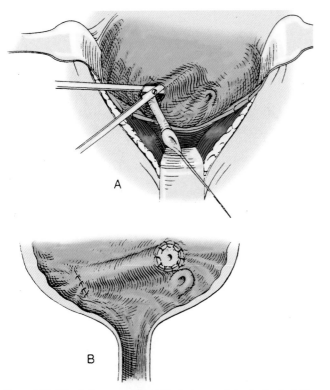

Figure 117–17. Cohen cross-trigonal technique, unilateral reimplantation. After the ureter is freed (**A**), a submucosal tunnel is made, with the new mucosal hiatus just above the contralateral ureteral orifice (**B**). (From Retik AB, Colodny AH, Bauer SB: Pediatric urology. In Paulson DF [ed]: Genitourinary Surgery, vol 2. New York, Churchill Livingstone, 1984, p 764.)

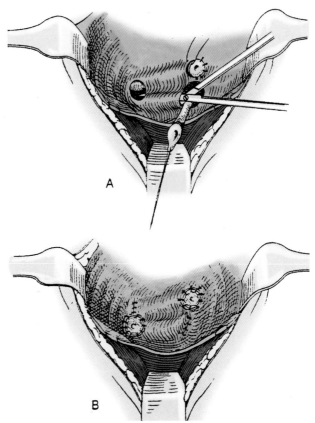

Figure 117–18. Cohen cross-trigonal technique, bilateral reimplant. **A,** The more superior ureter is tunneled transversely, with its new orifice just above the contralateral orifice. **B,** The other ureter is tunneled inferiorly, with its new orifice located at the inferior-most portion of the contralateral hiatus. (From Retik AB, Colodny AH, Bauer SB: Pediatric urology. In Paulson DF [ed]: Genitourinary Surgery, vol 2. New York, Churchill Livingstone, 1984, p 765.)

transversely, especially when the bladder wall is thickened. If the hiatus is excessively patulous, it can be reapproximated with one or more interrupted 3-0 polyglactin sutures to avoid the formation of a diverticulum (Ahmed and Tan, 1982). The hiatus should easily accommodate the tips of a large right-angle clamp alongside the ureter to avoid obstruction of the ureter.

4. The submucosal tunnel is developed with tenotomy scissors as previously described. When only one ureter is reimplanted, the tunnel is directed superior to the contralateral ureteral orifice. If both ureters are reimplanted, the tunnel for the more laterally displaced ureter is directed superior to the contralateral orifice. The second tunnel is directed toward the inferior edge of the orifice of the laterally displaced ureter. A common submucosal tunnel has been used successfully for bilateral reimplants (Androulakakis et al, 2003).

5. The ureter is spatulated and anastomosed to the bladder mucosa as described for the Politano-Leadbetter technique. The mucosa over the old hiatus is closed with 5-0 polyglactin suture.

6. Alternatively, the mucosal cuff of the ureteral orifice may be preserved and anastomosed to the bladder mucosa without spatulation.

7. The ureter is catheterized with a 5 French feeding tube to ensure patency, although continuous efflux of urine from the orifice provides the best assurance of patency.

8. Closure of the bladder and drainage are completed as described previously.

Extravesical Procedures

Lich and colleagues (1961) in the United States and Gregoir (1964) in Europe independently described the extravesical approach to ureteral reimplantation (Fig. 117–19). The technique became more popular after the modifications described by Daines and Hodgson (1971) and Zaontz et al (1987) popularized anchoring the ureter with advancement sutures. These modifications permit combined advancement of the ureter and lengthening of the tunnel proximally. In addition, anchoring sutures fix the ureter distally and thus maintain stability of the tunnel. The advantage of the extravesical technique is that the bladder is not opened and thus postoperative hematuria and bladder spasms are minimized. The technique is simple to learn and is readily taught.

The main concern with this technique has been the development of transient voiding inefficiency, which is seen in up to 20% (Fung et al, 1995; Lapointe et al, 1998; Lipski et al, 1998; Barrieras et al, 1999; Marotte and Smith, 2001) of

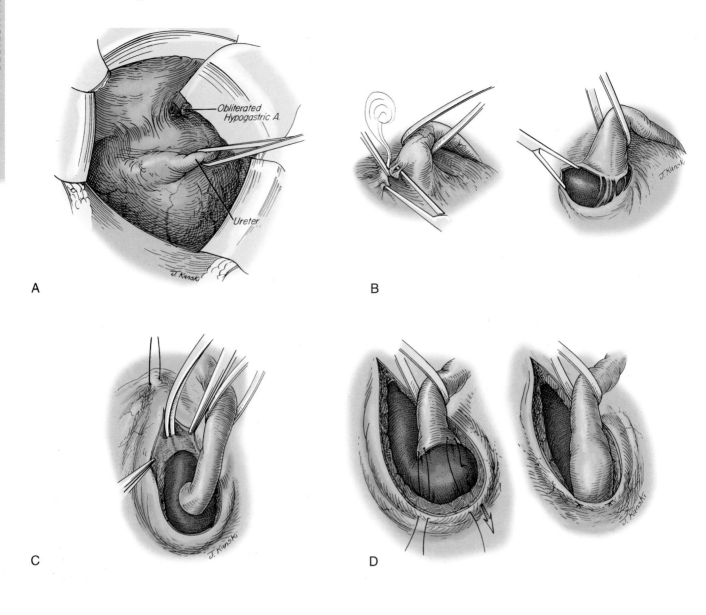

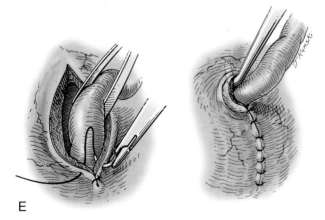

Figure 117–19. Modified Lich-Gregoir/detrusorrhaphy technique. **A,** The ureter is identified and gently grasped after ligation of the obliterated hypogastric artery. **B,** The ureter is circumferentially mobilized at its intersection with the bladder by incising the detrusor at the level of the ureteral hiatus. **C,** The serosal and muscular layers of the bladder (4 to 5 cm) are opened along a straight course cephalad and lateral from the ureterovesical junction to create the trough for reimplantation. A tacking suture aids in orientation. **D,** The bladder mucosa is elevated off muscle wall, and vest-type sutures are placed from the detrusor at the distal limit of dissection to the proximal ureteral adventitia and back again through same tissue planes. Tying of the vest sutures advances and anchors the ureter onto the trigone. **E,** Reapproximation of the detrusor creates a long submucosal tunnel and completes the repair. (From Peters C, Retik AB: Ureteral reimplantation including megaureter repair. In Marshall FF [ed]: Textbook of Operative Urology. Philadelphia, WB Saunders, 1996, pp 868-870.)

children who undergo bilateral extravesical reimplantation. The mechanism is thought to be due to disruption of the nerves to the bladder bilaterally, possibly because of excessive use of cautery during the detrusorotomy. The population most at risk appears to be boys younger than 3 years with bilateral high-grade reflux (Barrieras et al, 1999).

Leissner and associates (2001) used human cadavers to study the topography of the pelvic plexus in an effort to understand the mechanism of injury to the plexus as a result of extravesical reimplant surgery. They demonstrated that the main portion of the pelvic plexus is located approximately 1.5 to 2 cm dorsal and medial to the UVJ in adult cadavers. Smaller branches travel along the medial aspect of the ureter, outside the thin layer of tissue (the mesoureter) that surrounds the ureter. Based on their anatomic description, injury to the branches of the pelvic plexus is avoided if dissection of the distal ureter is carried out between the mesoureter and the ureteral adventitia. Yucel and Baskin (2003) further refined the description of the neuroanatomy of the distal ureter and UVJ by immunohistochemical analysis and three-dimensional imaging techniques in normal human fetuses (21 to 40 weeks' gestation). They confirmed localization of the nerves along the medial aspect of the ureter just outside Waldeyer's sheath. At the UVJ the nerves surround the ureter in a network-like fashion; distally, once the ureter enters the bladder, the nerves localize on the detrusor muscle distal and lateral to the ureter. From these two studies it is suggested that the incidence of voiding inefficiency observed after bilateral extravesical reimplantation depends on the surgical technique. The injury is limited to the smaller nerve branches rather than the actual pelvic plexus, which is located medially and posteriorly. The neural damage may be due to transection of the nerves, electrocautery, or neuropraxia from surgical trauma. Injury to the nerves may be prevented by limiting the dissection to the correct plane, just outside the ureteral adventitia, reducing the use and power of electrocautery, restricting the incision of the detrusor distal to the UVJ, and gentle handling of the tissues (David et al, 2004).

Patients in whom urinary retention develops and requiring insertion of a Foley catheter or intermittent catheterization are able to void within 1 to 2 weeks (Minevich et al, 1998a; Barrieras et al, 1999), thus indicating the reversibility of the neurologic lesion.

Approaching the Ureters

A Pfannenstiel incision is used as described earlier. It is best to have the bladder somewhat distended at this point to facilitate dissection of the peritoneum of the lateral bladder wall. The obliterated umbilical artery is identified. The ureter crosses medial to the point of origin of the obliterated umbilical artery from the internal iliac artery. This is an excellent anatomic reference point for identification of the distal ureter. Dividing the obliterated umbilical artery facilitates dissection and mobilization of the ureter. Some authors were concerned that injury to the bladder innervation might occur when the obliterated umbilical artery is divided. However, Lipski et al (1998) demonstrated that there was no difference between the two groups of patients regardless of whether the obliterated umbilical artery was divided. The peritoneum is meticulously reflected off the anterior surface of the ureter. To avoid injury to any of the branches of the pelvic plexus, it is recommended

that the surgeon stay close to the adventitia of the ureter during its dissection while being careful to not injure blood vessels running in the ureteral wall. A vessel loop is passed around the ureter and used as a handle. Dissection and mobilization of the ureter are carried distally to the point where it tunnels under the detrusor muscle.

Creation of the Extravesical Tunnel

With the bladder in its normal anatomic position, the course of the ureter along the posterior wall of the bladder is identified and marked for a distance of 5 cm. The bladder is reflected medially; a Dennis-Brown retractor is quite helpful for this procedure. The outlined course of the ureter is inspected. The peritoneal reflection may need to be gently lifted off the wall of the bladder. With the bladder retracted, the tunnel direction will appear to be pointing toward the anterior abdominal wall. It is important to have the bladder full and somewhat tense but not overstretched. The detrusor is incised with low-current electrical cautery (15 W) to create the new submucosal tunnel. Tenotomy scissors are then used to divide the detrusor fibers along the same line of the initial incision down to the bladder mucosa. Care should be taken to incise the detrusor fibers along one line, without wandering sideways, to facilitate lifting the detrusor off the mucosa with minimal disruption to the detrusor muscle and its innervation. Blood vessels are easily seen as one incises the detrusor fibers and are cauterized selectively with bipolar cautery. It is critical that all detrusor muscle bundles be divided before elevation of the detrusor flaps. When the last detrusor bundles have been divided, a **uniform** mucosal dome bulges out. This provides the surgeon with an excellent point of reference that the tunnel has been established in the correct plane.

The detrusor is dissected off the mucosa on either side of the incision to achieve a width slightly larger than the circumference of the ureter. This dissection is best carried out in a proximal-to-distal direction, with dissection around the ureter being left as the final step in creation of the tunnel.

There is a definite **avascular** plane between the muscle and the mucosa. The most efficient method to accomplish this dissection is to have the assistant grasp the detrusor bundles closest to the mucosa with two forceps and elevate the muscle off the mucosa. The surgeon gently depresses the mucosal bulge with one hand and uses the tenotomy scissors to sharply separate the muscle bundles off the mucosa, on either side, along the length of the tunnel. Injury to the mucosa during dissection of the tunnel is quite avoidable unless the bladder is thick walled and trabeculated. Inadvertent injury to the mucosa could be closed with 6-0 polyglactin figure-of-eight sutures. It is not necessary to create a wide tunnel unless the ureter is very dilated.

Particular attention is necessary when dissecting around the ureter. The detrusor fibers attached to the ureter are carefully divided while staying close to the ureter to avoid injury to any of the terminal nerve branches entering the bladder. The dissection is carried out along the lateral and medial attachments of the ureter but is not extended distally.

The original modification described by Zaontz et al (1987) for the extravesical procedure included incision of the detrusor distal to the ureteral orifice for 5 to 10 mm with advancement of the ureter via two vest sutures. Leissner and associates (2001) demonstrated that this particular aspect of the procedure may be responsible for injury to the bladder innervation at the trigonal area and may be the leading cause of urinary retention after bilateral extravesical reimplantation. Therefore, to avoid damage to the nerves, this maneuver should be avoided unless there is a paraureteral diverticulum that requires repair simultaneously (Jayanthi et al, 1995), and in such cases dissection of the detrusor distal to the ureter should be carried out in very limited fashion.

Once creation of the submucosal tunnel is complete, the bladder is decompressed before reapproximation of the detrusor. The ureter is positioned in the new tunnel and the detrusor reapproximated with interrupted 3-0 polyglactin suture. To achieve alignment of the tunnel it is best to place the most proximal suture first at the new ureteral hiatus and leave it untied and tagged on a mosquito snap. Tension applied to this suture straightens and elevates the detrusor flaps, thereby allowing the surgeon to reapproximate the detrusor without risk of injury to the ureter or the mucosa. The suturing commences at the most distal portion. The adventitia of the ureter may be incorporated in one or two of these sutures to stabilize the tunnel and prevent a diverticulum from forming at the most distal or proximal portion of it. After completion of the suture line the caliber of the hiatus should be tested with a right-angle clamp to ensure the absence of any constriction or compression of the ureter.

The bladder is refilled and the retractor is removed. The course of the ureter is reinspected to ensure the absence of any kinks in the retroperitoneum or any bulging of the mucosa at either end of the tunnel.

A Foley catheter is left in place for 24 to 48 hours; some authors recommended not leaving a catheter at all (Marotte and Smith, 2001). If an epidural caudal catheter is inserted for postoperative analgesia, it should be discontinued 6 to 12 hours before removal of the Foley catheter.

After being observed to void without problems, the child is discharged and scheduled to return for follow-up ultrasound and a VCUG, usually 3 months postoperatively.

Postoperative Evaluation

In expert hands, the success rate of ureteroneocystostomy in patients with low-grade primary VUR approaches 100%. As a result of these outstanding outcomes, several centers have evaluated the need for postoperative invasive imaging. Most agree that ultrasound is necessary at 6 to 12 weeks postoperatively. In a large study by Barrieras and coworkers, 723 renal units were evaluated. At 1 year postoperatively there was a significant difference between children who had undergone surgery for low-grade primary VUR (99% resolution) and those with high-grade reflux (94%). Thus, in patients who initially had low-grade primary reflux, normal preoperative and postoperative ultrasound findings, and no voiding dysfunction or recurrent UTI (Lavine et al, 2001), the success rate with uncomplicated ureteroneocystostomy approaches 100% (Bisignani and Decter, 1997; Bomalaski et al, 1997b; El-Ghoneimi et al, 1999; Barrieras et al, 2000; Grossklaus et al, 2001). Based on these reports, it has been suggested that the postoperative VCUG can be avoided in this group of patients. This recommendation should be individualized according to the family situation and the expertise of the center performing the surgery. Some families have dealt with reflux for several years and are anxious to know with certainty that the

reflux has resolved. In other families, the children are quite reluctant to undergo another VCUG, and in this situation it may be reasonable to not perform a postoperative study unless the child has a dysfunctional bladder or postoperative hydronephrosis or UTIs develop. However, the lower success rate for high-grade reflux would still support complete postoperative studies in most cases.

After ureteroneocystostomy, the presence of minimal ureteral dilatation and low-grade hydronephrosis on early postoperative ultrasound is not unusual (Bomalaski et al, 1997b; Barrieras et al, 2000). Indeed, this common finding should argue against performing such studies too early after surgery. On the other hand, persistence of this dilatation beyond 3 months or progression of it should be further investigated (Aboutaleb et al, 2003). Additionally, the development of new renal scars on late follow-up ultrasound, a discrepancy in renal growth, or recurrent UTIs may warrant complete radiologic reevaluation of the patient.

As discussed previously, children with renal scarring should have their blood pressure measured at every visit with their family physician.

COMPLICATIONS OF URETERAL REIMPLANTATION
Early Complications

Persistent Reflux. Early reflux after ureteroneocystostomy is not usually a significant clinical problem and commonly resolves by 1 year on repeat cystography. In the report by Barrieras and associates (2000), 49 of 723 renal units had reflux at 3 months, 11 of which were contralateral. At 12 months' follow-up, reflux had resolved spontaneously in 20 of the 38 ipsilateral and 8 of the 11 contralateral ureters. Persistent reflux at 1 year was more common in patients who had high-grade reflux preoperatively. In their study, 30% of patients undergoing surgery had high-grade reflux, and two thirds of those with persistent reflux at 1 year (12/18) were from that group. Thus, the majority of low-grade postoperative reflux detected on the initial VCUG at the 3-month follow-up point disappeared spontaneously, probably because of resolution of the bladder inflammation and improvement of the bladder dysfunction that may be present in the early postoperative period.

Contralateral Reflux. The issue of contralateral reflux has been the subject of several reports in the literature over the last 15 years, most of which are retrospective. Minevich and coworkers (1998b) and Burno and colleagues (1998) noted a very low incidence of contralateral reflux of 5.6% and 11.6%, respectively, after unilateral extravesical detrusorrhaphy. Diamond and colleagues (1996b), in a multicenter trial of 141 patients, reported an 18% incidence of contralateral VUR. These patients were analyzed according to grade of initial reflux, presence of a Hutch diverticulum or duplex system, and the surgical technique used to correct the reflux. There was no difference noted with the various surgical techniques, but there was a significant trend toward the development of contralateral reflux with the higher grades of ipsilateral corrected reflux and correction of reflux in duplex systems. They concluded that distortion of the contralateral hemitrigone was not a factor responsible for the contralateral reflux but rather the severity (grade V) of reflux and the presence of a duplex system put patients at risk for the development of contralateral reflux postoperatively. Conversely, Kumar and Puri (1997) reported on 495 children with unilateral reflux who had undergone subureteral Teflon injections. New contralateral reflux was diagnosed in only 37 children (7%). They were unable to find any correlation between the grade of preoperative ipsilateral reflux and postoperative contralateral reflux and suggested that the low incidence of new contralateral VUR may be due to the relative noninterference with the contralateral trigone afforded by endoscopic versus open reflux correction. They refuted the existence of the pop-off mechanism accounting for new contralateral reflux in their series because the risk for new contralateral reflux did not correlate with the preoperative reflux grade (grades IV and V). Sparr and associates (1998) reviewed a series of 143 patients undergoing conservative management in whom unilateral reflux was initially diagnosed but metachronous contralateral reflux subsequently developed. Contralateral reflux appeared in 33%, thus suggesting a different cause for the appearance of contralateral reflux unrelated to surgical correction. They speculated that the contralateral reflux was in fact synchronous (i.e., bilateral) but missed on the initial cystogram or that the natural history of unilateral or bilateral reflux may involve intermittent appearance and disappearance of VUR on one side.

Prophylactic bilateral reimplantation for unilateral reflux, to avoid contralateral reflux, is not warranted because of the high spontaneous resolution rates (Burno et al, 1998). Recommendations for management of contralateral reflux range from observation in the majority of cases to intervention for control of clinical pyelonephritis episodes. In asymptomatic children younger than 4 to 5 years, prophylactic antibiotics are warranted for postoperative contralateral reflux, particularly if one is to be consistent with the medical therapy for the previous ipsilateral reflux. If the child remains asymptomatic and free of infection, repeat VCUGs may not be necessary because contralateral reflux resolves spontaneously in the majority of children. In girls around the age of puberty, controversy persists regarding whether a VCUG and correction of reflux will become necessary at that point.

Obstruction. It is not unusual to detect a mild to moderate degree of hydronephrosis in the early postoperative period by ultrasound (see earlier), but it should resolve spontaneously with time. Acute postoperative obstruction may be related to technical issues such as twisting or kinking of the ureter in its new tunnel, intramural blood clots, or extramural compression by submucosal hematoma or edema at the site of anastomosis. Progressive, significant obstruction usually becomes apparent in the first 2 weeks after surgery. Such children typically have symptoms of acute ureteral obstruction, including acute abdominal pain, nausea, and vomiting. Although infection is less common, if it does occur, it is quite significant in the obstructed system. The diagnosis is readily made on ultrasound, and severe hydroureteronephrosis is confirmed by delayed function and excretion on renal scintigraphy. In more significant cases, drainage of the system by either retrograde insertion of a double-J stent or a percutaneous nephrostomy tube may be necessary. The nephrostomy tube should be internalized as early as possible to avoid a dry reimplant. Many of these cases resolve without requiring additional surgery.

Long-Term Complications

Obstruction

Progressive dilatation of the ureter and kidney after reimplantation surgery can be due to several factors and can be classified according to location of the obstructive lesion:

Suprahiatal. Twisting of the ureter and ischemia as a result of poor handling of the ureter are the most common causes of suprahiatal obstruction.

Hiatus. At the point of entry into the new hiatus, angulation of the ureter is most commonly due to a hiatus that is positioned too lateral or anterior such that when the bladder fills, the ureter is carried laterally and anteriorly, thereby resulting in the "high-reimplant" phenomenon. These ureters drain better when the bladder is empty. This situation may resolve spontaneously but on occasion requires stenting or redo surgery.

Tunnel. A submucosal tunnel that is not adequately developed can lead to compression of the ureter and resultant obstruction within the tunnel. The submucosal tunnel is obviously more difficult to develop in an abnormal bladder such as a PUV or neuropathic bladder. Developing a smooth capacious submucosal tunnel can be quite challenging because of irregularities created by the muscular hypertrophy, trabeculation, and cellule formation. Ischemia of the ureter and submucosal tunnel is another important factor that results from improper handling and subsequent devascularization of the ureter. Significant obstruction in the submucosal tunnel can be overcome by balloon dilatation and stenting for a period. If conservative measures are unsuccessful, redo reimplantation is required.

Orifice. Anastomosis of the ureter to the bladder and the new hiatal position is an important technical aspect of the reimplant procedure. The most vulnerable point for obstruction is the apex of the ureteral spatulation. The apical sutures must be placed with utmost care to ensure an adequate orifice caliber. Stenosis can also occur as a result of ischemic changes. Isolated obstruction of the orifice can be managed by dilatation and stenting. If the submucosal tunnel is of adequate length, endoscopic unroofing of the distal few millimeters, including the orifice, may relieve the obstruction while maintaining the antireflux mechanism.

Recurrent or Persistent Reflux

Failure of antireflux procedures in patients with primary low-grade reflux is extremely rare. Most failures occur in high-grade reflux because of an inadequate tunnel length–to–ureteral diameter ratio. Development of a short tunnel and failure to taper an excessively wide ureter are obvious important factors. Another significant cause of persistent or recurrent reflux is due to failure to recognize secondary reflux, especially that associated with neurogenic and PUV bladders. **Reflux in these situations is secondary to the poor storage or emptying characteristics of the bladder. These issues need to be addressed and optimized before attempting reimplant surgery.** In most situations, improving bladder storage or emptying (or both) with a combination of an anticholinergic and intermittent self-catheterization results in spontaneous resolution of secondary reflux (Agarwal et al,

1997). Proceeding with reimplantation surgery in the presence of an abnormal bladder results only in worsening of the ureteral dilatation and deposition of scar tissue in the pelvis, which would render future attempts at correcting the reflux even more difficult.

Redo Reimplantation

Redo reimplantation is technically more challenging and requires careful attention to detail and meticulous surgical technique. Dissection of the ureter and extensive mobilization are required to achieve an adequate submucosal tunnel. Careful dissection of the ureter is best accomplished by a combination of extravesical and intravesical mobilization as necessary. The ureter should be carefully evaluated and ischemic segments excised. Free bleeding from the divided distal end should be observed in addition to peristaltic activity to ensure normal musculature and blood supply. It is preferable to create a new hiatus and submucosal tunnel. If the ureter is shorter, a psoas hitch (Fig. 117–20) can be used to facilitate creation of the antireflux mechanism. The psoas hitch should be carried out with nonabsorbable suture before creation of the submucosal tunnel. The bladder is fixed to the psoas muscle sheath on either side of the iliac vessels to provide a stable posterior bladder wall. In children, the bladder can be mobilized sufficiently to bring it up almost to the bifurcation of the common iliac vessels, which may provide adequate bridging for a distal ureteral defect. A psoas hitch can be fashioned only on one side. Attempting a psoas hitch on both sides will not provide adequate length on either side and should thus be avoided. If both ureters are shortened, consider a psoas hitch on one side to achieve a satisfactory antireflux mechanism and a transureteroureterostomy for the other ureter.

Other techniques to consider for a short ureter include a Boari flap, in which a flap extending from the dome to the anterior wall of the bladder based on the posterior wall can be rotated proximally. The flap should be wide enough to allow creation of a submucosal tunnel and tubularization of this flap. In a short ureter a nipple valve can be created in associ-

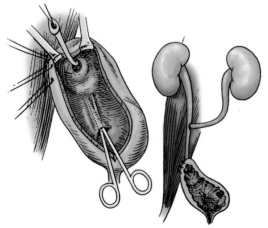

Figure 117–20. A psoas hitch can be used to effectively bridge significant ureteral defects. Its combination with transureteroureterostomy is ideal when both ureters are addressed in a reoperative setting. (From Keating MA, Retik AB: Management of failures of ureteroneocystostomy. In McDougal WS [ed]: Difficult Problems in Urologic Surgery. Chicago, Year Book, 1989, p 140.)

ation with a short submucosal tunnel. A nipple valve is particularly useful in dilated ureters and is fashioned by spatulating the ureter and folding it back onto itself.

In situations in which the ureter is significantly foreshortened, it can be replaced with a reconfigured segment of bowel as described by Pope and associates (1996). The colon or ileum is reconfigured similar to the Monti procedure. This technique offers important advantages over the classic tapered ileal ureter by allowing a long tube to be created from a short segment of colon without tapering, thus eliminating the metabolic consequences; additionally, the mesentery is in the center of the tube, which facilitates creation of the submucosal tunnel.

ENDOSCOPIC TREATMENT OF VESICOURETERIC REFLUX

In 1981, Matouschek first described the injection of polytetrafluoroethylene (PTFE) paste at the ureteral orifice to correct VUR. It was O'Donnell and Puri who popularized the technique in 1986 when they published their initial report on endoscopic correction of primary VUR in 103 ureters with a success rate of 75% after one injection. They coined the term STING (subureteric Teflon injection). This procedure became popular in many countries but never achieved widespread use in the United States because of lack of Food and Drug Administration (FDA) approval as a result of concern regarding the potential migration of PTFE particles (Malizia et al, 1984b; Aaronson et al, 1993). The ability to correct reflux in a large proportion of patients (the more recent studies report success rates approaching 90% after one injection of Deflux for low-grade primary reflux [Kirsch et al, 2004]) on an outpatient basis by using a simple procedure with minimal morbidity prompted the search for safer materials. One caveat when evaluating the reported results of endoscopic correction is to interpret with caution those reports in which the authors regard downgrading of reflux to grade I as a successful outcome. Because this would not be acceptable to most surgeons performing open surgery, the definition of success should be applied uniformly.

Because of the minimal morbidity of the procedure, the benefit of endoscopic injection in patients with newly diagnosed reflux has been evaluated by computer modeling with a view to reduce the morbidity and cost of repeated VCUGs and long-term antibiotics (Kobelt et al, 2003). Rigorous comparisons of various treatment approaches need to be undertaken, and **until the outcome of such studies is available, the indications for correction of reflux should remain unchanged regardless of whether reflux is corrected by open surgery, endoscopy, or laparoscopy.**

Two key challenges with endoscopic treatment of reflux are the reproducibility and durability of results. Long-term follow-up will determine whether endoscopic therapy, with the currently available materials, will stand the test of time or whether open surgery with its 95% to 99% success rate will remain the most cost-effective method of **permanently** correcting reflux.

Technique of Endoscopic Injection

The classic STING technique was described by O'Donnell and Puri (1984) (Fig. 117–21). Prophylactic antibiotic is usually

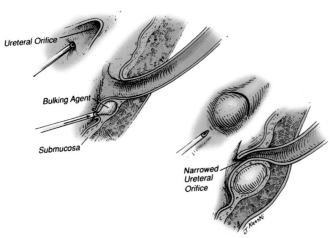

Figure 117–21. Principle of endoscopic treatment of reflux. A bulking agent is injected beneath the ureteral orifice with a needle. The buttress that is provided helps coapt the distal end of the ureter.

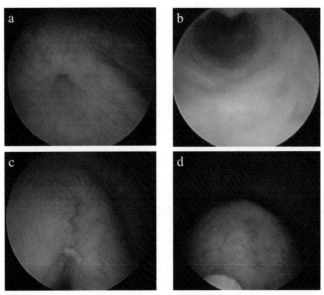

Figure 117–22. The classic STING technique. **A,** Appearance of the orifice before hydrodistention (**B**). **C,** The entry point of the needle is 2 mm distal to the 6-o'clock position. **D,** Appearance of the mound after completion of the injection.

administered with induction of anesthesia. Cystoscopy should be carried out before opening the materials in case the procedure is cancelled because of inflammatory changes in the bladder. If a rigid needle is used, an offset lens injection scope should be used. If a flexible needle is used, a standard 0- or 30-degree lens cystoscope can be used. The size of the needle varies depending on the viscosity of the material and ranges from 3.7 to 5 French. The viscosity of the material also determines whether injection of the material can be carried out with a regular syringe or requires a ratcheted metal syringe holder. A 3 French ureteric catheter may be introduced to lift the anterior wall of the ureter up and identify the axis of the tunnel. The needle is inserted with the bevel facing up at the 6-o'clock position. The original description by O'Donnell and Puri suggested entering the mucosa 2 to 3 mm distal to the UVJ and advancing the needle in the submucosal plane for a distance of 4 to 5 mm. For high-grade reflux and ureters without a submucosal tunnel, the Dublin group suggested inserting the needle directly inside the ureter to increase the length of the intravesical ureter (Chertin et al, 2003). Kirsch and coworkers (2004) popularized this approach (submucosal implantation within the intramural ureter) and reported better results for all grades of reflux than with the classic technique (92% versus 79% of ureters).

The accuracy of the needle entry point and needle placement is an important component for success of the procedure (Fig. 117–22). An improper puncture may not result in the desired mound formation and thus may not provide adequate support for the UVJ. If the needle requires repositioning, the implanted material may leak out of the first puncture site and result in failure of the procedure.

Injection should be carried out slowly. If the needle is positioned in the submucosal plane, the mound becomes apparent with the initial injection of 0.1 to 0.2 mL. This is a key point in the procedure; unsatisfactory mound formation and location after this initial injection indicate that the tip of the needle is not in the proper position. Repositioning of the needle by withdrawing it slowly and then advancing it while injecting, in addition to rotating the bevel gently (depending on the lateral location of the mound), should help achieve the desired effect. Once a volcano appearance with the ureteral

meatus on top of the mound is achieved, additional volume is injected until the ureteral orifice becomes crescent or slit shaped. The shape of the achieved mound was found to be a significant predictor of a successful outcome. Achieving a volcano-shaped mound was associated with an 87% success rate, whereas other morphologies were associated with only a 53% successful rate (Lavelle et al, 2005). With most materials the needle should be kept in place for 1 minute at the end of the injection to reduce extrusion of the material at the injection site. With Deflux this step is not essential. The bladder is emptied and the mound is inspected with an empty and a full bladder to ensure that adequate support of the ureter is present. Rarely, bleeding occurs at the puncture site and is best dealt with by emptying the bladder and applying gentle pressure with the tip of the scope until the bleeding stops. Cauterizing the area is not advisable because it results in sloughing of the mucosa and extrusion of the injected material. At the end of the procedure, lidocaine gel may be instilled in the urethra; catheter drainage is not necessary. In general, the child spends a brief amount of time in the recovery room, followed by discharge. All activities can be resumed immediately.

There is a significant learning curve with endoscopic correction of VUR (Kirsch et al, 2003). In a study by Herz and associates (2001), the importance of the learning curve was highlighted. In the first 6 months of their study the success rate was 46% in 18 children with 28 refluxing ureters. In the remaining 18 months of that study the overall correction rate was 93% in 56 children with 84 refluxing ureters after a single endoscopic injection. Although the technique is quite simple once learned, there are some technical nuances and details that require specific attention.

Follow-up

The child is maintained on antibiotics for 3 months, at which time a follow-up ultrasound and VCUG are obtained. If reflux is persistent, a repeat injection can be considered 6 months after the initial injection. If there is still no resolution, open surgery is recommended.

Most reports to date have not indicated any additional difficulty with open surgery after endoscopic correction with Deflux (Herz et al, 2001; Lackgren et al, 2001), although some have experienced difficulty with other substances. At open surgery the injected material either is not seen at all or is found well encapsulated but in a wrong plane or wrong location inside or outside the bladder. The material is easily removed en bloc and the open reimplant procedure carried out without difficulty.

Materials Used for Endoscopic Correction of Reflux

For an injectable biomaterial to be ideal, it must be nontoxic and stable without migration to vital organs, cause minimal local inflammation, and at the same time be well encapsulated by normal fibrous tissue and fibrocytes. The material should be easy to inject through a long needle that passes easily through most standard endoscopic instruments. It must be viscous enough to prevent leakage from the puncture site and maintain its injected volume and the mound shape after the normal process of exchange and excretion of any carrier molecules.

Several agents have been used for endoscopic correction of VUR. These materials can be classified as **particulate** or **degradable** and **autologous** or **nonautologous** (Table 117–7). The concern with particulate agents is migration and, with degradable agents, durability. Distant migration can occur by two mechanisms. Expansion of the injected bolus may lead to disruption of small vessels in the area of the distal ureter and trigone and result in the material gaining intravascular access. Particles smaller than 50 μm may bypass the pulmonary vascular bed and thus access the systemic circulation and reach other organs in the body. The second migration mechanism is via phagocytosis of the injected particles by tissue macrophages or blood-borne monocytes. Particle size determines whether phagocytosis can occur, and it is generally agreed that phagocytosis requires a particle less than 80 μm in diameter.

Nonautologous Materials

Polytetrafluoroethylene Paste (Teflon Paste). PTFE has been in use as a component of many biomaterials and

injectable agents for many years. It has been used for the manufacturing of vascular grafts, cardiac valves/implants, surgical sutures, cosmetic surgery, and patches for hernia repairs (Monaghan and Meban, 1991; Godin et al, 1995; Sayers et al, 1998; Briguori et al, 2001). Teflon paste was also used as an injectable agent for embolization of vessels (Weingarten and Kauffman, 1977), for injection of vocal cords (Kasperbauer, 1995), and as a bulking agent for urinary incontinence (Politano, 1992).

In 1981 Matouschek first reported on the use of Teflon paste as a bulking agent for correction of reflux. O'Donnell and Puri popularized this technique (O'Donnell and Puri, 1984; Chertin and Puri, 2002) and reported on its use in hundreds of patients with long-term follow up (Puri, 1995; Chertin et al, 2002). A large European multicenter survey reported on 6216 ureters in 4166 children with 10 years' follow-up and demonstrated a cure rate of 86% after one to four injections (Puri et al, 1995). The longest follow-up is available from Dublin: in 247 patients treated with Teflon paste with 11 to 17 years' follow-up, a sustained success rate of 95% with a 5% recurrence rate was reported (Chertin et al, 2002).

Teflon paste is relatively inexpensive; it is viscous and requires a ratcheted syringe for injection. Despite its widespread use in Europe, Teflon paste never gained FDA approval in the United States because of concern regarding distant migration of the PTFE particles. Malizia and associates (1984a, 1984b) demonstrated in experimental studies that the particles can migrate to regional lymph nodes and distant organs, including the lung and brain. Their findings were substantiated by several clinical reports confirming particle migration (Claes et al, 1989; Aaronson et al, 1993; Dewan and Fraundorfer, 1996; Steyaert et al, 2000). Particle migration is thought to be related to the small size of the Teflon paste particles, which range from 4 to 100 μm, with 90% of the particles being less than 40 μm.

With the availability of other, presumably safer injectable agents, PTFE has fallen totally out of favor and all but abandoned.

Cross-Linked Bovine Collagen. Apart from concern regarding allergy to bovine collagen in 3% of the population, this material is otherwise safe and causes minimal local inflammatory changes (Leonard et al, 1990). It is easily injectable through a 25-gauge needle with standard endoscopic equipment. The downside to cross-linked collagen is the fact that the results are not durable because of the variable degree of ingrowth of native fibroblast and replacement of the injectable collagen with native collagen (Leonard et al, 1990; Leonard et al, 1991; Frey et al, 1992). Despite the odd report of sustained effect (Reunanen, 1995), because of the inconsistency and questionable durability of cross-linked collagen (Haferkamp et al, 2000a; Haferkamp et al, 2000b), most centers have abandoned its use for correction of reflux.

Polydimethylsiloxane (Macroplastique). Polydimethylsiloxane (PDS) is a solid silicone elastomer that has been used as a soft tissue bulking agent. The injectable material is composed of a soft, flexible, highly textured implant of heat-vulcanized PDS suspended in a bioextractable carrier gel. The carrier gel is a water-soluble low-molecular-weight polyvinylpyrrolidone hydrogel (Povidone). The carrier gel is absorbed and replaced with host fibroblasts, which subse-

Table 117–7. Agents used for Endoscopic Correction of Vesicoureteral Reflux
Nonautologous Materials
Polytetrafluoroethylene (PTFE)
Cross-linked bovine collagen
Polydimethylsiloxane
Dextranomer hyaluronic copolymer (Deflux)
Autologous Materials
Chondrocytes
Fat
Collagen
Muscle

quently deposit collagen to encapsulate the implant and retain its size and shape. To minimize the risk of migration, PDS is engineered to create an elastomer instead of the less cross-linked silicone gels or non–cross-linked silicone oils. Although 76% of the particles are greater than 100 μm in diameter, **7% are less than 50 μm in diameter**. The smaller particles (Henley et al, 1995) and possible intramuscular injection of the agent are responsible for the migration of particles to the lungs, kidneys, brain, and lymph nodes demonstrated in animal models. Unlike Teflon paste, Macroplastique does not cause an intense local inflammatory response. In patients requiring open surgery after failed injection with Macroplastique, the injectable bolus was found to be encapsulated and easily removed without adherence to the ureter or bladder (Herz et al, 2001). Histologic examination of bladder muscle biopsy specimens and pelvic lymph nodes at the time of open surgery revealed a mild inflammatory reaction with no evidence of PDS particle migration in either the wall of the bladder or the draining lymph nodes.

The efficacy of PDS as a bulking agent for correction of reflux is well documented. Dodat and colleagues reported on the long-term outcomes of Macroplastique injections for correction of VUR. Results in 590 refluxing ureters in 389 patients who were injected with a minimum follow-up of 5 years revealed a sustained success rate of 79.4% (Dodat et al, 2004). Herz and coworkers (2001) demonstrated a success rate of 81% after a single injection and 90% after a second injection with a 12-month follow-up. Similarly, van Capelle and associates (2004) reported an 82.3% success rate in 311 ureters in 195 children over a 10-year period from two European centers.

The main advantage of PDS is that it is a permanent material that remains well encapsulated and causes minimal local inflammatory changes. Although it has a demonstrated long-term track record, PDS has yet to achieve FDA approval for correction of VUR in the United States, possibly because of concern regarding migration, particularly the proportion of particles that are smaller than 80 μm and the negative connotations associated with silicone implants.

Dextranomer/Hyaluronic Copolymer (Deflux). Dextranomer/hyaluronic copolymer (DX/HA) is formed from cross-linked dextranomer microspheres (80 to 250 μm in diameter) suspended in a carrier gel of stabilized sodium hyaluronate. DX/HA is biodegradable, the carrier gel is reabsorbed, and the dextranomer microspheres are capsulated by fibroblast migration and collagen ingrowth. DX/HA loses about 23% of its volume beyond 3 months of follow-up (Stenberg and Lackgren, 1995).

Deflux was first introduced by the Swedish group of Stenberg and Lackgren (1995), and it received FDA approval in 2001. Since then, there have been several clinical reports from Europe and the United States documenting success rates ranging from 68% to 89% (Lackgren et al, 2001; Puri et al, 2003; Kirsch et al, 2004; Lavelle et al, 2005). The 89% success rate was achieved by Kirsch and coworkers (2004) with an intraureteral injection technique. In a long-term follow-up study by Lackgren and associates (2001), 68% of 221 children monitored for a mean of 5 years maintained grade I VUR or less at the last VUCG. No significant long-term adverse effects were noted. In patients who fail endoscopic treatment with Deflux and proceed to open surgery, the bulking agent is noted

to have completely disappeared. Whether this disappearance represents a technical error in the injection technique or is due to complete reabsorption of the injectable agent remains unproved.

The appeal of Deflux is that it is a natural product that is easily administered without a ratcheted syringe through a smaller-gauge needle. It is currently the preferred agent for endoscopic correction in most centers; however, the durability of correction of VUR with Deflux remains to be proved.

Coaptite. Calcium hydroxyapatite is synthetic bone material. The particles have a uniform spherical shape and range in size from 75 to 125 μm. The material injects easily through a 21-gauge needle without the need for a ratcheted syringe. At the AUA meeting in 2002, Mevorach and colleagues presented the initial results in a clinical trial that included 98 patients and 155 ureters with grade II to IV reflux. Reflux resolved in 67% of the patients and 75% of the ureters. There are no published reports at this point, and the FDA is currently evaluating the clinical trials.

Autologous Materials

Fat, collagen, muscle, and chondrocytes have all been evaluated as bulking agents. The key advantage of these agents is that they are not foreign material, but the obvious disadvantage is the observed volume loss (up to 100% in the case of fat [Matthews et al, 1994]) and that they need to be harvested and expanded (in the case of chondrocytes and muscle) before injection. Autologous materials behave as a free graft at the injection site; therefore, reabsorption of the material is worrisome and may be responsible for the inconsistent results.

Chondrocytes. Atala and associates (1993, 1994) described the harvesting and expansion of chondrocytes in vitro and successful correction of VUR in animal models. Subsequently, human trials using chondrocytes harvested from the posterior auricular cartilage were conducted by Diamond and Caldamone (1999, 2001). The chondrocytes were grown in culture for 6 weeks, quantitated, concentrated, and then suspended in a mixture of sodium alginate and calcium sulfate solution for injection. At 3 months' follow-up, reflux was corrected in 57% (27/47) of the ureters, which improved to 86% after one or two repeat injections. At 1-year follow-up, reflux correction was maintained in 70% (32 of 46) of the ureters and 66% of the patients (19 of 29). At subsequent endoscopy, failures were attributable to volume loss and shifting of the subureteral mounds.

Recurrence of Vesicoureteral Reflux after Endoscopic Correction

The **true incidence** of recurrent VUR after successful endoscopic correction with any specific material is difficult to determine because a repeat VCUG is not obtained beyond the initial negative study except in the context of a research protocol.

Only a handful of series have reported long-term follow-up with repeat VCUG beyond the initial negative study. Chertin and coworkers (2002) reported a 5% recurrence rate with follow-up of up to 17 years for Teflon paste. A 13% recurrence rate with Deflux was reported by Lackgren and colleagues (2001) 2 to 5 years after an initial negative VCUG. The higher rate with Deflux, an absorbable agent, was not unexpected. In the absence of UTIs, the significance of confirming the long-term absence of VUR is less important. Furthermore, even if absorbable bulking materials were to lose volume or be reabsorbed completely over time, resolution of VUR may be maintained by growth of the child and maturation of the UVJ. The injectable agent may just have bought time for this process to conclude. The implications of recurrent reflux in young adulthood for these patients is inadequately defined at present.

LAPAROSCOPY AS APPLIED TO CORRECTION OF REFLUX

The laparoscopic approach to ureteral reimplantation should theoretically provide the success rate and durability of open surgery while avoiding its morbidity. Three procedures have been attempted laparoscopically: extravesical reimplantation, the Gil-Vernet procedure, and the Cohen cross-trigonal reimplantation.

In addition to the long operative times and steep learning curve, the initial experience with laparoscopic reimplantation identified significant technical challenges in creation of the submucosal tunnel while maintaining an intact bladder urothelium and in the suturing aspects of the procedures. Although a robot may assist with the suturing aspect, the current port size required is still not ideal for smaller children. The continued refinement of open reimplantation surgery, more recently dispensing with the use of postoperative bladder catheters and need for overnight hospital stay, will place even greater onus on the proponents of the laparoscopic approach to better define the ideal conditions for this minimally invasive technique.

The Gil-Vernet Procedure

In this procedure the trigonal mucosa is incised vertically and the two ureters are approximated into the midline with a single submucosal suture. This procedure has been performed transvesically with limited success. Okamura and associates (1999) and Cartwright and associates (1996) reported success rates of 59% and 62.5%, respectively. The recurrence of reflux is thought to be due to splitting of the trigone and lateral displacement of the ureters.

Laparoscopic Extravesical Reimplantation

Probably the most commonly reported procedure for laparoscopic correction of reflux, extravesical reimplantation has a steep learning curve; initial experiences described challenges with exposure of the ureter, trauma to the ureter, and difficulty developing the extravesical tunnel without injury to the urothelium, in addition to long operative times.

Separation of the urothelium from the detrusor is difficult laparoscopically because an adequately distended bladder protrudes into the limited pelvic working space and hinders the laparoscopic dissection. Additionally, the ability to adequately retract the incised detrusor edges to create a wider trough is limited because of the exposure and angles at which the instruments enter the abdomen.

Several modifications of the technique described by Lakshmanan and Fung (2000) have resulted in a more effective procedure with shorter operative time and outcomes that approximate those of open surgery.

Trocar Placement

A 5-mm, 0-degree laparoscope is inserted through the umbilicus. Three additional working ports are inserted in the lower part of the abdomen along the lines of a Pfannenstiel incision in the middle and on either end.

Ureteral Dissection

The ureter is best identified at the pelvic brim and followed distally. The overlying peritoneum is incised transversely. Ureteric catheters placed cystoscopically may aid in identification of the ureter in older patients. Once the ureter is identified, it can be grasped with Babcock forceps and freed from the surrounding tissues. In males, the peritoneal incision should be carried out caudal to the vas deferens so that the vas can be reflected with the peritoneum in a cephalad direction. A vessel loop or a Diamond-Flex retractor can be passed around the ureter and used as a holder.

Creation of the Tunnel

It is important to mark the direction of the tunnel with electrocautery while the bladder is semidistended in its normal position. A 4-0 Prolene traction suture is applied at the proximal end of the detrusor tunnel. This suture is passed through the abdominal wall on a straight needle and used to hitch the bladder, and then the needle is passed out again to provide external control to achieve the desired tension and elevation of the detrusor. The detrusor incision is carried out in a proximal-to-distal direction. The serosa is scored with cautery, but most of the dissection should be performed with scissors to prevent injury to the bladder innervation, as described for open extravesical reimplantation earlier in the chapter. Elevation of the detrusor flaps is more difficult in the laparoscopic procedure, and therefore a trough as wide as that developed with open surgery may not be achievable. The incision is continued distally around the ureter, with the distal attachments left intact. The mucosal bulge is not as obvious as in open surgery because the bladder is not as distended and is also compressed by the peritoneal insufflation.

Closure of the Myotomy (Detrusorrhaphy)

The ureter is positioned in the new tunnel and 3-0 polyglactin suture is placed at the most proximal end to stabilize the ureter and facilitate reclosure of the detrusor with interrupted sutures, starting at the ureteral orifice distally. Anchoring sutures are not required because the distal attachments of the ureter are left intact. After completion of the detrusorrhaphy, the bladder retraction suture is released and the bladder is filled. The ureter is observed in its new tunnel to confirm the absence of angulation or kinking. A catheter may be left in the bladder for 12 to 24 hours postoperatively.

The largest published series is that of Lakshmanan and Fung (2000), in which 71 ureters were reimplanted laparoscopically. Early in that series, three ureteral injuries occurred and required open reimplantation in two and stenting in one to drain a urinoma. The remaining patients are free of reflux and obstruction.

Endoscopic Cross-Trigonal Reimplantation

To avoid transgressing the peritoneum and the challenges associated with a small pelvis in children, other groups have developed a transvesical approach, similar to the Cohen cross-trigonal reimplant procedure, that involves carbon dioxide insufflation of the bladder (pneumovesicum).

Yeung and coworkers (2005) initially described performance of the procedure with standard laparoscopic instruments. Peters and Woo (2005) followed with a report describing a robotically assisted technique to facilitate creation of the submucosal tunnel and the ureteral anastomosis.

Port Placement

The patient is positioned supine with the legs separated to allow access to the urethra for cystoscopy and bladder catheterization intraoperatively. Cystoscopy is carried out and the bladder is distended with saline. A traction suture is passed percutaneously at the level of the bladder dome under cystoscopic vision to anchor the bladder wall to the abdomen and prevent it from pulling away when the camera port incision is made at the dome. A 5-mm port is then inserted under cystoscopic vision. The cystoscope is removed and a urethral catheter is inserted. CO_2 insufflation to a pressure of 10 mm Hg is started, and a 5-mm, 30-degree lens is inserted. Two additional 3-mm working ports are inserted on either side of the bladder under direct vision.

Dissection of the Ureter

A 5-cm segment of a 5 French feeding tube is inserted in the ureter and secured with 4-0 Prolene suture. The catheter facilitates handling and dissection of the ureter as described for the open Cohen procedure. Ureteral mobilization begins with the usual circumscribing incision with the hook electrocautery. The 3-mm endoscopic scissors are used to develop the plane of dissection, starting on the distal aspect of the ureter. The dissection is carried out circumferentially for a distance of 2 to 3 cm. The muscular defect in the ureteral hiatus is repaired with 4-0 absorbable suture.

Creation of the Submucosal Tunnel

An incision is made with the hook cautery at the site of the new ureteral orifice across the back wall of the bladder. The submucosal tunnel is started from the old hiatus toward the new hiatus with fine endo-scissors. A fine grasper is then inserted through the new hiatus, and the feeding tube is used to pull the ureter through the tunnel.

Ureteral Neocystostomy

The ureter is spatulated at the 6-o'clock position and anastomosed at the new location with 6-0 interrupted sutures. Peters and Woo (2005) described using a robot to facilitate the delicate suturing laparoscopically and improve the efficiency of the procedure.

The port sites in the bladder are closed and an indwelling urethral catheter is maintained for 24 hours.

Resolution of reflux was demonstrated in 15 of 16 patients in Yeung and colleagues' series and in 5 of 6 patients in the series of Peters and Woo.

MEGAURETER

The term megaureter (MGU) is simply a descriptive name that conveys the picture of a dilated ureter. It implies no particular unifying pathophysiologic principles but merely groups together a spectrum of anomalies associated with increased ureteral diameter. Because surgical solutions to the anomaly are reliable, the challenge arises in differentiating nonobstructive from obstructive variants and thus better defining the indications for surgery. This is analogous to the highly debated management of hydronephrosis caused by UPJ obstruction (Koff and Campbell, 1992), with which MGU may share similar pathophysiologic principles. **It is apparent by now that all dilatations of the urinary tract do not necessarily translate into physiologically significant obstructive processes with renal functional implications despite the anatomic distortion of the collecting system that they represent.**

Definition and Classification

Structurally, normal ureteral diameter is rarely greater than 5 mm (Cussen, 1971), and ureters wider than 7 to 8 mm can all be considered MGUs (Hellstrom et al, 1985). This measurement is somewhat arbitrary and may be subject to variation depending on the imaging modality and concomitant insults such as infection or inflammation (Hellstrom et al, 1987). The international classification presented by Smith (1977) and Stephens (1977) as a result of the joint meeting of the pediatric urology societies held in 1976 is the most comprehensive classification available and sets the basis for today's designations and categorization for management (Fig. 117–23, after King [1980]). As shown in Figure 117–23, **an MGU may be obstructed, refluxing, both refluxing and obstructed, or unobstructed and not refluxing, either from a primary (idiopathic) cause intrinsic to the ureter or secondary to specific pathologic processes such as outlet obstruction, neurogenic dysfunction, polyuria, or infection.** This practical division is of diagnostic and therapeutic importance and relies on a thorough evaluation of the urinary tract. Secondary causes should always be suspected because management would be directed at the specific problem and in many instances is quite different from interventions to treat primary MGU. Despite its widespread use and clinical utility, one of the persisting difficulties in categorizing a patient under this classification scheme is establishing the presence of obstruction. **If extrapolating the working definition used for UPJ obstruction—a restriction in urine flow that if left uncorrected, will lead to progressive renal deterioration (Koff, 1990)—differentiation between obstructed and unobstructed MGU can prove challenging.** Indeed, the concern for renal damage and irreversible loss of kidney function during prolonged observation has been the driving force behind the decision to surgically intervene in many cases.

Demographics and Clinical Findings

Primary MGU is a relatively common finding in neonates and infants referred for urologic evaluation. Prenatal ultrasound series suggest UVJ obstruction in up to 23% of patients with urinary tract dilatation (Brown et al, 1987). Primary MGU is

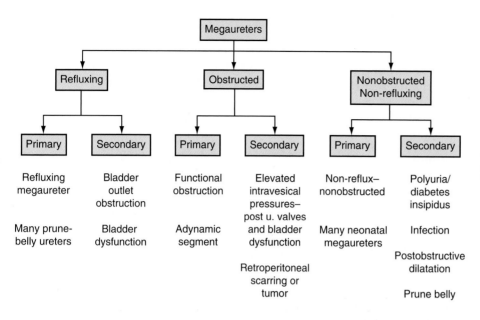

Figure 117–23. Three major classifications of megaureter based on primary and secondary causes. Not shown is the possible combination of reflux and obstruction.

two to four times more common in boys than girls, has a slight predilection (1.6 to 4.5 times) for the left side, and is bilateral in approximately 25% of patients (James et al, 1998; Shokeir and Nijman, 2000; Mouriquand et al, 2001). In up to 10% to 15% of children the contralateral kidney may be absent or dysplastic (Shokeir and Nijman, 2000), and concomitant obstruction of the ipsilateral UPJ area has been described on rare occasion (McGrath et al, 1987). There is no clear evidence for a hereditary predisposition, although some families with more than one affected member have been described (Shokeir and Nijman, 2000). The demographic characteristics of secondary MGU are presented elsewhere.

A growing number of cases are now being detected in utero with the diagnosis confirmed after birth. Clinically, patients have UTIs, abdominal pain, or hematuria. The diagnosis may be made later in life in some asymptomatic patients, either during imaging evaluation for an unrelated complaint or rarely at the time of surgery for another pathologic process. Patients with primary MGU are rarely initially seen with or progress to renal insufficiency.

Pathophysiology

The distal end of the ureter, as it becomes intramural and subsequently submucosal, rearranges the muscular layers in its wall. All layers become longitudinally oriented (Tanagho and Pugh, 1963; Hanna et al, 1976a), and the ureteral adventitia fuses to the bladder trigone by attachment to Waldeyer's sheath. Sympathetic and parasympathetic innervation to the distal ureter and UVJ area is believed to modulate primarily ureteral peristalsis; however, its exact role in regulating urine transport remains unclear. This anatomy is variable, depending on the type of MGU.

Primary Obstructive Megaureter

Even though the precise etiology of primary obstructive MGU remains unclear, it is generally agreed that the most common finding is an aperistaltic juxtavesical (adynamic) ureteral segment that prevents urine from flowing at an acceptable rate (Fig. 117–24). The predilection for distal ureteral involvement over other segments is unclear, but it

may be related to arrested development of the musculature in this segment, which is the last portion of the ureter to develop (Tanagho, 1973). Abnormal morphogenic events during other processes, such as formation of the intravesical antireflux mechanism, are other possibilities.

Several studies have examined the histologic and ultrastructural abnormalities that presumably alter distal ureteral function, including disorientation of the muscle fibers (Tanagho, 1973; MacKinnon, 1977), localized muscular hypoplasia or hypertrophy within the UVJ (Mackinnon et al, 1970; Tanagho et al, 1970), abnormal smooth muscle cells with more organelles and fewer myofilaments (Gosling and Dixon, 1978), mural fibrosis (McLaughlin et al, 1973) (Fig.

KEY POINTS: MEGAURETER

- MGU is a nonspecific term implying a spectrum of anomalies associated with pathologically excessive ureteral diameter.

- Primary (at the UVJ; adynamic segment) or secondary (e.g., bladder malfunction) causes influence management and must therefore be differentiated.

- Classification parameters include obstructing, nonobstructing, refluxing, and nonrefluxing.

- Nuclear diuretic renography is more challenging than in UPJ pathology and must include the ureter in the analysis.

- Indications for correction are often driven by serially increasing pelvicalyceal dilation, increasing ureteral diameter, or pyelonephritis and ureteral pyuria.

- Antibiotic prophylaxis should be used to protect the dilated ureter regardless of cause.

- Many cases of antenatally diagnosed MGU will resolve spontaneously.

APERISTALTIC DISTAL URETERAL SEGMENT
(PRIMARY MEGALOURETER)

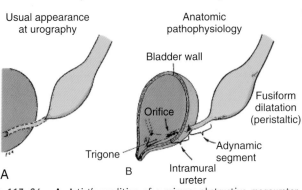

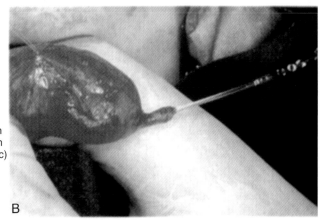

Figure 117–24. A, Artist's rendition of a primary obstructive megaureter. Ureteral dilation is depicted above a smaller-caliber adynamic segment, with transition point usually being a few millimeters above the bladder. (Courtesy of Dr A. P. McLaughlin III). **B,** Intraoperative photograph depicting the typical appearance of an obstructed megaureter. As frequently noted during surgery, there is rarely complete obliteration of the lumen.

117–25), and an excessive pattern of collagen deposition by light and electron microscopic studies (Gregoir and Debled, 1969; Notley, 1972; Hanna et al, 1976b; Pagano and Passerini, 1977; Medel and Quesada, 1985; Lee et al, 1992) (Figs. 117–26 and 117–27). Quantitative immunohistochemical analysis of collagen subtypes has demonstrated increases in collagen types I and III, with a predominance of type I collagen in primary obstructive MGU (Lee et al, 1998). The abnormal extracellular matrix deposition theoretically alters cell-to-cell junctions and disrupts myoelectrical propagation and peristalsis, a disturbance that is manifested by irregular wave patterns within these segments on ureteric profilometry—so-called ureteroarrhythmias (Shafik, 1996; Shafik, 1998). These disturbances can be further explained by abnormalities detected in acetylcholinesterase activity at the juxtavesical ureteral segment (immediately proximal to the constricted area) (Hofmann et al, 1986) and during the tissue's response to noradrenaline (Hertle and Nawrath, 1985), as well as in its autonomic innervation (Dixon et al, 1998). **Regardless of its cause, altered peristalsis prevents the free outflow of urine, and functional obstruction results.** As successive boluses of urine are unable to fully traverse the aberrant distal segment, urine accumulates and ureteral dilation

proximal to the abnormal segment develops. The proximal dilated segment also has an abnormal pattern of connective tissue elements (Notley, 1972; Hanna et al, 1977; Gosling and Dixon, 1978; Tokunaka and Koyanagi, 1982; Lee et al, 1992) and acquires an arrhythmic pattern with virtually no functional wave propagation. The resulting degree of ureteral dilatation is dependent on the volume of urine that accumulates proximally. Disruption in ureteral dynamics has obvious implications for the renal parenchyma if the pelvicalyceal system is unable to dampen the proximal pressure that can develop. Theoretically, it is possible that a compliant dilated ureter provides a larger reservoir and a lower-pressure buffering system than a similar, but higher obstructive process does (i.e., UPJ obstruction) (Shokeir and Nijman, 2000).

Other rare causes of primary obstructive MGU that should be considered include congenital ureteral strictures (Allen, 1970) (Fig. 117–28) and ureteral valves (Albertson and Talner, 1972; Jones et al, 1988).

Secondary Obstructive Megaureter

Secondary obstructive MGU most commonly occurs with neurogenic and non-neurogenic voiding dysfunction or infravesical obstruction such as PUVs. The ureter experi-

Figure 117–25. Even though normal ureteral muscular orientation is sometimes seen with megaureters (**A**), hypoplasia and atrophy of the smooth muscle layers is more common (**B**). (From McLaughlin AP III, Pfister RC, Leadbetter WF, et al: The pathophysiology of primary megaureter. J Urol 1973;109:805-811.)

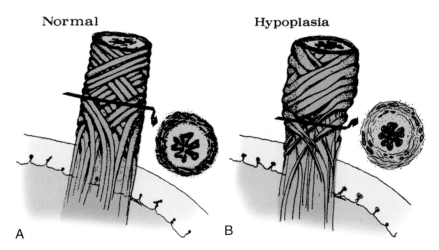

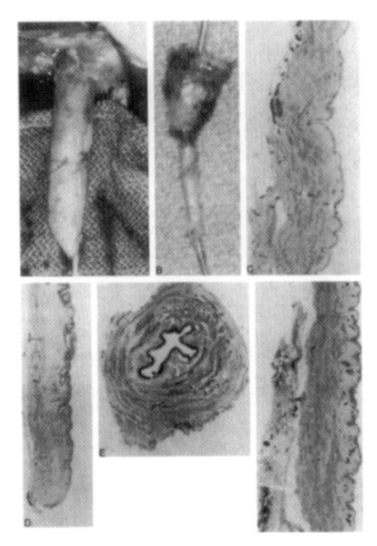

Figure 117-26. Primary obstructive megaureter. Light microscopic findings show various abnormalities. **A,** Operative exposure. **B,** Specimen. Note that the obstructed segment admits passage of a probe. **C,** No abnormality seen on longitudinal section. **D,** Reduced muscle bulk seen in some megaureters. **E,** Preponderance of circular muscle. **F,** Thickened adventitia. (From Hanna MK, Jeffs RD, Sturgess JM, et al: Ureteral structure and ultrastructure: Part II. Congenital ureteropelvic junction obstruction and primary obstructive megaureter. J Urol 1978;116:728.)

ences increasing difficulty with propulsion of urine when an elevated pressure differential of greater than 40 cm H_2O exists across the UVJ (McGuire, 1981). Progressive ureteral dilatation, decompensation of the UVJ, VUR, and subsequent renal damage can be expected if such pressures continue unchecked. The dilatation that occurs with most of these variants largely resolves once the cause of the elevated intravesical pressure is rectified. In other cases, the ureter remains permanently dilated from what appears to be altered compliance, a permanent insult to the organ's peristaltic mechanisms, fixed hypertrophy of the ureteral tissues, or some combination of these mechanisms. Transmural scarring from chronic UTI could be a contributing factor in some cases. Obstruction is not truly present within such ureters, but as the ureteral wall stiffens and loses compliance, its ability to protect the kidney is lessened and elevated intravesical pressure is projected proximally as a noncompliant column of fluid (Jones et al, 1988). Other obstructive causes of ureteral dilatation include ureteroceles, ureteral ectopia, bladder diverticula, periureteral postreimplantation fibrosis, neurogenic bladder, and external compression by retroperitoneal tumors, masses, or aberrant vessels.

Primary and Secondary Refluxing Megaureter

Because bladder filling and cyclic voiding can directly transmit pressure into the ureter, it is not difficult to envision this process progressively enlarging the ureter. With time, ureteral smooth muscle becomes a smaller component of the ureteral wall as deposition of collagen fibers is increased, and as a result the collagen–smooth muscle ratio is higher than that seen in normal ureters or primary obstructive MGU (Lee et al, 1992). A shift toward more type III collagen in this form of MGU also differs from primary obstructive MGU and normal ureteral specimens (Lee et al, 1998). The relative concentration of collagens I and III may have different effects on ureteral wall compliance, which may help explain the lower success rate of reimplantation of MGUs.

A refluxing MGU associated with prune-belly syndrome represents a special category and demonstrates rather particular gross, microscopic, and ultrastructural changes. These dilated and tortuous ureters exhibit wall thickening, which correlates with changes in the extracellular matrix and leads to poor dynamic characteristics and ineffective peristalsis. Quantitative histologic studies have identified massive

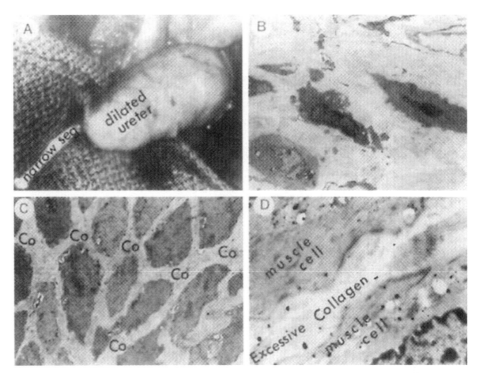

Figure 117-27. Primary obstructive megaureter: electron microscopic findings. **A,** Operative specimen. **B,** Muscle cell atrophy, absent nexus, and excessive ground substance and collagen in the intracellular space from a dilated ureter. **C,** Abnormal collagen fibers between muscle cells (×4000). **D,** Abnormality from a narrow ureter (×17,000). (From Hanna MK, Jeffs RD, Sturgess JM, et al: Ureteral structure and ultrastructure: Part II. Congenital ureteropelvic junction obstruction and primary obstructive megaureter. J Urol 1978;116: 728.)

replacement of the normal smooth muscle architecture with collagen, a progressive deposition that results in a high collagen–smooth muscle ratio (Gearhart et al, 1995). These changes are particularly evident in the wider, more distal ureter (Ehrlich and Brown, 1977), which characteristically shows the greatest dilation on imaging. Interestingly, both the caliber and histology of the more proximal segment of the ureter normalize as it approaches the kidney (Palmer and Tesluk, 1974). Although ureteral dilatation in prune-belly syndrome is suspected to result primarily from inefficient peristalsis, distal ureteral obstruction can occur in some cases (Cussen, 1971).

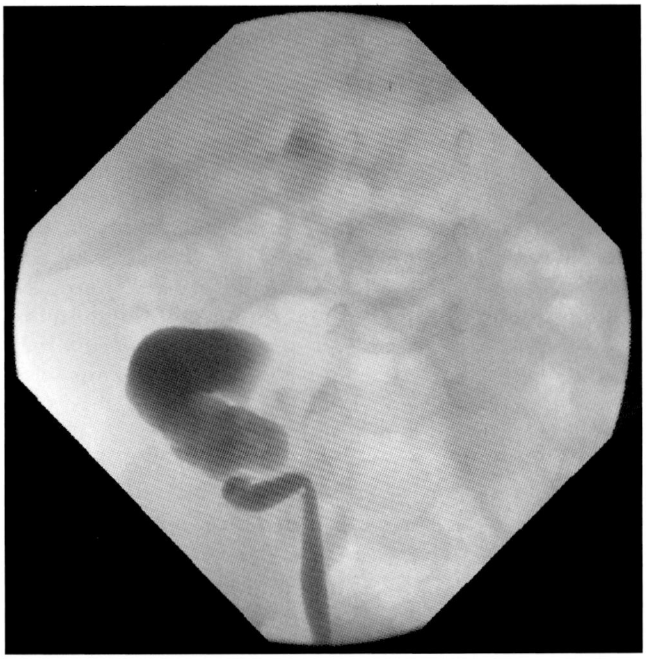

Refluxing Obstructed Megaureter

A small group of patients have an element of obstruction combined with reflux. In a series of more than 400 refluxing ureters, obstruction was present in approximately 2% (Weiss and Lytton, 1974). A dysgenetic distal ureteral segment that not only fails to coapt within the intramural tunnel but also results in ineffective peristalsis has been implicated. Many of these patients have an ectopic insertion of the ureter at the level of the bladder neck that allows for reflux of urine when relaxed and acts as a distal obstruction when muscle tone increases. Identification is important because management of obstruction differs from that of reflux alone.

Primary Nonobstructive, Nonrefluxing Megaureter

Most newborn MGUs fall in this category (Keating et al, 1989; Rickwood et al, 1992; Baskin et al, 1994). **To establish this diagnosis, VUR, UVJ obstruction, and secondary causes of dilatation must be ruled out. Clinically, this may not be straightforward in all cases, mostly because of pitfalls related to the definition of obstruction.** Explanations for the ureteral transformations that occur during development remain to be defined. However, a multifactorial cause with a basis in transitional renal physiology and ureteral development seems likely. The fetal kidney reportedly produces four to six times more urine before delivery than afterward as a

Figure 117-28. Retrograde ureterogram from a child with persistent, prenatally detected hydroureteronephrosis. On surgical exploration the child was found to have a congenital ureteral stricture.

result of differences in glomerular filtration, renal vascular resistance, and concentrating ability (Campbell et al, 1973; Hartnoll, 2003; Vanderheyden et al, 2003). When this polyuric state is associated with a relative transient distal obstruction, it can result in dilatation of the fetal ureter by virtue of its adynamic inability to transmit the increased volume load to the bladder. This situation is similar to normal ureters challenged with acquired high–urine output nephropathies. Persistent fetal folds (Fig. 117–29), delays in development of ureteral patency (Ruano-Gil et al, 1975), and immaturity of normal peristalsis are also plausible theories of obstruction. The less compliant, hyperreflexic bladder of infancy (Baskin et al, 1994) or a transient urethral obstruction that causes altered bladder compliance might also be implicated, especially in patients with bilateral abnormalities. Abnormal ureteral compliance and changes in configuration could also result from developmental differences in the deposition and orientation of matrix proteins, such as elastin and collagen (Escala et al, 1989). **A delay in the normal segmental maturation of the distal ureter has been postulated not only as an etiologic factor but also as a theory of spontaneous resolution over time (sometimes referred to as the maturational-delay hypothesis of primary MGU).** Nicotina and associates (1997) have proposed a correlation between segmental hypoplasia of the inner longitudinal muscle layer and abnormal levels of transforming growth factor-β (TGF-β) in the narrowed segments of primary MGUs. Autocrine overexpression of TGF-β may be the cause of delay in maturation of smooth muscle cells (Massague et al, 1986; Ewton et al, 1988; Florini and Ewton, 1988; Nilsen-Hamilton, 1990), whereas depletion of TGF-β may eventually lead to maturation into the normal "full-term" architecture of the distal ureter (Nicotina et al, 1997).

That this process is indeed related to subclinical obstruction is still a matter of debate. A newborn ureter appears to be a far more compliant conduit than that of an adult. The tortuous dilatations seen in response to distal obstruction in infants as compared with the "pipestem" response that occurs at older ages would suggest that the infant ureter accommodates the ever-increasing volume of urine by the formation of additional ureteral tissue, thereby adding to the hydrodynamic buffering capability of the infant MGU. **As a result, the kidneys of newborns are probably better protected from the pressure of any partial or transient distal ureteral obstruction that might form during development, with no detectable adverse effects on renal function.**

Secondary Nonobstructive, Nonrefluxing Megaureter

Nonobstructive, nonrefluxing MGUs are more common than once was recognized, and they often have an identifiable cause. During UTI, **significant ureteral dilatation can result from bacterial endotoxins that inhibit peristalsis.** Resolution is expected with appropriate antibiotic therapy (Retik et al, 1978). **Nephropathies and other medical conditions that cause significant increases in urinary output that overwhelm maximal peristalsis can also lead to progressive ureteral dilatation, even in a normal ureter, as a result of buffering the output from above. Such conditions include lithium toxicity, diabetes insipidus or mellitus, sickle cell nephropathy, and psychogenic polydipsia.**

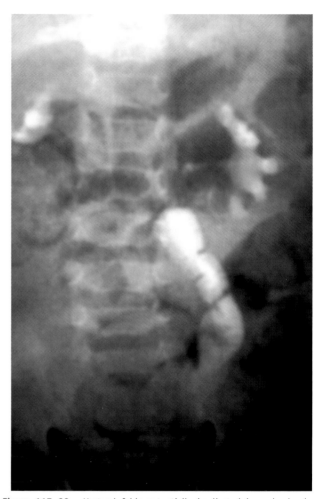

Figure 117–29. Ureteral folds potentially implicated in early developmental obstruction.

Evaluation

The routine practice of prenatal ultrasonography and improvements in ultrasound technology have led to an increase in detection of ureteral dilatation at an earlier age than previously diagnosed. **Ultrasound is the initial study obtained in any child with a suspected urinary abnormality. It usually distinguishes MGU from UPJ obstruction based on the presence or absence of a dilated ureter; provides useful anatomic detail of the renal parenchyma, collecting system, and bladder; and offers a baseline standard for the degree of hydroureteronephrosis to be observed in serial follow-up studies** (Fig. 117–30). Furthermore, ultrasound can detect associated abnormalities (e.g., ureteroceles [Shokeir and Nijman, 2002] and duplicated systems [Whitten et al, 2003]) and may even suggest ureteral ectopia in selected cases (Mathews et al, 1999; Vijayaraghavan, 2002). Even though techniques such as Doppler vascular evaluation with calculation of the renal resistive index and Doppler evaluation of ureteral jets have been used to suggest obstruction (Ordorica et al, 1993; Palmer and DiSandro, 1995; Shokeir et al, 1996; Shokeir et al, 1997a; Shokeir et al, 1997b; Strehlau et al, 1997; Patti et al, 2000; Cvitkovic Kuzmic et al, 2001), it must be remembered that the ultrasonography is purely a descriptive

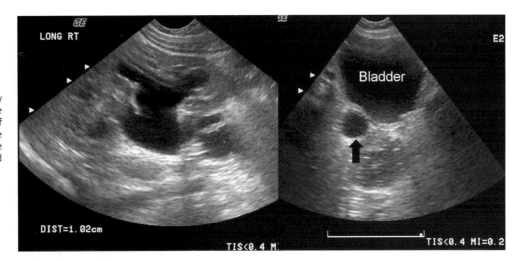

Figure 117–30. Ultrasound study in a patient with primary obstructive megaureter. Included is evaluation of the upper urinary tract (in this case labeled "Long RT"), as well as the pelvis. Note the dilated ureter behind the bladder (*arrow*).

imaging study and lacks the ability to quantify renal function or drainage.

Once ureteral dilatation is detected, a VCUG is subsequently obtained in most cases to rule out reflux. At the same time, a conventional fluoroscopic study allows for anatomic evaluation of the bladder and urethra, which can provide diagnostic clues to common causes of secondary MGU, such as neurogenic dysfunction or bladder outlet obstruction.

A study is also subsequently obtained to judge renal function and estimate the degree of obstruction, if any. A diuretic nuclear renal scan (renal scintigraphy) is currently the preferred imaging modality because it attempts to provide objective, reproducible parameters of function and obstruction. ^{99m}Tc-diethylenetriaminepentaacetic acid (DTPA) and ^{99m}Tc-mertiatide (also ^{99m}Tc-mercaptoacetyltriglycine [MAG-3]) are the radionuclides most commonly used to provide parameters of function and clearance.

However, the study has shortcomings in its ability to define obstruction or measure function. Differences in the mechanism of radionuclide renal clearance, tracer dosing, timing of the diuretic dose, the patient's level of hydration, and calculation of the area of interest are significant variables that must all be standardized to ensure valid comparison of test results (Conway, 1992; Conway and Maizels, 1992; Ebel, 1998). Defining the scanning area of interest, which should ideally include the lower ureter in all patients with MGU (Koff et al, 1984) (Fig. 117–31), is often highly subjective. The timing of diuretic administration and the classic parameters for $t_{[1/2]}$ values (originally defined for adult UPJ obstruction) remain largely empirical, especially in young patients. In addition, the tubules of a newborn kidney demonstrate a blunted response to diuretics. Therefore, whenever possible, it is preferable to defer the study for approximately 3 months after birth to allow for tubular maturation. Perhaps the most useful information is provided when there is no evidence of obstruction and in cases with preserved differential function. Fractional uptake of radionuclide within the first few minutes should be approximately equal if significant function is present. Ideally, these types of determinations offer functional correlates to hydroureteronephrosis by quantifying the effects of obstruction where it matters most, in the parenchyma rather than

within the collecting system, where slow rates of washout are to be expected because of dilatation. Nevertheless, **differentiating truly obstructive dilatations of the urinary tract from those that appear to represent no more than nonobstructive variants remains difficult.** Bilateral MGUs can be particularly challenging because they do not provide a normal side for comparison. Furthermore, neither kidney may function normally as a consequence of an earlier obstructive insult, even after the actual obstruction has resolved. Importantly, radionuclide scans can also be used to estimate glomerular filtration rates and absolute renal function by measuring the uptake of radionuclide early after its systemic administration. Correlation with glomerular filtration is high (Heyman and

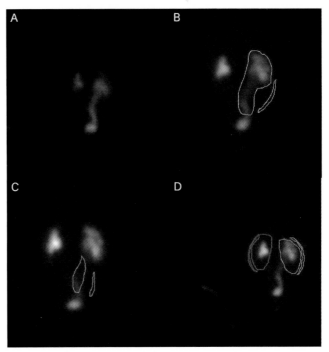

Figure 117–31. Diuretic renogram of the megaureter shown in Figure 117–30. **A,** Washout curve. **B** and **C,** Different areas of interest to calculate delayed washout. **D,** Equal function was present on early sequences.

Duckett, 1988). The percentage of the total dose filtered by the kidneys, or the extraction factor, can then be calculated and has been adopted by some institutions as a means of providing a more objective parameter for gauging significant obstruction.

Whitaker's perfusion test (Whitaker, 1973) and ureteral opening pressure (Fung et al, 1998) can also be used to evaluate obstruction, but their invasiveness and requirement for anesthesia are drawbacks in children. Although the Whitaker test requires a supraphysiologic flow rate that could potentially overcome the peristaltic flow capacity of a normal infant or child ureter, the modifications introduced by Fung and associates (1998) include calculating the infusion rate individually and within a physiologically relevant range, with obstruction identified when pressure within the pelvis increases above 14 cm H_2O. Even though the correlation between perfusion pressure and diuretic nuclear renography is poor, both studies can provide valuable information. Any discrepancy between these two studies is probably the result of measuring different physical parameters. In most situations, management can be planned with the aid of renal nuclear scans, with little additional data obtained by these invasive and somewhat complex tests (Kass et al, 1985). Exceptions include renal moieties with extremely poor function and cases in which the diuretic renogram is equivocal or difficult to interpret because of a very capacious collecting system.

Cystoscopy and retrograde imaging are infrequently performed as isolated diagnostic interventions. To avoid introducing infection into a dilated system, they are best performed at the time of surgical correction (Wunsch et al, 2000; Chowdhary et al, 2001).

Selected cases may also benefit from magnetic resonance urography. This impressive diagnostic modality can be coupled with dynamic contrast enhancement with gadolinium-DTPA to provide information that is functionally equal to nuclear scintigraphy while providing superb anatomic detail without the use of ionizing radiation (Fig. 117–32) (Perez-Brayfield et al, 2003). As it gains in popularity, concerns regarding cost, equipment limitations, sensitivity to patient motion, and the need for sedation must be addressed (Riccabona, 2004).

Management Recommendations

Today, through prenatal detection, the majority of children arrive with abnormalities that are totally asymptomatic, with only a minority having UTIs or pain. These two groups probably have different natural histories and should be considered separately. Because prenatal ultrasound is widely performed in many countries, the denominator has increased, and the clinical characteristics have changed. If left undetected, many prenatally detected MGUs might never become symptomatic or could lead to significant functional deterioration; indeed, many may normalize completely. These considerations raise questions with regard to surgical treatment. This is a common theme in pediatric urology and recalls the impact made by expectant management with serial ultrasound follow-up studies on redefining the natural history of MCDK and variants of UPJ obstruction (Ransley et al, 1990; Wacksman and Phipps, 1993; Menster et al, 1994; Woodward and Frank, 2002).

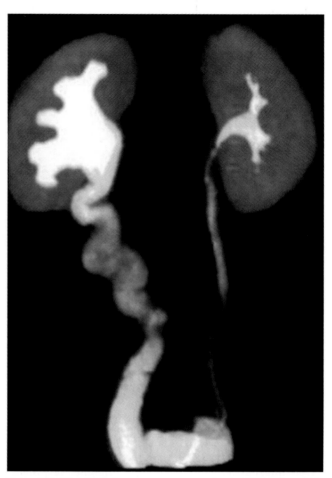

Figure 117–32. Magnetic resonance urogram showing obstruction at the right ureterovesical junction. (From Perez-Brayfield MR, Kirsch AJ, Jones RA, Grattan-Smith JD: A prospective study comparing ultrasound, nuclear scintigraphy and dynamic contrast enhanced magnetic resonance imaging in the evaluation of hydronephrosis. J Urol 2003;170:1330-1334.)

The therapeutic recommendations for MGUs that are truly obstructed and those that reflux are fairly well established. As previously stated, the challenge lies in differentiating primary obstructed MGU from the nonrefluxing, nonobstructed variants, especially in neonates. Given the constraints of the available diagnostic studies, such classification may not always be possible.

Primary Refluxing Megaureter

Routine surgical correction in newborns and infants with grade IV or V reflux is no longer appropriate. Instead, medical management is often the initial approach during infancy and is continued if a trend toward resolution is noted. Otherwise, surgery, which may include a consideration of endoscopic subureteric injection, is recommended for persistent high-grade reflux in older children, especially in the setting of recurrent pyelonephritis. In the rare infant for whom medical management has failed but who is considered too small for reconstructive surgery of a dilated ureter, distal ureterostomy for unilateral reflux or vesicostomy for bilateral disease may provide an ideal temporizing solution.

Secondary Refluxing or Obstructive Megaureter

Management of secondary MGUs is initially directed at their root cause. For example, impressive degrees of reflux and dilatation often improve with the ablation of urethral valves or medical management of neurogenic bladder. Other secondary causes, such as prune-belly syndrome or diabetes insipidus, require no more than observation alone. Chronic congenital dilation, regardless of its source, often imprints permanent dilatation on many collecting systems. As a result, some degree of nonobstructed hydroureteronephrosis usually persists, even after primary or secondary causes have been corrected. This dilation can be amplified with bladder filling, a finding that can pose a diagnostic dilemma because it mimics persistent or recurrent obstruction at the UVJ.

Primary "Dilated" Nonrefluxing Megaureter: Nonobstructive versus Obstructive

This topic is perhaps one of the most difficult to address in a patient with MGU. Deciding between surgery and expectant treatment sometimes becomes a function of clinical impression and experience. However, any haste in correcting MGU in a newborn is tempered by the realization that such repair represents a technical challenge in smaller infants. Even in experienced hands, the complication rate of surgery is higher than in older children (Peters et al, 1989; DeFoor et al, 2004). For example, repeat surgeries were required for 3 (7%) of 42 infants operated on before 8 months of age in one series (Peters et al, 1989). **In light of such clinical observations, most clinicians now believe that as long as renal function is not significantly affected and UTIs do not become a major problem, expectant management is preferred. Antibiotic suppression with close radiologic surveillance is appropriate in most cases.** Periodic urine culture and sonography every 3 to 6 months during the first year of life are appropriate. Diuretic nuclear renography is also sometimes repeated, especially in cases in which a trend toward improvement is not apparent. The duration between studies is extended once improvement in the degree of dilatation is seen. **When the hydroureteronephrosis is severe and shows no signs of improvement, in cases in which there is a documented decrease in renal function, or in patients with recurrent febrile infections despite prophylaxis, surgical correction is undertaken when technically feasible, usually between the ages of 1 and 2 years.** For the occasional newborn with massive dilatation, poor renal function (rare with MGUs), acute urine extravasation (Beetz et al, 2004), or recurrent infections, a distal cutaneous loop ureterostomy provides a simple, temporary, low-morbidity solution for poor drainage until the child is old enough to undergo reimplantation. Anecdotal alternative options for these patients include creation of a refluxing ureteral reimplantation (Lee et al, 2005) or temporary drainage with an internal ureteral stent (Shenoy and Rance, 1999). Definitive repair is also an option in experienced hands.

Clinical Correlates: Nonobstructive Megaureter

Past studies that have surgically addressed urinary tract obstruction or dilatation, or both, at the UPJ and UVJ suffer from two weaknesses: (1) they lack a diagnostic modality that allows for uniform and reliable differentiation of nonobstructive from obstructive dilatations, and (2) they are unable to predict the degree of renal recovery that might occur after surgical correction. In addition, data from surgical "correction" of urinary tract dilatation in neonates are confounded by a paradox peculiar to therapy at this age; that is, whereas truly obstructed kidneys often improve after surgery, unobstructed kidneys have been reported to increase relative uptake on renal imaging, thus making it difficult to determine whether surgical correction per se is responsible for improving renal function.

Antenatally diagnosed MGUs are different. Expectant treatment of this type of MGU is not novel, as evidenced in reports by Williams and Hulme-Moir (1970) and Pitts and Muecke (1974) more than 30 years ago. Keating and coworkers (1989) evaluated 23 units in 17 newborns managed by observation alone. Renal scintigraphy (DTPA) and assessment of function rather than drainage defined the parameters of obstruction. Comparative intravenous pyelography studies were also obtained in most patients. Notably, 20 (87%) of the 23 cases were deemed nonobstructive variants with no significant decrease in function and were monitored medically. None showed a decrease in renal function after an average follow-up period of 7 years, and the improvement in dilatation that occurred in most was impressive (Baskin et al, 1994) (Fig. 117–33). Others have noted the same phenomenon, although functional deterioration or breakthrough UTI occurred in 13 (16%) of 82 neonatal MGUs in the combined series of Rickwood and associates (1992) and Liu and colleagues (1994). More recent series have confirmed that over 70% of cases resolve spontaneously within 2 years of follow-up (McLellan et al, 2002; Shukla et al, 2005). This rate of improvement seems to be higher than the approximate 50% improvement seen in most series of UPJ obstruction. The fact that most prenatally diagnosed primary MGUs resolve spontaneously is not controversial. However, the rate of resolution, extent of follow-up, and predictive factors associated with resolution are still being investigated and remain a matter of debate. Shukla and coworkers (2005) have recently presented the long-term evaluation of a well-followed series in which a subgroup underwent reevaluation at a mean of 13.4 years. This report includes one asymptomatic patient with bilateral primary MGU who showed unilateral worsening function and increased hydroureteronephrosis because of loss of follow-up. Even though the evidence is limited, this issue requires further study and demands extended evaluation (perhaps up to adulthood), at least in patients with persistent dilation. Thus, for many families, conservative management mandates regular visits and radiologic evaluation. Currently, there is no established set of parameters that can be evaluated at the time of diagnosis that will accurately predict which patients will require surgical intervention or when spontaneous resolution will occur. McLellan and colleagues (2002) addressed these questions in a retrospective review of 54 patients prenatally diagnosed and monitored for an average of 25.8 months. Neither laterality nor gender had a significant effect on the rate of resolution. Mean initial ureteral diameter at initial postnatal evaluation was 0.8 cm in the group that resolved spontaneously versus 1.15 cm in the unresolved group and 1.32 cm in the surgically treated group, with sig-

SECTION XVII

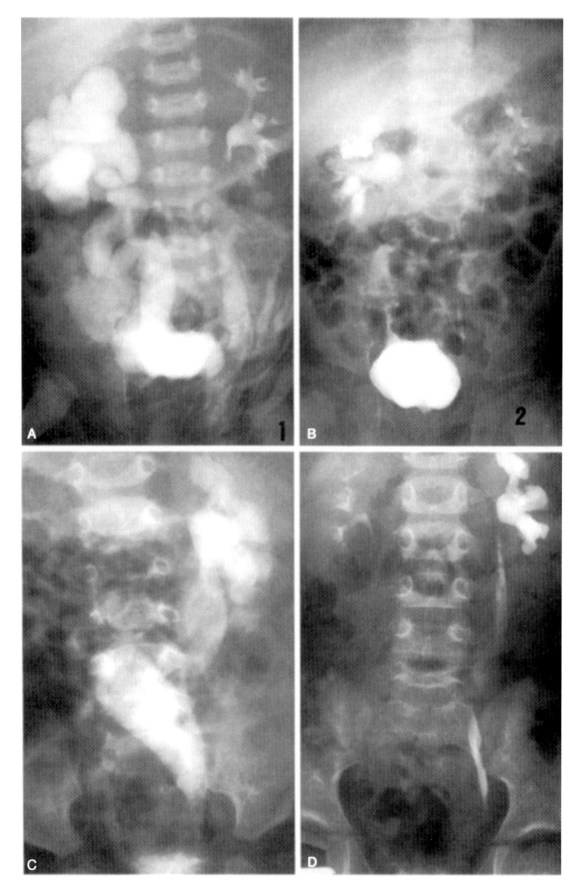

Figure 117–33. Neonatal megaureters managed expectantly. **A,** An excretory urogram at 3 weeks of age shows impressive dilatation of the right ureter. The renal scan documented good function but delayed drainage. **B,** Excretory urogram in same patient 2 years later. **C,** An excretory urogram demonstrates an impressively dilated left megaureter in a 6-week-old. **D,** Three years later, the appearance is almost normal.

INITIAL URETERAL DIAMETER

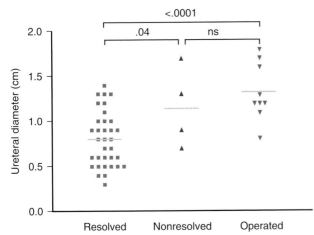

Figure 117-34. Distribution of retrovesical ureteral diameter in resolved, unresolved, and operated patients. *Horizontal bars* indicate *P* values in groups compared with the *t*-test. ns, not significant. (From McLellan DL, Retik AB, Bauer SB, et al: Rate and predictors of spontaneous resolution of prenatally diagnosed primary nonrefluxing megaureter. J Urol 2002;168:2177-2804.)

nificant overlap between the groups (Fig. 117–34). Interestingly, a significant correlation was described between the age at resolution and the grade of hydronephrosis at initial evaluation (defined on a scale from 1 to 5 and based on the appearance of the renal parenchyma, the renal pelvis anteroposterior diameter, and caliceal morphology). Grades 1 to 3 hydronephrosis resolved between the ages of 12 and 36 months, whereas grades 4 and 5 resolved at a mean of 48.5 months.

Surgical Options

Once it has been decided to embark on surgical correction, regardless of the cause of the MGU, the surgical objectives of ureteroneocystostomy are the same as for nondilated ureters. Ureteral tailoring (tapering or plication) is often necessary to achieve an adequate length-to-diameter ratio required for successful reimplantation. Narrowing of the ureter also theoretically enables its walls to coapt properly, thereby aiding effective peristalsis. Revising the distal segment intended for reimplantation is all that is usually required. The proximal segments of most MGUs regain tone once they are unobstructed. Children rarely have such massively dilated and tortuous ureters that straightening with removal of excess length and proximal revision becomes necessary, despite being free of infection and significant pelvicalyceal dilation (Hanna, 1979).

Two methods can be used to remodel MGUs. **Plication or infolding** (Kalicinski et al, 1977; Starr, 1979) **is useful for a moderately dilated ureter. Ureteral vascularity is preserved, and the revision can be taken down and redone if vascular compromise is suspected** (Bakker et al, 1988) (Fig. 117–35). **However, tissue bulk poses a problem with an extremely large ureter. Excisional tapering is preferred for a more severely dilated ureter or a ureter that is markedly thickened** (Hendren, 1969). Plication of ureters greater than 1.75 cm in diameter has been associated with more complications (Parrott et al, 1990). Remodeled MGUs have generally been reimplanted with standard cross-trigonal or Leadbetter-type techniques, but extravesical repairs can also be successfully done (Perovic, 1994). The success with reimplantation of remodeled MGUs, regardless of technique, is not as high as with nondilated ureters, yet the 90% to 95% success rate approximated in most series is commendable (Hendren, 1969; Retik et al, 1978; Parrott et al, 1990).

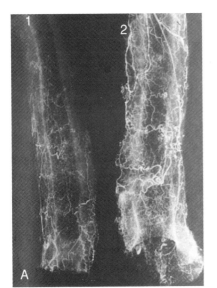
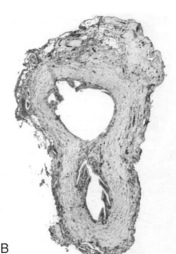
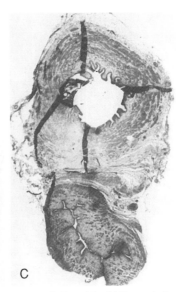

Figure 117-35. **A,** Comparison of microvasculature preservation in specimens obtained by excisional tapering (*left*) and by folding techniques (*right*). **B,** A histologic section of a folded ureter 3 weeks postoperatively shows no obliteration of the under-folded segment. **C,** The under-folded segment shows progressive obliteration at 3 months, although the lumen remains patent. (From Bakker HHR, Scholtameijer RJ, Klopper PJ: Comparison of 2 different tapering techniques in megaureters. J Urol 1988;140:1237.)

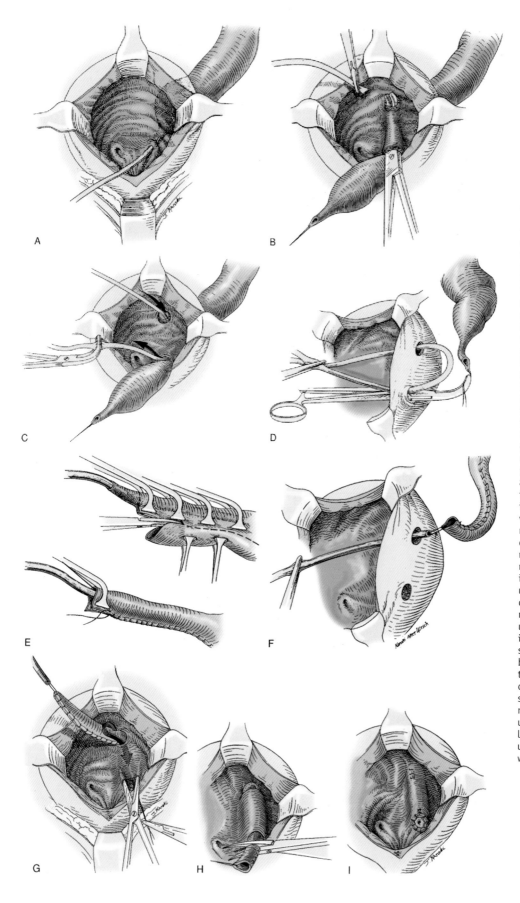

Figure 117–36. Technique for repair of megaureter. **A,** A No. 5 French feeding tube typically passes up a normal-caliber intravesical segment of primary obstructive megaureter. **B,** After the megaureter is freed from its intravesical and extravesical attachments, a blunt right-angle clamp is used to clear the peritoneum from the posterior and base of the bladder. If extravesical dissection is necessary, it is advisable to make the new hiatus before moving outside the bladder. A right-angle clamp is incised upon and spread. **C,** A fine red rubber catheter marks the new hiatus by being pulled from within the bladder to the outside and then through the old hiatus. **D,** A right-angle clamp is guided from within the bladder to the perivesical space, where it is identified and incised upon. The ureter is brought extravesically by grasping the traction suture in the ureter. **E,** Ureteral tailoring is completed. Tapering is done over a No. 8 French red rubber catheter in infants or a No. 10 French catheter in older children and adults. After vascularity is defined, special atraumatic clamps are placed over the catheter. Baby Allis clamps help retract the portion of ureter to be resected, which is usually lateral. It is important to not resect too much ureter. Running 5-0 polydioxanone or chromic suture is used to reapproximate the proximal two thirds of the ureter. Its distal third is closed with interrupted sutures to allow for shortening. **F,** The tailored ureter is brought back into the bladder through the new hiatus. **G,** After closing the original hiatus, a new submucosal tunnel is made to the new hiatus. **H,** The distal portion of ureter is resected to match the length of the tunnel. **I,** The revised ureter is anastomosed to the bladder with fine interrupted sutures.

Description of the Surgical Technique

After making a Pfannenstiel incision, the bladder is opened in the midline and the ureter dissected from its intravesical and extravesical attachments (Fig. 117–36). In some instances, it is possible to adequately mobilize the dilated ureter by staying within the bladder. In such cases, the maneuvers for reimplantation by either the Cohen or the Politano-Leadbetter method are repeated after ureteral tailoring. However, when very large ureters are being tapered, it is advisable to work outside the bladder if there is any difficulty with mobilization to better define and preserve the blood supply.

If a method of reimplantation similar to the Politano-Leadbetter technique is chosen, it is wise to make the new hiatus before moving extravesically. The hiatus is widened with a right-angle clamp and the peritoneum swept from the base of the bladder, again using the lighted suction-tip and Senn retractors. The clamp is incised upon and spread at an appropriate superior-medial location for the new hiatus. A red rubber catheter, which helps guide the ureter through its new hiatus, is engaged and carried extravesically and then back into the bladder, where it is snapped.

Dissection outside the bladder is begun by sweeping the lateral peritoneal attachments superiorly with a Kittner dissector. A right-angle clamp is used to pass the ureteral cuff stitch through the old hiatus to the perivesical space, and the ureter is brought extravesically.

The adventitia and blood supply to the lower ureter, which usually emanates medially, is carefully preserved. When working outside the bladder, it is helpful to divide the obliterated hypogastric (umbilical) artery to aid in the dissection and eliminate it as a possible source of obstruction. **Excessive mobilization plus removal of proximal kinks is unnecessary.**

After excision of any obstructive distal ureter or excessive length, ureteral tailoring is done over a 10 French red rubber catheter (8 French in an infant), unless the ureter is already snug over the catheter, in which case revision is unnecessary. Tailoring is achieved by one of the following methods:

Tapering (Fig. 117–37). The technique used is similar to that originally described by Hendren (1969). Baby Allis clamps are placed laterally to define redundant ureter while preserving

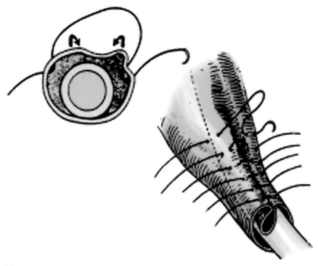

Figure 117–38. Ureteral plication is performed over the appropriate catheter, with interrupted 5-0 polyglycolic sutures placed in Lembert fashion (after Starr). (From Keating MA, Retik AB: Management of failures of ureteroneocystostomy. In McDougal WS [ed]: Difficult Problems in Urologic Surgery. Chicago, Year Book, 1989, p 131.)

the medial vascular supply. Atraumatic clamps are applied around the catheter, and excess ureter is excised. Excessive narrowing of the lumen should be avoided. A running, locking 6-0 polydioxanone suture is used to reapproximate the proximal two thirds of the tapered ureter. Interrupted sutures complete the repair to allow for any shortening that might be necessary. The proximal portion of the tailored ureter must remain outside the bladder after completion of the reimplantation with either tapering or plication. A dilated obstruction is likely if the entire tailored segment is located within the intravesical tunnel.

Starr Plication (Fig. 117–38). Ureteral redundancy is again defined by briefly applying atraumatic clamps to mark the extent of plication and preserve the best-vascularized portion of ureter. Starting proximally, the ureter is plicated with interrupted 5-0 polydioxanone sutures placed in Lembert fashion along the clamp impressions (Starr, 1979).

Kalicinski Plication (Fig. 117–39). Two 6-0 polydioxanone sutures are placed along the clamp impressions, one at the proximal extent of the proposed revision and the other at the new meatus. The ureter is divided longitudinally by weaving one suture through the ureter in running fashion along the clamp impression, thus creating two lumens. The ureter is then reduced by folding its nonfunctional portion over the catheterized lumen (Kalicinski et al, 1977).

The reimplantation is completed with either the cross-trigonal, Politano-Leadbetter, or extravesical technique. It is often helpful to secure the repair with a psoas hitch, especially in smaller children, patients who require a longer submucosal tunnel, and cases in which the surgeon is particularly concerned about angulation of the tailored ureter as it enters the bladder.

Tapered ureters are stented for 5 to 7 days. Stentograms are often unnecessary because leaks are rarely seen.

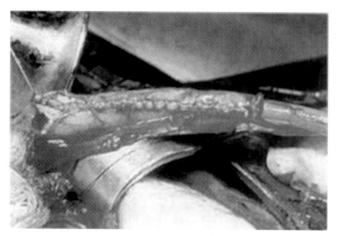

Figure 117–37. Megaureter after excision of the narrowed distal segment. The photograph shows excisional tapering being completed.

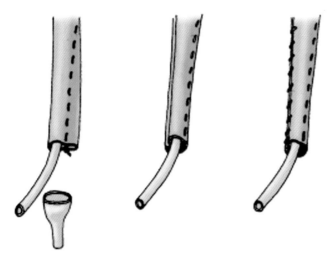

Figure 117–39. Ureteral folding technique. A running suture is longitudinally woven through the megaureter to create two lumens. This isolates the best-vascularized portion as a functional ureter (catheter within) and excludes redundancy. The redundant portion is then folded, and the two are tacked together with interrupted sutures. (From Kalicinski ZH, Kansy J, Kotarbinska B, et al: Surgery of megaureters: Modification of Hendren's operation. J Pediatr Surg 1977;12:183.)

Results and Complications

Reimplantation of MGUs is associated with the same complications (i.e., persistent reflux and obstruction) as reimplantation of nondilated ureters, but at increased rates. Complications can occur regardless of whether excisional tapering or a folding technique is used (Ehrlich, 1985; Daher et al, 1999; Fretz et al, 2004). Perdzynski and Kalicinski (1996) cited good results in 52 (93%) of 56 MGUs. Stenosis (two cases) and reflux (two cases) occurred in failures. Some authors have noted better results with obstructive MGU and higher rates of unresolved reflux after tailoring of refluxing variants (Johnston and Farkas, 1975; DeFoor et al, 2004), a finding that could be explained by the previously mentioned studies of Lee and coworkers (1998, 2005) in which abnormal collagen deposition in the refluxing variants may cause an intrinsically stiffer ureter and lessen surgical success. This has been attributed to a higher incidence of bladder dysfunction associated with the latter and to more significant abnormalities in their musculature. It has been suggested that extravesical reimplantation and excisional tapering can be performed with a high success rate in patients with primary obstructive MGU and that intravesical reimplantation can be reserved as a better option for children with voiding dysfunction or associated VUR (DeFoor et al, 2004).

On rare occasion, reflux persists despite ureteral tunnels deemed adequate intraoperatively in both tapered and normal-sized ureters. Postoperative VUR can occur in up to 5% of patients (Hendren, 1969; Kalicinski et al, 1977; Ehrlich, 1985; Peters et al, 1989; Parrott et al, 1990; Perdzynski and Kalicinski, 1996; Diamond and Parulkar, 1998; Daher et al, 1999; Fretz et al, 2004). Mild cases may improve with time. When associated with complications (e.g., recurrent episodes of pyelonephritis), surgical correction is indicated. Even though the experience is limited, subureteric injection therapy may be considered initially. Selected cases may proceed to open surgery, with the difficulties imposed by scarring and a potentially limited blood supply. If severe, the rigid distal ureter is incapable of normal peristalsis or appropriate coaptation during bladder contractions because of the intrinsic ureteral dysfunction caused by transmural scarring—factors that may limit the amount of ureter available for reconstruction. Transureteroureterostomy is ideal for unilateral disease (Mure et al, 2000). Bilateral cases can be approached by excising scarred distal ureter and creating exaggerated ureteral tunnels whose diameter-to-length ratio may exceed 10:1. In situ tailoring is another option for dilated ureters that continue to reflux after initial reimplantation. Vascularity is preserved and injury to the contralateral ureter avoided in unilateral cases (Diamond and Parulkar, 1998).

Ureteral obstruction is related to postoperative edema in many cases, and the edema generally resolves with time (up to 8 weeks) and requires temporary diversion (most commonly through a percutaneous nephrostomy and antegrade stenting). If persistent, the usual cause is ureteral ischemia, which requires revision and excision of the ischemic segment followed by reimplantation.

Special Situations

Dilated Duplex Ureter

Duplications of the ureters are seen with anomalies commonly associated with reflux or obstruction (or both) and result in dilatation of one or both ureters. Examples include ureteroceles and ectopic ureters. With salvageable renal function, a number of surgical options are available, depending on the cause, the degree of dilatation, and whether one or both ureters are abnormal. Ureteroureterostomy provides an ideal solution when only one ureter of a duplex system needs to be addressed. This procedure can be done above the bladder through a lower abdominal, extraperitoneal approach. Ureteropyelostomy is another option, but it leaves behind a segment of lower ureter unless a two-incision approach is used. When both ureters require correction, they can be mobilized within the bladder as a common sheath. One or both can then be tapered or plicated, depending on size. Tapering is performed on the side of the ureter (or ureters) away from the blood supply, which enters the adventitial septum between duplications (Weinstein et al, 1988). Reimplantation by a standard technique completes the repair. In cases in which there is no function, excision of the MGU is performed in concert with heminephrectomy. Because it is difficult to separate the distal segments of ureter, the common wall is usually left intact. After excision of lateral redundancy of the MGU, the lumen of any distal ureteral stump is closed distally at the bladder level if reflux is present. Newer laparoscopic approaches to pediatric urologic anomalies may expand the options for correction in these patients.

Adult Megaureter

Primary MGUs coincidentally found in adults have radiographic appearances that usually remain stable over many years (Heal, 1973; Pfister and Hendren, 1978). Fusiform dilatation of the distal ureteral spindle is the most common variant, although the entire ureter can be affected. Pyelocaliectasis is either absent or mild (Hanna and Wyatt, 1975).

It now appears that many perinatally diagnosed MGUs represent the anomaly at an earlier stage in its natural history and are precursors of the nonobstructive variants discovered serendipitously in adults. A small group of patients initially seen as adults have evidence of reduced renal function, recurrent infections, nephrolithiasis, or recurrent flank pain. Even though prenatal diagnosis and early intervention may decrease the size of this group even further, their delayed symptomatic condition may warrant surgical correction (Hemal, 2003).

SELECTED READINGS

Arant BS Jr: Medical management of mild and moderate vesicoureteral reflux: Followup studies of infants and young children. A preliminary report of the Southwest Pediatric Nephrology Study Group. J Urol 1992;148:1683-1687.

Birmingham Reflux Study Group: Prospective trial of operative versus nonoperative treatment of severe vesicoureteric reflux in children: Five years' observation. Birmingham Reflux Study Group. Br Med J (Clin Res Ed) 1987;295:237-241.

Connolly LP, Zurakowski D, Connolly SA, et al: Natural history of vesicoureteral reflux in girls after age 5 years. J Urol 2001;166:2359-2363.

Cooper CS, Chung BI, Kirsch AJ, et al: The outcome of stopping prophylactic antibiotics in older children with vesicoureteral reflux. J Urol 2000;163:269-272; discussion 272-273.

Edwards D, Normand IC, Prescod N, et al: Disappearance of vesicoureteric reflux during long-term prophylaxis of urinary tract infection in children. BMJ 1977;2:285-258.

Elder JS, Peters CA, Arant BS Jr, et al: Pediatric Vesicoureteral Reflux Guidelines Panel summary report on the management of primary vesicoureteral reflux in children. J Urol 1997;157:1846-1851.

Farhat W, McLorie G, Geary D, et al: The natural history of neonatal vesicoureteral reflux associated with antenatal hydronephrosis. J Urol 2000;164:1057-1060.

Ferrer FA, McKenna PH, Hochman HI, et al: Results of a vesicoureteral reflux practice pattern survey among American Academy of Pediatrics, Section on Pediatric Urology members. J Urol 1998;160:1031-1037.

Hodson CJ, Maling TM, McManamon PJ, et al: The pathogenesis of reflux nephropathy (chronic atrophic pyelonephritis). Br J Radiol 1975;13 (Suppl):1-26.

Hohenfellner K, Hunley TE, Yerkes E, et al: Angiotensin II, type 2 receptor in the development of vesico-ureteric reflux. BJU Int 1999;83:318-322

Kaefer M, Curran M, Treves ST, et al: Sibling vesicoureteral reflux in multiple gestation births. Pediatrics 2000;105:800-804.

Koff SA: Relationship between dysfunctional voiding and reflux. J Urol 1992;148:1703-1705.

Lebowitz RL, Olbing H, Parkkulainen KV, et al: International system of radiographic grading of vesicoureteric reflux. International Reflux Study in Children. Pediatr Radiol 1985;15:105-109.

Majd M, Rushton HG, Chandra R, et al: Technetium-99m-DMSA renal cortical scintigraphy to detect experimental acute pyelonephritis in piglets: Comparison of planar (pinhole) and SPECT imaging. J Nucl Med 1996;37:1731-1734.

Olbing H, Smellie JM, Jodal U, et al: New renal scars in children with severe VUR: A 10-year study of randomized treatment. Pediatr Nephrol 2003;18:1128-1131.

Podesta ML, Castera R, Ruarte AC: Videourodynamic findings in young infants with severe primary reflux. J Urol 2004;171:829-833; discussion 833.

Ransley PG, Risdon RA: The pathogenesis of reflux nephropathy. Contrib Nephrol 1979;16:90-97.

Roberts JA: Vesicoureteral reflux and pyelonephritis in the monkey: A review. J Urol 1992;148:1721-1725.

Smellie JM: Reflections on 30 years of treating children with urinary tract infections. J Urol 1991;146:665-668.

Smellie JM, Prescod NP, Shaw PJ, et al: Childhood reflux and urinary infection: A follow-up of 10-41 years in 226 adults. Pediatr Nephrol 1998;12:727-736.

Tamminen-Mobius T, Brunier E, Ebel KD, et al: Cessation of vesicoureteral reflux for 5 years in infants and children allocated to medical treatment. The International Reflux Study in Children. J Urol 1992;148:1662-16626.

118 Prune Belly Syndrome

ANTHONY A. CALDAMONE, MD • JOHN R. WOODARD, MD

Prune belly syndrome (PBS) represents a constellation of anomalies with variable degrees of severity. The three major findings are a deficiency of the abdominal musculature, bilateral intra-abdominal testes, and an anomalous urinary tract. The urinary tract is characterized by variable degrees of hydronephrosis, renal dysplasia, dilated tortuous ureters, an enlarged bladder, and a dilated prostatic urethra. Additional associated anomalies exist involving the respiratory tract, gastrointestinal tract, cardiac system, and musculoskeletal system. There is a broad spectrum of severity of the syndrome, with some children not surviving the newborn period and others being minimally affected. The single most important determinant of survival is usually the severity of the urinary tract anomaly, in particular, the degree of renal dysplasia.

The characteristic abdominal wall was first described by Frolich in 1839 and the full triad of anomalies by Parker in 1895. Osler's vivid description of the abdominal wall of an infant with the characteristic findings led to the term prune belly syndrome (Osler, 1901). Other names that have been applied to this syndrome include triad syndrome, Eagle-Barrett syndrome, and abdominal musculation syndrome (Eagle and Barrett, 1950; Greskovich and Nyberg, 1988).

The incidence of PBS has been reported to be 1 in 29,000 to 1 in 40,000 live births, similar to that of bladder exstrophy (Williams and Burkholder, 1967), **with 95% occurring in males** (Wheatley et al, 1996). Females with PBS have the abdominal wall deficiency and urinary tract dysmorphism without any gonadal anomaly (Rabinowitz and Schillinger, 1977; Reinberg et al, 1991b). A higher incidence is noted in twins, blacks, and children born to younger mothers. The incidence appears to be declining, possibly because of prenatal diagnosis and a decision to terminate the pregnancy.

GENETICS

The high male-to-female ratio, occasional occurrence in male siblings and cousins, and increased occurrence in twins suggest a genetic basis for PBS. Yet most cases are sporadic and have a normal karyotype. One in 23 children with PBS is the product of a twin pregnancy (Ives, 1974). However, the majority of reported twins have been discordant for PBS, evidence against a genetic etiology. It has been suggested that the etiology in twins may be due to an uneven distribution of mesenchymal tissue at a critical time of primitive streak development during the third week of embryogenesis (Coplen et al, 1996). There is a reported association with Turner's syndrome, monosomy 16, trisomy 13, and trisomy 18 (Amacker et al, 1986; Hoagland and Hutchins, 1987). A variety of inheritance patterns have been proposed, including X-linked recessive (Frydman et al, 1993), a two-step autosomal dominant mutation (Riccardo and Grum, 1977), and polygenetic transmission (Garlinger and Ott, 1974; Lockhart et al, 1979; Adeneyokunnu and Familusi, 1982). A report by Ramasamy and colleagues (2005) suggested a sex-influenced autosomal recessive mode of inheritance in familial PBS. The consensus, however, remains that an associated chromosomal abnormality is the exception rather than the rule, as most have a normal karyotype. Other reports have noted an association between PBS and Beckwith-Wiedemann syndrome (Silengo et al, 2002; Sinico et al, 2004).

EMBRYOLOGY

There have been several theories of the embryogenesis of PBS. However, because there is no experimental model that can be used to test these theories, the exact mechanism remains elusive. The four chief theories are (1) early in utero posterior urethral obstruction resulting in severe dilation of urinary tract and possible fetal ascites and oligohydramnios (Strumme, 1903; Pagon et al, 1979; Wheatley et al, 1996; Beasley et al, 1998); (2) primary defect in the lateral plate mesoderm, which is the precursor of the ureters, bladder, prostate, urethra, and gubernaculum (Ives, 1974; Gonzalez et al, 1990); (3) an intrinsic defect of the urinary tract leading to ureteral dilation and fetal ascites (Symonds and Driscoll, 1974; Monie and Monie, 1979; Smythe, 1981; Nakayama et al, 1984; Cazorlaet al, 1997); and (4) a yolk sac defect (Stephens, 1983; Stephens and Gupta, 1994). None of these theories have universal acceptance and there is some overlap between them.

CLINICAL FEATURES OF PRUNE BELLY SYNDROME

Genitourinary Anomalies

Kidneys

A spectrum of renal abnormalities extends from normal renal parenchyma to dysplasia (Fig. 118–1). The more severely dysplastic kidneys are generally associated with bladder outlet obstruction in which there has not been decompression through a patent urachus (Potter, 1972). **Dysplasia is present in 50% of cases; however, it may vary in degree and laterally** (Rogers and Ostrow, 1973; Stephens, 1983). **Renal dysplasia in PBS of the Potter type II and IV varieties is seen.** The Potter type II variety with few nephrons and parenchymal disorganization is more indicative of a renal mesenchymal defect, whereas the Potter type IV with cortical and tubular cysts is associated with outlet obstruction (Wigger and Blanc, 1977).

The renal collecting system is characteristically dilated, often to a severe degree. The degree of dilation, however, does not correlate with the degree of renal dysplasia. Calyceal morphology may be well preserved, even in the presence of massively dilated ureters and renal pelves (Berdon et al, 1977). Ureteropelvic junction obstruction can occur on a primary or secondary basis; however, nonobstructive hydronephrosis is the rule (Woodard and Parrott, 1978b). It is renal infection rather than obstruction that poses the greatest risk to renal function.

Ureters

The ureters are typically dilated, tortuous, and redundant (Fig. 118–2). The proximal (upper) portions of the ureters are usually less abnormal than the distal segments, although massive dilation and stenosis can occur at all levels. Histologic sectioning demonstrates a lack of smooth muscle cells and an increase in fibrous connective tissue. There generally are more normal-appearing smooth muscle cells in the proximal segments (Palmer and Tesluk, 1974; Stephens, 1983). This fact is critical when ureteral reconstruction is undertaken. The ratio of collagen to smooth muscle cells in prune belly ureters has been noted to be elevated, especially in refluxing ureters (Gearhart et al, 1995). A decreased number of thick and thin

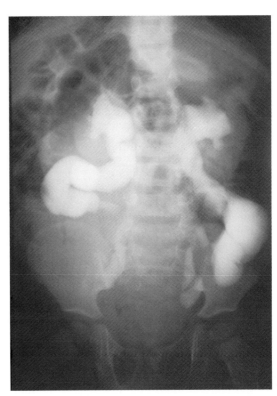

Figure 118–2. Excretory urogram of a patient with prune belly syndrome; note ureters displaced laterally and calyces relatively well preserved.

myofibrils noted on ultrastructural examination are thought to contribute to the poor peristalsis (Berdon et al, 1977; Stephens, 1983).

Vesicoureteral reflux is present in 75% of children with PBS (Berdon et al, 1977; Fallat et al, 1989) (Fig. 118–3). Obstruction is not common but has been reported at both the ureteropelvic and ureterovesical junctions (Wigger and Blanc, 1977; Moerman et al, 1982; Manivel et al, 1989).

These large ureters may have ineffective peristalsis because of poor ureteral wall coaptation. The ureteral conduction wave reaches a reduced smooth muscle cell population of poor contractile potential related to reduced myofibrils, often separated by patches of collagen with a resulting bolus of urine reaching more dilated ureteral segments as it progresses toward the bladder (Woodard and Smith, 1998). This can be seen fluoroscopically as ineffective peristalsis, resulting in upper tract stasis, which may lead to infection (Nunn and Stephens, 1961; Williams and Burkholder, 1967).

KEY POINTS: CLINICAL FEATURES

- Hydroureteronephrosis is often to a severe degree; however, the calyceal morphology may be well preserved.

- The proximal portion of the ureters has more normal muscle than the distal portions.

- The bladder is large with a pseudodiverticulum at the urachus and a wide bladder neck opening into a dilated prostatic urethra.

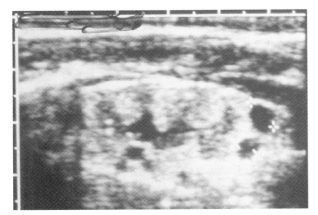

Figure 118–1. Ultrasound scan of a kidney of a newborn with prune belly syndrome demonstrating markedly echogenic renal parenchyma and cortical cysts indicative of renal dysplasia.

Bladder

The bladder usually appears massively enlarged with a pseudodiverticulum at the urachus (Fig. 118–4). **The urachus is patent at birth in 25% to 30% of children** (Lattimer, 1958; Wigger and Blanc, 1977; Stephens and Gupta, 1994). **Histologically, the bladder has an increased ratio of collagen to muscle fibers in the absence of obstruction** (Workman and Kogan, 1990). The wall is smooth, unlike that seen in obstructed bladders. The pelvic distribution of ganglion cells has been shown to be normal (Nunn and Stephens, 1961; Burke et al, 1969). Smooth muscle hypertrophy is seen, however, in the obstructed prune bladder (Perlmutter, 1976). Stephens demonstrated that the trigone is splayed with the ureteral orifices displaced laterally and superiorly, possibly contributing to the high incidence of reflux (Williams and Burkholder, 1967).

On voiding, the bladder neck opens widely into a dilated prostatic urethra (see Fig. 118–4). Urodynamic assessment generally shows normal compliance; however, there is a delayed first sensation to void and very large capacity (Snyder et al, 1976). The ability to empty the bladder is quite variable, with some emptying well and others carrying a significant postvoid residual. This is thought to be due to a relative outlet obstruction and the ability of the bladder to generate sufficient pressure with a detrusor contraction. When the relative outflow resistance prevents effective bladder emptying, the term unbalanced voiding is used (Snyder et al, 1976; Kinahan et al, 1992). **Despite these limitations, about 50% of prune belly patients void spontaneously with normal voiding pressures, normal flow rates, and low postvoid residuals** (Nunn and Stephens, 1961; Kinahan et al, 1992). However, as Kinahan and coworkers (1992) demonstrated, deterioration of balanced voiding can occur resulting in significant postvoid residuals, emphasizing the need for periodic assessment.

Prostate and Accessory Sex Organs

The dilation of the posterior urethra is due to prostatic hypoplasia probably related to abnormal mesenchymal-epithelial development (Stephens and Gupta, 1994). Histo-

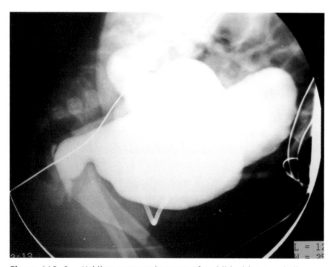

Figure 118–3. Voiding cystourethrogram of a child with prune belly syndrome demonstrating urethral atresia, urachal diverticulum, and vesicoureteral reflux.

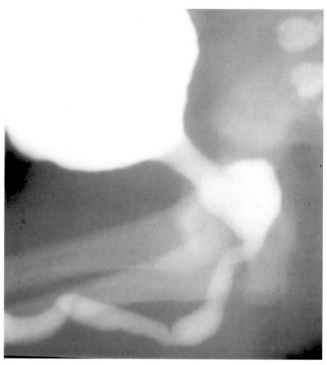

Figure 118–4. Voiding cystourethrogram of a child with prune belly syndrome demonstrating prostatic urethral enlargement related to a hypoplastic prostate.

logically, there are few prostatic cellular elements with a reduction of both epithelial and smooth muscle cells and an increase in connective tissue cells (Moerman et al, 1982; Popek et al, 1991; Stephens and Gupta, 1994). Various obstructive lesions of the distal posterior urethra have been described, such as urethral atresia, valves, urethral stenosis, urethral membrane, and urethral diverticulum, and are thought to occur in 20% of cases (Hoaglund and Hutchins, 1987). Stephens (1983) described an angulation of the urethra during voiding that he referred to as type IV valves, which results from lack of prostatic parenchymal tissue. Prostatic hypoplasia, the etiology of which is controversial, is thought to be a factor in the ejaculatory failure of PBS patients (Volmar et al, 2001). **The vas and seminal vesicles are often atretic, although either may be dilated or thickened** (Stephens and Gupta, 1994). **The epididymis may be poorly attached to the testis as is seen commonly in abdominal undescended testes. There may also be lack of continuity between the efferent ductules and the rete testis.** Ejaculation is usually in a retrograde fashion because of an incompetent bladder neck.

Anterior Urethra

Although the anterior urethra of the PBS child is usually normal, several anomalies of the anterior urethra have been reported, the most common being urethral atresia and megalourethra (Kroovand et al, 1982; Perrotin et al, 2001). **Unless it is associated with a patent urachus, urethral atresia is often lethal** (see Fig. 118–3). It has been postulated that urethral atresia or microurethra occurs because the urethra is unused rather than malformed. Spontaneous bladder rupture with fistula formation has also been reported (Reinberg et al, 1993).

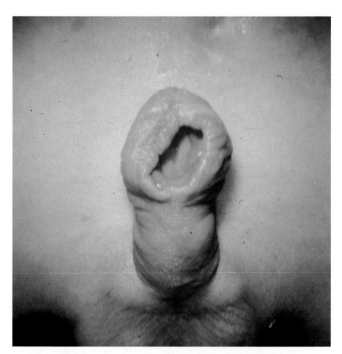

Figure 118-5. Scaphoid megalourethra of prune belly syndrome.

PBS is associated with two variations of megalourethra (Shrom et al, 1981; Mortensen et al, 1985). **The fusiform type is a deficiency of the corpus cavernosum as well as the spongiosum, and the scaphoid variety is a deficiency of the spongiosum only with preservation of the glans and corpora cavernosa (Fig. 118-5). With the scaphoid variety the ventral urethra dilates with voiding, whereas with the fusiform variety the entire phallus dilates with voiding.** The fusiform variety is thought to result from a mesenchymal deficiency of the urethral folds, whereas the scaphoid variety results from a mesenchymal deficiency of the urethral supportive tissues (Dorairajan, 1963). Megalourethra is more commonly see in PBS than any other syndrome (Appel et al, 1986). Transient in utero obstruction of the junction between the glanular and penile urethra has been proposed to cause megalourethra.

Testes

Bilateral intra-abdominal testes lying over the iliac vessels are the most typical findings. Although mechanical forces such as a distended bladder and intra-abdominal pressure have been implicated in maldescent of the testes (Kaplan, 1986; Hutson, 1988), the fact that some patients with the typical urinary tract and abdominal musculature anomalies (termed pseudoprune patients) may have descended testes raises some doubt about pure mechanical factors.

Pak and colleagues (1993) compared the histology of the testes in PBS patients with that of non–prune belly intra-abdominal testes as well as that of age-matched control subjects. **They found no difference in germ cell counts, Ad spermatogonia, and Leydig cells between PBS testes and non-PBS intra-abdominal testes. However, because germ cell counts in PBS patients younger than 1 year are similar to those of age-matched controls, the implication is that the**

environmental state of the abdomen is a major factor in their later spermatogenic potential (Nunn and Stephens, 1961; Coplen et al, 1996). This mirrors findings of Nunn and Stephens (1961) of normal germinal epithelium of fetal and newborn PBS testes. Alternatively, Orvis and coworkers (1988) noted decreased numbers of spermatogonia and Leydig cell hyperplasia in fetal PBS testes, implying an intrinsic testicular abnormality. Azoospermia was found in adult PBS patients, and no PBS patient has been reported to have fathered a child (Woodhouse and Snyder, 1985). More recently, Ross and associates (1998) have documented paternity in three adults with classical PBS, achieved by sperm retrieval techniques and intracytoplasmic sperm injection. The infertility is thought to be due to a combination of testicular histologic abnormalities, structural defects of the ducts, and prostatic abnormalities (Tayakkanonta, 1963).

Three cases of testis tumor have been reported (Woodhouse and Ransley, 1983; Sayre et al, 1986; Massad et al, 1991; Parra et al, 1991). Massad and coauthors (1991) described histologic testicular patterns similar to those in intratubular germ cell neoplasia in three infants. Although the risk of malignancy may be relatively low considering the lack of germinal epithelium (Uehling et al, 1984), it is clear that placement of the testis in the scrotum and long-term follow-up are necessary to reduce the risk of testicular malignancy and enhance detection.

Extragenitourinary Abnormalities

Of all children with PBS, 75% have non–urinary tract abnormalities (Geary et al, 1986). After the obvious abdominal wall defect, the most common are cardiac, pulmonary, and orthopedic (Table 118-1).

Table 118-1.	**Extragenitourinary Abnormalities**
Cardiac	Patent ductus arteriosus
	Ventricular septal defect
	Atrial septal defect
	Tetralogy of Fallot
Pulmonary	Lobar atelectasis
	Pulmonary hypoplasia
	Pneumothorax
	Pneumomediastinum
Gastrointestinal	Intestinal malrotation
	Intestinal atresias or stenosis
	Omphalocele
	Gastroschisis
	Hirschsprung's disease
	Imperforate anus
	Hepatobiliary anomalies
Orthopedic	Pectus excavatum, pectus carinatum
	Scoliosis
	Sacral agenesis (partial)
	Congenital hip subluxation or dislocation
	Genu valgum
	Talipes equinovarus
	Severe leg maldevelopment
Miscellaneous	Splenic torsion
	Adrenal cystic dysplasia

Modified from Woodard JR, Smith EA: Prune-belly syndrome. In Walsh PC, Retik AB, Vaughan ED Jr, Wein AJ (eds): Campbell's Urology, 7th ed. Philadelphia, WB Saunders, 1998:1991.

Abdominal Wall Defect

The appearance of the abdominal wall gives PBS of newborns their most characteristic feature (Fig. 118–6). Although in some cases the musculature of the abdominal wall may be totally absent (Manivel et al, 1989), most commonly there is uneven involvement with the medial and inferior muscular typically most deficient (Mininberg et al, 1973; Randolph, 1977). The appearance at birth is that of wrinkled, redundant skin with an abdomen that bulges in the flanks. One may be able to discern intra-abdominal organs through the thinned abdominal wall. **The most severely affected areas may have skin, subcutaneous fat, and a single fibrous layer on the peritoneum** (Mininberg et al, 1973; Baird and Sadovnick, 1987). **Randolph conducted electromyographic mapping and demonstrated the inferior and medial segments to be most consistently affected** (Randolph et al, 1981a). Electron microscopy has demonstrated a nonspecific pattern of myofilament disarray, Z-line disorganization, and mitochondrial proliferation (Afifi et al, 1972; Randolph et al, 1981b; Woodard and Smith, 1998). The fact that normal spinal anterior horn cells have been shown rules out a neuropathic etiology for the muscular deficiency (Nunn and Stephens, 1961). The muscular deficiency, however, is typically inconsistent and patchy.

As the child grows older, the abdomen becomes less wrinkled and takes on more of a pot-bellied appearance (Fig. 118–7). Gait is usually not affected, although it may be delayed, and the children tend to roll to their side and use their arms to sit from a supine position. The poor support of the

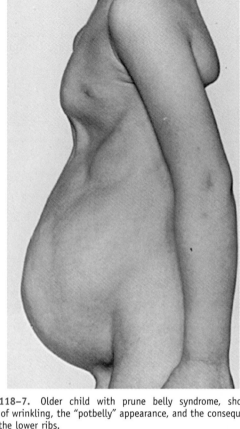

Figure 118–7. Older child with prune belly syndrome, showing the absence of wrinkling, the "potbelly" appearance, and the consequent deformity of the lower ribs.

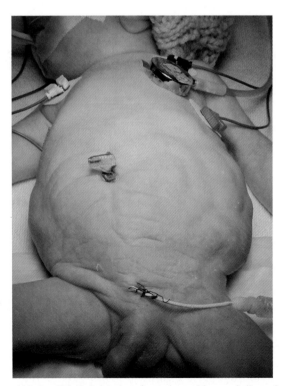

Figure 118–6. Wrinkled abdomen of a newborn with prune belly syndrome.

lower chest wall results in flaring of the costal margin (Woodard and Smith, 1998). These children are more vulnerable to respiratory illness as their cough effectiveness is compromised. In spite of these abdominal wall issues, Woodard and Smith (1998) reported good wound healing without a tendency toward infections or incisional hernias.

Cardiac Anomalies

Cardiac anomalies, such as patent ductus arteriosus, atrial septal defect, ventricular septal defect, and tetralogy of Fallot, occur in 10% of children with PBS (Adebonojo, 1973). Cardiac abnormalities at birth may take precedence over urologic issues.

Pulmonary

Pulmonary difficulties can be observed at any age in patients with PBS. **Pulmonary hypoplasia can result from severe oligohydramnios related to renal dysplasia or severe bladder outlet obstruction and may result in newborn demise. In addition, pneumothorax and pneumomediastinum can be seen with or without pulmonary hypoplasia** (Skoog, 1992). **Significant pulmonary difficulties have been reported in 55% of PBS survivors** (Geary et al, 1986). **The lack of ability to generate significant intra-abdominal pressure may contribute to pneumonia and lobar atelectasis** (Alford et al,

1978; Ewig et al, 1996). Acute respiratory illnesses or an anesthetic procedure can easily lead to respiratory insufficiency in the PBS patient, who may have underlying chronic bronchitis from repeated respiratory illnesses. Many patients demonstrate significant restrictive lung disease secondary to musculoskeletal abnormalities such as scoliosis, rib cage abnormalities, and compromised abdominal musculature (Coplen et al, 1996).

Gastrointestinal Abnormalities

In at least 30% of cases, gastrointestinal anomalies are observed. The majority of the anomalies result from incomplete rotation of the midgut giving way to a wide mesentery, which results in increased bowel mobility with intestinal malrotation, volvulus, atresias, and stenosis (Silverman and Huang, 1950; Wright et al, 1986). Splenic torsion related to abnormal mesenteric fixation has also been reported (Heydenrych and Du Toit, 1978; Teramoto et al, 1981). Omphalocele, gastroschisis, and anorectal abnormalities have been reported (Petersen et al, 1972; Morgan et al, 1978; Wilbert et al, 1978; Short et al, 1985; Walker et al, 1987). With a limited ability to generate intra-abdominal pressure, constipation becomes a lifelong problem and leads to acquired megacolon (Woodard and Smith, 1998).

Orthopedic

Orthopedic abnormalities, ranging in incidence from 30% to 45%, are second in frequency to those of the genitourinary tract and abdominal wall. Many of these abnormalities result from the compressive effects of oligohydramnios. Some think the musculoskeletal defects result from the abnormal mesenchymal development at 6 weeks of gestation (Loder et al, 1992). Green and colleagues (1993), however, pointed out that because many of the deformities are unilateral, oligohydramnios is the most likely etiology. Dimpling of the lateral aspect of the knees is a common finding in oligohydramnios. Oligohydramnios may also result in talipes equinovarus (26%), hip dysplasia (5%), and congenital scoliosis (4%) (Woodard and Smith, 1998). It has been proposed that a distended bladder that may impinge on the external iliac vessels may compromise the blood supply to the lower extremities and in severely affected cases result in lower extremity hypoplasia, absence, or amputation (Smith, 1913; Green et al, 1993).

PRESENTATION
Prenatal Diagnosis and Management

Prenatal ultrasonography has played a major role in the identification of congenital genitourinary abnormalities. Fetal hydronephrosis can be diagnosed accurately in the second trimester and is present in approximately 1% of all pregnancies. However, the etiology of the hydronephrosis cannot be accurately determined in all cases. Elder (1990) estimated that the accuracy of determining the etiology of fetal hydronephrosis varies from 30% to 85%.

In particular, PBS presents prenatally with findings similar to those of other causes of bladder outlet obstruc-

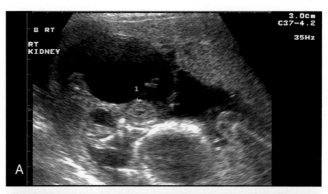
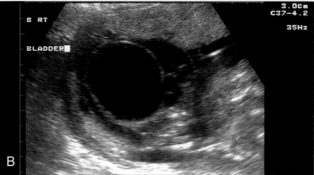

Figure 118–8. A, Prenatal ultrasound scan of a twin pregnancy with prune belly syndrome of one fetus, demonstrating a distended bladder and a small echogenic right kidney. **B,** Distended bladder with dilated loops of ureter and urinary ascites.

tion (Fig. 118–8A and B), **as in posterior urethral valves, or megacystis megaureter syndrome** (Kramer, 1983). **Although an accurate diagnosis of PBS has been made as early as 11 to 14 weeks of gestation** (Shimizu et al, 1992; Yamamoto et al, 2001), **the classical findings of hydroureteronephrosis, a distended bladder, and an irregular abdominal circumference are not consistently seen at 30 weeks** (Okulski, 1977; Bovicelli et al, 1980; Christopher et al, 1982; Shih et al, 1982). Early fetal ascites has been suggested to correlate with PBS (Scarborough et al, 1988). It is imperative to remember that the majority of patients with PBS do not have demonstrable urinary obstruction and that the degree of hydroureteronephrosis does not correlate with the postnatal renal function (Gadziala et al, 1982).

Whereas some have recommended in utero intervention for relief of urinary tract dilation and oligohydramnios (Gadziala et al, 1982; Glazer et al, 1982; Nakayama et al, 1984; Scarborough et al, 1988; Estes and Hanson, 1993; Leeners et al, 2000), others have recommended termination of pregnancy (Peschia et al, 1982). **It is difficult to justify the advocacy of pregnancy termination in light of our inability to diagnose precisely the etiology of prenatal hydronephrosis and inability to predict postnatal renal function on the basis of the degree of urinary tract dilation, except in rare cases of early and severe oligohydramnios.** Prenatal intervention has been applied to PBS with no proven benefit in terms of postnatal renal function (Elder et al, 1987; Sholder 1988;

Freedman 1999; Biard and Johnson, 2005; Blaicher et al, 2005). The only circumstances in which prenatal intervention may be justified are the rare situations of urethral atresia with progressive oligohydramnios (Steinhardt et al, 1990; Reinberg et al, 1993; Perez-Brayfield et al, 2001) or cases in which decompression of the urinary tract is necessary to prevent dystocia (Gadziala et al, 1982).

Neonatal Presentation

The appearance of the abdominal wall immediately suggests the diagnosis of PBS (see Fig. 118–6) whether or not the diagnosis was suspected prenatally. It should be remembered that other associated abnormalities, such as cardiac or pulmonary, often should take precedence over the urinary tract because in the absence of true bladder outlet obstruction as seen with urethral atresia the hydroureteronephrosis is not life threatening.

Spectrum of Disease

With the number of variable anomalies present in PBS, it is understandable that there is a wide spectrum of clinical presentations. There are three major categories of presentation in the neonatal period as described by Woodard (1985) (Table 118–2).

Category I consists of neonates who have experienced marked oligohydramnios as a result of renal dysplasia or severe bladder outlet obstruction with resultant pulmonary hypoplasia and skeletal abnormalities. Most infants with urethral atresia fall in this category. The exceptions to this are patients with urethral atresia and a patent urachus (Rogers and Ostrow, 1973). Those in this category, who are not stillborn, commonly succumb within a few days of life to pulmonary hypoplasia or later to renal failure. Approximately 20% of newborns with PBS die in the perinatal period (Woodard and Parrott, 1978b; Burbige et al, 1987; Fallat et al, 1989). It would be unusual for any urologic intervention in this category of patients to alter the course of events. Simple catheter drainage is all that is justifiable.

Category II demonstrates the full spectrum of the disorder with moderate or unilateral renal insufficiency and moderate to severe hydroureteronephrosis. **Pulmonary hypoplasia is not a prominent feature of this group of patients. The clinical course is that of stabilization of renal function at or somewhat below normal or progressive azotemia.** It is in this group of patients that significant controversy over management exists (Waldbaum and Marshall, 1970; Randolph, 1977; Woodard and Parrott, 1978b).

Category III consists of patients with mild features of the triad or incomplete forms of PBS. This category comprises the majority of PBS patients in whom hydroureteronephrosis is present to some degree but renal function is well maintained (Woodhouse et al, 1982; Woodard, 1998). **There is no evidence of pulmonary insufficiency.** There is little controversy that urologic intervention in the group is reserved for patients who demonstrate repeated urinary infections, probably related to urinary stasis or vesicoureteral reflux, or development of upper tract deterioration (Woodard and Smith, 1998). As previously noted, there is poor correlation between the extent of abdominal wall deficit and the degree of hydronephrosis or renal dysplasia, or both. This is also apparent in other variants of the syndrome. There are children with markedly dilated urinary tracts with minimal or no dysplasia and, therefore, normal renal function. Therefore, the appearance of the abdominal wall or the degree of hydronephrosis may have little bearing on the long-term prognosis of children with PBS.

Incomplete Syndrome

These are male patients who may not have all the features of the triad syndrome but share other features. **Most typically, these incomplete forms of the syndrome would lack the typical abdominal wall features but have the common uropathy and cryptorchidism. Many of these patients may go on to renal failure and, therefore require close observation, monitoring, and selective intervention.** Bellah reported a relatively high (8/15) tendency to progressive renal failure in his population of pseudoprune patients. This may be partially attributed to a delay in diagnosis in the absence of the obvious abdominal musculature deficiency, and, therefore, a tendency to present with recurring urinary tract infections (Bellah et al, 1996).

Adult Presentation

Patients with incomplete forms of PBS and specifically those who lack the abdominal wall features may present as late as adulthood with symptoms of renal failure and hypertension (Lee, 1977; Kerbl and Pauer, 1993). Although there have been isolated reports of adults with no history of urinary tract infections, most others who present in adulthood eventually develop urinary infections from the chronic urinary stasis associated with the syndrome (Culp and Flocks, 1954).

Female Syndrome

Five percent of PBS patients are female, most of whom have the abdominal wall deficiency and the abnormal urinary tract (Reinberg et al, 1991b). Rabinowitz and Schillinger (1977) reported female patients with the typical abdominal wall deficit and a normal urinary tract. In the series of Reinberg

Table 118–2.	Spectrum of Prune Belly Syndrome
Category	**Characteristics**
I	Renal dysplasia
	Oligohydramnios
	Pulmonary hypoplasia
	Potter's features
	Urethral atresia
II	Full triad features
	Minimal or unilateral renal dysplasia
	No pulmonary hypoplasia
	May progress to renal failure
III	Incomplete or mild triad features
	Mild to moderate uropathy
	No renal dysplasia
	Stable renal function
	No pulmonary hypoplasia

and colleagues (1991b), bladder outlet obstruction was commonly seen along with a 40% occurrence of anorectal anomalies similar to the statistics for the male; 40% did not survive the newborn period.

EVALUATION AND MANAGEMENT

The initial evaluation of the newborn with PBS requires a team consisting of a neonatologist, a nephrologist, and a urologist. As dictated, other specialists, particularly a cardiologist, may be indicated. Early orthopedic evaluation is also warranted. The major initial concern is that of management of cardiac and respiratory issues. An immediate chest radiograph is necessary to exclude commonly associated pulmonary abnormalities such as pneumothorax, pneumomediastinum, and pulmonary hypoplasia, which is commonly a result of oligohydramnios (Perlman and Levin, 1974). Early urologic intervention is indicated only for neonates with evidence of bladder outlet obstruction, in whom a percutaneous suprapubic tube can be inserted in the neonatal intensive care unit.

Initial evaluation of renal function and the urinary tract status is important but must be tempered by transitional neonatal physiology. Although an initial creatinine is important in establishing a baseline, it may be more reflective of mother's renal function, and, therefore, the trend in creatinine levels over the course of the early postnatal days or weeks is much more predictive of long-term renal function.

KEY POINTS: INITIAL MANAGEMENT

- A team consisting of neonatology, nephrology, urology, and other specialties such as cardiology is needed.

- A voiding cystourethrogram (VCUG) is indicated in the neonatal period if there is renal insufficiency or evidence of bladder outlet obstruction and only after antibiotic prophylaxis.

- A chest radiograph to evaluate for pneumothorax, pneumomediastinum, and pulmonary hypoplasia is needed.

- Baseline assessment of renal function should include renal and bladder ultrasonography, BUN, creatinine, and electrolytes.

- Circumcision is advisable in the absence of a structural penile abnormality.

- Early intervention is indicated for evidence of bladder outlet obstruction and preferably with a percutaneous suprapubic tube.

Serum, blood urea nitrogen (BUN), and electrolytes are needed to assess for the potential systemic acidosis and electrolyte imbalances that may be seen in renal insufficiency. It has been shown in multiple reports that a baseline creatinine of less than 0.7 mg/dL is predictive of adequate renal function through childhood, in the absence of repeated

insults from pyelonephritis (Geary et al, 1986; Reinberg et al, 1991a; Noh et al, 1999).

Early renal and bladder ultrasonography, once the newborn is stabilized, is necessary to assess the renal parenchyma for its thickness, density, and presence or absence of cortical cysts and degree of urinary tract dilation (see Fig. 118–1).

Avoidance of urinary infection is essential in light of the urinary stasis and often compromised baseline renal function. Circumcision is advisable in the absence of a structural penile abnormality to reduce the risk of infant urinary tract infections. Similarly, prophylactic antibiotic therapy is recommended, especially prior to urinary tract instrumentation, including the initial voiding cystourethrogram (VCUG). Although instrumentation without a defined purpose that may alter management should be avoided, a VCUG to assess the bladder outlet and bladder emptying ability, especially in the presence of renal insufficiency, is warranted (Woodard and Smith, 1998). The VCUG is needed in neonates with renal insufficiency to rule out bladder outlet obstruction as the etiology versus urinary stagnation. In up to 70% of children with PBS, vesicoureteral reflux is diagnosed (Berdon et al, 1977; Fallat et al, 1989). Any instrumentation should be carried out with strict attention to sterile technique to reduce the risk of inoculation of a static urinary system. One can avoid an early VCUG in the presence of normal renal function and evidence of adequate bladder drainage per urethra or a patent urachus.

As noted, neonates can be categorized on the basis of their spectrum of disease (see Table 118–1). There is little disagreement on the management of category I PBS patients. There is no evidence that anything beyond supportive care is justifiable; in particular, intervention in the urinary tract is not indicated beyond simple bladder drainage as their fate cannot be altered (Woodard and Smith, 1998).

At the other end of the spectrum, category III patients rarely require urologic intervention for the urinary tract as they are in a balanced state of hydronephrosis with good if not normal renal function. Early in infancy their cryptorchidism requires correction. Children in this category require regular monitoring of urinary tract dilation (ultrasonography) and renal function (serum creatinine).

Category II patients require individualization of evaluation and management based on the fact that within this category there are variable degrees of severity of each of the facets of PBS. There is, however, much controversy over their management. Evaluation of renal function or renal drainage, or both, is required in those with renal insufficiency. Excretory urography, while providing dramatic images of the urinary tract (see Fig. 118–3), does not provide sufficient information on comparative function. Renal parenchymal function is best assessed by a technetium-99m (^{99m}Tc) dimercaptosuccinic acid (DMSA) renal scan at 4 to 6 weeks of age to prevent difficulties in interpretation related to transitional neonatal physiology. Renal outflow obstruction is best assessed by ^{99m}Tc mercaptoacetyltriglycine (MAG3), which also provides an assessment of comparative renal function with massive hydronephrosis and resultant stasis. In the presence of poor renal function, assessment of renal outflow obstruction by nuclear scan techniques may be limited; therefore, selective use of the Whitaker antegrade perfusion test may be helpful.

Controversies in Management of Category II Prune Belly Syndrome

Aggressive surgical intervention was initially derived from early observations of the poor prognosis for category II infants as a group. Compilation of the cases reported in the literature between 1950 and 1970 by Waldbaum and Marshall (1970) revealed that 86% of the 56 accurately traceable patients had died, with or without surgical intervention. The obvious implication was that a more aggressive approach was necessary to improve the fate of the infant with PBS. **With the recognition that infection and progressive renal insufficiency are the factors that most often pose the greatest threat to quality of life and survival, surgical reconstruction to normalize the anatomy and function of the genitourinary tract was advocated. Early retailoring of the urinary system to reduce stasis and eliminate reflux or obstruction has included ureteral shortening, tapering, and vesicoureteral reimplantation and reduction cystoplasty.** Reconstruction is best delayed until the child is at least 3 months of age to allow for pulmonary maturation. This approach has been successful in achieving anatomic and functional improvement as evidenced by stable radiographic studies, stable creatinine values, and a reduced occurrence of infection (Walbaum and Marshall, 1970; Jeffs et al, 1977; Woodard and Parrott, 1978b; Randolph et al, 1981b). In the personal reconstructive experience of one of the authors (JW), 15 patients have maintained a normal creatinine level and only 2 have demonstrated moderate renal insufficiency, with follow-up ranging from 2 to 27 years.

An alternative approach of limited surgical intervention has also been applied. Proponents advocate close surveillance with medical management of bacteriuria and surgical intervention only in patients with proven obstruction or intractable infection. Opinions vary about the management of vesicoureteral reflux in the prune belly population, although there is no reason to believe that reflux in this population is any less important, and correction of high-grade reflux seems prudent. Success with minimal surgical intervention has been reported (Woodhouse et al, 1979; Duckett et al, 1980; Tank and McCoy, 1983; McMullin et al, 1988). Woodhouse and his associates reviewed a series of patients with PBS managed conservatively (Woodhouse et al, 1979). Nine of these 11 patients, who were monitored from infancy, remained well except for a few urinary tract infections for periods of up to 24 years. They were said to have normal voiding patterns and normal renal function. Certainly, patients in category III are candidates for this type of management.

The paucity of long-term data for category II patients, the probable variation in assignment of disease severity in treatment groups, and the variable natural history of the disease make comparisons of these retrospective studies difficult. **Spontaneous improvement in ureteral appearance and function may occur with normal growth and elongation of the ureters** (Duckett et al, 1980). **Also, some patients with gross abnormalities of the urinary collecting system have survived decades without medical attention** (Asplund and Laska, 1975; Lee, 1977; Texter and Koontz, 1980). **Yet, progressive uropathy is also well known to occur, and many patients with PBS ultimately require renal transplantation**

(Reinberg et al, 1989). Controversy will persist over category II patients until accurate application of a medical or surgical approach is possible based on distinct clinical features. Dénes and coworkers (2004) emphasize the individualization of care in their 17-year experience with 32 patients.

Surgical Management of the Prune Belly Syndrome Patient

Surgical management of children with PBS can be divided into three categories: urinary tract reconstruction, abdominal wall reconstruction, and orchidopexy. Urinary tract reconstruction is generally reserved for children with progressive or severe hydronephrosis, recurrent upper tract infections, true obstructive uropathy, and progressive renal failure. Temporary urinary diversion also has a role in the very young or the very ill child.

Supravesical Urinary Diversion

In certain instances the occurrence of repeated upper tract infections or deterioration of renal function dictates temporary urinary diversion. Although cutaneous vesicostomy usually provides adequate upper tract drainage and decompression, in rare instances more proximal diversion is indicated because of ureteropelvic or ureterovesical junction obstruction. Here a cutaneous pyeloplasty is advocated rather than proximal ureterostomy because it provides the best upper tract drainage and avoids sacrificing a normal proximal ureter that might be useful in later reconstruction.

Cutaneous Vesicostomy

Urinary diversion may be necessary as a temporary measure in children with acute renal failure, urinary sepsis, or bladder outlet obstruction from urethral atresia with limited patency of the urachus (Teramoto et al, 1981; Joseph, 1999). **When temporary urinary diversion is indicated, a cutaneous vesicostomy is the procedure of choice. This is best done by the Blocksom technique as described by Duckett** (Duckett, 1974; Duckett et al, 1986). If there is a large urachal diverticulum, it can be excised at that time. It is advisable to create a larger than normal stoma in the PBS patient, as stenosis is common, probably because of the decreased intra-abdominal pressure (Snow and Duckett, 1987).

Internal Urethrotomy

In the absence of urethral atresia, true anatomic obstruction of the urethra is rare in PBS. However, the normal resistance of the urinary sphincter has been implicated in "unbalanced" urethrovesical function contributing to large postvoid residuals. Snyder and Cukier proposed lowering urethral resistance by internal urethrotomy to improve bladder emptying (Snyder et al, 1976; Cukier, 1977). In patients studied by urodynamic flow rate profilometry, improved flow rates with reduced residual urine and improvement in the radiographic appearance of the upper tracts were found (Snyder et al, 1976; Woodhouse et al, 1979). Although sustained long-term success has not been demonstrated, internal urethrotomy should be considered in PBS children with high postvoid residuals, increasing hydroureteronephrosis, or vesicoureteral reflux with recurrent upper tract infections. Williams (1979) advocated utilizing an Otis urethrotome achieving a No. 24 to 30 Fr caliber with one or two incisions made anteriorly or anterolaterally; however, direct visual urethrotomy would seem preferable and should be performed at the distal end of the prostatic urethra (Smith and Woodard, 2002). It is interesting to note that internal urethrotomy does not result in incontinence in this population.

Reduction Cystoplasty

In many PBS patients, poor bladder contractibility leads to incomplete and infrequent emptying from the complicating urinary stasis and vesicoureteral reflux issues. This leads to the concept of reducing the size of the bladder and remodeling it into a more spherical shape to better direct the contractible forces (Perlmutter, 1976). A variety of approaches have been proposed, from simple excision of the urachal diverticulum to the excision of redundant mucosa with the creation of overlapping between flaps to improve contractibility (Williams and Parker, 1974; Woodard and Trulock, 1986). Over time, however, high bladder capacity and residual volumes seem to recur (Bukowski and Perlmutter, 1994). It seems, therefore, that reduction cystoplasty would be justified only to remove the larger urachal diverticulum or as part of a more extensive internal reconstruction. Intermittent catheterization through the urethra or through an appendicovesicostomy channel is likely to afford better long-term bladder emptying with reduction of residual urinary volumes (Joseph, 1999).

Anterior Urethral Reconstruction

On one end of the spectrum of urethral maldevelopment is urethral atresia, sometimes referred to as microurethra (see Fig. 118–3). Passerini-Glazel and colleagues (1988) reported on progressive gentle urethral dilation with good success. This technique may be utilized in situ or through and through in cases in which a vesicostomy has been performed (Fig. 118–9). As reported by Reinberg and coauthors (1993), however, this technique is not uniformly successful and one may require a more formal urethroplasty with skin flaps or grafts, or both.

Megalourethra in PBS may be either fusiform or scaphoid (Appel et al, 1986). This is best approached with a circumferential subcoronal incision and penile degloving (Fig. 118–10). The redundant urethra can be excised and the urethra reconstructed over an appropriately sized catheter. Alternatively, some of the urethra can be used to reinforce the urethroplasty, as in either form of megalourethra the spongiosum is deficient.

Ureteral Reconstruction

Ureteral remodeling remains controversial. It is best undertaken in children who demonstrated repeated nonsuppressible upper urinary tract infections or those with progressive upper tract deterioration. The goal of remodeling is to reduce urinary stasis. The key to success relies on meticulous surgical technique and preservation of the upper few centimeters of proximal ureter for reconstruction. Ureteral reimplantation into the abnormal bladder can be difficult in that the creation of a submucosal tunnel can be challenging (Woodard and Trulock, 1986). Woodard and his coworkers

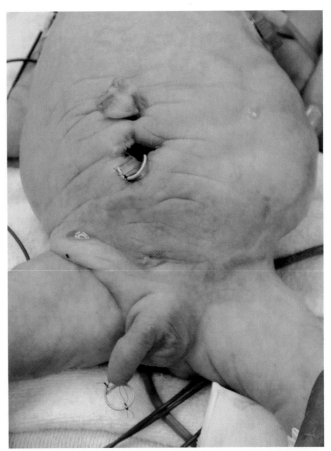

Figure 118–9. Prune belly syndrome patient with urethral atresia. Note vesicostomy and double J stent through the urethra for progressive dilation.

have demonstrated excellent success in this population when these procedures were performed in the neonatal period or in the older child (Woodard and Parrott, 1978b; Woodard, 1990). They no longer, however, recommend such extensive reconstructive surgery before the age of 3 to 6 months.

KEY POINTS: SURGICAL RECONSTRUCTION

■ Upper urinary tract reconstruction is controversial but clearly indicated for evidence of declining renal function in the presence of hydronephrosis, recurrent upper tract infections, or progression of the hydroureteronephrosis.

■ Orchidopexy is best performed early in life as this affords the most likely prospect of a successful single-stage procedure.

■ Abdominal wall reconstruction has demonstrated improved bladder emptying, a more effective cough, and improved defecation in addition to psychosocial benefits.

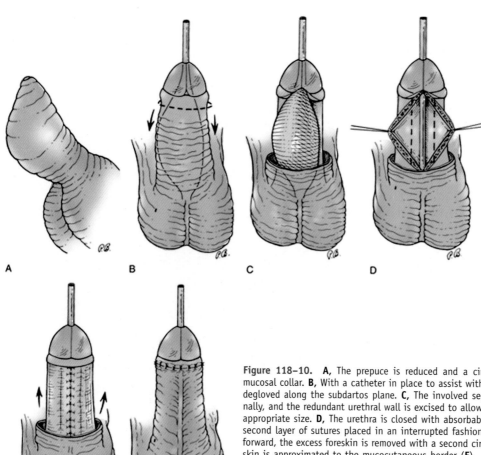

Figure 118–10. A, The prepuce is reduced and a circumcising incision is made, preserving a mucosal collar. **B,** With a catheter in place to assist with identification of the urethra, the penis is degloved along the subdartos plane. **C,** The involved segment of the urethra is opened longitudinally, and the redundant urethral wall is excised to allow tapering of the urethra over a catheter of appropriate size. **D,** The urethra is closed with absorbable running sutures and is bolstered with a second layer of sutures placed in an interrupted fashion if possible. **E,** The penile skin is brought forward, the excess foreskin is removed with a second circumferential incision, and the penile shaft skin is approximated to the mucocutaneous border (**F**).

Orchidopexy

The timing of orchidopexy is dictated by our current understanding of the need for early treatment of the undescended testis in non-PBS patients along with individual PBS patients' needs for either temporary or reconstructive surgery. Although the fertility potential of the PBS patient is known to be compromised, germ cells are present in the testes of infants with PBS. In addition, the prognosis for normal hormonal function at puberty is excellent. These factors, along with the potential risk of testicular carcinoma (Uehling et al, 1984; Massad et al, 1991), would justify early orchidopexy. As the testes are uniformly located in the abdomen, most commonly on a broad mesorchium overlying the iliac vessels (Coplen et al, 1996), standard inguinal approaches are not usually successful in achieving a satisfactory scrotal position. Four alternative approaches may be considered.

Transabdominal Orchidopexy. Woodard and Parrott as well as others noted that if an orchidopexy is done in the neonatal period and up to 6 months of age by a transabdominal approach, adequate spermatic vessel mobilization can usually be achieved for scrotal placement (Woodard and Parrott, 1978a, 1978b; Randolph et al, 1981a; Fallat et al, 1989).

Transabdominal bilateral orchidopexy at about 6 months of age is currently considered the approach of choice. This approach is often used in conjunction with other abdominal surgeries, either a vesicostomy, urinary tract reconstruction, or abdominal wall reconstruction (Fig. 118–11). In the absence of need for other abdominal surgeries, this can be accomplished laparoscopically.

Spermatic Vessel Ligation. When successful transabdominal orchidopexy cannot be accomplished in the first few months of life, the other options that may be considered are (1) Fowler-Stephens orchidopexy (Fowler and Stephens, 1959; Gibbons et al, 1979; Boddy et al, 1991; Kirsch, 1998), (2) staged Fowler-Stephens orchidopexy (Ransley et al, 1984; Bloom, 1991; Caldamone and Amaral, 1994; Docimo, 1995; Yu et al, 1995), and (3) microvascular autotransplantation (MacMahon et al, 1976; Wacksman et al, 1980; Boddy et al, 1991). A meta-analysis report by Docimo (1995) indicated comparative success rates of 67% and 77% for standard and staged Fowler-Stephens techniques, respectively. In a multi-institutional report of laparoscopic orchidopexy, Baker and colleagues (2001) noted a success rate of 81% for a standard Fowler-Stephens approach compared with 90% for a staged

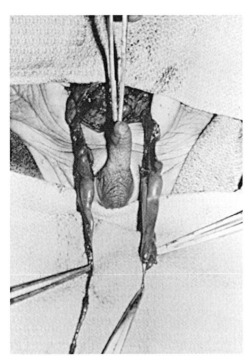

Figure 118–11. Operative photograph showing the ease with which the testes reach the scrotum after neonatal transabdominal mobilization of the spermatic cords.

approach. In a long-term follow-up report, Patil and associates (2004) reported a satisfactory outcome in PBS with a one- or two-stage Fowler-Stephens orchidopexy.

Reconstruction of the Abdominal Wall

Children with mild degrees of abdominal muscular deficiency may show improvement in the abdominal wall laxity as they mature. However, most others with moderate to severe degrees of abdominal wall laxity are left with a potentially psychologically crippling defect (Ehrlich et al, 1986; Parrott and Woodard, 1992). An elasticized corset can improve the external appearance when they are fully clothed; however, it is quite inconvenient to use. There is general agreement about the cosmetic benefit of abdominal wall reconstruction. However, whether it improves bladder, bowel, and pulmonary function is controversial (Smith et al, 1998; Woodard, 1998). Smith and colleagues demonstrated improved bladder emptying following abdominal wall reconstruction; however, some of their reconstructed patients underwent concomitant urinary tract remodeling as well. Potential effects include a more effective cough and improvement in defecation. The timing of abdominal wall reconstruction should be dictated by the need for other surgical interventions, particularly if upper urinary tract remodeling is necessary. If upper tract remodeling is not anticipated, the abdominal wall can be addressed at any time and has been done as young as 6 months of age along with transabdominal orchidopexy (Smith and Woodard, 2002). However, if the procedure is done in infancy, one must be prepared to place the infant on a respirator postoperatively for a period of time. Of the following techniques, the consensus currently is that the Monfort and Ehrlich techniques provide the best functional and cosmetic results.

Randolph Technique

Randolph and coworkers (1981) first popularized a technique for abdominal wall reconstruction based on electromyographic mapping, which indicated that the most severely affected area of the abdomen is the infraumbilical regions and the lateral and supraumbilical regions are generally least affected. This technique makes a transverse incision from the 12th rib to the pubic symphysis to the opposite 12th rib with a full-thickness removal of the skin, lower abdominal musculature, and peritoneum and the healthy fascia is then approximated to the anterior iliac spines, pubic tubercle, and inferior fascia. Although this technique is successful in establishing a waistline, lateral abdominal bulging often persists. Of the 16 patients reported, 9 had excellent cosmetic results and there was some residual protuberance in 7 (Fallat et al, 1989).

Ehrlich Technique

The technique described by Ehrlich utilized a vertical midline incision and allows preservation of the umbilicus on a vascular pedicle from the inferior epigastric artery (Ehrlich et al, 1986; Ehrlich and Lesavoy, 1993). The skin and subcutaneous tissues are elevated off the muscle and fascial layers and an overlapping, pants over vest, advancement of each side to the contralateral flank is performed, preserving the less affected lateral muscles and fascia.

Monfort Technique

Monfort described a technique that is vertically oriented similar to that of Ehrlich's approach; however, an elliptically oriented incision is used to isolate the redundant skin (Monfort et al, 1991). The incision extends from the tip of the xiphoid to the pubis. A second incision is made around the umbilicus to preserve it in situ (Fig. 118–12). The skin and subcutaneous tissue are dissected off the attenuated fascia and muscle with the dissection extending laterally to the anterior axillary line. Vertical fascial incisions are made lateral to the superior epigastric arteries, leaving a central fascial bridge. If intra-abdominal surgery is necessary, excellent exposure to the urinary tract or abdominal testes is afforded through these lateral fascial incisions. The lateral fascial is then advanced over the central fascial bridge from both sides, alleviating the redundancy and increasing the thickness of the abdominal wall (Fig. 118–13).

Furness and coauthors (1998) described a modified midline approach with less abdominal wall dissection that avoids entering the peritoneum, which may be useful if intra-abdominal surgery is not planned. A modification of the Monfort technique utilizes laparoscopy to protect the abdominal contents (Franco, 2005).

LONG-TERM OUTLOOK

The nadir creatinine during infancy has proved to be a useful predictor of long-term renal function. If the nadir value is less than 0.7 mg/dL, renal function tends to be stable during childhood unless there is further renal compromise by pyelonephritis (Geary et al, 1986; Reinberg et al 1991b; Noh et al 1999). The importance of urinary tract monitoring by periodic cultures and prompt treatment of urinary tract

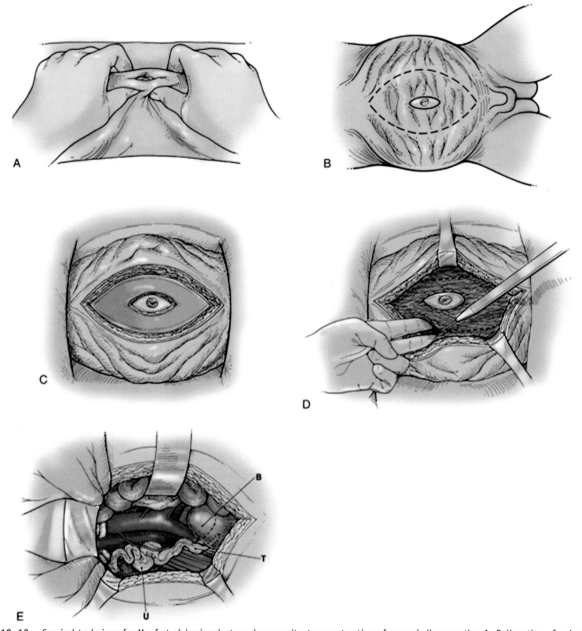

Figure 118–12. Surgical technique for Monfort abdominoplasty and concomitant reconstruction of prune belly uropathy. **A,** Delineation of redundancy by tenting up abdominal wall. **B,** Skin incisions are outlined with a separate circumscribing incision to isolate the umbilicus. **C,** Skin (epidermis and dermis only) is excised with electrocautery. **D,** Abdominal wall central plate is incised at the lateral border of the rectus muscle on either side, from the superior epigastric to the inferior epigastric vessels, creating a central musculofascial plate. **E,** Adequate exposure is provided for concomitant transperitoneal genitourinary procedures.

Continued

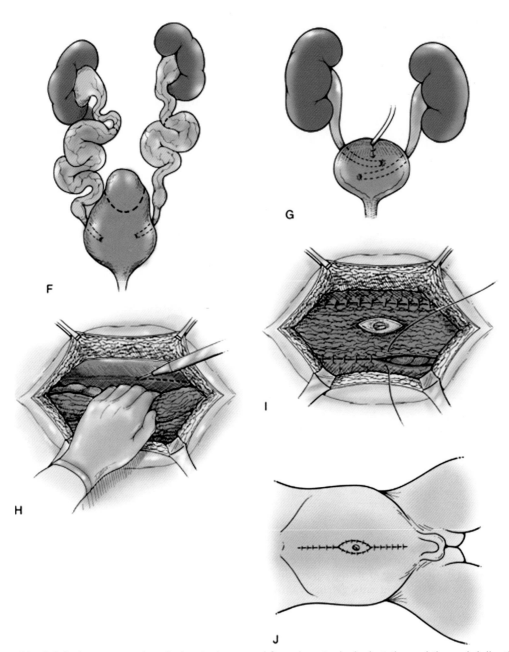

Figure 118–12, cont'd. F, Only the more normal proximal ureter is preserved for vesicoureteral reimplantation, and the urachal diverticulum is excised. **G,** Transtrigonal ureteral reimplantation is performed with or without ureteral tapering as necessary. The bladder is closed in two layers, and ureteral stents (not shown) and a cystostomy tube are employed. **H,** Completion of abdominoplasty by scoring of the parietal peritoneum overlying the lateral abdominal wall musculature with electrocautery. **I,** The edges of the central plate are sutured to the lateral abdominal wall musculature along the scored line. **J,** Lateral flaps are brought together in the midline, with closed suction drains placed between the lateral flaps and the central plate. Skin is brought together in the midline, enveloping the previously isolated umbilicus. (From Woodard JR, Perez LM: Prune-belly syndrome. In Marshall FF [ed]: Operative Urology. Philadelphia, WB Saunders, 1996.)

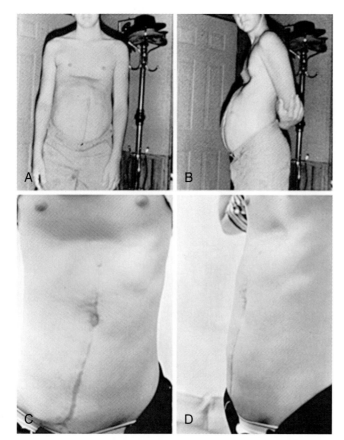

Figure 118–13. **A** and **B,** Anterior and lateral views of the abdomen of a 14-year-old boy who underwent major surgical remodeling of the urinary tract during early infancy with good results. Note typical abdominal configuration. **C** and **D,** Anterior and lateral views of the same boy 1 month after undergoing abdominoplasty with the technique described by Monfort.

infections cannot be overemphasized. **Unfortunately, the risk of infection is constant in the setting of urinary tract dilation and stasis. As many as 30% of patients, generally those with impaired renal function at initial evaluation, develop chronic renal failure during childhood or adolescence**

(Geary et al, 1986). Renal transplantation is necessary for these patients to ensure normal growth and development, and success with transplantation in prune belly patients can be expected to equal that in other age-matched groups (Reinberg et al, 1989). Normal growth can be expected in most of the patients with normal renal function, although growth retardation in the absence of renal compromise was observed in one third of patients in one series (Geary et al, 1986). A normal pattern of secondary sexual development can be expected (Woodhouse and Snyder, 1985). Although primary fertility is not expected in the PBS population, fertility with assisted reproductive techniques may be feasible in those having had successful early orchidopexy.

The overall outlook for the PBS patient, both for survival and for quality of care, has improved considerably, largely through advances in medical, surgical, and urodynamic management. The key to management of the PBS patient is individualization of care, as some require major urologic reconstruction and others little if any reconstruction. Long-term surveillance of the urinary tract is essential as functional dynamics can change over time.

SUGGESTED READINGS

Monfort G, Guys JM, Bocciardi A, et al: A novel technique for reconstruction of the abdominal wall in the prune belly syndrome. J Urol 1991;146:639.

Noh PH, Cooper CS, Zderic SA, et al: Prognostic factors in patients with prune belly syndrome. J Urol 1999;162:1399-1401.

Reinberg Y, Manivel JC, Fryd D, et al: The outcome of renal transplantation in children with the prune belly syndrome. J Urol 1989;142:1541.

Smith CA, Smith EA, Parrott TS, et al: Voiding function in patients with prune belly syndrome after Monfort abdominoplasty. J Urol 1998;159:80-89.

Stephens FD, Gupta D: Pathogenesis of the prune belly syndrome. J Urol 1994;152:2328-2331.

Woodard JR, Smith EA: Prune belly syndrome. In Walsh PC, Retik AB, Vaughan ED Jr, Wind AJ (eds): Campbell's Urology. Philadelphia, WB Saunders, 1998:1917-1938.

Woodhouse CR, Ransley PG, Innes Williams D: Prune belly syndrome—Report of 47 cases. Arch Dis Child 1982;57:856-859.

Exstrophy-Epispadias Complex

JOHN P. GEARHART, MD • RANJIV MATHEWS, MD

THE EXSTROPHY-EPISPADIAS COMPLEX

The exstrophy-epispadias complex of genitourinary malformations can be as simple as a glandular epispadias or an overwhelming multisystem defect such as cloacal exstrophy (Fig. 119–1). This chapter deals with the diagnosis and modern management of the exstrophy-epispadias complex.

Historical Aspects

In older texts, the first account of bladder exstrophy was ascribed to Assyro-Babylonian sources dating from the first and second millennia BC. At that time, birth anomalies in both humans and animals were carefully recorded on tablets for their importance as omens, based on their interpretation by divination experts. Feneley and Gearhart (2000) examined Assyro-Babylonian descriptions of congenital anomalies from cuneiform texts at the British Museum in London. Although references to anomalies involving the external genitalia were frequent (e.g., hermaphroditism, absence of external genitalia, unilateral and bilateral undescended testes), references to renal and bladder anomalies were few and difficult to interpret medically. Duplication and laterality of anomalies were described in detail owing to their distinct significance, but malformations in combination were not recorded. On the basis of these studies performed with a prominent Assyriologist, a definitive description of bladder or cloacal exstrophy was not corroborated. **The first recorded case of epispadias is attributed to the Byzantine Emperor Heraclius** (AD 610 to 641) and the first description of bladder exstrophy to Schenck in 1595 (Feneley and Gearhart, 2000).

Incidence and Inheritance

The incidence of bladder exstrophy has been estimated as between 1 in 10,000 and 1 in 50,000 (Lattimer and Smith, 1966) live births. However, data from the International Clearinghouse for Birth Defects monitoring system estimated the incidence to be 3.3 cases in 100,000 live births (Lancaster, 1987). The male-to-female ratio of bladder exstrophy derived from multiple series is 2.3:1 (Shapiro et al, 1984). However, two series reported a 5:1 to 6:1 male-to-female ratio of exstrophy births (Ives et al, 1980; Lancaster, 1987).

The risk of recurrence of bladder exstrophy in a given family is approximately 1 in 100 (Ives et al, 1980). Shapiro and coworkers (1984) conducted a questionnaire of pediatric urologists and surgeons in North America and Europe and identified the recurrence of exstrophy and epispadias in only 9 of approximately 2500 indexed cases. Lattimer and Smith (1966) cited a set of identical twins with bladder exstrophy and another set of twins in whom only one child had exstrophy. Shapiro's series identified five sets of male and female nonidentical twins in whom only one twin was affected with exstrophy; five sets of male identical twins in whom both twins were affected; one set of identical male twins in whom only one twin was affected; and three sets of female identical twins in whom only one twin had the exstrophy anomaly

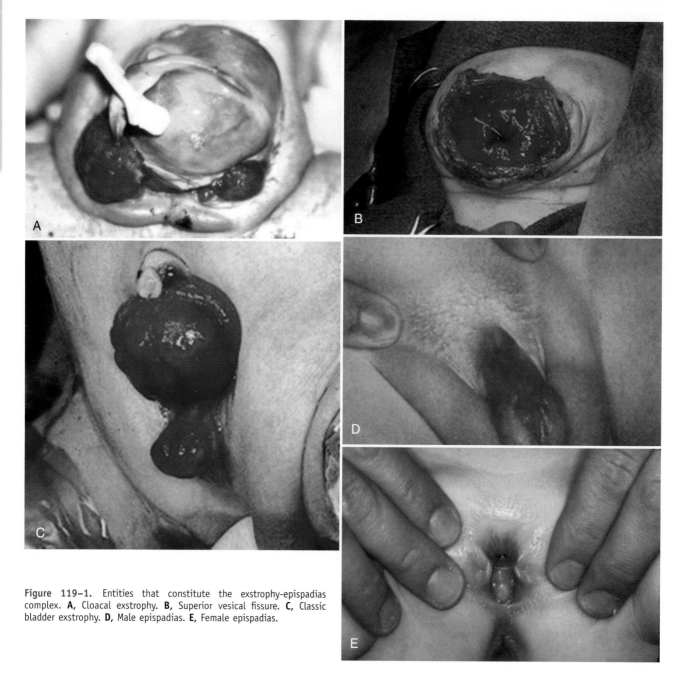

Figure 119–1. Entities that constitute the exstrophy-epispadias complex. **A,** Cloacal exstrophy. **B,** Superior vesical fissure. **C,** Classic bladder exstrophy. **D,** Male epispadias. **E,** Female epispadias.

(Shapiro et al, 1984). Evidence by Reutter and coworkers has demonstrated six families with two occurrences of exstrophy-epispadias complex, one in which the proband was the product of a consanguineous union and four discordant twin pairs. Also, Boyadjiev and colleagues (2004a) found four multiplex families (2.7%) in a cohort of 151 families with the exstrophy-epispadias complex. There were three twin pairs, two of which were monozygotic, and concordance was present in only one of the twin pairs. Consanguinity was present in one family. The inheritance pattern of bladder exstrophy in a literature review by Clemetson (1958) identified 45 women with bladder exstrophy who produced 49 offspring. None of their offspring demonstrated features of the exstrophy-epispadias complex.

Bladder exstrophy or epispadias was not reported until the 1980s in the offspring of parents with the exstrophy-epispadias complex. Shapiro and colleagues (1984) described two women with complete epispadias who gave birth to sons with bladder exstrophy. They also reported that another woman with bladder exstrophy gave birth to a son with bladder exstrophy. The inheritance of these three cases of bladder exstrophy was identified in a total of 225 offspring (75 boys and 150 girls) produced by individuals with bladder exstrophy and epispadias. **Shapiro and colleagues (1984) determined that the risk of bladder exstrophy in the offspring of individuals with bladder exstrophy and epispadias is 1 in 70 live births, a 500-fold greater incidence than in the general population.** Boyadjiev (2004) studied sibling data from 200 families and found 259 unaffected children in addition to the probands with exstrophy. Twenty-six probands had first-, second-, or third-degree relatives with congenital anomalies unrelated to the exstrophy-epispadias complex, most of which were midline defects and oral clefts. Four probands had a total of seven biologic children that were unaffected. In a multinational review of exstrophy patients (Lancaster, 1987), two interesting trends were found: (1) bladder exstrophy tends to occur in infants of younger mothers, and (2) an increased risk at higher parity is observed for bladder exstrophy but not for epispadias. Boyadjiev's (2004) data, however, differ from these trends, indicating that the average maternal age was 34 years and the average paternal age was 32 years. In addition, 49% of probands were born from first pregnancies. This change may represent societal changes indicating advancing maternal age for first pregnancies and increasing utilization of assisted reproductive techniques in first pregnancies.

Exploration of possible etiologies for the exstrophy-epispadias complex continues. A report from Israel indicated a 10-fold increase in exstrophy births to mothers who had received large doses of progesterone in the early part of the first trimester. Wood and colleagues (2003) reported on a sizable series of children with exstrophy conceived using assisted reproductive techniques. A 7.5-fold increase in incidence was noted when in vitro fertilization was utilized. These two reports indicate a role for hormonal changes in the etiology of the exstrophy-epispadias complex. Genetic studies to identify a genetic locus for the exstrophy-epispadias complex

are under way. Boyadjiev and coauthors (2004b) have reported finding a breakpoint disruption in the 5′ region of the *CASPR3* gene on chromosome 9. This observation is the first to suggest a possible genetic basis for development of the exstrophy-epispadias complex.

Embryology

Bladder exstrophy, cloacal exstrophy, and epispadias are variants of the exstrophy-epispadias complex (see Fig. 119–1). The cause of this complex is thought to be the failure of the cloacal membrane to be reinforced by ingrowth of mesoderm (Muecke, 1964). The cloacal membrane is a bilaminar layer situated at the caudal end of the germinal disk that occupies the infraumbilical abdominal wall. Mesenchymal ingrowth between the ectodermal and endodermal layers of the cloacal membrane results in formation of the lower abdominal muscles and the pelvic bones. The cloacal membrane is subject to premature rupture, and, depending on the extent of the infraumbilical defect and the stage of development during which the rupture occurs, bladder exstrophy, cloacal exstrophy, or epispadias results (Ambrose and O'Brien, 1974).

After mesenchymal ingrowth occurs, the urorectal septum grows in a caudal direction and divides the cloaca into a bladder anteriorly and a rectum posteriorly (Fig. 119–2). Distally, the septum meets the posterior remnant of the bilaminar membrane, which eventually perforates and forms the urogenital and anal openings. The paired genital tubercles

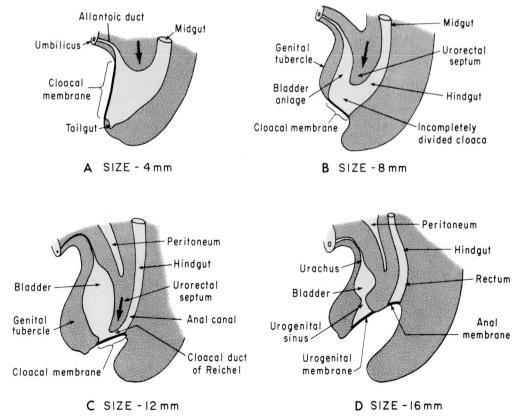

Figure 119–2. Development of the cloaca and cloacal membrane in the 4- to 16-mm embryonic stages. Caudal growth of the urorectal septum leads to separation of the anterior urogenital sinus from the posterior rectum.

migrate medially and fuse in the midline, cephalad to the dorsal membrane before perforation.

The theory of embryonic maldevelopment in exstrophy held by Marshall and Muecke (1968) is that the basic defect is an abnormal overdevelopment of the cloacal membrane, which prevents medial migration of the mesenchymal tissue and proper lower abdominal wall development. The timing of the rupture of this defective cloacal membrane determines the variant of the exstrophy-epispadias complex that results. This theory is supported by Muecke's work in the chick embryo and by the high incidence of expected central perforations, resulting in the preponderance of classic exstrophy variants. Classic exstrophy accounts for more than 50% of the patients born with this complex (Muecke, 1964; Marshall and Muecke, 1968). Martinez-Frias and coworkers (2001) using epidemiologic factors of low birth weight, twinning, single umbilical artery, and associated defects postulated that exstrophy of the cloaca and exstrophy of bladder are two different expressions of a primary developmental field defect with cloacal exstrophy being an early defect. However, this precept conflicts with data from Bruch and coauthors (1996), who presented a patient who was shown on repeated antenatal ultrasonography to have cloacal membrane rupture after the 18th week of gestation and had cloacal exstrophy.

Other plausible theories concerning the cause of the exstrophy-epispadias complex exist. Abnormal development of the genital hillocks caudal to the normal position, with fusion in the midline below rather than above the cloacal membrane, has been embraced by other investigators (Patton and Barry, 1952; Ambrose and O'Brien, 1974). Another interesting hypothesis that remains controversial describes an abnormal caudal insertion of the body stalk, which results in a failure of interposition of the mesenchymal tissue in the midline (Mildenberger et al, 1988). As a consequence of this failure, translocation of the cloaca into the depths of the abdominal cavity does not occur. A cloacal membrane that remains in a superficial infraumbilical position represents an unstable embryonic state with a strong tendency to disintegrate (Johnston and Kogan, 1974). The lack of ability of the Meucke hypothesis to explain the absence of the ileocecal region of the digestive system and the superior mesenteric blood supply of the exstrophied intestinal region has led to a suggestion that there may be involvement of the allantois in the development of cloacal exstrophy (Zarabi and Rupani, 1985). Absence of migration, ascent, or alignment of the allan-tois with the yolk sac with its persistence at the dome of the cloaca can be used to explain the bowel abnormalities noted in cloacal exstrophy. Maldevelopment of the bony pelvis rather than soft tissue defects has been suggested to be the inciting issue for the development of exstrophy. Beaudoin and colleagues (1997) have suggested that lack of "rotation" of the pelvic ring primordium prevents structures attached to the pelvic ring from joining in the midline, allowing herniation of the bladder to occur. The cause of this inadequate rotation remains elusive. Stec and coworkers (2003) were able to demonstrate that the anatomic microstructure of the pelvic ring in exstrophy was similar to that in age-matched control subjects.

CLASSIC BLADDER EXSTROPHY
Anatomic Considerations

Exstrophy of the bladder is part of a spectrum of anomalies involving the urinary tract, the genital tract, the musculoskeletal system, and sometimes the intestinal tract. In classic bladder exstrophy, most anomalies are related to defects of the abdominal wall, bladder, genitalia, pelvic bones, rectum, and anus. Because of the involved nature of this defect, the deficits are described here as they affect each system.

Skeletal Defects

Formerly, classic bladder exstrophy was thought only to show the characteristic widening of the pubic symphysis caused by malrotation of the innominate bones in relation to the sagittal plane of the body along both sacroiliac joints. In addition, there was an outward rotation or eversion of the pubic rami at their junction with the iliac bones. More recently, Sponseller and associates (1995), using computed tomography (CT) of the pelvis with three-dimensional (3-D) reconstruction, have further characterized the bone defect associated with both classic bladder exstrophy and cloacal exstrophy. **In reviewing a large group of patients with exstrophy of the bladder, using pelvic CT scans and age-matched controls, Sponseller and coworkers (1995) found that patients with classic bladder exstrophy have a mean external rotation of the posterior aspect of the pelvis of 12 degrees on each side, retroversion of the acetabulum, and a mean 18 degrees of external rotation of the anterior pelvis, along with 30% shortening of the pubic rami, in addition to the previously described diastasis of the symphysis pubis (Fig. 119–3).** In

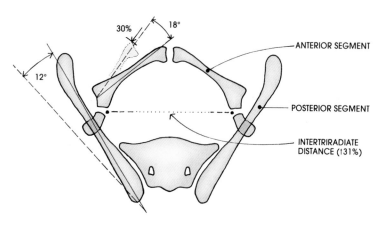

Figure 119–3. Pelvic bone abnormalities noted in classic bladder exstrophy. The posterior bone segment is externally rotated (12 degrees mean on each side) but the length is unchanged. The anterior segment is externally rotated (18 degrees mean on each side) and shortened by 30%. The distance between the triradiate cartilage is increased by 31%.

long-term follow-up there was a foot progression angle of 20 to 30 degrees of external rotation beyond the normal limits seen in early childhood, but this rotation improved with age. Likewise, patients with cloacal exstrophy not only had pelvic deformities to a greater degree but also had asymmetry of the preceding parameters between the right and left sides of the pelvis, malformation of the sacroiliac joints, and occasional dislocations of the hip (Sponseller et al, 1995).

Data from Stec and associates (2001a) using 3-D models from CT scans have provided further insight into the bone defect of children born with classic bladder exstrophy. Using age-matched controls, they found that the sacroiliac joint angle (before closure) was 10 degrees larger in the exstrophy pelvis, being 10 degrees more toward the coronal plane than sagittal (Fig. 119–4). Also, the bony pelvis in exstrophy has 14.7 degrees more inferior rotation than in healthy patients. Lastly, the sacrum in exstrophy patients has a 42.6% larger

volume and 23.5% more surface area than in controls. These new findings will help with planning better osteotomies and better reduction of both the pubic diastasis and pubic long-term undergrowth in these patients.

These rotational deformities of the pelvic skeletal structures contribute to the short, pendular penis seen in bladder exstrophy. Outward rotation and lateral displacement of the innominate bones also account for the increased distance between the hips, waddling gait, and outward rotation of the lower limbs in these children, which in itself causes little disability and usually corrects to some degree over time. Data from Sponseller and colleagues (2001) show an increased incidence of premature osteoarthritis of the hip in adult patients who were closed without an osteotomy. Although these findings do not affect function, periodic radiologic evaluation of the pelvis and lumbosacrum should be performed in adult life.

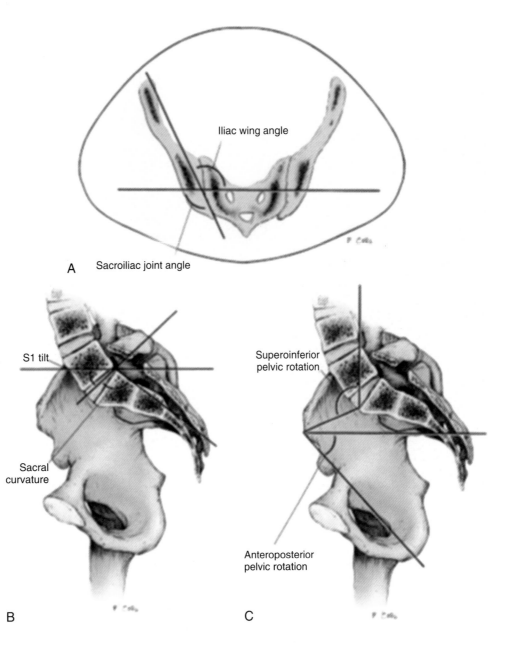

Figure 119–4. Sacroiliac joint angles prior to closure in children with classic exstrophy 10 degrees larger than normal controls. The bony pelvis has 14.7 degrees inferior rotation compared with normal controls. (From Stec AA, Pannu HK, Tadros YE, et al: Evaluation of the bony pelvis in classic bladder exstrophy using 3 D CT—Further insights. Urology 2001; 58:1030.)

Spinal abnormalities have frequently been noted in children with cloacal exstrophy, but incidence in bladder exstrophy had not been studied. A study of 299 children with bladder exstrophy indicated spinal variations without clinical significance (spina bifida occulta, lumbarization or sacralization of vertebrae) in 11%, uncomplicated scoliosis in 2.7%, and spinal dysraphism in 4% including myelomeningocele, lipomeningocele, scimitar sacrum, and hemivertebrae, but only one patient demonstrated any evidence of neurologic dysfunction (Cadeddu et al, 1997). Thus, although present in classic bladder exstrophy, symptomatic spinal anomalies appear rare.

Pelvic Floor Defects

Stec and colleagues (2001b), using 3-D models created from CT scans of children with classic bladder exstrophy and normal age-matched controls, found that the puborectal slings were supporting two times more body cavity area than normal. The levator ani group is positioned more posteriorly in exstrophy patients, with 68% located posterior to the

rectum and 32% anterior (versus 52% posterior and 48% anterior in healthy controls) (Fig. 119–5). The levators are also rotated outward 15.5 degrees, and in the coronal aspect the levators are 31.7 degrees more flattened than normal. This deviation from normal makes the exstrophy puborectal sling more flattened than its normal conical shape. There was no significant difference in the length or thickness of these muscles between patients with exstrophy and normal controls.

These new insights further elucidate the entire exstrophy defect, especially in regard to pelvic reconstruction. Interest in development of continence after primary closure in some patients has led to further investigation of the pelvic floor anatomy. Differences in orientation and anatomy of the pelvic floor musculature may directly affect development of continence following closure alone. The successful application of 3-D magnetic resonance imaging (MRI) in anorectal anomalies has led to its use for the anatomic definition of the pelvic floor musculature in exstrophy. A comparison of 3-D MRI in children with exstrophy prior to closure and in normal controls indicated that the levator ani group was less dome shaped

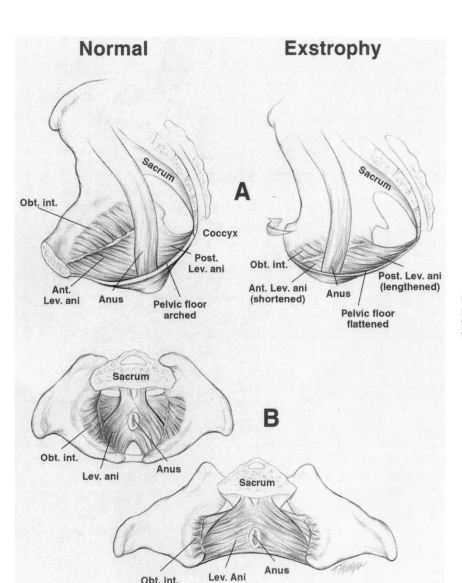

Figure 119–5. Pelvic floor changes in the patient with exstrophy; levator ani group is positioned more posteriorly (68% located posterior to the rectum) compared with normal controls.

and more irregular in those with exstrophy (Williams et al, 2004). Also, there was no relationship between the amount of pubic diastasis and the extent of disproportionate curvature of the levator ani group. In addition, Halachmi and coauthors (2003) reported on the postoperative appearance of the pelvic floor with 3-D MRI. In two patients who had some degree of continence, the intrasymphyseal distance was noted to be shortest, the angle of the levator ani divergence sharpest, and the bladder neck most deeply positioned in the pelvis. Gargollo and others (2004), reporting on a series of patients who had MRI before and after exstrophy closure, noted that the puborectalis angle in those with dry intervals was decreased compared with that prior to closure. These two studies correlate well with earlier findings of Gearhart and coworkers (1993) showing that in the adult patients who were dry the puborectalis angle was less than 65 degrees. These data reinforce the necessity for aggressive dissection and posterior placement of the posterior urethra and bladder and the role for osteotomy and pelvic fixation.

Abdominal Wall Defects

The triangular defect caused by the premature rupture of the abnormal cloacal membrane is occupied by the exstrophy bladder and posterior urethra. The fascial defect is limited inferiorly by the intrasymphyseal band, which represents the divergent urogenital diaphragm. This band connects the bladder neck and posterior urethra to the pubic ramus on anatomic study. The anterior sheath of the rectus muscle has a fanlike extension behind the urethra and bladder neck that inserts into the intrasymphyseal band. Investigations into the relationship of the rectus muscle and fascia to the urogenital diaphragm (Wakim and Barbet, 2002) have found no gross or histologic evidence of the presence of the striated sphincter. However, clear evidence of bladder musculature extending laterally to the pubis was found where it interdigitates with fibers from the rectus fascia forming the fibrous urogenital diaphragm (Wakim and Barbet, 2002). Gearhart and colleagues (1991) have shown the importance of radical incision of these fibers lateral to the urethral plate down to the level of the inferior pubic ramus and levator hiatus for the bladder and posterior urethra to be placed in a deep pelvic position. Data from failed exstrophy closures show these fibers to be intact in many patients at the time of reclosure.

At the upper end of the triangular fascial defect is the umbilicus. In bladder exstrophy, the distance between the umbilicus and the anus is always foreshortened. Because the umbilicus is situated well below the horizontal line of the iliac crest, there is an unusual expanse of uninterrupted abdominal skin. Although an umbilical hernia is usually present, it is usually of insignificant size. The umbilical hernia is repaired at the time of the initial exstrophy closure. Omphaloceles, although rarely seen in conjunction with bladder exstrophy, are frequently associated with cloacal exstrophy. Omphaloceles associated with classic bladder exstrophy-epispadias complex are usually small and can be closed at the time of bladder closure.

The frequent occurrence of indirect inguinal hernias is attributed to a persistent processus vaginalis, large internal and external inguinal rings, and lack of obliquity of the inguinal canal. **Connolly and coauthors** (1995), **in a review of 181 children with bladder exstrophy, reported inguinal hernias in 81.8% of boys and 10.5% of girls.** At the time of closure of the bladder exstrophy, these hernias should be repaired by excision of the hernial sac and repair of the transversalis fascia and muscle defect to prevent recurrence or a direct inguinal hernia. The contralateral side should also be explored because the incidence of synchronous or asynchronous bilaterality is very high.

Anorectal Defects

The perineum is short and broad and the anus is situated directly behind the urogenital diaphragm; it is displaced anteriorly and corresponds to the posterior limit of the triangular fascial defect. The anal sphincter mechanism is also anteriorly displaced and should be preserved intact in case internal urinary diversion is required in future management.

The divergent levator ani and puborectalis muscles and the distorted anatomy of the external sphincter contribute to varying degrees of anal incontinence and rectal prolapse. Anal continence is usually imperfect at an early age. In rare patients, the rectal sphincter mechanism may never be adequate to control the liquid content of the bowel. Rectal prolapse frequently occurs in untreated exstrophy patients with a widely separated symphysis. It is usually transient and easily reduced. Prolapse virtually disappears after bladder closure or cystectomy and urinary diversion. The appearance of prolapse in an infant is an indication to proceed with definitive management of the exstrophied bladder. **If rectal prolapse occurs at any time after exstrophy closure, posterior urethral/bladder outlet obstruction should be suspected, and immediate evaluation of the outlet tract by cystoscopy should be performed** (Baker and Gearhart, 1998).

Male Genital Defect

The male genital defect is severe and is probably the most troublesome aspect of the surgical reconstruction, independent of the decision whether to treat with modern staged closure, combined closure, or a form of urinary diversion (Fig. 119–6). Formerly, it was thought that the individual corpora cavernosa were of normal caliber but appeared shorter because of the wide separation of the crural attachments, the prominent dorsal chordee, and the shortened urethral groove. **However, Silver and colleagues** (1997b) **described the genital defect for the first time in bladder exstrophy in greater detail. MRI was used in adult men with bladder exstrophy and compared with results for age- and race-matched controls. They found that the anterior corporal length of male patients with bladder exstrophy was almost 50% shorter than that of normal controls** (Fig. 119–7). However, although the posterior length of the corporal body was the same as in age-matched controls, the diameter of the posterior corporal segment was greater than in normal controls. It was also found on MRI that the diastasis of the symphysis pubis increased the intrasymphyseal and intercorporal distances but the angle between the corpora cavernosa was unchanged because the corporal bodies were separated in a parallel fashion. Therefore, the penis appears short not only because of the diastasis of the pubic symphysis, as thought in the past, but also because of marked congenital deficiency of anterior corporal tissue (Silver et al, 1997b).

A functional and cosmetically pleasing penis can be achieved when the dorsal chordee is released, the urethral

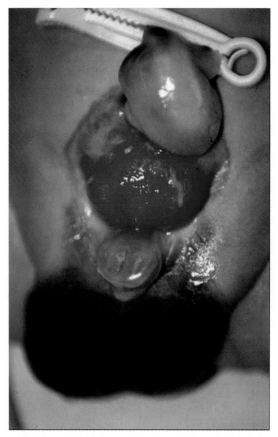

Figure 119–6. Newborn male with classic bladder exstrophy. Note the dorsal chordee, short urethral plate, and flattening of the scrotum.

groove lengthened, and the penis somewhat lengthened by mobilizing the crura in the midline. Patients with a very small or dystrophic penis should be considered for sex reassignment only after other opinions have been obtained and the parents have been counseled about the implications of this step.

In a study by Gearhart and associates (1993c), **13 adult men born with bladder exstrophy were evaluated with MRI of the pelvis to evaluate the size and configuration of the prostate and sex accessory organs. The volume, weight, and maximum cross-sectional area of the prostate appeared normal compared with published control values** (Fig. 119–8). However, in none of the patients did the prostate extend circumferentially around the urethra, and the urethra was anterior to the prostate in all patients. Except for studies to document the presence of the prostate gland or its size, data do not exist concerning the function of the prostate gland in the patient with exstrophy. Silver and coworkers (1997a) reported free and total prostate-specific antigen levels for a group of adult men with bladder exstrophy. Although they were measurable, they were below the upper limits of established age-specific reference ranges for normal men. The vas deferens and ejaculatory ducts are normal in the exstrophy patient, provided they are not injured iatrogenically. Also, the mean seminal vesicle length in men with exstrophy was normal compared with published controls. Additional evaluation of the puborectalis muscle group was undertaken, and these muscles were found to be widely separated and provided lateral support of the prostate with a narrower puborectalis angle in those who were continent and had undergone prior iliac osteotomy.

Autonomic innervation of the corpus cavernosum is provided by the cavernous nerves. These autonomic nerves are displaced laterally in patients with exstrophy (Schlegel and Gearhart, 1989). These nerves are preserved in almost all exstrophy patients as potency is preserved after surgery.

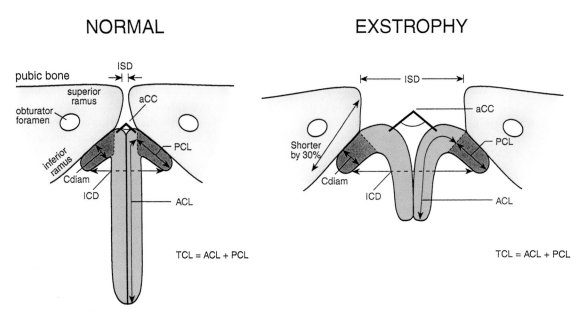

Figure 119–7. Separation of the pubic bones in men with classic exstrophy combined with the congenital deficiency of the anterior corporal tissue leads to the shorter appearance of the penis. aCC, corpora cavernosa sustended angle; ACL, anterior corporal length; Cdiam, corpus cavernosum diameter; ICD, intercorporal distance; ISD, intersymphyseal distance; PCL, posterior corporal length; TCL, total corporal length.

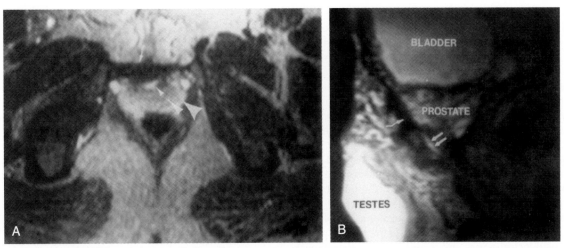

Figure 119–8. **A,** Axial T2-weighted image of the midprostate in a 20-year-old continent patient with bladder exstrophy. *Small arrowhead,* lumen of the urethra; *medium arrowhead,* transitional zone; *large arrowhead,* peripheral zone. *Curved arrow,* fibrous band of the intersymphyseal bar. **B,** Sagittal T2-weighted image through the midprostate gland shows anterior urethra *(double arrows)* and posterior prostate gland. Intersymphyseal fibrous band *(curved arrow)* extends along the entire length of the prostate.

However, retrograde ejaculation may occur after bladder closure and later bladder neck reconstruction.

Testis function has not been studied in a large group of postpubertal exstrophy patients, but it is generally believed that fertility is not impaired by testicular dysfunction. The testes frequently appear undescended in their course from the widened separated pubic tubercles to the flat, wide scrotum. Most testes are retractile and have an adequate length of spermatic cord to reach the scrotum without the need for orchiopexy.

Female Genital Defects

Reconstruction of the female genitalia presents a less complex problem than in the male (Fig. 119–9). **The vagina is shorter than normal, hardly greater than 6 cm in depth, but of normal caliber. The vaginal orifice is frequently stenotic and displaced anteriorly, the clitoris is bifid, and the labia, mons pubis, and clitoris are divergent. The uterus enters the vagina superiorly so that the cervix is in the anterior vaginal wall. The fallopian tubes and ovaries are normal.** The clitoral halves should be joined and the two ends of the labia minora joined to make a fourchette at the time of primary closure. Vaginal dilatation or episiotomy may be required to allow satisfactory intercourse in the mature female. The defective pelvic floor may predispose mature females to the development of uterine prolapse, making uterine suspension necessary. This usually occurs after childbirth but can occur in the nulliparous patient. When studied in a large adult female population, 10 of 56 women developed uterine prolapse at a mean age of 16 years. Six patients had been managed with reconstruction that included a posterior iliac osteotomy (Mathews et al, 2003a). Mean age at the time of osteotomy was 2.1 years. The use of the modern combined anterior innominate and vertical iliac osteotomy early in life may lead to reduction in the incidence of later prolapse.

Urinary Defects

At birth, the bladder mucosa may appear normal; however, ectopic bowel mucosa, or an isolated bowel loop, or more

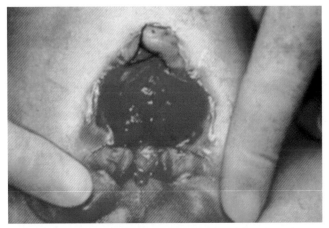

Figure 119–9. Newborn girl with classic bladder exstrophy. Notice the open urethral plate, bifid clitoral halves, and anterior displacement of the vaginal orifice.

commonly a hamartomatous polyp may be present on the bladder surface. If the bladder mucosa is not frequently irrigated with saline and protected from surface trauma by the interposition of some form of protective membrane before closure, cystic or metaplastic changes in the mucosal surface of the bladder may occur.

The size, distensibility, and neuromuscular function of the exstrophied bladder, as well as the size of the triangular fascial defect to which the bladder muscles attach, affect the decision to attempt repair. In the past several years, multiple basic science studies have been published that further delineate the exact nature of the exstrophied bladder in the newborn. **One of the first papers to characterize the neuromuscular function of the bladder was published by Shapiro and colleagues (1985). In their work, muscarinic cholinergic receptor density and binding affinity were measured in control subjects and in patients with classic bladder exstrophy. The density of the muscarinic cholinergic receptors in both the control and exstrophy groups were similar, as was the** binding affinity of the muscarinic receptor. Therefore, it was thought by the authors that the neurophysiologic composition of the exstrophied bladder is not grossly altered during its anomalous development. Studies have investigated both the neural innervation of the newborn exstrophy bladder and its muscle and collagen content. Lee and coworkers (1996) looked at bladder biopsies obtained from 12 newborns with bladder exstrophy, compared with age-matched controls, and found an increase in the ratio of collagen to smooth muscle in the newborns with bladder exstrophy. In addition, using anticollagen antibodies, they evaluated various types of collagen in these bladders. Compared with normal control bladders, there was no statistical difference in the amount of type I collagen in the bladders of newborns with exstrophy at initial closure, but there was a threefold increase in type III collagen. Peppas and associates (1999) found, in patients who gained adequate bladder capacities and were awaiting bladder neck reconstruction, that the ratio of collagen to smooth muscle decreased markedly after a successful closure and infection-free follow-up. Lais and coworkers (1996) reported similar findings, but they measured the ratio of smooth muscle to collagen and found it increased after a successful closure.

In an extension of the studies just cited, Mathews and coworkers (1999b) looked at the number of myelinated nerves per field in the newborn bladders of normal subjects and those with exstrophy. The average number of myelinated nerves per field was reduced in the exstrophy bladders compared with controls, and the difference was statistically significant. This reduction in nerve fibers appears to be the result of a lack of small fibers with preservation of larger nerve fibers. In light of the findings already mentioned, it is believed that bladder exstrophy in a newborn probably represents an earlier stage in bladder development.

In a large study by Rosch and colleagues (1997) **from Germany, multiple immunocytochemical and histochemical markers were examined in patients with epispadias or classic bladder exstrophy. These studies involved indirect immunocytochemistry for vasoactive intestinal polypeptide (VIP), neuropeptide Y (NPY), substance P (SP), calcitonin gene–related product (CGRP), protein gene product (PGP) 9.5, and nicotinamide adenine dinucleotide phosphate diaphorase (NADPHd). No evidence of bladder muscle dysinnervation was found morphologically in any cases of classic bladder exstrophy.** Cases of bladder exstrophy after failed reconstruction had muscle innervation deficiencies that increased subepithelial and intraepithelial innervation. Therefore, although a newborn with bladder exstrophy may have a maturational delay in bladder development, these bladders have the potential for normal development after a successful initial closure.

When the bladder is small, fibrosed, inelastic, and covered with polyps, functional repair may be impossible (Fig. 119–10). Novak and colleagues (2004) investigated the pathology and malignant potential of the polyps found in these small bladders. Two types of polyps were observed, with some overlap in findings: fibrotic and edematous. Both were associated with overlying squamous metaplasia in approximately 50% of cases. Varying degrees of von Brunn's nests, cystitis cystica, and cystitis glandularis were noted. Cystitis glandularis was noted in a higher percentage of secondary closures. Because of the potential risk of adenocarcinoma

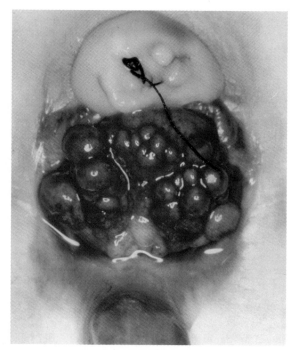

Figure 119–10. Small inelastic bladder template covered with polyps, unsuitable for primary closure.

associated with cystitis glandularis, future surveillance of these patients with urine cytology and cystoscopy as they enter adulthood is recommended. The more normal bladder may be invaginated, or it may bulge through a small fascial defect, indicating the potential for satisfactory capacity after successful initial closure. **Also, not until examination under anesthesia can the true defect be adequately evaluated because bladders that appear small in the nursery may have a good bit of bladder sequestered below the fascial defect. The depth of this extension often cannot be appreciated unless the infant is totally relaxed under anesthesia.**

Bladder function was assessed in a group of continent exstrophy patients with normal reflexive bladders. Normal cystometrograms were obtained in 70% to 90% of cases (Toguri et al, 1987). Diamond and associates (1999), looking at 30 patients with bladder exstrophy at various stages of reconstruction, found that 80% of patients had compliant and stable bladders before bladder neck reconstruction. After bladder neck reconstruction, approximately half of the patients maintained normal bladder compliance and a lesser number maintained normal stability. The authors believed that compliance and stability were impaired after bladder neck reconstruction and that 25% of patients with exstrophy may maintain normal detrusor function after reconstruction. In an earlier paper by Hollowell and colleagues (1993), 13 of 21 children revealed involuntary contractions and only 4 revealed stable bladders before bladder neck reconstruction. Also, 7 of 21 had increased pressures (greater than 10 cm H_2O), suggesting decreased compliance. The difference in findings between these two urodynamic studies is difficult to explain from an experimental perspective. However, standardized methods of bladder neck repair do not exist, and these differences may be reflected in the different urodynamic findings after bladder neck repair in these two groups of patients.

Several interesting aspects of the microstructure of the bladder in children with bladder exstrophy were noted by Mathews and coauthors (2004) using specimens obtained from children with bladder exstrophy at various stages of reconstruction (newborn bladder closure, bladder neck reconstruction, augmentation cystoplasty). At the cellular level, important differences were noted. Caveoli, which are important intracellular structures involved in cell-cell signaling, were found to be normal in the patients with a successful closure and improvement in bladder capacity and significantly lacking in the patients who required eventual augmentation cystoplasty (Fig. 119–11). In addition, the ultrastructure of cells in the patients in whom closure failed was noted to be abnormal.

The urinary tract is usually normal, but anomalous development does occur. Horseshoe kidney, pelvic kidney, hypoplastic kidney, solitary kidney, and dysplasia with megaureter are all encountered in these patients. The ureters have an abnormal course in their termination. The peritoneal pouch of Douglas between the bladder and the rectum is enlarged and unusually deep, forcing the ureter down laterally in its course across the true pelvis. The distal segment of the ureter approaches the bladder from a point inferior and lateral to the orifice, and it enters the bladder with little or no obliquity. **Therefore, reflux in the closed exstrophy bladder occurs in 100% of cases, and subsequent surgery is usually required at the time of bladder neck reconstruction. If excessive outlet resistance is gained at the time of either initial closure or combined epispadias and bladder exstrophy closure and recurrent infections are a problem even with suppressive antibiotics, ureteral reimplantation is required before bladder neck reconstruction.** Dilatation of the distal ureter frequently occurs on ultrasound and pyelogram studies and is a result of edema, infection, and fibrosis of the terminal ureter acquired after initial closure.

Prenatal Diagnosis

Currently, the prenatal diagnosis of bladder exstrophy is difficult to delineate. Often, a diagnosis of omphalocele or gastroschisis is made and the exstrophy condition is overlooked. Ultrasound evaluation of the fetus, by means of high-resolution real-time units, allows a thorough survey of the fetal anatomy, even during routine obstetric ultrasound examinations (Gearhart et al, 1995a). Several groups have outlined important criteria for the diagnosis of classic bladder exstrophy prenatally. In these reviews, the absence of a normal fluid-filled bladder on repeated examinations suggested the diagnosis, as did a mass of echogenic tissue on the lower abdominal wall (Mirk et al, 1986; Verco et al, 1986). **In a review of 25 prenatal ultrasound examinations with the subsequent birth of a newborn with classic bladder exstrophy** (Gearhart et al, 1995a), several observations were made: (1) absence of bladder filling, (2) a low-set umbilicus, (3) widening pubis ramus, (4) diminutive genitalia, and (5) a lower abdominal mass that increases in size as the pregnancy progresses and as the intra-abdominal viscera increases in size (Fig. 119–12).

The application of 3-D ultrasonography and fetal MRI has improved the antenatal diagnosis of bladder and cloacal exstrophy. The main reason for the prenatal diagnosis of bladder exstrophy is so that the parents can be counseled regarding the risks and benefits and other aspects of the condition. After appropriate counseling, arrangements can be made for delivery of the baby in a specialized exstrophy center where immediate reconstruction of the exstrophy can occur. Presentations from various centers have shown that the sooner the bladder is closed, the more likely it is that the bladder will grow and will not require augmentation. Delivery in a specialized exstrophy center allows the parents to be exposed to the expertise of multiple disciplines, including the

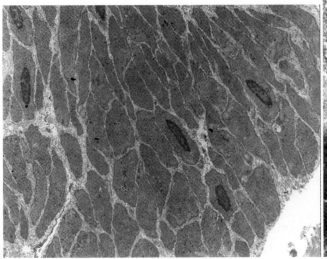
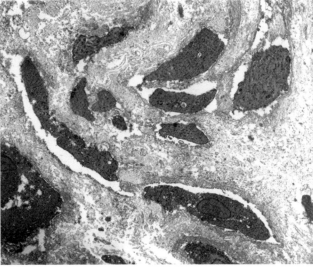

A   B

Figure 119–11. Ultrastructural changes noted in the exstrophic bladder. **A,** Normal muscle and nerve profiles in the newborn bladder. **B,** Following failure of prior closure, significant deterioration is noted with increased intercellular collagen and degenerating muscle and few nerve profiles. (From Mathews RI, Wills M, Perlman E, et al: Neural innervation of the newborn exstrophy bladder: An immunohistological study. J Urol 1999b;162:506.)

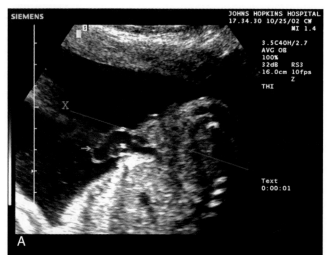

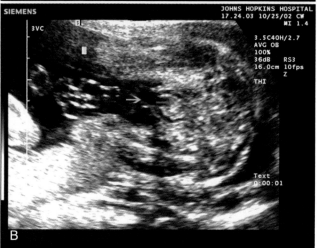

Figure 119–12. Prenatal ultrasound scan demonstrating bladder exstrophy. **A,** Longitudinal view showing the low-set umbilicus *(cyan arrow)*, lack of intra-abdominal bladder, and lower abdominal mass *(red arrow)*. **B,** Transverse view through the plane (X) in A shows presence of the umbilicus *(cyan arrow)* and the upper edge of the bladder plate that appears hyperechoic *(red arrow)*.

Jeffs et al, 1972; Williams and Keaton, 1973; Gearhart and Jeffs, 1989b). **Although this procedure was successful, it has been significantly modified to include bladder, abdominal wall closure, and urethral closure onto the penis in the newborn period with bilateral innominate and vertical iliac osteotomy, if indicated; epispadias repair at 6 months to 1 year of age; and bladder neck reconstruction along with antireflux procedure at age 4 to 5 years, when the child has achieved an adequate bladder capacity for bladder neck reconstruction and is motivated to participate in a postoperative voiding program** (Gearhart and Jeffs, 1998) (Table 119–1).

Other methods of treatment of the newborn with bladder exstrophy have been offered. Grady and Mitchell (1999) proposed combining bladder exstrophy closure with epispadias repair in the newborn period. Baka-Jakubiak (2000) recommended newborn exstrophy closure alone and combined bladder neck reconstruction and epispadias repair when the child reaches a satisfactory age for participation in a voiding program. Schrott and colleagues (1984) recommended bladder closure, ureteral reimplantation, epispadias repair, and bladder neck reconstruction in the newborn period. Lastly, Stein and coworkers (1999) recommended ureterosigmoidostomy in the newborn period with abdominal wall and bladder closure. This chapter deals mainly with the author's preference of the modern staged reconstruction of bladder exstrophy (MSRE), comparing the techniques and outcomes with the other repairs mentioned.

Evaluation and Management at Birth

At birth, although the bladder mucosa is usually smooth, pink, and intact, it is also sensitive and easily denuded. In the delivery room the umbilical cord should be tied with 2-0 silk close to the abdominal wall so that the umbilical clamp does not traumatize the delicate mucosa and cause excoriation of the bladder surface. The bladder can then be covered with a nonadherent film of plastic wrap (e.g., Saran Wrap) (Fig. 119–13) to prevent sticking of the bladder mucosa to clothing or diapers. In addition, each time the diaper is changed the

all-important psychological support these young parents need when a child with a birth defect of this magnitude is delivered.

SURGICAL RECONSTRUCTION OF BLADDER EXSTROPHY

Sweetser and associates (1952) initially described a staged surgical approach for bladder exstrophy. Four to 6 days before bladder closure, bilateral iliac osteotomies were performed. Epispadias repair was performed as a separate procedure. The continence procedure was limited to freeing the fibers from the intrasymphyseal band and wrapping this band around the urethra at the time of closure to increase outlet resistance.

The initial staged approach to functional bladder closure included three separate stages: bladder, abdominal wall, and posterior urethral closure; bladder neck reconstruction and antireflux procedure; and later epispadias repair. This approach was recommended for most cases of exstrophy reconstruction beginning in the early 1970s (Cendron, 1971;

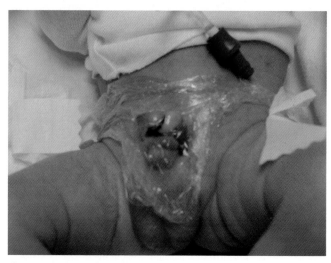

Figure 119–13. Use of plastic wrap to keep bladder plate moist prior to closure.

Table 119-1. Initial Presentation and Management of Exstrophy of the Bladder

Age	Problem	Possible Solution
Initial Presentation		
0-72 hr	Classic exstrophy with reasonable capacity and moderate symphyseal separation; long urethral groove; mild dorsal chordee.	I: Midline closure of bladder, fascia, and symphysis to level of posterior urethra; no osteotomy. In *very* select cases combined bladder closure and epispadias repair.
0-72 hr	Above-mentioned findings with short urethra and severe dorsal chordee.	II: Close as in I, adding lengthening of dorsal urethral groove by paraexstrophy skin (cautiously).
0-72 hr	Above-mentioned findings with very wide separation of symphysis or late presentation of patient (beyond 72 hr up to 1–3 yr) for initial treatment.	Osteotomy (combined anterior and vertical iliac) and closure as in I or II.
0-2 wk	Male, penis duplex or extremely short.	Consider female sex of rearing and closure as in I or II (very rare).
0-2 wk	Very small, nondistensible bladder patch.	Prove by examination under anesthesia, then nonoperative expectant treatment awaiting internal or external diversion or delayed closure if bladder plate grows.
Incontinent Period after Initial Closure		
1 mo-4 yr	Infection with residual resulting from outlet stenosis.	Urethral dilatation, occasional meatotomy or bladder neck revision.
	Infection, grade III reflux, with pliable outlet resistance.	Continuous antibiotic suppression with plan for early ureteroneocystostomy.
	Partial dehiscence at bladder neck or partial prolapse of bladder (both prevent bladder capacity increase).	Reclosure of bladder neck with osteotomy (with epispadias repair if older than 6 mo of life).
Epispadias Repair Continence		
6 mo-1 yr	Closed bladder with incontinence, normal ultrasound and good penile size and length of urethral groove.	Epispadias repair after preparation with testosterone.
	Epispadias penis, short with severe chordee, before bladder neck reconstruction.	Correction of chordee, lengthening of urethral groove, and epispadias repair, prepare with testosterone.
4-5 yr	Epispadias repair, capacity greater than 85 mL, child ready to be dry and be involved in voiding program.	Proceed to bladder neck plasty and ureteroneocystostomy.
4 yr or older	Completed repair of bladder, bladder neck, and epispadias with dry interval but wet pants.	Patience, biofeedback, oxybutynin chloride (Ditropan), imipramine, and time (up to 2 yr).
	Above-mentioned problems with marked stress incontinence and good bladder capacity.	Wait—may require bladder neck revision or endoscopic injection or possible artificial sphincter.
	Small-capacity bladder unchanged by time, epispadias repair, or attempted bladder neck reconstruction	Consider augmentation cystoplasty and bladder neck transection/reconstruction; acceptance of intermittent catheterization with abdominal or urethral access may be necessary.
4-7 yr	Late presentation of untreated exstrophy, unsuitable for closure.	Consider temporary diversion by colon conduit with plan to undivert to bladder using bladder to form urethra and conduit for augmentation; in patients older than 5 yr, artificial sphincter or continent diversion can be considered.
4-7 yr	Small closed exstrophy unsuitable for bladder neck reconstruction or augmentation.	Consider permanent external or internal diversion; internal diversion direct by ureterosigmoidostomy or indirect by colocolostomy; evaluate day continence of anal sphincter and nighttime seepage before surgery or continent neobladder.
5-15 yr	Closed exstrophy with epispadias repaired with uncontrolled stress or dribbling incontinence.	Consider (1) revision of bladder neck reconstruction, (2) endoscopic injection, (3) augmentation and bladder neck revision, (4) artificial sphincter with omental wrap, and (5) continent diversion.
10-20 yr	Closed bladder with inadequate penis.	Consider penile lengthening, urethral reconstruction using free graft, pedicle grafts, and tissue transfer.
10-20 yr	Diverted exstrophy with inadequate penis.	As above-mentioned recommendations or penile lengthening without urethral reconstruction (prostatic fistula at base).

plastic wrap should be removed, the bladder surface irrigated with sterile saline, and clean plastic wrap placed over the bladder surface area.

The distraught parents need reassurance at this stage. Counseling of the parents and decisions regarding eventual therapy should begin prenatally if the condition is diagnosed by prenatal ultrasonography. The parents should be educated by a surgeon with a special interest and experience in managing cases of bladder or cloacal exstrophy. An exstrophy support team should be available and should include a pediatric orthopedic surgeon, pediatric anesthesiologist, social workers, nurses with special interest in bladder exstrophy, and

a child psychiatrist with expertise and experience in genital anomalies. The Association of Bladder Exstrophy Children is available and has a website for parents and family members to obtain further information about the bladder exstrophy condition. In addition, should the parents desire, websites are available in some major exstrophy centers for further information.

Although it is true that parents need to be educated as fully as possible about the exstrophy condition, this is especially true regarding the sex of rearing in males with bladder exstrophy. We have seen several families who were made even more distraught by being told that their child had ambiguous genitalia in addition to bladder exstrophy and that the child would need a change of gender. The need for changing the sex of rearing in classic bladder exstrophy is almost nonexistent in the male infant.

Cardiopulmonary and general physical assessment measures can be carried out in the first few hours of life. Radionuclide scans and ultrasound studies can provide evidence of renal structure, function, and drainage, even in the first few hours of life before the patient undergoes closure of the exstrophy defect.

Circumstances may be less than ideal at birth. A thorough neonatal assessment may have to be deferred until transportation to a major children's medical center can be arranged. In these days of modern transportation, no child is ever more than a few hours away from a neonatal center with full diagnostic and consultative services. During travel the bladder should be protected by a plastic membrane, as in the nursery, to prevent damage to the delicate newborn bladder mucosa.

Selection of Patients for Immediate Closure

Successful treatment of exstrophy with functional closure demands that the potential for success in each child be carefully considered at birth. The size and the functional capacity of the detrusor muscle are important considerations for the eventual success of functional closure. Correlation between apparent bladder size and the potential bladder capacity must not be confused. In minor grades of exstrophy that approach the condition of complete epispadias with incontinence, the bladder may be small yet may demonstrate acceptable capacity, either by bulging when the baby cries or by indenting easily when touched by a sterile gloved finger in the operating room with the child under anesthesia. **Sometimes a good bit of previously unappreciated bladder can be discovered behind the fascia under examination with anesthesia** (Gearhart and Jeffs, 1998). Once the bladder is relieved of surface irritation and repeated trauma, the small bladder can enlarge and increase in capacity with the absence of sphincter activity and with minimal outlet resistance. The exstrophied bladder that is estimated at the time of birth to have a capacity of 5 mL or more and demonstrates elasticity and contractility can be expected to develop useful size and capacity after successful bladder, posterior urethral, and abdominal wall closure with early epispadias repair (Gearhart and Jeffs, 1998).

Modern Staged Reconstruction of Bladder Exstrophy

Over the past two decades, modifications in the management of functional bladder closure have contributed to a dramatic increase in the success of the procedure. **The most significant changes in the management of bladder exstrophy have been (1) early bladder, posterior urethral, and abdominal wall closure, usually with osteotomy; (2) early epispadias repair; (3) reconstruction of a continent bladder neck and reimplantation of the ureters; and, most important, (4) definition of strict criteria for the selection of patients suitable for this approach.** The primary objective in functional closure is to convert the bladder exstrophy into a complete epispadias with the urethra well onto the penis. The resultant inconti-

nence with balanced posterior outlet resistance not only preserves renal function but also stimulates bladder growth. Typically, epispadias repair is now performed between 6 months and 12 months of age, after testosterone stimulation. Bladder neck repair usually occurs when the child is 4 to 5 years of age, has an adequate bladder capacity, and, most important, is ready to participate in a postoperative voiding program.

Bladder, Urethral, and Abdominal Wall Closure

Various steps in primary bladder closure are illustrated in Figure 119-14. A strip of mucosa 2 cm wide, extending from the distal trigone to below the verumontanum in the male and to the vaginal orifice in the female, is outlined for prostatic and posterior urethral reconstruction in the male and adequate urethral closure in the female. The male urethral groove may be adequate, in which case no transverse incision of the urethral plate need be performed for urethral lengthening (see Fig. 119–14A). We tend not to incise a urethral plate unless the length of the urethral groove from the verumontanum to the urethral glans is so short that it interferes with eventual penile length and reduces dorsal angulation. If so, the urethral groove is lengthened after the manner of Johnston (1974) or Duckett (1977). The drawings in Figure 119–14B and C show marking of the incision just above the umbilicus, down the junction of the bladder and paraexstrophy skin, to the level of the urethral plate.

An appropriate plane is entered just above the umbilicus, and a plane is established between the rectus fascia and the bladder (see Fig. 119–14D). The umbilical vessels are doubly ligated and incised and allowed to fall into the pelvis. The peritoneum is taken off the dome of the bladder at this point so that the bladder can be placed deep into the pelvis at the time of closure. The plane is continued caudally down between the bladder and rectus fascia until the urogenital diaphragm fibers are encountered bilaterally. The pubis is encountered at this junction, and a double-pronged skin hook can be inserted into the bone at this time and pulled laterally to accentuate the urogenital diaphragm fibers and help the surgeon radically incise these fibers between the bladder neck, posterior urethra, and pubic bone (see Fig. 119–14E). Gentle traction on the glans at this point shows the insertion of the corporal body on the lateral inferior aspect of the pubis. These urogenital diaphragm fibers are taken down sharply with electrocautery down to the pelvic floor in their entirety (see Fig. 119–14F). If this maneuver is not performed adequately, the posterior urethra and bladder will not be placed deeply into the pelvis, and when the pubic bones are brought together, the posterior vesical unit will be brought anteriorly into an unsatisfactory position for later reconstruction.

If the decision is made at this point that the urethral groove is to be transected, the groove is cut distal to the verumontanum with continuity maintained between the thin, mucosal, non–hair-bearing skin adjacent to the posterior urethra and bladder neck and the skin and mucosa of the penile skin and glans. Flaps in the area of the thin skin are subsequently moved distally and rotated to reconstruct the urethral groove, resurfacing the penis dorsally. The corporal bodies are not brought together at this juncture because later

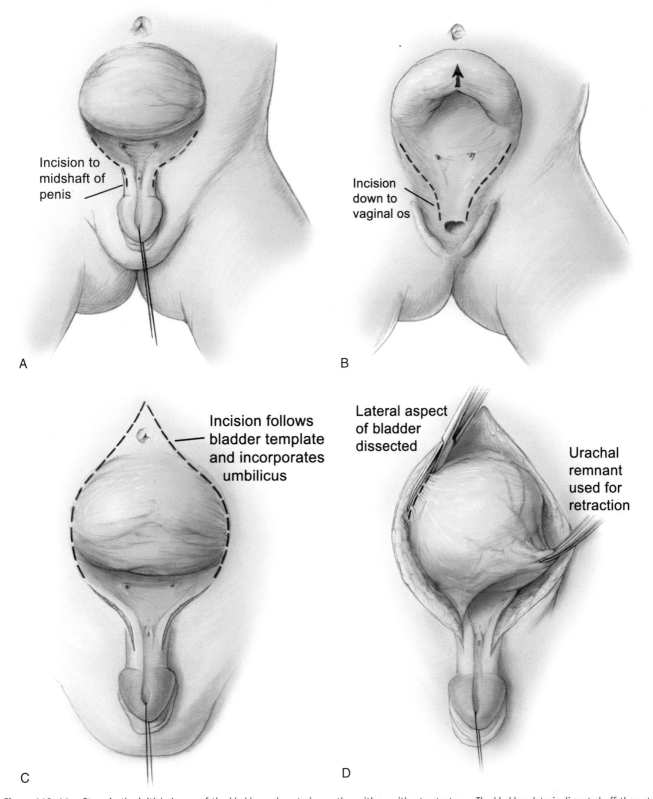

Figure 119–14. Steps in the initial closure of the bladder and posterior urethra with or without osteotomy. The bladder plate is dissected off the anterior abdominal wall. **A,** Initial incision around the bladder plate in the male. **B,** Initial incision around the bladder plate in the female. **C,** Incision follows the bladder template and includes the umbilicus. **D,** Dissection of the lateral aspect of the bladder from the abdominal wall. *Continued*

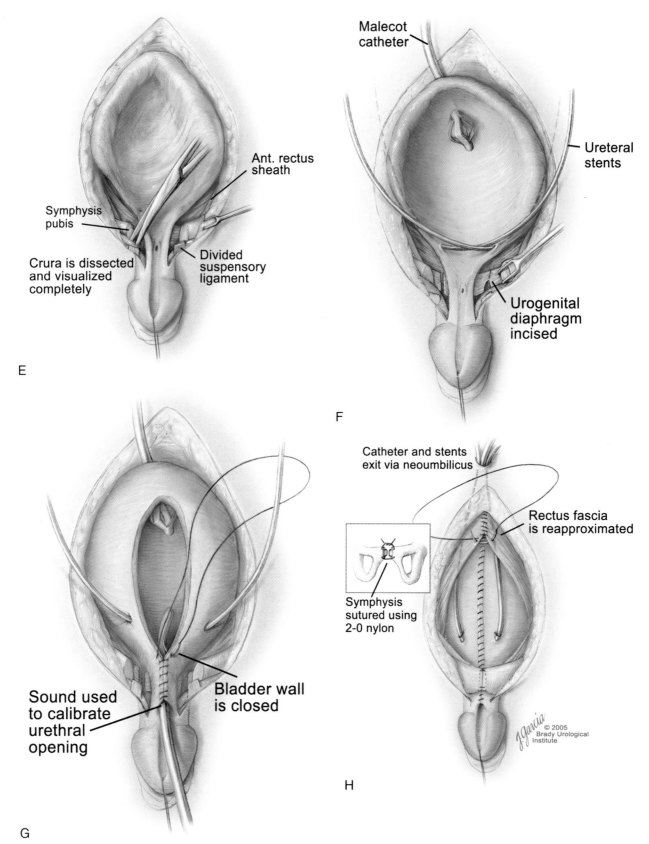

E, Dissection of the crura from the symphysis pubis.
- Symphysis pubis
- Ant. rectus sheath
- Crura is dissected and visualized completely
- Divided suspensory ligament

F
- Malecot catheter
- Ureteral stents
- Urogenital diaphragm incised

G
- Sound used to calibrate urethral opening
- Bladder wall is closed

H
- Catheter and stents exit via neoumbilicus
- Rectus fascia is reapproximated
- Symphysis sutured using 2-0 nylon

© 2005
Brady Urological Institute

Figure 119–14, cont'd. **E,** Dissection of the crura from the symphysis pubis. **F,** Division of the urogenital diaphragm fibers. Note stents and suprapubic tubes in place in the bladder. **G,** Initial layer of the bladder closure. Urethral meatus is calibrated to 14 Fr size. Stents are brought out of the bladder. **H,** Pubic approximation is performed with No. 2 nylon mattress suture (see inset). Abdominal wall closure is completed. Suprapubic tube and stents are brought out through the neoumbilicus.

Cantwell-Ransley epispadias repair will require the urethral plate to be brought beneath the corporal bodies. If the urethral plate is left in continuity, it must be mobilized up to the level of the prostate in order to create as much additional urethral and penile length as possible. Further urethral lengthening can be performed at the time of epispadias repair.

Penile lengthening is achieved by exposing the corpora cavernosa bilaterally and freeing the corpora from their attachments to the suspensory ligaments on the anterior part of the inferior pubic rami. **However, because Silver and colleagues (1997b) showed that there is a 50% shortage of length of the corporal bodies in exstrophy versus normal controls, any penile length that is obtained is more correction of chordee and change in angulation of the penis rather than true penile lengthening.** The wide band of fibers and muscular tissue representing the urogenital diaphragm is detached subperiosteally from the pubis bilaterally (see Fig. 119–14F). Reluctance to free the bladder neck and urethra well from the inferior ramus of the pubis moves the neobladder opening cephalad should any separation of the pubis occur during healing, thus increasing the chance of bladder prolapse. The mucosa and muscle of the bladder and urethra are then closed well onto the penis in the midline anteriorly (see Fig. 119–14G). This accommodates a No. 10 to 12 Fr sound comfortably. The size of the opening should allow enough resistance to aid in bladder adaptation and to prevent prolapse but not enough outlet resistance to cause upper tract changes. The posterior urethra and bladder neck are buttressed with a second layer of local tissue if possible. The bladder is drained by a suprapubic nonlatex Malecot catheter for a period of 4 weeks. The urethra is not stented in order to avoid necrosis with accumulation of secretions in the neourethra. Stents provide drainage during the first 10 to 14 days after closure as swelling caused by the pressure of closure of a small bladder can obstruct the ureters and give rise to obstruction and transient hypotension. If there are no problems with the stents during healing, we leave the stents in as long as 2 to 3 weeks.

When the bladder and urethra have been closed and the drainage tubes placed, pressure over the greater trochanters bilaterally allows the pubic bones to be approximated in the midline. Horizontal mattress sutures are placed in the pubis and tied with a knot away from the neourethra (see Fig. 119–14H). Often, we are able to use another stitch of No. 2 nylon at the most caudal insertion of the rectus fascia onto the pubic bone. This maneuver adds to the security of the pubic closure. A V-shaped flap of abdominal skin at a point corresponding to the normal position of the umbilicus is tacked down to the abdominal fascia, and a drainage tube exits this orifice. The method described by Hanna (1986) is our most commonly performed procedure. Before and during the procedure, the patient is given broad-spectrum antibiotics in an attempt to convert a contaminated field into a clean surgical wound. Nonreactive sutures of polyglycolic acid (Dexon/Vicryl) and nylon are used to avoid an undesirable stitch reaction or stitch abscess.

Osteotomy

Pelvic osteotomy performed at the time of initial closure confers several advantages, including (1) easy approximation of the symphysis with diminished tension on the abdominal wall closure and elimination of the need for fascial flaps; (2) placement of the urethra deep within the pelvic ring, enhancing bladder outlet resistance; and (3) bringing the large pelvic floor muscles near the midline, where they can support the bladder neck and aid in eventual urinary control** (Fig. 119–15). After pubic approximation with osteotomy, some patients show the ability to stop and start the urinary stream, experience dry intervals, and in some cases become completely continent (Gearhart and Jeffs, 1991a). In a review of a large number of patients referred to our institution after failed exstrophy procedures, it was found that a majority of the patients who had partial or complete dehiscence of the bladder or major bladder prolapse had not undergone a prior osteotomy at the time of initial bladder closure (Gearhart et al, 1993b). We recommend performing bilateral transverse innominate and vertical iliac osteotomy when bladder closure is performed after 72 hours of age (Fig. 119–16). In addition, if the pelvis is not malleable or if the pubic bones are more than 4 cm apart at the time of initial examination under anesthesia, osteotomy should be performed, even if closure is done before 72 hours of age. A well-coordinated surgery and anesthesia team can perform osteotomy and proceed to bladder closure without undue loss of blood or risk of prolonged anesthesia in the child. However, it must be realized that osteotomy together with posterior urethral and bladder closure and abdominal wall closure is a 5- to 7-hour procedure in these infants.

If the patient is less than 72 hours old and examination under anesthesia reveals that the pubic bones are malleable and able to be brought together easily in the midline by medial rotation of the greater trochanters, the patient can undergo closure without osteotomy. However, no chances should be taken with a decision of this magnitude. If there is any doubt, an osteotomy should be performed.

The most frequently used osteotomy today is the bilateral anterior innominate and vertical iliac osteotomy, popularized by Gearhart, Sponseller, and coworkers in 1996 (Gearhart et al, 1996b). This approach improves the ease of symphyseal approximation in the patient with exstrophy compared with posterior approaches, which require turning the patient. In our experience, this osteotomy is superior to the pubic mobilization seen with simple bilateral transverse anterior innominate osteotomy or even pubic ramotomy. With the ease of approximation obtained with this combined osteotomy, tension on the midline abdominal closure is lessened and the rates of bladder dehiscence and bladder prolapse are markedly decreased (Gearhart and Jeffs, 1998). In addition, pelvic closure allows approximation of the levator ani to strengthen the puborectalis sling, with positioning of the bladder neck and posterior urethra deep within the pelvic ring and improved continence rates. **Besides the ease of approximation, combined osteotomy was developed for three reasons: (1) osteotomy is performed with the patient in the supine position, as is the urologic repair, thereby avoiding the need to turn the patient; (2) the anterior approach to this osteotomy allows placement of an external fixator device and intrafragmentary pins under direct vision; and (3) the cosmetic appearance of this osteotomy is superior to that of the posterior iliac approach** (Gearhart et al, 1996b).

Although our experience with posterior iliac osteotomy is not associated with any failures after initial closure, the

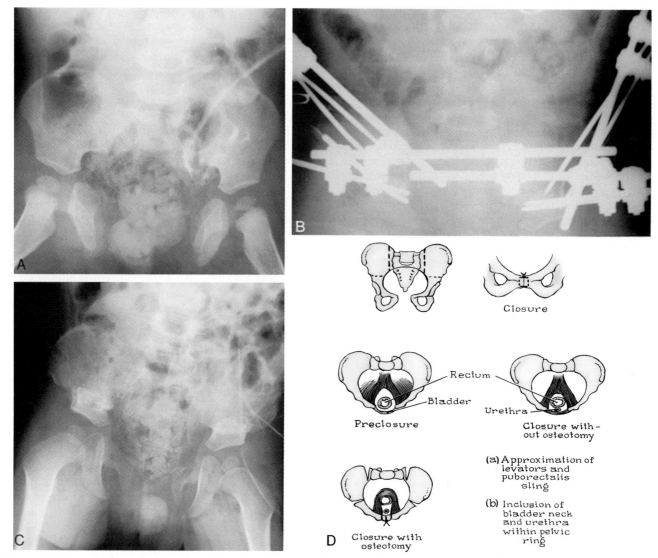

Figure 119–15. **A,** Eight-month-old patient with classic bladder exstrophy closed at birth without osteotomy with complete dehiscence. Patient was initially seen at 8 months of age. **B,** Patient after having undergone anterior innominate and vertical iliac osteotomy and placement of intrafragmentary pins and external fixator. **C,** The same patient 4 months after removal of external fixator and pins. Successful closure was achieved. **D,** The technique of combined osteotomy showing incision sites.

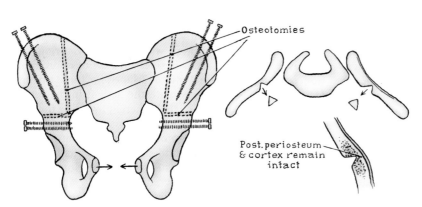

Figure 119–16. Depiction of the new combined transverse innominate and vertical iliac osteotomy indicating intrafragmentary pin placement sites and bone approximation.

mobility of the pubis was disappointing, there was occasional malunion of the ileum, the blood loss was greater in the posterior approach, and, most important, the need to turn the patient intraoperatively from the prone to the supine position was always worrisome. Initially, the experience with osteotomy was in patients who had failed to benefit from initial exstrophy closure with or without iliac osteotomy or pubic ramotomy (Sponseller et al, 1991). The results of the new approach with combined horizontal transverse innominate osteotomy and vertical iliac osteotomy were so satisfactory that the approach is now being used in all primary closures of bladder exstrophy that require pelvic osteotomy (Gearhart et al, 1996b).

Combined osteotomy is performed by placing the patient in the supine position, preparing and draping the lower body below the costal margins, and placing soft absorbent gauze over the exposed bladder. The pelvis is exposed from the iliac wings inferiorly to the pectineal tubercle and posteriorly to the sacroiliac joints. The periosteum and sciatic notch are carefully elevated, and a Gigli saw is used to create a transverse innominate osteotomy exiting anteriorly at a point halfway between the anterior-superior and anterior-inferior spines (see Fig. 119–16). This osteotomy is created at a slightly more cranial level than that described for a Salter osteotomy in order to allow placement of external fixator pins in the distal segments. In addition to the transverse osteotomy, the posterior ileum may be incised from the anterior approach in an effort to correct the deformity more completely. This is important because anatomic studies have shown that the posterior portion of the pelvis is also externally rotated in patients with exstrophy, and as patients age they lose elasticity of the sacroiliac ligaments. For this part of the osteotomy, an osteotome is used to create a closing wedge osteotomy vertically and just lateral to the sacroiliac joints. The proximal posterior iliac cortex is left intact and used as a hinge (see Fig. 119–16). This combination osteotomy easily corrects the abnormalities in both the anterior and posterior segments of the pelvis.

Two fixator pins are placed in inferior osteotomized segment, and two are placed in the wing of the ileum superiorly. Radiographs are obtained to confirm pin placement, soft tissues are closed, and the urologic procedure is performed

(see Fig. 119–15). At the end of the procedure, the pelvis is closed with a suture between the two pubic rami. The external fixators are then applied between the pins to hold the pelvis in a correct position. In a newborn with less than optimal amounts of cancellous bone, only one pin is placed inferiorly and superiorly in the wing of the ileum, whereas older children have two pins in each bone wing.

Radiographs are taken 7 to 10 days after surgery to look for complete reduction of the symphyseal diastasis. If this diastasis has not been completely reduced, the right and left sides can be gradually approximated by means of the fixator bars over several days. Longitudinal skin traction is used to keep the legs still (Fig. 119–17). The patient remains supine in traction for approximately 4 weeks to prevent dislodgement of tubes and destabilization of the pelvis. The external fixator is kept on for 4 to 6 weeks, until adequate callus is seen at the site of the osteotomy (see Fig. 119–15B and C). Postoperatively, in newborns who undergo closure without osteotomy in the first 48 to 72 hours of life, the baby is immobilized in modified Bryant's traction in a position in which the hips have 90 degrees of flexion. When modified Bryant's traction is used, the traction is employed for 4 weeks (Fig. 119–18). A horizontal mattress suture of No. 2 nylon is placed between the fibrous cartilage of the pubic rami and tied anteriorly to the pubic closure at the time of bladder closure. **Evidence obtained by Sussman and associates (1997) from biomechanical testing in an intact piglet pelvic model revealed that all methods of pubic approximation were weak compared with the intact symphysis. However, the best technique with the strongest load-to-failure ratio was a No. 2 nylon horizontal mattress suture.** Should this suture work loose or cut through the tissues during healing, the anterior placement of a knot in the horizontal mattress suture ensures that it will not erode into the urethra and interfere with the bladder or urethral lumen.

Complications of Osteotomy and Immobilization Techniques

Complications of immobilization can include failure of the closure and skin breakdown with resultant ulceration.

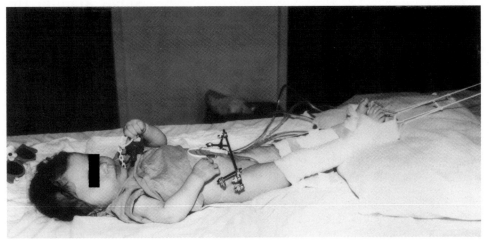

Figure 119–17. Fifteen-month-old patient following reclosure of bladder exstrophy with external fixator in place and modified Buck's traction.

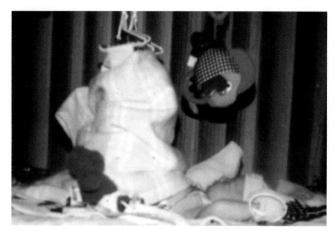

Figure 119–18. Newborn closure without osteotomy with patient in modified Bryant's traction.

Meldrum and colleagues (2003) reviewed a series of 86 patients in whom initial exstrophy closure failed. Most had been immobilized with a "mummy wrap" or spica cast. Successful closure was noted in 97% of those immobilized with an external fixator and modified Buck's traction. In addition, in those failing initial closure, six had severe skin ulcerations from the mummy wrapping or spica cast, and two of these children required later skin grafting.

Sponseller and colleagues (2001) reported on a total of 86 combined bilateral anterior innominate and vertical iliac osteotomies performed in 88 children. Ten of these children had cloacal exstrophy, and 72 had bladder exstrophy with at least 2 years of clinical follow-up (mean 4.8 years). Complications included seven cases of transient left femoral nerve palsy, which resolved fully by 12 weeks after surgery. There were no cases of right femoral nerve palsy, although the same surgeon performed the same technique on both sides. Patients with transient femoral nerve palsy were at bed rest for the first 6 to 8 weeks; a knee immobilizer was needed for the remaining 6 weeks until resolution. Other complications included three cases with delayed ileal union, one case of superficial infection of the ileal femoral incision that required irrigation and débridement, one case of transient right thigh abductor weakness, one infection of the ileum around a pin site requiring irrigation and débridement, and one case of transient right peroneal palsy. Almost all patients had skin inflammation around the pins, particularly those in the proximal (iliac crest) segments. This was always controlled with the use of oral antibiotics. One child with classic exstrophy had bladder prolapse after primary bladder closure and combined osteotomies. Another child with classic exstrophy developed wound dehiscence after primary closure and pelvic osteotomy secondary to a respiratory virus and severe associated respiratory distress. In addition, data of Nelson and coworkers (2005) indicate that bilateral innominate and posterior iliac osteotomy can be safely performed in children who have had prior osteotomies for reconstruction.

Whichever type of osteotomy is used, pelvic ring closure not only allows midline approximation of the abdominal wall structures but also allows the levator ani and puborectalis muscles to lend potential support to the bladder outlet, thus increasing resistance to urinary outflow (see Fig. 119–15D)

(Sponseller et al, 1991; Gearhart et al, 1993b, 1996b; Schmidt et al, 1993; McKenna et al, 1994). Furthermore, a continence procedure can be performed later on the bladder neck and urethra deep within the closed pelvic ring at a distance from the surface without independent movement of the two halves of the pubis. The urethra and bladder neck are set more deeply in the true pelvis, in a more normal relationship than when acutely angulated.

When good callus formation is seen on radiography, the fixating device and pins are removed with the patient under light sedation. The age of the patient plays a role in the amount of correction of the diastasis that is maintained over time. On review of the previously described types of osteotomy, both classic and cloacal exstrophy patients gained approximation, although the former group gained greater correction toward normal (Gearhart et al, 1996b). Greater postoperative diastasis as well as less optimal bone density in the newborn contributes to the greater difficulty in obtaining and maintaining closure of the pelvic bone deformity over time.

It is our impression that partial recurrence of diastasis in classic exstrophy occurs by two mechanisms. First, the pelvis may partially derotate owing to early loosening of pins before the time of osteotomy healing; this is seen mostly in infants. In the older child, increased bone density allows more rigid external fixation and thus better maintenance of the corrected position. Second, there is long-term undergrowth of the ischiopubic segment, which has been shown to be 33% smaller than normal in the adult with exstrophy, as the pelvis grows. Pubic diastasis increases with growth in the patient with uncorrected exstrophy. Therefore, even with some loss of approximation, significant correction remains in comparison to the unoperated state. We regard the main role of osteotomy to be relaxation of tension on the bladder, posterior urethra, and abdominal wall repair during healing. Therefore, we use osteotomy rarely in newborns and young infants because ligament laxity allows the pelvis to be closed without tension. However, it becomes essential in the older child with a failed exstrophy repair, in the patient with cloacal exstrophy, and in a newborn with a wide diastasis and excellent bladder template. **In patients undergoing combined exstrophy closure and epispadias repair, osteotomy allows the pubis to be joined, making it easier for the corpora to be brought over the closed proximal urethra** (Gearhart et al, 1998).

Small Bladder Unsuitable for Closure

A small, fibrotic bladder patch that is stretched between the edges of the small triangular fascial defect without elasticity or contractility cannot be selected for the usual closure procedure (Gearhart and Jeffs, 1998) (see Fig. 119–10). **Examination with the patient under anesthesia may at times be required to assess the bladder adequately, particularly if considerable edema, excoriation, and polyp formation have developed between birth and the time of assessment. Decisions regarding the suitability of bladder closure or the need for waiting should be made only by surgeons with a great deal of experience in the exstrophy condition** (Gearhart and Jeffs, 1998). Neonatal closure, even when the bladder is small, can allow assessment of bladder potential, provides an initial step in genital reconstruction, and is helpful in reassuring the family. Some conditions preclude primary closure, including penoscrotal duplication, ectopic bowel within the extruded bladder (a relative contraindication), a hypoplastic bladder, and significant bilateral hydronephrosis.

In a review by Dodson and associates (2001) of cases at our institution, it was found on initial judgment that the bladder was too small for closure in 20 patients evaluated at birth. After a period of time when the bladder had grown sufficiently, closure was undertaken. Long-term follow-up revealed that 50% of these patients were dry after bladder neck reconstruction and 50% required other adjunctive procedures. **Ideally, waiting for the bladder template to grow for 4 to 6 months in the child with a small bladder is not as risky as submitting a small bladder template to closure in an inappropriate setting, resulting in dehiscence and allowing the fate of the bladder to be sealed at that point.** If the bladder does not grow to sufficient size after 4 to 6 months, other options include excision of the bladder and a nonrefluxing colon conduit or ureterosigmoidostomy. Another alternative involves urinary diversion with a colon conduit and placing the small bladder inside to be used later for the posterior urethra in an Arap-type procedure. Lastly, if the bladder is small and the presentation is for late primary closure, bladder augmentation, ureteral reimplantation, and an outlet procedure, in addition to a continent urinary stoma, can be considered.

OTHER MODERN APPROACHES TO EXSTROPHY RECONSTRUCTION

Although the modern staged repair of exstrophy (MSRE) currently enjoys widespread popularity, other methods have been described for the primary reconstruction of exstrophy. This section describes some of these reconstructive methods and their application in children with exstrophy.

Warsaw Approach

First described by Baka-Jakubiak in 2000, this procedure involved closing the bladder posterior urethra, pubis, and abdominal wall at the time of primary closure with or without osteotomy but always with appropriate immobilization. When the bladder had achieved suitable capacity (more than 70 mL) and the child was interested in continence, bladder neck repair was performed along with epispadias repair. Baka-Jakubiak has used this approach in 73 boys with classic exstrophy and complete epispadias. The intersymphyseal band is routinely divided to allow better visualization of the bladder neck and posterior urethra region. An additional proposed benefit of this procedure is that the bladder neck and posterior urethral unit is straighter at the second procedure and this allows easier catheterization and cystoscopy following reconstruction. A 10% complication rate, mainly urethral fistula or stricture, was noted in this procedure.

Surer and colleagues (2001b) published a series of 19 patients using this methodology (17 boys with exstrophy and 2 with complete epispadias). All of these patients were referred at an older age following initial bladder closure at another institution, and many had an osteotomy at the initial reconstruction. A modified Cantwell-Ransley repair was the technique used for epispadias reconstruction (see later) and a

modified Young-Dees-Leadbetter bladder neck reconstruction. Urethrocutaneous fistula was the main complication noted in 8%, and dorsal chordee persisted in three patients, requiring reoperation.

Erlangen Approach

This approach is clearly the most involved of any of the primary closure techniques. Not only is bladder closure performed, but the ureters are reimplanted. In addition, bilateral "wings" of detrusor are rolled together as a bladder neck and the bladder above this is closed. The epispadias repair is performed at the same time, and the pelvic girdle is brought together followed by abdominal wall closure. This method is truly a "complete repair" as it accomplishes all of the facets of exstrophy reconstruction in a single procedure. Surgical repair is, however, performed at 8 to 10 weeks of age, when the infant is larger and has had the opportunity to be medically stabilized (Rosch et al, 2001).

Seattle Approach (Complete Repair)

Developed by Mitchell, the complete repair combines the standard bladder closure with the "penile disassembly" technique for epispadias repair in an effort to decrease the number of procedures required for reconstruction and potentially provide continence without the need for formal bladder neck reconstruction (Grady and Mitchell, 1999). The urethral plate is dissected from the corporal bodies and the urethra and the bladder plate are moved posteriorly into the pelvis. Mitchell emphasizes the importance of dissecting the perineal membrane from the pubis, allowing the bladder and posterior urethra to be set deep into the pelvis. This feature is common to all properly performed exstrophy reconstructions but was not emphasized in prior descriptions. The dissection of the urethral plate from the corpora leaves 60% to 75% of patients with hypospadias (Hafez et al, 2004), and 50% of children require ureteral reimplantation in the first year of life (Grady and Mitchell, 1999).

Combined Bladder Closure and Epispadias Repair

The modern staged repair of bladder exstrophy has yielded consistently good cosmetic and functional results, and the utilization of osteotomy has improved the potential for successful initial closure and later continence. **In an effort to decrease costs, decrease the morbidity associated with multiple operative procedures, and possibly affect continence, there has been interest in performing single-stage reconstruction or combining procedures in appropriately selected patients.** This technique was first described by Lattimer (1960) but was abandoned in the 1970s because of high complication and failure rates. The technique was revisited by Gearhart and Jeffs (1991a) for failed exstrophy closures and more recently by Grady and Mitchell for newborn patients (1999). In the combined exstrophy and epispadias repair, bladder closure is combined with the modified Cantwell-Ransley epispadias repair (Gearhart et al, 1998; Baird et al, 2004). This technique can be applied to both delayed primary closure and failed closures.

As with the complete repair, many require early ureteral reimplantation, but none were made hypospadiac.

Results have now emerged in groups of boys undergoing single-stage reconstruction (bladder closure and epispadias repair) in infancy (Gearhart et al, 1998; Baird et al, 2004). In our opinion, this technique should be limited to boys of older age (older than 4 to 6 months) because of evidence indicating that potential complication of these combined procedures is significant loss of penile and corporal tissue that makes further reconstruction problematic (Husmann et al, 2004). Patients should be carefully selected, and utilization of these extensive procedures by the occasional exstrophy surgeon is not recommended. **Selection should take into account phallic size and length, depth of the urethral groove, and size of the bladder template in those with delayed primary closures, as well as perivesical and urethral scarring in those who have undergone a prior failed closure** (Gearhart and Jeffs, 1991; Gearhart et al, 1998; Baird et al, 2004).

Management after Primary Closure

The initial step of the MSRE converts a patient with exstrophy into one with complete epispadias and incontinence. **Before removal of the suprapubic tube, 4 weeks after surgery, the bladder outlet is calibrated by a urethral catheter or a urethral sound to ensure free drainage. A complete ultrasound examination is obtained to ascertain the status of the renal pelves and ureters, and appropriate urinary antibiotics are administered as all patients have reflux after closure.** Residual urine is estimated by clamping the suprapubic tube, and specimens for culture are obtained before the patient leaves the hospital and at subsequent intervals to detect infection and ensure that the bladder is empty. If the initial ultrasound examination shows good drainage, upper tract imaging by ultrasonography is repeated 3 months after discharge from the hospital and at intervals of 6 months to 1 year during the next 2 to 3 years to detect any upper tract changes caused by reflux, infection, or obstruction. Prophylactic antibiotics should be continuous because all patients with bladder exstrophy, once closed, have vesicoureteral reflux. If a useful continence interval has resulted from the initial closure, a further operation for incontinence may not be required; however, this situation is quite unusual. In our experience with more than 85 primary closures, this has occurred in three patients, all of whom were girls. After the conversion from exstrophy to complete epispadias with incontinence, the bladder gradually increases in capacity as inflammatory changes in the mucosa resolve.

Cystoscopy and cystography at yearly intervals are used to evaluate the degree of reflux noted in almost 100% of patients and to provide an estimate of bladder capacity (Gearhart and Jeffs, 1998). Even in a completely incontinent patient, bladder capacity gradually increases to a point at which the bladder can be distended at cystography to its true capacity. This must be done under anesthesia in young children because the values obtained differ markedly from those obtained when trying to fill the bladder of a crying, squirming infant on an x-ray table (Gearhart and Jeffs, 1998). If the bladder has not achieved a capacity of at least 30 mL by 1 to 2 years, concern must be voiced to the parents about the overall ability of the bladder to undergo a continence proce-

dure. Currently, the only parameters available to predict overall success are the size of the bladder template at birth and a successful primary closure with absence of infections.

Should bladder outlet resistance be such that urine is retained within the bladder and reflux and ureteral dilatation develop with infected urine, it may be necessary to dilate the urethra or to begin intermittent catheterization (Baker et al, 1999). Sometimes the posterior urethral obstruction can be such that it requires a transurethral incision of the stricture to maintain an adequate posterior urethral outlet. If bladder outlet resistance persists and infections continue, an antireflux procedure may be required as early as 6 months to 1 year after initial closure (Mathews and Gearhart, 2001). If severe upper tract changes occur, surgical revision of the bladder outlet by advancing skin flaps into the orifice or even patching the stricture may be necessary to prevent scarring and further obstruction. As mentioned previously, transurethral incision of the urethral stricture to obtain a balanced outlet should be tried before surgical revision. Judgment is required to know when to avoid attempts at functional closure and to know when to return to urinary diversion as a means to preserve renal function. This change of plan is seldom necessary if an adequate outlet has been constructed at the initial closure and if careful attention has been paid to the details of follow-up of the bladder and posterior urethra. An important caveat is that if there are recurrent urinary tract infections and if the bladder is distended on ultrasonography, cystoscopy should be performed and the posterior urethra should be carefully examined anteriorly for erosion of the intrapubic stitch, which may be the cause of the recurrent infections (Baker et al, 1999). If the intrapubic stitch is seen in the posterior urethra, a small suprapubic incision should be made and the stitch should be removed, or, if it can be grasped, it should be removed transurethrally. Husmann and colleagues (1990) have shown very acceptable levels of upper tract function after primary closure as long as prophylactic antibiotics were used after initial closure and elevated urinary residuals were kept below 50 mL.

Penile and Urethral Closure in Exstrophy

Epispadias Repair

Historically, bladder neck reconstruction was performed before penile and urethral reconstruction. However, an increase in bladder capacity in patients with extremely small bladder capacities after epispadias repair prompted a change in the management program (Gearhart and Jeffs, 1989a) (Fig. 119–19). In a group of patients with a small bladder capacity after initial closure, there was a mean increase of 55 mL in males in only 22 months after epispadias repair. However, with MSRE, the epispadias repair is now performed at about 6 months of age in all patients. With this modification, possibly all patients can achieve an appropriate capacity at the time when they are ready physically and mentally to undergo bladder neck reconstruction. Because most boys with exstrophy have a somewhat small penis and a shortage of available penile skin, all patients undergo testosterone stimulation before urethroplasty and penile reconstruction (Gearhart and Jeffs, 1987).

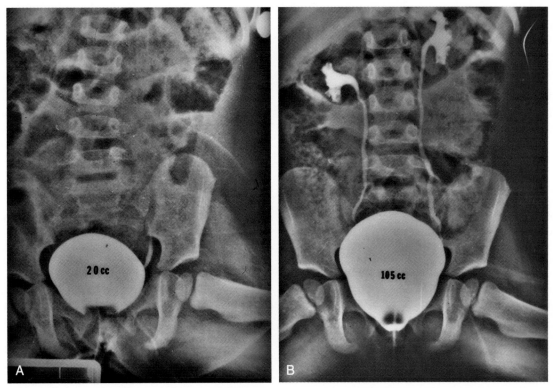

Figure 119–19. **A,** Initial cystogram under anesthesia showing small bladder capacity after bladder closure. **B,** Improvement in bladder capacity noted following urethroplasty.

Many techniques have been described for reconstruction of the penis and urethra in patients with classic bladder exstrophy. Current methods of epispadias repair in bladder exstrophy are the Cantwell-Ransley repair (1989), the modified Cantwell-Ransley repair (1992, 1995), and the penile disassembly technique described by Mitchell and Bagli (1996) (Ransley et al, 1989; Gearhart et al, 1992, 1995c; Mitchell and Bagli, 1996).

Regardless of the surgical technique chosen for reconstruction of the penis in bladder exstrophy, four key concerns must be addressed to ensure a functional and cosmetically pleasing penis. These concerns are (1) correction of dorsal chordee, (2) urethral reconstruction, (3) glandular reconstruction, and (4) penile skin closure.

Although it is possible to achieve some penile lengthening with release of chordee at the time of initial closure, it is often necessary to perform formal penile elongation with release of chordee at the time of urethroplasty in exstrophy patients. Data of Silver and associates (1997b) clearly showed that this is more an apparent lengthening of the penis than a true lengthening because the anterior corporal bodies in exstrophy patients have 50% less length than those of age-matched controls in adult life. Certainly, all remnants of the suspensory ligaments and old scar tissue from the initial bladder closure must be excised. Also, further dissection of the corpora cavernosa from the inferior pubic ramus can be achieved. It is often surprising how little is accomplished in freeing the corporal bodies from the pubis at the time of initial exstrophy closure (Gearhart, 1991).

Lengthening of the urethral groove is also essential. Whether or not paraexstrophy skin flaps are used at the time of bladder closure, further lengthening is needed. This can range from something as simple as Cantwell's original procedure to transection of the urethral plate and replacement of the genital tissue. However, in modern techniques of epispadias repair, replacement of the urethra is not typically performed. In the penile disassembly technique described by Mitchell and Bagli (1996), the urethral plate is dissected completely from the glans; in over 70% of patients it is not long enough to reach the tip of the penis and as a result hypospadias is present with further reconstruction needed at another setting (Hafez et al, 2004). **We believe that because of the marked length disparity in male children with exstrophy compared with normal males, complete detachment of the urethra from the glans is an unnecessary step in light of the small amount of length that is obtained with this maneuver and the near certainty of creating hypospadias, which requires an additional surgical procedure.**

Chordee

Besides lengthening of the urethral groove, dorsal chordee must be addressed. To release dorsal chordee, one may lengthen the dorsomedial aspect of the corpora by incision and anastomosis of the corpora themselves (Gearhart et al, 1992). Also, length can be gained by placement of a dermal graft to allow lengthening of the dorsal aspect of the corpora (Woodhouse, 1986). Another technique to improve dorsal chordee before urethroplasty is shortening or medial rotation of the ventral corpora (Koff and Eakins, 1984). However, most of these techniques, especially grafting, are reserved for patients who are seen in adolescent and adult years for epispadias surgery with the need for some increased penile length and correction of residual chordee.

Urethral Reconstruction

Urethral reconstruction is an important aspect of external genital reconstruction in exstrophy. This can be accomplished by many previously reported methods. Tubularization of the dorsal urethral groove as a modified Young urethroplasty has been abandoned in our practice because of the high incidence of urethrocutaneous fistula and the less than optimal cosmetic appearance of the penis (Lepor et al, 1984). In the past, interposition of a free graft of genital or extragenital skin, or even bladder mucosa, has been used (Hendren, 1979). In addition, ventral transverse island flaps and double-faced island flaps have been used with some success for urethral reconstruction in exstrophy patients (Thomalla and Mitchell, 1984; Monfort et al, 1987). However, modern techniques of epispadias repair associated with bladder exstrophy utilize tubularization of the urethral plate, moving the urethral plate under the corporal bodies after closure to lessen the incidence of urethrocutaneous fistula and also to give the penis a more downward deflection and more easily catheterizable urethral channel (Surer et al, 2001a).

Penile Skin Closure

If skin closure continues to be a problem in genital reconstruction, owing to the paucity of skin associated with this condition, a Z-plasty incision and closure at the base of the penis prevents skin contraction and upward tethering of the penis. The ventral foreskin can be split in the midline and brought to the dorsum as lateral preputial flaps for coverage of the penile shaft. If the flaps are a bit asymmetrical, a staggered dorsal suture line results, with less upward tethering. Alternatively, a buttonhole can be created in the ventral foreskin and simply transposed to the dorsum for additional penile skin coverage.

Modified Cantwell-Ransley Repair

Our preference for urethroplasty and penile reconstruction, if the urethral groove has adequate length, is the modified Cantwell-Ransley repair (Gearhart et al, 1992, 1995c, 2004) (Fig. 119–20). Currently, in the modern applications of the staged reconstruction of bladder exstrophy, epispadias repair is performed when the child is 6 months to 1 year of age. The modified Cantwell-Ransley procedure is begun by placing an island stitch through the glans as a traction stitch. Incisions are made over two parallel lines marked previously on the dorsum of the penis that outline an 18-mm-wide strip of urethral mucosa, extending from the prostatic urethral meatus to the tip of the penis (see Fig. 119–20A). For this procedure, a deep vertical incision is made in the urethral plate distally. The incision is then closed with 6-0 polyglycolic sutures in a transverse fashion (see Fig. 119–20B to D). This procedure flattens the distal urethral plate and advances the urethra to the tip of the phallus so that it will be in excellent glandular position when the glandular wings are closed over the reconstructed urethra. Glandular mucosal areas of the dorsal glans are excised adjacent to the urethral strip and thick glandar flaps are constructed bilaterally (Fig. 119–20F). Lateral skin flaps are mobilized and undermined. A Z-incision of the suprapubic area permits wide exposure and division of the suspensory ligaments and old scar tissue from initial exstrophy closure (Fig. 119–20F).

Ventral penile skin is taken down to the level of the scrotum (see Fig. 119–20E). Care is taken to preserve the mesentery to

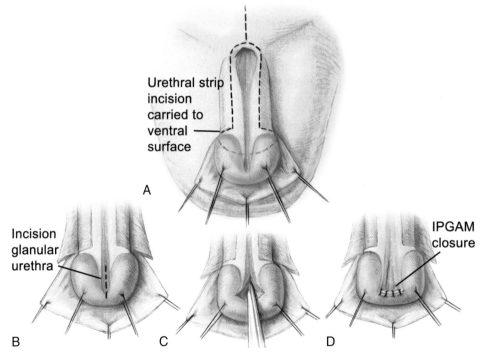

Urethral strip incision carried to ventral surface

A

Incision glanular urethra

B

C

IPGAM closure

D

Figure 119–20. Modified Cantwell-Ransley epispadias repair. **A,** Initial incision line extending around the urethral plate and the coronal sulcus. **B** to **D,** Performance of the IPGAM procedure to bring the urethral meatus to the tip of the glans. *Continued*

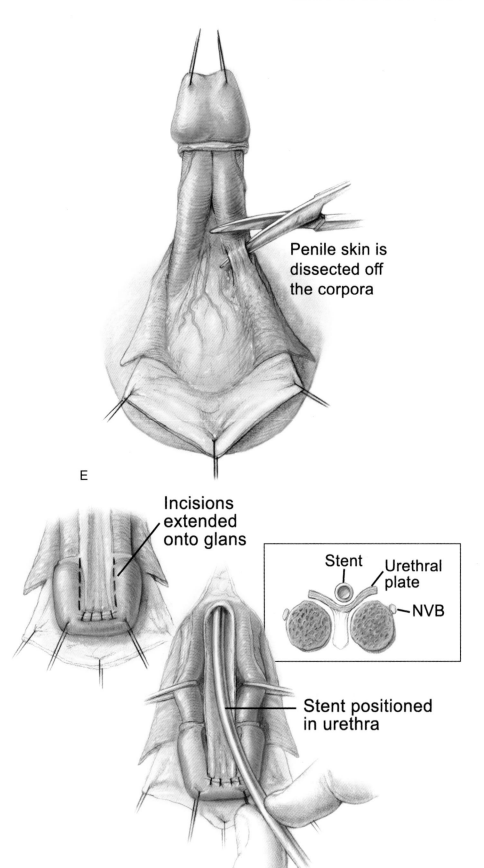

Figure 119–20, cont'd. **E,** Dissection of the foreskin on the ventral aspect of the penis. **F,** The corpora are dissected off the urethral plate and parallel incisions made into the glans to create glans wings. Note the lateral position of the neurovascular bundles (inset).

Continued

Penile skin is dissected off the corpora

E

Incisions extended onto glans

Stent

Urethral plate

NVB

Stent positioned in urethra

F

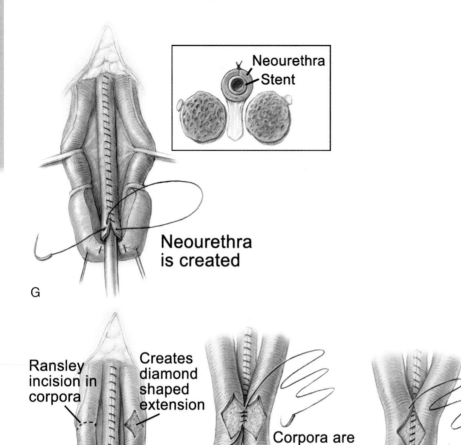

G

Neourethra
Stent

**Neourethra
is created**

Ransley
incision in
corpora

Creates
diamond
shaped
extension

**Corpora are
sutured in the
midline**

**Resulting in extended
corporal length and
ventral displacement
of neourethra**

H

Figure 119–20, cont'd. **G,** The urethra is tabularized using a continuous running suture. **H,** Approximation of the corpora using the incisions in the corpora if indicated. **I,** Corpora approximated above the urethra to provide an anatomically ventral location of the urethra (see inset). **J,** Glans is reconstructed in two layers. *Continued*

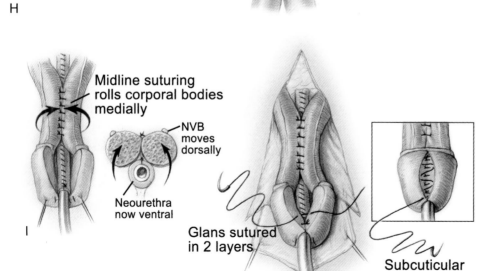

**Midline suturing
rolls corporal bodies
medially**

NVB
moves
dorsally

Neourethra
now ventral

I

**Glans sutured
in 2 layers**

**Subcuticular
closure**

J

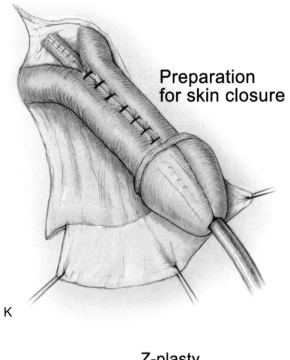

Preparation
for skin closure

K

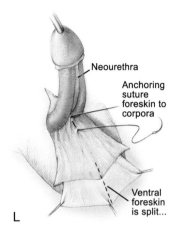

Neourethra

Anchoring
suture
foreskin to
corpora

Ventral
foreskin
is split...

L

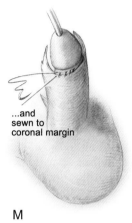

...and
sewn to
coronal margin

M

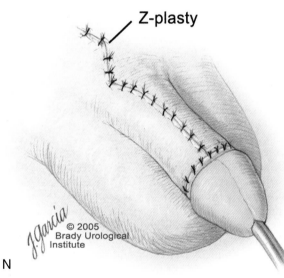

Z-plasty

© 2005
Brady Urological
Institute

N

Figure 119–20, cont'd.   K, Preparation for skin closure. **L,** Suture is placed at the base of the penis to locate the foreskin on the shaft of the penis as well as to provide area of distinction between the penis and the scrotum. **M,** Foreskin is sewn to the coronal sulcus. **N,** Completion of the repair with resurfacing of the penis and use of a proximal Z-plasty incision to provide downward penile deflection.

the urethral plate, which arises proximally and extends upward between the corporal blood supply to the urethral plate. Dissection of the corpora is begun ventrally with dissection on the surface of Buck's fascia covering the corporal bodies. The plane is followed closely until one exits on the dorsum of the penis between the corpus spongiosum and the corporal body, first on one side and then on the other (see Fig. 119–20F and G). The loops are placed around the corporal bodies and the dissection is extended proximally on the corpora to dissect the urethral plate free from the corporal bodies up to the level of the prostate. Although one might expect difficulties when dissecting proximally where the paraexstrophy skin flaps had been sutured to the urethral plate, this has not been encountered in our experience, and

dissection is kept just on the corporal bodies while proceeding proximally. The urethral plate is also dissected distally past the level of the junction of the glans with the corporal bodies. In this manner, adequate mobilization is obtained, and it is not difficult to bring the corporal bodies over the urethra at the level of the corona. This almost separates the penis into three components, the two corpora and the urethral plate (see Fig. 119–20F). However, complete penile disassembly is not undertaken, and the distalmost 1-cm attachment of the mucosa plate to the glans is left intact (Surer et al, 2001a; Gearhart et al, 2004).

The neurovascular bundles, situated between Buck's fascia and the corporal wall, are typically left intact in young patients if rotation of the corporal bodies over the urethra effectively straightens the penis. If not, the neurovascular bundles are dissected free from the corporal bodies, with vessel loops being placed around these structures so that the neurovascular bundles will not be compromised when incisions are made in the corpora and the corpora are rotated medially over the neourethra (see Fig. 119–20H). After the corporal bodies are incised or rotated over the urethra, the urethral strip is closed in a linear manner from the prostatic opening to the glans over a No. 8 Fr silicone stent with 6-0 polyglycolic sutures. After this is accomplished, incisions are made in the corporal bodies at the point of maximum curvature, opening a diamond-shaped effect in the erectile tissue (see Fig. 119–20H). The corpora are then closed over the neourethra with two running sutures of 5-0 polydiaxone, and the diamond-shaped defects in the adjacent area of the corpora are sutured to each other. This procedure effectively displaces the urethra ventrally in a normal position. This not only causes the downward deflection of the penis but also allows some additional length by dorsal rotation and approximation of the corporal bodies over the neourethra. After the urethra has been transferred to the ventrum, further sutures of 4-0 polyglycolic acid are placed between the corporal bodies to bury the urethra further, especially at the level of the junction of the glans and the corporal bodies at the corona (see Fig. 119–20I).

The glans wings are then closed over the glandular urethra using subcuticular sutures of 5-0 polyglycolic acid, and the glans epithelium is closed with 6-0 polyglycolic acid sutures (see Fig. 119–20I). The ventral skin is then brought up and sutured to the ventral edge of the corona, and the flaps are fashioned to provide adequate coverage and lengthening of the dorsum of the penis. The skin is reapproximated with interrupted 5-0 or 6-0 polyglycolic sutures (see Fig. 119–20K to M). A Z-plasty at the base of the penis is closed with interrupted 5-0 or 6-0 polyglycolic acid sutures. A silicone stent is left indwelling in the neourethra to provide drainage for 10 to 12 days (see Fig. 119–20N).

Postoperative Problems

Postoperative pain and bladder spasms after extensive external genital reconstructive surgery require a combined effort of the pediatric anesthesia pain service and the surgical service. Controlling bladder spasms is paramount because they are associated with urinary extravasation and fistula formation. All of our patients have a caudal epidural catheter placed at the time of surgery to help with postoperative pain control and bladder spasms. In addition, oxybutynin is started immediately after surgery to decrease the incidence of bladder spasms and enhance the patient's comfort. At the time of discharge, the plastic dressing on the penis is left intact and the child is discharged with narcotics, antispasmodics, and appropriate broad-spectrum antibiotic coverage.

Female Genitalia

We reconstruct the mons and external genitalia at the time of initial exstrophy closure. Although this adds a bit of time to the operation, once the pubic bones are brought into apposition with osteotomy it is quite easy to reconstruct the female external genitalia.

The bifid clitoris is denuded medially and brought together in the midline at the time of closure along with labia minora

reconstruction by creating a fourchette. A good closure with an attractive mons area and reconstruction of the female genitalia gives the parents a sense of well-being and markedly enhances the overall appearance of the female child born with bladder exstrophy (see Fig. 119–9).

Continence and Antireflux Procedure

Bladder capacity is measured with the child under anesthesia with a gravity cystogram at the 1-year anniversary of the initial closure (Gearhart and Jeffs, 1998). Formerly, it was believed that if the bladder capacity was 60 mL or higher, bladder neck reconstruction could be planned (Gearhart and Jeffs, 1998). However, Chan and colleagues (2001) found that, in selected exstrophy patients who underwent closure, epispadias repair, and bladder neck reconstruction at our institution, a median bladder capacity of 85 mL was more common in the group who were completely dry after bladder neck reconstruction. Most of these children were 4 to 5 years of age and were ready emotionally, maturationally, and intellectually to participate in a postoperative voiding program. Continence and antireflux procedures performed at our institution are illustrated in Figure 119–21. The bladder is open through a transverse incision at the bladder neck with a vertical extension. The later midline closure of this incision is the width of the bladder neck and enlarges the vertical dimension of the bladder, which in exstrophy is often short (see Fig. 119–21A). A Cohen transtrigonal ureteral reimplantation or a cephalotrigonal reimplantation is performed to move the ureter across the bladder, above the trigone, or to direct the ureter cephalad up onto the edge of the trigone (see Fig. 119–21B and C) (Canning et al, 1992). In addition, if the ureters are low on the trigone, there is a need to move the ureteral hiatus higher on the trigone. The hiatus is simply cut in a cephalad direction, and cross-trigonal reimplants are performed at the upper aspect of the trigone (see Fig. 119–21C).

The continence procedure is begun by selecting a posterior strip of mucosa 15 to 18 mm wide and 30 mm long that extends distally from the midtrigone to the prostate or posterior urethra (see Fig. 119–21D). Bladder muscle lateral to the mucosal strip is denuded from the mucosa. It is often helpful at this juncture to use one or two epinephrine-soaked sponges to aid in the control of bleeding and the visualization of the denuded area. Tailoring of the denuded lateral muscle triangles is aided by multiple small incisions on the free edge bilaterally that allow the area of the reconstruction to assume a more cephalad position (see Fig. 119–21E). **These muscle flaps not only are smaller but also are not incised transversely at their cephalad extent as described in the original Young-Dees procedure. We believe that, if these flaps are incised medially at the cephalad border only where they join the floor of the bladder, there is a significant risk of denervation and ischemia that will harm the bladder neck repair. The basic premise is to create a mucosa-lined tube inside a muscular funnel that narrows from its junction with the floor of the bladder that extends caudally.** The edges of the mucosa and underlying muscle are closed with interrupted sutures of 4-0 polyglycolic acid (see Fig. 119–21F). The adjacent denuded muscle flaps are overlapped and sutured firmly in place with a 3-0 polydiaxone suture to provide reinforcement of the bladder neck and urethral reconstruction (see Fig.

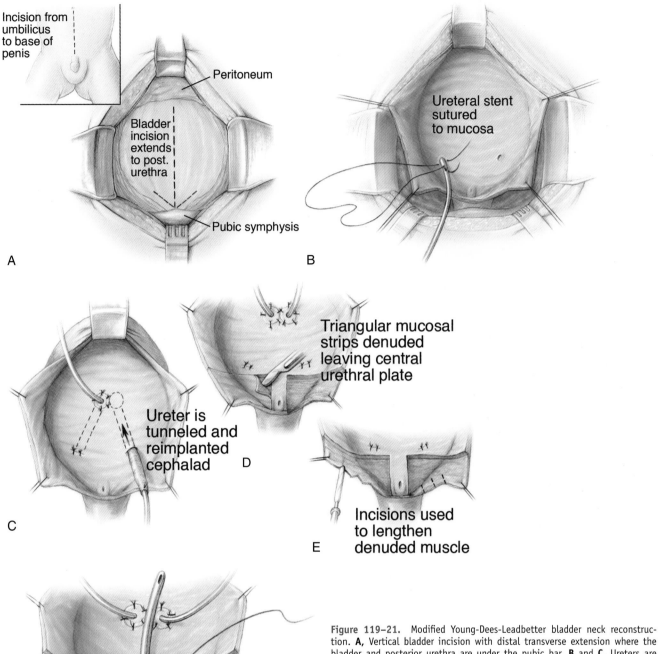

Incision from umbilicus to base of penis

Peritoneum

Bladder incision extends to post. urethra

Pubic symphysis

A

Ureteral stent sutured to mucosa

B

Ureter is tunneled and reimplanted cephalad

C

D Triangular mucosal strips denuded leaving central urethral plate

E Incisions used to lengthen denuded muscle

Tubularization of mucosal strip

F

Figure 119–21. Modified Young-Dees-Leadbetter bladder neck reconstruction. **A,** Vertical bladder incision with distal transverse extension where the bladder and posterior urethra are under the pubic bar. **B** and **C,** Ureters are identified, mobilized, and reimplanted in a cephalotrigonal position. **D** and **E,** Segments of mucosa are excised from either side of a median strip (1.5 cm × 3 cm) that will form the neourethra. Short incisions in the muscle will permit extension of the bladder neck. **F,** Urethra is tabularized using a continuous running suture. *Continued*

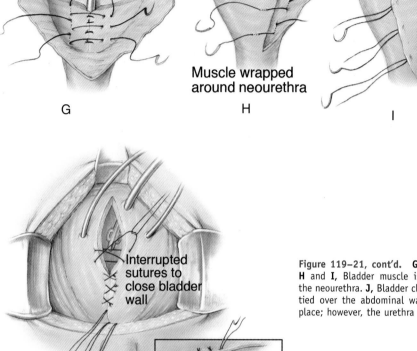

G

Muscle wrapped around neourethra

H

I

Interrupted sutures to close bladder wall

Suspension sutures tied over rectus fascia

J

Figure 119–21, cont'd. G, Posterior urethra and bladder neck are reconstructed. **H** and **I,** Bladder muscle is brought together in a double-breasted fashion over the neourethra. **J,** Bladder closure is completed and the distal suspensory sutures are tied over the abdominal wall (see inset). Suprapubic tube and stents are left in place; however, the urethra is left unstented.

119–21G to I). A No. 8 Fr urethral stent may be used as a guide during urethral reconstruction, but it is removed after the bladder neck reconstruction is completed. After the bladder neck repair is completed, the repair is suspended to the rectus fascia (see Fig. 119–21J; see inset).

Very radical dissection of the bladder, bladder neck, and posterior urethra is required, not only within the pelvis but also from the posterior aspect of the pubic bar to provide enough mobility for the bladder neck reconstruction. This maneuver allows adequate bladder neck narrowing and tightening of the bladder neck repair and subsequent anterior suspension of the newly created posterior urethra and bladder neck. If visualization of the posterior urethra is problematic, the intrasymphyseal bar can be cut, thus providing a widened field of exposure. The intrasymphyseal bar is approximated with 2-0 sutures of polydioxanone. If the intrasymphyseal bar is cut, mobility of the child should be restricted in the postoperative period to allow proper healing of the intrasymphyseal bar.

Postoperative Care

Ureteral stents are placed in the reimplanted ureters and brought out through the wall of the bladder, and the bladder is drained by suprapubic tube, which is left indwelling for a 3-week period. **At the end of 3 weeks the suprapubic tube is clamped and the patient is allowed to attempt to void. Initially, the tube should not be clamped for over 1 hour. If voiding does not occur, the child is given an anesthetic and a No. 8 Fr Foley catheter is placed.** This is left in place for 5 days, then removed, and another voiding trial is begun. This part of the postoperative period is most demanding on the patient, family, and surgeon. Some children require several catheter placements before voiding is initiated. If the child can empty the bladder satisfactorily, the suprapubic tube is removed. Frequent bladder and renal ultrasound examinations are required in the first few months after bladder neck repair.

Combined Bladder Exstrophy and Epispadias Repair

Combined closure of exstrophy and epispadias repair is considered in patients who have closure delayed beyond the newborn period or in patients in whom initial newborn closure fails. This procedure follows the initial aspects (Fig. 119–22A to J) of closure of bladder exstrophy and the poste-

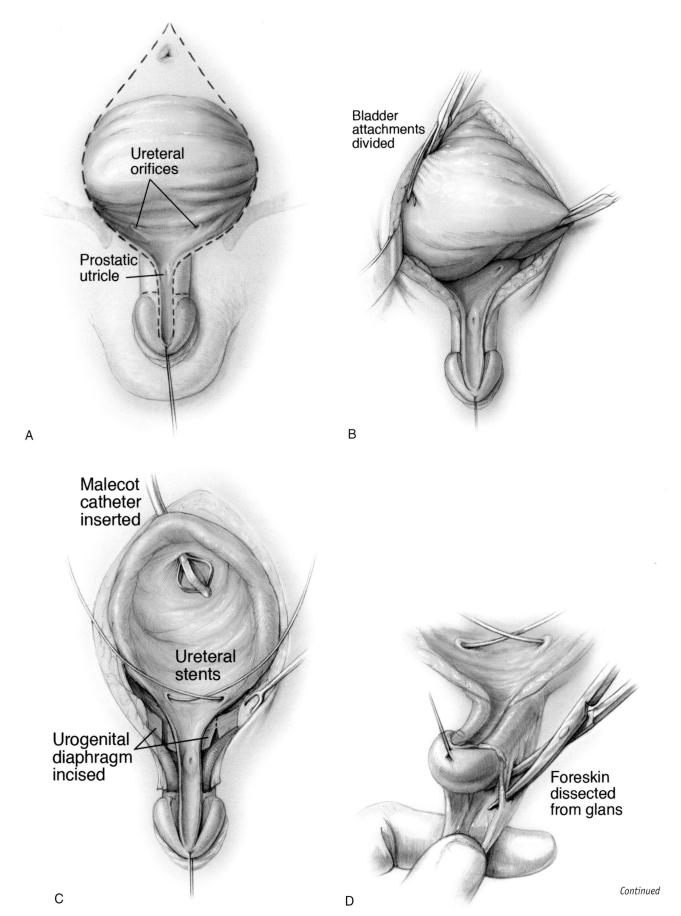

Figure 119–22. Combined bladder closure and epispadias repair. **A,** Initial incision extends around bladder and includes the urethral plate. **B,** Bladder is dissected off the lateral abdominal wall. **C,** Stents are placed in the ureters and suprapubic tube is placed. Urogenital fibers are divided. **D,** Foreskin is dissected off the shaft of the penis.

Continued

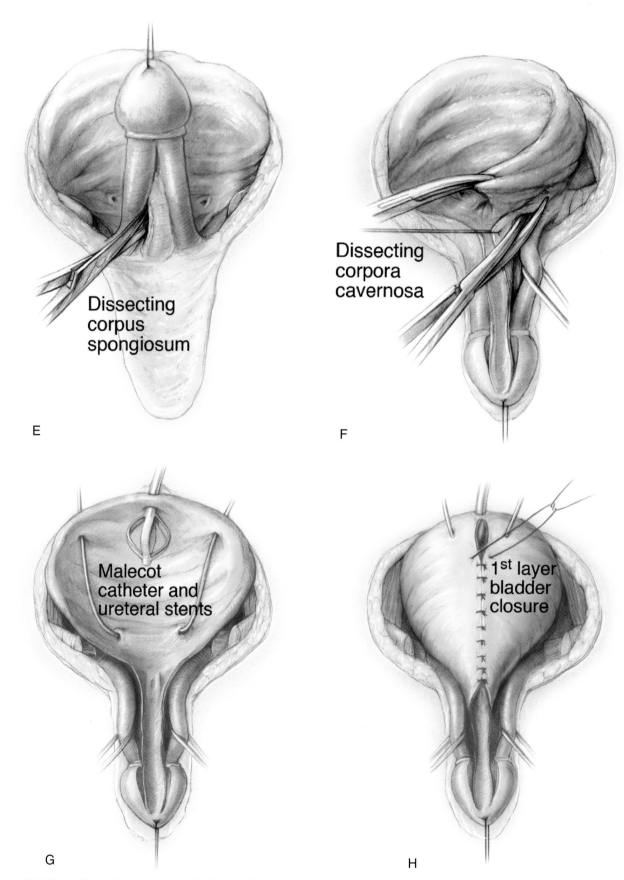

Figure 119–22, cont'd. **E,** Corpus spongiosum is dissected, leaving a ventral vascularized pedicle. **F,** Corpora are dissected proximally toward the bladder. **G,** Completed dissection of the urethral plate and corpora. **H,** Bladder closure is completed.

Continued

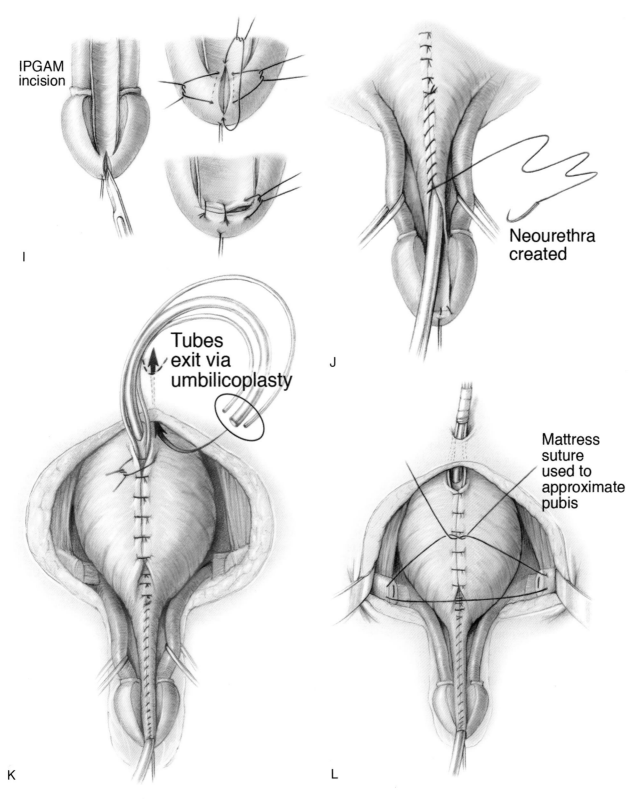

I, IPGAM incision
J, Neourethra created
Tubes exit via umbilicoplasty
K
Mattress suture used to approximate pubis
L

Figure 119–22, cont'd. **I,** IPGAM incision and closure performed at the distal end of the urethral plate. **J,** Urethral plate is tabularized using a continuous running suture. **K,** Second layer of bladder closure completed and suprapubic tube and stents brought out through umbilicoplasty. **L,** Pubic bones are approximated and **(M)** initial layer of abdominal wall closure is completed. Corpora are closed over the urethral closure (see Cantwell-Ransley repair, Fig. 119-20).   *Continued*

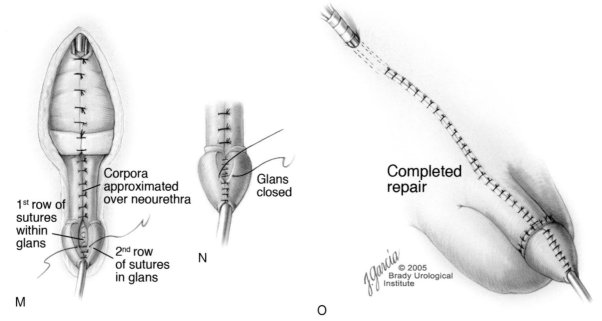

1st row of sutures within glans

Corpora approximated over neourethra

2nd row of sutures in glans

Glans closed

M

N

Completed repair

© 2005
Brady Urological Institute

O

Figure 119–22, cont'd. **N,** Glans closure is completed. **O,** Completed penile and abdominal wall skin closure. Urethral stent is omitted in children having initial closure but is left in place in those undergoing reclosure.

rior urethra as described for the staged reconstruction (Gearhart et al, 1998; Baird et al, 2004). Evaluation of the bladder template is performed by inverting the bladder into the abdomen with a sterile gloved finger. This allows evaluation of the extent of the urethral plate, which may be larger than noted on visual inspection of the abdominal wall defect. Extent of bladder polyposis and scarring is also noted. In addition, the urethral plate is examined for its length and depth and the presence of scarring from any prior attempt at repair. All patients receive preoperative testosterone to enhance penile size and testosterone cream to the urethral plate and bladder neck if prior surgery has led to scarring. The operative procedure begins and proceeds as with a standard closure of the bladder, posterior urethra, and abdominal wall, with only a few variations (see Fig. 119–22B and C). One major difference is that great care must be used to resect any remnants of the urogenital diaphragm fibers (see Fig. 119–22C). It is surprising how frequently these fibers are still intact in patients undergoing reclosure after failure of the initial operative procedures.

If adequate dissection has been performed, the entire posterior urethra-bladder unit can be moved posteriorly into the pelvis. Once the bladder and posterior urethra are adequately dissected, attention can be given to dissection of the penis, corporal bodies, and urethral plate. This part of the procedure (see Fig. 119–22D to I) progresses much as in a standard epispadias repair and exstrophy closure.

After dissection of the penis and corporal bodies, the urethral plate is dissected off the corpora except for the distal 0.5 to 1 cm (see Fig. 119–22G). A No. 2 nylon suture is then placed in a horizontal mattress fashion in the pubis and used to bring the pelvis together (see Fig. 119–22L). If a child older than 1 year is being managed with osteotomy, the fixator pins may be used to assist with rotation of the pelvis medially into place.

In young children, the lack of ossified bones prohibits this maneuver. Approximation of the pubic tubercles allows the corpora to rotate significantly medially so that they can easily be brought over the closed urethral plate (see Fig. 119–22M).

Penile and glans reconstruction is completed with appropriate skin coverage using reverse Byars flaps or, in some cases, a Nesbit turnover flap (see Fig. 119–22N to O). A small suction drain is placed next to the bladder closure, and the abdominal wall closure is completed. A No. 8 Fr Silastic stent is used to stent the urethra for 7 to 10 days. The external fixating device is then attached to the intrafragmentary pins and tightened.

External fixation of the pelvis is maintained for 4 to 6 weeks in children with primary closure and for 6 weeks in those undergoing reclosure of the bladder. **Follow-up is much the same as with standard exstrophy closure and includes monitoring of residual urines and upper tract imaging with ultrasonography before removal of the suprapubic tube.** Although some of our patients have achieved long-term continence after these procedures, most require bladder neck reconstruction when bladder capacity is deemed adequate and the child is able to participate in a postoperative voiding program (Gearhart et al, 1998).

MODERN STAGED REPAIR OF EXSTROPHY: OUTCOMES AND RESULTS

The use of functional bladder closure in bladder exstrophy has resulted in dramatic improvements in the success of reconstruction. Several series (Chisholm, 1979; Mollard, 1980; Ansell, 1983) have demonstrated the success and applicability of the staged functional closure approach to bladder exstrophy. Other series (Conner et al, 1988; Husmann et al, 1989a)

Table 119–2. Urinary Continence after Functional Bladder Closure*

Series	Number of Closures Evaluated	Patients Who Became Continent
Perlmutter et al (1991)	15	77%
Mollard et al (1994)	73	69%
McMahon et al (1996)	33	70%
Lottmann et al (1998)	57	67%
Chan et al (2001)	90	90%[†]

*Includes only personal series (one or two surgeons only) repairing continence rates greater than 6%.
[†]74% dry day and night, 16% dry for >3 hr during day with some wet nights.

Table 119–3. Complications and Corrective Surgical Procedures in 90 Primary Bladder Closures*

Item	Number
Complication	
Bladder prolapse	3
Outlet obstruction	3
Bladder calculi	4
Renal calculi	2
Wound dehiscence	1
Stitch erosion	3
Procedure	
Repair prolapse/dehiscence	4
Cystolithopaxy	4
Urethrotomy	3
Nephrolithotomy	2
Removal of intrapubic stitch	3

*All closed primarily at the Johns Hopkins Hospital.
From Chan DY, Jeffs RD, Gearhart JP: Determinates of continence in the bladder exstrophy population after bladder neck reconstruction. Urology 2001;165:1656.

have shown acceptable continence rates with preservation of renal function. More recent series (Perlmutter et al, 1991; Mollard et al, 1994; McMahon et al, 1996; Gearhart and Jeffs, 1998; Lottmann et al, 1998) have documented continued improvements in outcomes, acceptable urinary continence, and preservation of renal function in a majority of patients (Table 119–2).

A large series by Surer and colleagues (2001b) has demonstrated the importance of a successful primary closure. Sixty-eight patients (57 males; 11 females) were referred for bladder neck reconstruction after primary closure elsewhere. Twenty percent had pelvic osteotomy at the time of the initial repair. The majority of patients were closed in the first 72 hours of life. Mean bladder capacity at the time of bladder neck reconstruction was 121 mL. Eighty-three percent are continent and voiding per urethra. This application of modern staged repair with primary closure by one surgeon and follow-up reconstruction by a second surgeon shows convincingly that a successful initial closure is one of the most important determinants of eventual bladder capacity and compliance regardless of who originally performed the repair.

Initial Closure

In a series by Chan and associates (2001), 90 patients with bladder exstrophy who were referred to our pediatric urology service between 1975 and 1997 were evaluated. Complications from bladder closure and additional surgical procedures required to correct these complications are presented in Table 119–3. **The importance of a successful initial closure is emphasized by Oesterling and Jeffs** (1987) **and by Husmann and colleagues** (1989a), **who found that the onset of eventual continence was quicker and the continence rate higher in those who underwent a successful initial closure with or without osteotomy. In addition, Gearhart and associates** (1996a) **reported on 23 patients with bladder exstrophy who underwent more than two failed attempts at closure. If a patient underwent two closures, the chances of having an adequate bladder capacity for bladder neck reconstruction was 60%, and the chance of successful continence was 30%. Patients who had undergone three closures had only a 40% chance of obtaining an adequate bladder capacity and less than a 20% chance of being continent of urine.** In the evaluation of this group of selected exstrophy patients, it was found that at the time of initial closure 19 of 23 patients had no form of osteotomy. Six of the patients had obtained

bladder capacity suitable for bladder neck reconstruction; three were dry, and three were incontinent. Bladder size was inadequate in nine patients after being monitored for bladder growth. The chance of obtaining an adequate bladder capacity and eventual continence after more than one closure attempt is markedly diminished. These less than satisfactory results underline the paramount importance of a secure abdominal wall, posterior urethra, and bladder closure in these complex cases. Lastly, the importance of early initial closure was emphasized by data from Husmann and colleagues (1989a) showing that only 10% of the patients who undergo bladder closure before 1 year of age but 40% of those who have the procedure at a later age require eventual augmentation.

Epispadias Repair

Although urinary incontinence remains the most significant problem for patients with classic bladder exstrophy and epispadias, anxiety about inadequate and unattractive genitalia still poses the greatest concern to male patients. Formerly, the modified Young repair was the most commonly used technique at our institution to repair the epispadiac penis (Lepor et al, 1984). Because of the tortuosity of the urethra, high fistula rate, and significant dorsal chordee associated with this repair, a modification of the Cantwell-Ransley procedure was adopted as a new repair technique. We began using the modified Cantwell-Ransley repair in patients with classic exstrophy or epispadias in 1988 and have reported our early experience (Gearhart et al, 1992; Gearhart et al, 1995c; Gearhart et al, 2004).

Since 1988, the modified Cantwell-Ransley repair has been performed for 93 male patients with either classic bladder exstrophy (79 patients) or epispadias (14 patients) (Surer et al, 1999). At the time of surgery, the patients' age ranged from 1 to 18 years with an average age of 2.6 years. Over the past 2 years, however, the mean age at the time of epispadias repair decreased to 1.2 years. Of the 79 patients with bladder exstrophy, 31 had a short urethral groove requiring paraexstrophy skin flaps for penile lengthening at the time of initial bladder exstrophy closure. Of the 14 epispadiac patients, 11 had penopubic and 3 had penile epispadias at presentation.

This technique was used for primary urethroplasty in 65 patients with bladder exstrophy and 12 with epispadias. The modified Cantwell-Ransley repair was used as a secondary procedure after failed urethroplasty in 4 patients with exstrophy and 2 with epispadias and was combined with reclosure of bladder exstrophy in 10 patients. Early epispadias repair was performed when the patients were 6 months to 1 year of age. However, because of concerns about getting the urethra deeper under the corpora at the glandular level, beginning in 1994 we further modified the Cantwell-Ransley repair by detaching the mucosal plate from the corona except for the distal 0.5 to 1 cm of the plate. Intramuscular testosterone enanthate in oil was given to all children at a dose of 2 mg/kg at approximately 5 weeks and again at 2 weeks before surgery.

This series has been expanded to include 129 patients with a mean follow-up of 88 months (Gearhart et al, 2004). One hundred twenty patients had a horizontal or downward-angled penis while standing. The incidence of urethrocutaneous fistula in the immediate postoperative period was 16% and at 3 months it was 12%. Nine patients developed a urethral stricture of the proximal anastomotic site, and 12 had minor skin separation of the dorsal skin closure. Cystoscopy with catheterization in 120 patients revealed an easily negotiable channel in all. Eight patients required further penile straightening surgery. Fifteen patients older than 16 years had engaged in satisfactory intercourse, and all reported orgasms and ejaculation with a straight penis on erection. One patient reported that his penis was shorter following surgery.

Modern penile reconstructive techniques should create a straight and functional penis with a glanular meatus, an easily catheterizable neourethral channel (if needed), and an acceptable cosmetic appearance. Many adolescents considered their odd-appearing genitalia with a short, widened penis to be a greater psychosocial problem than incontinence, and therefore every effort should be made to restore the penis to a normal condition. Historically, most repairs of the epispadiac penis came from Cantwell's original description in 1895. In 1989, Ransley and associates introduced a concept to release dorsal chordee by incision and anastomosis of the dorsomedial aspect of the corpora over the urethra and urethral meatotomy at the distal end of the glans, to move the meatus to a more normal position and secure good direction of the urinary stream (IPGAM). Ransley's group have reported their long-term experience with 95 patients in whom the modified Cantwell-Ransley repair was used: fistula occurred in only 4% of patients and a urethral stricture in only 5% (Kajbafzadeh et al, 1995).

Dissection of the urethral strip to inside the glans penis provides a ventral position of the urethra and the glans and submerges the urethra well below the corpora at the glans level. This approximation of raw surface of glanular tissues dorsally over the urethra is clearly why the incidence of fistula in the area of the corona is very rare compared with the Young repair. Fistulas in our patients usually appear at the base of the penis, where the urethra comes up proximally between the corporal bodies. In modern exstrophy reconstructive techniques, most surgeons try to preserve the urethral plate at the time of exstrophy closure. Interestingly, we do not find a significant difference for fistula formation between those in whom paraexstrophy skin flaps were used at the time of initial closure and those in whom they were not. Despite the positive findings with regard to fistula formation, the use of paraexstrophy skin flaps has been noted to be associated with the development of strictures. Use of these flaps is therefore limited to selected patients in whom penile lengthening cannot be achieved with standard techniques.

Some authors have advised even more aggressive techniques than those proposed originally by Cantwell. Mitchell and Bagli (1996) described a complete penile disassembly technique in which the epispadiac phallus is completely disassembled into three components: the urethral plate and the right and left hemicorporal glandular bodies. A group of 10 patients with follow-up of 57 months were reported to be very happy with the horizontal direction of the penis. There were three fistulas after surgery, but these were in two patients who had undergone secondary repair. A multicenter report on the use of this repair in a total of 17 boys found that 3 of the 17 had a urethrocutaneous fistula, two of which closed spontaneously (Zaontz et al, 1998). One patient had a complete dehiscence, but all boys with intact repairs had straight erections, an orthotopic meatus, and a satisfactory appearance. In a series of 42 males from Egypt, undergoing this repair, the fistula rate was 2.4%, but in 10% ischemic glandar changes were noted (Hammouda, 2003).

In our opinion, none of the current epispadias repairs offers any significant gain in penile length by removal of the entire urethral plate from the glans or even the use of a free graft. Data reported by Silver and colleagues (1997b) clearly showed that, although anterior corporal length is significantly less in patients with exstrophy, the posterior corporal length is normal. These findings suggest that penile lengthening procedures at the time of epispadias repair improve apparent penile length and straighten the penis but do not transfer additional tissue (i.e., length) to the corporal bodies. We have observed with increasing experience that the modified Cantwell-Ransley repair effectively corrects corporal chordee and adds some penile length. It can be hoped that dorsal penile curvature, which is often seen during the growth spurt at puberty, will be resisted. In the patients in whom corporal rotation is used without corporal incision and anastomosis, the neurovascular bundle is left intact and not dissected from its bed. However, if incision and anastomosis are needed, mobilization of the neurovascular bundle is required. Typically in our experience, incision and rotation are used only for older patients with marked chordee. Although review of findings reveals that almost all penises are straight or deflected downward, many of these patients are still young children. The long-term assessment of penile and urethral reconstruction in exstrophy patients by the modified Cantwell-Ransley repair has shown that in patients with bladder exstrophy and epispadias there is some increase in penile length, and a relatively straight penis with an adequate urethral caliber, which is adequate to void and ejaculate through, can be achieved with minimal morbidity. These findings compare favorably with the series by Mesrobian and coworkers (1986) of 18 patients who underwent primary closure with a straight penis and downward angulation in 85% of patients. In a follow-up study of a group of postpubertal patients, those authors found that 86% of patients with a straight penis could achieve satisfactory intercourse when the penis was angulated downward (Mesrobian et al, 1986).

Bladder Neck Repair

Bladder neck reconstruction results in the exstrophy population have been reported by several groups. Some large experiences have come from the European groups in Lyon and Paris. Mouriquand and associates (2003) reported on 80 children with bladder exstrophy and 25 with incontinent epispadias. Follow-up ranged from 1 to 11 years. Forty-five percent of the group with exstrophy and 52% of those with epispadias had a dry interval greater than 3 hours. Although the continence rate was very low, many of the exstrophy patients were not closed until 6 to 12 months of age. Also, many had their epispadias repair after bladder neck reconstruction, a factor known to influence both eventual capacity and continence. Lottmann and colleagues (1998) presented a long-term follow-up study of Cendron's exstrophy patients who underwent complete reconstruction. With the Young-Dees repair they were able to achieve urinary continence in 71% of male patients and 53% of females. Overall continence was 65% with a mean follow-up of 12 years after bladder neck repair. Also, Jones and colleagues (1993), using their modification of the Young-Dees repair, reported 64% of patients dry and 18% partially dry in a group that included children with exstrophy, epispadias, and myelomeningocele. Series from North America using mainly the classic Young-Dees-Leadbetter repair reported continence rates ranging from 60% to 82% (Husmann et al, 1989a; Mergurian et al, 1991; Perlmutter et al, 1991; Franco et al, 1994; McMahon et al, 1996; Chan et al, 2001; Cole et al, 2003). **The most important long-term factor gleaned from a review of all these series is the fact that bladder capacity at the time of bladder neck reconstruction is a very important determinant of eventual success.**

Records of 90 patients who underwent all stages of bladder exstrophy reconstruction at our institution between 1975 and 1997 were reviewed by Chan and colleagues (2001). Sixty-two patients with bladder neck reconstruction were available for analysis after exclusion of 21 patients awaiting bladder neck reconstruction, 3 female patients who achieved continence without bladder neck repair, 3 patients with recent bladder neck repair, and 1 patient lost to follow-up. The current voiding status of each patient was obtained from parental or patient interview or direct observation by the nursing and physician staff. The patients were categorized as spontaneous voiding not on intermittent catheterization and were assigned a status of (1) completely dry day and night; (2) socially continent, being dry at least 3 hours during the day with occasional nighttime wetting; or (3) wet, being dry for less than 3 hours during the day and wet at night (Table 119–4).

Of the 62 patients who underwent bladder neck repair, 47 were male and 15 were female. The median age for primary closure was 9 days, and the mean was 4 months. The average age at bladder neck reconstruction was 4 years, and these patients had a median bladder capacity of 85 mL at the time of bladder neck repair. Of the 62 patients observed for over 1 year, 46 (74%) were continent and voiding urethrally without the need for augmentation or intermittent catheterization. Ten patients (16%) had social continence with only occasional

Table 119–4. Urinary Continence after 62 Initial Bladder Neck Reconstructions

Result*	Average Daytime Dry Interval (hr)	Patients	
		Number	Percentage
Continent (dry day and night)	3	46[†]	74
Social continence (dry >3 hr daytime, occasional nighttime wetness)	3	10	16
Wet	<3	4	10

*Two patients required diversion after bladder neck reconstruction for upper tract changes.
[†]Voiding per urethra without intermittent catheterization.

nighttime accidents, two required diversion for continence after failed bladder neck repair, and four were wet. The renal units of all patients who underwent bladder neck reconstruction were evaluated by intravenous pyelography or ultrasonography postoperatively on multiple occasions to assess the preservation of renal function after the continence procedure. One patient had reflux and hydronephrosis after bladder neck reconstruction and bilateral ureteral reimplantation and developed pyelonephritis on the left with mild scarring. A dimercaptosuccinic acid (DMSA) scan of this patient revealed nearly symmetrical renal function. Conservative management of vesicoureteral reflux over time led to the resolution of the reflux in this patient. No other patient developed significant upper tract pathology. There were no other major complications (e.g., ureteral obstruction). Bladder outlet obstruction required cystoscopy and placement of a urethral catheter in 18 patients and prolonged suprapubic drainage for voidings in 12 patients.

The findings in this series were that continence was more likely in patients who underwent initial bladder closure before 72 hours of age or after 72 hours of age with an osteotomy. These results agree with those of Husmann and associates (1989a), who found that patients who underwent delayed closure without osteotomy showed a significantly lower rate of continence (10%). There was another revealing factor in this study. Although it was previously thought that a bladder capacity of 60 mL was adequate for successful bladder neck reconstruction, in this highly selected group of patients who underwent closure, epispadias repair, and bladder neck repair at our institution the continence rate was higher in those who had a median bladder capacity of 85 mL at the time of bladder neck repair. In addition, the data from Surer and colleagues indicated that in a group of 68 patients undergoing bladder neck reconstruction with a mean bladder capacity of 121 mL, long-term voided continence was achievable in 83%. Therefore, bladder capacity determined under anesthesia before bladder neck reconstruction continues to be an important predictor of eventual urinary continence.

A continence procedure should be deferred until the bladder reaches a capacity of 85 mL and the child is motivated to be dry and to participate in a postoperative voiding program. In our particular series, the age at the time of bladder neck reconstruction was not as important as the capacity before bladder neck repair. The onset of continence is a very interesting phenomenon in this group of exstrophy patients. **The vast majority of patients achieve daytime continence in the first year after bladder neck reconstruction.** A few patients gain a longer daytime interval during the second year after bladder neck repair. However, patients who are not dry after 2 years are considered incontinent. The onset of nighttime continence varies but often takes longer than the time needed to achieve daytime continence and can be 2 to 3 years. Caione and coworkers (1999) showed that use of desmopressin acetate (DDAVP) can increase the number of dry nights in these patients.

Urodynamic evaluation after exstrophy reconstruction by Dave and colleagues (2001) showed that patients with good continence after bladder neck reconstruction had higher maximal cystometric capacity and compliance than those who remained incontinent. Unstable contractions, however, were seen in both groups. Dave and colleagues (2001) also reported that patients with higher end filling pressure had a higher incidence of nonobstructive hydronephrosis even if they were continent. These findings, in addition to those of Bolduc and others (2002), indicate the necessity for follow-up into adulthood after successful reconstruction.

OTHER EXSTROPHY REPAIRS: OUTCOMES
Warsaw Approach

The long-term reported outcomes of this repair include 36 patients with classic exstrophy and 37 with epispadias. Eighty-nine percent of patients with epispadias were continent during the day, but more than 40% were still wet at night. Seventy-five percent of patients with classic exstrophy had daytime continence, but nine had occasional wet nights. Eleven boys required short-term intermittent catheterization, which was easily performed by the patient and family. All but two began voiding within 3 to 5 months, and only two have continued with intermittent catheterization. Complications in seven boys included two urethrocutaneous fistulas and five urethral strictures (Baka-Jakubiak, 2000). All of these responded to urethral dilatation or endoscopic incision. There were no instances of abdominal wall dehiscence or glanular or corporal loss. Ureteral reimplantation was not performed at the time of bladder neck reconstruction and epispadias repair, but many patients required later reimplantation for gradually worsening hydronephrosis.

Compared with this experience, Mathews and coauthors (2003b) reported on a group of patients who had ureteral reimplantation performed at the time of bladder neck reconstruction and epispadias repair. None of these patients developed reflux or worsening hydronephrosis. Baka-Jakubiak recommends performance of this combined procedure if the bladder capacity is documented to be above 100 mL and the penis is large enough for epispadias repair. Follow-up urodynamic studies demonstrated the presence of normal detrusor function in most, although some patients developed high voiding pressures and some had poor detrusor contractility. If poor detrusor contractility was noted, prolonged intermittent catheterization was required and high voiding pressures were managed with anticholinergic therapy. Most patients were

managed later in life, and the standard addition of ureteral reimplantation at the time of reconstruction should probably be universally performed.

Erlangen Approach

Popularized by Rosch and colleagues (2001), who have reported on 100 patients, this technique has been utilized in both newborns and failed closures. Ninety-one children with exstrophy (69 boys and 22 girls) and nine with complete epispadias (7 boys and 2 girls) have had this procedure performed. The complete single-stage repair was performed in 47 children and included pelvic closure without osteotomy, bladder neck reconstruction, an antireflux procedure, and epispadias repair using the Cantwell-Ransley technique. An additional 53 patients had primary reconstruction elsewhere and then had bladder neck reconstruction and epispadias repair performed. Continence was defined as dryness for more than 3 hours and no nocturnal enuresis. Partial continence was defined as dry for 1 to 3 hours or greater than 3 hours with occasional stress incontinence or wet nights. Patients dry for less than 1 hour were considered incontinent. Among the patients undergoing single-stage repair (47 patients), 83% are continent, 35 of 39 voiding per urethra, 2 on clean intermittent catheterization (CIC), and 3 on CIC following augmentation. Four patients are partially continent and two are dry on desmopressin. Four patients are incontinent and three have had continent diversion. Of 53 patients who had primary closure elsewhere, 55% are continent and 7 have been augmented. Fourteen are partially continent and 10 are incontinent, 4 of whom have had continent diversion. No prolapse or dehiscence was reported, but six patients developed urethrocutaneous fistulas. None of the patients had loss of the glans or corpora or major soft tissue losses. The authors have emphasized the superiority of this repair for primary rather than failed closures.

Seattle Approach (Complete Repair)

Grady and Mitchell (1999) reported that with the use of the complete repair several patients in their series of 18 children had a continent interval (i.e., dry for 2 hours during the day). They reported that 50% of patients have required reimplantation during the first year of life because of uncontrollable upper tract infections and significant upper tract dilatation. Borer and colleagues (2004) found a continence rate of 20% with most patients requiring later bladder neck reconstruction. Further, most patients had a median of four surgical procedures after primary repair in infancy. Another study by Alpert and associates (2004) indicated that penopubic fistulas in males were noted in 42% of patients. El-Sherbiny and others (2002) found the incidence of hypospadias using this technique to be 59%, and those undergoing newborn closure developed a 60- to 90-minute dry interval on follow-up.

Husmann and Gearhart (2004) and Gearhart and Baird (2004) have reported soft tissue losses following reconstruction with this technique. These have included loss of the glans, corpora, corpora and glans, and the urethral plate following repair. Hammouda (2003) reported ischemic changes in 5 of his initial 10 patients, and 2 of these patients suffered loss of the glans. Although all exstrophy reconstruction has potential for serious complications, the soft tissue losses of the penis associated with this technique are a formidable challenge for later reconstruction. This procedure should therefore be performed only by experienced exstrophy surgeons.

Combined Closure Results

In an updated series of 38 boys with classic bladder exstrophy who underwent combined closure and epispadias repair either as a secondary closure or as a delayed primary closure at a mean age of 26.5 months (Baird et al, 2004), urethrocutaneous fistula was noted in 6 of 28 patients who underwent Cantwell-Ransley repair, 3 of 8 who had a Young repair, and 1 patient who had an island flap repair, at the time of bladder closure. The urethrocutaneous fistula resolved spontaneously in seven boys and required reoperative closure in three boys. Four patients developed a urethral stricture and two required a full-thickness skin graft for reconstruction. The other two boys were managed with direct vision internal urethrotomy.

At the time of evaluation, three boys were dry for longer than 3 hours after bladder closure and epispadias repair alone. Nineteen boys had gone on to modified Young-Dees-Leadbetter bladder neck reconstruction. Twelve of the 19 were totally dry day and night. Continent urinary diversion has been performed in six reclosure patients and is being considered in a further four. Eleven boys were awaiting the development of an adequate bladder capacity for bladder neck reconstruction; one was waiting for augmentation and continent stoma construction.

The combination of epispadias repair and bladder closure can be safely performed (Gearhart et al, 1991, 2000; Baird et al, 2004). However, when complications occur they can significantly affect the potential of the bladder. This approach, when successful, may have a positive influence on bladder capacity or even continence and may lead to a reduction in the number of procedures required for reconstruction. Data from the combined approach for exstrophy reconstruction are still early, and its use by the novice exstrophy surgeon should be discouraged. As experience is gained, these procedures may eventually take their place in the surgeon's armamentarium for exstrophy reconstruction.

As newer techniques are proposed and evolve to take their place in the armamentarium of the exstrophy surgeon, their results need comparison with the current "gold standard" of modern staged repair. Modern staged repair has been shown to provide secure bladder closure and a cosmetic penile appearance and, when successful, provides the patient with the best potential for eventual voided continence with upper tract preservation. The widespread utility and success of this repair were demonstrated by Surer and coworkers (2001), who reported on 68 classic exstrophy patients who were referred after successful primary closure. Most were closed early and had developed excellent bladder capacities at the time of bladder neck reconstruction; 83% were continent and voiding per urethra. This group, closed by multiple surgeons with bladder neck reconstruction by a second surgeon, shows that the modern staged repair is a reliable and reproducible technique in varied settings. It may eventually be replaced as the standard for reconstruction, but longer follow-up is required for the newer reconstructive techniques.

EXSTROPHY RECONSTRUCTION FAILURES
Failed Closure

After any form of repair, failures can manifest as complete bladder dehiscence, bladder prolapse, or neourethral stricture and obstruction. Meldrum and associates (2005) reported on a select group of children who failed exstrophy reconstruction prior to referral to a tertiary care facility. In the cohort of 101 children, 51 had primary surgical management performed by a fellowship trained pediatric urologist, 18 by a general urologist, 6 by a pediatric surgeon, and 9 by an unknown surgeon. Following successful reclosure, 38 patients eventually developed adequate bladder capacity for bladder neck reconstruction, and only 26% (10) eventually achieved dryness. These data emphasize the need for initial successful reconstruction and suggest that individuals undertaking this reconstruction should be comfortable with the complexity of repair. It is prudent for the surgeon who may see only a few patients with this condition to consider referral of these complex management situations to a center where special expertise and experience exist.

Dehiscence, which may be precipitated by incomplete mobilization of the pelvic diaphragm and inadequate pelvic immobilization postoperatively, wound infection, abdominal distention, or urinary tube malfunction, necessitates a 6-month recovery period before a second attempt at closure can be made (Gearhart and Jeffs, 1991a; Gearhart et al, 1993b) (Fig. 119–23A). Dehiscence and prolapse have also been reported following the complete repair and may be associated with glandar, corporal, urethral plate, and other major soft tissue loss (Fig. 119–23B) Tension-free reclosure with osteotomy and immobilization are important factors in initial and subsequent closures. Unfortunately, the chance of obtaining adequate bladder capacity for bladder neck plasty and eventual continence after multiple closures is markedly diminished (Gearhart et al, 1996a). Similarly, bladder prolapse is considered a failure and requires bladder reclosure or revision (Fig. 119–23C). In a patient with significant bladder prolapse or dehiscence, at the time of secondary closure we combine epispadias repair with bladder, posterior urethra, and abdominal wall closure (Gearhart et al, 1998). The patient is given testosterone enanthate intramuscularly 5 weeks and 2 weeks before surgical repair and undergoes an osteotomy with concomitant bladder, urethral, and abdominal wall closure. Major soft tissue loss that is seen following complete repair requires extensive preoperative planning and may require use of buccal mucosal or full-thickness grafts or tissue expansion (Gearhart and Baird, 2004a).

Baird and coauthors (2004) reported on 38 boys undergoing combined exstrophy closure and epispadias repair along with osteotomy. Thirty of these boys had failed prior reconstruction. Complications in this group were limited to urethrocutaneous fistulas and urethral strictures. Twelve of 19 boys who have subsequently had bladder neck reconstruction are continent. Six boys have required and four await continent diversion. Eleven boys are awaiting adequate capacity for bladder neck reconstruction. Although the results after reclosure are not as good as those obtained with a successful primary closure, they are respectable and may obviate the

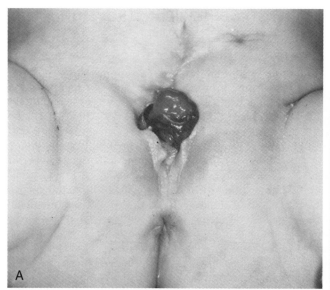
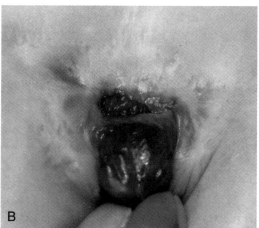

Figure 119–23. **A,** Complete dehiscence of bladder closure in a child who had reconstruction without osteotomy. **B,** Dehiscence of a patient who had bladder closure using the complete reconstruction technique.

need for bladder augmentation. Neourethral stricture is often associated with paraexstrophy skin flap use, pubic suture reaction, erosion, or the use of urethral stents. This may be somewhat subtle; however, warning signs consist of urinary tract infections, detectable increased bladder volumes on ultrasonography, bladder stones, prolonged dry intervals, and unexplained rectal prolapse. In a review by Baker and colleagues (1999), posterior urethral obstruction was found in 41 patients. Most episodes occurred within 60 days after primary closure. If diversion was used for longer than 6 months, the ultimate fate of the bladder was augmentation. If diversion was used for less than 6 months, most reconstructions were ultimately bowel free. Ultimately, posterior urethral obstruction after exstrophy closure markedly decreased the success of any repair. This complication presents a significant risk to the upper urinary tract and should be detected early.

Although all closed exstrophy bladders have vesicoureteral reflux, upper tract deterioration is the ultimate fate of significant outlet obstruction. At this point the management includes urethral dilation (incision), open urethroplasty, or upper tract diversion. If renal function is compromised, the choice must achieve unquestionable free drainage to allow the upper tracts and kidneys to recover fully. Further bladder neck or urethral reconstruction should not be performed until the posterior urethral stricture is clearly repaired and free drainage has been achieved.

Despite satisfactory closure, some bladders never achieve adequate capacity to act as functional bladders. It has become clear that multiple bladder closures, bladder prolapse, dehiscence, bladder calculi, recurrent infections, and vesicostomy have a negative impact on the potential of the exstrophy bladder (Silver et al, 1997b). We have used transurethral injection of collagen around the bladder neck to increase outlet resistance and stimulate the bladder to grow. However, in our hands this has not been as successful as reported by Caione and colleagues (Caione et al, 1993a; Caione et al, 1993b) from Italy. If the bladder does not grow to a sufficient size for

bladder neck reconstruction, bladder augmentation is recommended in this situation. If the bladder neck or urethra or both are problematic, a catheterizable continent stoma with or without bladder neck plasty or transection is performed, along with augmentation (Gearhart et al, 1995b).

Failed Bladder Neck Repair

If urinary continence, defined as a 3-hour dry interval, is not achieved within 2 years after bladder neck reconstruction, failure to achieve dryness has resulted. Occasionally, the dry interval is nearly acceptable for daytime dryness (i.e., longer than 2 hours). In these situations, collagen injections into the bladder neck can move the dry interval up to 3 hours, but more than one injection may be required (Ben-Chaim et al, 1995a). Data from Lottmann with the use of dextranomer implant (Deflux) have shown improvement in the dry interval when used following partial success with bladder neck reconstruction. Some successes have been seen with repeated Young-Dees-Leadbetter repair if the bladder neck is patulous, the bladder capacity is adequate, and urodynamic evaluation reveals a stable bladder (Gearhart et al, 1991). A majority of bladder neck failures require eventual augmentation or continent diversion. The artificial urinary sphincter has been used with some success in patients who have a good bladder capacity. However, in most of these failures the bladder capacity is small and augmentation is required. At the time of reoperative surgery, either the bladder neck is transected proximal to the prostate with a Mitrofanoff substitution or a continence procedure is performed, such as an artificial sphincter or collagen injection, or both. In our extensive experience with failed bladder neck reconstructions, most of the patients have had several surgeries and need to be dry. In such cases, the most suitable alternative is bladder neck transection, augmentation, and a continent urinary stoma (Gearhart et al, 1995b; Hensle et al, 1995).

Delayed urinary continence has been reported at the onset of puberty in some males and has been attributed to prostatic growth. On MRI, the prostate of exstrophy patients is clover shaped and absent anteriorly, and its mean weight and maximal cross section and volume are normal (Gearhart et al, 1992). Therefore, it is doubtful that growth of this abnormally configured prostate can have much impact on later urinary continence after failed bladder neck repair.

Failed Genitourethral Reconstruction

Common complications of modern epispadias repair include urethrocutaneous fistula formation. This has been reported in as few as 4% and as many as 19% of cases (Kajbafzadeh et al, 1995; Surer et al, 2000). Urethral tortuosity with difficult catheterization or strictures are uncommon with modern epispadias repair. Since the application of the penile disassembly for epispadias reconstruction, newer, more significant complications have been noted (Hammouda, 2003). Gearhart and Baird (2004b) have reported loss of the glans, corpora, or both in addition to loss of penile skin and the urethral plate. Whether this is secondary to surgical misadventure, vagaries in the blood supply of the penis, or the intrinsic difficulties in the procedure remains a topic of debate. Reconstruction of these complications has required additional techniques including tissue expansion, full-thickness skin grafting, buccal mucosal grafting, and other complex techniques. In some patients with significant losses, tissue engineering may eventually provide the material for final cosmetic reconstruction.

At an older age, unsightly penile scars and a short phallus may prompt further surgical intervention. Scar excision can be closed in a plastic fashion if enough penile skin is available. Otherwise, flaps or full-thickness skin grafts can be used. In severe cases, tissue expanders can be placed under the penile skin and gradually inflated over 6 weeks to allow more penile skin and obviate the need for grafting. Freeing all scar tissues and suspensory ligament tissue can maximize available penile length. A dorsal dermal corporal graft or ventral corporal plication or rotation may additionally help lengthen as well as correct any chordee. However, it must be recognized that the exstrophy penis, when compared with age- and race-matched controls, is congenitally deficient in anterior corporal tissue as assessed by MRI (Silver et al, 1997b). Therefore, overly aggressive attempts at penile lengthening may result only in corporal denervation and devascularization without additional lengthening.

Alternative Techniques of Reconstruction

Not all children with bladder exstrophy are candidates for staged functional closure or other primary repair at initial evaluation because of a small bladder plate or significant hydronephrosis. Additional reasons for seeking other methods of treatment include failure of initial closure with a small remaining bladder or failure of continence surgery, or both. Excluding the patients in whom initial treatment fails, this discussion deals with options available when modern staged functional closure or combined repair is not chosen by the surgeon or for other reasons has not been suitable.

Ureterosigmoidostomy

Whichever urinary diversion is chosen, the upper tracts and renal function are initially normal. This allows the reimplantation of normal-sized ureters in a reliable, nonrefluxing manner into the colon or other suitable reservoir. Historically, ureterosigmoidostomy was the first form of diversion to be popularized for patients with exstrophy. Although the initial series was associated with multiple metabolic problems, results improved markedly with newer techniques of reimplantation (Zarbo and Kay, 1986; Koo et al, 1996). Ureterosigmoidostomy is favored by some because of the lack of an abdominal stoma. **However, this form of diversion should not be offered until one is certain that anal continence is normal and after the family has been made aware of the potential serious complications, including pyelonephritis, hyperkalemic acidosis, rectal incontinence, ureteral obstruction, and delayed development of malignancy** (Spence et al, 1979; Duckett and Gazak, 1983). More recently, ureterosigmoidostomy has been proposed again as an initial treatment of bladder exstrophy with acceptable continence and renal preservation on follow-up of 10 years or longer.

Stein and associates (1999) treated a group of 128 patients with bladder exstrophy-epispadias with the Mainz technique for ureterosigmoidostomy. The Mainz Sigma Pouch is constructed and the ureters reimplanted in a nonrefluxing manner. The abdominal wall is reconstructed and the bladder is closed as a seminal receptacle above the prostate. The penis is then reconstructed at a later date. D'elia and coauthors (2004) reported on 26 patients with the exstrophy-epispadias complex who showed excellent continence rates with long-term upper tract preservation when compared with standard ureterosigmoidostomy. Continence was achieved in 95% of patients with a rectal reservoir. Their recommendation for treatment in a number of patients with severely impaired renal function was that a colonic conduit was the best method of choice for diversion. In the patients with a normal or slightly dilated upper tract and intact anal sphincters, a Mainz rectal reservoir was recommended. Although the group from Mainz reported no cancer in a long-term follow-up study of patients who underwent ureterosigmoidostomy, the risk for malignancy still exists and must be carefully considered in a young child. Patients who have had mixing of urine and feces at any time during reconstruction remain at high risk for the development of cancers (Smeulders and Woodhouse, 2001). Bladder exstrophy patients who have failed an initial reconstruction and have polyposis at the time of repeated closure may also be at higher risk for the later development of malignancy (Novak et al, 2004). This is especially true in today's very mobile society, in which careful long-term follow-up may be difficult to guarantee.

Other Forms of Diversion

Alternative techniques of urinary diversion in bladder exstrophy have been described. Maydl (1894) described a method of trigonosigmoidostomy. Boyce and Vest (1952) reported their results on long-term follow-up with these patients. Overall, renal function was normal in 91% and all children achieved daytime continence. A long-term report of Boyce's series by Kroovand and Boyce (1988) showed that most of the patients had stable upper tracts, minimal leakage, and no electrolyte imbalances or malignant changes in the vesical rectal reservoir.

Lastly, the procedure of Heitz-Boyer and Houvelaque (1912) included diverting the ureters into an isolated rectal segment and pulling the sigmoid colon through the anal sphincter just posterior to the rectum. Taccinoli and colleagues (1977) reviewed 21 patients with bladder exstrophy who had undergone this procedure with follow-up of 16 years. They reported 95% fecal and urinary continence, with no urinary calculi, electrolyte abnormalities, or postoperative mortality. Ureterorectal strictures developed in three patients and required surgical revision.

Continent Urinary Diversion in the Exstrophy Patient

In modern pediatric urology there is usually very little need for incontinent urinary diversion in the patient with bladder exstrophy. In a young child with a bladder that is too small to close, or in a failed closure where the bladder template is too small to reclose, we recommend a nonrefluxing colon conduit. This protects the kidneys from vesicoureteral reflux, and undiversion can be performed when clinically indicated at an older age.

Advances in the reconstruction of the lower urinary tract in the past several years have been applied to the patient with exstrophy. Most commonly, further reconstruction in required in the patient in whom bladder neck reconstruction has failed. If a patient does not meet the criteria for bladder neck reconstruction (i.e., inadequate bladder capacity or inability to conform to a voiding regimen), deferring surgery is advisable. Patients in whom bladder neck reconstruction fails are most often destined to augmentation cystoplasty and continent urinary diversion. Surer and colleagues (2003) reported on 91 patients with the exstrophy-epispadias complex who underwent continent urinary diversion. Eight patients had bladder exstrophy, eight had cloacal exstrophy, and three had complete epispadias. The majority had undergone prior failed bladder neck reconstruction (n = 62). Seventy-nine patients (87%) had exstrophy closure prior to referral, 53 had also undergone bladder neck reconstruction, and 29 patients had never reached adequate capacity for bladder neck reconstruction. Ten of the 53 patients had undergone one prior attempt, 35 had two prior attempts, and 8 had three prior attempts at bladder neck reconstruction. A combined augmentation cystoplasty, continent urinary diversion, and bladder neck closure was performed in 59 patients (65%) and reaugmentation and continent urinary diversion was performed in 18 children. Ileocystoplasty was utilized in 41 patients, and sigmoid cystoplasty was performed in 30 patients. The appendix was used as the continent urinary diversion in 67 patients. Continence using intermittent catheterization through the stoma was achieved in 93% of children with the most common complication reported being that of bladder stones, noted in 26%.

Continence can be achieved in most patients with exstrophy following failure of bladder neck reconstruction. This continence is typically obtained through augmentation cystoplasty and revision of the bladder neck reconstruction or closure. If a patient is unlikely to develop adequate capacity for eventual bladder neck reconstruction, moving early to continent urinary diversion is preferable.

KEY POINTS: BLADDER EXSTROPHY— PRIORITIES IN MANAGEMENT

- Size and quality of bladder template
- Extent of pubic diastasis and malleability of the pelvis
- Need for osteotomy
- Length and width of urethral plate
- Penile size
- Associated anomalies

CLOACAL EXSTROPHY

Cloacal exstrophy includes a spectrum of abnormalities but is primarily an anterior abdominal wall defect. A reported incidence of 1:200,000 to 1:400,000 makes this one of the rarer urologic abnormalities (Hurwitz et al, 1987). Although prior reports have suggested a male/female ratio of 2:1 (Gearhart and Jeffs 1998), a large study by Boyadjiev and colleagues (2004) indicated that the sex ratio may be 1:1. Most cases are sporadic, and isolated incidences of unbalanced translocations have been reported to be potentially causative (Thauvin-Robinet et al, 2004); however, one report noted recurrence in siblings, perhaps indicating a more multifactorial etiology. Associated defects of the neurospinal axis, intestinal tract, and urogenital and skeletal systems are frequently noted. When neurospinal defects and omphalocele coexist with cloacal exstrophy, the term OEIS complex (omphalocele, exstrophy, imperforate anus, spinal defects) has been used (Keppler-Noreiul, 2001). Advances in critical care of children have resulted in most patients surviving into adult life and modified the focus to improving quality of life (Mathews et al, 1998).

Anatomic Considerations

The classic constellation of anomalies that are noted in children with cloacal exstrophy includes exstrophy of the bladder, complete phallic separation, wide pubic diastasis, exstrophy of the terminal ileum between the two halves of the bladder, a rudimentary hindgut, imperforate anus, and the presence of an omphalocele. Many children have associated spinal defects, and various lower extremity malformations may be noted (Loder and Dayioglu, 1990; Jain and Weaver, 2004) The urogenital anomalies in cloacal exstrophy are similar to those seen with classic bladder exstrophy (see earlier), although they are typically of greater severity.

Neurospinal Abnormalities

Abnormalities of the spinal cord or vertebral column, or both, have been noted in 85% to 100% of children with cloacal exstrophy (Appignani et al, 1994; McLaughlin et al, 1995). Although most patients have lumbar myelodysplasia (80%), thoracic defects may be noted in 10% with the remaining having sacral defects. In a large series of 34 patients from a single center with cloacal exstrophy and associated spinal defects, Mathews and coworkers (1998) noted lipomeningocele in 17, myelomeningocele in 8, and spina bifida and isolated cord tethering in 7 and 2 patients, respectively. The nearly universal incidence of spinal abnormalities has led some authors to suggest MRI for all patients with a diagnosis of cloacal exstrophy (Cohen, 1991). Spinal ultrasound evaluation, which is easily performed, has been noted to be comparable to MRI for the diagnosis of spinal anomalies in infants with cloacal exstrophy (Dick et al, 2001). Karrer and colleagues (1988) noted that only one in five children with spinal dysraphism noted on ultrasonography had a sacral abnormality visible on the skin surface.

The embryologic basis for the neurospinal defects associated with cloacal exstrophy has been postulated to be secondary to problems with the disruption of the tissue of the dorsal mesenchyme rather than failure of neural tube closure (McLaughlin et al, 1995). Alternatively, it has been suggested that the defects that lead to the formation of cloacal exstrophy may lead to the developing spinal cord and vertebrae being pulled apart (Cohen, 1991). Functional deficits can range from patients who have almost normal sensation of the pelvis and lower extremity to patients who are wheelchair bound. The presence of a clinically significant neurologic anomaly was found to affect negatively the development of continence (Husmann et al, 1999) and led to a significant reduction in continence when compared with patients with

bladder exstrophy. Only 1 of 13 neurologically impaired patients in this series developed voided continence.

The neuroanatomic dissections performed by Schlegel and Gearhart (1989) further indicate that the neuroanatomic landmarks in the infant with cloacal exstrophy are different from those in the normal newborn with the autonomic bladder innervation being derived from a more medial location (Fig. 119–24). This potentially puts the nerve supply in jeopardy during initial bladder dissection and reconstruction and may leave the bladder neuropathic following reconstruction (Husmann et al, 1999). **Innervation to the duplicated corporal bodies arises from the sacral plexus, travels in the midline, perforates the interior portion of the pelvic floor, and courses medially to the hemibladders** (Schlegel and Gearhart, 1989). Innervation abnormalities were also noted at a histologic level in the studies by Rosch and colleagues. When compared with those in patients with bladder exstrophy, the neural elements identified on immunohistochemical evaluation were found to show significant structural abnormalities.

Skeletal System Abnormalities

Anomalies of the skeletal system are universally noted in children with cloacal exstrophy. The pelvic defects that are seen with classic bladder exstrophy are noted with greater severity in the patient with cloacal exstrophy. Sponseller and associates (1995), studying patients with the exstrophy complex,

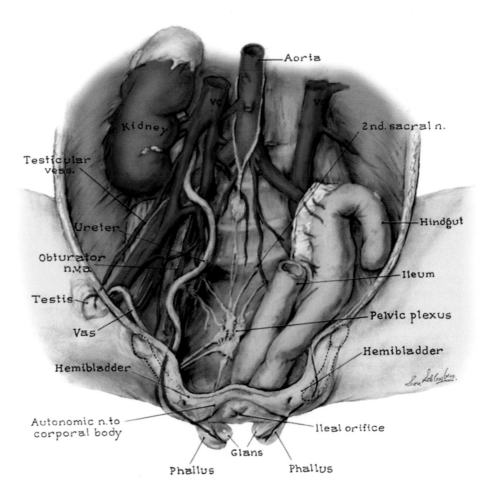

Figure 119–24. Internal view of a patient with cloacal exstrophy. Pudendal vessels, nerves, and other vessels and autonomic innervation of the corporal bodies are demonstrated. Internal structures of the pelvis along with duplication of the vena cava in this dissected specimen are also shown.

noted that the posterior segment of the pelvis in children with cloacal exstrophy was angled farther posteriorly and there was a greater likelihood of asymmetry between the two sides. Similarly, the anterior segment of the pelvis had more severe degrees of external rotation. The actual length of the bone segments, however, was similar between those with cloacal and classic exstrophy. The interpubic distance (diastasis) in children with cloacal exstrophy was noted to be almost twice that of children with classic bladder exstrophy. Malformation of the sacroiliac joints and side-to-side asymmetry were also noted. These issues become of increasing importance, and most children with cloacal exstrophy require osteotomy for successful reconstruction. Stec and colleagues (2003) noted that, microscopically, the bones in children with cloacal exstrophy were similar to those in normal controls and were developing at a similar rate, indicating that the potential for growth was also similar.

Vertebral anomalies that were not associated with myelodyplasia were noted in 8 of 37 children with cloacal exstrophy (Mathews et al, 1998). Loder and Dayioglu (1990) noted vertebral anomalies in three of five children with cloacal exstrophy. Absence or shortening of limbs was also noted, as were clubfoot malformations. **Skeletal and limb anomalies were also reported by Diamond (1990) in 12% to 65% of cases.** The vast majority were clubfoot deformities, although absence of feet, severe tibial or fibular deformities, and congenital hip dislocations were commonly noted in this group of patients. A similar high incidence of foot abnormalities and greater than normal abduction of the hips was noted in a study by Greene and coworkers (1998).

Intestinal Tract Abnormalities

Gastrointestinal tract anomalies occur in virtually all patients with cloacal exstrophy. **In Diamond's series (1990), the incidence of omphalocele was 88%, and a majority of all series reported an incidence of 95% or greater.** In the series reported by Mathews and colleagues (1998), 100% had an omphalocele. Omphaloceles do vary in size and usually contain small bowel or liver, or both. Immediate closure of the omphalocele defect in the newborn period is advised to prevent subsequent rupture.

Hurwitz and colleagues (1987), in a large review of cloacal exstrophy patients, reported a 46% incidence of associated gastrointestinal tract anomalies, with malrotation, duplication anomalies, and anatomically short bowel occurring with equal frequency. A hindgut remnant of varying size is also noted in most patients. Hurwitz noted a 23% incidence of short gut syndrome, which is compatible with the 25% incidence reported by Diamond (Hurwitz et al, 1987; Diamond, 1990). It now seems well accepted that short gut syndrome may occur in the presence of normal small bowel length, suggesting absorptive dysfunction and emphasizing the absolute need to preserve as much large bowel as possible. If not utilized for incorporation into the fecal stream, the hindgut remnant may be preserved for use in urogenital tract reconstruction (Mathews et al, 1998).

Genitourinary Abnormalities

Müllerian anomalies have been frequently noted in conjunction with cloacal exstrophy. **The most commonly reported müllerian anomaly was uterine duplication, seen in 95% of patients** (Diamond, 1990). The vast majority of these patients had partial uterine duplication, predominantly a bicornate uterus. Vaginal duplication occurred in 65% of cases, and vaginal agenesis was seen in 25% to 50% of patients. In a report by Hurwitz and colleagues (1987), cases of complete duplication of the uterus and fallopian tubes associated with both vaginal duplication and vaginal agenesis were noted. Gearhart and Jeffs (1991b) recommended preservation of all müllerian duplication anomalies for possible utilization in reconstructing the lower urinary tract.

Upper urinary tract anomalies occurred in 41% to 60% of patients in Diamond's review. The most common anomalies were pelvic kidney and renal agenesis, both occurring in up to one third of patients. Hydronephrosis and hydroureter were common, occurring in one third of patients. Multicystic dysplastic kidneys and fusion anomalies were seen less frequently. Ectopic ureters draining to the vasa in the male and into the uterus, vagina, or fallopian tubes in the female were also reported (Diamond, 1990). A similar incidence of upper tract defects was noted by Mathews and colleagues. Ureteral duplication, congenital stricture, and megaureter were also reported.

Genital anomalies in the male have typically included complete separation of the two phallic halves and accompanied separation of the scrotal halves. Asymmetry of these structures can also be seen and provide additional challenges to successful reconstruction. Testes may be noted in the scrotum but are frequently noted to be undescended, and associated inguinal hernias are a common finding. Girls typically have widely divergent clitoral halves.

The lower urinary tract is typically composed of two exstrophied hemibladders flanking the exstrophied intestinal segment. Each bladder half usually drains the ipsilateral ureter and is closely related to the ipsilateral phallic segment. Variations of anatomy, however, are frequently seen and every patient has unique anatomic features.

Additional System Anomalies

Life-threatening cardiovascular and pulmonary anomalies are rarely seen in cloacal exstrophy. Reported cases included two patients with cyanotic heart disease and one with aortic duplication. A bilobed lung was reported in two patients and an atretic right upper lung in one. Also, Schlegel and Gearhart (1989) reported caval duplication in their anatomic dissection of a patient with cloacal exstrophy.

Because of the complexity and the multisystem nature of cloacal exstrophy, Hurwitz and coauthors (1987) have devised a grid for the clarification of anatomy in each patient and to permit planning for reconstruction (Fig. 119–25). This permits the standard form of cloacal exstrophy to be separated from variants and allows the soft tissue components of the defect to be described systematically.

Prenatal Diagnosis

Since its initial description in the early 1980s, further refinements in the prenatal diagnosis of cloacal exstrophy have occurred (Meizner and Bar-Ziv, 1985). These authors indicated that the three main criteria used to identify the diagnosis were a large midline infraumbilical anterior abdominal wall defect, lumbosacral myelomeningocele, and failure to

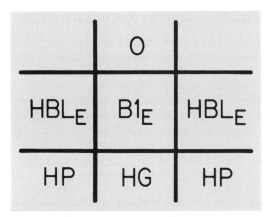

Figure 119–25. Coding grid used to describe cloacal exstrophy and its variants. O, omphalocele; HBL$_E$, hemibladder; B1$_E$, everted bowel; HP, hemiphallus; HG, hindgut. (From Hurwitz RS, Manzoni GA, Ransley PG, Stephen FD: Cloacal exstrophy: A report of 34 cases. J Urol 1987;138:1060.)

visualize the urinary bladder. Chitrit and colleagues (1993) reported the diagnosis of monozygotic twins with cloacal exstrophy detected during antenatal ultrasound screening. Since these initial reports, there have been only occasional case reports of prenatal diagnosis of cloacal exstrophy, and only 15% of patients with this anomaly have been diagnosed by prenatal ultrasonography, according to the literature. With the marked improvements in survival of patients with cloacal exstrophy in the last 20 years and the common application of fetal ultrasonography, early diagnosis may permit appropriate prenatal counseling for parents and expedite postnatal care.

Austin and colleagues (1998) reviewed 20 patients with this abnormality, expanded on the diagnostic findings, and proposed major and minor criteria for the prenatal diagnosis of cloacal exstrophy, based on the frequency of occurrence rather than the severity of individual findings. A criterion was considered major if it was present in more than 50% of cases. The gestational age at diagnosis of cloacal exstrophy ranged from 15 to 32 weeks (mean, 22 weeks). Major diagnostic criteria included nonvisualization of the bladder in 91%, a large midline infraumbilical anterior wall defect or a cystic anterior wall structure in 82%, an omphalocele in 77%, and a myelomeningocele in 68%. Minor criteria included lower extremity defects in 23%, renal anomalies in 23%, ascites in 41%, widened pubic arches in 18%, narrow thorax in 9%, hydrocephalus in 9%, and a single umbilical artery in 9%. Hamada and coauthors (1999) reported a single case in which ultrasonography revealed a wavy cordlike segment of soft tissue protruding from the anterior abdominal wall of the fetus below the umbilicus. This was found to be prolapsed terminal ileum, which resembled the trunk of an elephant. The authors suggested that this sonographic image be added to the criteria described by Austin and associates (1998) for making a prenatal diagnosis of cloacal exstrophy.

Universal use of antenatal ultrasonography has permitted diagnosis of cloacal exstrophy to be made at a time when parental counseling may lead to possible pregnancy termination. Extensive parental counseling regarding the significant anatomic anomalies that constitute the complex is appropriate in conjunction with psychological support.

Table 119–5. Modern Staged Functional Reconstruction of Cloacal Exstrophy

Immediate Neonatal Assessment

  Evaluate associated anomalies
  Decide whether to proceed with reparative surgery

Functional Bladder Closure (Soon after Neonatal Assessment)

  One-stage repair (few associated anomalies)
    Excision of omphalocele
    Separation of cecal plate from bladder halves
    Joining and closure of bladder halves and urethroplasty
    Bilateral anterior innominate and vertical iliac osteotomy
    Gonadectomy in males with unreconstructible phallus
    Terminal ileostomy/colostomy
    Genital revision if needed
  Two-stage repair
    First stage (newborn period)
      Excision of omphalocele
      Separation of cecal plate from bladder halves
      Joining of bladder halves
      Gonadectomy in male with unreconstructible phallus
      Terminal ileostomy/colostomy
    Second stage
      Closure of joined bladder halves and urethroplasty
      Bilateral anterior innominate and vertical iliac osteotomy
      Genital revision if needed

Anti-incontinence/Reflux Procedure (age 4-5 yr)

  Bladder capacity ≥85 mL (small select group of patients):
    Young-Dees-Leadbetter bladder neck reconstruction
    Bilateral Cohen ureteral reimplantations
    Bowel and/or stomach segment used to augment bladder
      or
    Continent diversion with abdominal/perineal stoma

Vaginal Reconstruction

  Vagina constructed or augmented using colon, ileum, or full-thickness skin graft

SURGICAL RECONSTRUCTION OF CLOACAL EXSTROPHY

The initial successful reconstruction of cloacal exstrophy was reported by Rickham (1960). Survival in the 1970s remained at about 50%; however, the institution of intensive postnatal care led to improvement in survival in the 1980s to almost 100%.

Evaluation and Management at Birth

Immediate management is directed to the medical stabilization of the infant. Complete physical examination and determination of the various anatomic defects present allow short- and long-term management strategies to be created (Table 119–5). This initial planning stage should include decisions about gender assignment. The bowel and bladder segments are kept moist with protective plastic dressings as with bladder exstrophy (Gearhart and Jeffs, 1998). Presence of neurospinal abnormalities requires immediate neurosurgical evaluation. Consultations from social work, pediatric orthopedic surgery, and other disciplines should be obtained. Evaluation of the genitalia and gender assignment should be made by a gender assignment team, including a pediatric urologist, pediatric surgeon, pediatrician, pediatric endocrinologist, and child psychologist or psychiatrist. Gender assignment decisions should be made in conjunction with appropriate parental counseling and involvement. In a large medical center with experience in dealing with complex malformations, these multiple consultations should be done in a short period of time. If there are medical concerns, delayed closure after initial intestinal diversion is appropriate (Mathews et al, 1998).

Gender Assignment

Because of the significant separation of the corpora of the penis and scrotum and the reduction in corporal size noted in boys with cloacal exstrophy, early reports had recommended universal gender reassignment of boys (46,XY) with cloacal exstrophy to functional females (Tank and Lindenaur, 1970). To this end, bilateral orchiopexy was combined with phallic reconstruction as a functional clitoris and early or delayed vaginoplasty. Reiner (2004) has reported on 29 males with cloacal exstrophy who had gender reassignment to female. Psychosexual evaluation indicated that all of these patients had a marked male shift in psychosexual development despite having no pubertal hormonal surges. A comparison of patients with cloacal exstrophy and other cloacal anomalies at the Great Ormond Street, however, indicated no difference in social or behavioral competence or psychological problems. Gender assignment was not associated with childhood psychological, emotional, or behavioral problems (Baker Towell and Towell, 2003). Schober and coauthors (2002), reporting on 14 children who had undergone early gender reassignment, indicated that although patients had masculine childhood behavior, they had a feminine gender identity. Currently, however, most authors recommend assigning gender that is consistent with karyotypic makeup of the individual if at all possible (Fig. 119–26). This policy can be supported by a report indicating that the histology of the testis at birth is normal (Mathews et al, 1999a). Furthermore, with evolution of techniques for phallic reconstruction, a functional and cosmetically acceptable phallus can now be constructed (Husmann et al, 1989b).

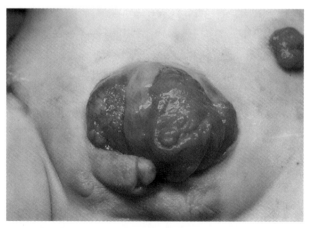

Figure 119–26. A 46,XY child with cloacal exstrophy with a dominant right hemiphallus. This child was reconstructed and reared as male.

Immediate Surgical Reconstruction

Cloacal exstrophy patients should undergo carefully planned and individualized reconstructions (Ricketts et al, 1991; Lund and Hendren, 1993; Mathews et al, 1998). For infants with spinal dysraphism and myelocystocele, neurosurgical consultation should be obtained and closure undertaken as soon as the infant is medically stable. After closure of the myelocystocele, long-term follow-up is mandatory to evaluate for subtle changes in the neurologic evaluation that could herald cord tethering. Symptomatic spinal cord tethering can be seen in up to 33% of children (McLaughlin et al, 1995).

Neonatal omphalocele closure is recommended to prevent untimely rupture and is typically combined with intestinal diversion. Formerly, initial attempts focused on ileostomy with resection of the hindgut remnant. **Since the recognition of the metabolic changes that occur in patients with ileostomy, an attempt is always made to use the hindgut remnant to provide additional length of bowel for fluid absorption** (Husmann et al, 1989a: Mathews et al, 1998). Enlargement of the hindgut remnant and increased water absorption have been noted in children who have had this segment incorporated into construction of a fecal colostomy. The hindgut segment may be anastomosed in an isoperistaltic or retroperistaltic fashion to increase motility and generate formed stool. Children who have anal stenosis and not imperforate anus may have the capability for later continence and may be treated with a pull-through procedure (Ricketts et al, 1991). If the hindgut remnant is not used for bowel reconstruction, it should be left as a mucus fistula to be used for later bladder augmentation or vaginal reconstruction (Lund and Hendren, 1993; Mathews et al, 1998). If gastrointestinal reconstruction is combined with bladder closure, approximation of the pubis, usually with osteotomies, is beneficial in reconstruction of the pelvic ring and increases the potential for successful bladder and abdominal wall closure (Mathews et al, 1998). Some authors have suggested that gastrointestinal reconstruction after initial fecal diversion be delayed for 1 to 2 years of observation (Soffer et al, 2000). After this time, radiographic evaluation is performed to determine residual colonic length. If near-normal colonic length is noted, a pull-through procedure is performed. If there is short colon but the patient is able to make solid stool, the patient may still be a candidate for pull-through procedures. Patients who are unable to make solid stool are typically managed with a permanent fecal stoma.

At the initial stage of omphalocele closure, if it is determined that bladder and abdominal wall closure may not be accomplished, the bladder halves are approximated in the midline without further dissection and the defect converted to a bladder exstrophy (Ricketts et al, 1991; Mathews et al, 1998). This permits abdominal distention to allow enlargement of this bladder plate for later closure. If the hindgut segment is not utilized in the initial reconstruction of the bowel, it is left as a mucus fistula.

Urinary Reconstruction

Modern Staged Reconstruction

The staged management of the urinary tract follows that utilized for the management of bladder exstrophy (Gearhart and

Jeffs, 1991b). Once the bladder halves have been approximated posteriorly, the lateral edges are separated from the abdominal wall and brought together in the midline. As in the patient with classic exstrophy, placement of the bladder and posterior urethra deep into the pelvis remains a key factor in the successful surgical reconstruction of the urinary tract. Inguinal hernias that are noted should be repaired at the time of closure. In genetic females and in genotypic male subjects undergoing gender reassignment, reconstruction should be performed to improve the appearance of the genitalia.

Reconstruction of the external genitalia in the immediate postnatal period is performed to make the infant appear more congruent with the gender assigned. The psychiatric studies of children who have had gender assignment have fueled interest in male gender assignment if adequate unilateral or bilateral corporal tissue is present (Reiner, 2004). Histologic studies indicate normal histology in the testes of male subjects who have had gender reassignment despite the presence of cryptorchidism (Mathews et al, 1999a). Results of phallic reconstruction in male patients with minimal or no penile tissue in the past have been disappointing. For male-to-female reassignment, initial female genital reconstruction should bring the phallic halves together in the midline as a clitoris.

However, in instances with adequate corporal tissue, either unilaterally or bilaterally, epispadias repair can be performed at around age 1 using the standards identified for the staged reconstruction. Vaginal reconstruction can be performed early in the genetic female patient. In gender-converted male patients who require reconstruction of a neovagina, delayed reconstruction is appropriate. Reconstruction may be performed by using a preserved hindgut segment or expanded perineal skin. Long-term dilatation of the neovagina may be required.

Pubic approximation permits abdominal wall closure and usually requires osteotomy and fixation with postoperative traction. External fixation and traction are typically maintained for 6 to 8 weeks to permit healing.

Role of Osteotomy

Infants who are medically stable may be considered for urinary tract reconstruction in the immediate postnatal period. Osteotomy is indicated in all children with cloacal exstrophy at the time of bladder closure because of the wide diastasis that is invariably present (Mathews et al, 1998). Osteotomy allows the pelvic ring, bladder, and abdominal wall to be closed without undue tension on the closure. Reduction in dehiscence and postoperative ventral hernias has been noted in patients treated with osteotomy. In a large series reported by Ben-Chaim and associates (1995c), significant complications occurred in 89% of patients who underwent closure of the cloacal exstrophy without osteotomy but in only 17% of patients who underwent osteotomy at the time of initial cloacal exstrophy closure. Interestingly, the patients who underwent osteotomy and those who did not were similar in terms of size of the omphalocele, presence of myelomeningocele, and time of primary closure. However, it is not surprising that osteotomy had no effect on eventual continence of patients with cloacal exstrophy.

Currently, combined anterior innominate and vertical iliac osteotomies are routinely used at our institution (Silver et al, 1999). This approach does not require the patient to be repo-

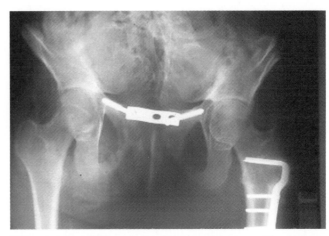

Figure 119-27. Pubic approximation and maintenance with a stainless steel plate in a child with cloacal exstrophy.

sitioned on the operating table before commencing bladder and abdominal wall closure. In addition, this method obviates the use of a posterior approach and any complication of the procedure related to the spinal or back closure. **In a series of five patients with extreme pubic diastasis greater than 10 cm, Silver and colleagues (1999) described initial pelvic osteotomy and gradual pelvic closure of the fixator for 1 to 2 weeks, followed by abdominal wall closure and bladder closure.** Closure was successful in all patients without technical problems or complications. This technique of staged pelvic closure may provide reliable initial secondary repair in patients with cloacal exstrophy in whom one-stage pelvic closure is not feasible, even with pelvic osteotomy. An interpubic stainless bar has been added to permit stabilization of the pubic approximation and maintain the reduction in diastasis (Fig. 119–27) (Mathews et al, 2005). Because of the possible asymmetry that can be noted in the pelvic bones, care must be used when performing osteotomies and fixation. In patients who have lower extremity abnormalities, providing postoperative traction can also be challenging.

Single-Stage Reconstruction

Grady and Mitchell (1999) have reported using a single-stage reconstruction in cloacal exstrophy—a procedure similar to that done for bladder exstrophy. Delay in urinary tract reconstruction has also been advised by these authors if there is a large omphalocele or other medical instability. In this situation, the conversion to a bladder exstrophy and subsequent reconstruction of the bladder and penis as a single step is performed. Among the small number of patients who have had this type of management strategy, occasional patients have been reported to be able to have voided continence. As with staged reconstruction, some patients have required augmentation cystoplasty for continence.

Techniques to Create Urinary Continence

Urinary continence is possible in most children but usually requires bladder augmentation and the use of intermittent catheterization. Multiple series by Gearhart and Jeffs (1991b),

Mitchell and associates (1990), and Hendren (1992) have shown the applicability of modern techniques for lower tract reconstruction to help these patients achieve urinary continence. Enhancement of bladder capacity may be performed using a hindgut segment, if available; ileum; or stomach. Continence appears to be more difficult to achieve in male patients who undergo gender reassignment, and a continent stoma may be most applicable in this special group of patients (Mathews, 1998). In genetic female patients, successful continence has been achieved after Young-Dees-Leadbetter bladder neck reconstruction, but the vast majority of patients have required intermittent catheterization (Husmann et al, 1999). Similar findings were reported in a series by Mitchell and associates (1990). Husmann and colleagues (1999) reported that the success rate of Young-Dees-Leadbetter bladder neck reconstruction in the cloacal exstrophy population was closely related to the presence of coexisting neurologic abnormalities.

Urinary continence can be achieved in these individuals in many ways. An orthotopic urethra can be constructed from local tissue, vagina, ileum, stomach, or ureter. A catheterizable stoma can be constructed from ileum when enough bowel is present and fluid loss is not a problem. The bladder may be augmented with unused hindgut, ileum, or stomach. However, surgery to provide a continent urinary reservoir should be delayed until a method of evacuation can be taught and the child is old enough to participate in self-care. The choice between a catheterizable urethra and an abdominal stoma depends on the adequacy of the urethra and bladder outlet, interest and dexterity of the child, and orthopedic status regarding the spine, hip joints, braces, and ambulation. In a series by Gearhart and Jeffs (1991b) and in another series by Mitchell and associates (1990), multiple techniques were used to produce continence in patients with cloacal exstrophy. An innovative approach is required to find a suitable solution for each individual patient according to the patient's bladder size and function and mental, neurologic, and orthopedic status. With the advent of modern pediatric anesthesia and intensive care, the newborn survival rate is high. Improving survivorship makes reconstructive techniques applicable in a large percentage of patients born with this condition.

LONG-TERM ISSUES IN CLOACAL EXSTROPHY

Because survival has become almost universal, the focus has changed in cloacal exstrophy to improving quality of life. Improvement in functional outcomes has become the mainstay of improving the quality of life. Patients presenting with significant neurologic defects need intensive management to provide improvement in quality of life. In this population, management of the bowel with permanent diversion and using continent catheterization channels for urinary management provide independence and promote improvement in self-esteem. When neurologic issues are minimal or absent, bowel pull-through and voided continence would be ideal. Ricketts and associates (1991) have presented a continence score that can be used in this group of children. Using a six-point scoring system to determine bowel and bladder continence (6 = best; 0 = worst), they evaluated 12 patients who

had been managed over time. They had seven patients with a continence score of 1 (colostomy and incontinent bladder) and only one patient who had a score of 5 (enema program and a continent bladder), attesting to the difficulties presented with surgical reconstruction.

Some children have required permanent ileostomy for management of their gut. Husmann and colleagues (1989) noted that patients undergoing permanent ileostomy, in comparison with terminal colostomy, had greater initial morbidity; however, bowel adaptation appeared to occur by age 3 years with resolution of the short gut syndrome in most. If patients with terminal ileostomy were aggressively managed with hyperalimentation, growth characteristics in the two groups were very similar.

Attempts at phallic reconstruction in the past had minimal success because of the diminutive nature of the corpora in boys and the wide pubic separation. Modern reconstructive surgical techniques may allow some boys to have complete phallic reconstruction performed with forearm grafts. Fertility appears to be universally compromised in boys, but girls have normal fertility and pregnancy has been reported. Girls have higher degrees of cervical prolapse when compared with their counterparts with bladder exstrophy.

Summary

Evolution in management of cloacal exstrophy has permitted near-universal survival with significant improvement in cosmetic and functional outcomes. Debate continues regarding the issue of gender reassignment, and long-term data are still accruing on the best strategy for management. Continence can be achieved with appropriate reconstruction and the use of intermittent catheterization. Despite the extensive malformations noted, many patients have gone on to live fruitful lives.

KEY POINTS: CLOACAL EXSTROPHY— PRIORITIES IN MANAGEMENT

- Medical stabilization
- Gender assignment
- Colonic functionalization
- Separation of bladder from the gastrointestinal tract
- Functional genital reconstruction

EPISPADIAS

Epispadias varies from a mild glanular defect in a covered penis to the penopubic variety with complete incontinence in males or females. It is most commonly noted as a component of bladder and cloacal exstrophy.

Male Epispadias

Isolated male epispadias is a rare anomaly, with a reported incidence of 1 in 117,000 males. Most male epispadias patients (about 70%) have complete epispadias with incon-

tinence (Gearhart and Jeffs, 1998). Epispadias consists of a defect in the dorsal wall of the urethra. The normal urethra is replaced by a broad, mucosal strip lining the dorsum of the penis extending toward the bladder, with potential incompetence of the sphincter mechanism. The displaced meatus is free of deformity, and occurrence of urinary incontinence is related to the degree of the dorsally displaced urethral meatus (Gearhart and Jeffs, 1998). The displaced meatus may be found on the glans, penile shaft, or in the penopubic region. All types of epispadias are associated with varying degrees of dorsal chordee. In penopubic or subsymphyseal epispadias, the entire penile urethra is opened and the bladder outlet may be large enough to admit the examining finger, indicating obvious gross incontinence (Fig. 119–28A). To a lesser extent than those with classic bladder exstrophy, patients with epispadias have a characteristic widening of the symphysis pubis caused by outward rotation of the innominate bones. This separation of the pubis causes divergent penopubic attachments that contribute to the short, pendular penis with dorsal chordee. Therefore, the penile deformity is virtually identical to that observed in bladder exstrophy. The reported male-to-female ratio of epispadias varies between 3:1 (Dees, 1949) and 5:1 (Kramer and Kelalis, 1982a).

Kramer and Kelalis (1982a) reviewed their experience with 82 male patients with epispadias. Penopubic epispadias occurred in 49 cases, penile epispadias in 21, and glandular epispadias in 12. Urinary incontinence was observed in 46 of 49 patients with penopubic epispadias, in 15 of 21 patients with penile epispadias, and in no patient with glandular epispadias. The goals of the treatment of complete male epispadias include creation of normal urinary control and establishment of a straight, cosmetically acceptable penis of adequate length that is functional for normal sexual intercourse. It has been postulated that complete male epispadias is similar to classic bladder exstrophy except that in complete epispadias the bladder is closed and bladder closure procedures are not required.

Associated Anomalies

Anomalies associated with complete epispadias are usually confined to deformities of the external genitalia, diastasis of the pubic symphysis, and deficiency of the urinary continence mechanism. The only renal anomaly observed in 11 cases of epispadias was agenesis of the left kidney (Campbell, 1952). In a review by Arap and associates (1988), 1 case of renal agenesis and 1 ectopic kidney occurred among 38 patients.

The ureterovesical junction is inherently deficient in complete epispadias, and the incidence of reflux has been reported in a number of series to be between 30% and 40% (Kramer and Kelalis, 1982a; Arap et al, 1988). In a review by Ben-Chaim and colleagues (1995b) of a series of 15 patients with complete male epispadias treated at our institution, a lower rate of vesicoureteral reflux was noted compared with male patients with classic bladder exstrophy (100% versus 82%, respectively); the rate of inguinal hernias (33%) was also significantly lower. A possible explanation for the lower incidence of reflux in complete male epispadias is that the pouch of Douglas is not as enlarged and deep. Therefore, the distal ureter enters the bladder in a more oblique fashion than in classic exstrophy (Gearhart and Jeffs, 1998).

Surgical Management

The objectives of repair of penopubic epispadias include achievement of urinary continence with preservation of the upper urinary tracts and the reconstruction of cosmetically acceptable genitalia. The surgical management of incontinence in penopubic epispadias is virtually identical to that in closed bladder exstrophy.

Young (1922) reported the first cure of incontinence in a male patient with complete epispadias. Since this initial

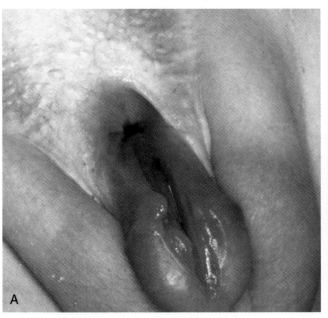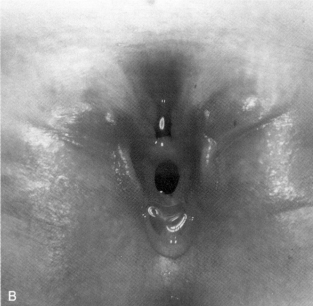

Figure 119–28. **A,** Three-month-old boy with complete epispadias. **B,** Six-month-old girl with complete female epispadias.

report, continence following surgical reconstruction has progressively improved (Burkholder and Williams, 1965; Kramer and Kelalis, 1982a; Arap et al, 1988; Peters et al, 1988; Mollard et al, 1998). In patients with complete epispadias and good bladder capacity, epispadias and bladder neck reconstruction can be performed in a single-stage operation. Urethroplasty formerly was performed after bladder neck reconstruction (Kramer and Kelalis, 1982a; Arap et al, 1988). However, improvements in bladder capacity in the small bladder associated with exstrophy (Gearhart and Jeffs, 1989a) and that associated with epispadias (Peters et al, 1988) have led us to perform urethroplasty and penile elongation before bladder neck reconstruction. A small, incontinent bladder with reflux is hardly an ideal situation for bladder neck reconstruction and ureteral reimplantation. Before bladder neck reconstruction there was an average increase in bladder capacity of 95 mL within 18 months after epispadias repair in the patients with an initial small bladder capacity and a continence rate of 87% after the continence procedure (Peters et al, 1988). **In a series by Ben-Chaim and colleagues (1995b) composed exclusively of patients with complete male epispadias, bladder capacity increased by an average of 42 mL within 18 months after urethroplasty.** Nine (82%) of 11 patients were dry day and night after an average of 9 months.

In epispadias, as in the bladder exstrophy, bladder capacity is the predominant indicator of eventual continence (Richey et al, 1988). Arap and coworkers (1988) reported higher continence rates in patients who had an adequate bladder capacity before bladder neck reconstruction than in those with inadequate capacity (71% versus 20%, respectively). In addition, in Arap's group of patients with complete epispadias, most obtained continence within 2 years, similar to results in patients with classic bladder exstrophy.

A firm intrasymphyseal band typically bridges the divergent symphysis, and an osteotomy is not usually performed. The Young-Dees-Leadbetter bladder neck plasty, Marshall-Marchetti-Krantz suspension, and ureteral reimplantation are performed when the bladder capacity reaches approximately 80 to 85 mL, which usually occurs between 4 and 5 years of age. Genital reconstruction procedures in epispadias and exstrophy are similar. The following reconstructive maneuvers must take place: release of dorsal chordee and division of the suspensory ligaments; dissection of the corpora from their attachments to the inferior pubic ramus; lengthening of the urethral groove; and lengthening of the corpora, if needed, by incision and anastomosis or grafting or by medial rotation of the ventral corpora in a more downward direction.

Urethral reconstruction in complete epispadias has been performed in many ways. A transverse island flap was used by Monfort and colleagues (1987). The urethra, once reconstructed, can be positioned between and below the corpora (Cantwell, 1895; Ransley et al, 1989; Gearhart et al, 1992; Gearhart et al, 1995c). Mitchell and Bagli (1996) reported their experience with a complete penile disassembly technique, and a multicenter experience with the technique was later reported in a total of 17 patients from four institutions (Zaontz et al, 1998). Chordee was reliably corrected, erectile function was preserved, the urethra was eventually situated in a cosmetic fashion, and satisfactory cosmesis was achieved. Ransley and Surer and their associates reported excellent results using the modified Cantwell-Ransley procedure, saving cavernocavernostomy for patients with very severe chordee and especially those in the older age group (Kajbafzadeh et al, 1995; Surer et al, 2000). For detailed description of the surgical reconstruction, see the previous discussion in the section for bladder exstrophy.

Achievement of urinary continence after epispadias repair in patients with isolated epispadias is summarized in Table 119–6. A majority of these patients underwent reconstruction by means of a Young-Dees-Leadbetter bladder neck plasty. Urinary continence was obtained in 82% of male patients (Ben-Chaim et al, 1995b). As in the exstrophy population, repair of the epispadiac deformity results in an increase of outlet resistance and possible increase in bladder capacity before bladder neck reconstruction. Although both complete epispadias and bladder exstrophy patients achieve improvement in bladder capacity after epispadias repair, the mean increase in overall capacity is higher in those with complete epispadias. This increase in bladder capacity may account for increased continence in this group compared with the classic bladder exstrophy population. **Clinically, these bladders are more supple, easier to mobilize, and more amenable to bladder neck reconstruction.** Ben-Chaim and colleagues (1995b) reported that the mean time to initial continence following bladder neck reconstruction was 90 days in patients with complete male epispadias compared with 110 days in those with bladder exstrophy. These results suggest that, for patients with complete epispadias, bladder capacity before reconstruction and the rate of achieving continence afterward are better than for patients with bladder exstrophy. The reason

Table 119–6. Urinary Continence after Bladder Neck Reconstruction (BNR) in Patients with Complete Epispadias					
Item	**Ben-Chaim et al (1995b)**	**Gearhart et al (1993a)**	**Kramer and Kelalis (1982a)**	**Arap et al (1988)**	**Burkholder and Williams (1965)**
No. patients	15	11	53	38	27
Males					
No. treated with BNR	11	—	32*	21	17
No. with surgically corrected incontinence	9	—	22	15	8
Percentage with surgically corrected incontinence	82	—	69	71	47
Females					
No. treated with BNR	0	9	8	9	10
No. with surgically corrected incontinence	0	8	8	7	7
Percentage with surgically corrected incontinence	0	87	88	77	70

*All complete female epispadias cases.

might be that the bladder is not exposed in utero and does not have any scarring from prior closure; therefore, its potential for expansion is higher.

It was formerly thought that the effect of urethral lengthening and prostatic enlargement might be significant in complete epispadias by increasing outlet resistance if continence was not perfect as the child became older. Earlier in a series by Arap and associates (1988), the establishment of continence had no relation to puberty and usually occurred within 2 years, usually preceding puberty by several years. In the series reported by Ben-Chaim and coworkers (1995b), as stated previously, all patients obtained daytime continence at a mean of 9 months after bladder neck reconstruction, and 9 (82%) of 11 patients attained total day and night continence. All patients voided spontaneously. After a mean follow-up of 7 years, all patients maintained normal upper tracts and kidney function. All of them had cosmetically pleasing genitalia, as judged by parents, patients, and physicians, and experienced normal erections. A 36-year-old patient was married and had fathered three children. Many of the patients were younger than 16 years of age and had not yet become sexually active.

Results of urethroplasty in epispadias have been reported in a number of publications (Mesrobian et al, 1986; Ransley et al, 1989; Kajbafzadeh et al, 1995; Zaontz et al, 1998). In a modern series of modified Cantwell-Ransley repairs reported by Surer and colleagues (2000), the incidence of postoperative fistula in the 3-month period after surgery was 19%, and the incidence of urethral stricture formation was less than 10%. Catheterization and cystoscopy could easily negotiate the neourethral channel in all patients who underwent a modified Cantwell-Ransley epispadias repair. In another modern series reported by Mollard and coworkers (1998), the continence rate was 84% and the fistula rate was less than 10%. In Mollard's series with long-term follow-up, patients had normal erections; the vast majority had regular sexual intercourse, and most had normal ejaculation or had fathered children. Most of Surer's patients were quite young, and assessment of genital reconstruction must be deferred until these patients are sexually mature and active (2000). In a large series of Hammouda and associates (2003) using the penile disassembly technique, 6% of boys were made hypospadiac and 1% had partial glandar loss. Although many methods of epispadias repair exist, meticulous follow-up of the urethra, selection of patients, and surgical experience remain the milestones of success. Lastly, Ransley and colleagues (Kajbafzadeh et al, 1995) obtained very good results using a modified Cantwell-Ransley repair in a large number of patients with epispadias. The fistula rate was 4%, and the urethral stricture rate was 5.3%.

In a different approach to the treatment of incontinence associated with epispadias reported by Duffy and Ransley (1998), 12 boys age 3 to 7 years underwent endoscopic submucosal injection of plastic microspheres. All patients had undergone a modified Cantwell-Ransley epispadias repair before injection. The procedure was performed 24 times, with a total volume of 83 mL of material injected into 59 sites in the posterior urethra. Mean follow-up was 10.8 months. Three patients (25%) were rendered completely dry, the degree of incontinence was improved in six, and there was no change in three. The authors offered this as an alternative to bladder

neck reconstruction in patients with primary epispadias. Ben-Chaim and coworkers (1995a) reported that submucosal injection of collagen in the bladder neck area can have a role in improving stress incontinence when the patient with complete epispadias has incomplete urinary control or as an adjunct after bladder neck reconstruction.

Kramer and associates (Mesrobian et al, 1986) reported the success of genital reconstruction in epispadias, with good long-term follow-up ending with a straight penis angled downward in almost 70% of patients, with normal erectile function. Of this group, 80% had satisfactory sexual intercourse, and of 29 married patients, 19 had fathered children. These results were mirrored in the long-term follow-up study of Mollard and associates (1998).

A carefully constructed and well-planned approach to the management of urinary incontinence in genital deformities associated with complete epispadias should provide a satisfactory cosmetic appearance, normal genital function, and preservation of fertility potential in most patients.

Female Epispadias

Female epispadias is a rare congenital anomaly; it occurs in 1 of every 484,000 female patients (Gearhart and Jeffs, 1998). We use the classification of Davis (1928), which describes three degrees of epispadias in female patients. In the least degree of epispadias, the urethral orifice simply appears patulous. In intermediate epispadias, the urethra is dorsally split along most of the urethra. In the most severe degree of epispadias, the urethral cleft involves the entire length of the urethra and sphincteric mechanism and the patient is rendered incontinent (see Fig. 119–28B). The genital defect is characterized by a bifid clitoris. The mons is depressed in shape and coated by a smooth, glabrous area of skin. Beneath this area, there may be a moderate amount of subcutaneous tissue and fat, or the skin may be closely applied to the anterior and inferior surface of the symphysis pubis. The labia minora are usually poorly developed and terminate anteriorly at the corresponding half of the bifid clitoris, where there may be a rudiment of a preputial fold. These external appearances are most characteristic: on minimal separation of the labia, one sees the urethra, which may vary considerably, as mentioned previously. The symphysis pubis is usually closed but may be represented by a narrow fibrous band. The vagina and internal genitalia are usually normal.

Associated Anomalies

The ureterovesical junction is inherently deficient in cases of epispadias, and the ureters are often laterally placed in the bladder with a straight course so that reflux occurs. The incidence of reflux is reported to be 30% to 75% (Kramer and Kelalis, 1982b; Gearhart et al, 1993). Because there is no outlet resistance, the bladder is small and the wall is thin. However, after urethral reconstruction, the mild urethral resistance created allows the bladder to develop an acceptable capacity for potential later bladder neck reconstruction.

Surgical Objectives

Objectives for repair of female epispadias parallel those devised for male patients: (1) achievement of urinary continence, (2) preservation of the upper urinary tracts, and (3)

reconstruction of functional and cosmetically acceptable external genitalia.

Operative Techniques

With the patient in the lithotomy position, the defect of the female epispadias with incontinence is apparent (Fig. 119–29A). The two halves of the clitoris are widely separated, and the roof of the urethra is cleft between 9 o'clock and 3 o'clock positions. The smooth mucosa of the urethra tends to blend cephalad with the thin, hairless skin over the mons. The urethral incision is begun at the cephalad extent of the vertical incision at the base of the mons and is brought inferiorly through the full thickness of the urethral wall at the 9 o'clock and 3 o'clock positions (see Fig. 119–29B). Sutures can be placed in the urethra to permit downward traction on the urethra so that the roof of the urethra is excised to a level near the bladder neck (Fig. 119–29C). Often, one finds the dissection proceeding under the symphysis. An inverting closure of the urethra is then performed over a 12 or 10 Fr Foley catheter. Suturing is begun near the bladder neck and progresses distally until closure of the neourethra is accomplished (Fig. 119–29D). Attention is then given to denuding the medial half of the bifid clitoris and the labia minora so that proper genital coaptation can be obtained.

After this is done, fat from the mons and subcutaneous tissue can be used to cover the suture line and obliterate the space in front of the pubic symphysis (see Fig. 119–29E and F). The two halves of the clitoris and labia minora are brought together using interrupted sutures of 6-0 polyglycolic acid. The corpora may be partially detached from the anterior ramus of the pubis to aid in the urethral closure. Also, bringing these tissues together may contribute by adding resistance to the urethra. Mons closure is further aided by mobilizing subcutaneous tissue laterally and bringing it medially to fill any prior depression that remains (see Fig. 119–29G). The subcutaneous layer is closed with 4-0 polyglactin suture in an interrupted fashion (see Fig. 119–29H). The skin is closed with interrupted sutures of 6-0 polypropylene (see Fig. 119–29I to K). A 10 Fr catheter is left indwelling for 5 to 7 days. Should the patient undergo simultaneous bladder neck reconstruction, a Foley catheter is not left in the urethra and the patient is placed in the supine position for the abdominal part of the procedure.

Achievement of a satisfactory cosmetic appearance of the external genitalia and urinary continence in the female child with epispadias represents a surgical challenge. Many operations have been reported to control continence in the epispadias group, but the results are disappointing. These procedures include transvaginal plication of the urethra and bladder neck, muscle transplantations, urethra twisting, cauterization of the urethra, bladder flap, and Marshall-Marchetti vesicourethral suspension (Stiles, 1911; Davis, 1928; Marshall et al, 1949; Gross and Kresson, 1952). These procedures may increase urethral resistance, but they do not correct incontinence or the malformed anatomy of the urethra, bladder neck, and genitalia.

The challenge of the small bladder in the female epispadias patient is comparable to a situation seen in some patients with closed bladder exstrophy. The small, incontinent bladder, with or without reflux, is hardly an ideal setting for a successful bladder neck reconstruction and ureteral reimplantation. A

third of all incontinent epispadias patients have a bladder capacity of less than 60 mL, in our experience and that of Kramer and Kelalis (1982b). Bladder augmentation, injection of polytetrafluoroethylene (Teflon) in the bladder neck area, and simultaneous bladder neck reconstruction and bladder neck augmentation have been offered as a solution to this challenge. However, primary closure of the epispadiac urethra in children with closed exstrophy was found to increase bladder capacity without causing hydronephrosis, and this approach has been applied to male and female patients with epispadias (Peters et al, 1988; Gearhart and Jeffs, 1989a; Ben-Chaim et al, 1995b). Although we typically perform urethral and genital reconstruction at about 1 year of age, we advocate delaying bladder neck reconstruction until the child is 4 to 5 years old. Not only does this delay allow the bladder to increase in capacity, it also allows the child to accept essential instructions for toilet training, which is critical to achieving satisfactory continence in the postoperative state.

Surgical Results

The continence rate of 87.5% in our female patients is comparable to that of Hanna and Williams (1972), who found a 67% continence rate in female patients with good bladder capacity, and that of Kramer and Kelalis (1982b), who reported an 83% continence rate in patients with adequate bladder capacity. All of the authors' patients seen for primary treatment have achieved a capacity in excess of 80 mL.

Hendren (1981) and Kramer and Kelalis (1982b) showed that genitourethral reconstruction can be accomplished with satisfactory results. At our institution, patients who underwent prior urethral and genital reconstruction had a mean bladder capacity at bladder neck reconstruction of 121 mL, making the bladder suitable for the reconstruction and eventual continence without the use of augmentation cystoplasty or need for intermittent catheterization.

The time interval to achieve continence in our patients was a mean of 18 months for those who underwent genitourethral and bladder neck reconstruction in one procedure and 23 months for those who underwent preliminary urethroplasty and genital reconstruction after bladder neck reconstruction. In a series by Klauber and Williams (1974), the mean interval to acceptable continence was 2.25 years. Also, in a series by Kramer and Kelalis (1982b), some patients became continent within a short period, whereas complete continence was delayed for several years in others. The time delay for achieving continence may represent increased pelvic muscular development, as suggested by Kramer and Kelalis (1982b). In regard to the interval to continence, no advantage appears to be gained by preliminary urethroplasty. However, we believe that the advantage gained by increased bladder capacity at the time of bladder neck reconstruction outweighs any advantage gained by a combined approach.

Exstrophy Complex and Variants

Exstrophy complex includes a spectrum of anomalies ranging from epispadias to cloacal exstrophy. Many variations in anatomy and types of defects have been noted. Because there is probably a common embryologic origin for all of these defects, they all share many or some of the defects noted in the three major components of the complex—

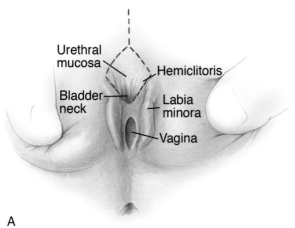

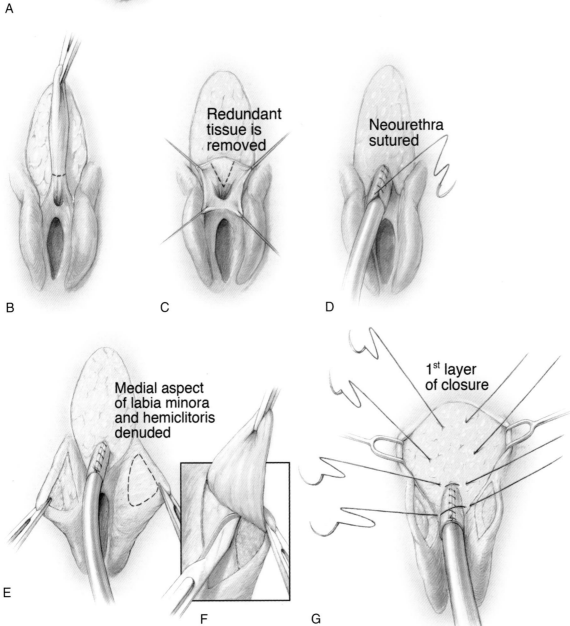

Figure 119–29. **A,** Typical appearance of female epispadias with initial incisions outlined. **B,** Excision of the glabrous skin of the mons. **C,** Tapering of the urethra with a dorsal resection of a wedge of tissue. **D,** Reconstruction of the urethra over a catheter with running suture. **E** and **F,** Medial aspect of the labia minora and clitoris. **G,** Initial layer of mons closure.   *Continued*

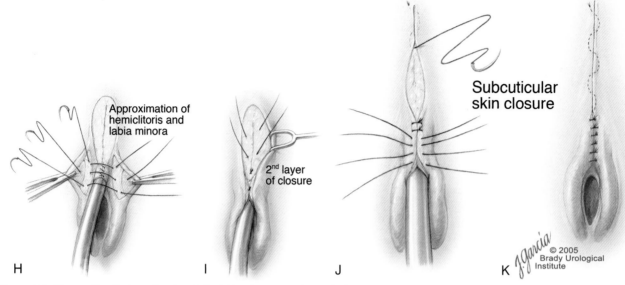

Subcuticular
skin closure

© 2005
Brady Urological
Institute

H   I   J   K

Figure 119–29, cont'd. **H,** Approximation of the labia minora over the urethral reconstruction. **I,** Second layer of mons closure. **J,** Creation of clitoral hood. **K,** Completion of mons closure.

<table>
<tr><td colspan="2">

KEY POINTS: EPISPADIAS— PRIORITIES IN MANAGEMENT

</td></tr>
</table>

- Length and width of the urethral plate in the male
- Length and width of the urethral plate and genitalia relationships in the female
- Bladder size
- Bladder neck involvement
- Associated anomalies

skeletal, urinary, and genital. The presence of a characteristic musculoskeletal defect of the exstrophy anomaly with no major defect in the urinary tract has been named "pseudo-exstrophy" (Marshall and Muecke, 1968). Predominant characteristics include an elongated, low-set umbilicus and divergent rectus muscles that attach to the separated pubic bones (Fig. 119–30). In this variant, the mesodermal migration has been interrupted in its superior aspect only, thus wedging apart the musculoskeletal elements of the lower abdominal wall without obstructing the formation of the genital tubercle.

In the superior vesical fissure variant of the exstrophy complex, the musculature and skeletal defects are exactly the same as those in classic exstrophy; however, the persistent cloacal membrane ruptures only at the uppermost portion, and a superior vesical fistula results that actually resembles a vesicostomy. Bladder extrusion is minimal and is present only over the normal umbilicus (see Fig. 119–1B).

Duplicate exstrophy occurs when a superior vesical fissure opens but there is later fusion of the abdominal wall and a portion of the bladder elements (mucosa) remains outside (Fig. 119–31). Three cases were reported by Arap and Giron (1986) in which the patients had classic musculoskeletal defects and two of the three were continent. Of the two male patients, one had an associated complete epispadias and the other had a completely normal penis. Therefore, the external genital manifestations in duplicate exstrophy can be quite variable.

In addition to pseudoexstrophy, superior vesical fissure, and duplicated exstrophy, isolated occurrences of a fourth entity, "covered exstrophy," have been reported (Cerniglia et al, 1989). This has also been referred to as split symphysis variant. A common factor in these patients is the presence of musculoskeletal defect associated with classic exstrophy but no significant defect of the urinary tract. Chandra and associates (1999) reported a covered exstrophy with incomplete duplication of the bladder. However, in most cases of covered exstrophy (Narasimharao et al, 1985; Cerniglia et al, 1989), there has been an isolated ectopic bowel segment present on the inferior abdominal wall near the genital area, which can be either colon or ileum with no connection with the underlying gastrointestinal tract and only epispadias in the male. A patient seen at our institution had the standard appearance of most split symphysis variants, and one could actually see the bladder through a thin membrane of lower abdominal skin. Although all of the classic musculoskeletal defects of exstrophy were present, there was no isolated ectopic bowel segment present on the lower abdominal wall (Fig. 119–32).

SEXUAL FUNCTION AND FERTILITY IN THE EXSTROPHY PATIENT
The Male Patient

Reconstruction of the male genitalia and preservation of fertility were not primary objectives in early surgical management of bladder exstrophy. **Sporadic instances of pregnancy**

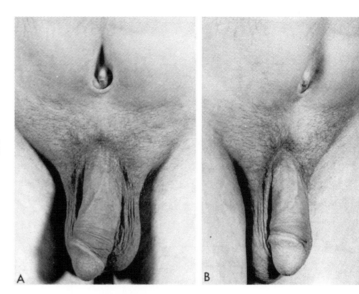

Figure 119–30. Pseudoexstrophy in an adult male patient. Musculoskeletal deformity characteristic of the exstrophy complex is present, but the urinary tract is intact.

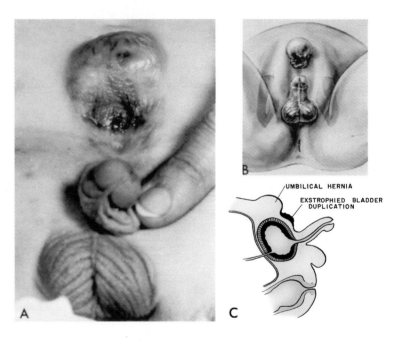

Figure 119–31. Duplicate exstrophy in a boy with an intact lower urinary tract.

or the initiation of pregnancy by males with bladder exstrophy have been reported. In two large exstrophy series, male fertility was documented. Only 3 of 68 men in one study (Bennett, 1973) and 4 of 72 in another (Woodhouse et al, 1983) had successfully fathered children. In a large series of 2500 patients with exstrophy and epispadias (Shapiro et al, 1984), there were 38 males who had fathered children.

Hanna and Williams (1972) compared semen analyses in men who had undergone primary closure and ureterosigmoidostomy. A normal sperm count was found in only one of eight men after functional closure and in four of eight men with diversion. The difference in observed fertility potential is probably attributable to iatrogenic injury to the verumontanum during functional closure or bladder neck reconstruction. Retrograde ejaculation may also account for low sperm counts after functional bladder closure. **In a long-term study from our institution, Ben-Chaim and associates (1996)**

found that 10 of 16 men reported they ejaculated a few cubic centimeters of volume, 3 ejaculated only a few drops, and 3 had no ejaculation. Semen analysis was obtained in four patients: three had azoospermia and one had oligospermia. The average ejaculated volume of the patients who had sperm counts was 0.4 mL. In another large series by Stein and colleagues (1994) from Germany, the authors found that none of the patients who had reconstruction of the external genitalia could ejaculate normally, nor had they fathered children. Five patients who did not undergo reconstruction had normal ejaculation, and two had fathered children. The conclusion was that male patients with genital reconstruction and closure of the urethra demonstrated high risk of infertility.

Assisted reproductive techniques have been applied to the exstrophy population. **Bastuba and coworkers (1993) reported pregnancies achieved with the use of assisted reproductive techniques. Regardless of the method of**

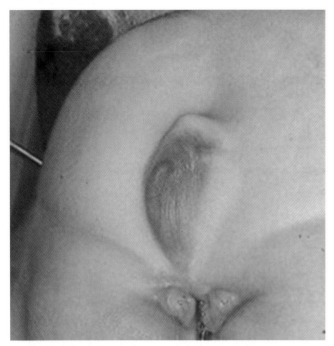

Figure 119–32. Skin-covered exstrophy in a female patient. Note urethral sound in the bladder and the subcutaneous position below the skin of the abdominal wall. No bowel is sequestered on the abdominal wall as has been reported in some patients with this variant.

reconstruction of the external genitalia and bladder neck, newer techniques such as gamete intrafallopian transfer (GIFT) or intracytoplasmic sperm injection (ICSI) can be used to assist these patients in their goal of pregnancy achievement. Use of GIFT or ICSI in 13 boys with exstrophy led to successful pregnancy with no instances of exstrophy in any of the offspring.

Sexual function and libido in exstrophy patients are normal (Woodhouse, 1998). The erectile mechanism in patients who have undergone epispadias repair appears to be intact because 87% of boys and young men in the Hopkins series experienced erections after repair of epispadias (Surer et al, 2000). Poor or absent ejaculation may occur after genital reconstruction. Complete absence of ejaculation is rare, but the emission that does occur may be slow and may occur for several hours. Milking the urethra in an antegrade fashion from proximal to distal has provided pregnancy in some cases (Woodhouse, 1999). In papers from both Woodhouse (1998) and Ben-Chaim and colleagues (1996), most patients reported satisfactory orgasm; half of the men and all of the women described intimate relationships as serious and long term. In the series by Ben-Chaim, the only patients who had no ejaculation were two patients who had undergone cystectomy. Overall, it seems from the experience in England, Germany, and the United States that most men with exstrophy achieve erection and have a reasonable sex life.

The Female Patient

Further reconstruction of the female genitalia, if needed, may be necessary during adolescent years. In our experience, the external genitalia are fully reconstructed at the time of initial exstrophy closure because with the use of osteotomy a nice

mons pubis can be created and the bifid clitoris and labia can easily be brought together in the midline. **Vulvoplasty is sometimes indicated in patients before they become sexually active or start using tampons. In Woodhouse's experience (1999), most patients required vaginoplasty before intercourse could take place.** Woodhouse reported successful intercourse in all of his patients, but three found it painful. Stein and associates (1995) from Germany reviewed a large series of patients with exstrophy and found that a cut-back vaginoplasty was required before intercourse in 23 patients. We have also seen several patients who have not had vulvoplasty, have two clitoral halves, have a normal sex life and normal orgasm, and desire no surgical repair of this condition.

Mathews and coauthors (2003a) reported on a large series of girls and women with the exstrophy complex. All girls older than 18 years indicated that they had normal sexual desire and many were sexually active. Mean age for commencement of sexual activity was 19.9 years. Although a few patients complained of dyspareunia, most indicated normal orgasms. Some patients indicated that they restricted sexual activity because of the cosmetic appearance of their external genitalia. Mons plasty is therefore very important to obtain a cosmetically pleasing appearance either in infancy or in adolescence because hair-bearing skin and fat should be used to cover the midline defect. As mentioned earlier, we perform this procedure at the time of initial closure. It certainly can be done in adolescence with the use of rhomboid flaps, as popularized by Kramer and colleagues (1986).

Obstetric Implications

Review of the literature reveals 45 women with bladder exstrophy who successfully delivered 49 normal offspring. The main complication after pregnancy was cervical and uterine prolapse, which occurred frequently (Krisiloff et al, 1978). Burbage and coworkers (1986) described 40 women ranging from 19 to 36 years of age who were treated in infancy for bladder exstrophy; 14 pregnancies in 11 of these women resulted in 9 normal deliveries, 3 spontaneous abortions, and 2 elective abortions. Uterine prolapse occurred in 7 of the 11 patients during pregnancy. All had undergone prior permanent urinary diversions. Spontaneous vaginal deliveries were performed in those women, and cesarean sections were performed in women with functional bladder closures to eliminate stress on the pelvic floor and to avoid traumatic injury to the urinary sphincter mechanism (Krisiloff et al, 1978). With modern reconstructive techniques, successful pregnancies have been reported in female patients who have undergone continent urinary diversion (Kennedy et al, 1993).

Woodhouse and associates (1999) reported prolapse in a number of patients, and it was said to be a considerable problem to correct. Seven patients had total prolapse, one of whom had never had intercourse or a pregnancy. Woodhouse believes that prolapse may occur in up to half of patients after pregnancy. In a report from Mathews and coauthors (2003a), vaginal and uterine prolapse was noted commonly and even quite early in life (mean age 16 years). Uterine suspension provided only modest success for the prevention of recurrent prolapse. Stein and colleagues (1995), in a large exstrophy series from Germany, found that uterine fixation was required to correct prolapse in 13 patients with long-term follow-up of more than 25 years. The anterior displacement of the vaginal os and the marked posterior displacement of the dorsorectalis sling with its deficient anterior component were postulated as reasons for prolapse. It is hoped that the modern use of osteotomy with resultant recreation of the pelvic floor will help to reduce the incidence of this entity.

Regardless of the method of repair, the uterus must be anchored in such a way that it is fixated in the pelvis and less susceptible to prolapse. Some authors have advocated fixation of the uterus to the anterior abdominal wall in childhood; this, they say, prevents prolapse but still allows normal pregnancy. Woodhouse (1999) believed that, although prophylactic surgery may be helpful, once prolapse occurs, anterior fixation is insufficient to correct uterine prolapse in the exstrophy patient.

LONG-TERM ADJUSTMENT ISSUES

Interest has increased in long-term adjustment issues in patients with bladder exstrophy. Children with exstrophy undergo multiple reconstructive surgeries and have potential problems with respect to urinary incontinence and sexual dysfunction. However, the ultimate outcome would be better measured by how these children adjust overall in society. The severe nature of the exstrophy disorder could predict that this birth defect could have substantial psychological implications. Parental reaction to the child's medical condition may change the way the parents interact with the child. Incontinence may have a negative impact on social function and self-esteem. Multiple hospitalizations may interfere with the ability to be like other children. Concerning the potential medical and psychological implications of this anomaly, children born with exstrophy may be at increased risk for difficulties.

However, there has been a limited amount of information in the literature concerning this condition and its treatment and whether or not it has a deleterious effect on children and their families. Montagnino and coworkers (1998) evaluated younger children who performed more poorly and had disturbed behavior, specifically in skills related to function in school. Children who achieved continence after the age of 5 years were more likely to have problems with acting-out behavior. There were no differences in adjustment based on male or female sex, bladder versus cloacal exstrophy, type of continence strategy, or gender reassignment versus no reassignment. **The conclusions of this long-term study were that children with exstrophy do not have clinical psychopathology** (Montagnino et al, 1998). There was acting-out behavior rather than depression or anxiety, suggesting that improved outcomes may be achieved through a focus on normal adaptation rather than potential psychological stress. In addition, earlier achievement of continence through reconstructive efforts is potentially of psychological benefit.

Reiner (1999) studied 42 children with exstrophy and presented preliminary results suggesting that these patients tend to have more severe behavioral and developmental problems than children with other anomalies, significant body distortion, and self-esteem problems. Reiner has recommended early intervention with the exstrophy patient and family and continuation with long-term psychiatric support into adult life. In a study from Europe, Feitz and associates (1994) found a more positive picture when they evaluated 11 women and 11 men with exstrophy, of whom 9 women (82%) and 10 men (91%) did not manifest any clinical levels of psychological stress. The authors concluded that these adults had a positive attitude toward life. With the use of structured instruments and appropriate evaluation and interviews, Reiner (2004) indicated that all 20 patients evaluated met criteria for at least one anxiety disorder. Older patients experienced waning of anxiety associated peer discovery of incontinence following successful surgical reconstruction, and all noted intensified sexual activity with age.

Being born with exstrophy does not result in childhood psychopathology. **Children with exstrophy exhibit some tendency toward increased problems with acting out or lack of attainment of age-appropriate adaptive behavior** (Montagnino et al, 1998; Reiner, 1999). Therefore, all experts in childhood psychology tend to agree that counseling should come from the nursing and medical staff early in the exstrophy condition. Likewise, the patient and parents should be served by an experienced exstrophy support team, and psychological support and counseling should be extended into adult life.

SUGGESTED READINGS

Ansell JE: Exstrophy and epispadias. In Glenn JF (ed): Urologic Surgery. Philadelphia, JB Lippincott, 1983, p 647.

Chan DY, Jeffs RD, Gearhart JP: Determinates of continence in the bladder exstrophy population after bladder neck reconstruction. Urology 2001;165:1656.

Dodson J, Jeffs RD, Gearhart JP: The small exstrophy bladder unsuitable for closure. J Urol 2001;165:1656.

Gearhart JP, Ben-Chaim J, Jeffs RD, et al: Criteria for the prenatal diagnosis of classic bladder exstrophy. Obstet Gynecol 1995;85:961.

Gearhart JP, Stec A, Tadros YE, et al: Pelvic floor anatomy in classic bladder exstrophy: First insights. J Urol 2001;166:1444.

Grady R, Mitchell ME: Complete repair of exstrophy. J Urol 1999;162:1415.

Husmann DA, McLorie GA, Churchill BM: Closure of the exstrophic bladder: An evaluation of the factors leading to its success and its importance on urinary continence. J Urol 1989a;142:522.

Mathews R, Jeffs RD, Reiner WG, et al: Cloacal exstrophy: Improving the quality of life—The Johns Hopkins experience. J Urol 1998;160:2552.

Meldrum KK, Baird, AD, Gearhart JP: Methods of pelvic and extremity immobilization following bladder exstrophy closure: Associated complications and impact on surgical success. Urology 2003;62:1109.

Sponseller PD, Bisson, L, Jani L, et al: Anterior innominate osteotomy in repair of bladder exstrophy. J Bone Joint Surg Am 2001;83:184.

120 Surgical Techniques for One-Stage Reconstruction of the Exstrophy-Epispadias Complex

RICHARD W. GRADY, MD • MICHAEL E. MITCHELL, MD

BACKGROUND

COMPLETE PRIMARY EXSTROPHY REPAIR

RESULTS

SUMMARY

Until the 20th century, no effective surgical remedy was available to consistently ameliorate the morbidity associated with bladder exstrophy. The subsequent popularization of urinary diversion allowed many patients with exstrophy the opportunity for more normal lives. At the same time, some surgeons continued to strive for a more anatomic approach to the surgical treatment of patients with the exstrophy-epispadias complex. Although a myriad of operations for exstrophy have been proposed and attempted, these operations for exstrophy may be broadly characterized into two approaches. The first approach includes operations designed to remove the exstrophic bladder and replace it with a form of urinary diversion. The second approach includes anatomically oriented procedures designed to reconstruct the bladder either in multiple stages or in a single stage. Surgeon preference, patient anatomy, previous surgical procedures, availability of tertiary care facilities, and access to medical care all play a role in which operative procedures are chosen for a particular patient. No standard of care exists for this patient population. Because of the complexity of care involved with the exstrophy-epispadias complex and the rarity of this congenital defect, specialists with an interest in the exstrophy-epispadias complex usually manage these patients most effectively.

In the late 1980s, an anatomic approach to exstrophy repair that combined bladder reconstruction with bladder neck remodeling and epispadias repair was initiated by Mitchell (Grady et al, 1999). This operation evolved out of a technique developed for the treatment of epispadias—the complete penile disassembly technique (Mitchell and Bagli, 1996). This approach allowed the tissue deformation in exstrophy to return more closely to an anatomically oriented position. We have used this approach—the disassembly technique with complete primary repair of exstrophy (CPRE) or Mitchell technique—exclusively for the surgical treatment of newborns with exstrophy since 1990. This technique or its principles may also be employed in reoperative or delayed repairs for exstrophy.

BACKGROUND

Efforts to reconstruct the genitourinary system have been tried for over 100 years. Trendelenburg (1906) attempted to reconstruct an exstrophic bladder to achieve urinary continence at the turn of the last century. This was the first time in modurn history that a surgeon had tried to do this; Trendelenburg approached this by reconfiguring the bladder in as anatomically normal a position as he could achieve. He used sacroiliac disarticulation and emphasized the importance of pubic reapproximation in front of the reconstructed bladder to achieve continence and prevent dehiscence. This patient ultimately did not gain continence despite initial urinary control after his operation. Such discouraging results led to abandonment of the functional reconstruction of exstrophy by most surgeons. The treatment of choice became cystectomy and urinary diversion with ureterosigmoidostomy. To this day ureterosigmoidostomy remains the preferred treatment in some areas of the world, because it offers a reliable means to achieve urinary continence for patients who may not have reliable access to health care facilities or who have not achieved urinary continence despite attempts at functional reconstruction (Stein et al, 1999).

During the early to middle portion of the last century some surgeons, however, continued to attempt functional reconstruction for children with exstrophy despite the popular use of urinary diversion. Unfortunately, successful results with anatomic reconstruction were sporadic. Young reported a successful primary bladder closure in 1942 when he achieved urinary continence after reconstructing the exstrophic bladder of a young girl. Since Young's report, other investigators intermittently achieved a satisfactory result with a one-stage reconstructive effort to repair the exstrophied bladder. Ansell, an early advocate for primary reconstruction of the newborn with exstrophy, reported on a one-stage closure in 1971 with a successful outcome in a newborn female. He eventually reported 28 cases closed in this fashion (Ansell, 1979). Montagnani (1982) also described a one-stage functional bladder reconstruction in two female babies aged 8 and 13 months. His bladder reconstruction procedure included innominate osteotomy, bladder closure, an antireflux procedure, and narrowing of the bladder outlet followed by pubic reapproximation. Continence was achieved in one of the two patients. The second patient required further bladder neck reconstruction to achieve continence. Fuchs and associates (1996) achieved urinary continence in 8 of 15 patients who underwent a single-stage repair. Other large series of patients who underwent single-stage reconstruction in the 1960s and 1970s noted lower continence rates of only 10% to 30%. Specifically, continence rates ranged from 0% to 45%, with an average of 17% for single-stage reconstruction in these older series (Ezell and Carlson, 1970; Marshall and Muecke, 1970; Cendron, 1971; King and Wendel, 1972; Engel, 1973; Williams and Keeton, 1973; Megalli and Lattimer, 1973, Johnston and Kogan, 1974). Renal damage was as high as 90% in these series, generally because of bladder outlet obstruction (Cukier and Ott, 1971; King and Wendel, 1972).

Because of these complications and the low rate of urinary continence, reconstructive surgical efforts were subsequently directed toward staged bladder reconstruction, an approach pioneered and advocated by Dr. Robert Jeffs as well as others from the 1970s to the 1990s (Jeffs, 1977; Saltzman et al, 1985). More recently, new techniques of single-stage reconstruction for exstrophy have been advocated by Mitchell, Fuchs, Kelly, and others that appear to be safer than techniques used in the past. Continence rates in these series approach or equal those reported in series using a staged surgical reconstruction approach (Fuchs et al, 1996; Grady and Mitchell, 1999).

The single-stage anatomic approach offers many advantages. It offers the possibility to correct the penile, bladder, and bladder neck abnormalities in one setting. These new techniques also have a lower complication rate than reported in older series of single-stage reconstruction efforts. Finally, urinary continence can be achieved for many of these patients without the need for further bladder neck reconstruction.

Currently, the Mitchell or CPRE technique appears to be the most widely used single-stage anatomic approach to exstrophy. Kelly (1995) proposed a technique that differs from the CPRE technique in its plane of dissection. In an effort to preserve the periurethral and pelvic floor muscles, Kelly's technique initiates the plane of dissection subperiosteally on the bony pelvis to bring the exstrophic structures medially. The method proposed by Fuchs and associates (1996) combines the standard techniques used in a staged approach to exstrophy into one setting, including ureteral reimplantation, Young-Dees bladder neck repair, epispadias repair, and abdominal wall closure.

The advantages of a primary repair technique for exstrophy that may largely be performed in one stage are recognizable intuitively over urinary diversion or a multiple-staged approach. However, the mechanism to achieve a functional result without staging has been slow to evolve; it has clearly been based on the efforts of many surgeons interested in this difficult challenge.

COMPLETE PRIMARY EXSTROPHY REPAIR
Disassembly Technique
Considerations

Complete primary repair of exstrophy (Mitchell technique) is optimally performed in the newborn period (Fig. 120–1), when primary reconstruction is technically easier than when performed in an older patient. It also offers the theoretical advantage that supports normal bladder development based on normal filling and emptying, which should ultimately improve the potential for bladder healing, function, and continence. The bony pelvis also remains pliable in the newborn period so that osteotomies may be avoided in some cases; however, we are presently leaning to osteotomies in most patients (Chan et al, 2001).

This technique effectively relocates the bladder, bladder neck, and urethra posteriorly, thus positioning the proximal urethra within the pelvic diaphragm in an anatomically normal position. This takes advantage of the pelvic muscles and support structures in securing urinary continence. Posterior positioning of the bladder neck and elongation of the proximal urethra also helps to reapproximate the pubic symphysis and to create a more anatomically normal muscular pelvic diaphragm.

CPRE reduces anterior tension on the urethra and abdominal wall because the urethra is separated from its attachments to the underlying corporeal bodies and pelvic diaphragm. Left attached, the urethra will be anteriorly tethered; this will

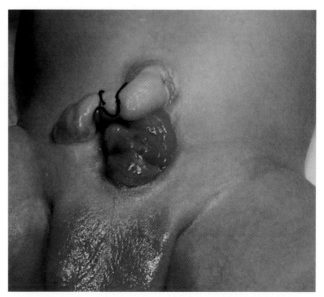

Figure 120–1. Newborn male with classic bladder exstrophy.

prevent posterior placement of the proximal urethra and bladder neck in the pelvis. Tension reduction increases the success of initial primary bladder closure. It also reduces the tension on the corporeal bodies that contributes to dorsal chordee and deflection in males with exstrophy/epispadias. Combining the epispadias repair with primary closure allows for the most important aspect of primary closure—division of the intersymphyseal ligament or band (anterior portion of the pelvic diaphragm) located posterior to the urethra in these patients (Figs. 120–2 and 120–3). This allows for posterior positioning of the bladder, bladder neck, and urethra in a more anatomically normal position. The goal of the complete primary repair approach is to combine the elements of a staged anatomic reconstruction in a single operation (i.e., bladder closure, epispadias repair, and achievement of urinary continence).

Preoperative Care

After delivery, the umbilical cord should be ligated with silk suture rather than a plastic or metal clamp to prevent trauma to the exposed bladder plate. We believe it is important to protect the exstrophic bladder against the elements by whatever means are available. We advocate hydrated gel dressings such as Vigilon. This type of dressing is easy to use, keeps the bladder plate from desiccating, and stays in place to allow handling of the infant with minimal risk of trauma to the bladder. The exposed bladder may be covered with plastic wrap as an acceptable alternative. Dressings should be replaced daily and the bladder should be irrigated with normal saline with each diaper change. Other authors have advocated the use of a humidified air incubator to minimize bladder trauma (Churchill et al, 1997).

We also recommend the routine use of the following:
1. Intravenous antibiotic therapy in the preoperative and postoperative period. This decreases the chance for infection.
2. Preoperative ultrasonography to assess the kidneys and to establish a baseline examination for later ultrasonographic studies
3. Preoperative spinal sonographic examination if sacral dimpling or other signs of spina bifida occulta are noted on physical examination
4. Pelvic computed tomography with three-dimensional reconstructions to assess pubic diastasis (minimally a kidney-ureter-bladder view).

Operative Considerations

In the newborn period, we perform primary exstrophy closure using general inhalation anesthesia. We advise against the use of nitrous oxide during primary closure because it may cause bowel distention, which decreases surgical exposure during the operation and increases the risk of wound dehiscence. Some advocate the use of nasogastric tube drainage to decrease abdominal distention in the postoperative period (Gearhart, 1999). We have not routinely used nasogastric suction in most patients but do routinely use a one-time caudal block to reduce the inhaled anesthetic requirement during the operation.

For patients older than 3 days, or newborns with a wide pubic diastasis, we perform anterior iliac osteotomies. Osteotomies assist closure and enhance anterior pelvic floor support, which may improve later urinary continence (Aadalen et al, 1980; Ben-Chaim, 1995).

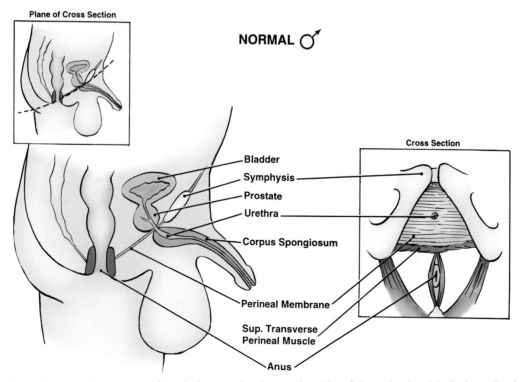

Figure 120–2. Schematic cross-sectional drawing of a male demonstrating the normal position of the urethra in pelvic diaphragm in relation to the urethral diaphragm and intersymphyseal ligaments.

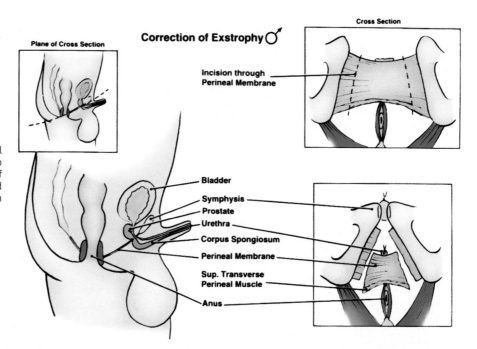

Figure 120–3. Schematic cross-sectional drawing demonstrating the approximation to anatomically normal posterior positioning of the bladder, bladder neck, and urethra achieved after complete disassembly has been performed.

KEY POINTS: OPERATIVE CARE

Factors that are important in the operative period include the following:

- Use of osteotomies in selected cases and for newborn closures more than 24 to 48 hours after birth

- Ureteral stenting catheters placed intraoperatively for use in the postoperative period to divert urine

- Avoidance of abdominal distention

- Use of intraoperative antibiotics

KEY POINTS: POSTOPERATIVE CARE

Postoperative factors that appear to directly impact the success of initial closure include the following:

- Postoperative immobilization

- Use of postoperative antibiotics

- Ureteral stenting catheters

- Adequate postoperative pain management

- Avoidance of abdominal distention

- Adequate nutritional support

- Secure fixation of urinary drainage catheters

Postoperative Care

The patient must be immobilized to decrease lateral stresses on the closure after any primary reconstructive procedure for exstrophy. A number of options exist for this purpose. We prefer to use a spica cast for immobilization. A spica cast for 4 weeks to prevent external hip rotation and optimize pubic apposition can facilitate early discharge and home care (Fig. 120–4). Modified Buck's traction has been used by many groups for 3 to 4 weeks. A posterior lightweight splint can be used in newborns when the child is out of traction to facilitate home care and early removal of traction. We have stopped using Buck's traction because spica casts are easier for the families to care for at home. External fixation devices have also been advocated by several centers and provide effective immobilization. Fixator pins for these devices should be cleaned several times a day to reduce the chance for infection. Internal fixation may be necessary in older patients. "Mummy wrapping" may be unreliable and should not be used routinely (Gearhart, 1999).

Because of the high incidence of vesicoureteral reflux, we prescribe low-dose suppressive antibiotic therapy for all newborns after bladder closure (Lowe and Jeffs, 1983;

Husmann et al, 1989). This is continued until the vesicoureteral reflux is corrected or it resolves spontaneously.

Surgical Technique—Bladder Exstrophy

Initial Dissection

After standard preparation of the surgical field, we place 3.5 Fr umbilical artery catheters into both ureters and suture them in place with 5.0 chromic suture and outline the planned lines of dissection (Figs. 120–5 and 120–6). Initial dissection begins superiorly and proceeds inferiorly to separate the bladder plate from the adjacent skin and fascia. We use fine-tipped electrocautery (Colorado tip) during this dissection. The umbilical cord usually needs to be mobilized on its vessels in a cephalad direction such that the resulting umbilicus will be at the level of a line drawn between the two iliac crests. The relocated umbilicus will also be the cutaneous site for bringing out the suprapubic tube. All dissection in classic exstrophy patients should be extraperitoneal.

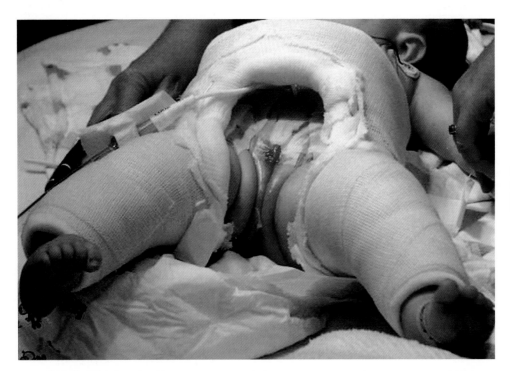

Figure 120–4. The use of the spica cast to maintain immobilization in the postoperative period after use of the CPRE technique.

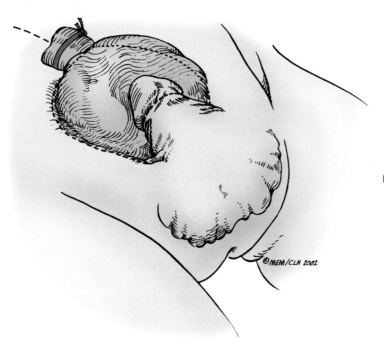

Figure 120–5. Initial lines of dissection: ventral perspective.

Penile/Urethral Dissection

To aid in dissection, traction sutures are placed into each hemiglans of the penis. These sutures are placed at the beginning of the operation and are initially oriented transversely in the hemiglans. The sutures will rotate to a parallel vertical orientation as the corporeal bodies rotate medially after dissection of the corporeal bodies and the urethral wedge (urethral plate plus underlying corpora spongiosa) from each other.

We begin the penile dissection along the ventral aspect of the penis as a circumcising incision. This should precede dissection of the urethral wedge from the corporeal bodies because it is easier to identify Buck's fascia ventrally. We develop the initial plane of dissection just above Buck's fascia. Buck's fascia stops at the corpus spongiosum ("urethral plate") during the dissection. So, as the dissection progresses medially, the plane shifts subtly from above Buck's fascia to just above the tunica albuginea. Dorsally, methylene blue or brilliant green helps differentiate urothelium from squamous epithelium. Injection of the surrounding tissues with 0.25% lidocaine and 1:200,000 U/mL epinephrine also improves

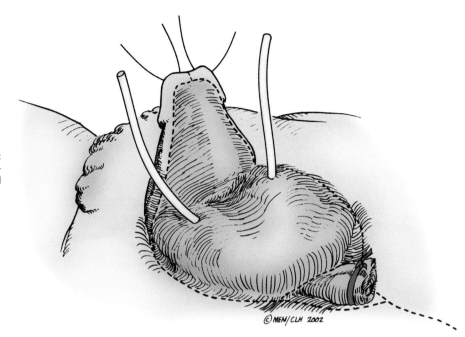

Figure 120–6. Initial lines of dissection: dorsal perspective. Lines at bladder neck indicate approximate tailoring that may be needed at bladder neck.

©MEM/CLH 2002

hemostasis, which assists the dissection. The margins of the dorsal urethra are usually obvious. The surgeon must take care not to narrow the urethral wedge because this will be tubularized later. Urethral wedge dissection is carried proximally to the bladder neck. Careful lateral dissection of the penile shaft skin and dartos fascia from the corporeal bodies is paramount because the neurovascular bundles are located laterally on the corpora of the epispadic penis. The lateral dissection of the penis is always superficial to Buck's fascia because the neurovascular bundles are located laterally (lateral to the urethral plate) in the epispadic penis. Medially, under the urethral wedge, the dissection plane is on the tunica albuginea of the corpora cavernosa.

Complete Penile Disassembly

As described by Bagli and Mitchell (1996), the penis is surgically disassembled into three components—the right and left corporeal bodies with their respective hemiglans and the urethral wedge (urothelium with underlying corpora spongiosa). This is done primarily to provide exposure to the intersymphyseal band and to allow adequate proximal dissection. It is easiest to initiate the dissection proximally and ventrally (on the underside of the corpora cavernosa) (Fig. 120–7). The plane of dissection should be carried out at the level of the tunica albuginea on the corpora. After a plane is established between the urethral wedge and the corporeal bodies, this dissection is carried distally to separate the three components from each other (Fig. 120–8). This maximizes the degree of freedom for the best repair. The corporeal bodies may be completely separated from each other because they exist on a separate blood supply. It is important to keep the underlying corpora spongiosa with the urethral plate; the blood supply to the urethral plate is based on this corporeal tissue, which should appear wedge-shaped after its dissection from the adjacent corpora cavernosa. The urethral/corporeal spongiosal component will later be tubularized and placed ventral to the corporeal bodies. Para-exstrophy skin flaps should not

be used for urethral lengthening because this maneuver may devascularize the distal urethra. However, because the bladder and urethra are moved posteriorly into the pelvis as a unit, division of the urethral wedge should never be necessary. However, in some cases, a male patient will be left with a hypospadias that will require later surgical reconstruction (short distal urethra).

Proximal Dissection

Proximal dissection of the urethral wedge from the corporeal cavernosa bodies facilitates exposure of the intersymphyseal ligament, which must be incised. The dissection may be carried into the pelvis following the planes along the medial aspects of the corporeal bodies (Fig. 120–9). Deep incision of the intersymphyseal ligaments posterior and lateral to each side of the urethral wedge is absolutely necessary to allow the bladder to achieve a posterior position in the pelvis (Fig. 120–10). This dissection should be carried until the pelvic floor musculature becomes visible (i.e., the intersymphyseal ligament is completely incised). Computed tomography of the pelvis demonstrates that these ligaments lie posterior to the bladder neck and urethra. Failure to adequately dissect the bladder and urethral wedge from surrounding structures will create anterior tension along the urethral plate and prevent posterior movement of the bladder in the pelvis.

Primary Closure

Once the bladder and urethral wedge are adequately dissected from the surrounding tissues, the majority of the procedure is done and the closure is straightforward and anatomic. The importance of recognizing the proper location of the bladder neck is key (in boys proximal to the verumontanum and in girls just distal to the trigone). The bladder plate is broadened in this area. Before reapproximating the bladder, a suprapubic tube is placed and brought out through the umbilicus. We then perform a primary closure of the bladder using a three-layer closure with absorbable suture (i.e., Monocryl and

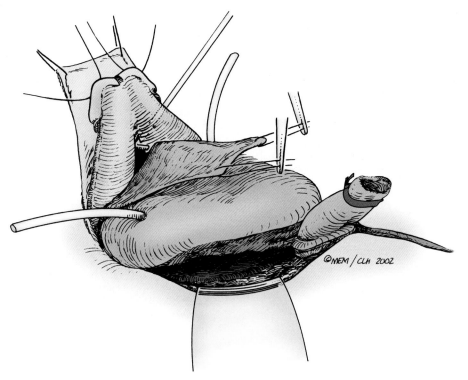

Figure 120–7. Disassembly of urethral wedge from corporeal bodies.

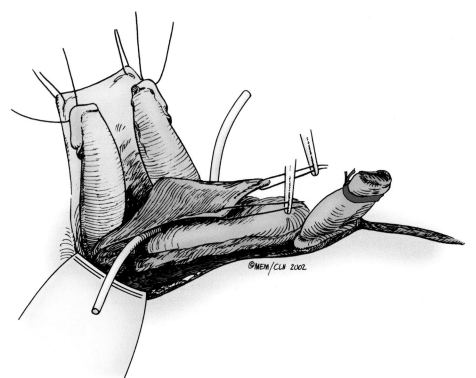

Figure 120–8. Distal separation of corporeal bodies.

Vicryl) suture. The urethra is tubularized using a two-layer running closure with monofilament and Vicryl suture as well (Fig. 120–11). The tubularized urethra is then placed ventral to the corpora in an anatomically normal position.

We then reapproximate the pubic symphysis using "0" polydiaxonone interrupted figure-of-eight sutures. Knots are anterior to prevent suture erosion into the bladder neck

(Fig. 120–12). Rectus fascia is reapproximated using a running 2-0 polydioxanone suture (e.g., PDS). Penile shaft skin is reconfigured using either a primary dorsal closure or reversed Byars flaps if needed to provide dorsal skin coverage. Skin covering the abdominal wall is reapproximated using a two-layer running closure of absorbable monofilament suture.

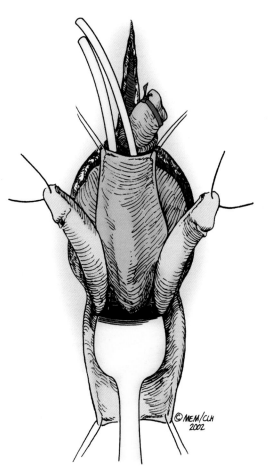

Figure 120–9. Perineal view of dissection of corporeal bodies from urethral wedge.

The corporeal bodies will tend to rotate medially with closure when the lateral margins of Buck's fascia of each corpora cavernosa are approximated. This rotation will assist in correcting the dorsal deflection and can be readily appreciated by observing the vertical lie of the previously horizontally placed glans traction sutures. Occasionally, significant discrepancies in the dorsal and ventral lengths of the corpora will require dermal graft insertion. However, this is rarely needed in the newborn closure. The corpora are reapproximated with fine interrupted suture along their dorsal aspect.

The urethra can then be brought up to each hemiglans ventrally to create an orthotopic meatus (Fig. 120–13). The glans is reconfigured using interrupted mattress sutures of polydioxanone followed by horizontal mattress sutures of 7-0 monofilament suture (e.g., Maxxon) to reapproximate the glans epithelium. The neourethra is matured with 7-0 braided polyglactin suture (e.g., Vicryl) similar to our standard hypospadias repair. We also will perform glans tissue reduction to create a conical-appearing glans. In roughly half of our cases, the urethra lacks enough length to reach the glans. In this situation the urethra may be matured along the ventral aspect of the penis to create a hypospadias (Fig. 120–14). This can be corrected at a later date as a second-stage procedure. We often leave redundant shaft skin ventrally in these patients to assist in later penile reconstructive procedures.

Modifications of the CPRE Technique

In an effort to improve the results of the CPRE technique, several authors have reported modifications. Caione and colleagues (2000) described the use of an electrical muscle stimulator during deep pelvic dissection to preserve and reconfigure the periurethral muscle complex. Long-term

Figure 120–10. Diversion of intersymphyseal band and deep pelvic dissection.

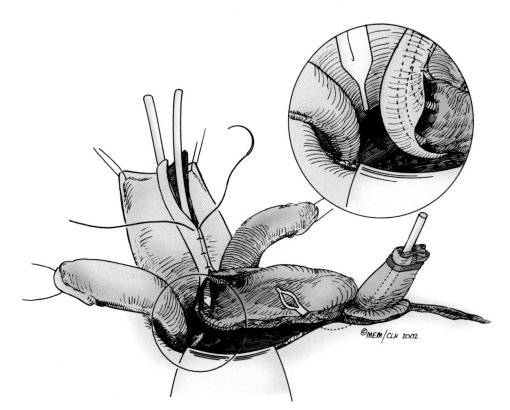

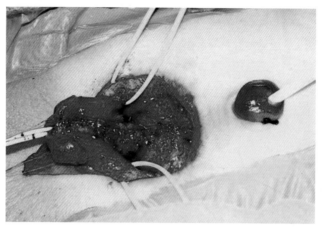

Figure 120–11. Closure of bladder.

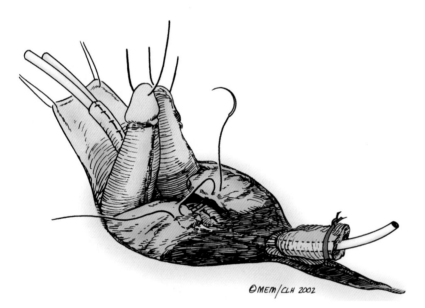

©MEM/CLH 2002

Figure 120–12. Reapproximation of pubis symphysis. Note medial rotation of glans.

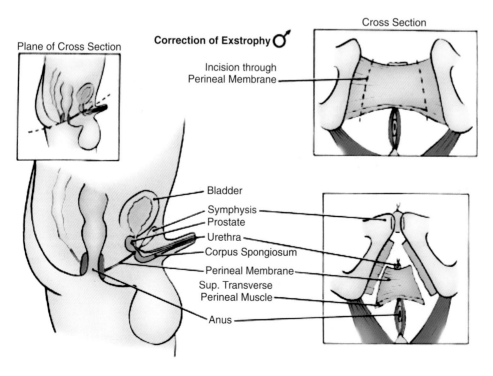

Plane of Cross Section

Correction of Exstrophy ♂

Cross Section

Incision through
Perineal Membrane

Bladder
Symphysis
Prostate
Urethra
Corpus Spongiosum
Perineal Membrane
Sup. Transverse
Perineal Muscle
Anus

Figure 120–13. Schematic drawing of ventral positioning of the urethra. This allows the bladder and urethra to be positioned posteriorly in an anatomically more normal location.

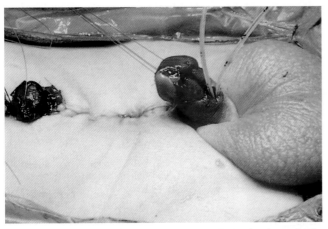

Figure 120–14. Midshaft hypospadias can occur during the closure for the complete primary exstrophy repair because the urethra is too short after the bladder has been positioned posteriorly in the pelvis.

results of this patient series have not yet been reported; preliminary results are promising.

Others have described a modification of the penile disassembly technique preserving the connection between the distal urethral wedge and the corporeal bodies to decrease the incidence of hypospadias (El-Sherbiny and Hafez, 2005).

Female Technique

The principles of repair are analogous for boys and girls. We prefer to perform the reconstructive surgery during the neonatal period (Fig. 120–15).

Initial Dissection

The lines of initial dissection are depicted in Figure 120–16. We tailor the bladder neck dissection in an effort to clearly define the bladder neck. As in boys, the bladder neck, urethra, and vagina are mobilized as a unit. We perform this dissection with a tungsten-tipped electrocautery (Colorado tip) to min-

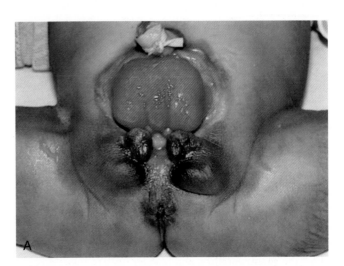

Figure 120–15. **A,** Newborn female with classic bladder exstrophy. Note exstrophic bladder, vaginal vault, clitoral bodies, urethral wedge. **B,** Cross-sectional view of female exstrophy.

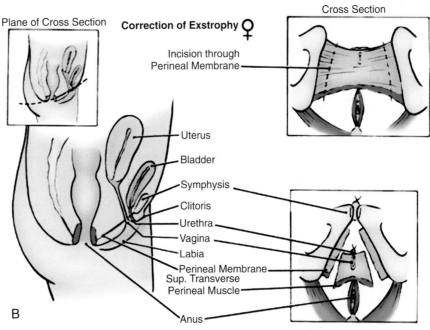

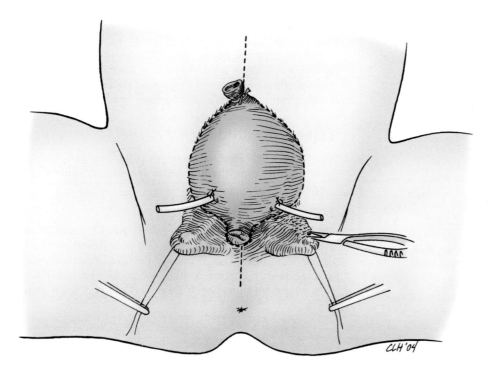

Figure 120–16. Initial lines of dissection. The dissection is carried around the vaginal vault inferiorly.

imize tissue damage while achieving hemostasis. The appropriate plane of dissection is found anteriorly along the medial aspect of the bifid clitoris and proceeds posteriorly along the lateral aspect of the vaginal vault (Fig. 120–17). The vagina is mobilized with the urethral plate and bladder neck. The urethra and bladder neck should not be dissected from the anterior vaginal wall, because this will compromise the blood supply to the urethra.

Proximal Dissection

During the posterior lateral dissection, the intersymphyseal band will be encountered and should be deeply incised to allow the vagina, urethra, and bladder neck to move posteriorly. The posterior limit of the dissection is reached when the pelvic floor musculature is exposed. The proximal urethra can be lengthened to some degree with parallel incisions in the bladder plate to the trigone.

Primary Closure

After adequate dissection the vagina and urethra are moved posteriorly in the perineum with a YV-plasty. The urethra is then tubularized using a two-layer closure of absorbable suture (Fig. 120–18). Before the urethral closure, we routinely place a suprapubic tube to provide postoperative urine drainage (Fig. 120–19). The bladder, bladder neck, and urethra should be positioned deeply in the pelvis and traverse the pelvic diaphragm (Fig. 120–20). The pubic symphysis is then reapproximated using two "0" polydioxanone figure-of-eight sutures (Fig. 120–21).

As in the repair in the boy, osteotomies may be necessary when a wide pubic diastasis prevents a low-tension reapproximation of the pubic symphysis. We use anterior diagonal iliac osteotomies in these situations. The rectus fascia can then be closed in the midline. We mature the neourethra with 5-0 Vicryl sutures and reapproximate the already denuded bifid

clitoris medially so that they fuse together after suturing with 7-0 Maxxon suture. The labia majora is advanced posteriorly to the perineum at this time to improve cosmesis of the external genitalia (Fig. 120–22). A Z-plasty skin closure can be employed as well.

Cloacal Exstrophy

When possible we perform a one-stage closure for patients with cloacal exstrophy using components of the CPRE technique described previously. More commonly, we have applied the principles of the CPRE technique in a sequential fashion for children with cloacal exstrophy with the sequence taking place over a period of months. The decision to proceed with one-stage closure versus staged reconstruction must be weighed carefully. The importance of including surgeons experienced in the care of these patients cannot be overemphasized. Factors that affect a decision to proceed with a single-stage reconstruction include the size of the omphalocele, the extent of the pubic diastasis, and coexisting medical conditions (Husmann et al, 1999). A large omphalocele, in particular, will make single-stage closure hazardous.

When it is not possible to perform a single-stage reconstructive approach for these infants, we prefer to separate the hindgut in its entirety from the exstrophic bladder and then reapproximate the bladder plates. This essentially re-creates the anatomy of classic bladder exstrophy. Once the infant has recovered sufficiently to tolerate another surgical procedure, we proceed with functional reconstruction of the bladder, bladder neck, and genitalia using the CPRE technique (Plaire and Mitchell, 2000).

In a staged or primary approach to cloacal exstrophy using CPRE principles, the steps are as follows. Initially, after the child is stabilized, the omphalocele is repaired. If the omphalocele is not closed because of increased abdominal

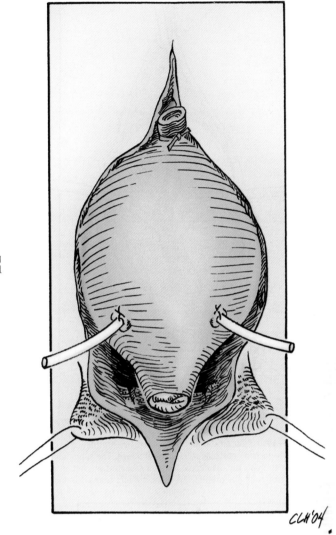

Figure 120–17. The appropriate plane of dissection is found anteriorly along the medial aspect of the bifid clitoris and proceeds posteriorly along the lateral aspect of the vaginal vault.

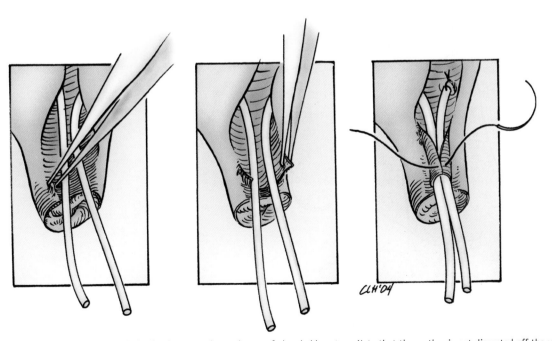

Figure 120–18. The urethra is then tubularized using a two-layer closure of absorbable suture. Note that the urethra is not dissected off the vaginal vault because this may compromise the blood supply to the urethra.

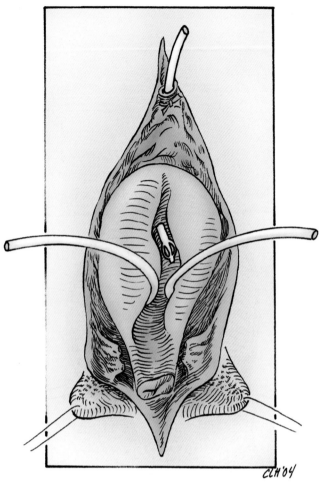

Figure 120–19. Prior to the urethral closure, we routinely place a suprapubic tube to provide postoperative urine drainage. The suprapubic tube is brought out through the umbilicus. Ureteral catheters are left in place and brought out through the urethra. All tubes are left to gravity drainage.

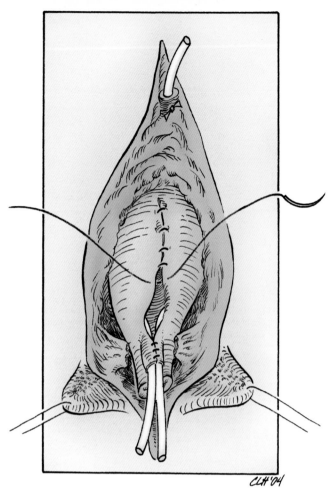

Figure 120–20. The bladder, bladder neck, and urethra should be positioned deeply in the pelvis and traverse the pelvic diaphragm.

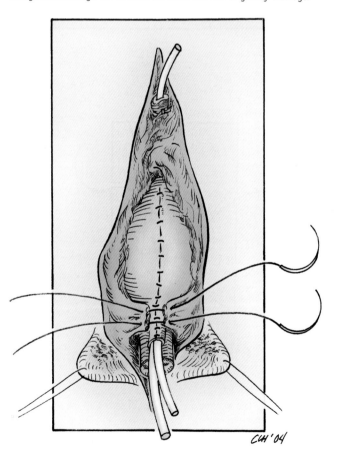

Figure 120–21. Reapproximation of pubis symphysis using interrupted sutures. Lateral dissection may be required to reapproximate the rectus fascia in the midline.

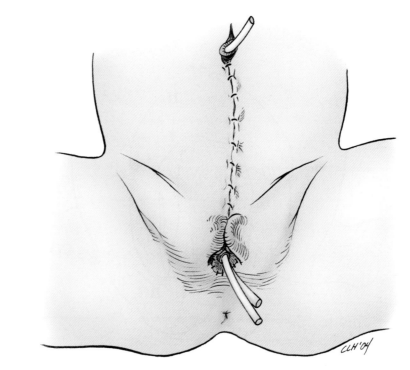

Figure 120–22. Skin closure.

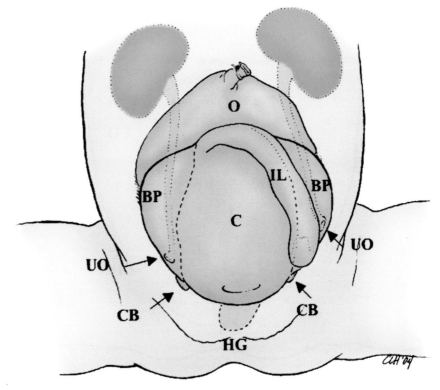

Figure 120–23. Drawing of cloacal exstrophy. *Dashed line* represents line of excision of cecum (C) from bladder plates (BP) and hindgut (HG) from the perineum. Note the omphalocele (O), ileum (IL), corporeal bodies (CB), and ureteral orifices (UO).

pressure or tension, other options exist. A Silastic silo closure may be used as a delayed closure of the abdominal hernia or permit the omphalocele to form an eschar and contract. The primary goal of the initial procedure is to convert the cloacal exstrophy (Fig. 120–23) into a classic bladder exstrophy. The hindgut and intussuscepted ileum and cecum are separated from the bladder plates, reduced, and repaired (Fig. 120–24).

A colostomy is created. Hindgut reconstruction varies depending on individual patient characteristics. Options include (1) incorporation in the gastrointestinal tract and (2) removal if not viable and/or conversion to a mucous fistula. The hindgut segment may be used in the future for an anorectoplasty, bladder augmentation, or vaginal reconstruction. We separate the hindgut segment from between the bladder plates

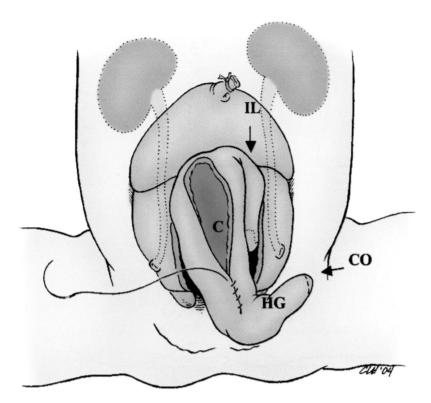

Figure 120–24. Hindgut removal. The cecum (C) has been separated from the bladder plates and closed. The hindgut is prepared for a colostomy (CO). The ileum has been placed posteriorly (IL).

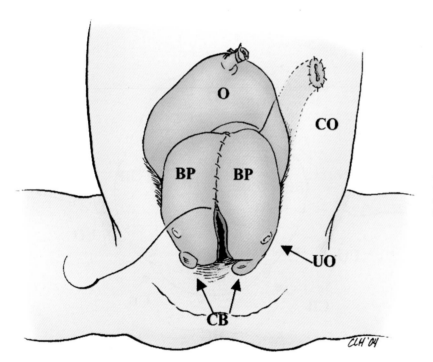

Figure 120–25. Conversion to classic exstrophy. After complete removal of the hindgut and cecum, the bladder plates (BP) are reapproximated posteriorly. The omphalocele (O) could be closed to convert to classic bladder exstrophy. UO, ureteral orifices; CB, corporeal bodies.

and place it in continuity with the rest of the intestines when possible.

The bladder plates are reapproximated in the midline with a running 3-0 polydioxanone suture. The omphalocele is repaired and closed, giving an appearance of a classic exstrophy (Fig. 120–25).

After conversion to a classic bladder exstrophy appearance, CPRE may be attempted if (1) the patient is hemodynamically stable, (2) the omphalocele is small, (3) the pubic diastasis is not wide, and (4) pulmonary function is adequate to tolerate increased abdominal pressure. If the patient develops increased intra-abdominal pressures during preliminary efforts to reapproximate the bladder using CPRE principles or preliminary efforts to reapproximate the bony pelvis that compromise ventilatory pressures, causes ischemia or excessive tension to the midline closure, or compromises lower extremity blood flow, then it is prudent to stop and reconstruct the bladder in a classic exstrophy configuration for future repair using CPRE principles.

Reconstruction is performed when the patient is stable. While the child is awaiting closure, the bladder plate is again covered with a nonabrasive hydrophilic dressing. The CPRE technique is used to complete the reconstruction. The technique has been previously described (Grady and Mitchell, 1999; Plaire and Mitchell, 2000). Complete penile disassembly and division of the intersymphyseal band are crucial to allow for appropriate posterior positioning of the bladder and urethra (Fig. 120–26). After the bladder and urethra are positioned within the pelvis, reconstruction of the bladder, penis, abdomen, and pelvis is anatomic (Fig. 120–27). Osteotomies are performed during this portion of the procedure. Osteotomies are almost always necessary to assist in closure and posterior positioning of the urinary tract.

Because of the wide pubic diastasis in cloacal exstrophy, pubic reapproximation often requires iliac osteotomies even if the closure is performed within the first 48 hours of life. We determine the need for osteotomies by assessing the lower extremities and external genitalia for ischemia during pubic reapproximation before osteotomies are performed. We have used osteotomies to assist in the reconstruction of the majority of these patients. Other authors prefer to avoid the use of osteotomies because they believe that osteotomies make the abdominal closure more difficult. This has not been our experience.

RESULTS
Bladder Exstrophy Series

Between 1989 to 2004, at our institution 18 boys and 13 girls with bladder exstrophy (n = 31) and 5 boys and 2 girls with

Figure 120–26. A, Complete penile disassembly. The bladder (B) is mobilized from the abdominal wall. Traction sutures are placed into each hemiglans. The dissection of the corporeal bodies (CB) begins ventrally along Buck's fascia to provide access to the intersymphyseal band. **B and C,** Deep division of the intersymphyseal band (IS) posterior and lateral to the urethral wedge (UW) is crucial to the proximal dissection of the corporeal bodies (CB) and posterior positioning of the bladder in the pelvis. The urethral wedge is the urethral plate and corpus spongiosum separated from the corpus cavernosum (CC). The blood supply of the urethral wedges is from the corpus spongiosum. The dissection begins proximally and moves distally. After complete disassembly the urethral wedges are joined.

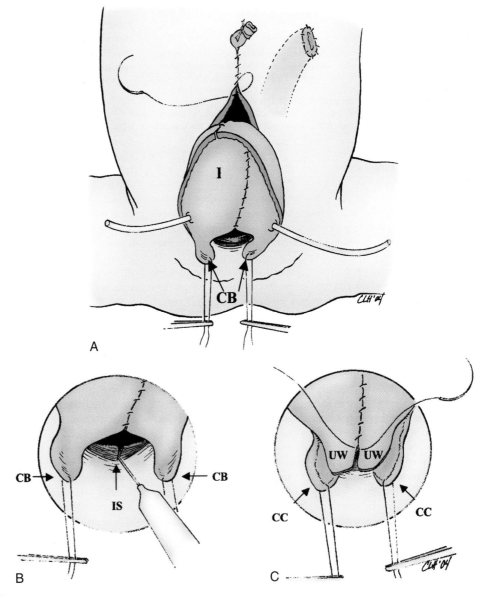

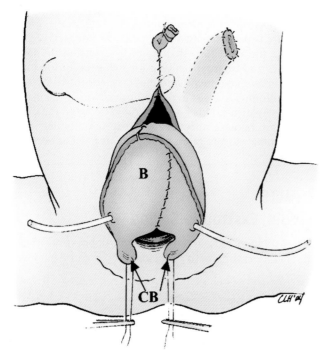

Figure 120–27. Anatomic closure. After the bladder (B) and urethral wedge are completely mobilized, the remainder of the closure is anatomic. A suprapubic tube is placed and ureteral catheters are brought out the urethra. Primary closure of the bladder is done in three layers and that of the urethra in two layers. The urethra is placed ventral to the corpus cavernosum. The pubic symphysis is reapproximated, rectus fascia is closed, and penile skin coverage is completed. Lower extremity and external genitalia ischemia are assessed. Osteotomies are usually required to assist in closure. CB, corporeal bodies.

cloacal exstrophy (n = 7) have undergone the disassembly technique with complete primary repair as a primary procedure. Twenty-three patients underwent this procedure during the first day of life.

Median operative time for this procedure was 5.2 hours for boys with classic exstrophy or epispadias (range: 4 hours 10 minutes to 9 hours 53 minutes) and 3.9 hours for girls (range: 2 hours 40 minutes to 4 hours 53 minutes). Osteotomies were performed for 7 boys and 2 girls in this series. Median operative time for boys who underwent osteotomies at the time of CPRE was 7 hours 25 minutes compared with 4 hours 10 minutes for CPRE alone. The operative time for the 2 girls who underwent simultaneous CPRE and osteotomies was 6 hours 5 minutes versus a median operative time of 3 hours 50 minutes for the girls in the series who had CPRE alone. Six of 7 children with bladder exstrophy in this series repaired after 48 hours of life underwent osteotomies during the initial operation by orthopedic surgeons at our institution. Median estimated blood loss was 49 mL (range: 5 to 150 mL). The average estimated blood loss for CPRE alone was 30 mL. One girl in whom closure was done initially after 48 hours in this series later underwent osteotomies during a repair of a urinary cutaneous fistula several weeks after her initial repair.

Twenty-two of 31 children with classic exstrophy and epispadias are old enough to be evaluated for urinary continence. We defined day-time continence as 2-hour dry intervals with volitional voiding. Day-time continence for the entire group equaled 77%. Seventeen children (9 boys and 8 girls) with classic exstrophy are included in this group. Day-time continence rates are 76% for both boys and girls with bladder exstrophy in this series. Twenty-two percent (2/9) of the boys and 37% (3/8) of the girls with bladder exstrophy achieved primary day-time continence without the need for further bladder neck reconstruction.

To achieve urinary continence, one child in this series has undergone intestinocystoplasty because of a bladder capacity and compliance that was not adequate to achieve urinary continence with bladder neck reconstruction alone. Seven children have Mitrofanoff channels. We usually constructed these channels at the time of bladder neck reconstruction to aid in postoperative management. Four children in this series continue to use these channels to assist in bladder emptying in addition to voiding on their own. One child relies exclusively on clean intermittent catheterization through the Mitrofanoff channel.

Five children with penopubic epispadias (n = 2) or female epispadias (n = 3) have also been repaired with the complete disassembly technique. Of this group, 1 boy and 3 girls have achieved day-time continence. One girl with epispadias in this series has achieved day-time continence primarily. Three children with epispadias have undergone bladder neck reconstruction.

Day-time urinary continence was achieved after bladder neck reconstruction in 8 of 14 children with exstrophy and 3 with epispadias in this series. Three required bladder neck injections for continence. This technique moves the anterior tissue of the bladder neck superiorly onto the bladder and allows the proximal urethra and bladder neck to be narrowed. It has been described previously (Jones et al, 1993). Some of these children underwent this procedure in conjunction with ureteral reimplantation with the primary indication for surgical intervention being breakthrough urinary tract infections, despite the use of suppressive antibiotic therapy. Preoperative urodynamic studies were not routinely done in this patient group as a consequence. However, no patient who achieved urinary continence in this series after bladder neck reconstruction has subsequently become incontinent secondarily.

All the children in this series underwent preoperative renal and bladder ultrasonographic evaluation. None of these children had evidence of hydronephrosis before CPRE. After surgery, 34 renal units demonstrated no hydronephrosis. Twenty-five renal units demonstrated mild hydronephrosis. Eight renal units demonstrated moderate hydronephrosis and 4 renal units showed severe hydronephrosis. Mild and moderate hydronephrosis was transient in 14 of 16 units with mild hydronephrosis and 5 of 6 renal units with moderate hydronephrosis. We evaluated the 2 renal units with severe hydronephrosis with diuretic nuclear renography. Renography with furosemide (Lasix) demonstrated delayed washout in both cases. One of these children did undergo balloon dilation of the ureterovesical junction because of concerns of a possible stricture at that location. Subsequently, the hydronephrosis in both cases was believed to be due to a combination of bladder outlet obstruction (and vesicoureteral reflux in one case). These children were placed on clean intermittent catheterization. The hydronephrosis has subsequently improved for both children. One of the children has undergone ureteral reimplantation and no longer requires catheterization.

As with any other form of anatomic reconstruction for exstrophy, vesicoureteral reflux (VUR) is common after bladder closure using a complete primary repair technique. VUR is seen in the majority of patients in our series. All patients with VUR are maintained on suppressive antibiotic therapy. However, febrile urinary tract infections despite suppressive antibiotic therapy have necessitated neoureterocystostomy in many of our patients with VUR.

Since the advent of the CPRE technique, several centers have used this technique both for newborn exstrophy repair and delayed or re-do cases. Caione and his coworkers (2000) used the CPRE technique to reconstruct 13 patients with exstrophy. They modified the technique that was described earlier by reconfiguring the periurethral muscle complex using a muscle stimulator. Kropp and Cheng (2000) applied the principles of CPRE to the repair of seven girls who presented with variants of the exstrophy-epispadias complex. Hammouda and Kotb (2003) reported a series of 33 cases. They achieved continence in 72% of the patients in their series with minimal complications, thus mirroring the results at our institution. Hammouda (2003) has also used the complete penile disassembly technique for 42 patients with excellent functional results. El-Sherbiny and colleagues (2002) have used the CPRE technique after failed initial closure as well. In this patient population, the technique appeared safe to use although success was less in the subgroup of patients who were repaired in a delayed fashion or after initial failed closure.

Cloacal Exstrophy Series

Seven patients with cloacal exstrophy have been repaired using the CPRE technique. One patient underwent combined omphalocele repair and CPRE in one stage. Six patients were converted to a classic exstrophy appearance and then closed using CPRE principles within 18 to 180 (mean: 70) days of the first operation. There was one mortality in this series. Two of 6 patients developed moderate (n = 1) or severe (n = 1) postoperative hydronephrosis. Three of six patients had vesicoureteral reflux. Six patients report dry intervals and spontaneous voids before toilet training. Three patients report stress urinary incontinence; 2 patients have been treated with bladder neck injections, and 1 has undergone bladder neck reconstruction and construction of a nonorthotopic catheterizable channel for clean intermittent catheterization (Mitrofanoff). One patient reports complete dryness after toilet training. One child has undergone bladder augmentation.

Complications

As is the case with any operation, operative complications can occur after CPRE. These include urethrocutaneous fistula formation. Fistula formation occurs most commonly at the penopubic junction. In the setting of newborn closure, fistulas may occur in up to 6% of cases. The vast majority of these close spontaneously (Hammouda and Kotb, 2003). In delayed cases or when used after initial failure, the CPRE technique resulted in fistula formation in up to 50% of cases—all of which closed spontaneously (El-Sherbiny et al, 2002).

Dehiscence of the primary closure can also occur. After CPRE, if the bladder and urethra have been adequately dissected, fascial dehiscence should not jeopardize the bladder and urethral closure. This is in marked contrast to the devastating consequences of wound dehiscence after a staged primary closure.

Hypospadias can occur when the CPRE technique is used to repair the exstrophy-epispadias complex. In some series, it occurs in over 50% of the male patients (El-Sherbiny et al, 2002; Hafez and El-Sherbiny, 2005). Hypospadias results because the inherently short urethra found in the exstrophy patient will not reach the glans when the urethra, bladder neck, and bladder are moved deep into the pelvis. Some surgeons have modified the original technique by leaving the distal urethra attached to the distal corporeal bodies in an effort to avoid hypospadias (Perovic 1999). Others have used standard hypospadias repair techniques to correct this condition. Hafez and El-Sherbiny (2005) reported a series of 22 boys. In their hands, they found better results using a tubularized vertical island flap or Mustarde technique in comparison to a Theirsch-Dupley urethroplasty in this admittedly small patient group. Emir and colleagues (2002) have described the use of vertical parameatal based skin flaps to achieve an orthotopic meatus. Pippi-Salle and Chan (1999) described a case in which they believed hypospadias was avoided by using an interrupted suture line to reapproximate the urethra.

Following CPRE, some patients will develop bladder and kidney infections. They should be appropriately evaluated to ensure they have no evidence of outlet obstruction. We routinely maintain our patients on suppressive antibiotic therapy if they have VUR.

Other complications that have been reported after CPRE are atrophy of the corpora cavernosa and of the urethra (Gearhart, 2001). This can occur if the blood supply to the corporeal bodies or urethral wedge is damaged during dissection and has been described after the initial stage of a staged reconstruction as well (Hanna and Williams, 1972). Furthermore, severe asymmetry and hypoplasia of the corpora have been observed in patients with atypical exstrophy. In experienced hands, these complications are unusual. These complications do underscore the importance of involving surgeons experienced in the surgical management of these patients in their care.

SUMMARY

The CPRE technique represents a logical extension of previous efforts at anatomic exstrophy reconstruction beginning with Trendelenburg's attempts at the turn of the century. The CPRE technique also incorporates principles of the modified Cantwell-Ransley repair and orthopedic reconstruction. The key features of this single-stage technique largely involve an extended dissection that is facilitated by separating the corporeal bodies from each other. This extended dissection occurs along anatomic planes and allows the bladder and urethra to move posteriorly into a more normal anatomic position. Bladder reconstruction of the exstrophic patient remains a challenge. The CPRE technique will not replace the surgical skills and experience needed to effectively care for these patients. It does, however, offer the promise of improving the care of these patients by streamlining the operations these children require and by hastening their time to continence.

Acknowledgments

The authors would like to thank Cheryl Herndon for her superb artwork to help us illustrate the CPRE technique. We would also like to thank Dr. Richard Lee who diligently recorded the results of the CPRE technique in patient with cloacal exstrophy and Michele Roedel who served as our research coordinator from 2000-2005 in the Section of Pediatric Urology.

SUGGESTED READINGS

Ansell JS: Surgical treatment of exstrophy of the bladder with emphasis on neonatal primary closure: Personal experience with 28 consecutive cases treated at the University of Washington hospitals from 1962 to 1977: Techniques and results. J Urol 1979;121:650-653.

Gearhart JP: Bladder exstrophy: Staged reconstruction. Curr Opin Urol 1999;9:499-506.

Grady RW, Mitchell ME: Complete primary repair of exstrophy. J Urol 1999;162:1415-1420.

Husmann DA, McLorie GA, Churchill BM: Closure of the exstrophic bladder: An evaluation of the factors leading to its success and its importance on urinary continence. J Urol 1989;142:522-524; discussion 542-543.

Jeffs RD: Functional closure of bladder exstrophy. Birth Defects Orig Artic Ser 1977;13:171-173.

Kelly JH: Soft tissue repair of vesical exstrophy. Pediatr Surg Int 1995;10;298-304.

Trendelenburg F: The treatment of ectopia vesicae. Ann Surg 1906;44:981-989.

Young H: Exstrophy of the bladder: The first case in which a normal bladder and urinary control have been obtained by plastic operations. Surg Gynecol Obstet 1942;74:729-737.

121 Bladder Anomalies in Children

DOMINIC FRIMBERGER, MD • BRADLEY P. KROPP, MD, FAAP

BLADDER AND URACHAL DEVELOPMENT

CLASSIFICATION OF BLADDER ANOMALIES

SUMMARY

Although anomalies of the urogenital tract are among the most commonly diagnosed antenatal malformations, the incidence of all congenital bladder anomalies is low (Carrera et al, 1995). Additionally, bladder anomalies are often a reaction to infravesical obstruction or part of a more serious disorder rather than a true isolated structural malformation. Bladder anomalies can be severe, cause urinary obstruction, and even lead to renal failure. Early detection and intervention is crucial to prevent future decompensation of the genitourinary tract. Anomalies can be detected prenatally or postnatally using ultrasound but often require voiding studies for definite diagnosis. In this chapter we review congenital bladder abnormalities in the prenatal and postnatal period and focus on malformations not caused by infravesical obstruction. A discussion of the initial presentation, diagnosis, and current treatment options for the different entities is presented along with a classification based on the prenatal and postnatal presentations of bladder anomalies.

BLADDER AND URACHAL DEVELOPMENT

A comprehensive understanding of the embryologic development of the bladder and urachus is mandatory to correctly interpret the prenatal and postnatal findings and to counsel the parents toward the optimal management.

Between the 4th and 6th weeks of gestation, the urorectal septum divides the endodermal cloaca into a ventral urogenital sinus and a dorsal rectum. The cranial part of the urogenital sinus is continuous with the allantois and develops into the bladder and pelvic urethra. The caudal portion gives rise to the phallic urethra in males and the distal vagina in females. Unlike in males, the entire female urethra is derived from the pelvic part of the urogenital sinus. The allantois develops as an extraembryonic cavity from the yolk sac and connects with the cranioventral portion of the cloaca, the future bladder. Around the 4th to 5th month of gestation, the allantoic duct and the ventral cloaca involute as the bladder descends into the pelvis. The descent causes the allantoic duct to elongate because it does not grow with the embryo. This epithelialized fibromuscular tube continues to become narrower until it is obliterated into a thick fibrous cord, the urachus (Moore, 1982). The obliterated urachus becomes the median umbilical ligament and connects the apex of the bladder with the umbilicus (Nix et al, 1958).

Normal Antenatal Sonographic Findings of the Bladder

The fetal bladder presents as an elliptical structure filled with anechoic fluid within the pelvis. It is bordered laterally by the umbilical arteries. The pubic bones mark the anterior border, and the rectosigmoid indicates the posterior border. The bladder wall thickness should not exceed 3 mm, and the mucosa and musculature present with a similar echogenicity to other structures in the pelvis (McHugo and Whittle, 2001). **The bladder can be visualized in about 50% of cases in the fetal pelvis at the 10th week of gestation, concurrent with the onset of urine production** (Green and Hobbins, 1988). **The detection rate increases with fetal age to 78% at 11 weeks, 88% at 12 weeks, and almost 100% at 13 weeks** (Rosati and Guariglia, 1996). Compared with abdominal ultrasound, transvaginal ultrasound increases the quality of the obtained images as well as the detection rate. Because the fetal bladder empties every 15 to 20 minutes, a second ultrasound in the same setting is mandatory in case of nonvisualization of the bladder. The bladder's diameter increases during the first trimester but should not be more than 6 to 8 mm (Sebire et al, 1996).

The fetal sex, the amount of amniotic fluid, and the appearance of the umbilical cord become increasingly important in the interpretation and differential diagnosis of abnormal bladder findings. Fetal sex is difficult to determine before week 14 and should not be based on the presence or absence of a phallus but on the visualization of testes (Efrat et al, 1999). The measurement of amniotic fluid as an indicator of fetal urine production is a critical portion of every antenatal ultrasound. Until 16 weeks of gestation, the amniotic fluid is mainly consistent with placental transudate, at which time it changes to predominantly fetal urine (Takeuchi et al, 1994). The umbilical cord should contain two arteries and one vein without evidence of a fluid-filled urachus (Bronsthein et al, 1990).

CLASSIFICATION OF BLADDER ANOMALIES

Bladder anomalies can present either as abnormal findings during prenatal ultrasound or postnatally due to symptoms or as a part of an unrelated workup.

It is difficult to classify bladder anomalies due to the large variety of possible malformations, the relatively low incidence of the anomalies, and the common association with other congenital anomalies. Therefore, it seems reasonable to classify the different presentations into two main groups:

- Prenatally detected
  - Dilated
  - Nondilated
- Postnatally detected
  - Urachal abnormalities
  - Bladder diverticulum
  - Bladder duplication
  - Other bladder anomalies

Prenatally Detected Bladder Anomalies

The fetal bladder can either appear dilated, hypoplastic, or absent on ultrasound. If the bladder is dilated, the condition can either be due to obstruction or caused by incomplete emptying of the bladder itself without evidence of a mechanical obstruction. In nondilated conditions, the bladder is either completely absent or is unrecognizable as a fluid-filled structure due to incomplete formation.

Dilated Fetal Bladder

In the first trimester, the fetal bladder is considered to be dilated if larger than 7 mm on ultrasound evaluation. If, on subsequent ultrasound studies, the bladder continues to retain urine and shows no evidence of urine cycling, concern regarding obstruction should be raised. If the amniotic fluid does not increase, this may indicate the progression to oligohydramnios. Determination of the sex of the child is very important because of the male gender predominance of certain diseases such as posterior urethral valves or prune-belly syndrome. It can be difficult to distinguish in utero if the dilatation is due to obstruction. In a retrospective study, Kaefer and colleagues (1997) described 15 patients with marked bladder dilatation in utero, 8 with and 7 without obstruction. All of the obstructed cases presented with moderate to severe oligohydramnios and a marked increase in renal echogenicity, whereas all but one of the nonobstructed bladders had normal amniotic fluid levels and regular renal echogenicity. **Therefore, fetuses with nonobstructive dilatation appear to pass enough urine to maintain renal function and adequate amniotic fluid levels throughout the pregnancy** (Mandell et al, 1992).

Urethral Anomalies and External Bladder Outlet Obstruction. Dilatations of the fetal bladder caused by anatomic obstructions are mostly due to urethral anomalies or external obstruction. Urethral anomalies include congenital urethral strictures, anterior and posterior urethral valves, and urethral atresia. Compression of the bladder outlet region can be due to obstructing syringoceles, a sacrococcygeal teratoma or pelvic neuroblastoma, an anterior sacral myelomeningo-cele, or rectal anomalies. The observed bladder changes are due to mechanical obstruction and affect bladder development at a critical time, which can lead to bladder wall hypertrophy and remodeling (Pagon et al, 1979; Beasley et al, 1988; Stephens and Gupta, 1994).

Prune-Belly Syndrome and Neurogenic Bladder Disease. Affected patients do not demonstrate any sign of obstruction on postnatally performed voiding studies or cystoscopic evaluations, except when urethral atresia is also present. In this case the presentation is similar to posterior urethral valve patients. However, it is possible that the largely distended bladder, as in prune-belly syndrome, is caused by a transient obstruction in utero, and in some cases the presence of urethral atresia has been noted with the prune-belly syndrome. Another possibility for the distention is the presence of neurologic disorders leading to an inability to empty the bladder in utero.

Congenital Megacystis

The term *megacystis* is often used to describe any condition leading to a distended fetal bladder in utero without referring to the cause of the dilation. Historically, congenital megacystis was thought to be caused by bladder neck obstruction, leading to massive bilateral vesicoureteral reflux (VUR) and a thin bladder wall (Williams 1957; Paquin et al, 1960). Even the describing authors recognized that surgical interventions at the bladder neck level did not change the future outcome. Harrow (1967) revisited the subject and recognized that all patients had normal urethras and complete emptying of their bladders on voiding cystourethrography. Therefore, the observed reflux is not an aftereffect of obstruction but rather the cause of the bladder dilatation from continuous recycling of the urine between the upper tract and bladder. Congenital megacystis is defined currently as a dilated, thin-walled bladder with a wide and poorly developed trigone. The wide gaping ureteral orifices are displaced very laterally, causing massive reflux (Fig. 121–1). Bladder contractility is normal, although a majority of the urine refluxes into the ureters with each void. No neurogenic abnormalities are described. Most patients are recognized prenatally and should be placed on prophylactic antibiotics after birth (Mandell et al, 1992). Correcting the reflux often restores normal voiding dynamics and should be performed after 6 months of age. Reduction cystoplasty can be performed but is usually unnecessary (Burbige et al, 1984). Although the bladder is large enough to accommodate the tapered ureters even in a young infant, the operation can be very difficult owing to the bladder wall's thinness.

Congenital megacystis has been recognized in association with microcolon-intestinal hypoperistalsis syndrome. This syndrome is a rare congenital disorder characterized by a dilated, nonobstructive urinary bladder and hypoperistalsis of the gastrointestinal tract. The syndrome can be identified by antenatal ultrasound by the appearance of a largely dilated bladder. It has been reported mostly in females and is usually considered lethal (Srikanth et al, 1993; Lashley et al, 2000).

Nondilated or Absent Fetal Bladder

To truly diagnose an absent fetal bladder on ultrasound, the examination has to be repeated after 15 to 20 minutes to rule out that the fetus had not simply emptied the bladder.

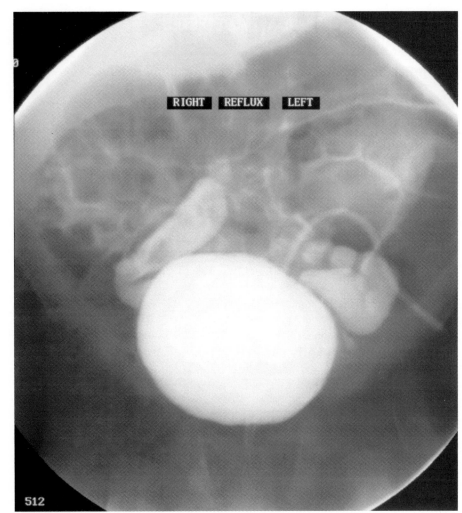

Figure 121–1. Megacystis. VCUG image of congenital megacystis with associated reflux.

Cloacal and Bladder Exstrophy. Bladder exstrophy conditions are characterized by the presence of a bladder template only. Therefore, it can be suspected in the absence of regular bladder filling during fetal ultrasound. Bladder exstrophy can be distinguished from bladder agenesis by the bladder template on the lower abdominal wall, which, along with the amniotic fluid level, remains normal throughout the pregnancy (Mirk et al, 1986; Gearhart et al, 1995).

Bladder Hypoplasia. The bladder can be hypoplastic due to inadequate filling or storing of urine during fetal life. Although the bladder is formed during fetal development and can be detected on antenatal ultrasound throughout pregnancy, it never reaches an adequate capacity. Conditions caused by inadequate bladder outlet resistance (e.g., severe epispadias), separation defects (e.g., urogenital sinus abnormalities), abnormalities of renal development (e.g., bilateral renal dysplasia or agenesis), or urine bypassing the bladder (e.g., ureteral ectopia) can all lead to underdevelopment of the fetal bladder. Some of these bladders grow once the malformation is corrected; however, later bladder augmentation is often required to reach adequate capacity (Gearhart, 2002).

Bladder Agenesis. Embryologic development of bladder agenesis remains difficult to explain. The division of the cloaca into the urogenital sinus and the anorectum apparently is regular, because the hindgut is usually normal. Therefore, the defect can either be due to atrophy of the cranial part of the urogenital sinus or to a failure to incorporate the mesonephric ducts and ureters into the trigone (Krull et al, 1988). The absence of the bladder is often associated with neurologic, orthopedic, or other urogenital anomalies, such as renal dysplasia or agenesis or absence of the prostate, seminal vesicles, penis, and vagina (Aragona et al, 1988). It is a very rare anomaly; only 16 live births have been reported of the 45 known cases in the English literature. All but 2 were female (Adkes et al, 1988; Gopal et al, 1993; Di Benedetto et al, 1999). The defect is only compatible with life if the ureters drain ectopically into normally developed müllerian structures in the female or in the rectum in males. In surviving infants, the diagnosis can be confirmed by retrograde ureteronephrograms via the ectopic openings. Renal function can be preserved after creation of a ureterosigmoidostomy or external stoma (Glenn, 1959; Berrocal et al, 2002).

KEY POINTS: PRENATALLY DETECTED BLADDER ANOMALIES

- Prenatally detected bladder anomalies can be categorized into dilated and nondilated anomalies.

- Dilated bladders can be caused by anatomic or functional obstruction.

- They are commonly associated with severe anomalies, are often the cause for oligohydramnios, and can require fetal or immediate postnatal intervention to prevent fetal demise.

- Nondilated anomalies are associated with the most severe forms of congenital urologic malformations, such as bladder and cloacal exstrophy.

- Usually normal amniotic fluid levels are found.

- Bladder agenesis is only compatible with life if the ureters drain ectopically.

Postnatally Detected Bladder Anomalies

The malformations in this group can be diagnosed by antenatal ultrasound. However, most patients are diagnosed postnatally due to symptomatic disease or during workup for a nonrelated disease. Malformations listed in the prenatally detected group usually severely affect fetal development, are often associated with other malformations, and require prenatal or postnatal interventions. Postnatal detected defects, on the other hand, usually do not affect fetal development and generally can be treated with conservative measures or a single surgical intervention. Bladder anomalies in the infant or child are suspected in cases of urinary tract infections, hematuria, voiding difficulties, anatomic malformations and masses, or umbilical site drainage.

Urachal Anomalies

Understanding the embryologic development of the urachus and its unique location is the key to understanding congenital urachal anomalies. The urachus is located preperitoneal in the center of a pyramid-shaped space. This space is lined by the obliterated umbilical arteries, with its base on the anterior dome of the bladder and the tip directed toward the umbilicus (Fig. 121–2). The urachal length varies from 3 to 10 cm. It has a diameter between 8 to 10 mm and can connect with one or both obliterated umbilical arteries. Microscopically, three layers can be identified. An inner layer consisting of either transitional or cuboidal epithelial cells is surrounded by a layer of connective tissue, and a smooth muscle layer in continuity with the detrusor muscle comprises the outer layer. Because the urachus is surrounded by the umbilicovesical fascia, disease processes usually remain contained inside the pyramid-shaped space (Hammond et al, 1941). The urachus can remain either completely open or obliterate partially, leading to the formation of cystic structures at any site throughout its course.

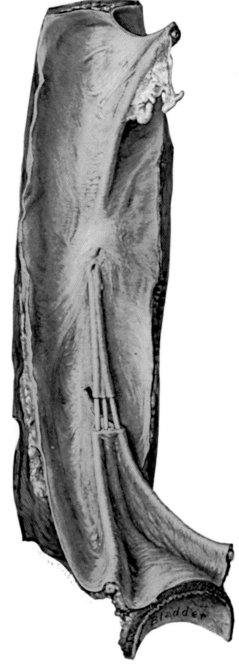

Figure 121–2. Urachal anatomy. (From Cullen TS: Embryology, Anatomy and Diseases of the Umbilicus. Philadelphia, WB Saunders, 1916.)

Four different urachal anomalies have been described (Fig. 121–3):
1. Patent urachus (50%)
2. Umbilical-urachus sinus (15%)
3. Urachal cyst (30%)
4. Vesicourachal diverticulum (3% to 5%)

Patent Urachus

Patent urachus is explained by nondescent of the bladder or, more commonly, failure of the epithelial-lined urachal canal to obliterate (Gearhart, 2002). Bladder obstruction during

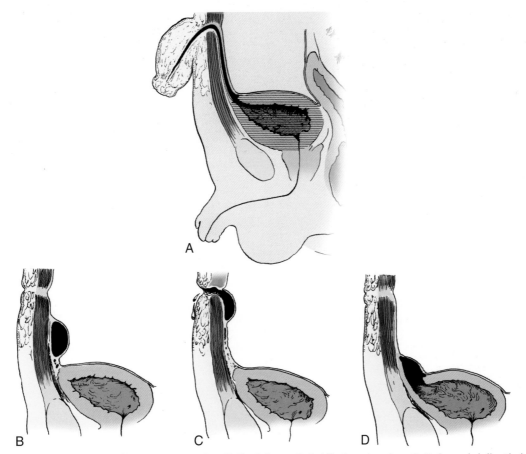

Figure 121–3. Urachal anomalies. **A,** Patent urachus. **B,** Urachal cyst. **C,** Umbilical-urachus sinus. **D,** Vesicourachal diverticulum.

fetal development has been blamed for the urachus remaining tubular. The fact that urachal patency is often absent with severely obstructed bladders in utero, however, casts doubt on this theory. Additionally, only up to 14% of patients with a patent urachus have postnatal confirmation of in-utero bladder obstruction (Schreck and Campbell, 1972; Mesrobian et al, 1997). **It seems possible that obliteration of the urachus may be independent from the level of bladder distention.** Therefore re-tubularization, rather than primary patency, might be the cause for urinary drainage from the umbilicus. This theory is supported by reports of umbilical urinary fistulas in acquired bladder obstructions later in life (Schubert et al, 1983; Berman et al, 1988).

A patent urachus is suspected in the neonatal period by continuous or intermittent drainage of fluid from the umbilicus. The most common organisms cultured from the umbilical drainage include *Staphylococcus aureus, Escherichia coli, Enterococcus,* and *Citrobacter* and, rarely, *Proteus* species (Mesrobian et al, 1997). Additional presentations include an enlarged or edematous umbilicus and delayed healing of the cord stump (Razvi et al, 2001; Schiesser et al, 2003). The diagnosis is confirmed by the demonstration of the fluid-filled canal on longitudinal ultrasound or filling with contrast medium on retrograde fistulogram or voiding cystourethrography (VCUG) (Fig. 121–4) (Mesrobian et al, 1997). Computed tomography (CT) can aid in the diagnosis but is usually dependent on the bladder's filling status. **It is important to differentiate the condition from a patent omphalomesen-**

teric duct. The presence of both anomalies in the same patient is rare (Mendoza et al, 1968).

Management of an infected urachus with abscess formation includes initial drainage under antibiotic coverage. Once the infection has subsided, complete excision of the patent urachus, including a bladder cuff, is required (Nix et al, 1958). It is important to remove all anomalous tissue. This avoids recurrences or stone formation and prevents the rare event of later transformation into a malignant adenocarcinoma (Blichert-Toft and Nielsen, 1971; Sheldon et al, 1984; Goldman et al, 1988; Upadhay and Kukkady, 2003).

Traditionally, the patent urachus is surgically excised using a transverse or midline infraumbilical incision. Before surgery, a balloon catheter is used to distend the bladder. In infants, a small transverse subumbilical incision is often possible because the bladder dome is still high. A feeding tube or small catheter is placed into the patent urachus for better intra-operative identification. The urachus can be incised in a circumscript manner, without removing the umbilicus for cosmetic reasons. The rectus fascia is incised in a longitudinal fashion, the muscles spread apart, and the dome of the distended bladder identified. The urachus is identified and isolated, and a vessel loop is placed. The dissection continues extraperitoneally toward the umbilicus until the previously incised umbilical portion is free and can be pulled into the surgical field. It is then removed. A bladder cuff including the urachal insertion is marked and excised using electrocautery. The bladder is closed in a watertight fashion in two layers. The

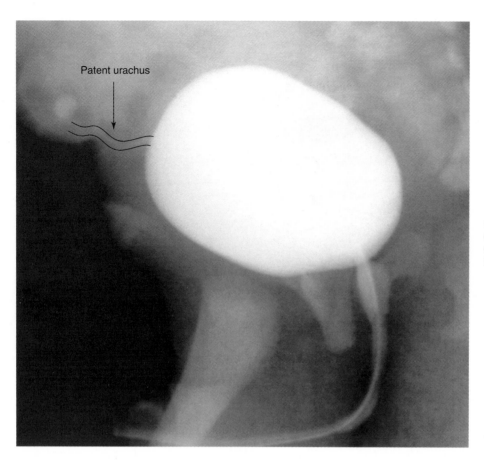

Patent urachus

Figure 121–4. Patent urachus. VCUG image of patent urachus in a newborn. Retrograde contrast filling of patent canal with contrast pooling in umbilicus.

catheter can be left in place overnight and removed the following morning.

Alternatively, urachal remnants can be removed laparoscopically. This can be done even in children younger than 6 months of age (Fahlenkamp et al, 1995; Cadeddu et al, 2000; Khurana and Borzi, 2002). Khurana and Borzi (2002) described their laparoscopic experience with four children between 5 months and 10 years of age and found the procedure to be safe in children of all ages. Technically, they suggested a three-port approach, with the camera port in the midline between the umbilicus and the xiphoid and two working ports on either side in the upper quadrant. The advantage of the laparoscopic technique is the good visualization of the course of the urachus and the bladder dome. However, the laparoscopic techniques require an intraabdominal approach and pose the potential risk of spilling infected or malignant material into the abdominal cavity.

Umbilical-Urachus Sinus

In this situation, the urachus obliterates at the bladder level but remains open at the umbilical site, causing a continuously draining sinus. The presentation is similar to that of the patent urachus. The diagnosis is made by sinogram. The caudal part of the urachus is filled with desquamated epithelial cells, and no connection to the bladder can be identified. The presence of a persistent omphalomesenteric duct has to be considered. This would present as a Meckel diverticulum connected to the umbilicus. These structures can be very difficult to differentiate from an umbilical-urachus sinus because no connection to the bladder or bowel can be seen on a sinogram. However, the surgical approach to both anomalies requires the complete excision of all tissue. Unlike urachal structures, omphalomesenteric remnants can show gastric or small bowel mucosa on histologic examination.

Urachal Cyst

There is no communication of the cyst with the bladder or umbilicus. However, the fluid-filled cyst can drain through the umbilicus or into the bladder intermittently. Urachal cysts are found more commonly in the distal part of the urachus and present more commonly in adults than in infants or children (Cilento et al, 1998). The cyst material consists of desquamated epithelial cells. These cells can become infected; *S. aureus* has been identified as the most common organism (Mesrobian et al, 1997).

Once infected, urachal cysts can present as umbilical abscess formation or bladder infections. Additional symptoms include localized lower abdominal pain, voiding symptoms, or even a painful and palpable mass. The diagnosis is confirmed by ultrasound, demonstrating the localized cyst between the anterior abdominal wall and the peritoneum. In a case of massive infection or difficult presentation, CT can clarify the anatomy and extent of disease (Berrocal et al, 2002). If unrecognized, the infected cyst can perforate into the bladder (Maruschke et al, 2003) or peritoneal cavity. This can cause peritonitis and formation of an enteric fistula (Ohgaki et al,

2003; Quek et al, 2003). Treatment consists of draining the infected cyst, followed by complete excision of the urachal remnant structures.

Vesicourachal Diverticulum

The urachus obliterates almost completely, except at the level of bladder apex. Here it forms a diverticulum of varying size. These lesions are usually nonsymptomatic and found incidentally on nonrelated radiographic workups. Although the diverticulum can enlarge in size in case of urinary obstruction, they rarely cause problems because they tend to have a large opening and drain into the bladder well. There have been reports of stone formation and urinary infections, especially in the case of a narrowed neck, resulting in the need for intervention.

KEY POINTS: URACHAL ANOMALIES

- Urachal anomalies are usually detected postnatally due to umbilical drainage.

- Infected urachal remnants are initially treated with drainage and antibiotics, followed by surgical excision.

- Conservative treatment with observation is justified in asymptomatic cases due to possible spontaneous resolution.

- Imaging possibilities include ultrasound, CT, and VCUG. Nonresolved urachal remnants should be excised owing to the increased risk of later adenocarcinoma.

Bladder Diverticulum

Bladder diverticula are caused by infravesical obstruction, are iatrogenic after bladder surgery, or are a congenital defect. Independent from the cause, all diverticula develop as herniation of bladder mucosa between defects of bladder smooth muscle fibers. The neck of the resulting diverticulum depends on the size of the muscular defect. The incidence is reported to be low, with 1.7% in a selected pediatric population of children undergoing radiographic evaluation for symptomatic disease (Blane et al, 1994). In adult males the incidence tends to be much higher owing to the increased occurrence of infravesical obstruction. The true incidence in children is difficult to evaluate because many of the congenital diverticula remain asymptomatic and are probably never detected.

In his landmark article from 1961, Hutch describes two kinds of diverticula at the ureteral hiatus:

1. **Primary paraureteral diverticula** are seen in smooth-walled bladders, occur isolated with no other diverticula, are intermittent, and occur in children with no infravesical obstruction.

2. **Secondary paraureteral diverticula** are found in trabeculated bladders as one of many diverticula in the bladder, are always present, and are caused by infravesical obstruction.

Primary diverticula arise as a localized herniation of bladder mucosa through the ureteral hiatus between the intravesical ureter and the roof of the ureteral hiatus. These primary diverticula are also known as *congenital diverticula* and are most likely caused by a congenitally deficient bladder wall (Fig. 121–5). Some authors have implied an isolated defect in Waldeyer's sheet; however, congenital diverticula often occur on one side only and a unilateral defect seems unlikely (Stephens, 1963). Congenital diverticula are often

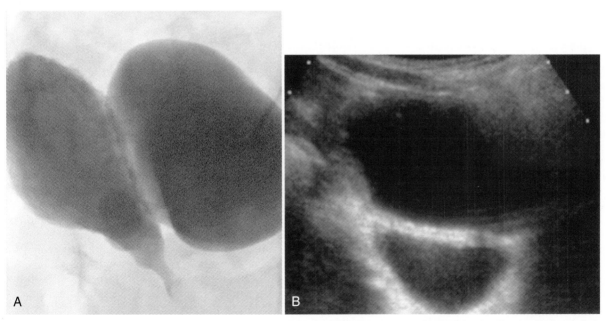

Figure 121–5. Primary paraureteral diverticulum. **A,** VCUG image of large primary paraureteral diverticulum. **B,** Ultrasound image of the same diverticulum.

found in children with generalized connective tissue diseases such as Ehlers-Danlos, Williams Elfin-Facies, or Menkes' syndromes (Babbitt et al, 1979; Daly and Rabinovitch, 1981; Levard et al, 1989). These diverticula can be resected if symptomatic; however, because of the impaired healing in patients with connective tissue disease, recurrence and wound healing complications are more common.

Secondary paraureteral diverticula are acquired and develop due to existing infravesical obstruction. The resulting increased infravesical pressure forces the bladder mucosa to bulge between the muscle fibers. These diverticula are usually just one of many "pop off" mechanisms that can occur throughout the bladder. These diverticula can also be caused by weakening in the bladder muscle by infection (Barrett et al, 1976) or development of a muscular defect after bladder surgery (Sheu et al, 1998).

In both types of paraureteral diverticula, Waldeyer's sheet eventually becomes damaged as the diverticulum expands in size. The increasing diverticulum pulls the intravesical ureter out of its anchored position, causing dysfunction of the ureterovesical junction. Eventually, the enlarged diverticulum can become responsible for ureteral obstruction. This has even been associated with renal dysplasia (Amar, 1972; Livne and Gonzales, 1985).

Paraureteral diverticula or diverticula located in the lower part of the bladder can become so large that they compress the bladder neck or posterior urethra. The resulting bladder outlet obstruction starts a vicious circle by continuously filling and expanding the diverticulum. This increases the obstructing and subsequently causes complete urinary retention (Sheldon and Essig, 1994; Zia-Ul-Miraj, 1999).

Bladder diverticula can be detected on prenatal ultrasound (Gaudet et al, 1999) but are mostly discovered during workup for infection, hematuria, incontinence, or obstruction. They can be suspected during ultrasound examination, especially if the bladder is viewed in different filling stages. The gold standard remains VCUG, which will reveal possible accompanying VUR. If no VUR is present, an intravenous pyelogram with oblique views can help determine the relationship of the ureter with the diverticulum if there is hydronephrosis. Alternatively, nuclear renal studies can be used to obtain information concerning anatomy, kidney function, and ureteral obstruction. It is important to remember that congenital diverticula can have a dynamic nature and might not be present on every study. Radiographic studies may need to be repeated in cases of continuous clinical suspicion.

Small, asymptomatic congenital diverticula detected during unrelated workups can be treated conservatively with regular observation. Many surgeons tend to recommend excision of paraureteral diverticula if they are accompanied by VUR. **Girls will show spontaneous resolution of their diverticula in association with VUR more frequently than boys.** In his review of 304 patients with VUR, Amar (1972) confirmed the lesser resolution rate in boys. He attributed it to higher voiding pressures even without the presence of infravesical obstruction.

In acquired bladder diverticula, the infravesical obstruction has to be eliminated first. After bladder outlet resistance is normalized, the bladder can reshape and diverticulectomy might become unnecessary. If symptomatic, the diverticulum should be excised. The ipsilateral ureter should be reimplanted if it is near or included in the diverticulum. This traditionally has been performed intravesically; however, the procedure can be safely performed via an extravesical approach (Jayanthi et al, 1995; Yu, 2002). Laparoscopic excision also has been successfully performed in a 6-year-old child (Kok et al, 2000). Endoscopic subureteral injection of dextranomer/hyaluronic acid (Deflux) has been used for the correction of VUR, even in the presence of a primary paraureteral diverticulum (Perez-Brayfield et al, 2004).

KEY POINTS: BLADDER DIVERTICULUM

- Bladder diverticula can be detected on prenatal ultrasound, but the gold standard remains VCUG, which will reveal possible accompanying VUR.

- Primary diverticula arise as a localized herniation of bladder mucosa at the ureteral hiatus and are most likely caused by a congenitally deficient bladder wall.

- Secondary paraureteral diverticula are acquired and develop due to existing infravesical obstruction.

- Symptomatic diverticula, especially in conjunction with VUR, should be treated surgically.

Bladder Duplication

Duplication of the bladder and urethra can be complete or incomplete. It can occur in either the coronal or the sagittal plane. Abrahamson (1961) attempted to classify the various bladder duplication anomalies and found complete duplication in the sagittal plane the most common. In incomplete duplications, the two bladder halves communicate and are usually drained by a single urethra. In complete duplications, the two bladders are fully separated entities with normal mucosa and a full-thickness musculature wall divided by a peritoneal fold (Fig. 121–6). Although the size and quality of each entity can be different, they are usually supplied with their own ureter and are drained by an individual urethra and external meatus (Esham and Holt, 1980). In rare cases, one bladder can lack a urethra. This leads to ipsilateral renal dysplasia via complete obstruction (Cheng and Maizels, 1996). Both bladders may possess a sufficient continence mechanism, or one side is compromised, causing incontinent episodes.

Associated duplication anomalies of the external genitalia have been reported in up to 90% of cases; associated duplication anomalies of the lower gastrointestinal tract have been reported in up to 42% of cases (Kossow and Morales, 1973). Duplicated vaginas can be connected to a separate unicornuated uterus. Duplicated penises are supplied with an individual urethra. Additional urologic abnormalities such as VUR, renal ectopia, or dysplasia are commonly found. Association with other nonurologic congenital anomalies are more frequent in sagittal than in coronal duplications. Multiple manifestations have been described, including gastrointestinal malformations, duplications of the spine, spina bifida conditions, and various fistula formation between the urogenital and gastrointestinal tracts (Berrocal et al, 1999). In duplication variations of the classic cloacal-bladder exstrophy

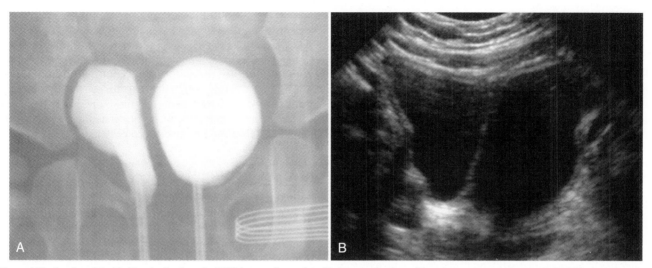

Figure 121–6. Complete bladder duplication. **A,** VCUG image of complete bladder duplication with catheters inserted into each individual urethra. Note the size discrepancy. **B,** Ultrasound image of the same patient.

complex, patients present with an exstrophic bladder and urethra in addition to a closed regular intra-abdominal bladder (Perren and Frey, 1998).

The embryologic development of the various duplication anomalies remains poorly understood. Complete duplication of the bladder and hindgut is thought to occur because of partial twinning of the tail portion of the embryo (Ravitch and Scott, 1953). It also is suggested that the development of a sagittal fissure on the cloacal plate occurs when the urorectal septum separates the urogenital from the digestive sinus (Bellagha et al, 1993).

The wide range of anatomic manifestations of duplicate bladders explains the different time points and modes of presentation. With associated malformations of the gastrointestinal or external genital tracts, the diagnosis is often made in the newborn period. However, many children are not diagnosed until recurrent infections or incontinence initiates a urologic workup. Although similarities exist, each case is different and warrants individual management. **Complete preoperative diagnostic evaluations with karyotype, ultrasound, intravenous pyelography, video-urodynamic studies, genitography, and gastrointestinal tract imaging are useful to determine the anatomic situation.** VCUG and nuclear renal scans can supply additional information regarding VUR and renal function. Complete understanding of the various anomalies can be very difficult. Often the final treatment plan has to be deferred until the time of endoscopic and surgical exploration of the malformation. Initial treatment is directed toward renal preservation and prevention of infections by relieving possibly obstructed genitourinary tracts. Long-term goals include achieving continence and reconstructing the internal and external genitalia. Incomplete duplications may not require surgical procedures if both bladder halves are sufficiently drained by a common urethra. In complete duplications, the two bladders can be combined into one. If both sphincter complexes are competent, the distal urethras are connected. If one is incompetent, the corresponding bladder neck can be closed and the connected urethra excised. Duplicated vaginas are combined in the midline, and a vulvoplasty

is performed. The urogenital duplications can also be left uncorrected if the patient is asymptomatic; Gastol and colleagues (2000) reported two successful pregnancies in a 26-year-old woman. Because of the rarity of the disease and the large variety of presentations, the surgeries must be individualized and should be performed in centers experienced in complex urogenital reconstruction.

KEY POINTS: BLADDER DUPLICATION

- Bladder duplication is often associated with duplication anomalies of the external genitalia and lower gastrointestinal tract.

- Initial treatment is directed toward renal preservation and prevention of infections by relieving possibly obstructed genitourinary tracts.

- Long-term goals include achieving continence and reconstructing the internal and external genitalia.

- Because of the rarity of the disease and the large variety of presentations, the surgeries must be individualized.

Other Bladder Anomalies

Nephrogenic Adenoma

Nephrogenic adenoma of the urinary bladder is a rare benign tumor mostly found in adults. Sporadic case reports in children describe the lesion as a reaction to infection, lithiasis, or trauma or as occurring in response to surgery. Heidenreich and colleagues (1999) found a significant predominance of girls compared with boys (5:1) typically presenting with hematuria or irritative bladder symptoms. The diagnosis is established after cystoscopy with biopsy. Treatment consists of transurethral fulguration or resection and can be combined with long-term antibiotic prophylaxis.

Although malignant transformation has not been reported, tumor recurrence developed in 80% of the children with a latency period of 4 years.

Eosinophilic Cystitis

Eosinophilic cystitis in children is sporadically described in case reports with a predominance in boys. The etiology remains unclear and the histopathologic examination includes inflammatory cells with numerous eosinophils throughout all layers of the bladder wall (Tsakiri 2004). Presenting symptoms include dysuria, hematuria, suprapubic pain, and urinary retention. It can be detected on ultrasound, but the diagnosis is made by cystoscopy with transurethral biopsy of the lesion. Immunologic diseases as well as allergies have been suggested to be causative for the development of the lesions. In his large review of 135 cases, van de Ouden (2000) found transurethral resection combined with corticosteroids, antihistaminics, or antibiotics to be most successful for all age groups. In neonates and young children the disease can be self limited and observation is justified (Al-Omar et al, 2005).

Bladder Hemangioma

These benign vascular tumors are mostly seen in association with Klippel-Trenaunay syndrome and can be solitary or in multiple locations throughout the bladder. The leading symptom is macrohematuria, and the vascular tumors are found during cystoscopy. Treatment consists of neodymium:yttrium-aluminum-garnet laser irradiation of the affected areas (Kato et al, 2000).

SUMMARY

Isolated congenital bladder anomalies are very rare. Most published information relies on case reports of various malformations and their individualized management. Many of the detected anomalies are due to infravesical obstruction or are part of a syndrome affecting other parts of the genitourinary or nonurologic systems. Prenatal ultrasound allows early detection of bladder changes and has vastly influenced the prenatal and postnatal management of the described malformations. However, owing to the rarity of the various presentations, large series with adequate follow-up are missing. Management and treatment remain individualized. Severe anomalies are often difficult to understand, and treatment should be centralized in specialized centers.

Acknowledgments

We thank Dr. Faridali G. Ramji, Associate Professor and Director of the Fellowship Program in the Department of Radiology at the Children's Hospital of Oklahoma, Oklahoma University Medical Center for providing the figures, and the Imaging Technologists in the Department of Radiology at the Children's Hospital of Oklahoma, Oklahoma University Medical Center for assisting with the image formatting.

SUGGESTED READINGS

Abrahamson J: Double bladder and related anomalies: Clinical and embryological aspects and a case report. Br J Urol 1961;33:195-212.

Berrocal T, Lopez-Pereira P, Arjonilla A, Gutierrez J: Anomalies of the distal ureter, bladder and urethra in children: Embryologic, radiologic and pathologic features. RadioGraphics 2002;22:1139-1164.

Gearhart JP, Ben-Chaim, Jeffs RD, et al: Criteria for the prenatal diagnosis of classic bladder exstrophy. Obstet Gynecol 1995;85:961.

Harrow BR: The myth of the megacystis syndrome. J Urol 1967;98:205.

Hutch JA: Saccule formation at the ureterovesical junction in smooth walled bladders. J Urol 1961;86:390-399.

Kaefer M, Peters CA, Retik AB, Benacerraf BB: Increased renal echogenicity: A sonographic sign for differentiating between obstructive and nonobstructive etiologies of in utero bladder distension. J Urol 1997;158(3 pt 2):1026-1029.

Mesrobian HG, Zacharias A, Balcom AH, Cohen RD: Ten years of experience with isolated urachal anomalies in children. J Urol 1997;158:1316-1318.

122 Posterior Urethral Valves and Other Urethral Anomalies

ANTHONY J. CASALE, MD

POSTERIOR URETHRAL VALVES
Description, Classification, and Embryology

Congenital obstruction of the urethra is one of the most devastating anomalies to occur in the urinary tract and one of the few that are life-threatening in the neonatal period. These lesions usually result in lifelong disabilities with incontinence and decreased renal function despite optimal medical management. The condition of posterior urethral valves is still relatively common and makes up the majority of congenital urethral obstructions.

Langenbeck is credited with first reporting congenital obstruction of the prostatic urethra in 1802 (Dewan et al, 1999). Despite this observation, it was left for Hugh Hampton Young, more than a century later, to define the condition and name it posterior urethral valves (Young et al, 1919). His remarkably accurate observations were made with only gross pathologic dissection and with the primitive cystoscopic instruments of his day (Fig. 122–1). Young observed the anatomic variability of the anomaly and developed a classification that is still used today.

The term *valves* is unfortunate because it implies function. This obstructive membrane has no active function and is not a developmental stage in the embryology of the urethra. It is simply a passive barrier to urine flow. Young adopted this term when he found that a urethral sound would pass easily from the urethral meatus into the bladder in a retrograde manner while the same sound (or urine for that matter) would not pass antegrade out of the bladder and down the urethra. This unidirectional access through the urethra suggested to Young the function of a one-way valve, and he described the condition as such.

Posterior urethral valves occur in 1 in 8,000 to 25,000 live births and make up 10% of urinary obstructions diagnosed in utero (Atwell, 1983; Thomas and Gordon, 1989; Casale, 1990). The diagnosis has been made on average in 1 in 1250 fetal ultrasound screenings (Gunn et al, 1995). There are reported cases of congenital urethral obstruction in girls, but the classic posterior urethral valves occur only in boys (Nesbit, 1964). The incidence of posterior urethral valves is dropping in some populations because of the effects of prenatal diagnosis and subsequent termination of affected fetuses. In one report, fetuses with diagnosed valves were electively terminated in 46% of cases (Cromie et al, 2001).

Despite several alternative proposals, Young's classification is still most commonly used (Dewan, 1993). He described three types of posterior urethral valves:

Type I. In the most common type there is a ridge lying on the floor of the urethra, continuous with the verumontanum, which takes an anterior course and divides into two fork-like processes in the region of the bulbomembranous junction. These processes are continued as thin membranous sheets, directed upward and forward which may be attached to the urethra throughout its entire circumference. In the majority of cases of this general type the fusion of the valves anteriorly is not complete, there existing at this point a slight separation of the folds. However, in a few of the cases . . . the anterior fusion is complete while a cleft exists between the folds posteriorly.

It has been proposed that all boys with valves originally have complete fusion along the anterior urethra, leaving only an

3583

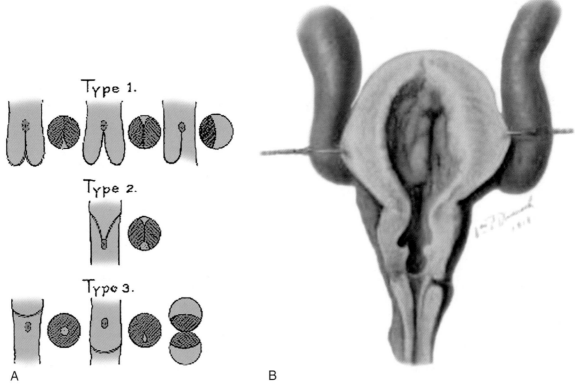

Figure 122–1. **A,** Young's original figures from his 1919 article. He described three types of posterior urethral valves and diagrammed them. **B,** William P. Didusch drew this pathologic dissection that shows the features of posterior urethral valves, the thickened bladder wall with an elevated bladder neck, and enlarged posterior urethra. The two valve leaflets of type I valves are seen. The ureters are massively dilated. (From Young HH, Frontz WA, Baldwin JC: Congenital obstruction of the posterior urethra. J Urol 1919;3:289.)

open channel along the posterior urethral wall. The frequently observed cleft in the membrane may be iatrogenic, caused by instrumentation or catheterization that erodes the valve tissue in the anterior midline and splits the valve in two leaflets (Robertson and Hayes, 1969; Dewan et al, 1992).

Young's type I valves make up 95% of all posterior urethral obstructions. The thickness of the valves varies from rigid, thick tissue to thin, almost transparent membranes (Fig. 122–2). The valve itself is made of a fibrous stroma covered on each side by transitional epithelium. There is no muscle within the valve. The degree of obstruction also varies widely and, in turn, the amount of damage to the urinary tract.

The embryology of posterior urethral valves is speculative but may be related to an abnormal insertion of the mesonephric ducts into the fetal cloaca. Evidence supporting this theory lies in the fact that patients with type I valves lack plicae colliculi, mucosal folds found in the normal male urethra that are believed to represent a remnant of the normal pathway of migration of the mesonephric ducts toward the verumontanum (Stephens, 1983).

Young described a type II valve as arising from the verumontanum and extending along the posterior urethral wall toward the bladder neck. This description was based on the similar appearance of these folds to the membranes found in type I. These type II folds are not obstructive and probably result from hypertrophy of muscles of the superficial trigone and prostatic urethra in response to high voiding pressure from distal obstruction. They can be seen in response to many obstructive conditions, such as urethral strictures, posterior urethral valves, anterior urethral valves, and detrusor-sphincter dyssynergia. These type II folds are no longer referred to as valves.

Young described the type III valve as a membrane lying transversely across the urethra with a small perforation near its center (Fig. 122–3). The membrane is distal to the verumontanum and sometimes is elongated, like a windsock, reaching the bulbous urethra (Field and Stephens, 1974). Type III valves make up only 5% of the total. Young described them as follows:

> There is a third type which has been found at different levels of the posterior urethra and which apparently bears no such relation to the verumontanum as the types just considered. . . . This obstruction was attached to the entire circumference of the urethra, there being a small opening in the center. Incomplete varieties of this type have been described, the most common being a more or less crescentic or semicircular fold crossing the urethra and being attached either to the roof or floor.

The embryologic origin of type III valves has been attributed to incomplete dissolution of the urogenital portion of the cloacal membrane. Type III valves present in the same manner and are managed in the same way as the more common type I, although there is some evidence that type III valves have a worse prognosis (Rosenfeld et al, 1994).

The inheritance of posterior urethral valves is poorly understood and may involve several genes (Livne et al, 1983).

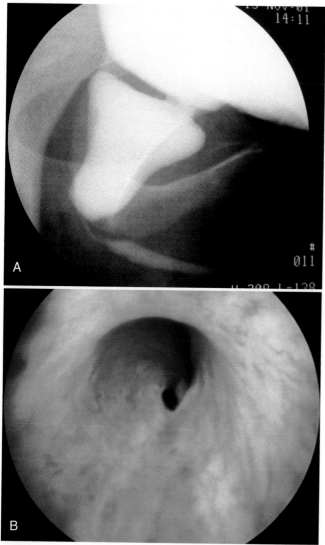

Figure 122–2. **A,** Voiding cystourethrogram demonstrates a typical type I posterior urethral valve with a dilated posterior urethra, elevated bladder neck, and valve leaflets obstructing the flow of contrast material from the bladder. **B,** This cystoscopic image from the distal urethra shows the valve leaflets forced into the lumen with the bladder full, illustrating their obstructive effect.

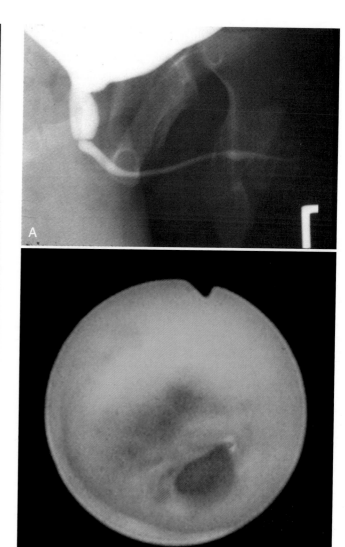

Figure 122–3. **A,** Voiding cystourethrogram demonstrates a typical type III posterior urethral valve with a transverse septum crossing the urethra at a right angle distal to the verumontanum. **B,** A cystoscopic image from the distal urethra shows the thin membrane and a small off-center opening.

Valves have occurred in siblings, in twins, and in successive generations (Farkas and Skinner, 1976; Hanlon-Lundberg et al, 1994; Morini et al, 2002). The timing of valve development is also speculative, but it would appear that they become obstructive during or after the eighth week of life, by which time the prostatic urethra has developed from the urogenital sinus (Mitchell and Close, 1996).

Pathophysiology

The effects of congenital obstruction of the urethra are reflected in the entire urinary tract above the level of obstruction. Proximal urethra, prostate, bladder neck, bladder, ureters, and kidneys are all affected and suffer various forms of damage (Table 122–1).

Lower Urinary Tract

The injury to the lower urinary tract appears to be caused by high-pressure urine storage and voiding (McConnell, 1989; Keating, 1994). **Histologic examination of the bladder of fetuses with posterior urethral valves shows hypertrophy and hyperplasia of the detrusor muscle along with increased connective tissue.** The ratio of muscle to connective tissue is the same as in normal bladders, but there is conflicting evidence that the type of collagen within the bladder is altered (Kim et al, 1991; Ewalt et al, 1992). Some bladder findings in neonates, such as wall thickness and poor compliance, will improve after relief of obstruction, but the valve bladders seldom if ever achieve normal function.

High voiding pressures distend and thin the prostatic urethra. The storage capacity of the prostatic urethra some-

Table 122–1.	Damage due to Posterior Urethral Valves	
Organ	**Effect**	**Natural History**
Lung	Pulmonary hypoplasia	May be fatal in newborns If infant survives, there are few long-term problems

Kidney
  Glomerular injury
    Obstructive uropathy
	Reversible renal insufficiency	Usually improves with initial treatment but can recur with bladder dysfunction

Dysplasia	Irreversible renal insufficiency	Permanent level of renal damage that limits growth; leads to progressive renal failure and hypertension
Tubular injury	Inability to limit sodium and water loss	Progressive with age; nephrogenic diabetes insipidus
Bladder	Poor sensation, hypercontractility, low compliance, and eventual myogenic failure all may contribute to incontinence and poor emptying	Bladder problems are lifelong and change with age
Ureters	Poor contractility and inability to coapt and transport urine	Most will improve initially, but most have chronic hydronephrosis

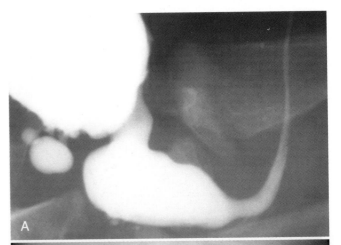

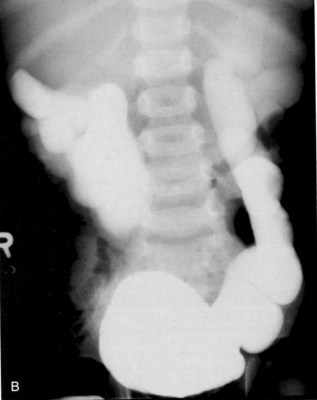

Figure 122–4. **A,** Voiding cystourethrogram shows a posterior bladder diverticulum near the base of the bladder and an extremely high bladder neck. A catheter passed blindly can fail to pass over the bladder neck and coil in the dilated posterior urethra. **B,** Massive vesicoureteral reflux in a boy with valves.

times exceeds that of the bladder because of the relative lack of muscle there. The verumontanum is distorted, and the ejaculatory ducts may be dilated from refluxing urine. The bladder neck is rigid and hypertrophied (Fig. 122–4). This high bladder neck was once mistaken as another cause of obstruction and was surgically incised to facilitate bladder emptying. Unfortunately, this practice often resulted in total incontinence. We now understand the appearance of the bladder neck to be a result of distal obstruction and not an obstructive lesion itself. Bladder neck appearance and function usually improve after the obstructive valves are destroyed.

Upper Urinary Tract

Ureteral damage is usually severe. The appearance and function of the ureters are markedly abnormal. The ureteral wall is thickened and the lumen massively dilated. The ureter is at the mercy of the ureterovesical junction. If this junction functions to prevent reflux, the ureter and kidney are somewhat protected from the complete force of the bladder contractions. If the junction allows reflux, the entire pressure of the thickened and hypercontractile bladder is transmitted directly to the upper tract with severe consequences. Virtually all valve patients have hydroureteronephrosis, and this can be the result of obstruction from the valves, the ureterovesical junction, or both. Whereas reflux is variable, hydroureteronephrosis is a constant in these patients. Severely dilated ureters coapt poorly and contract weakly if at all (Gearhart et al, 1995). The propulsion of urine down the

ureter is diminished in the infant, and this ureteral dysfunction may persist throughout life despite relief of distal obstruction.

The nature of the renal injury in boys with posterior urethral valves is complex and appears to have two distinct components. Some damage, described as obstructive uropathy, is caused by persistent high pressure. It is ongoing and can be progressive, but it is potentially reversible with relief of high pressures. Other damage, termed renal dysplasia, may be the result of either increased pressure during the development of the kidney or abnormal embryologic development. **Renal dysplasia is not reversible, and therefore the degree of dysplasia is critical in determining eventual renal function in valve patients.**

Dysplasia is, in fact, a histologic diagnosis and depends on identification of a fundamental disorganization of the renal parenchyma on a cellular and tissue level. The elements of dysplasia include embryonic tubules, cartilage, cysts, and mesenchymal connective tissue. The particular type of dysplasia in valve patients is termed microcystic and can be observed primarily in the peripheral cortical zone of the kidney.

The exact cause of dysplasia is a matter of continued debate. Beck and Glick demonstrated that dysplasia could be produced by early urinary obstruction in lambs (Beck, 1971; Glick, 1983). Maizels and colleagues (1983) also produced a form of dysplasia in chicken embryos by obstructing the fetal urinary tract. There is ample evidence that a form of dysplasia can be induced by early fetal urinary obstruction and resultant high intra-renal urinary pressure.

On the other hand, Stephens and Henneberry have demonstrated that dysplasia may be found in patients who do not seem to have a history of obstruction but instead have abnormal ureteral development (Henneberry and Stephens, 1980). In patients with severe vesicoureteral reflux, the ureteral orifice is usually in an abnormal position. These patients frequently demonstrate renal dysplasia, and the degree of dysplasia is proportional to how much the position of the ureter deviates from normal. **Stephens postulated that this dysplasia is the result of a faulty ureteral bud arising in an abnormal position along the mesonephric duct.** Since the ureteral bud induces the development of the kidney, it follows that an abnormal bud may induce an abnormal kidney.

Dysplasia therefore occurs in association with obstruction and with reflux, seemingly unrelated conditions. Both theories are plausible and not exclusive. Whatever the cause, dysplasia is the defining factor in long-term renal function in most patients with valves. Since this type of renal damage is not reversible, the extent of dysplasia will ultimately determine the growth and functional potential of the infant's kidneys. **There are a number of other related factors that may contribute to declining renal function in valve patients, including infection, persistent obstruction, hypertension, hyperfiltration of damaged parenchyma, and perhaps high-protein diet, but none is as important as the degree of dysplasia** (Brenner et al, 1982; Klahr, 1989; Farnham et al, 2005).

All posterior urethral valve patients have a degree of associated obstructive uropathy. Obstructive uropathy involves both glomerular injury and tubular injury. Glomerular injury occurs when high pressures result in decreased renal perfusion and filtration. These changes are partially reversible when pressures are dropped and obstruction is relieved. The potential for recovery is thought to be time sensitive, and early relief of obstruction should favor recovery. Some degree of scarring and fibrosis within the parenchyma persists, but unlike dysplasia, obstructive uropathy usually improves with treatment.

Tubular damage from increased urinary pressure results in failure to concentrate and acidify the urine. This occurs in up to 59% of valve patients and sometimes occurs in patients without evidence of glomerular injury (Parkhouse and Woodhouse, 1990; Dinneen et al, 1995). Concentrating defects in the form of nephrogenic diabetes insipidus lead to increased urine output independent of the patient's state of hydration. Patients are at risk for electrolyte imbalances and dehydration due to inability to conserve sodium and water even in the face of dehydration (Gonzales, 1978). Pathologically, large urine output also stresses the ureters and bladder and contributes to persistent hydroureteronephrosis and bladder dysfunction. **Tubular damage worsens with age despite early relief of obstruction in many patients, and resultant high urine volumes contribute to the deterioration of renal and bladder function in late childhood.**

Vesicoureteral Reflux and Dysplasia and Pop-off Mechanisms

Hoover and Duckett (1982) identified the relationship between valves, reflux, and dysplasia. In comparing refluxing and nonrefluxing kidneys, they recognized that valve infants with unilateral reflux had markedly different renal function. **Reflux was consistently associated with dysplastic and damaged kidneys.** They postulated that the reflux allowed the high bladder pressures to focus on the refluxing kidney, sparing and protecting the nonrefluxing kidney. The vesicoureteral reflux and dysplasia relationship is found in 13% of valve patients, and interestingly, the refluxing kidney is on the left in 92%.

The proposed mechanism of this protection is that the refluxing collecting system acts as a pressure pop-off valve. They thought that the protected kidney would ultimately lead to a better long-term prognosis than for boys without unilateral reflux. The long-term protective effect of vesicoureteral reflux and dysplasia has not been as helpful as originally thought, and longitudinal studies have shown in patients with vesicoureteral reflux and dysplasia that by mid-childhood, serum creatinine concentration was only 30% of normal and glomerular filtration rate was significantly decreased compared with that of normal children (Cuckow et al, 1997). Other types of pop-off pressure systems include bladder diverticula, urinomas, and urinary ascites (Rittenberg et al, 1988). The protective effect of these clinical situations is highly variable.

KEY POINTS: PATHOPHYSIOLOGY

- Posterior urethral valves damage the entire urinary tract proximal to the valve.

- Pulmonary hypoplasia is the most common cause of mortality in valve patients.

- Most renal damage occurs early in fetal life.

- Bladder dysfunction is usually a lifelong problem resulting in incontinence and poor emptying.

- Persistent hydronephrosis is common and may be due to either ureteral or bladder dysfunction.

- Reflux usually improves and often resolves after valve ablation.

Clinical Presentation

In the past, boys with posterior urethral valves presented with a variety of symptoms and at various ages (Hendren, 1971). **They ranged from newborns with life-threatening renal and pulmonary conditions to older children with minor voiding dysfunction.** In general, the symptoms are age dependent; the more severely affected boys present earlier in life (Dinneen and Duffy, 1996).

Neonates

Today, most patients with posterior urethral valves are diagnosed with prenatal ultrasonography. Obstruction leads to decreased fetal urine output and results in oligohydramnios. The observation of marked hydroureteronephrosis, a distended bladder, and a thickened bladder wall in utero strongly supports the diagnosis of valves. The urologist often has been consulted long before delivery, and intervention has been undertaken in utero in some cases.

Pulmonary Hypoplasia. The most severe clinical problem facing the neonate with posterior urethral valves is pulmonary hypoplasia. The babies are often cyanotic and require respiratory support at delivery. Pulmonary hypoplasia is a direct result of oligohydramnios and accounts for most of the mortality today (Churchill et al, 1990). The exact etiology of the pulmonary hypoplasia is unclear, but a contributing factor is physical restriction of fetal breathing motion (Landers and Hanson, 1990). The lack of amniotic fluid to surround and buffer the baby from intra-abdominal pressure leads to a small chest cavity and prevents chest wall breathing motion and normal musculoskeletal development. Amniotic fluid may be important in development of the fetal pulmonary tree by providing needed intraluminal pressure, volume, and flow. In addition, the amniotic fluid may provide some cellular or molecular stimulus to the developing lung. The result of oligohydramnios is often life-threatening, and some infants succumb despite heroic measures. The mortality of valves has decreased significantly during the past two decades with development of better methods to manage pulmonary hypoplasia by neonatologists. It is rare to have a baby die today with the quality of pulmonary support available in the newborn intensive care unit (Gibbons et al, 1993).

Renal Insufficiency. In addition to pulmonary distress, the newborn with posterior urethral valves usually presents with signs of severe systemic illness, such as intrauterine growth retardation, failure to thrive, lethargy, and poor feeding. The infants may be pale and have poor muscle tone. They may demonstrate the classic signs of oligohydramnios, such as Potter's facies and bowed and deformed limbs with pressure dimples over knees and elbows from intrauterine pressure. Examination of the abdomen may reveal masses due to hydroureteronephrosis and a distended bladder. The infant may suffer from extensive edema and urinary ascites. The caregivers may notice a diminished force of urinary stream, but this sign is not reliable to predict valves (Smith and Duckett, 1996). If they are not diagnosed in utero, the most severely affected valve patients present as newborns. Urinary tract infection or urosepsis often precipitates evaluation and diagnosis.

Ascites. Forty percent of neonatal ascites is caused by urinary conditions (Adzick et al, 1985). Urinary ascites occurs when high intraluminal pressure forces urine to extravasate from the kidney, usually across a renal fornix. Urine then enters the retroperitoneum and travels across the peritoneum as a transudate (Fig. 122–5). If it is aspirated from the peritoneal cavity, the ascites or extravasated urine contains electrolyte and creatinine levels similar to those of serum. The urine within the peritoneum is subject to the large absorptive mesothelial surface that quickly normalizes these values, masking the identity of ascitic fluid as urine. The diagnosis of urinary ascites may be difficult and may require definitive upper tract drainage in the form of nephrostomy tubes to establish the cause of the ascites and allow its resolution. **Urinary ascites in the case of distal obstruction may serve to lower urinary pressures and offer some protection to the developing kidneys** (Conner et al, 1988).

Patil and colleagues (2003) reviewed a large group of 615 valve patients and analyzed the protective effect of ascites compared with unilateral and bilateral urinomas. The authors found that the kidney associated with a unilateral urinoma is often impaired. Bilateral urinomas are associated with good renal function, but urinary ascites alone has a poorer prognosis. The glomerular filtration rate of patients with urinary ascites alone was 29 mL/min per 1.73 m^3 compared with 36 mL for boys with unilateral urinoma alone, 74 mL for boys with urinoma plus ascites, and 104 mL for bilateral urinomas.

Older Children

The majority of boys who present later in life do so with urinary tract infection or voiding dysfunction. With a better understanding of functional voiding disorders, valves are now an uncommon cause of minor voiding dysfunction (Pieretti, 1993). Because of widespread prenatal ultrasonography, it is now rare to see a new patient with posterior urethral valves past the neonatal period. Whereas boys who present later in life are generally thought to have more normal urinary tracts, this is not a uniform finding. One series reported that patients who presented at school age suffered renal insufficiency in 35% of cases (Bomalaski et al, 1999).

Initial Diagnostic Evaluation

Ultrasonography

The widespread use of maternal ultrasonography in the past 25 years in the United States has resulted in at least 80% of women undergoing ultrasound screening during pregnancy. Posterior urethral valves is the third most common antenatal genitourinary diagnosis made today and accounts for 10% of all fetal uropathy (Thomas and Gordon, 1989). It was reported that two thirds of patients with valves presented on fetal ultrasound examination during the 1990s, but this percentage has continued to rise (Greenfield, 1997). The quality and availability of ultrasound technology continue to improve and with it our ability to image the fetus.

Ultrasonography is sensitive in detecting fetal hydronephrosis, but the specific diagnosis of posterior urethral valves is more difficult. The differential diagnosis of bilateral hydronephrosis includes posterior urethral valves, prune-belly

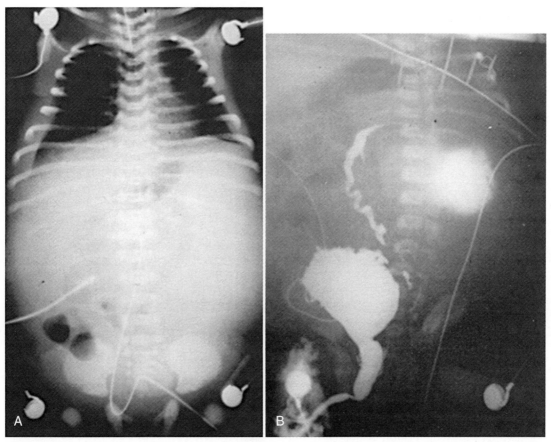

Figure 122-5. A, Abdominal radiograph shows the ground-glass appearance of an infant with ascites. **B,** Voiding cystourethrogram demonstrates reflux of contrast material, which is then seen extravasating into a urinoma and later flowing into the abdominal cavity as urinary ascites. (From Gonzales ED: Posterior urethral valves and other ureteral anomalies. In Walsh PC, Retik AB, Vaughan ED, Wein AJ, eds: Campbell's Urology, 8th ed. Philadelphia, WB Saunders, 2002.)

syndrome, bilateral ureteropelvic junction obstruction, bilateral high-grade vesicoureteral reflux, bilateral ureterovesical junction obstruction, congenital urethral atresia, and anterior urethral obstruction. Valves were correctly diagnosed in only 66% of 18 fetuses that were identified with hydronephrosis (Skolder et al, 1988). In a review of 42 patients with valves, only 45% were detected on antenatal ultrasonography (Dinneen et al, 1993).

The timing of screening for fetal uropathy is an important factor in accuracy. There is compelling evidence that valves may be missed if the screening ultrasound examination is done before 24 weeks of gestation (Jee et al, 1993; Hutton et al, 1994). In Dinneen's series, 92% of the 36 patients scanned before 24 weeks of gestation were not detected. The classic ultrasound findings in patients with valves include bilateral hydroureteronephrosis, distended bladder, dilated posterior urethra, and thickened bladder wall. The "keyhole" sign of a dilated bladder above a dilated prostatic urethra is also helpful. Bladder wall thickness is an important diagnostic sign (Fig. 122–6). The findings of an excessively thick bladder wall and a distended bladder indicate distal obstruction (Kaefer et al, 1997b).

Renal echogenicity is another parameter that may aid in the diagnosis of valves. Increased echogenicity predicted an obstructive process in a study of fetuses with bilateral

hydroureteronephrosis and distended bladders (Kaefer et al, 1997a). Patients with a nonobstructive process, such as megacystis-megaureter association, failed to demonstrate increased echogenicity, whereas 87.5% of valve patients had increased echogenicity at a mean gestational age of 26 weeks. The same predictive value was found with oligohydramnios. Any male fetus with bilateral hydroureteronephrosis, decreased amniotic fluid, and distended bladder should be considered to have posterior urethral valves until proved otherwise. The ultrasound findings of a neonate with posterior urethral valves are identical to those of a fetus.

Voiding Cystourethrography

Voiding cystourethrography (VCUG) remains the most important study in diagnosis of posterior urethral valves because it defines the anatomy and gross function of the bladder, bladder neck, and urethra. When the diagnosis of valves is in question, VCUG should be performed as soon as possible. On imaging of the bladder and upper tracts of children with neuropathic bladder, urethral stricture, anterior urethral obstruction, and posterior urethral valves may all appear identical. Images of the urethra during voiding are necessary to make the correct diagnosis. It is not necessary to remove the catheter during voiding to observe the valves (Ditchfield et al, 1995).

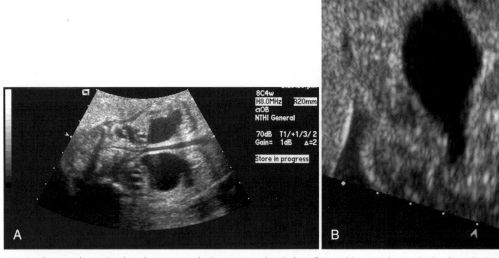

Figure 122–6. **A,** Ultrasound examination shows severe hydroureteronephrosis in a fetus with posterior urethral valves. **B,** Fetal ultrasound examination demonstrates a severely thickened bladder wall with a distended bladder and posterior urethra. These two fluid collections, a larger one above the smaller one, produce the "keyhole" sign indicative of posterior urethral valves.

In posterior urethral valves, the bladder is thickened and trabeculated. VCUG often demonstrates bladder diverticula and severe vesicoureteral reflux. From the lateral projection, the bladder neck is elevated and the proximal urethra is dilated, and the actual valve structure is often visible. **Vesicoureteral reflux is present in at least 50% of valve patients at the time of diagnosis** (Churchill et al, 1990) (Fig. 122–7). The incidence of reflux has been found to be higher in neonates than in older children. Since most valve patients are now discovered in utero, the incidence of reflux may continue to increase compared with historical studies. There is an 80% incidence of reflux on the left side in patients with unilateral reflux for no apparent reason (Hoover and Duckett, 1982).

Ultrasound imaging of the posterior urethra from the perineum has been suggested as a noninvasive way to diagnose valves (Good et al, 1996). Valve leaflets can be visualized on ultrasound examination; bladder wall thickness and posterior urethral diameter before and during voiding were increased in valve patients. Whereas this application has little to add to the newborn evaluation, it can be used to evaluate older children without catheterization.

Radionuclide Renal Scan

In addition to VCUG and renal ultrasonography, the radionuclide renal scan has become an important part of the evaluation. Mercaptoacetylglycine (MAG3) is the most useful agent for this imaging because it provides functional data and adequate imaging of both the parenchyma and collecting system. Scans provide differential renal function and some insight about drainage of the upper urinary tracts. In patients with reflux, the bladder must be emptied during the entire study with a catheter to avoid artificial enhancement of renal func-

KEY POINTS: DIAGNOSIS AND EVALUATION

- Most cases of posterior urethral valves are diagnosed on antenatal ultrasound screening.

- VCUG with urethral imaging is the key study in the diagnosis of valves.

- Evaluation of the infant's renal function often takes several days to allow maternal effects on serum chemistries to resolve.

- Urodynamics are necessary in understanding bladder function throughout life.

- Nuclear renal scans and in some cases Whitaker perfusion tests are needed in some patients to evaluate persistent hydroureteronephrosis.

tion by reflux of the isotope from the bladder. If the catheter cannot keep the bladder empty through gravity, it may be necessary to aspirate it with a syringe during the study.

Laboratory Evaluation

Initial laboratory evaluation of the newborn with valves is usually misleading because of the effects of maternal renal function mediated through the placenta. It will take at least 48 hours for the serum levels of creatinine and blood urea nitrogen to accurately represent the child's intrinsic renal function. Creatinine, blood urea nitrogen, and electrolyte

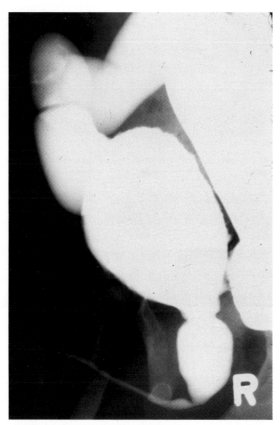

Figure 122–7. Voiding cystourethrogram reveals massive vesicoureteral reflux in an infant with posterior urethral valves.

values should be determined twice daily for the first few days of life until they plateau. Serum bicarbonate, sodium, and potassium concentrations are critical factors to monitor.

Initial Management of Posterior Urethral Valves

Bladder Drainage

Initial management of all patients with posterior urethral valves requires the immediate establishment of urinary catheter drainage from the bladder. This should be performed even if the diagnosis has not been confirmed by VCUG. Neonates can be catheterized with a 3.5 or 5 French pediatric feeding tube. Foley catheters have been used with success, but there have also been reports that the balloon causes irritation and resultant bladder spasms. The bladder may be extremely irritable, and the presence of any catheter can cause spasms so severe as to obstruct the flow of urine into the bladder (Noe and Jerkins, 1983; Jordan and Hoover, 1985). Adequate drainage must be established and documented either by irrigation of the catheter or by bladder imaging. Because it is difficult to pass the catheter over the elevated bladder neck and to avoid placing the catheter in the dilated prostatic urethra instead of the bladder, a one-shot cystogram is often advisable to aid and document proper catheter placement.

The ill newborn with posterior urethral valves is usually in the hands of the neonatal service for the management of the most threatening issues, such as pulmonary hypoplasia and renal insufficiency. It is in these areas that improvement of medical management has decreased early mortality in valve babies (Nakayama et al, 1986). These infants may require maximal ventilatory support, extracorporeal membrane oxygenation, dialysis, parenteral nutrition, control of hypertension, and a host of other care needs provided by neonatology and pediatric nephrology services (Gibbons et al, 1993).

Valve Ablation

After successful initial bladder drainage and when the patient's medical condition has stabilized, the next step is to permanently destroy the valves. In the past, destruction of valves was done by open surgery, or patients were managed with long-term suprapubic tube drainage (Gonzales et al, 1990). Both of these early therapies can lead to unacceptable complications, such as incontinence, stones, and infection (Churchill et al, 1983).

Today, a number of successful surgical techniques are available to disrupt or destroy posterior urethral valves, including hooks, balloon catheters, and valvulotomes (Deane et al, 1988; Kolicinski, 1988; Cromie et al, 1994; Chandna et al, 1996; Chertin et al, 2002). One of the more common methods uses the Whitaker hook. This instrument looks like a crochet hook and has been used successfully to cut valves either blindly or with fluoroscopic control (Whitaker and Sherwood, 1986). **New smaller pediatric cystoscopes with improved optics are favored today because of the ability to perform the procedure under direct vision.** A Bugbee electrode or a pediatric resectoscope with a hook or cold knife can be used to incise the valves (Fig. 122–8). A number of authors report use of a cystoscope and laser to disrupt valves (Ehrlich and Shanberg, 1988; Biewald and Schier, 1992; Gholdoian et al, 1998). Although most surgeons incise the valves from a retrograde position viewed through the urethra, others have found that an antegrade approach through a vesicostomy or suprapubic puncture of the bladder is helpful (Zaontz and Firlit, 1985).

Originally, surgeons attempted to completely resect the valves. This practice produced frequent complications of urethral stricture from electrosurgical and instrument damage to the urethra. Modern, appropriately sized cystoscopic equipment and limited use of electrosurgery have reduced the incidence of urethral injury to 5% (Nijman and Scholtmeyer, 1991). Today, the goal is not to remove the valves but to incise them so that they are not suspended across the urethra, obstructing urine flow. Well-placed incisions can disrupt their integrity and allow the valves to lie freely along the walls of the urethra when the child voids. The exact point of incision can vary. Some surgeons prefer the 12-o'clock position; others prefer incisions at 4- and 8-o'clock, and others all three. Although most valves are thin and do not bleed at surgery, it is sometimes preferable to leave a catheter in place for 24 hours after incision. The valve remnants resolve after incision, and there is often no evidence of them on later cystoscopic examination.

Cutaneous Vesicostomy

If the infant is too small for safe instrumentation for valve ablation, a cutaneous vesicostomy can be performed as a temporary measure (Fig. 122–9). Temporary vesicostomy

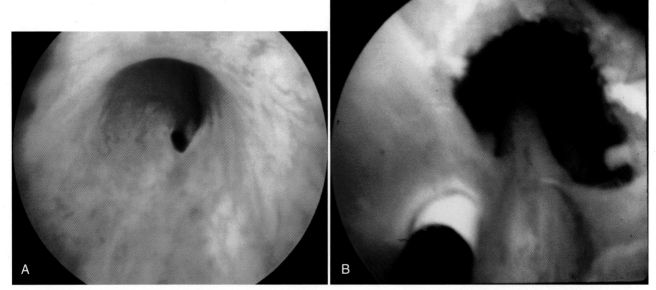

Figure 122-8. Cystoscopic photographs made from the distal urethra show the posterior urethral valves before ablation (**A**) and after ablation (**B**). The ureteral catheter has been passed through a perforation in the valve leaflet.

drainage allows the urologist to incise the valves later when the patient is older and healthier. The vesicostomy has proved to be a safe and efficient treatment, with long-term results in preserving renal function and somatic growth equal to those of primary valve ablation (Walker and Padron, 1990; Narasimhan et al, 2004). The vesicostomy provides adequate drainage of the upper tracts in more than 90% of cases (Krahn and Johnston, 1993). Vesicostomy itself is not without complication, however, and one study reported an 8.6% reoperation rate (Noe and Jerkins, 1985). There has been concern that vesicostomy would cause permanent loss of bladder volume, but this has not proved to be true, and vesicostomy does not significantly affect bladder capacity (Jayanthi et al, 1995). Some authors report that compliance may be decreased in vesicostomy bladders compared with those treated with primary ablation (Kim et al, 1996; Podesta et al, 2000). **In general, primary ablation is the preferred surgical procedure to treat posterior urethral valves and vesicostomy is reserved for very small or very ill infants. Vesicostomy remains an excellent alternative treatment in these difficult situations.**

Upper Tract Diversion

In the past, initial management of posterior urethral valves relied on upper tract diversion with ureterostomy or pyelostomy (Johnston, 1963). Diversion was effective in decompressing the upper tracts and controlling infection. Infants with high urinary diversion, however, often faced difficult urinary reconstructive problems later in life. In addition, high diversion produces stomas that present chronic management problems with incontinence. Even with these difficulties, urinary diversion provided the best management available for valve patients for many years.

With the development of new cystoscopic equipment, Johnston (1966) demonstrated that endoscopic ablation could be performed safely and with good initial results. Once the option of primary valve ablation was available, there then followed a long and thorough debate about the relative merits of initial upper tract diversion versus primary valve ablation.

Since both approaches yield good initial control of infection and adequate decompression of the upper urinary tract in most cases, the controversy focused on long-term results and measured renal function, bladder function, and somatic growth in each group. There are conflicting data about ultimate renal function and somatic growth. Krueger and associates (1980) presented data supporting ureterostomy from the large Toronto experience. They found that patients initially diverted had better eventual renal function and somatic growth. On the other hand, Reinberg, Duckett, and Hendren presented data supporting the conclusion that there is no significant difference in the long-term outcomes between the two initial treatments (Hendren, 1978; Duckett and Norris, 1989; Reinberg et al, 1992a). More study may help clarify the situation, but the current consensus is that neither initial treatment is superior in promoting renal function and somatic growth.

Despite early concerns that a bladder left without urine flow by proximal diversion would deteriorate from disuse, more recent data have shown that most of these bladders do not lose significant function. After upper tract diversion, urodynamics have shown that bladder capacity is preserved in 80% and compliance in 69% (Lome et al, 1972; Tanagho, 1974; Ghanem and Nijman, 2005). Primary valve ablation may give the best chance for optimal bladder rehabilitation because of the ability of the bladder to cycle, but temporary supravesical diversion remains a reasonable alternative in the complex valve patient and usually leads to a marginal if any decrease in long-term bladder function (Close et al, 1997; Podesta et al, 2002). In support for preservation of function in the defunc-

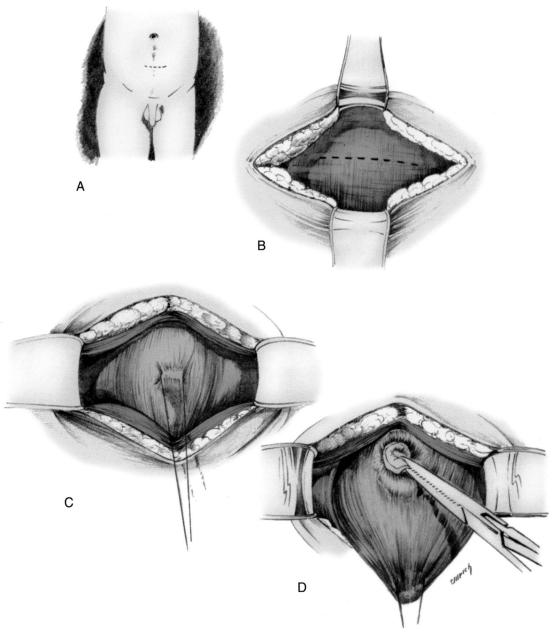

Figure 122–9. Blocksom technique for performance of cutaneous vesicostomy. **A,** After the bladder is filled, a transverse incision is made at the upper limit of the filled bladder and near the midpoint between pubis and umbilicus. **B,** A transverse incision is made in the rectus fascia. **C** and **D,** The bladder is mobilized with a stay stitch and blunt dissection to free the peritoneum away from the bladder dome.   *Continued*

tionalized bladder is a review of urodynamics in 32 valve patients that produced data showing that boys who had undergone temporary diversion actually had larger functional capacities, better compliance, and less instability than those who underwent primary valve ablation (Kim et al, 1996). The valve bladder and its problems appear to be inconsistently influenced by primary treatment, either ablation or diversion.

The current consensus is that both approaches eventually yield similar results and that infants who undergo initial upper tract diversion are at the disadvantage of needing more surgical procedures. Today, upper tract diversion is usually limited to those patients who fail to respond to bladder-level drainage. The specific clinical situation for upper tract diversion in posterior urethral valves today develops when bladder-level drainage is insufficient to prevent infection or to drain the upper tracts adequately. The decision to perform upper tract diversion relies on renal function, infection, and, to a lesser extent, degree of hydronephrosis. Kidney development and growth in early life are critical, and neonatal kidneys may potentially recover function and continue to develop during this period (Mayor et al, 1975; Hayslett, 1983). It is compelling to place these damaged kidneys in the best possible physiologic situation to recover,

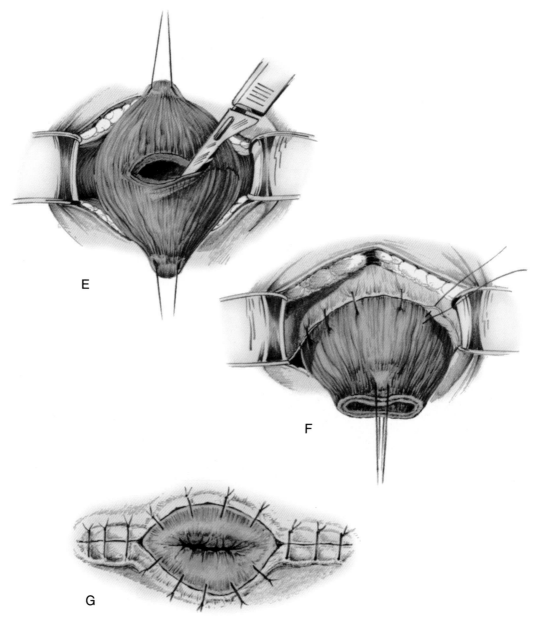

Figure 122–9, cont'd. E, A transverse incision is made into the bladder. **F,** The bladder is sewn to the rectus fascia, placing these sutures 1 cm away from the edge of the bladder incision. **G,** The bladder wall is sewn flush to the skin. (From Gonzales ED: Posterior urethral valves and other ureteral anomalies. In Walsh PC, Retik AB, Vaughan ED, Wein AJ, eds: Campbell's Urology, 8th ed. Philadelphia, WB Saunders, 2002.)

but this must be balanced with the knowledge that although upper tract diversion does initially improve renal function and drainage, there is no evidence that it offers any long-term advantage over primary ablation.

After the bladder has been adequately decompressed, the decision of whether to perform upper tract diversion is one of clinical judgment. Since hydronephrosis usually takes months to improve significantly, renal function is a better early parameter to follow. If the serum creatinine concentration drops below 2.0, it is safe to rely on improved bladder drainage for additional kidney improvement. If the creatinine concentration remains above 2.0 after 10 days of adequate bladder decompression and if hydronephrosis is unimproved, upper tract diversion may be considered. The type of diver-

sion remains the surgeon's choice, and there are proponents of high loop ureterostomy, ring ureterostomy, pyelostomy, and end ureterostomy (Sober, 1972; Williams and Cromie, 1975; Novak, 1978) (Fig. 122–10). The type of upper tract diversion I prefer is a low loop ureterostomy because it provides adequate drainage, places the stoma under the diaper, and offers the most logical and simple reconstruction later.

If upper tract diversion is performed, reconstructive surgery to internalize the urinary tract should be delayed until the bladder and upper tracts have improved as much as can be expected. My practice has been to undivert the child at the age of 2 or 3 years and to fully evaluate the bladder function before the need for transplantation. If the patient is destined to reach end-stage renal disease, reconstruction may be delayed until

KEY POINTS: MANAGEMENT OF POSTERIOR URETHRAL VALVES

- Immediate catheter drainage is the initial management in all patients thought to have valves.

- Primary valve ablation is the preferred initial surgical treatment in most patients.

- If the infant is too small or ill for endoscopic valve ablation, a vesicostomy is an excellent form of temporary diversion and provides drainage of the urinary tract.

- Initial management of hydronephrosis and reflux is valve ablation and observation with antibiotic prophylaxis.

- Bladder and renal function are often unstable in valve patients and usually change throughout life, requiring lifelong monitoring.

transplantation can be performed (Sheldon et al, 1992). On the other hand, I have found it to be advantageous to have the urinary tract fully functional long before the need for transplantation. It is imperative to establish an efficient method to empty the bladder, by either voiding or intermittent catheterization, before undiversion and transplantation.

Management of Vesicoureteral Reflux

Between 50% and 70% of patients with posterior urethral valves will have vesicoureteral reflux at the time of diagnosis (Hulbert and Duckett, 1992). Scott (1985) studied 46 affected boys with valves and found reflux in 72% of patients and in 53% of ureters. Bilateral reflux occurred in 32% of this study group.

Reflux in posterior urethral valves is considered secondary to bladder outlet obstruction so that the initial management of reflux is relief of obstruction. Reflux resolves after valve ablation in between 20% and 32% of refluxing ureters (Scott, 1985). Most reflux resolves within several months, but some can take as long as 3 years. Reflux is more likely to resolve when it is associated with a better functioning kidney. Hassan and coworkers (2003) found that reflux resolved in only 10% of kidneys with less than 20% split renal function in a series of 73 boys with valves. Children with initial bilateral reflux are more likely to have reflux resolve than are those with unilateral reflux. As for any child with vesicoureteral reflux, they must be maintained on prophylactic antibiotics to prevent infection.

If persistent high-grade reflux is a clinical problem because of urinary tract infections or incontinence, bladder function and drainage must be reviewed. Inadequate emptying and high storage pressures are the usual causes of persistent reflux (Fig. 122–11). **Surgery to repair reflux in valve patients must be undertaken with great care, and reimplantation of ureters into a valve bladder that has not been**

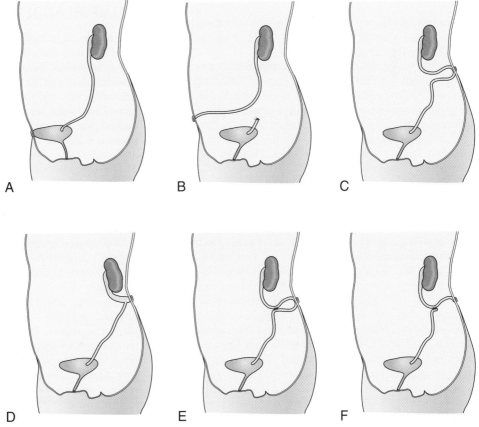

Figure 122–10. The variety of urinary tract diversions useful in posterior urethral valves. **A,** Vesicostomy. **B,** Distal ureterostomy. **C,** Proximal loop ureterostomy. **D,** Cutaneous pyelostomy. **E,** Ring ureterostomy. **F,** Sober Y ureterostomy. (From Glassberg KI, Horowitz M: Urethral valves and other anomalies of the male urethra. In Belman AB, King LR, Kramer SA, eds: Clinical Pediatric Urology, 4th ed. London, Martin Dunitz, 2002:899-945.)

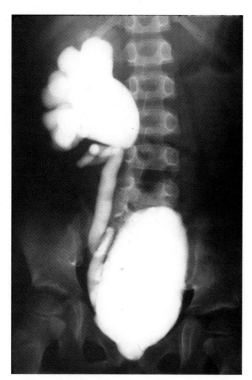

Figure 122–11. Voiding cystourethrogram shows persistent high-grade vesicoureteral reflux in a boy with posterior urethral valves. Note the large-capacity, mildly trabeculated bladder.

Management of Hydronephrosis

Almost all patients with posterior urethral valves have severe hydroureteronephrosis at diagnosis. Scott (1985) found hydronephrosis in 96.5% of valve patients, and it was bilateral in 78%. Hydronephrosis may or may not be associated with reflux. Like reflux, hydronephrosis is a secondary phenomenon in valve patients, and like reflux, it often resolves once the primary pathologic process, obstruction, is relieved. **Nonrefluxing hydronephrosis resolves in 49% of patients and may do so rapidly after valve ablation.** This leaves a significant population of valve patients with persistent hydronephrosis for years despite adequate bladder emptying (Johnston and Kulatilake, 1971). Hulbert and Duckett (1988) found that 25% of valve patients have dilated upper tracts 5 to 15 years after successful valve ablation.

The majority of patients with persistent hydronephrosis do not have obstruction at either the bladder outlet or the ureterovesical junction. Whitaker (1973) developed his antegrade perfusion test specifically to examine chronic hydronephrosis in valve patients and to document pressures within the upper urinary tract and across the ureterovesical junction. Tietjen and associates (1997) also used the Whitaker test to evaluate 25 valve patients with persistent hydronephrosis and found only 8% of patients to have an element of obstruction at the ureterovesical junction. The majority of patients with hydronephrosis had a measured mean perfusion pressure of only 3 cm H_2O (normal is less than 15 cm H_2O). The ureterovesical junction may be functionally obstructed before ablation of the valves, but this usually resolves with bladder rehabilitation (Glassberg, 1982).

VALVE BLADDER SYNDROME

The terms *valve bladder* and *full valve bladder* were coined by Mitchell to describe a chronic condition in patients with valves in which, despite successful valve ablation, intrinsic bladder dysfunction leads to deterioration of the upper urinary tracts and incontinence (Mitchell, 1982). **The combination of poor sensation, high bladder volumes, and poor compliance produces storage pressures high enough to prevent adequate drainage of the upper tracts.** These boys are comfortable with large bladder volumes at high pressures. They frequently have overflow incontinence and void infrequently and incompletely. Videourodynamics are necessary to diagnose this condition, and there is a direct correlation of abnormal urodynamics indicating poor compliance and detrusor overactivity with poor renal function (Ghanem et al, 2004). Initial management is usually timed voiding, but if this does not successfully lower pressures and empty the bladder, α blockers or clean intermittent catheterization can be used (Austin et al, 1999).

Glassberg (2001) has suggested that proactive urodynamic directed bladder management might improve long-term bladder outcome. Koff and associates (2002) also proposed that valve bladder syndrome is not a permanent state due to prenatal bladder damage but an induced condition due to a combination of polyuria, impaired bladder sensation, and residual urine volume. Bladder decompensation in response to this situation results in increasing residual urine, upper tract dilation, and renal injury. They proposed intermittent

adequately rehabilitated will lead to a high failure and complication rate (Hulbert and Duckett, 1992; Warshaw et al, 1985; El-Sherbiny et al, 2002a).

The first step in evaluation of persistent reflux is to repeat VCUG to look for persistent valve remnants. If no remnants are found, urodynamics are needed to evaluate the bladder. If the bladder function is adequate and persistent reflux remains a problem, surgery to correct reflux may be necessary. Ureteroneocystostomy is usually limited to the situation in which infections cannot be controlled and bladder function is adequate.

High-grade reflux is often associated with severe dysplasia and nonfunction in the associated kidney in valve patients. In the past, these nonfunctional kidneys and dilated collecting systems were removed early in life. **It has become evident that there is no urgency to remove these units as long as they do not lead to recurrent infection.** They are best retained until the bladder has been rehabilitated as much as possible. The dilated collecting system could possibly be used as a ureteral augmentation if bladder volume or pressure warrants (Bellinger, 1993). Ureter is the best material available for augmentation cystoplasty since it is lined with urothelium and the ureteral muscle will not contribute to high pressures from detrusor contractions (Landau et al, 1994). It is also possible to leave these nonfunctional units in place and successfully repair the reflux (Kim et al, 1997). This is a reasonable alternative when faced with the need for reimplantation surgery on the contralateral side.

catheterization with continuous nocturnal bladder emptying. They found a significant improvement of hydronephrosis in 10 boys with valves treated in this manner. Holmdahl and colleagues (2003) also studied 35 boys with valve bladder and found that intermittent catheterization not only improved glomerular filtration rate but also improved bladder compliance and capacity more than expected for age and compared with valve patients who did not catheterize.

Glassberg and associates (1982) categorized the hydronephrotic upper tracts of valve patients into three types: those that drain independent of bladder volume, those that drain efficiently only with the bladder empty, and those that are obstructed independent of bladder volume. Duckett applied this classification to 100 valve patients and found only four cases of true obstruction of the upper tracts independent of bladder dysfunction, and all had undergone ureteral reimplantation (Smith and Duckett, 1996).

Evaluation of persistent hydronephrosis in valve patients is complex and may require measurement of voided volumes to evaluate the relationship between renal tubular competence and bladder function, videourodynamics to evaluate the ability of the bladder to hold and empty adequate volumes at acceptable pressures, ultrasonography to evaluate degree of hydronephrosis, Lasix renography to evaluate relative renal function and induced drainage, and Whitaker perfusion test to measure intrarenal pressures at a given drainage rate. Access to all of these modalities is necessary to choose proper management of the valve patient with persistent hydronephrosis. Most children with persistent hydronephrosis do not need surgical therapy outside of valve ablation and attention to bladder function.

Management of Bladder Dysfunction

Posterior urethral valves affect no organ more consistently and profoundly than the bladder. The degree of damage varies considerably, and it is the rare patient who does not suffer significant lifelong bladder dysfunction. The bladder causes two types of long-term problems for the valve patient: interference with upper tract drainage and incontinence. The abnormal bladder subjects the upper tracts to a form of obstruction at two points of life, in the newborn period and late in childhood. At birth, the bladder is thick and trabeculated with saccules and diverticula. It contracts with great force, and compliance is low. Although urodynamics are difficult to perform in infants, particularly in the presence of reflux and diverticula, the bladder can be seen on imaging to undergo strong contractions. This stage of bladder dysfunction can persist for months despite successful valve ablation. Late in childhood, the bladder is less contractile but displays poor compliance, and this along with poor sensation leads to the valve bladder syndrome discussed earlier. Both the hypercontractile bladder of infancy and the rigid bladder of late childhood inhibit upper tract drainage.

Incontinence is a major problem for valve patients. A review of 100 patients revealed that 81% had delayed day and night continence at 5 years of age (Smith et al, 1996). Another large series discovered that only 53% were dry by the age of 12 years (Churchill et al, 1990). This problem improves in most by 20 years of age, but the delay in attaining continence causes painful difficulties during adolescence

(Parkhouse et al, 1988). In the past, incontinence was thought to be due to sphincter injuries and bladder neck dysfunction, but today this problem is thought to be multifactorial and due to a combination of poor bladder sensation, poor bladder compliance, detrusor instability, and polyuria. **Renal tubular damage, which progresses during childhood, leads to inability to conserve sodium and free water and can lead to nephrogenic diabetes mellitus and urine volumes up to several liters per day. These exaggerated volumes can overcome any bladder's functional ability, especially one with limited potential.**

Peters identified three urodynamic patterns in boys with valves: myogenic failure, detrusor hyperreflexia, and decreased compliance/small capacity (Peters et al, 1990). Myogenic failure usually occurs in older children and leads to overflow incontinence and incomplete bladder emptying. Management includes timed voiding, double voiding, α blockers, and intermittent catheterization. The urinary frequency and urge incontinence due to detrusor hyperreflexia are managed with anticholinergic medications. Anticholinergics may also help those patients with small, poorly compliant bladders but may not be sufficient to prevent the need for augmentation cystoplasty to provide adequate urine storage necessary for continence and upper tract drainage. Inappropriate use of anticholinergic medications may induce iatrogenic myogenic failure; therefore, they should be used only with urodynamic monitoring (Misseri et al, 2002).

Holmdahl and colleagues (1996) studied valve patients with urodynamics for many years to assess changes in bladder function. **They found that the functional patterns outlined by Peters overlap in the majority of patients and that the dominant pattern changed with age. They concluded that these patterns are stages of development.** In infants, poor compliance dominates; in older children, instability from hypercontractility is the dominant pattern; in postpubertal boys, myogenic failure becomes the norm. The valve bladder is surely one in constant transition during childhood. Urodynamics are necessary to track changes and to alter management in these patients throughout the first two decades of life (Kim et al, 1997).

Boys with valves who present later in childhood frequently have only voiding complaints and a more functional urinary tract. In a study of 70 children who presented at the average age of 7.5 years, Schober and coworkers (2004) found that ablation of valves will dramatically improve symptoms of urinary frequency and diurnal and nocturnal enuresis. Despite this improvement, most boys will continue to have a degree of hydronephrosis and some voiding difficulties.

Management of Glomerular Injury and Renal Function

The primary goal of management in posterior urethral valves is to preserve renal function and to maximize renal growth and development. Renal injury in posterior urethral valves includes two initial glomerular insults: dysplasia and obstructive uropathy. Dysplasia is by far the most important since it is irreversible and not only produces a level of renal insufficiency at diagnosis but also limits future growth and development of the kidney. Obstructive uropathy may produce ongoing injury and is potentially reversible. It is mandatory to provide low-pressure storage and drainage of urine to prevent further renal damage.

Other threats to glomerular function come from persistent or progressive obstruction and infection. Hyperfiltration has been recognized in animal models as a cause of additional injury, but its importance in humans remains undocumented (Brenner et al, 1982). As somatic growth makes additional demands on the kidneys, valve patients can experience proteinuria, hypertension, and progressive loss of renal function (Tejani et al, 1986; Burbige and Hensle, 1987; Parkhouse et al, 1988; Farnham et al, 2005). Poorly controlled hypertension also can add to renal deterioration. Consistent and regular urologic care with monitoring of bladder function and infection will place the kidneys in the best position to grow and develop to their full potential.

ANTENATAL DIAGNOSIS AND MANAGEMENT

The incidence of urologic anomalies detected on ultrasonography may be as high as 1 in 200 fetuses (Dillon and Ryall, 1998). The most common cause of bilateral hydronephrosis in male fetuses is posterior urethral valves. **Most valve patients are diagnosed by prenatal ultrasonography, and the ability to image the fetus continues to improve with the technology of ultrasound.** The accuracy of ultrasound diagnosis is proportional to fetal age, and valves may be missed in scans done before 24 weeks of gestation (Skolder et al, 1988; Abbott et al, 1998). The differential diagnosis of a male fetus with bilateral hydroureteronephrosis and a distended bladder includes prune-belly syndrome and severe reflux. Bladder wall thickness is impressively increased only with valves. Fetal urine parameters may also be useful in predicting renal damage in utero. **Aspirated fetal bladder urine with high sodium content and isosthenuria compared with serum values suggests poor renal function and that fetal intervention would not be helpful from a renal standpoint** (Glick et al, 1985).

Valves have emerged as the only urologic anomaly to be considered for antenatal intervention. Fetal intervention, although championed in the 1980s, has become rare because of a lack of objective evidence that it alters renal development (Reinberg et al, 1992b; Freedman et al, 1999). Whereas antenatal decompression of the urinary tract and the subsequent restoration of amniotic fluid are usually accomplished by placement of a vesicoamniotic shunt, there have also been reports of fetal valve ablation (Quintero et al, 1995) (Fig. 122–12).

Restoration of the volume of amniotic fluid can be a lifesaving maneuver because of its effect on pulmonary function (Harrison et al, 1982). For optimal results, this intervention must be performed during the appropriate stage of pulmonary development, later than 20 weeks and before 32 weeks. Oligohydramnios earlier than 20 weeks is usually incompatible with life because of pulmonary hypoplasia; and if it is diagnosed later than 32 weeks, early delivery is preferable to fetal intervention. The decision to undertake fetal intervention must weigh the potential benefit for the fetus against the risk of complications to both fetus and mother that

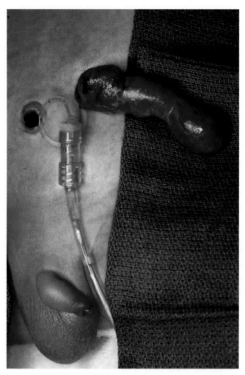

Figure 122–12. This boy had a vesicoamniotic shunt placed at 18 weeks of gestational age. The shunt has been attached to a drainage bag in the intensive care unit. The structure extending from the shunt site is herniated omentum. There is a significant risk of abdominal wall hernia at the shunt site.

occurred in 44% of those cases reviewed by the International Fetal Surgery Registry (Elder et al, 1987).

PROGNOSTIC INDICATORS OF RENAL FUNCTION

There are four basic predictors of renal function in patients with posterior urethral valves: ultrasound appearance, serum chemistries, age at diagnosis, and presence of reflux. Ultrasound appearance, age at diagnosis, and presence of reflux can be determined at diagnosis, but serum chemistries require some time to develop.

Ultrasound appearance is a method of estimating the amount of dysplasia present in the kidneys. Dysplasia, strictly speaking, is a histologic diagnosis of tissue disorganization and includes fibrosis and cysts. This disorganization appears more echogenic on ultrasound examination and may be obvious by comparing the kidney to the liver and spleen as controls (Sanders et al, 1988). Kidneys that are considerably brighter than the liver usually contain significant dysplasia. Loss of the normal corticomedullary junction normally visible on ultrasound examination has also been correlated with poor long-term renal function (Hulbert et al, 1992).

Age at diagnosis may be helpful in predicting prognosis. In the past, infants who presented before 1 year of age had a worse prognosis than those who presented later in life. Older boys usually present with voiding difficulty and were long considered to represent the least affected of valve patients, but recent evidence has shown that some suffer significant renal damage (Pieretti, 1993; El-Sherbiny et al, 2002b). One study of boys who presented after 5 years of age revealed that 35% had renal insufficiency and 10% reached end-stage renal disease (Bomalaski et al, 1999). In a review of 70 boys who presented at the mean age of 7.5 years, Schober and colleagues (2004) found that all had a normal serum creatinine concentration.

Today, with most infants diagnosed antenatally and having improved prenatal care, mortality of newborns with valves has decreased from almost 50% to between 3% and 10% (Williams, 1954; Churchill et al, 1990). Despite this improvement in mortality, the long-term outcome in terms of renal function has not been improved. Even early prenatal diagnosis has not led to improved renal function. This probably relates to the timing of the renal damage and that it occurs before our ability to diagnose the problem.

Reflux in valve patients carries a poor prognosis. Johnston (1979) reviewed a series of valve patients in which the mortality was 57% in patients with bilateral reflux, 17% with unilateral reflux, and 9% with no reflux. Many other authors have noted the grave effect of bilateral reflux on patients with posterior urethral valves (Parkhouse et al, 1988; Churchill et al, 1989). The commonly accepted explanation is that the incompetent ureterovesical junction that allows free reflux into the kidney also transmits the high pressures generated by the bladder. On the other hand, Stephens and others believe that severe reflux is associated with dysplasia primarily because the ureteric bud is abnormal and in turn induces an abnormal kidney.

The final prognostic factor is based on serum chemistries and relies on serial measurements of renal performance over time. Warshaw and associates (1985) reported that a nadir creatinine of 0.8 mg/dL or less during the first year of life is a good predictor of long-term renal function. Conner and Burbige (1990) found the same relationship with a nadir creatinine level of 1.0 mg/dL during the first year of life. Early renal function may be a helpful predictor as well. Denes and coworkers (1997) described 32 patients with posterior urethral valves treated with immediate drainage. Serum creatinine concentration was measured at diagnosis, after 4 days of drainage, and in the first year of life. After a mean of 10 years, the authors found that patients fell into two groups, one with a glomerular filtration rate of more than 70 mL/1.73 m^2, and the other with a glomerular filtration rate of less than 70 mL/1.73 m^2. The group with worse long-term function had initial creatinine concentration of 3.6 mg/dL, post-drainage creatinine concentration of 2.4, and 1-year nadir of 1.7. The group with better long-term renal function had initial creatinine concentration of 1.3 mg/dL, post-drainage creatinine concentration of 0.6, and 1-year nadir of 0.4. The most powerful tools yet proposed in predicting outcomes in posterior urethral valves may lie at the genetic or molecular level (Woolf et al, 2004).

TRANSPLANTATION IN VALVE PATIENTS

Obstructive uropathy is the most common cause of end-stage renal disease in children and accounts for 16.3% of children presenting for transplantation (Seikaly et al, 2001). **The most common condition producing this degree of dysfunction is posterior urethral valves.** Up to 50% of boys with posterior urethral valves will reach end-stage renal disease in their lifetime. Most of these will need dialysis or transplantation during the first two decades of life. Since renal transplantation allows a better quality of life and optimal somatic growth, it is the preferred method of managing end-stage renal disease in children and adolescents. The damaged bladder of valve patients presents a technical challenge for renal transplantation, and abnormal bladder function has been considered a threat to the success of transplantation.

Early transplant series in children with valves demonstrated significantly decreased success in transplant graft survival and in graft function compared with those who suffered end-stage renal disease due to reflux nephropathy (Churchill et al, 1988; Reinberg et al, 1988). The principal cause of graft failure was chronic rejection, and the relationship between bladder function and rejection was not apparent. Valve patients are known to have decreased bladder compliance and increased storage pressures, but in the absence of obstructive hydronephrosis or infection, these factors can be managed successfully to protect the kidney.

More recent data have shown improved results; some series demonstrated good graft survival but a statistically significant increase in serum creatinine levels compared with controls (Bryant et al, 1991; Salomon, 1997). Still others have found no significant difference between valve patients and others in either graft survival or renal function (Groenewegen et al, 1993; Ross et al, 1994; DeFoor et al, 2003; Mendizabal et al, 2005). Since the lower urinary tract is markedly abnormal in valve patients, it is not surprising that urologic complications are higher than in patients with normal bladders. Urethral strictures, stones, and urinary retention were among the urologic complications that occurred in 19% of valve patients undergoing transplantation (Ross et al, 1994). Mochon and coworkers (1992) found an increased risk of urinary tract infection in valve patients compared with others after transplantation, but this relationship may have been present before transplantation, and it did not affect graft function.

It is safe to say that renal transplantation is an important part of management of some valve patients and that success rates are high. It must be undertaken with the knowledge that urinary tract management may be more complex and complications more common than with other children undergoing transplantation. Careful urodynamic evaluation of bladder function before transplantation is vital, and the patient may need intermittent catheterization or augmentation cystoplasty to function safely with the new kidney (Zaragoza et al, 1993; Indudhara et al, 1998; Koo et al, 1999; Salomon et al, 2000; Mendizabal et al, 2005).

ANTERIOR URETHRAL VALVES

Anterior urethral obstruction is rare compared with posterior urethral valves. Although these obstructive structures may be called valves, they often occur in the form of a diverticulum of the urethra, with one wall acting as an obstructive "valve" (Tank, 1987) (Fig. 122–13). There are also some reported cases of urethral flaps or valves in the anterior urethra (DeCastro et al, 1987; Scherz et al, 1987). The first case was reported in 1906, and the total number in the literature is small (Watts, 1906; Williams and Retik, 1969; Firlit et al, 1978).

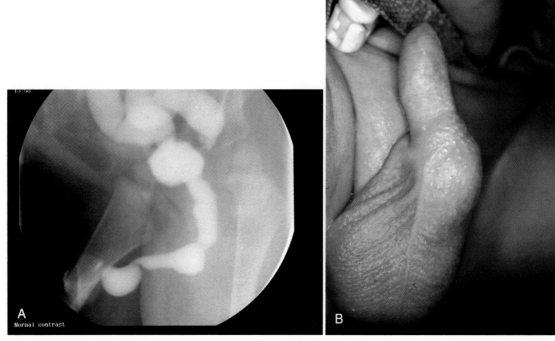

Figure 122–13. A, Voiding cystourethrogram shows a severe case of anterior urethral valves. The bladder is almost empty, and there is massive reflux. The valve is in the form of a diverticulum. **B,** The filled diverticulum can sometimes be seen as a mass on the penis that resolves between voids. Pressing on the mass may express urine for some time after voiding.

Anterior urethral diverticula typically occur where there is a defect of the corpus spongiosum, leaving a thin-walled urethra. This segment of urethra balloons during voiding and causes a mass that is sometimes visible along the ventral wall of the penis. The mass resolves as urine drains from it between voids; when it is full, urine can be expressed from the diverticulum by applying pressure (Fig. 122–14). The distal edge of the diverticulum forms a flap that obstructs the flow of urine, and the effects of anterior urethral valves can be as damaging to the urinary tract as those of the posterior urethra. The embryology of these structures remains unclear, but they seem to be unrelated to the development of posterior urethral valves.

Boys with anterior urethral valves often present later in childhood with infection, straining to void, or incontinence. One third present with voiding symptoms, a third with antenatal hydronephrosis, and the remainder with a visible diverticulum (Van Savage et al, 1997). The degree of obstruction can be severe and produce pressures as high as with posterior urethral valves. Spontaneous rupture of the fetal bladder in anterior urethral valves has been reported (Merrot et al, 2003).

Diagnosis depends on VCUG or cystoscopy. It may be difficult to pass a catheter into the bladder because the catheter often easily enters the diverticulum and becomes trapped. **Treatment is similar to that of posterior urethral valves in that relief of obstruction is the most important goal.** In severely ill children or young infants, a vesicostomy is a good option for temporary drainage, allowing the urinary tract to decompress and delaying urethral repair until conditions are optimal (Rushton et al, 1987).

Treatment of anterior urethral valves may include transurethral incision to allow free flow of urine or open urethral reconstruction. If the diverticulum is small or there is a urethral flap, transurethral incision is preferred; but if the diverticulum is large, it will usually cause pooling of urine and repeated infection. The best option is an open excision of diverticulum and repair of the urethra. This can be difficult surgery and requires catheter drainage to facilitate urethral healing.

The long-term outcomes of anterior urethral obstruction are similar to those of the posterior urethra. In general, the severity of obstruction, degree of hydronephrosis, and incidence of renal failure are usually better in anterior urethral valves. Less than 5% of patients with anterior urethral valves have reached end-stage renal disease compared with more than 30% of those with posterior urethral valves (Kaplan and Scherz, 1992).

CONGENITAL URETHRAL STRICTURE

Congenital urethral strictures are rare anomalies that produce the same pathologic and clinical problems as posterior urethral valves (Currarino and Stephens, 1981). They occur in the posterior urethra and lead to oligohydramnios, bilateral hydroureteronephrosis, and distended bladder (Narborough et al, 1990) (Fig. 122–15). Initial treatment in the newborn is almost always vesicostomy. Since these strictures are usually too long to be incised and too tight to be dilated with sounds, they may be dilated gradually with increasingly larger catheters with good results (Passerini-Glazel et al, 1988).

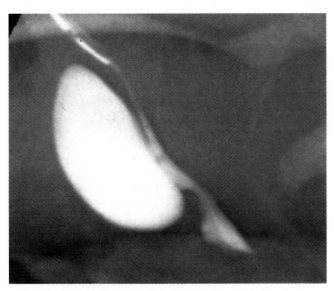

Figure 122–14. Voiding cystourethrogram demonstrates an anterior urethral diverticulum trapping urine during voiding.

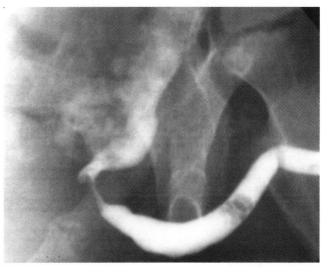

Figure 122–15. Voiding cystourethrogram shows a congenital urethral stricture. These rare conditions cause a clinical situation similar to posterior urethral valves.

URETHRAL POLYPS

Urethral polyps are rare anomalies of the male urethra. Patients with urethral polyps usually present with intermittent voiding complaints such as hematuria, stranguria, and dysuria (Raviv et al, 1993; Walsh et al, 1993). Unlike urethral valves, polyps do not produce extensive damage to the urinary tract. They usually occur in the prostatic urethra near the bladder neck and may be mobile on a long stalk. Anterior urethral polyps have been reported (Coleburn and Hensle, 1991).

The polyps are usually diagnosed on VCUG, and the diagnosis is confirmed by cystoscopy (Fig. 122–16). They are benign but may be confused with rhabdomyosarcoma of the prostate. Benign urethral polyps are usually solitary; the polypoid form of rhabdomyosarcoma usually presents with multiple polyps and a mass extending beyond the bladder or prostate. Transurethral resection is curative in urethral polyps (Gleason and Kramer, 1994).

URETHRAL DUPLICATION

Duplication of the urethra is a rare anomaly. There are a variety of types and several classification systems (Effmann et al, 1976; Woodhouse and Williams, 1979) (Fig. 122–17). In practice, urethral duplications are so rare that they are usually described by anatomic landmarks. Most occur in the same sagittal plane, and these can be divided into either dorsal or ventral. Some more rare duplications occur in the same horizontal plane and the urethras lie next to one another, one left and one right. This horizontal type may be associated with duplicated phallus or complete bladder duplication (Woodhouse and Williams, 1979). Some patients present with incontinence or infection, but most are discovered in infancy on examination by the mother or pediatrician.

Dorsal urethral duplication occurs when there is a normal urinary meatus, dorsal chordee of the penis, and a second epispadiac meatus along the dorsal aspect of the

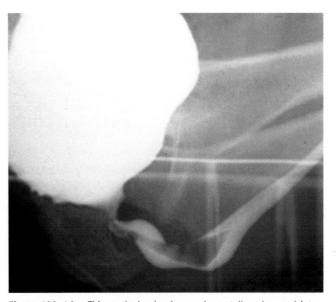

Figure 122–16. This urethral polyp is on a long stalk and caused intermittent dysuria and straining to void.

penis (Fig. 122–18). The foreskin may be incomplete dorsally, and the epispadiac meatus can occur anywhere along the midline of the penis (Sharma et al, 1987). **The normal urethra is the ventral one that ends on the glans.** The epispadiac duplicate urethra may be blind ending or extend to the bladder (Fig. 122–19). If it communicates with the bladder, the patient may be incontinent. These patients may have a widened symphysis pubis similar to epispadias or exstrophy.

Ventral urethral duplications are extremely rare, and they may also be complete or incomplete with a blind-ending urethra. There may be a normally placed urethra on the glans and a second along the ventral aspect of the penis or even along the perineum. The dorsal urethra may be of normal

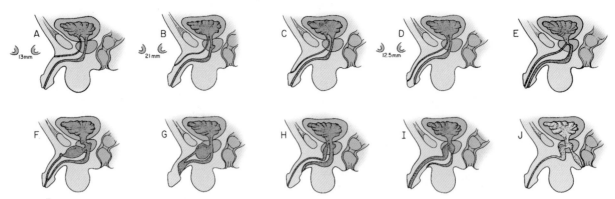

Figure 122–17. Variations of urethral duplications in the sagittal plane. Each of these drawings shows the ventral urethra as the functional one as it passes through the prostate and sphincter. (From Colodny A: Urethral lesions in infants and children. In Gillenwater JT, Howards SS, Duckett JW, eds: Adult and Pediatric Urology, 2nd ed. St. Louis, Mosby–Year Book, 1991:2013.)

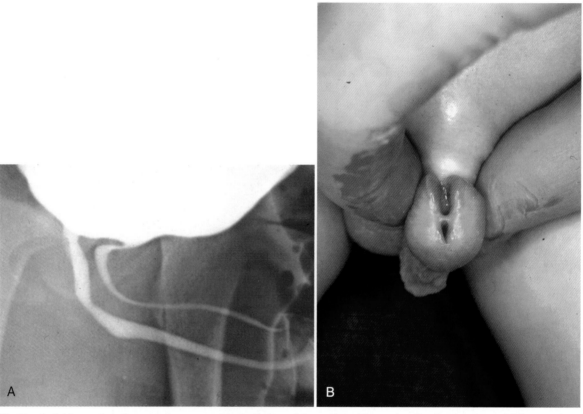

Figure 122–18. **A,** Voiding cystourethrogram shows a complete duplication of the urethra with an epispadiac dorsal segment. **B,** The ventral urethra is in the center of the glans and the dorsal urethra ends in the dorsal glans cleft in an epispadiac location.

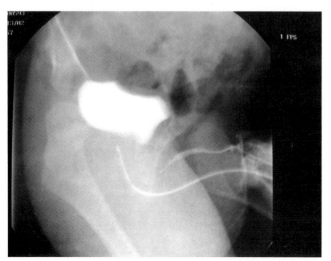

Figure 122–19. This urethral duplication has a blind-ending dorsal segment that ends under the pubis.

caliber or narrow. The ventral urethra is considered the more normal because it usually passes out of the bladder neck and sphincter (Salle et al, 2000). The Y duplication occurs when the prostatic urethra splits into two channels with one extending to the glans and the more functional ventral one coursing to the perineum near the rectum.

Diagnosis of urethral duplication depends on the type of anomaly. If the duplication is complete, VCUG will demonstrate both urethras during voiding (Hoekstra and Jones, 1985). If the duplication is blind ending, a retrograde injection of contrast material and cystoscopy may be required to delineate the anatomy (Podesta et al, 1998).

Management of urethral duplication varies with symptoms and the severity of the anomaly. Some patients do not require treatment if they are free from infection and incontinence. Simple accessory duplicate urethras may be fulgurated with a Bugbee electrode and allowed to scar and close (Holst and Peterson, 1988). Others need to be excised to make the patient dry and to prevent infection. If both urethras are functional and end adjacent to one another on the glans, the septum between the two can be excised at the meatus, giving the patient a single urinary meatus. The most complex Y fistulas may require extensive urethroplasties with tissue transfer, such as buccal mucosa grafts (Ortolano and Nasrallah, 1986).

SUGGESTED READINGS

Churchill BM, McLorie GA, Khoury AE, et al: Emergency treatment and long-term follow-up of posterior urethral valves. Urol Clin North Am 1990;17:343.

Close CE, Carr MC, Burns MW, Mitchell ME: Lower urinary tract changes after early valve ablation in neonates and infants: Is early diversion warranted? J Urol 1997;157:984.

Dinneen MD, Duffy PG: Posterior urethral valves. Br J Urol 1996;78:275.

Freedman AL, Johnson MP, Smith CA, et al: Long-term outcome in children after antenatal intervention for obstructive uropathies. Lancet 1999; 354:374.

Ghanem MA, Wolffenbuttel KP, De Vylder A, et al: Long-term bladder dysfunction and renal function in boys with posterior urethral valves based on urodynamic findings. J Urol 2004;171:2409.

Hassan JM, Pope JC, Brock JW, et al: Vesicoureteral reflux in patients with posterior urethral valves. J Urol 2003;170:1677.

Holmdahl G, Sillen U, Hanson E, et al: Bladder dysfunction in boys with posterior urethral valves before and after puberty. J Urol 1996;155:694.

Indudhara R, Joseph DB, Perez LM, Diethelm AG: Renal transplantation in children with posterior urethral valve revisited: A 10-year follow-up. J Urol 1998;160:1201.

Narasimhan KL, Kaur B, Chowdhary SK, et al: Does mode of treatment affect the outcome of neonatal posterior urethral valves? J Urol 2004;171:2423.

Young HH, Frontz WA, Baldwin JC: Congenital obstruction of the posterior urethra. J Urol 1919;3:289.

Voiding Dysfunction in Children: Non-Neurogenic and Neurogenic

C. K. YEUNG, MD • JENNIFER D. Y. SIHOE, MD • STUART B. BAUER, MD

Non-Neuropathic Dysfunction of Lower Urinary Tract

C. K. YEUNG, MD • JENNIFER D. Y. SIHOE, MD

Our increasing understanding and recognition of non-neurogenic lower urinary tract dysfunction as a cause of various urologic disorders in childhood has had a profound influence on our management strategies over the past decade. What was known as primary or idiopathic, such as primary vesicoureteric reflux or primary nocturnal enuresis, is often associated with underlying bladder dysfunctions evident on urodynamics and resolves with successful correction of the bladder physiology (Koff and Murtagh, 1983; Homsy et al, 1985; Watanabe et al, 1994; Yeung et al, 1998, 1999). Conversely, failure of recognition and treatment of the associated problem can result in persistence or even further deterioration.

The understanding of the spectrum of dysfunction of the bladder and even of normal bladder physiology in infants and young children is complex. Not only are the dynamics and functional disturbances of the lower urinary tract very different from those in adults, but the evolution in normal bladder-sphincteric function during growth and maturation in children poses continuous changes (Yeung, 1995; Yeung et al, 1995a; Sillen et al, 1996; Holmdahl, 1997). More confusingly, one type of bladder dysfunction may often progress with time and evolve imperceptibly into another, without a sharp distinction between the different stages. This is further confounded by a lack of age- and sex-specific normal reference values for various urodynamic parameters, especially for the very young age groups (Yeung et al, 1995a).

Recent advances and development in the use of urodynamic techniques specially designed for infants and young children have allowed more accurate assessment of bladder function and provided much better understanding of bladder pathophysiology. This has allowed for better recognition of functional disorders as well as to provide a scientific basis for their therapy (Hjalmas, 1988; Perez et al, 1992; Bauer, 1997; Nørgaard et al, 1998). In view of the important association of bladder dysfunctions with various common urologic disorders, urologists should be acquainted with the spectrum of dysfunction and the techniques to facilitate proper diagnosis and treatment.

NORMAL BLADDER FUNCTION IN INFANTS AND CHILDREN
Anatomy and Innervation of Bladder

The bladder is a very unique organ of the human body in that not only does it carry a dual function of both storage and emptying of urine but has a complex innervation of voluntary and involuntary control of function. Understanding of the functional anatomy of the lower urinary tract stems from extensive postmortem studies carried out over decades (Gosling et al, 1981; Gosling, 1985; DeLancey, 1988; de Groat, 1993; Zvara et al, 1994.)

The bladder is an abdominal organ and, when full, can be readily palpable in infants and young children due to a shallow pelvis (Wiegel, 1990). The bladder wall consists of three layers: mucosa, detrusor, and adventitia. **The detrusor consists of a meshwork of smooth muscle fibers arranged into a single functioning unit with an ability to elicit nearly maximal active tension over a wide range of length.** This allows the bladder to fill with urine from the upper tract at low pressures (compliance) (Mattiasson, 1994). The ability of the bladder to store urine (reservoir function) is determined by the concomitant activity of the detrusor muscle and the bladder outlet (consisting of the bladder neck, proximal urethra, and striated muscle of the pelvic floor) (de Groat, 1993).

The bladder sphincter (external and internal) plays a major role in urinary continence by closure of the bladder neck and proximal urethra. The anatomy of the external urinary sphincter consists of a cylindrical structure, which is accentuated anteriorly and thinned out or actually absent posteriorly, thus giving a characteristic horseshoe or omega shape on cross section. It has an inner layer of smooth and an outer layer of striated muscle, extending from the apex of the prostate to invest the length of the membranous urethra in males. In the females this is less well developed and extends from the bladder neck to the mid urethra. The internal sphincter, however, has not been well delineated anatomically. It has generally been accepted that it consists of smooth muscle fibers continuing from the bladder base and trigone that traverse inferiorly through the bladder neck to extend toward the proximal urethra. Its existence has been better delineated on radiologic and urethral pressure measurement studies. During micturition, the bladder base, bladder neck, and proximal urethra can be shown to contract simultaneously as a unit, producing a funneling effect that opens up the bladder outlet with initiation of voiding.

Little, too, is known about the natural course of development or maturation of the structure as well as function of the sphincter mechanism. **Literature suggests that immature detrusor-sphincter coordination, manifested as detrusor hypercontractility and interrupted voiding, commonly occurs in the first 1 to 2 years of life causing some degree of** **functional bladder outflow obstruction** (Sillen et al, 1992; Yeung et al, 1998). In a postmortem study of the ontogeny of the external urinary sphincter in human fetuses, infants, and young children, Kokoua and colleagues (1992) found significant age-related differences in the histologic structure of the sphincter as compared with that in adults. Striated muscle fibers of the sphincter first appeared at around 20 weeks of gestation, then became arranged in a concentric pattern as a closed ring, fused posteriorly to form a tail-like structure that was directed to the perineal body. Posterior splitting of the striated sphincter, starting first caudally and progressively in a cephalad manner then occurred during the first year of life, coinciding in parallel with gradual resorption of the "tail," to eventually giving way to a mature omega-shaped structure. Because a complete closed ring of striated sphincteric muscle was present up to 1 year of age in over 40% of cases, it may well be conjectured that this could be related to the high intravesical pressures and interrupted voiding that are commonly observed during urodynamic studies in infants (Sillen et al, 1992; Yeung et al, 1995a, 1998).

Activation, coordination, and integration of various parts of the bladder-sphincteric complex involves both the central somatic and autonomic nervous systems through three sets of peripheral nerves: sacral parasympathetic (pelvic nerve), thoracolumbar sympathetic (hypogastric nerves and sympathetic chain), and sacral somatic nerves (primarily the pudendal nerve) (de Groat, 1993; Mattiasson, 1994) (Fig. 123–1).

Parasympathetic nerve fibers run in the pelvic nerve (S2 to S4) to supply the pelvic and vesical plexuses before entering the bladder. Parasympathetic ganglia are found within these plexuses and in the bladder wall. Sympathetic nerves arise from segments T10 to L2 of the spinal cord and go to the inferior mesenteric ganglion through the sympathetic trunk. From the inferior mesenteric ganglion the nerve fibers pass to the pelvic plexus and bladder through the hypogastric nerves. There is also sympathetic innervation originating from T10 to L2 supplying the detrusor and urethral sphincter (Bradley et al, 1974). The somatic nervous system (pudendal nerve) supplies the periurethral pelvic floor musculature (Mattiasson, 1994). The sensory and motor nerves carried by all three nerves innervate both the bladder and urethral sphincter. They originate from parasympathetic ganglia located in the second, third, and fourth segments of the sacral spinal cord (Bradley et al, 1974). Within the spinal cord, information from bladder afferents is integrated with that from other viscera and somatic sources and projected to the brain stem centers that coordinate the micturition cycle (Harrison and Abrams, 1994).

Development of Normal Bladder Function and Micturition Control

Urodynamic studies on normal infant bladders have shown that bladder function in young children is very different from that in adults. During the first 2 to 3 years of life there is progressive development from an initially indiscriminate infantile voiding pattern to a more socially conscious and voluntary or adult type of micturition. This is achieved through an active learning process whereby the child acquires the ability to voluntarily inhibit or initiate voiding at socially convenient times.

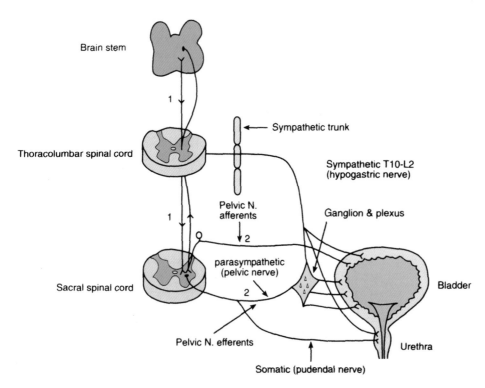

Figure 123–1. Diagram to illustrate the innervation of the bladder-sphincter complex. (From Yeung CK: Pathophysiology of bladder dysfunction. In Gearhart JP, Rink RC, Mouriquand PDE [eds]: Pediatric Urology. Philadelphia, WB Saunders, 2001.)

This natural evolution of bladder control entails an intact nervous system and depends on at least three main events occurring in parallel: **(1) a progressive increase in bladder functional storage capacity; (2) maturation of voluntary control over the urethral striated muscle sphincter; and, perhaps most importantly, (3) development of direct volitional control over the bladder-sphincteric unit so that the child can voluntarily initiate or inhibit the micturition reflex.** This process can also be influenced by an awareness of the accepted social norms in families during toilet training (Yeung, 2001).

Change in Bladder Functional Parameters

Voiding Frequency. During the third trimester of pregnancy, the fetus is voiding at the rate of approximately 30 times every 24 hours (Goellner et al, 1981). However, immediately after birth, this drops dramatically for the first few days of life only to increase again after the first week to reach a peak by weeks 2 to 4 to an average of once per hour. Subsequently this rate declines again to 10 to 15 times per day between 6 and 12 months and to 8 to 10 times per day by 2 to 3 years (Goellner et al, 1981; Yeung, 1995; Holmdahl et al, 1996). This **reduction in voiding frequency observed during the first few years of life** appears to be related mainly to an increase in bladder capacity in parallel to body growth, which is proportionately greater than simultaneous increase in urine volume production (Yeates, 1973; Koff, 1997). By the age of 12, the voiding pattern is very similar to that in an adult and usually comprises 4 to 6 voids per day (Fig. 123–2).

Bladder Capacity, Voided Volume, and Emptying Efficiency. The increase in bladder capacity with the growth of the child is a crucial step in the development of bladder function and urinary continence. **An adequate reservoir function for urine storage is necessary to meet the increased rate of**

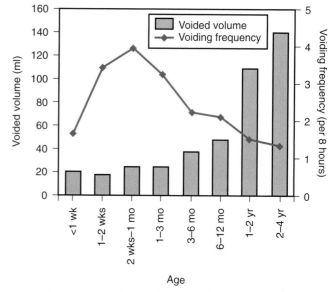

Figure 123–2. Changes in voided volume and micturition frequency from neonates to early infancy.

urine production and decreased voiding frequency in the growing child.

Several studies have shown that functional bladder capacity at a certain age can be accurately estimated and expressed as a function of age with no difference in sex. For young infants it can be expressed as follows (Holmdahl et al, 1996):

$$\text{Bladder capacity (mL)} = 38 + 2.5 \times \text{Age (mo)}$$

For older children, the most widely accepted formula includes Koff's formula (Koff, 1983):

$$\text{Bladder capacity (mL)} = [\text{Age (yr)} + 2] \times 30$$

Or similarly, Hjalmas' formula (1988):

$$\text{Bladder capacity (mL)} = 30 + [\text{Age (yr)} \times 30]$$

In parallel to the increase in bladder capacity, **the mean voided volume of each micturition increases with age.** Of note, urodynamic studies have shown that a significant proportion of infants with incomplete maturation of detrusor-sphincter coordination before the age of 1 are still able to achieve satisfactory bladder emptying (over 80% efficacy) (Yeung, 1995, 1998; Yeung et al, 1995a; Holmdahl et al, 1996; Bachelard et al, 1999; Sillen et al, 2000).

Detrusor Pressure at Voiding. There are limited studies on detrusor pressures at voiding in normal infants due to the technical difficulties involved in performing urodynamic studies in young infants and an ethical consideration in justifying doing so. From the data we have in a natural filling cystometric study of infants with normal lower urinary tracts (as indicated by a normal micturating cystourethrogram) and who had undergone either dismembered pyeloplasty for pelviureteric junction obstruction or nephrectomy for dysplastic kidney, we have documented **significantly higher maximum detrusor pressures with micturition (Pdetmax) than in normal adults.** It was also noted that male infants voided with significantly higher pressures than females (mean Pdetmax: 118 vs. 75 cm H_2O, respectively, $P < .03$) (Yeung et al, 1995a, 1995b, 1998). Similar findings were reported in healthy, asymptomatic infant siblings of children with vesicoureteric reflux (Bachelard et al, 1999).

Studies have also shown that these high detrusor pressures noted during micturition were mainly observed only during the first year of life and decreased progressively with age. Furthermore, an interrupted or "staccato" type of urinary stream was noted in over half of the patients (Yeung et al, 1995a, 1995b, 1998). This was demonstrated by fluctuations of the detrusor pressure when it reached maximum during voiding and resumption of urinary stream in conjunction with a sharp fall in the detrusor pressure. The high detrusor pressures during voiding are thought to represent variations between individual infants in the maturation process of detrusor and sphincter coordination during the first 1 to 2 years of life (Yeung et al, 1995a, 1998; Holmdahl et al, 1996; Bachelard et al, 1999; Sillen et al, 2000).

We have further confirmed this finding using video-cystometry under fluoroscopy combined with natural-fill urodynamics and perineal electromyography (EMG) in infants with history of urinary tract infections (UTIs). Periods of increase in perineal or sphincteric EMG activities were noted during voiding and associated with a sudden cessation of urinary flow with a simultaneous isometric rise or high peak of detrusor pressure. In contrast, resumption of urinary flow was associated with relaxation of the external urinary sphincter and a paradoxical drop in detrusor pressure. Also, the detrusor pressure associated with the initiation of urinary flow was usually significantly lower than the maximal detrusor pressure during micturition (Pdetmax) and the Pdetmax was significantly higher than those recorded in normal adults (Fig. 123–3).

Evolution of Normal Micturition Control

Traditionally, it has been assumed that micturition in newborns and young infants occurs automatically with a full

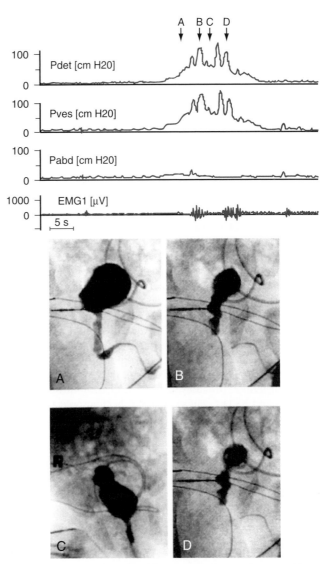

Figure 123–3. Interrupted voiding pattern due to detrusor-sphincter dyscoordination as revealed by urodynamic study with simultaneous perineal electromyographic (EMG) monitoring and videocystourethrography. *Arrows with letters in top graph* correspond to urethrograms at bottom. **A,** Urinary flow started. **B,** Premature sphincteric contraction and urethral closure as evidenced by the urethrogram and increase in sphincteric EMG activities, leading to a sharp spike of detrusor pressure (isometric increase) associated with a paradoxical abrupt cessation of urinary flow. **C,** Urinary flow resumed in parallel with sphincter relaxation. **D,** Repeated sphincteric contraction leading to another sharp increase in detrusor pressure and paradoxical interruption of urinary flow. P abd, abdominal pressure; P det, detrusor pressure; P ves, intravesical pressure. (From Yeung CK: Pathophysiology of bladder dysfunction. In Gearhart JP, Rink RC, Mouriquand PDE [eds]: Pediatric Urology. Philadelphia, WB Saunders, 2001.)

bladder by a simple spinal cord reflex, with little or no mediation by the higher neural centers and that, with progressive maturation, voluntary inhibition of the bladder emptying reflex is achieved by adulthood. A delay in the normal maturation of bladder control was attributed to certain conditions such as primary nocturnal enuresis and hence the traditional belief that all enuretics would get better with age. However, more recent studies have indicated that this is an oversimplification of what actually occurs. **Even in full-term** fetuses and newborns, it has been shown that micturition is modulated by higher centers. Ohel and colleagues (1995) showed that intrauterine micturition almost exclusively occurs while the fetus is awake rather than randomly distributed over various behavioral (sleep/arousal) states. Furthermore, it has been observed that micturition in a full-term fetus can be elicited by vibroacoustic stimulation, all of which indicates that the micturition reflex is probably under higher neural control even at near gestational term (Zimmer et al, 1993). Further extensive modulation occurs during the postnatal period.

Studies on normal neonates using ambulatory bladder monitoring techniques in conjunction with polysomnographic recordings have shown that even in newborns, micturition does not occur during sleep (Yeung et al, 1995a). During sleep the bladder is normally quiescent and stable with lack of facilitation of detrusor contractions whereas during wakefulness marked detrusor overactivity is observed. Clear electroencephalographic (EEG) evidence of cortical arousal or actual awakening occurs in response to bladder distention and sleeping infants are noted to wake up before bladder activity returns and voiding occurs. However, this arousal period may often be transient with the infant crying or moving for a brief period, micturating, and then going back to sleep without being noticed to have awakened. This wakening response to bladder distention probably involves more complicated neural pathways and higher centers than has been appreciated until now (Fig. 123-4).

These results also correlate with recent animal studies showing a sophisticated integration of preexisting central and peripheral neural pathway in micturition control at birth with remodulation occurring in the early postnatal period (Maggi et al, 1986; Thor et al, 1989). Extensive studies using experimental animals by de Groat have indicated that early postnatal maturation of bladder function probably occurs at different levels: (1) changes in the properties of detrusor muscle; (2) developmental modifications in the peripheral innervation of the bladder; and (3) alterations in central synaptic circuitry and neuroplasticity in the parasympathetic reflex pathways to the bladder (de Groat et al, 1993, 1998;

Araki and de Groat 1997; Sugaya et al, 1994, 1997). Recordings of spontaneous activity in bladder smooth muscle in neonatal rats showed much larger amplitude and more synchronous rhythmic contractions compared with those observed in adult rats (Sugaya and de Groat, 1994). This suggests that there is a progressive reduction in intercellular communication between detrusor smooth muscle cells, resulting in less spontaneous activities and hence more efficient urine storage, during early postnatal development. In addition, peripheral and central neural mechanisms also change extensively during this period. In cats (and some other species) micturition during the newborn period is dependent on an exteroreceptive somatovesical reflex triggered when the mother licks the perineum of the kittens (de Groat et al, 1993, 1998; Araki and de Groat 1997). This somatovesical reflex, processed in the sacral spinal cord, disappears in older animals but may reappear after spinal cord injury. Further neuroanatomic studies have indicated that spinal bladder reflexes are mediated via interneurons located immediately adjacent to, and synapsing with, the sacral preganglionic neurons (Sugaya et al, 1997). This interneuron-preganglionic neuron synaptic transmission is very efficient immediately after birth but is very abruptly downregulated during the third postnatal week when the mature supraspinal micturition reflexes start to appear (Araki and de Groat, 1997). Transection of the spinal cord prevents this downregulation, indicating that the higher neural centers play an important role in this synaptic remodeling, which contributes to postnatal development of micturition reflexes.

During the second or third year of life there is progressive development toward a socially conscious continence and a more voluntary or adult type of micturition control. The child becomes more aware of the sensation of bladder distention and the urge to urinate, as well as the social norm and embarrassment associated with urinary incontinence. Through an active learning process, the child acquires the ability to voluntarily inhibit and delay voiding until a socially convenient time and then actively initiate urination even when the bladder is not very full and allow it to proceed to completion. **This natural evolution of micturition control mechanisms depends on an intact neural pathway and awareness of social norms as well as multiple other factors, including the gradual increase in functional bladder capacity, maturation of detrusor-sphincter coordination, and progressive development of voluntary control over the whole bladder-sphincteric-perineal complex.** The final steps are usually achieved at around the age of 3 to 4 years, when most children have developed the adult pattern of urinary control and will be dry both day and night. The child has learned to inhibit a micturition reflex and postpone voiding and voluntarily initiate micturition at socially acceptable and convenient times and places. This development of continence and voluntary micturition is also dependent on behavioral learning and can be influenced by toilet training, which in turns depends on the cognitive perception of the maturing urinary tract. It is understandable therefore that this series of complex events is highly susceptible to the development of various types of dysfunctions.

Neurologic control of normal micturition occurs at different levels of the central nervous system (CNS), from the spinal cord with the "sacral micturition center," to the brain stem

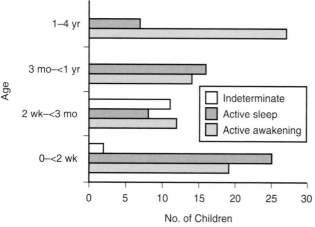

Figure 123-4. Incidence of micturition during different sleep states, according to age group.

with the "pontine micturition center," the cerebellum, basal ganglia, limbic system, thalamus and hypothalamus, and cerebral cortex (Blaivas, 1982; McLorie and Husmann, 1987; de Groat 1993; Fernandes et al, 1994). It should be noted that the bladder is unique among other visceral organs in that its function is under the control of both the somatic and the autonomic nervous system. Besides acetylcholine and norepinephrine, various other neurotransmitters, including prostaglandin substance P, opioid peptides, vasoactive intestinal peptide, and neuropeptide Y are involved during bladder stimulation (Fernandes et al, 1994). Simple manipulation of adrenergic and cholinergic receptors may only partially abolish the effect of neural stimulation, which explains why pharmacologic blockage of the classic neurotransmitters (acetylcholine and norepinephrine) alone may fail to elicit the expected full clinical response.

Transitory Detrusor-Sphincter Discoordination in Infancy

Studies have shown that in making the transition from an infantile to an adult pattern of micturition control, all children may transiently display some degree of abnormal bladder-sphincteric function (Koff, 1997). For instance, it has been clearly shown that a significant proportion of normal infants exhibit prominent detrusor-sphincter discoordination and interrupted voiding during the first 1 to 2 years of life. This is manifested by a discoordinated and interrupted urine flow, which may even be brought to a complete stop for 1 to 2 minutes before restarting, producing a pattern of repeated small voidings in quick succession (Yeung et al, 1995a, 1995b, 1998). **Urodynamic findings show association with high voiding pressures and interruption of flow but no impairment of overall bladder emptying.** However, this type of dysfunction resolved with a period of successful toilet training and was only transitory or intermittent and does not persist. One must therefore be very cautious in the assessment of young children with apparent voiding dysfunctions and should be able to resist the temptation to overinterpret intermittent or transient symptoms as pathologic and hence overinvestigate. However, if voiding dysfunctions are persistent well beyond the period of toilet training, especially if associated with urinary complications such as recurrent urosepsis, then the possibility of underlying anatomic and neurologic causes must be considered and duly evaluated.

EPIDEMIOLOGY AND CLASSIFICATION OF NON-NEUROPATHIC BLADDER-SPHINCTER DYSFUNCTION IN CHILDREN

Epidemiology and Prevalence

Non-neuropathic bladder-sphincteric dysfunction in children is probably more common than what meets the eye but often they only present to us when UTI, vesicoureteric reflux, or urinary incontinence is manifested. It has been reported that 15% of 6-year-old children suffer this condition (Hoebeke, 2002).

Categorization of Non-Neuropathic Bladder-Sphincter Dysfunction in Children

Various conditions have been described under the category of non-neuropathic bladder-sphincter dysfunction, but it must be emphasized that these conditions should not be viewed rigidly as separate and distinct entities but rather as transitional phases of a complex sequence of events. For instance, a girl with dysfunctional voiding may start with having detrusor instability associated with sphincter and pelvic floor overactivity, then gradually evolve to develop fractionated voiding with increasing post-micturition residues, and finally develop bladder decompensation and the "lazy bladder" syndrome (van Gool et al, 1992). It must also be emphasized that use of the term *non-neuropathic* is based purely on the fact that no obvious and identifiable neurologic lesions can be identified. However, conditions such as the urofacial syndrome complex (Ochoa syndrome) and the Hinman syndrome behave almost identically to the typical neuropathic bladder-sphincter dysfunctions. It is indeed conceivable that they do have an organic underlying neurologic cause, although the exact neuroanatomic lesion has not yet been identified. Therefore, the distinction between neuropathic and non-neuropathic bladder dysfunctions may not be as clear as traditionally thought.

In adults, lower urinary tract function has been well understood and standardization of terminology has been established by a committee working under the International Continence Society (ICS) since the early 1970s (Bates et al, 1976a, 1976b, 1979). In contrast, neural control over the bladder-sphincter unit in children is age dependent and is much more variable and complex. Definitions of normal versus abnormal lower urinary tract function have therefore been far less standardized. Various classifications for bladder dysfunctions in children have been described over the past few decades (Lapides, 1970; Bellinger, 1996; Wein, 1998). To avoid confusion, the classification proposed by the International Children's Continence Society in 1997, with a standardized set of terminology and definitions for different lower urinary tract dysfunctions, will be adopted (Nørgaard et al, 1998).

Etiologic Classification of Bladder Dysfunction

Dysfunction of the lower urinary tract in children can be secondary to derangement of nervous control, disorders of detrusor and sphincteric muscle function, structural abnormalities, and other unclassified conditions (Nørgaard et al, 1998).

Derangement of Nervous Control. These include:
- Congenital malformations of CNS (e.g., myelomeningocele, spina bifida occulta, caudal regression syndrome, tethered cord syndrome)
- Developmental disturbances (e.g., mental retardation, dysfunctional voiding, urge syndrome)
- Acquired conditions (e.g., cerebral palsy, progressive degenerative diseases of the CNS associated with spasticity, transverse myelitis, multiple sclerosis, vascular malformations, trauma of the spinal cord)

Disorders of Detrusor and Sphincteric Muscle Function. These include:

- Congenital conditions (e.g., muscular dystrophy, neuronal dysplasia [megacolon-megacystis syndrome])
- Acquired conditions (e.g., chronic bladder distention, fibrosis of detrusor and bladder wall)

Structural Abnormalities. These include:
- Congenital conditions (e.g., bladder exstrophy, epispadias, cloacal anomaly, ureteroceles, posterior urethral valves and other urethral anomalies, prune belly syndrome)
- Acquired conditions (e.g., traumatic stricture or damage to the sphincter or urethra)

Other Unclassified Conditions. These include:
- Giggle incontinence
- Hinman syndrome
- Ochoa syndrome (urofacial syndrome)

Functional Classification of Bladder Dysfunction

This is based on the functional state of the bladder-sphincteric complex with respect to detrusor activity, bladder sensation, bladder compliance and capacity, and urethral function both during the filling and the voiding phase of cystometry (Nørgaard et al, 1998) (Fig. 123–5).

During the Filling (Storage) Phase

Detrusor Activity

Normal or Stable. Bladder volume increases during filling without significant rise in detrusor pressure or no involuntary contractions despite provocation.

Overactive. This is characterized by phasic involuntary detrusor contractions, which may occur either spontaneously or on provocation by alterations of posture, coughing, walking, jumping, and other triggering procedures. Overactive detrusor function can be further divided into unstable and hyperreflexic. The term unstable is used when the contractions are unrelated to any underlying neurologic disorder.

Alternatively, the term detrusor instability can also be used. The exact pathogenesis for detrusor instability has not been resolved. Various underlying causes have been proposed: (1) failure of maturation of CNS control mechanisms; (2) low detrusor levels of inhibitory vasoactive intestinal peptide; (3) abnormal enkephalin-mediated inhibitory neurotransmission; (4) denervation hypersensitivity; and (5) alterations in the properties of the detrusor myocytes (Wein and Barrett, 1992; Harrison et al, 1994; Brading, 1997). Unstable detrusor contractions are frequently found in children with both diurnal and nocturnal enuresis (Bauer et al, 1980; Nørgaard et al, 1998). However, the precise relationship between an unstable detrusor contraction exhibited on a cystometrogram and different types of urinary incontinence is still debated (Nørgaard et al, 1998). Children with an unstable bladder typically present with a sudden urge to void that can only be partially suppressed. Often a girl with unstable bladder will squat down on the heel of one foot, demonstrating the pathognomonic sign of Vincent's curtsy.

***Detrusor hyperreflexia* is defined as overactivity due to disturbance of the neural control mechanisms.** Thus, the term *detrusor hyperreflexia* should only be used when there is objective evidence of a relevant neurologic disorder.

Bladder Sensation. This can be normal, increased (hypersensitive), reduced (hyposensitive), or absent.

Bladder Capacity. This can be normal, high, or low.

Compliance. This can be normal, high, or low. During normal bladder filling little or no pressure change occurs, but there are no standardized reference ranges for compliance in children.

Urethral Function

Normal. Positive urethral closure pressure is maintained during filling, even in the presence of increased abdominal pressure (guarding reflex) but decreases immediately before micturition to allow flow.

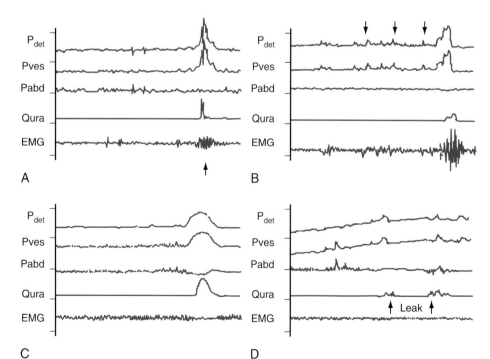

Figure 123–5. Various bladder functional patterns. **A,** Dyssynergic patterns with an increase in sphincteric EMG activities during micturition *(arrow)*, leading to an interrupted urinary flow. **B,** Overactive bladder, characterized by frequent unstable detrusor contractions *(arrows)* during the filling phase. **C,** Normal female micturition pattern; note the pelvic floor relaxation as evidenced by a drop in abdominal pressure during micturition. **D,** Bladder with low (poor) compliance as evidenced by a rapid increase in intravesical pressure during filling, often associated with urinary leakage *(arrows)*. EMG, electromyogram; Pabd, abdominal pressure; Pdet, detrusor pressure; Pves, intravesical pressure; Qura, uroflow. (From Yeung CK: Pathophysiology of bladder dysfunction. In Gearhart JP, Rink RC, Mouriquand PDE [eds]: Pediatric Urology. Philadelphia, WB Saunders, 2001.)

Incompetent. Leakage of urine occurs in the absence of detrusor contraction despite urethral closure.

During the Voiding (Emptying) Phase
Detrusor Activity

Normal. **Voiding is achieved by voluntarily initiated detrusor contraction that is sustained and cannot usually be suppressed voluntarily until at least after the age of 4 years.** Complete bladder emptying is achieved in the absence of bladder outlet obstruction;

Underactive. Detrusor contraction is of inadequate magnitude and/or duration to effect bladder emptying with a normal time span. The term should be reserved for describing detrusor activity during micturition because it is not readily visible during the filling phase of the cystometrogram. It is often observed in the overdistended postobstructive bladder.

Acontractile. This is due to an abnormality of nervous control and denotes the complete absence of centrally coordinated contractions.

Urethral Function

Normal. The urethra opens to allow bladder emptying.

Obstructive. This may be due to sphincteric overactivity or mechanical obstruction due to obstructive urethral lesions such as congenital obstructive posterior urethral membrane or syringoceles (Dhillon et al, 1993; Dewan and Goh, 1995).

Dysfunctional Elimination Syndrome

The association of constipation with urologic pathologic processes has been described in the literature since the 1950s, but it was only over the past decade that clinicians have paid more attention to this relationship and recognized its existence with the term *dysfunctional elimination syndrome* (DES). This term is used to reflect the broad spectrum of functional disturbances that may affect the urinary tract, including that of functional bowel disturbances, and can be classified as follows:

- Functional disorder of filling: overactive bladder, overdistention of bladder or insensate bladder, which may be associated with fecal impaction or rectal distention with infrequent call to stool.
- Functional disorder of emptying: over-recruitment of pelvic floor activity during voiding causing interrupted and/or incomplete emptying also associated with defecation difficulties due to nonrelaxation of puborectalis, pain on defecation, or even anismus (Bower et al, 2005).

Koff and colleagues (1998) showed that the pattern of **DES significantly influenced clinical outcome of ureteric reimplantation surgery for vesicoureteral reflux (VUR) in children.** Children with constipation had the highest likelihood of developing a breakthrough UTI and thus require surgery. DES also had an adverse effect on the rate of spontaneous reflux resolution with the children requiring an average of 1.6 years longer to outgrow reflux than in children without DES. For those requiring surgery, both the results and postoperative complications seemed to be negatively influenced by DES. Postoperative UTIs developed in 78% of children with DES. All children who had persistent reflux, recurrent reflux after 2 years, and contralateral reflux after unilateral reimplantation had DES.

Loening-Baucke (1997) looked at resolution of urinary incontinence and UTIs in children after treatment of their constipation. This study showed that after successful treatment of constipation, 89% of those with day-time incontinence and 63% with night-time incontinence became dry. None of the children who had UTI had recurrence after treatment of constipation.

It therefore seems from these data that management of the underlying dysfunction should be given priority in the treatment protocol of children with conditions such as VUR, incontinence, and UTI, because successful management may significantly improve outcome. Thus more attention should be paid to evaluate for the presence of functional bowel disturbances even in cases of urologic pathologic processes.

BLADDER-SPHINCTER DYSFUNCTION DURING BLADDER FILLING
Overactive (Unstable) Bladder, Urge Syndrome, and Urge Incontinence

The term *unstable bladder* has often been used rather loosely without a precise definition. **Traditionally, the infant bladder has been described as unstable or uninhibited, but recent studies using prolonged natural filling bladder monitoring techniques have shown that to the contrary, the bladder is normally quiescent and stable even in newborns** (Yeung et al, 1995a). Clinically, the condition of "unstable bladder" is best exhibited by urge syndrome with or without urge incontinence. The syndrome, characterized by frequent attacks of sudden and imperative sensations of urge, due to detrusor overactivity during the filling phase, is more prevalent in girls. This burning sensation or urge to void occurs even with small bladder capacities. The unstable contractions are often counteracted by voluntary contraction of the pelvic floor muscles in an attempt to externally compress the urethra (hold maneuvers) exhibited as squatting (Vincent's curtsey sign) in many cases (Vincent, 1966; Van Gool and de Jonge, 1989). However, despite this move, urge incontinence can still occur with frequent urine leakage onto the underpants. Urge incontinence usually consists of small quantities of urine loss and occurs most often in the afternoon or when the child is preoccupied in play or other activities and is not alert enough to contract the pelvic floor in response to the urge sensation. Children with urge syndrome have small bladder capacities for age and often choose to drink extremely little to escape from the social embarrassment of frequent imperative urges to go to the toilet and from urinary incontinence but have otherwise complete relaxation of the pelvic floor musculature in most instances. In addition, habitual voluntary pelvic floor contraction to counteract every urge to void also may often lead to inappropriate postponement of defecation, constipation, and fecal soiling (Vincent, 1966; O'Regan et al, 1986). This should not be confused with encopresis in children with behavioral problems.

Functional Urinary Incontinence

This can be defined as the **involuntary loss of urine, due to a failure of control of the bladder-sphincteric unit,** which is frequent enough to constitute a social or hygienic problem, and in the absence of underlying anatomic causes (Nørgaard et al, 1998). Apart from urge incontinence that is associated with detrusor overactivity and urge syndrome as just described, other forms of functional urinary incontinence exist as a result of failure of the bladder storage and/or sphincteric control mechanisms. *Stress incontinence* represents the involuntary leakage of urine occurring at times when the intravesical pressure exceeds the bladder outlet or urethral resistance, in the absence of measurable detrusor contraction. Unlike in adults and particularly in elderly women, true stress incontinence is extremely uncommon in neurologically normal children and is in general not associated with any demonstrable urodynamic abnormalities. It should therefore be differentiated from urge incontinence and detrusor overactivity. Insufficient bladder outlet or urethral resistance is usually not a main factor. Because the amount of urine leakage in most patients is usually small, the incontinence may at times be only scarcely discernible. It is possible therefore that the actual incidence of this condition may be underestimated. Nygaard and colleagues showed that 28% of a group of young nulliparous female athletes reported urine loss during their sports activity and that the impact forces transmitted from the lower limbs to the pelvic floor may play a role in its etiology (Nygaard et al, 1994, 1996).

Giggle Incontinence

Giggle incontinence is usually seen in girls and is characterized by involuntary and typically unpredictable wetting during giggling or laughter. In contrast to stress incontinence, it produces a much larger volume of urine leakage, often amounting to complete bladder emptying. Similar to stress incontinence, however, cystometry may be completely normal or occasionally demonstrate some detrusor overactivity. Treatment is notoriously difficult but sometimes a course of anticholinergic drugs may help to ameliorate the symptoms. There are also suggestions that this is a centrally mediated and hereditary disorder that may respond to CNS stimulants such as methylphenidate (Sher and Reinberg, 1996).

BLADDER-SPHINCTER DYSFUNCTION DURING BLADDER EMPTYING
Dysfunctional Voiding

Dysfunctional voiding is characterized by incomplete relaxation or overactivity of the pelvic floor muscles during micturition. It can manifest in different patterns depending on the degree of functional outflow obstruction caused as well as the status of the detrusor activity. As outlined earlier, the underlying bladder-sphincteric dysfunction may evolve progressively and change with time through a transitional phase of a complex sequence of events of bladder functional development.

Staccato and Fractionated Voiding

In *staccato voiding* the urinary stream is often delayed after the onset of detrusor contraction and is typically interrupted, resulting in a few small squirts of urine passed in quick succession. The interrupted voiding is caused by periodic bursts of pelvic floor muscle activities during micturition, resulting in the characteristic abrupt elevation or spikes of voiding pressures, coinciding with paradoxical cessation of urinary flow. The flow time is usually prolonged and bladder emptying is often incomplete, resulting in increased postmicturition residues and hence a predisposition to UTIs.

Fractionated voiding **is characterized by infrequent and incomplete emptying secondary to detrusor inactivity.** Micturition occurs in several small, discontinuous fractions due to poor and unsustained detrusor contractions, leaving significant postvoid residual urine volumes. Abdominal straining is usually evident as an effort to improve bladder emptying. However, this is often paradoxically counteracted by a reflex increase in activities of the pelvic floor muscles that is triggered by an increase in intravesical pressure. The bladder capacity is usually large for age and may gradually increase as the condition further progresses, and overflow incontinence may ultimately develop.

Infrequent Voiding and "Lazy Bladder" Syndrome

These two conditions are described together as they represent a spectrum of disease that more commonly occurs in girls. At one end of the spectrum, the *lazy bladder syndrome* is **generally regarded as the endpoint of long-standing dysfunctional voiding culminating in a fully decompensated system.** As a result of the chronic functional bladder outflow obstruction, there is a gradual deterioration in detrusor contractility and emptying efficiency. Postmicturition residual urine and bladder capacity progressively increase, eventually developing into a large, floppy bladder with very inefficient emptying. The child uses abdominal straining as the main driving force for bladder emptying, and detrusor contractions are small and unsustained with very low pressures and at times being completely undetectable using conventional cystometry. **Because urge sensation is either absent or diminished, voiding is very infrequent and occasionally the child may not void for 8 to 10 hours or even longer if engaged in activities.** The typical presentation of a child with *infrequent voiding syndrome* is where the mother always complains that the child never voids unless told to do so. The resultant large volume of postmicturition residual urines predispose to recurrent UTI, which often constitutes the primary complaint bringing the child to the pediatric urologist. Overflow incontinence is usually evident, which may be further associated with constipation and/or fecal soiling. Urodynamic studies typically reveal a large capacity bladder, with very high compliance on filling. Detrusor contractions are noticeably absent and voiding is associated with increased abdominal pressures, resulting in a very fractionated flow pattern. Electromyography often shows increased activity in the pelvic floor muscle with each abdominal strain.

Hinman's Syndrome and Occult Neuropathic Bladder

Hinman, Allen, and Dorfman first coined the terms *non-neurogenic neurogenic bladder* or *subclinical neurogenic bladder,* and later *Hinman syndrome,* to describe a presumably **acquired form of bladder-sphincteric dysfunction in children that was characterized by a combination of bladder decompensation with incontinence, poor emptying, and recurrent urinary infections** (Dorfman et al, 1969; Hinman and Baumann, 1973; Allen, 1977; Hinman, 1986). **Most children also have significant bowel dysfunction,** including encopresis, constipation, and fecal impaction. In British literature the condition is often referred to as "occult neuropathic bladder" after the article by D. Innes Williams (Williams, 1975). The condition has all the clinical and urodynamic features typical of neuropathic bladder dysfunction but no neurologic pathology can be demonstrated. Hinman and Baumann (1973) initially hypothesized that the condition could be ascribed to acquired psychologically abnormal behavior with voluntary discoordination between the detrusor muscle and the pelvic floor-external urethral sphincter complex during voiding. This notion, however, has not received strong support from later studies, and controversies still exist as to whether a very subtle or occult spinal pathologic process can occur to account for an isolated bladder neuropathy in a child who does not exhibit other somatic neurologic deficits and has normal magnetic resonance imaging of the spinal cord. Urodynamic studies often revealed marked sphincteric overactivity and abrupt contractions of the pelvic floor as the child attempted to control incontinence from uninhibited bladder contractions. In its severe form, the bladder-sphincter dysfunction can cause full-blown bladder decompensation with day- and night-time wetting, large postmicturition residual urine volumes, recurrent UTIs, and significant damage to the upper urinary tracts (Dorfman et al, 1969; Hinman and Baumann, 1973; Williams et al, 1975; Allen, 1977; Hinman 1986, 1997; Jayanthi et al, 1997). Imaging studies often reveal profound changes in the upper urinary tracts, with about two thirds of the children developing hydroureteronephrosis and over half having VUR. Nearly every patient has a grossly trabeculated, large-capacity bladder with a considerable volume of postmicturition residual urine. Treatment should therefore entail measures to control infection and to restore normal bladder storage and emptying function. Because of the great similarities to neuropathic bladder dysfunction, the management strategy in these children generally follows very similar principles for the former condition.

Another piece of indirect evidence that a very subtle or occult neurologic lesion may account for some cases of "non-neurogenic neurogenic" bladder-sphincteric dysfunction is the *Ochoa (urofacial) syndrome.* **Children with this syndrome exhibit all the classic features of dysfunctional voiding, including urinary incontinence, recurrent UTIs, constipation, reflux, and upper tract damage, but they also have a peculiar painful or apparently crying facial expression during smiling** (Ochoa and Gorlin, 1987; Ochoa, 1992). The condition has an autosomal recessive inheritance, and the gene has been located on chromosome 10. Urodynamic studies characteristically showed a sustained contraction of the external sphincter during voiding. The resulting severe bladder-sphincter dysfunction is often associated with a dismal outcome. Of the 66 children reported by Ochoa, 33% had renal functional impairment, 26% had hypertension, and 24% had end-stage renal failure. Five patients received renal

transplantation, and 17 died (Ochoa, 1992). Because the neural ganglia controlling the facial muscles are situated very close to the pontine micturition center, it is tempting to speculate that a small genetically predetermined, congenital neurologic lesion in this area may be responsible for both the peculiar facial expression and the bladder dysfunction. Further studies in this direction may help to resolve some of the continuing dilemma.

Postvoid Dribbling

Postvoid dribbling refers to involuntary leakage of urine immediately after voiding. Typically this refers to post–toilet-trained girls who dribble soon after standing up after a void and are otherwise normal with no other associated urinary symptoms. In these circumstances it **may be a result of vesicovaginal reflux whereby urine is trapped in the vagina during voiding and once the child stands, the urine begins to dribble out.** When in doubt, it can be confirmed by performing a micturating cystourethrogram. The condition is harmless and tends to resolve with age, but the child may also be taught to empty her vagina by simply voiding with her thighs apart and leaning forward after voiding before getting up.

DYSFUNCTIONAL ELIMINATION SYNDROME, CONSTIPATION, AND BLADDER DYSFUNCTION

It has long been recognized that children with dysfunctional voiding and recurrent UTIs often have associated bowel dysfunction, including constipation, fecal impaction, and encopresis. However, only recently has the term *dysfunctional elimination syndrome* been given to recognize the existence of this relationship. Studies have been performed to explain how constipation and chronic rectal dilatation may interfere with the normal function of the lower urinary tract, resulting in bladder dysfunction, reflux, and UTIs (Yazbeck et al, 1987; O'Regan et al, 1997). **The close proximity of the rectum to the posterior wall of the bladder makes it possible that any gross distention of the rectum by impacted feces can result in mechanical compression of the bladder and bladder neck, leading to urinary obstruction** (Shopfner, 1968; O'Regan et al, 1997). **In addition, it has been observed that large fecal impaction may induce significant detrusor instability and other bladder dysfunctions, which in turn will result in the urge syndrome, UTI, and reflux** (Shopfner, 1968; Yazbeck et al, 1987, O'Regan et al, 1997). O'Regan and associates (1985, 1986) have reported a high incidence of enuresis in children with UTI and constipation. It has been noted that in constipated enuretic children who had detrusor instability, treatment of concomitant constipation resulted in cessation or improvement of enuresis. Animal studies have also revealed an increased predisposition to bacteriuria in rats with surgically induced fecal retention (Breda et al, 1975). The evidence available so far therefore strongly suggest that there is an important relationship between constipation, detrusor instability, reflux, UTI, and enuresis. Proper attention to associated bowel dysfunction should therefore form an integral part of the overall management in children with bladder dysfunctions.

RELATIONSHIP BETWEEN BLADDER-SPHINCTER DYSFUNCTION, VESICOURETERAL REFLUX, AND RECURRENT URINARY TRACT INFECTIONS

Impairment in the functions of the lower urinary tract often coexists with recurrent UTIs and VUR, without any identified neurologic or other causal pathology (Koff and Murtagh, 1983; Griffiths and Scholtmeijer, 1987; Sillen et al, 1992; Chandra et al, 1996; Yeung et al, 1998). Incidence of higher intravesical pressure, detrusor overactivity, detrusor sphincter dyssynergia, or incomplete voiding has been reported in a significant proportion of children with VUR; and, vice versa, micturating cystourethrograms performed in children with bladder dysfunctions often find concomitant VUR. **The most common abnormalities of the lower urinary tract found to coexist with VUR are predominantly detrusor overactivity and uncoordinated detrusor sphincter function during micturition.** These abnormalities may occur secondary to urinary infection or can be acquired during the period when voluntary control of micturition is being established. Although the bladder instability can occur in most children with VUR, it is unlikely to have its role in initiating VUR (Koff and Murtagh, 1984). However, **reflux from incompetence of the ureterovesical junction may be worsened by detrusor instability** (Stephens, 1979). The urethral sphincteric dysfunction or discoordination is characterized urodynamically by obstruction during voiding owing to involuntary constriction of the urinary sphincter and is believed to be the normal response of the individual to an uninhibited bladder contraction while attempting not to void (Scholtmeijer and Griffiths, 1990; Koff, 1992; Homsy, 1994; Scholtmeijer and Nijman, 1994). It is considered as the most serious dysfunction, because it has been reported that patients with this dysfunction often have bilateral high-grade reflux and injured upper renal tracts (Griffiths and Scholtmeijer, 1987; Orellana et al, 2004). The discoordinated bladder also regularly decompensates, and a significant number of children with moderate or severe VUR were reported to have overdistended bladder with weak contractions and high capacity (Hjalmas et al, 1994; Koff et al, 2002; Garat Barredo et al, 2004).

Previous studies showed that infants with UTI and VUR have a high prevalence of high voiding detrusor pressure (Sillen et al, 1992, 1996; Yeung et al, 1998) (Fig. 123–6). **Male refluxers are characterized by considerably higher maximum voiding pressures associated with detrusor hypercontractility, which may represent a more pronounced form of detrusor-sphincter dyssynergia, as compared with age-matched female refluxers and normal nonrefluxing infants.** In contrast, in the majority of female refluxing infants no detrusor hypercontractility was noted and instead they often displayed a urodynamic pattern with normal voiding pressures and relatively large bladder capacity with or without emptying inefficiency and postmicturition residues. The finding of higher voiding detrusor pressure in male infants compared with female infants may be attributed to higher urethral resistance of the longer male urethra and smaller urethral meatus and anatomic difference in the configuration of external sphincter. Studies have also shown that high intravesical pressure significantly contributes to the development and severity of VUR. It was shown that infants with bilateral high-grade VUR had significantly higher voiding detrusor pressures and higher prevalence of detrusor overactivity than those with lower grade or unilateral VUR (Chandra and Maddix, 2000).

It has been further shown that the spontaneous resolution of VUR may be delayed in the presence of abnormal dynamics of the bladder (Godley et al, 2001; Sofia et al, 2004). Bladder dysfunction was shown to have a powerful relationship with the nonresolution of high-grade infant VUR. It is generally accepted that bladder dysfunction delays the spontaneous resolution of reflux in older children (Taylor, 1982; Koff and Murtagh, 1984). Studies have also shown that there is a strong correlation between recurrent infections and nonresolution, which probably reflects the fact that most infections were seen in infants and children with bladder dysfunction. Therefore, recurrent infections can be regarded as a marker of bladder dysfunction, indicating an investigation of bladder function (Sofia et al, 2004).

Moreover, successful treatment of the underlying bladder dysfunction resulted in marked increase in the rate of spontaneous resolution of reflux and significant reduction in recurrent UTIs. It is therefore of paramount importance that early detection and proper management of underlying lower urinary tract abnormalities are crucial in the treatment of VUR in infants and children. The first step in management in those children presenting postnatally with VUR or UTI should be a detailed evaluation of bladder function to choose an appropriate treatment modality and to prevent renal deterioration.

Why do children who have VUR have such a high incidence of bladder dysfunction? The correlation of this maturational lag in the bladder function and development of the CNS is the other untouched area of investigation. A similar association between gastroesophageal reflux and cerebral palsy is now well studied, and effective surgical treatment protocol has evolved over the past 2 decades.

EVALUATION OF NON-NEUROPATHIC BLADDER-SPHINCTER DYSFUNCTION
History

The majority of children with non-neuropathic bladder-sphincter dysfunction typically present after toilet training with symptoms of either night-time or day-time urinary incontinence or both. Occasionally they can be recognized at an earlier age when the child presents for investigation of UTIs or VUR. In any case, it is important to obtain a detailed history from the child and guardian. This should include relevant questions to exclude neurologic and congenital abnormalities. Bowel dysfunction can coexist in the form of encopresis, constipation, and fecal impaction and should be noted during history taking. The urinary history should focus on symptoms related to both the storage and evacuation of urine.

Voiding Diary

A voiding diary is used to record daily fluid intake and urine output at home under normal conditions. When properly

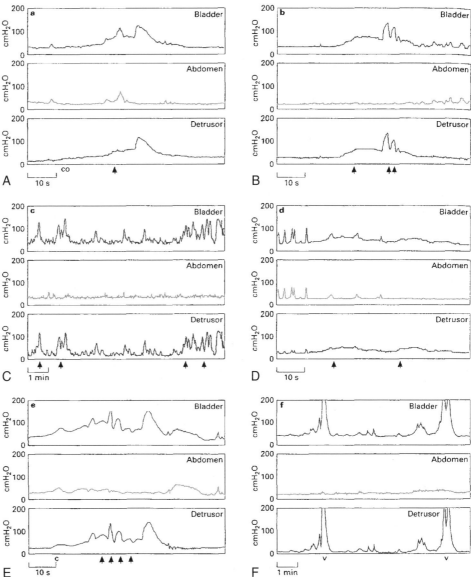

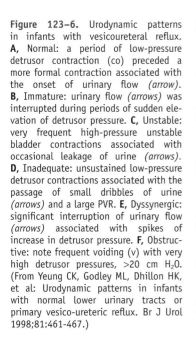

Figure 123–6. Urodynamic patterns in infants with vesicoureteral reflux. **A,** Normal: a period of low-pressure detrusor contraction (co) preceded a more formal contraction associated with the onset of urinary flow (arrow). **B,** Immature: urinary flow (arrows) was interrupted during periods of sudden elevation of detrusor pressure. **C,** Unstable: very frequent high-pressure unstable bladder contractions associated with occasional leakage of urine (arrows). **D,** Inadequate: unsustained low-pressure detrusor contractions associated with the passage of small dribbles of urine (arrows) and a large PVR. **E,** Dyssynergic: significant interruption of urinary flow (arrows) associated with spikes of increase in detrusor pressure. **F,** Obstructive: note frequent voiding (v) with very high detrusor pressures, >20 cm H₂0. (From Yeung CK, Godley ML, Dhillon HK, et al: Urodynamic patterns in infants with normal lower urinary tracts or primary vesico-ureteric reflux. Br J Urol 1998;81:461-467.)

filled in, it can be very informative and give clues to the underlying dysfunction. The number of voidings per day, the distribution of voids during the day, and each voided volume is recorded. It can also record any episodes of urgency and leakage. It is a useful tool to help identify those who may warrant further studies as well as in follow-up of patients (Fig. 123–7).

Physical Examination

Physical examination is usually normal in children with non-neuropathic bladder-sphincter dysfunction, but careful examination is required to exclude those who may require further neurologic evaluation. Occasionally, in an otherwise normal child, one may find a palpable bladder on abdominal examination in cases of decompensated bladders. Abnormalities of the lower spine should be sought specifically to exclude the possibility of an occult spinal dysraphism. Lesions such as an asymmetrical gluteal fold, hairy patch, dermovascular malformation, or lipomatous abnormality of the sacral region should prompt further imaging evaluation. The external genitalia may be examined to exclude any obvious anatomical problems that can explain the urinary symptoms in question. Rectal examination may reveal fecal impaction or distended rectum in those with chronic constipation. In the absence of any positive findings on examination, further investigations may be warranted.

Laboratory Investigations

Laboratory investigations are generally not routinely required unless the child presents with complications such as UTIs. However, to complement a full workup, urinalysis may be performed to rule out bacteriuria and glucosuria. Serum and urine osmolality may be looked at in cases of nocturnal enuresis to assess renal concentrating ability.

(1) Please use measuring jar to measure voiding volume (ml) each time (3) Please observe for any 'urge', 'wet' or 'incontinence' symptoms

(2) Please record drinking volume in a whole day (ml) (4) Please measure voiding and drinking volume for two whole days before follow up and bring the chart back to see doctor

Name: _____ Date: / /

Time	Urge	Wet	Incontinence	Voiding / CIC Vol. (ml)	Drink Vol. (ml)
	(Please put a "√" in the appropriate box)				
07:00	√			275	345
08:00					
09:00					230
10:00					
11:00					
12:00					
13:00	√			260	375
14:00		√			
15:00					
16:00					300
17:00	√			245	
18:00					
19:00					400
20:00	√			340	
21:00					
22:00					
23:00	√			175	
00:00					
01:00					
02:00					
03:00					
04:00					
05:00					
06:00					
Total				1275	1650

Date: / /

Time	Urge	Wet	Incontinence	Voiding / CIC Vol. (ml)	Drink Vol. (ml)
	(Please put a "√" in the appropriate box)				
07:00	√			250	345
08:00					
09:00					
10:00					300
11:00					
12:00	√			250	
13:00					
14:00					400
15:00					
16:00					
17:00	√			300	
18:00					
19:00					275
20:00					
21:00	√	√		145	
22:00					200
23:00	√			100	
00:00					
01:00					
02:00					
03:00					
04:00					
05:00					
06:00					
Total				1045	1520

Figure 123–7. Examples of frequency–volume chart.

Ultrasonography

Ultrasonography is often the first-line investigation in children with non-neuropathic bladder-sphincter dysfunction because it is a simple, readily available, and noninvasive tool that is able to provide information both on anatomic and functional problems when performed by experienced pediatric radiologists.

Ultrasonography has been increasingly used in the study of the pelvic floor musculature. In boys, the external sphincter, puborectalis, and bulbocavernosus have been observed to contract during a hold maneuver. In girls, lengthening of the urethra and movement of the bladder neck in the direction of the symphysis is seen. However, in **patients with non-neuropathic bladder-sphincter dysfunction, approximately one third of the children were unable to elicit movement of the pelvic floor or had paradoxical movement.** The clinical significance of this remains unclear, but when introduced to a period of urotherapy and pelvic floor rehabilitation, marked improvement of symptoms had been reported. Similarly, ultrasonography has been employed in the study of bladder neck mobility. Studies have shown that in a proportion of girls with hyperlaxity of joints, coughing or straining would result in a wide opening of the bladder neck and urethra. In this group of girls, urotherapy would prove difficult and occasionally some would go on to require surgery to the bladder neck (de Jong, 2005). Ultrasound can provide a noninvasive means to monitor this subgroup of children not responsive to standard urotherapy.

More recently, ultrasound has been used to measure bladder parameters used in calculating a bladder volume and wall thickness index (BVWI). This BVWI can be classified into normal, thick, or thin according to the measured parameters. Our studies have shown that these classifications corresponded closely to urodynamic findings of underlying bladder dysfunctions and can act as a reliable tool to guide for further invasive investigations (Yeung et al, 2004).

Other Imaging Studies

Radiologic examination of the spine may be necessary to rule out any neurogenic causes of bladder-sphincter dysfunction.

A micturating cystourethrogram may be performed in patients to rule out VUR. Information on the bladder emptying efficiency may be obtained and the status of the urethra can be assessed to exclude any outflow obstruction.

Urodynamic Studies

Urodynamic studies are employed to describe the physiologic parameters involved in the bladder mechanics during filling and voiding.

Uroflowmetry

All urodynamics should be preceded by or combined with a uroflow study. When performing uroflowmetry, the child must experience normal desire to void for it to be representative and repeated recordings should be performed. Preferably, the voiding should be observed and correct sitting or standing position ascertained. **In children, normal flow rates are different from in adults and there is usually a poor correlation between maximal flow rate (Qmax) and outflow resistance because the detrusor is able to exert much stronger contractions to counteract any increased resistance.** It is therefore important to study the pattern of the flow curve in addition to the flow rates in children. The precise shape of the flow curve is determined by detrusor contractility, the presence of any abdominal straining, and the bladder outlet. The normal pattern is that of a smooth *bell* shape. A *tower*-shaped curve produced by an explosive voiding contraction is seen in overactive bladders, and a low *plateau*-shaped curve is representative of an outlet obstruction. A *staccato* pattern is seen with sphincteric overactivity during voiding with peaks and troughs throughout voiding, and an *interrupted* flow is seen in acontractile or underactive bladders. When combined with cystometry and perineal EMG studies, further information on the different spectrum of functional bladder outflow obstructions can be analyzed (Nijman, 1997).

Conventional Fill Urodynamic Studies

This involves more sophisticated instruments and becomes more invasive to the patient, requiring a bladder catheter introduced transurethrally or suprapubically. The use of suprapubic catheterization has been suggested as a better alternative to transurethral catheterization. Although it may be considered more invasive, it is much more physiologic than to try to void with a catheter in the urethra, particularly in children. Not only is it obstructive to flow but the trauma of placing the catheter just before the investigation may cause significant discomfort. For suprapubic catheterization, a 6-Fr double-lumen catheter is placed suprapubically under sedation and left in situ for 24 hours before commencement of the urodynamic study.

The suprapubic catheter is connected to a computer system and used to measure intravesical pressure. Another catheter is placed in the rectum to measure intra-abdominal pressure surrounding the bladder. By subtracting the latter from the intravesical pressure, we can calculate the detrusor pressure. Sphincteric activity can also be measured with simultaneous perineal EMG recordings. All the measured data are directly fed into a computer for analysis and display of graphical measurements. The urodynamic study looks at both the filling and voiding phases of the bladder. Bladder filling and storage is described according to bladder sensation, detrusor activity, bladder compliance, and bladder capacity. Pressure flow studies are carried out during the voiding phase.

Traditionally, the bladder is filled artificially with water or normal saline to speed up the procedure. The child is asked to indicate his or her desire to void if old enough to do so and then void into a specially designed seat with an uroflowmeter attached. The investigator observing the study should also make note of any events occurring during the study, for example, any large movements of the patient, coughing, or, in particular, any urinary dribbling.

By combining cystometry with fluoroscopy, video-urodynamics can be performed with fluoroscopic images of the bladder, bladder neck, and urethra captured. Conventional fill urodynamics is performed in the usual manner with the child in a specially designed chair with a uroflowmetry device in the fluoroscopy suite. Fluoroscopic images are taken during filling and during voiding. This has the added advantage of being able to observe the shape of the bladder during filling and voiding, observing for signs of VUR as well as the configuration of the urethra and pelvic floor.

Natural Fill Urodynamic Studies

More recently, studies have shown that the nonphysiologic filling of the bladder during conventional fill urodynamics, even at low filling rates, can lead to misrepresentations of true bladder activity during normal situations. Therefore, natural fill urodynamic studies may be performed whereby the child is asked to drink to allow the bladder to fill up on its own rate. Urodynamic studies in children with urge syndrome usually reveal detrusor overactivity associated with a small bladder capacity but may occasionally be normal with incontinence only barely perceptible, particularly if conventional fill cystometry rather than natural filling cystometry is used. It appears that the **artificial filling may inhibit the detrusor response and attenuate its maximum contractile potential, rendering detrusor instability much less pronounced and undetectable.** Therefore, natural fill cystometry is the preferred technique in children or, better still, the combined use of artificial and natural filling urodynamic studies is helpful to accurately delineate the underlying bladder dysfunction (Yeung et al, 1995b).

Ambulatory Urodynamic Studies

The unfamiliar hospital and urodynamic laboratory environment as well as the presence of a urodynamics investigator can sometimes cause significant distress, particularly to young children. To overcome this, an ambulatory urodynamic study may be performed. This study is performed with ambulatory equipment strapped to the child and relies on infrared telemetry while the investigator sits behind a one-way mirror (Yeung, 1998).

The system consists of an ambulatory urodynamic recorder with a specially designed built-in extension board that converts digital pressure signals to a modulated infrared wave. Two external infrared leads are connected to the output and fixed to the clothing of the patient (Fig. 123–8). The optimal emission from the recorder has a 10-m range and completes the circuit of the infrared on-line link by cable to the computer. Direct "line-of-sight" from the transmitter to the receiver is unnecessary because the infrared signals reflect from the walls of the room before reaching the receiver. For very active and uncooperative patients, more than one receiver connected in parallel with the power unit and computer can be used at the same time to enhance signal collection. The first receiver to receive valid signals transmits the data to the computer and inhibits the other receivers simultaneously (Fig. 123–9).

During the investigation the infant can conduct normal activities, be totally mobile, and be accompanied by one or

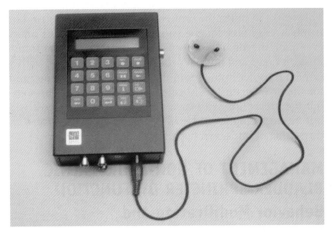

Figure 123–8. The ambulatory urodynamic recorder with the external infrared leads mounted in a plastic holder that can be attached to the patient. (From Yeung CK: Continuous real-time ambulatory urodynamic monitoring in infants and young children using infrared telemetry. Br J Urol 1998:81;76-80.)

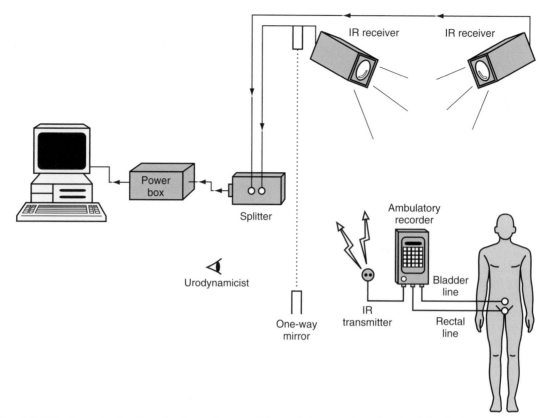

Figure 123–9. Schematic diagram to show the setup for continuous real-time ambulatory urodynamics using infrared telemetry. (From Yeung CK: Continuous real-time ambulatory urodynamic monitoring in infants and young children using infrared telemetry. Br J Urol 1998:81;76-80.)

both of the parents undisturbed in a private cubicle. From an adjoining room the hidden investigator observes and records the patient's activities, including urinary dribbling and micturition, through a one-way mirror, while real-time on-line pressure signal displays are monitored continuously on the computer. Only natural fill studies are possible by this means. Overall, it allows for a continuous monitoring of bladder function under near natural conditions for the child.

More recently, the Bluetooth system has been introduced. This works in much the same way as the infrared system but is much less bulky for the patient to carry around. It offers even more freedom of movement with a much longer transmission range and more reliable reception. If coupled with a camera recorder in the room the child is in, there is no need for the investigator to sit behind a one-way mirror throughout the procedure. With such advances in technology, it will not be surprising if urodynamics can soon be performed in the setting of one's own home!

MANAGEMENT OF NON-NEUROPATHIC BLADDER-SPHINCTER DYSFUNCTION
Behavior Modification and Standard Urotherapy

Urotherapy is a nonpharmacologic and nonsurgical combination of cognitive, behavioral, and physical therapy with an aim to normalize micturition pattern and prevent further **functional disturbances of the lower urinary tract.** The children and their parents are educated on proper voiding mechanics, and the specific problem is explained to them to provide motivation for improvement. Specific instructions are then given as to how and when to void. Children are assessed and taught correct sitting or standing positions for voiding. They are taught how to relax the pelvic floor and avoid straining. Their drinking and voiding habits are studied and modified accordingly to include proper hydration with timed voiding. A proper assessment of their bowel function is imperative to successful management. To achieve good results, strong patient support with adequate motivation of both the child and the parents are essential.

Biofeedback and Pelvic Floor Rehabilitation

Biofeedback is based on the concept of building self-perception on detrusor contractions and pelvic floor relaxation in the patient. By combining uroflowmetry with real-time monitoring, the child is able to see how well he or she is voiding. It also helps the child understand what can be altered with voluntary control and with relaxation of the pelvic floor. Biofeedback as a treatment modality for children with dysfunctional voiding is based on this concept and has proven to be highly effective either on its own or in combination with standard urotherapy (Figs. 123–10 to 123–12).

Neuromodulation, Acupuncture, and Other Treatment Modalities

Recent studies reported that transcutaneous electrical nerve stimulation (TENS) is a simple, cost-effective, noninvasive treatment modality for the management of a wide variety of lower urinary tract disorders with few side effects. The mechanisms of action of the reported techniques remain unclear, but symptomatic improvements are common. Some reports indicate changes in urodynamic parameters during transcutaneous stimulation, suggesting that the TENS therapy was capable of inhibiting detrusor contractions. The beneficial effects of TENS over the sacral dermatomes (S2-S3) in patients with lower urinary tract symptoms associated with detrusor overactivity have been reported. **The use of low-frequency electrical current to inhibit detrusor activity in adults is common and appears to modulate excitatory and inhibitory components of bladder control.** Such studies provide the rationale for the application of TENS therapy to modulate detrusor function in patients with functional detrusor dysfunction.

Traditional acupuncture has also reported high efficacy in the treatment of nocturnal enuresis with low relapse rate. Reports have used acupoints innervated by sacral segments S2-S4, and stimulation involved both manual and electrical stimulation. However, its use in the pediatric population remains limited by the intrinsic fear of needling in children with subsequent lack of cooperation (Bower et al, 2005).

Bowel Management

The principles of bowel management include rectal emptying of impacted stool and the maintenance of regular soft stools. A reliable bowel habit pattern can only be established when the child is able to achieve pain-free defecation of soft stool. An initial cleanout of the bowel can be achieved by oral laxatives and rectal enemas on a regular basis until complete disimpaction of the rectum. Occasionally, high colonic washouts may be necessary to achieve a good result. Only when this has been achieved should the second stage of management commence, which involves prevention of further stool accumulation with continuation of regular oral laxatives and/or stool softeners as well as dietary modification. Correct toileting posture and correct recruitment of abdominal muscles in the defecation process aids in the effectiveness of bowel emptying. However, success of a bowel management program can only be achieved with sound support from the family. Parental education is necessary so that the parents can help reinforce and encourage correct toileting habits at home.

Medications

Pharmacologic control of the lower urinary tract can either act via the CNS or peripherally. Several CNS regions have been identified to be involved with micturition control, including the cortex, pontine tegmentum, medulla, and spinal structures. All these regions are modulated by several different neurotransmitters, which have become targets for drug treatment. **However, many of the drugs developed with CNS action are not sufficiently selective to effect only the lower urinary**

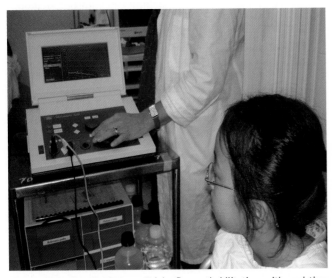

Figure 123–10. Urotherapy. Pelvic floor rehabilitation with real-time biofeedback monitoring.

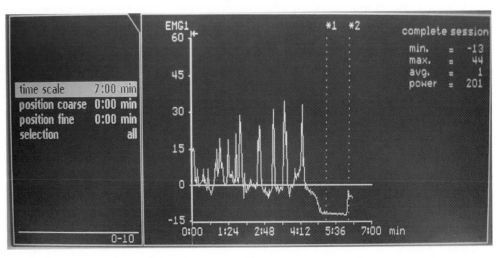

Figure 123–11. Urotherapy. Example of real-time pelvic floor rehabilitation biofeedback tracing showing voluntary contraction and relaxation of pelvic muscles.

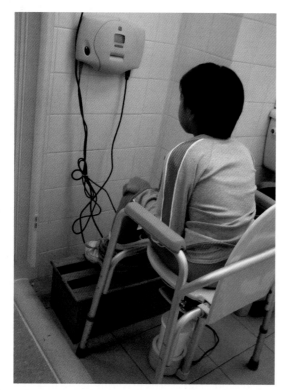

Figure 123–12. Urotherapy. Biofeedback with real-time uroflowmetry.

tract, hence the possibility of these drugs causing adverse drug reactions. Pharmacologic targets for treating bladder dysfunction may be aimed at the bladder, urethra, ganglia, or peripheral nerves. **The main targets for drug therapy are receptors or ion channels known to be involved in bladder contraction** (e.g., muscarinic receptors, L-type calcium channels). More recently, research has been focused more on alternative neurotransmission and modulation of afferent signaling from the lower urinary tract.

Antimuscarinic Agents

These agents are the **gold standard in treatment of overactive bladders.** Muscarinic receptors are found in the human detrusor muscle, and bladder contractions are initiated by stimulation of these receptors with the release of acetylcholine from cholinergic nerves. The main action of antimuscarinics is on the M1 and M3 receptor subtypes, which are thought to be responsible for the pathogenesis of detrusor overactivity. Antimuscarinics, such as oxybutynin, **act by reducing the frequency and intensity of involuntary contractions, resulting in an increase in the functional bladder capacity.** The clinical efficacy depends on various factors, such as receptor affinity, pharmacokinetics, and the specificity for the bladder. Latest developments have focused on receptor specificity and the ratio of efficacy to side effects. **The nonselective pattern of activity and penetration of the blood-brain barrier are known to induce systemic and central side effects.**

α-Adrenergic Blockers

The body of the bladder receives relatively sparse innervation by noradrenergic nerves. The density of noradrenergic nerves increases markedly toward the bladder neck, where the smooth muscle receives a dense noradrenergic nerve supply, particularly in males. **The normal response to norepinephrine is relaxation of the detrusor and contraction of the bladder neck. α-Adrenergic blockers are therefore used in patients with evidence of bladder neck dysfunction for relaxation of the bladder neck.**

Other Medications

Tricyclic antidepressants such as imipramine have been found to be effective for increasing urine storage by both decreasing the detrusor contractility and increasing outlet resistance. However, the precise mechanism of action is not well explained. Their possible effect on the bladder outlet has been described by inhibition of norepinephrine reuptake producing α-adrenergic stimulation. These agents are associated with a high incidence of side effects, and their use should be judicious.

β-Adrenergic agonists can cause significant increases in bladder capacity but can also cause significant cardiovascular side effects.

Parasympathicomimetics, calcium antagonists, potassium channel openers, and prostaglandin inhibitors have all been described for use with effect on the bladder, but these are rarely used in children, either owing to their unfavorable side effects or to a lack of proven efficacy.

Clean Intermittent Catheterization

Clean intermittent catheterization may become necessary in children with decompensated bladders or lazy bladder syndrome where bladder emptying efficiency is compromised and upper urinary tract dilatation may exist. Regular emptying of the bladder to achieve low-pressure emptying improves detrusor contractility and bladder emptying function. Therefore, a regular clean intermittent catheterization program can allow for bladder retraining. Some of these children may be able to eventually be weaned from use of this procedure.

Surgery

When conservative management with nonpharmacologic and pharmacologic treatment fails, surgical approaches may need to be considered. **Bladder augmentation may be performed to help produce a low-pressure system with increased bladder capacity.** Augmentation may be performed using intestinal segments such as colon, ileum, or stomach. However, the complications that may ensue must be considered, including mucus production, electrolyte imbalance, and even possible metaplasia/malignancy.

Surgical means have also been employed to reduce urethral/sphincteric pressure as an alternative to α-adrenergic blockers. Recent studies have focused on the use of balloon dilatation of the bladder neck and botulinum A toxin injection into the urethral urinary sphincter in children with non-neuropathic bladder-sphincter dysfunction with very promising results. However, these methods seem to require repeated attempts and the long-term effect and efficacy have yet to be presented.

NOCTURNAL ENURESIS
Etiologic Factors

Primary nocturnal enuresis is a common disorder among children. Despite extensive research there is still significant controversy regarding its etiology, and it is now generally accepted that multiple pathologic factors are probably involved. Among others, a common finding is that the nocturnal urine output in many enuretic children is in excess of the bladder reservoir capacity during sleep at night (Nørgaard et al, 1985; Hjalmas, 1997, 1998). **Nocturnal polyuria can be either absolute, which is usually associated with a derangement of the circadian rhythm of antidiuretic hormone secretion, or relative, due mainly to a reduced functional bladder capacity during sleep at night.** However, whether it is an increased urine pro-

duction or a reduced bladder capacity that results in the mismatch between nocturnal bladder capacity and the amount of urine produced during sleep at night there must be a simultaneous arousal failure in response to bladder fullness before bedwetting can occur.

Bladder-Sphincter Dysfunction

The exact role of bladder dysfunction in the pathogenesis of primary nocturnal enuresis has until recently remained largely controversial. Whereas some workers have observed markedly reduced functional bladder capacities among enuretic children compared with age-matched nonenuretic controls, others have previously reported that enuretic episodes were triggered by a full bladder and that bladder capacities in the enuretic chil-

VOIDING CYSTOMETRY—PEDIATRIC #5

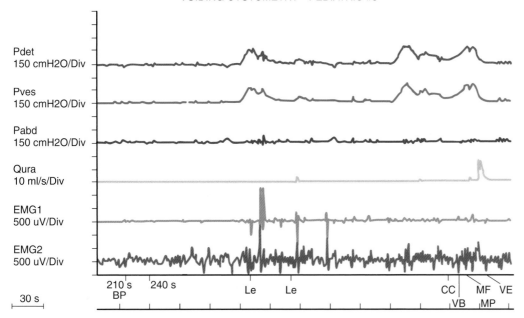
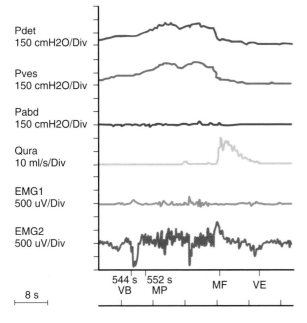

Figure 123–13. Urodynamic tracing showing primary bladder neck dysfunction characterized by a marked delay in initiation of flow after onset of detrusor contraction, often associated with high detrusor pressure but minimal pelvic EMG activities.

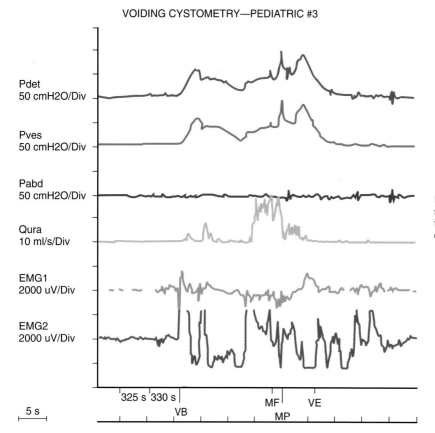

VOIDING CYSTOMETRY—PEDIATRIC #3

Pdet
50 cmH2O/Div

Pves
50 cmH2O/Div

Pabd
50 cmH2O/Div

Qura
10 ml/s/Div

EMG1
2000 uV/Div

EMG2
2000 uV/Div

325 s 330 s   MF VE
VB   MP

5 s

Figure 123–14. Urodynamic tracing showing detrusor-sphincter dyssynergia characterized by marked staccato or interrupted voiding, often associated with DO and/or evidences of increased EMG activities.

dren were completely normal (Starfield, 1967; Nørgaard, 1989; Jarvelin et al, 1990). Recent studies have, however, very convincingly proven that in a **significant proportion of children with severe nocturnal enuresis, especially those who were refractory to conservative treatment and failed to respond to desmopressin therapy, there was a marked reduction in functional bladder capacities when compared with age-matched normal controls** (Watanabe, 1994; Kirk et al, 1995; Rushton et al, 1996; Eller et al, 1998; Yeung et al, 1999). Furthermore, it has been shown that other types of bladder dysfunctions, notably dysfunctional voiding, bladder instability, and marked detrusor hypercontractility with extremely high voiding pressures suggestive of an obstructive pattern are not uncommon among enuretic children (Yeung et al, 1999). More recently, it has been shown on urodynamics that 73% of adults with primary nocturnal enuresis had some form of functional bladder outflow obstruction classified as (1) primary bladder neck dysfunction (Fig. 123–13), (2) detrusor-sphincter dyssynergia (Fig. 123–14), and (3) dysfunctional voiding (Fig. 123–15) (Yeung et al, 2004).

Sleep Arousal Disturbance and Brain Stem Dysfunction

More recently, the involvement of the central nervous system in the etiology of childhood nocturnal enuresis has been assessed. **Enuretic boys were shown to be more difficult to arouse than age-matched controls. The arousal inability in patients with nocturnal enuresis may relate to either elevated arousal thresholds or the presence of spontaneous uninhibited bladder contractions.**

There is also cumulating evidence that a small functional bladder capacity and detrusor overactivity may play an important role in the pathophysiology of nocturnal enuresis and can further provide reliable predictive clues to the treatment response. Most interestingly, **overnight studies in enuretic children with simultaneous sleep electroencephalographic and cystometry have revealed marked detrusor instability only after sleep at night but not during wakeful periods during the day** (Watanabe et al, 1994; Yeung et al, 1999). This can result in a marked reduction in the nocturnal functional bladder capacity (Watanabe et al, 1994; Rushton et al, 1996; Eller et al, 1998; Yeung et al, 1999). Because this pattern has not been observed in normal non-enuretic subjects even during the newborn period, one may hypothesize that this could be due to a small neurologic lesion affecting a tiny area surrounding the vicinity of the pontine micturition center, the posterior hypothalamus (responsible for secretion of antidiuretic hormone), and the locus coeruleus (which is thought to play an important role in the initiation of cortical arousal and release of norepinephrine) (Yeung et al, 1995a, 1998, 1999).

Despite the high prevalence of underlying bladder dysfunction among patients with severe, refractory primary nocturnal enuresis, many have no identifiable day-time urinary symptoms, including incontinence, frequency, and urgency. A detailed urodynamic study would, however, reveal detrusor instability in 30% to 90% of patients. Our experience has shown that many enuretic children with reduced functional bladder capacity have learned, either consciously but more probably subconsciously, to restrain fluid intake during the day as an attempt to avoid the social inconvenience of urinary

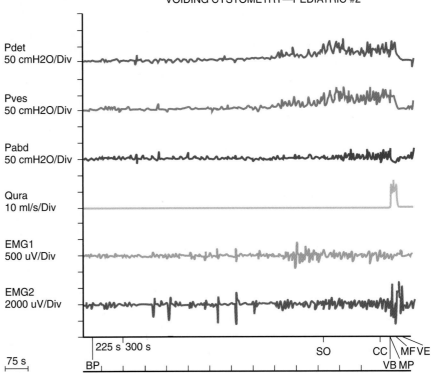

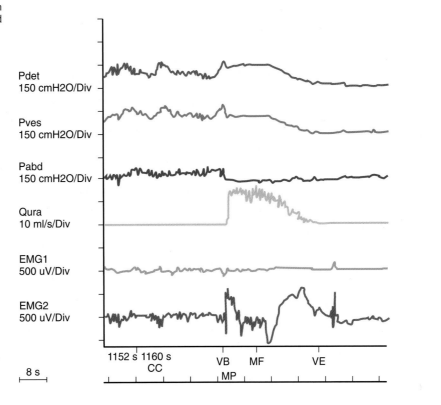

Figure 123–15. Urodynamic tracing showing dysfunctional voiding characterized by abdominal/pelvic straining (holding maneuver) immediately prior to initiation of micturition, often associated with DO and evidence of increased pelvic EMG activities.

frequency and urge incontinence. This could often be easily spotted by a detailed home-recorded voiding diary by an extraordinarily low fluid intake and infrequent, small volume voiding. By giving these patients a standard fluid intake and then asking them to repeat a home recording of micturition frequency and urinary volume, one could quite easily obtain a highly reliable estimation of the functional bladder capacity and hence identify those patients with reduced bladder capacities (Rittig et al, 1997; Yeung et al, 1999).

Relationship between Bladder and Brain Dysfunctions (The Bladder-Brain Dialogue)

Previous studies on nocturnal enuresis have shown elevated auditory awakening theshold and sensory gating dysfunction in patients. As micturition, sleep/arousal, and information processing share a common neural pathway in brain stem-thalamus-cortex reticular ascending system, it is postulated that a relationship exists between brain and bladder function. More recent studies further support this. A deficiency of prepulse inhibition of startle has been reported in enuretic children such that prestimulation 120 ms before the main stimulus resulted in significantly less inhibition of the blink reflex among enuretic children than in healthy controls. Prepulse inhibition is based on an inhibition of the startle pathway by the pedunculopontine tegmental nucleus, which lies in close proximity to the pontine micturition center in the brain stem. It has been postulated that a deficient prepulse inhibition and reduced ability to inhibit micturition during sleep might both originate from a common dysfunction in the pontine tegmentum. This suggests that a relationship may exist between nocturnal bladder function and brain stem functions in humans (Ornitz et al, 1999, 2000; Diao et al, 2005).

Furthermore, it has also been shown that after successful treatment of nocturnal enuresis in these children both the sleep arousal threshold and the prepulse inhibition of startle improved. This suggests that the brain stem dysfunction may be a secondary effect to the underlying bladder dysfunction, further supporting the "bladder-brain dialogue" concept whereby there is a bidirectional communication between the bladder and the brain.

SUMMARY

Despite extensive clinical and animal research, it is perhaps embarrassing to admit that the exact neurologic mechanisms of the development of micturition control from newborn to infancy and later childhood, as well as the pathophysiologic pathways that are involved in various types of bladder dysfunction, have as yet remained largely unclear. It is, however, certain that the bladder and the brain "talk" with each other all the time as early as in the fetus and that there are extremely rapid and extensive changes and modulation of micturition reflexes during the early postnatal period, leading to copious potentials for developmental errors and voiding dysfunctions. Over the past decade we have learned that both normal as well as abnormal bladder function is much more dynamic than we had previously believed. New investigative tools and research

have allowed us to study in much greater detail and precision the various components, including neurologic, muscular, urodynamic and hormonal mechanisms, that may intricately interact to produce different patterns of bladder dysfunctions and their relentless, dynamic changes.

KEY POINTS: NON-NEUROPATHIC DYSFUNCTION OF LOWER URINARY TRACT

- The bladder has dual function (storing and emptying) as well as dual innervation (central somatic and autonomic nervous systems).
- There is evidence that micturition is modulated by higher neural centers even in full-term fetuses and newborns and that micturition almost always occurs during wakefulness.
- In the transition from an infantile to adult bladder, detrusor-sphincteric discoordination may be a normal transient phenomenon that resolves after toilet training.
- The natural evolution of micturition control involves the gradual increase in functional bladder capacity, maturation of detrusor-sphincter coordination, and progressive development of voluntary control over the whole bladder-sphincteric-perineal complex.
- Bladder dysfunctions during filling include overactive bladders, urge syndrome, functional urinary incontinence, and giggle incontinence.
- Bladder dysfunctions during emptying include dysfunctional voiding, staccato voiding, infrequent voiding, Hinman syndrome, Ochoa syndrome, and postvoid dribbling.
- It is now well recognized that dysfunctional voiding often has associated bowel dysfunction and together this is known as the dysfunctional elimination syndrome.
- Vesicoureteral reflux may be secondary to underlying bladder dysfunction, particularly in girls. Treatment should aim at correcting the voiding dysfunction before contemplating surgery.
- A significant proportion of children with severe nocturnal enuresis have marked reduction in functional bladder capacities.
- The majority of patients with nocturnal enuresis are found to have underlying bladder dysfunction.
- Studies have shown that brain stem dysfunction may be related and secondary to underlying bladder dysfunction in patients with nocturnal enuresis.
- Treatment may consist of behavioral modification, standard urotherapy, biofeedback, pelvic floor rehabilitation, neuromodulation, bowel management, drug therapy, and/or surgery.

SUGGESTED READINGS

Harrison SCW, Abrams P: Bladder function. In Sant GR (ed): Pathophysiologic Principles of Urology. London, Blackwell Scientific Publications, 1994, pp 93-121.

Hjalmas K, Arnold T, Bower W, et al: Nocturnal enuresis: An international evidence based management strategy [Review Article]. J Urol 2004;171: 2545-2561.

Koff SA, Wagner TT, Jayanthi VR: The relationship among dysfunctional elimination syndromes, primary vesicoureteral reflux and urinary tract infections in children. J Urol 1998;160:1019-1022.

Nørgaard JP, van Gool JD, Hjalmas K, et al: Standardization and definitions in lower urinary tract dysfunction in children. International Children's Continence Society. Br J Urol 1998;81(Suppl 3):1-16.

Yeung CK: The normal infant bladder. Scand J Urol Nephrol Suppl 1995;173:19-23.

Yeung CK: Pathophysiology of bladder dysfunction. In Gearhart JP, Rink RC, Mouriquand PDE (eds): Pediatric Urology. Philadelphia, WB Saunders, 2001, pp 453-469.

Yeung CK, Godley ML, Ho CKW, et al: Some new insights into bladder function in infancy. Br J Urol 1995;6:235-240.

Neuropathic Dysfunction of the Lower Urinary Tract

STUART B. BAUER, MD

URODYNAMIC EVALUATION

NEUROSPINAL DYSRAPHISMS

CENTRAL NERVOUS SYSTEM INSULTS

At least 25% of the clinical problems seen in pediatric urology are the result of neurologic lesions that affect lower urinary tract function. As pediatric urology developed in the latter half of the 20th century, urinary diversion initially was the mainstay of treatment for these children with either intractable incontinence or normal or abnormal upper urinary tracts (Smith, 1972). The advent of clean intermittent catheterization (CIC) in the early 1970s by Lapides and associates (1972), refinements in techniques of urodynamic studies in children (Gierup and Ericsson, 1970; Blaivas et al, 1977; Blaivas, 1979), and the development of surgical modalities in conjunction with CIC to manage incontinence dramatically changed the way this group of children was traditionally managed. Along with this change came a greater understanding of the pathophysiology of the many diseases that affect children primarily. With the increased reliability of data collection, the applicability of urodynamic testing expanded so much that most pediatric urologic centers consider functional assessment of the lower urinary tract an integral element in the evaluation process and as important as radiographic visualization in characterizing and managing these abnormal conditions (McGuire et al, 1981; Bauer et al, 1984). The natural outcome of early functional investigation has been the advocacy of proactive or early aggressive management in the children who are at risk for urinary tract deterioration based on specific hostile urodynamic parameters (Perez et al, 1992; Edelstein et al, 1995; Kaufman et al, 1996). This has resulted in (1) a statistically significant decrease in upper urinary tract deterioration, compared with those children followed expectantly in the past, and (2) a dramatic

reduction in the need for augmentation cystoplasty (Wu et al, 1997; Kaefer et al, 1999; Bauer, 2000). Furthermore, there is now evidence that molecular changes occur intracellularly when prophylactic treatment is begun as early as possible (Park et al, 1999; Ohnishi et al, 2000). Because urodynamic testing has become such an integral part of any discussion of the subject, this chapter first defines the testing process as it applies to children, outlines its pitfalls and advantages, and then elaborates on the various neurologic abnormalities that are prevalent in children. For purposes of minimizing ambiguity the terminology used in this chapter is based on the International Continence Society (ICS) standardization of terminology documents (Abrams et al, 2002; Abrams et al, 2003).

URODYNAMIC EVALUATION

Before a urodynamic study is performed, it is important for the child and the family to have full knowledge of the procedure. Therefore, an explanation of the test and a questionnaire are sent to each family before the appointment. A booklet is provided so that parents will know what to expect and can explain the test to their child, or the child can read about it if he or she is old enough. Attempts are made to minimize anxiety in children who are able to understand what will happen by providing reasons for specific portions of the test and explaining exactly what the child will experience. The questionnaire tries to elicit information about the mother's pregnancy history, the child's birth and development, his or her current bladder and bowel habits, and any other information that might be pertinent at the time of the procedure.

Rarely is any premedication given either orally or intramuscularly, but the child is conscientiously attended to in order to minimize his or her fears. Parents are instructed to make sure the child has a bowel movement the night before the study. If the child is on a bowel management program, it is administered the night before. If no specific program is adhered to, either an oral or rectal cathartic is given the evening before. EMLA cream, a topical anesthetic, is applied to the perineum about 45 minutes before the electromyography (EMG) needle is inserted to record sphincter activity. If possible, the child is instructed to come to the urodynamic suite with a full bladder to obtain an initial representative uroflow. The time of the child's previous urination (or catheterization) is noted to calculate an average rate of urine production per unit of time. In addition, this information allows the nurse to record a reliable residual urine volume when catheterizing the child after voiding. The flowmeter is located in a private bathroom that contains a one-way mirror so that voiding can be viewed unobtrusively. This allows the investigator to see what position the child assumes and whether a Credé or a Valsalva maneuver is employed by the child to help empty the bladder.

Next, the nurse reviews the test and shows the child all the equipment in an attempt to make the patient feel as comfortable as possible. The child is catheterized with either a No. 7 Fr or a No. 11 Fr triple-lumen urodynamic catheter (Cook Urological Inc, Spencer, IN)—the smaller, the better—after a small amount of liquid lidocaine (Xylocaine) (1%) has been injected into the urethra and held in place for a moment or two. First, the intravesicular pressure is recorded. Then the bladder is drained and the residual urine is carefully measured, yielding a pressure at residual volume (Kaefer et al, 1997a). Sometimes it is necessary to aspirate the catheter to get accurate information on the volume of residual urine, especially if the bladder is underactive (particularly if the child is taking anticholinergic medication) or has been previously augmented and secretes mucus (because it may not drain completely after insertion of a catheter).

A small balloon catheter is passed into the rectum at this time to measure intra-abdominal pressure during the cystometrogram to identify artifacts of motion and monitor increases in abdominal pressure during the filling and emptying phases of the study (Bates et al, 1970; Bauer, 1979). Having an empty rectal vault helps maintain the catheter in place. Detrusor overactivity and straining to empty can be clearly differentiated by this maneuver.

Before the bladder is filled, a urethral pressure profile is sometimes obtained by infusing saline through the side-hole channel at a rate of 2 mL/min as the catheter is withdrawn at a rate of 2 mm/s (Yalla et al, 1980). Another way of determining maximal urethral closure pressure is by measuring the leak point pressure at various stages of bladder filling as well as with a bladder contraction or Valsalva maneuver (Ghoniem et al, 1990; Homma et al, 1999). When the maximum resistance is known, the catheter is positioned so that the urethral pressure port is located at that or any other point of interest. This area can then be monitored throughout the urodynamic study.

Urethral pressure profilometry (UPP) measures the passive resistance of a particular point within the urethra to stretch (Gleason et al, 1974). Many factors contribute to this resistance, including the elastic properties of the tissues surrounding the lumen and the tension generated by the smooth and skeletal muscles of the urethra, which are constantly changing during the micturition cycle (Fig. 123–16) (Abrams, 1979; Evans et al, 1979). Therefore, the static urethral pressure profile is a measure of resistance in a specific set of circumstances (Yalla et al, 1979). It is difficult to extrapolate data obtained when the bladder is empty and apply it to periods when the bladder is full, is responding to increases in abdom-

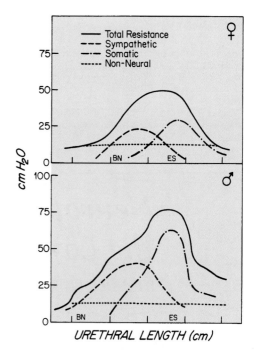

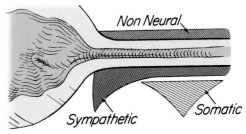

Figure 123–16. Components of urethral wall tension according to their geographic distribution and effect along the urethra in males and females. BN, bladder neck; ES, external sphincter. (From Bauer SB: Urodynamic evaluation and neuromuscular dysfunction. In Kelalis PP, Kin LR, Belman AB [eds]: Clinical Pediatric Urology, 2nd ed. Philadelphia, WB Saunders, 1985, vol 1, pp 283-310.)

inal pressure, or is in the process of emptying (Fig. 123–17). Failure to recognize this fact leads to false assumptions and improper treatment. For these reasons many centers have eliminated urethral pressure measurements in favor of monitoring detrusor leak point pressure (the subtracted detrusor pressure at which the child leaks when the bladder is filled to its functional or maximal capacity).

External urethral sphincter EMG is performed using a 24-gauge concentric needle electrode (Diokno et al, 1974; Blaivas et al, 1977b) inserted perineally in boys or paraurethrally in girls and advanced into the skeletal muscle component of the sphincter until individual motor unit action potentials are seen or heard on a standard EMG recorder. Alternatively, perineal electrodes (Maizels and Firlit, 1979) or abdominal patch electrodes (Koff and Kass, 1982) have been used to record the bioelectric activity in the sphincter muscle. Disagreements exist concerning the accuracy of these surface electrode measurements, compared with those obtained with needle electrodes, particularly during voiding. The intactness of sacral spinal cord function is easily measured with needle electrodes by (1) looking at the characteristic waveform of individual

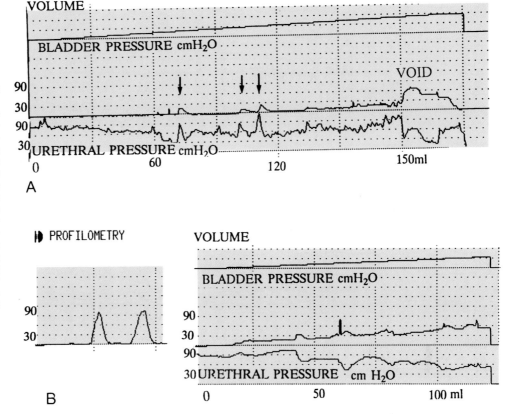

Figure 123–17. **A,** Urodynamic study in an 8-year-old boy with enuresis with the urethral pressure profilometry (UPP) port of the multichannel urodynamic catheter positioned in the mid urethra. Note that urethral resistance is adequate at the start of filling but that it decreases just before and then increases with each uninhibited contraction (arrows). At capacity, the resistance is very high but then it equals bladder pressure during voiding. **B,** A 7-year-old girl with myelomeningocele has a very good level of resistance when UPP is performed initially. During bladder filling, with the catheter positioned in the mid urethra, urethral resistance drops from 90 to 58 cm H_2O at capacity.

motor unit action potentials when the patient is relaxed and the bladder is empty, (2) performing and recording the responses to bulbocavernosus and anal stimulation and to Credé and Valsalva maneuvers, (3) asking the patient to voluntarily contract and relax the external sphincter, and (4) seeing the reaction of the sphincter to filling and emptying of the bladder (Fig. 123–18) (Blaivas et al, 1977a; Blaivas, 1979b).

The rate of bladder filling per minute is selected by first calculating the child's predicted or known capacity and then dividing the result by 10 in order to fill the bladder slowly. The average capacity in milliliters for a child older than 2 years of age is determined by adding 6 to half of the child's age in years and multiplying the result by 30; for children under 2 years, it is determined by adding 2 to twice the child's age and multiplying the result by 30 (Kaefer et al, 1997b). In children with myelodysplasia, the average bladder capacity fits the following formula: 24.5 × age in years + 62 (Palmer et al, 1997). It has been shown that more rapid filling rates may yield falsely low levels of detrusor compliance and may minimize an overactive detrusor (Turner-Warwick 1975; Joseph, 1992). In an attempt to avoid this problem, the bladder is filled slowly with saline warmed to 37° C (Chin-Peuckert et al, 2004). When it is important to determine very mild degrees of a poorly compliant detrusor, even slower rates of filling are used to measure its true incidence (Kerr et al, 1994; Yeung et al, 1995; Zermann et al, 1997). Some investigators have recorded pressure at residual volume to measure natural filling pressure as the most accurate means of denoting poor compliance (Kaefer et al, 1997a; Walter et al, 1998). During filling, it is helpful to try to divert the child's attention by asking unrelated questions,

reading a story aloud, or showing a movie or cartoon. If the examiner wishes to elicit detrusor overactivity, the child is asked to cough (Mayo, 1978); alternatively, a cold solution may be instilled at a rapid rate.

The study is not considered complete until the child urinates and voiding pressures are measured in those children who urinate on their own. The small size of the urodynamic catheter does not seem to affect micturition pressures adversely, even in very young children. The normal voiding pressure varies from 55 to 80 cm H_2O in boys and from 30 to 65 cm H_2O in girls (Blaivas et al, 1977b; Blaivas, 1979a; Gierup et al, 1979). Infants tend to have higher voiding pressures than older children. Sometimes it is difficult to get the child to void; patience and time are needed in this situation. Placing a bedpan under the buttocks of the child who is supine or dripping tepid water on the genital area often stimulates the child sufficiently to begin urinating. Having the child listen to the audio channel of the EMG amplifier machine while he or she tightens and/or relaxes the sphincter provides a means of biofeedback training to get the child to void. Once the child has voided, it is important to do the following:

- Analyze the pressure curve to determine whether the contraction is sustained until voiding is complete.
- Determine whether abdominal pressure has been used to facilitate the emptying process.
- Listen to changes in EMG activity of the sphincter to determine whether it remained quiet throughout the voiding process.
- Note whether the flow rate curve was bell shaped, intermittent, or prolonged.
- Measure the voided volume.

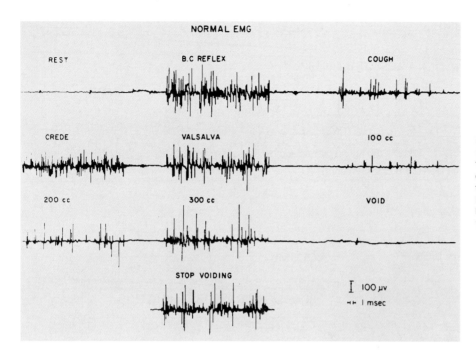

Figure 123–18. Normal reaction of the external urethral sphincter on electromyogram to all the sacral reflexes and to bladder filling and emptying. (From Bauer SB: Urodynamic evaluation and neuromuscular dysfunction. In Kelalis PP, Kin LR, Belman AB [eds]: Clinical Pediatric Urology, 2nd ed. Philadelphia, WB Saunders, 1985, vol 1, pp 283-310.)

- Calculate whether the patient voided to completion.
- Observe whether an after-contraction occurred.

Video-urodynamics has gained popularity since its introduction in 1970 (Bates et al, 1970). Visualization of the bladder and bladder neck during filling and of the urethra during voiding has added a dimension for more accurately integrating all aspects of lower urinary tract function and characterizing an abnormality (Glazier et al, 1997). Incompetency of the bladder neck or pelvic floor or the location of any posterior urethral obstruction can be correlated with pressure measurements and external urethral sphincter EMG activity recorded simultaneously (Zerin et al, 1990). Sometimes, aberrations noted on pressure monitoring of sphincter EMG tracings can be confirmed, enhancing these findings (Passerini-Glazel et al, 1992; Weerasinghe and Malone, 1993). Ambulatory urodynamics has become available and feasible in children with the development of microtransducers mounted on small catheters positioned in the bladder (McInerney et al, 1991; Kulseng-Hanssen and Klevmark, 1996). Data can be stored up to 24 hours at a time and analyzed later. When combined with techniques to monitor wetness, it can be a very effective way to determine the cause of incontinence (Webb et al, 1991). There are many difficulties and artifacts inherent with this technique (Heslington and Hilton, 1996), but over time it may provide the most accurate way to evaluate lower urinary tract function in a natural setting (Bristow and Neal, 1996).

Often, because it is appropriate to see the effects of drug administration, studies are repeated under similar circumstances several weeks to months later. This is especially true when one is trying to treat poor detrusor compliance or overactivity medically. To determine the maximal effect, the usual dose of most drugs is taken 2 to 3 hours before the test is performed a second time. The most commonly used drugs that affect lower urinary tract function are listed in Table 123–1, along with their appropriate dose ranges.

Table 123–1. Drugs That Affect Lower Urinary Tract Function

Type	Dosage	
	Minimum	Maximum
Cholinergic		
Bethanechol (Urecholine)	0.7 mg/kg tid	0.8 mg/kg qid
Anticholinergic		
Propantheline (Pro-Banthine)	0.5 mg/kg bid	0.5 mg/kg qid
Oxybutynin (Ditropan)	0.2 mg/kg bid	0.2 mg/kg qid
Glycopyrrolate (Robinul)	0.01 mg/kg bid	0.03 mg/kg tid
Hyoscyamine (Levsin)	0.03 mg/kg bid	0.1 mg/kg tid
Tolterodine (Detrol)	0.01 mg/kg bid	0.04 mg/kg bid
Sympathomimetic		
Phenylpropanolamine (alpha)	2.5 mg/kg tid	2.5 mg/kg qid
Ephedrine (alpha)	0.5 mg/kg tid	1.0 mg/kg tid
Pseudoephedrine (alpha)	0.4 mg/kg bid	0.9 mg/kg tid
Sympatholytic		
Prazosin (alpha) (Minipress)	0.05 mg/kg bid	0.1 mg/kg tid
Phenoxybenzamine (alpha)	0.3 mg/kg bid	0.5 mg/kg tid
Propranolol (beta)	0.25 mg/kg bid	0.5 mg/kg bid
Smooth muscle relaxant		
Flavoxate (Urispas)	3.0 mg/kg bid	3.0 mg/kg bid
Dicyclomine (Bentyl)	0.1 mg/kg tid	0.3 mg/kg tid
Other		
Imipramine (Tofranil)	0.7 mg/kg bid	1.2 mg/kg tid

NEUROSPINAL DYSRAPHISMS
Myelodysplasia

The most common cause of neurogenic bladder dysfunction in children is abnormal development of the spinal canal and internecine spinal cord. Formation of the spinal cord and vertebral column begins at about the 18th day of gestation. Closure of the canal proceeds in a caudal direction from the cephalad end and is complete by 35 days. The exact mechanism that results in closure and what produces a dysraphic state are yet to be elucidated, but numerous factors have been implicated. The incidence was reported as 1 per 1000 births in the United States (Stein et al, 1982), but there has been a definite decrease in this rate in the past 20 years (Laurence, 1989; Lary and Edmonds, 1996; CDC, 2004; Williams et al, 2005). With the advent of prenatal screening, many affected fetuses are being identified and the pregnancies terminated before 16 weeks of gestation, thereby lowering the number of children born with this disease (Palomaki et al, 1999). If spina bifida is already present in one member of a family, there is a 2% to 5% chance that a second sibling will be conceived with the same condition (Scarff and Fronczak, 1981). The incidence doubles when more than one family member has a neurospinal dysraphism (Table 123–2). Therefore, when the disease is already present in a family, the Medical Research Council Vitamin Study Group recommends that women of childbearing age take 4000 µg (4.0 mg) of folic acid per day beginning at least 2 months before the time they plan on becoming pregnant (Committee on Genetics, American Academy of Pediatrics, 1999). There is strong evidence that folate deficiency can lead to a myelodysplastic abnormality de novo; therefore, maternal ingestion of 400 µg of folate per day in all women of child-bearing age can reduce the incidence of spina bifida by 50% (Laurence et al, 1981; MRC Vitamin Study Research Group, 1991; Czeizel and Dudas, 1992; Centers for Disease Control and Prevention, 2004). It is now mandatory that enriched grain products be fortified with folic acid (U.S. Food and Drug Administration, 1996). Since these recommendations have been followed worldwide, there has been a reduction in neural tube defects in the United States (Williams et al, 2005) and elsewhere (Botto et al, 2005). In some cases, however, despite increased folic acid intake, women may still give birth to a child with spina bifida owing to antibodies that have developed in response to the increased folate ingestion, thus negating its salutary effect (Rothenberg et al, 2004).

Pathogenesis

Myelodysplasia is an all-inclusive term used to describe the various abnormal conditions of the vertebral column that affect spinal cord function. More specific labels for each abnormality include the following: a *meningocele* occurs when just the meninges but no neural elements extend beyond the confines of the vertebral canal; in a *myelomeningocele,* neural tissue, either nerve roots or portions of the spinal cord, has evaginated with the meningocele (Fig. 123–19); the term *lipomyelomeningocele* denotes that fatty tissue has developed with the cord structures and both are extending with the

Table 123–2. Familial Risk of Myelodysplasia in the United States per 1000 Live Births	
Relationship	*Incidence*
General population	0.7–1.0
Mother with one affected child	20–50
Mother with two affected children	100
Patient with myelodysplasia	40
Mother older than 35 years	30
Sister of mother with affected child	10
Sister of father with affected child	3
Nephew who is affected	2

protruding sac. **Myelomeningocele accounts for more than 90% of all open spinal dysraphic states** (Stark, 1977). Most spinal defects occur at the level of the lumbar vertebrae, with the sacral, thoracic, and cervical areas, in decreasing order of frequency, less affected (Bauer et al, 1977) (Table 123–3). An overwhelming number of meningoceles are directed posteriorly, but on rare occasions they may protrude anteriorly, particularly in the sacral area. Usually the meningocele is made up of a flimsy covering of transparent tissue, but it may be open and leaking cerebrospinal fluid. For this reason urgent

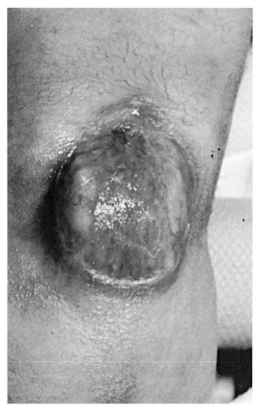

Figure 123–19. Typical appearance of a newborn with an open myelomeningocele.

Table 123–3.	**Spinal Level of Myelomeningocele**
Location	**Incidence (%)**
Cervical–high thoracic	2
Low thoracic	5
Lumbar	26
Lumbosacral	47
Sacral	20

repair is necessary, with sterile precautions being followed in the interval between birth and closure. In 85% of affected children, there is an associated Arnold-Chiari malformation, in which the cerebellar tonsils have herniated down through the foramen magnum, obstructing the fourth ventricle and preventing the cerebrospinal fluid from entering the subarachnoid space surrounding the brain and spinal cord.

In the past several years, several centers in the United States have begun closing the defect in fetuses between 19 and 25 weeks of gestation in an attempt to improve the neurologic defect in these children (Adzick et al, 1998; Bruner et al, 1999; Holzbeierlein et al, 2000). Thus far, this procedure has not altered the incidence of abnormal findings in the lower extremities (Farmer et al, 2003) or on urodynamic assessment in the postnatal period (Koh et al, 2003), but, surprisingly, aqueduct obstruction and, consequently, hydrocephalus has not occurred at birth to the same incidence or extent (Johnson et al, 2003). **It is possible that leakage of cerebrospinal fluid from the open spinal column accounts for herniation of the posterior brain stem down the foramen magnum, leading to the development of hydrocephalus.**

The neurologic lesion produced by this condition can be variable, depending on what neural elements, if any, have everted with the meningocele sac. The bony vertebral level often provides little or no clue to the exact neurologic level or lesion produced. The height of the bony level may differ from the highest extent of the neurologic lesion for one to three vertebrae in either direction (Bauer et al, 1977). Furthermore, there may be differences in function from one side of the body to the other at the same neurologic level and from one neurologic level to the next owing to asymmetry of the affected neural elements. It is important to remember that no two children have the same neurourologic defect. In addition, in 20% of affected children a vertebral bony or intraspinal abnormality occurs more cephalad than the vertebral defect and meningocele, and this can affect function in those portions of the cord. Children with thoracic or upper lumbar meningoceles often have complete reconstitution of the spine in the sacral area, and these individuals frequently have intact sacral reflex arc function involving the sacral spinal roots (in our series of patients with high-level lesions, 74% of newborns and 54% of older children were affected thusly) (Pontari et al, 1995). In fact, it is more likely that children with upper thoracic or cervical lesions will have just a meningocele and no myelomeningocele. Children with neurologic deficits at S1 or lower may also manifest a variety of findings on urodynamic testing, ranging from normal function to upper and/or lower motor neuron lesions involving either the bladder and/or the external urethral sphincter (Dator et al, 1992). Approximately 10% of newborns with myelomeningocele exhibit no abnormality on urodynamic testing (Tarcan et al, 2001). Finally, the

differing growth rates of the vertebral bodies and the elongating spinal cord add a dynamic factor in the developing fetus that further confounds the picture (Lais et al, 1993). Twenty-four percent of children with normal lower urinary tract function at birth develop upper motor neuron changes over time (Tarcan et al, 2001). Superimposed on all this is the Arnold-Chiari malformation, which can have a profound effect on the brain stem and pontine mesencephalic center, areas that are involved in control of lower urinary tract function.

Therefore, **the neurologic lesion produced by this condition influences lower urinary tract function in a variety of ways and cannot be predicted just by looking at the spinal abnormality or the neurologic function of the lower extremities.** Even careful assessment of the sacral area may not provide sufficient information to make a concrete inference. As a result, urodynamic evaluation in the neonatal period is now the standard of care at most pediatric centers in the United States, because it not only provides a clear picture of the function of the sacral spinal cord and lower urinary tract but also has predictive value in infants at risk for future urinary tract deterioration and progressive neurologic change (McGuire et al, 1981; Van Gool et al, 1982; Bauer, 1984b; Sidi et al, 1986). The advent of hostility scores and the reliability of urodynamic risk factors has led many clinicians to initiate prophylactic therapy in those newborns considered to be at risk for urinary tract deterioration (Perez et al, 1992). There are some, however, who do not consider urodynamic testing an important factor but rely solely on physical examination and radiologic assessment to direct their decision-making process (Hopps and Kropp, 2003), a concept not shared by many.

Newborn Assessment

Ideally, it would be best to perform urodynamic testing immediately after the infant is born, but the risk of spinal infection and the exigency for closure have not made this a viable option. It was accomplished in one study, however, and the results showed that 1 in 30 children (3.2%) experienced a change in neurologic status as a result of the spinal canal closure (Kroovand et al, 1990). Therefore, **renal ultrasonography and measurement of residual urine are performed as early as possible after birth,** either before or immediately after the spinal defect is closed. Urodynamic studies are delayed until it is safe to transport the child to the urodynamic suite and place him or her on the back or side for the test. If the infant cannot empty the bladder after a spontaneous void or with a Credé maneuver, CIC is begun even before urodynamic studies are conducted. If the Credé maneuver is effective in emptying the bladder, it is performed on a regular basis instead of using CIC until the lower urinary tract can be fully evaluated. The normal bladder capacity in the newborn period is 10 to 15 mL; therefore, a residual urine of less than 5 mL is acceptable. Other tests that should be performed in the neonatal period include a urinalysis and culture, serum creatinine determination, and a careful neurologic examination of the lower extremities.

Once the spinal closure has healed sufficiently, a renal ultrasonogram and renal scan are performed to reassess upper urinary tract architecture and function. Next, voiding cystourethrography (VCUG) and urodynamic study are conducted. **These studies meet several objectives: they** provide baseline information about the radiologic appearance of the upper and lower urinary tracts as well as the condition of the sacral spinal cord and the central nervous system (CNS); they provide information that can be compared with findings on subsequent assessments, so that early signs of deterioration of urinary tract function and drainage, or of progressive neurologic denervation, can be detected; they help to identify infants at risk for urinary tract deterioration as a result of a poorly compliant or overactive detrusor or outflow obstruction from detrusor-sphincter dyssynergia (DSD), which predetermines the need to initiate prophylactic measures before any deterioration in upper urinary tract structure and function actually takes place; and they help the physician to counsel parents about the child's future bladder and sexual function (McGuire et al, 1981; Bauer et al, 1984; Bauer, 1984a; Sidi et al, 1986; Lais et al, 1993).

KEY POINTS: EVALUATION OF THE NEWBORN WITH NEUROGENIC BLADDER DYSFUNCTION

- Renal ultrasonography and measurement of residual urine are performed as early as possible after birth.

- Initial evaluation can be compared with findings on subsequent assessments, so that early signs of deterioration of urinary tract function and drainage, or of progressive neurologic denervation, can be detected.

- Infants at risk for urinary tract deterioration as a result of a poorly compliant or overactive detrusor or outflow obstruction from detrusor-sphincter dyssynergia need to be identified.

- This determines the need to initiate prophylactic measures before any deterioration in upper urinary tract structure and functions take place.

- Fifteen to 20 percent of newborns have an abnormal urinary tract on radiologic examination when first evaluated.

- Three categories of lower urinary tract dynamics may be detected: synergic (26%), dyssynergic with and without poor detrusor compliance (37%), and complete denervation (36%).

Findings

Fifteen to 20 percent of newborns have an abnormal urinary tract on radiologic examination when first evaluated (Bauer, 1985); 3% have hydroureteronephrosis secondary to spinal shock, probably from the spinal canal closure (Chiaramonte et al, 1986), and 15% have abnormalities that developed in utero as a result of abnormal lower urinary tract function in the form of outlet obstruction (Bauer, 2003).

Urodynamic studies in the newborn period have shown that 63% of infants have bladder contractions. This is also true for an equivalent number of children with upper lumbar

or thoracic lesions in whom the sacral spinal cord is spared, 50% of whom have detrusor overactivity (Pontari et al, 1995). Thirty-seven percent have a noncontractile detrusor with compliance during filling that is either good (20%) or poor (17%) in this subgroup (Bauer et al, 1984; Bauer, 2003). EMG assessment of the external urethral sphincter demonstrates an intact sacral reflex arc with no evidence of lower motor neuron denervation in 40% of newborns; partial denervation is seen in 24%; and complete loss of sacral cord function is noted in 36% (Lais et al, 1993; Bauer, 2003).

A combination of bladder contractility and external sphincter activity results in **three categories of lower urinary tract dynamics: synergic (26%), dyssynergic with and without poor detrusor compliance (37%), and complete denervation (36%)** (Fig. 123–20) (Bauer et al, 1984; Sidi et al, 1986; Bauer, 2003). DSD occurs when the external sphincter fails to decrease or actually increases its activity during a detrusor contraction or a sustained increase in intravesical pressure as the bladder is filled to capacity (Blaivas et al, 1986). Frequently, a poorly compliant bladder with high intravesical pressure occurs in conjunction with dyssynergic sphincter, resulting in a bladder that empties only at high intravesical pressure (Van Gool et al, 1982; Sidi et al, 1986). Synergy is characterized by complete silencing of the sphincter during a detrusor contraction or when capacity is reached at the end of filling. Voiding pressures are usually within the normal range. Complete denervation is noted when no bioelectric potentials are detectable in the region of the external sphincter at any time during the micturition cycle or in response to sacral stimulation or a Credé maneuver.

The categorization of lower urinary tract function in this way has been extremely useful because it reveals which children are at risk for urinary tract changes, who should be treated prophylactically, who need close surveillance, and who can be monitored at greater intervals. Within the first 3 years of life, 71% of newborns with DSD had urinary tract deterioration on initial assessment or subsequent studies, whereas only 17% of synergic children and 23% of completely denervated individuals developed similar changes (Fig. 123–21). The infants in the synergic group who showed deterioration did so only after they converted to a dyssynergic pattern of sphincter function. Among the infants with complete denervation, the ones who showed deterioration were those who had increased levels of urethral resistance, presumably caused by fibrosis of the skeletal muscle component of the external sphincter. Therefore, it appears that outlet obstruction is a major contributor to the development of urinary tract deterioration in these children (Fig. 123–22). Poor detrusor compliance plays an important role in this regard, especially when outlet resistance exceeds 40 cm H_2O (McGuire et al, 1981; Landau et al, 1994; Tanaka et al, 1999). Detrusor compliance seems to be worse in children with high levels of outlet resistance (Ghoniem et al, 1989). Bloom and colleagues (1990) and then Park and associates (2001) noted an improvement in compliance when outlet resistance was reduced after gentle urethral dilation in these children; however, the reasons for this change are unclear, and the long-term effect of this maneuver on ultimate continence and lower urinary tract function remains uncertain.

It may be that detrusor filling pressures need to be looked at in a more critical way to determine whether they are an

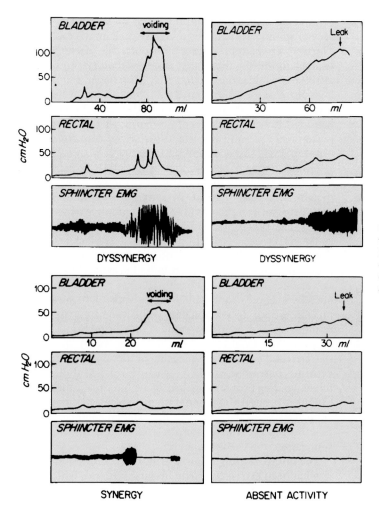

Figure 123–20. Various patterns of urodynamic findings on electromyography (EMG) in newborns with myelodysplasia. Note that a hypertonic detrusor with a nonrelaxing sphincter is also labeled dyssynergy. (From Bauer SB: Early evaluation and management of children with spina bifida. In King LR [ed]: Urologic Surgery in Neonates and Young Infants. Philadelphia, WB Saunders, 1988, pp 252–264.)

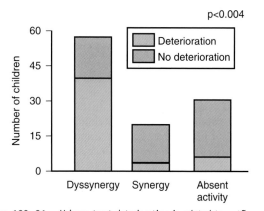

Figure 123–21. Urinary tract deterioration is related to outflow obstruction and is most often associated with dyssynergy. Children with synergy converted to dyssynergy, and patients with complete denervation developed fibrosis with a fixed high outlet resistance in the external sphincter, before any changes occurred in the urinary tract. (From Bauer SB: Early evaluation and management of children with spina bifida. In King LR [ed]: Urologic Surgery in Neonates and Young Infants. Philadelphia, WB Saunders, 1988, pp 252–264.)

important factor in upper urinary tract deterioration. **Landau and colleagues (1994) developed the concept of low detrusor filling pressure (less than 30 cm H$_2$O)** at specific volumes adjusted for age, and not at maximal capacity. Applying this idea, they noted significantly improved sensitivity in predicting upper urinary tract deterioration. The ability to predict accurately which newborns are at risk for urinary tract deterioration prompted the initiation of prophylactic therapy with CIC and anticholinergic drugs (Geranoitis et al, 1988; Kasabian et al, 1992). Long-term success has been achieved in preventing reflux and hydronephrosis and in reducing the need for augmentation cystoplasty, from between 27% and 41% to between 11% and 17% (Edelstein et al, 1995; Wu et al, 1997; Kaefer et al, 1999). Others believe that aggressive observation and prompt intervention yields similar long-term results with less morbidity from catheterization (Teichman et al, 1994), but only time will delineate which avenue of treatment is most efficacious (Tanaka et al, 1999; Hopps and Kropp, 2003).

Recommendations

Because expectant treatment has revealed that infants with outlet obstruction in the form of DSD are at

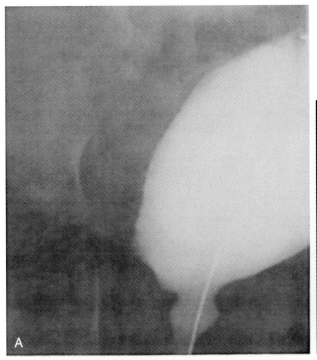

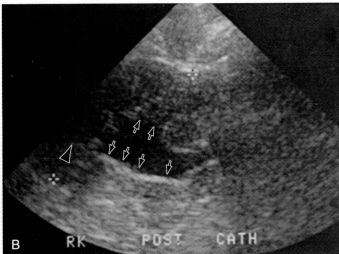

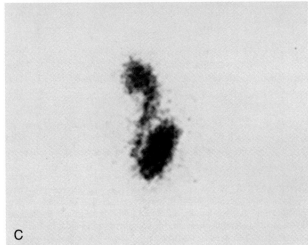

Figure 123–22. **A,** A voiding cystourethrogram in a newborn girl with dyssynergy and elevated voiding pressures demonstrates no reflux and a smooth-walled bladder. Her initial renal echogram was normal. She was started on clean intermittent catheterization and oxybutynin chloride (Ditropan) but did not respond. Within 1 year, she developed right hydronephrosis (**B,** *arrows*) and severe reflux on a radionuclide cystogram (**C**).

considerable risk for urinary tract deterioration, the idea of treating these children prophylactically has emerged as an important alternative. When CIC is begun in the newborn period, it is easy for parents to master, even in uncircumcised boys, and for children to accept as they grow older (Joseph et al, 1989). Complications such as meatitis, epididymitis, and urethral injury are rarely encountered, and urinary infections occur in fewer than 30% (Kasabian et al, 1992), although asymptomatic bacteriuria can be seen in almost 70% (Schlager et al, 2001).

CIC alone or in combination with anticholinergic agents, when detrusor filling pressures exceed 40 cm H_2O and voiding pressures are higher than 80 to 100 cm H_2O, resulted in an incidence of urinary tract deterioration of only 8% to 10% (Geranoitis et al, 1988; Kasabian et al, 1992; Edel-

stein et al, 1995). This represents a significant drop in the occurrence of detrimental changes compared with children observed expectantly (McGuire et al, 1981; Bauer et al, 1984; Sidi et al, 1986; Teichman et al, 1994; Wu et al, 1997). Oxybutynin hydrochloride is administered in a dose of 1.0 mg per year of age every 12 hours to help lower detrusor filling pressures. In neonates and children younger than 1 year of age, the dose is lowered to less than 1.0 mg in relation to the child's age at the time and increased proportionately as the age approaches 1 year. Side effects have not been manifest when oxybutynin is administered according to this schedule (Joseph et al, 1989; Kasabian et al, 1992). On rare occasions when an overactive or poorly compliant bladder fails to respond to these measures, augmentation cystoplasty may be needed with cutaneous vesicostomy almost

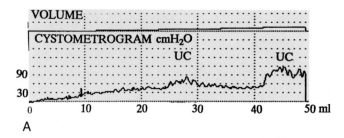

A

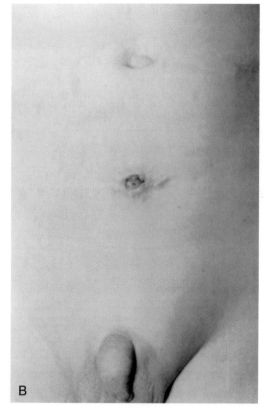

KEY POINTS: MANAGEMENT PRINCIPLES

- Bladder pressures should be maintained below 30 cm H_2O as much as possible to prevent urinary tract deterioration.

- CIC alone or in combination with anticholinergic agents, when detrusor filling pressures exceed 30 to 40 cm H_2O and voiding pressures are higher than 80 to 100 cm H_2O, can reduce the incidence of urinary tract deterioration.

- The neurologic lesion in myelodysplasia is a dynamic disease process in which changes take place throughout childhood.

- Sequential urodynamic testing on a yearly basis beginning in the newborn period and continuing until the child is 5 years old provides a means of monitoring these children.

- Vesicoureteral reflux occurs in 3% to 5% of newborns with myelodysplasia.

- The indications for antireflux surgery are not very different from those applicable to children with normal bladder function.

Figure 123–23. **A,** A 6-month-old boy with a myelomeningocele and detrusor sphincter dyssynergy fails to lower bladder filling and detrusor contractile pressures on oxybutynin. UC, uninhibited contraction. **B,** Because the lower ureters showed increasing dilation on ultrasonography, in addition to this poor response to medication in lowering intravesical pressure, a vesicostomy was performed.

never required (Fig. 123–23) (Duckett, 1974; Mandell et al, 1981).

Neurologic Findings and Recommendations

It has been documented that **the neurologic lesion in myelodysplasia is a dynamic disease process in which changes take place throughout childhood** (Epstein, 1982; Reigel, 1983; Venes and Stevens, 1983; Oi et al, 1990), especially in early infancy (Spindel et al, 1987) and later at puberty (Begger et al, 1986), when the linear growth rate accelerates again. When a change is noted on neurologic, orthopedic, or urodynamic assessment, radiologic investigation of the CNS often reveals (1) tethering of the spinal cord (Fig. 123–24), (2) a syrinx or hydromyelia of the cord, (3) increased intracranial pressure due to a shunt malfunction, or (4) partial herniation of the brain stem and cerebellum. Children with completely intact or only partially denervated sacral cord function are particularly vulnerable to progressive changes. Today, magnetic resonance imaging (MRI) is the test of choice because it reveals anatomic details of the spinal column and CNS (Just et al, 1990). However, it is not a functional study and when used alone it cannot provide exact information about a changing neurologic lesion.

Sequential urodynamic testing on a yearly basis beginning in the newborn period and continuing until the child is 5 years old provides a means of carefully monitoring these children to detect signs of change, thus offering the hope that early detection and neurosurgical intervention may help to arrest or even reverse a progressive pathologic process. Changes occurring in a group of newborns monitored in this

manner involved both the sacral reflex arc and the pontine-sacral reflex interaction (Fig. 123–25) (Lais et al, 1993). Most children who undergo such changes tend to do so in the first 3 years of life (Phuong et al, 2002) (Fig. 123–26). Twenty-two of 28 children in whom the neurologic picture became worse underwent a second neurosurgical procedure; 11 of them had a beneficial effect from the surgery and showed improvement in urethral sphincter function (Lais et al, 1993). Infants with only sacral level deficits have a 47% risk of deterioration (Dator et al, 1992). Even children with normal neurourologic function at birth have a 32% risk of developing a tethered spinal cord with the development of DSD with or without detrusor overactivity (Tarcan et al, 2001).

As a result of these developments, **it is recommended that all infants with myelodysplasia be monitored according to**

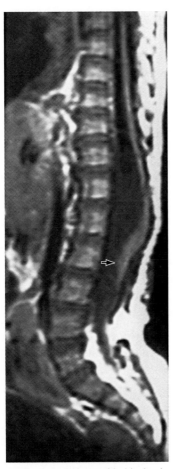

Figure 123–24. MR image in a 9-year-old girl who developed a tethered cord after myelomeningocele repair reveals the conus opposite the L3-4 vertebrae (*arrow*).

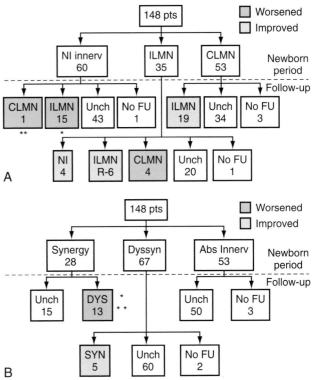

Figure 123–25. The changes in innervation of the purely sacral (**A**) and pontine-sacral (**B**) reflex arc pathways that occurred in a group of children with myelodysplasia who were monitored with sequential urodynamic studies beginning in the newborn period. ILMN, incomplete lower motor neuron lesion; CLMN, complete lower motor neuron lesion; NL, normal innervation; Unch, unchanged; FU, follow-up; DYS, dyssynergy; Syn, synergy. In **A**, the *double asterisk* indicates 1 patient changed from synergy to dyssynergy and the *single asterisk* indicates 4 of 15 patients so changed. In **B**, the *single asterisk* indicates 1 patient changed from normal to partial and then complete denervation and the *double asterisk* indicates 4 patients changed from normal to partial denervation. (From Lais A, Kasabian NG, Dyro FM, et al: Neurosurgical implications of continuous neuro-urological surveillance of children with myelodysplasia. J Urol 1993;150:1879-1883.)

the guidelines set forth in Table 123–4. It is not enough to look at just the radiologic appearance of the urinary tract; scrutiny of the functional status of the lower urinary tract is important as well. In addition to the reasons cited previously, it may be necessary to repeat a urodynamic study if the upper urinary tract dilates secondary to impaired drainage from a poorly compliant detrusor.

Management of Reflux

Vesicoureteral reflux occurs in 3% to 5% of newborns with myelodysplasia, usually in association with poor detrusor compliance, detrusor overactivity, or DSD (Flood et al, 1994). It is rare to find reflux in any neonate without these urodynamic findings (Bauer, 1984b; Geranoitis et al, 1988; Edelstein et al, 1995). If left untreated, the incidence of reflux in these infants at risk increases with time until 30% to 40% are afflicted by 5 years of age (Bauer, 1984a; Seki et al, 1999). Prophylactic treatment that lowers detrusor filling and voiding pressures with anticholinergic agents and empties the bladder by means of CIC significantly reduces this rising incidence of reflux (Edelstein et al, 1995).

In children with reflux grades 1 to 3 (International Classification) who void spontaneously or have complete lesions with little or no outlet resistance and empty their bladder

Table 123–4. Surveillance in Infants with Myelodysplasia*

Sphincter Activity	Recommended Tests	Frequency
Intact–synergic	Postvoid residual volume	q 4 mo
	IVP or renal echo	q 12 mo
	UDS	q 12 mo
Intact–dyssynergic[†]	IVP or renal echo	q 12 mo
	UDS	q 12 mo
	VCUG or RNC[‡]	q 12 mo
Partial denervation	Postvoid residual volume	q 4 mo
	IVP or renal echo	q 12 mo
	UDS[§]	q 12 mo
	VCUG or RNC[‡]	q 12 mo
Complete denervation	Postvoid residual volume	q 6 mo
	Renal echo	q 12 mo

IVP, intravenous pyelogram; echo, sonogram; UDS, urodynamic study; VCUG, voiding cystourethrogram; RNC, radionuclide cystogram.
*Until age 5 years.
[†]Patients receiving intermittent catheterization and anticholinergic agents.
[‡]If detrusor hypertonicity or reflux is already present.
[§]Depending on degree of denervation.

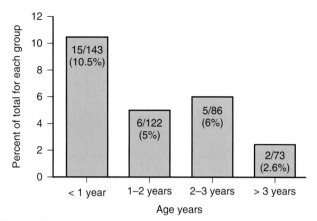

Figure 123–26. The propensity for a change in urethral sphincter innervation is greatest in the first year of life. (From Lais A, Kasabian NG, Dyro FM, et al: Neurosurgical implications of continuous neuro-urological surveillance of children with myelodysplasia. J Urol 1993;150:1879-1883.)

completely, management consists solely of prophylaxis with antibiotics to prevent recurrent infection. In children with high-grade reflux (grade 4 or 5), CIC is begun to ensure complete emptying. Children who cannot empty their bladder spontaneously, regardless of the grade of reflux, are treated with CIC to empty the bladder efficiently. Children with poor detrusor compliance with or without hydroureteronephrosis are also started on anticholinergic agents to lower intravesical pressure and ensure adequate upper urinary tract decompression (Flood et al, 1994). When reflux is managed in this manner there has been a dramatic response, with reflux resolving in 30% to 55% of individuals (Kass et al, 1981; Bauer, 1984b; Joseph et al, 1989; Flood et al, 1994 Agarwal et al, 1997; Hopps and Kropp, 2003). Although bacteriuria can be seen in as many as 56% of children on CIC it is not harmful except in the presence of high-grade reflux, because symptomatic urinary infection and renal scarring rarely occur with lesser grades of reflux (Kass et al, 1981; Cohen et al, 1990).

Credé voiding should be avoided in children with reflux, especially those with a reactive external sphincter. In this circumstance, the Credé maneuver results in a reflex response in the external sphincter that increases urethral resistance and raises the pressure needed to expel urine from the bladder (Barbalais et al, 1983) (Fig. 123–27). This has the effect of aggravating the degree of reflux and accentuating its water-hammer effect on the kidneys. Vesicostomy drainage (Duckett, 1974; Mandell et al, 1981) is rarely required today but is reserved for those infants (1) who have such severe reflux that CIC and anticholinergic medication fail to improve upper urinary tract drainage, (2) whose parents cannot adapt to the catheterization program, or (3) who are not good candidates for augmentation cystoplasty (Morrisroe et al, 2005).

The indications for antireflux surgery are not very different from those applicable to children with normal bladder function. They include recurrent symptomatic urinary infection while receiving adequate antibiotic therapy and appropriate catheterization techniques; persistent hydroureteronephrosis despite effective emptying of the bladder and lowering of intravesical pressure; severe reflux

with an anatomic abnormality at the ureterovesical junction; reflux that persists into puberty; and the presence of reflux in any child undergoing surgery to increase bladder outlet resistance. Although some clinicians do not advocate reimplanting ureters in patients with low-grade reflux who are undergoing augmentation cystoplasty to lower intravesical pressure, this concept is not universally accepted (Nasrallah and Aliabadi, 1991).

Jeffs and colleagues (1976) were the first to show that **antireflux surgery can be very effective in children with neurogenic bladder dysfunction as long as it is combined with measures to ensure complete bladder emptying.** Before this observation was made, the results of ureteral reimplantation were so dismal that most physicians treating these children advocated urinary diversion as a means of managing reflux (Smith, 1972; Cass, 1976). Since the advent of CIC, success rates for antireflux surgery have approached 95% (Kass et al, 1981; Woodard et al, 1981; Bauer et al, 1982; Kaplan and Firlit, 1983). Bilateral surgery for unilateral disease need not be done, because contralateral reflux does not occur postoperatively (Bauer, 1984a). The endoscopic injection of Deflux (microspheres containing dextranomer in sodium hyaluronic solution) has altered the management of reflux in children with myelomeningocele, but its long-term salutary effects are yet to be appreciated (Elder et al, 2004; Schlussel, 2004).

Continence

Urinary continence is becoming an increasingly important issue that demands attention at an early age as parents try to mainstream their handicapped children. It has been shown that children who are continent have higher ratings in self confidence and social acceptance than boys and girls who are wet; thus, this issue becomes paramount as the children grow up and are mainstreamed into society (Moore et al, 2004). **Initial attempts at achieving continence include CIC and drug therapy designed to maintain low intravesical pressures and a reasonable level of urethral resistance** (Figs. 123–28 and 123–29). Although these measures can be initiated on a trial-and-error basis, it is more efficient to use exact treatment protocols based on specific urodynamic findings. As a result, urodynamic testing is performed if initial attempts with CIC and oxybutynin fail to achieve continence. Without urodynamic studies it is hard to know whether (1) a single drug is effective, (2) the dose should be increased, (3) a second drug should be added to the regimen, or (4) alternative methods of treatment (i.e., augmentation cystoplasty) should be contemplated.

At this point, if poor detrusor compliance or overactivity have not been dealt with effectively, another anticholinergic agent may be combined with or given instead of oxybutynin (see Table 123–1). Glycopyrrolate is the most potent oral anticholinergic drug available today, but it may have the typical belladonna-like side effects common to all these drugs. Tolterodine, a newly approved anticholinergic drug, is equally effective as oxybutynin in reducing hyperreflexia and improving compliance but with fewer side effects, especially constipation (Goessl et al, 2000). Hyoscyamine produces fewer side effects still, but its potency is less. Intravesical instillation of oxybutynin has been proven to be successful in lowering detrusor pressures and has fewer side effects compared with oral administration; serum concentrations may reach similar

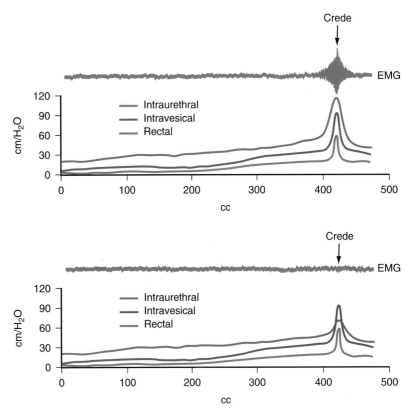

Figure 123–27. When the external sphincter is reactive *(top graph)*, a Credé maneuver produces a reflex increase in electromyographic (EMG) activity of the sphincter and a concomitant rise in urethral resistance, resulting in high "voiding" pressure. A child whose sphincter is denervated and nonreactive *(bottom graph)* will not have a corresponding rise in EMG activity, urethral resistance, or voiding pressure. A Credé maneuver here will not be detrimental. (From Bauer SB: Early evaluation and management of children with spina bifida. In King LR [ed]: Urologic Surgery in Neonates and Young Infants. Philadelphia, WB Saunders, 1988, pp 252-264.)

KEY POINTS: CONTINENCE IN NEUROGENIC BLADDER DYSFUNCTION

■ Initial attempts at achieving continence include CIC and drug therapy designed to maintain low intravesical pressures and a reasonable level of urethral resistance.

■ If urodynamic testing reveals that urethral resistance is inadequate to maintain continence, α-sympathomimetic agents are added.

■ Surgery becomes a viable option when drug therapy fails to achieve continence.

■ If bladder neck or urethral resistance is insufficient to allow adequate storage capacity, several operations are available to improve this continence mechanism.

■ Continent urinary diversion with closure of the bladder neck (or compression via a fascial sling) has been used to provide a better quality of life for those with intractable urethral incompetence.

---

levels regardless of the route of intake (Greenfield and Fera, 1991; Massad et al, 1992). Inconvenience of administration, however, seems to preclude its long-term use (Kasabian et al, 1994). Trospium chloride, a recently approved quaternary ammonium compound with antimuscarinic activity that has

a high binding affinity for muscarinic receptors M1, M2, and M3 but not nicotinic or cholinergic receptors, holds promise because it has a more direct effect on detrusor function with fewer systemic side effects than anticholinergic agents (Rovner, 2004; Doroshyenko et al, 2005; Kim et al, 2005).

Mechanical treatments, such as botulinum toxin A injected into the detrusor muscle, have effectively paralyzed the bladder for varying periods of time in myelodysplastic children and may become a viable option in the future with refinements of technique (Schulte-Baukloh et al, 2002; Riccabona et al, 2004).

If urodynamic testing reveals that urethral resistance is inadequate to maintain continence because either the sphincter fails to react to increases in abdominal pressure or its resistance drops with bladder filling (see Fig. 123–17B), α-sympathomimetic agents are added to the regimen (see Table 123–1); phenylpropanolamine is the most effective drug in this regard.

Surgery becomes a viable option when this program of drug therapy fails to achieve continence. In general, surgical intervention is not considered until the child is about 5 years of age and ready to start school. A persistent poorly compliant or overactive detrusor may be treated with either enterocystoplasty (Mitchell and Piser, 1987; Sidi et al, 1987; Hernandez et al, 1994), autoaugmentation (Cartwright and Snow, 1989a, 1989b), or a combination thereof (Duel et al, 1998). Sigmoid, cecum, and small intestine, in that order, have been used to enlarge the bladder. Although the ileocecal segment is a favored source for bladder replacement in adults, it is avoided in children with myelodysplasia because remov-

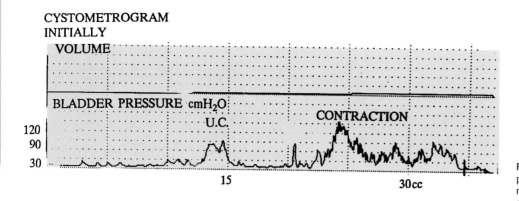

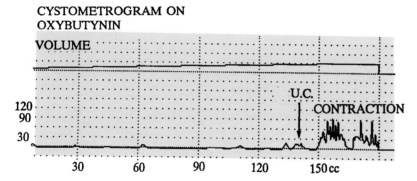

Figure 123–28. Oxybutynin is a potent anticholinergic agent that dramatically delays detrusor contractions and lowers contraction pressure, as demonstrated on these two graphs. U.C., uninhibited contraction.

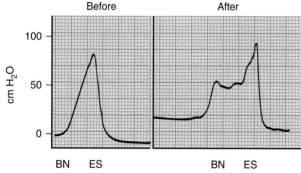

Figure 123–29. α-Sympathomimetic agents potentially have their greatest effect in the bladder neck region, where the highest concentration of α-receptor sites exists. They can raise outlet resistance and improve continence in many individuals. BN, bladder neck; ES, external sphincter.

ing it might aggravate the bowel dysfunction that is so often a factor in these children. Detubularization of the bowel is needed to minimize the intrinsic contractions of the intestinal segment and prevent it from causing intractable incontinence once it has been added to the bladder (Goldwasser et al, 1987; Hinman, 1988). When gastrocystoplasty was widely advocated as a means to augment the bladder it appeared to be ideal because it had fewer intrinsic contractions; the diamond-shaped patch did not have to be reconfigured so there are fewer suture lines; the spherical reservoir created by the patch seemed to be the most efficient way to store urine; it provided an acid milieu and thus caused fewer side effects such as

urinary infection and stones (Kaefer et al, 1998); and it had little or no mucus secretion, which led to repeated urinary infections (Adams et al, 1988; Atala et al, 1993).

Concerns have surfaced about gastric segments because they can cause hyponatremic hypochloremic metabolic alkalosis (Gosalbez et al, 1993) or the hematuria dysuria syndrome (Nguyen et al, 1996). As a result, some surgeons have advocated peeling the detrusor muscle off the dome of the bladder, leaving the mucosa intact, and augmenting this bladder with demucosalized intestine (Gonzalez et al, 1994) or stomach (Nguyen et al, 1996). However, this too has not yielded a uniform long-term success rate in providing a bladder of adequate capacity and good compliance (Carr et al, 1999). Except for children with progressive or end-stage renal failure, gastrocystoplasty has not been recommended as a routine form of augmentation (Leonard et al, 2000; Plaire et al, 2000).

With the long view of the retrospectoscope it is becoming evident that augmentation cystoplasty with any segment of the gastrointestinal tract can lead to long-term consequences in acid-base balance, vitamin B_{12} deficiency, fat absorption, renal function, bone metabolism, growth retardation, recurrent urinary tract infection, stone formation, and even cancer risk (Gilbert and Hensle, 2005). Consequently, there is considerable interest in developing new techniques for replacing the bladder without the need for bowel substitution (i.e., tissue engineered autologous augments). (See also Chapter 17, "Tissue Engineering and Cell Therapy.")

If bladder neck or urethral resistance is insufficient to allow adequate storage capacity, several operations are available to improve this continence mechanism. Bladder neck reconstruction can be undertaken in a variety of ways, including the Young-Dees or Leadbetter procedures (Young, 1919; Dees, 1949; Leadbetter, 1964) or the Kropp approach (Kropp and Angwafo, 1986), modified by Salle to make catheterization easier (Salle et al, 1994). A fascial sling procedure that suspends the bladder neck and buttresses it against the undersurface of the pubis has been advocated enthusiastically by several clinicians (McGuire et al, 1986; Raz et al, 1988; Peters et al, 1989). Artificially derived material, small intestine submucosa (SIS) (Colvert et al, 2002), and a rectus muscle "fascial" wrap around the bladder neck (Walker et al, 2000) have been as effective as rectus fascia in increasing bladder neck resistance and their effectiveness does not seem to diminish over time (Elder, 1990; Castellan et al, 2005). Even though it is applicable to males it has not been as effective as in females (Nguyen et al, 2001; Castellan et al, 2005). Each of these operations, however, necessitates the use of CIC to empty the bladder postoperatively. It is most effective when combined with augmentation cystoplasty to ensure an adequate reservoir with good compliance (Castellan et al, 2005). The artificial sphincter (Barrett and Furlow, 1982; Light and Scott, 1983; Light et al, 1983) also increases bladder outlet resistance, and its mechanism of action allows emptying at low urethral pressures. Any patient who can empty his or her bladder before the device is implanted should be able to do so afterward without the need for CIC. In fact, this is the only bladder neck procedure that allows for spontaneous voiding yet is compatible with CIC when needed (Herndon et al, 2003). Poor detrusor compliance can develop postoperatively if the preoperative cystometrogram is not carefully scrutinized for signs of increased filling pressure (Woodside and McGuire, 1982; Bauer et al, 1986), and this may lead to progressive renal failure if not treated in a timely fashion with medication or augmentation cystoplasty (Bauer et al, 1993). Long-term results with the artificial sphincter have shown that it is a viable option in children with neurogenic bladder dysfunction (Bosco et al, 1991; Levesque et al, 1996; Kryger et al, 1999; Kryger et al, 2001; Herndon et al, 2003).

In an attempt to avoid many of the complications associated with these invasive procedures, there was initial enthusiasm for glutaraldehyde cross-linked bovine collagen injected endoscopically around the bladder neck to increase urethral resistance (Ben-Chiam et al, 1995). Although early reports were encouraging, longer-term assessment has been discouraging, with many patients requiring repeated injections to stay dry (Perez et al, 1996; Silveri et al, 1998; Guys et al, 2001). Atala and associates developed a self-sealing, detachable membrane balloon that can be placed submucosally at the bladder neck to improve outlet resistance (Yoo et al, 1997). Initial results revealed improved continence (Diamond et al, 1999), but no long-term data are available. Currently, Deflux injections at the bladder neck are being advocated as a bulking agent to enhance bladder outlet resistance (Caione and Capozza, 2002; Misseri et al, 2005) but again no long-term data are available.

Urinary diversion, once considered a panacea for children with myelodysplasia, has turned out to be a Pandora's box of new clinical problems (Schwarz and Jeffs, 1975; Shapiro et al, 1975). Pyelonephritis and renal scarring, calculi, ureterointestinal obstruction, strictures of the conduit, and stomal stenosis are often encountered in children who are monitored on a long-term basis. Although antirefluxing colon conduits seem to have fewer complications, they are still not ideal. In the past 15 years very successful attempts have been made to reverse urinary tract diversions in children who probably would not undergo urinary diversion today (Hendren, 1973, 1990). Few children undergo urinary diversion now; if they do, it is in association with a continent stoma.

Continent urinary diversion with closure of the bladder neck (or compression via a fascial sling) has been used to provide a better quality of life for those with intractable urethral incompetence despite bladder outlet surgery or to make it easier to catheterize those individuals who cannot easily catheterize themselves via their native urethra (MacNeily et al, 2005).

Several operations have been devised, but the ones that achieved the most publicity initially were the Kock pouch in adults (Kock, 1971; Skinner et al, 1987) and the Indiana reservoir in children (Rowland et al, 1987). **Mitrofanoff (1980) created a continence mechanism by tunneling one end of the vermiform appendix into the bladder, as if reimplanting the ureter to prevent reflux, with the other end being brought out through the skin as a catheterizable stoma. This principle has been extended to the ureter.** After the ureter is transected at the pelvic brim, a proximal transureteroureterostomy is performed and the cut end of the distal segment is brought to the skin as a stoma (Duckett and Snyder, 1986); the continence mechanism is provided by the intramural detrusor tunnel of the ureter. Other narrow structures (e.g., fallopian tube, a rolled strip of stomach, a tapered or reconfigured ileal segment) have been implanted either into the native bladder or along the tinea of a detubularized portion of sigmoid or cecum acting as a urinary reservoir (Woodhouse et al, 1989; Reidmiller et al, 1990; Bihrie et al, 1991; Montie et al, 1997). The success rate for achieving continence has been excellent, approaching 85%, primarily owing to the flap valve effect of the intramural tunnel (Hinman, 1990; Watson et al, 1995; Kaefer et al, 1997; Gerharz et al, 1998). For this reason, it is now the preferred method for continent urinary diversion (Harris et al, 2000).

Sexuality

Sexuality in this population is becoming an increasingly important issue as more individuals reach adulthood and want to marry or to have meaningful long-term relationships with the opposite sex (Cromer et al, 1990). Investigators are looking into the concerns, fears, self-imagery, and desires of teenagers and young adults, and at the ability of males to procreate and females to bear children (Bomalaski et al, 1995). However, few studies are available that look critically at sexual function in these patients. It is important to remember that sexual development depends on socialization and the ability of the child to make friends and discuss shared experiences and thoughts. Mental handicaps, poor manual dexterity, lack of education regarding normal and abnormal sexual function, invasion of personal privacy, and overprotective parents often prevent independent behavior and, as a result, lead to poor understanding of sexual issues (Joyner et al, 1998; Woodhouse, 2005).

In several studies, researchers interviewed groups of teenagers and reported that **28% to 40% of them had had one or more sexual encounters and almost all of them had a desire to marry and ultimately to bear children** (Cromer et al, 1990; Palmer et al, 1999). In one study, 72% of male subjects claimed they were able to have an erection, and two thirds of these were able to ejaculate (Decter et al, 1997). Other studies revealed that 70% to 80% of myelodysplastic women were able to become pregnant and to have an uneventful pregnancy and delivery, although urinary incontinence in the latter stages of gestation was common in many, as was delivery by cesarean section (Laurence and Beresford, 1975; Cass et al, 1986; Bomalaski et al, 1995; Arata et al, 2000). In the same studies, 17% to 39% of male subjects claimed that they were able to father children and another 25% had a good prognosis for fathering them (Laurence and Beresford, 1975; Bomalaski et al, 1995; Decter et al, 1997). It is more likely that men will have problems with erectile and ejaculatory function because the sacral spinal cord is frequently involved, whereas reproductive function in women, which is under hormonal control, is not affected. Men with neurologic lesions at S1 or lower are likely to have normal or adequate reproductive sexual function, but only 50% of those with lesions above that level have adequate function (Woodhouse, 1994, 2005). Poor semen quality (Reilly and Oates, 1992) and Sertoli cell only histology on testis biopsy (Glass and Soni, 1999) have been reported as reasons (in addition to erectile dysfunction) for infertility in males with spina bifida.

Sexuality or the ability to interact with the opposite sex in a meaningful and lasting way is just as important as knowledge of one's precise sexual function. **The degree of sexuality is inversely proportional to the level of neurologic dysfunction** (Joyner et al, 1998; Palmer et al, 1999). Until recently, however, this subject has been taboo (Decter et al, 1997). Sexual identity, education, and social mores have been taken out of the realm of secrecy and are now openly discussed and taught to handicapped people. **However, parents of children with spina bifida are more overprotective than parents of normal children and are less willing to grant autonomy to them for adequate peer and sexual development** (Holmbeck et al, 2002); this tends to lead to less self-assurance regarding social interaction with the opposite sex and diminished sexual identity. Boys reach puberty at an age similar to the age for normal males, whereas breast development and menarche tend to start as much as 2 years earlier than usual in myelodysplastic girls. The cause of this early hormonal surge is uncertain, but it may be related to changes in pituitary function in girls secondary to hydrocephalus (Hayden, 1985).

Bowel Function

There is no unanimity regarding the ideal bowel management program for myelodysplastic children. The external anal sphincter is innervated by the same (or similar) nerves that modulate the external urethral sphincter, whereas the internal anal sphincter is influenced by more proximal nerves from the sympathetic nervous system. In addition, the internal anal muscle reflexively relaxes in response to anal distention. Consequently, **bowel incontinence is frequently unpredictable and is not associated with the attainment of urinary conti-** nence; it is often related to the consistency of fecal material and how rapidly the anal area refills after an evacuation, the degree of intactness of sacral cord sensation and motor function, and reflex reactivity of the external anal sphincter muscle (Younoszai, 1992).

KEY POINTS: BOWEL FUNCTION

■ Bowel incontinence is frequently unpredictable and is not associated with the attainment of urinary continence.

A majority of pediatricians managing these children believe that a regular and efficient bowel emptying regimen is paramount and mandatory. Most programs begin at about 1 year of age, but the best method of attaining these objectives is still controversial. Usually the children are placed on diets that are intended to create formed but not severely constipated stool. Roughage in the form of fruits and bran and stool softeners (in older children) are given to achieve this goal. Suppositories that help evacuate the rectum are used on a regular basis to help train the lower bowel to fill and empty. Some physicians believe that enemas are more effective in evacuating a greater portion of the lower bowel, but one problem with them is the difficulty of retaining the solution when the anal sphincter muscle is lax. Biofeedback training programs to strengthen the external anal sphincter are no more effective than a good bowel management program in attaining fecal continence (Loening-Baucke et al, 1988). Whereas electrostimulation of the bowel has had a variable effect in fecal continence, ranging from 0% to 36% (Marshall and Boston, 1997; Palmer et al, 1997), intravesical bladder stimulation has had a more pronounced effect on bowel continence (Han et al, 2004). When a carefully constructed bowel regimen is adhered to, most children with myelomeningocele can achieve some degree of fecal continence (Myers, 1984), but the uncertainty of accidents always makes this a tenuous situation. Often the urinary incontinence is effectively managed with CIC, drugs, and/or surgery but episodes of fecal soiling remain a problem, particularly in socially minded adolescents (Hayden, 1985; Krogh et al, 2003). When diet, medications, and manual evacuation fail to achieve predictable bowel emptying without soiling, a continent cutaneous pathway from the lower abdominal wall to the cecum may be created using the vermiform appendix; this is called the ACE procedure, for *Antegrade Continence Enema* (Griffiths and Malone, 1995). When the appendix is unavailable, a small segment of the bowel may be reconfigured to act as a conduit. Enemas consisting of either Golytely, saline, or tap water, sometimes in combination with bisacodyl are instilled daily or every other day to evacuate the colon. Cleansing the colon in this manner has resulted in complete continence in 89% of children in whom it has been tried (Squire et al, 1993; Gerharz et al 1997; Yerkes et al, 2002). Older children readily become independent in managing their bowel function leading to improved self-esteem and sociability (Bau et al, 2001; Aksnes et al, 2002)

Lipomeningocele and Other Spinal Dysraphisms

Diagnosis

There is a group of congenital defects that affect the formation of the spinal column but do not result in an open vertebral canal (James and Lassman, 1972) (Table 123–5). They occur once in 4000 live births, but with the ease of MRI screening of children with suspected lesions, the incidence of these defects is increasing (Bruce and Schut, 1979). In a study just published the incidence of lipomeningocele in families was calculated to be 0.043% (Sebold et al, 2005). These lesions can be very subtle and have no obvious outward signs, but in more than 90% of children there is a cutaneous abnormality overlying the lower spine (Anderson, 1975; Pierre-Kahn et al, 1997). This varies from a small dimple or skin tag to a tuft of hair, a dermal vascular malformation, a very noticeable subcutaneous lipoma, or an asymmetrically curving gluteal cleft (Fig. 123–30). In addition, on careful inspection of the legs, one may note a high arched foot or feet; alterations in the configuration of the toes with hammer or claw digits; a discrepancy in muscle size, shortness, and decreased strength in one leg compared with the other, typically at the ankle; and/or a gait abnormality, especially in older children (Dubrowitz et al, 1965; Weissert et al, 1989; Jindal and Mahaptra, 2000). Absent perineal sensation, back pain, and secondary incontinence after a period of dryness are common symptoms in older children and young adults (Linder et al, 1982; Yip et al, 1985; Weissert et al, 1989). Lower urinary tract function is abnormal in 40% to 90% of affected older individuals, with the incidence of an abnormality increasing proportionally with age (Mandell et al, 1980; Koyangi et al, 1997; Pierre-Kahn et al, 1997; Sarica et al, 2003). The child may experience difficulty with toilet training, urinary incontinence after an initial period of dryness once toilet trained (especially during the pubertal growth spurt), recurrent urinary infection, and/or fecal soiling. Occasionally, some patients without an obvious back lesion escape detection until they develop urinary (66%) or lower extremity (19%) symptoms or back pain (14%) after puberty caused by delayed traction on the spinal cord (Satar et al, 1995).

Findings

When these children are evaluated in the newborn period or early infancy, **the majority have a perfectly normal neurologic examination** (Atala et al, 1992). Urodynamic testing, however, reveals abnormal lower urinary tract function in about one third of infants younger than 18 months of age (Keating et al, 1988) (Fig. 123–31). Such studies may provide

Table 123–5.	Types of Occult Spinal Dysraphisms

Lipomeningocele
Intradural lipoma
Diastematomyelia
Tight filum terminale
Dermoid cyst/sinus
Aberrant nerve roots
Anterior sacral meningocele
Cauda equina tumor

the only evidence of a neurologic injury involving the lower spinal cord (Keating et al, 1988; Foster et al, 1990; Atala et al, 1992, Satar et al, 1997; Nogueira et al, 2004). When present, the most likely abnormality is an upper motor neuron lesion characterized by an overactive detrusor and/or hyperactive sacral cord reflexes (Fone et al, 1997; Pierre-Kahn et al, 1997); mild forms of DSD are rarely noted. Lower motor neuron signs with denervation potentials in the sphincter or an acontractile detrusor occur in only 10% of young children.

In contrast, practically all individuals older than 3 years of age who have not been operated on or in whom an occult dysraphism has been belatedly diagnosed have either an upper or lower motor neuron lesion or a combination thereof, on urodynamic testing (92%) (see Fig. 123–31) or neurologic signs of lower extremity dysfunction (Yip et al, 1985; Kondo et al, 1986; Keating et al, 1988; Atala et al, 1992; Satar et al, 1997; Nogueira et al, 2004). When such children were observed expectantly from infancy after the diagnosis was made, 58% deteriorated within 2 years (Andar et al, 1997; Cornette et al, 1998). There does not seem to be a preponderance of one type of lesion over another (i.e., upper vs. lower motor neuron); each occurs with almost equal frequency, and often the child shows signs of both (Hellstrom et al, 1986; Kondo et al, 1986). In one study of children older than 3 years of age, 43% had denervation in the sphincter and 52% detrusor areflexia, with a total of 81% having an abnormality (Satar et al, 1995).

KEY POINTS: LIPOMENINGOCELE AND OTHER SPINAL DYSRAPHISMS

- There is a group of congenital defects that affect the formation of the spinal column but do not result in an open vertebral canal.

- In contrast, practically all individuals older than 3 years of age who have not been operated on or in whom an occult dysraphism has been belatedly diagnosed have either an upper or lower motor neuron lesion or a combination thereof.

- The majority have a perfectly normal neurologic examination.

- Early detection and early intervention can both reverse the progression of the lesion, which does not happen in the older child.

Pathogenesis

Various occult spinal dysraphic lesions produce different neurourologic findings. When they do cause an abnormality, lipomas of the cauda equina invariably cause an upper motor neuron lesion (70%), alone or in combination with a lower motor neuron deficit (30%) (Satar et al, 1997). The split cord syndrome results in an isolated upper or lower motor neuron lesion in 25% each or a combined lesion in 50% (Proctor et al, 2000).

The reason for this difference in neurologic findings may be related to (1) compression on the cauda equina or sacral

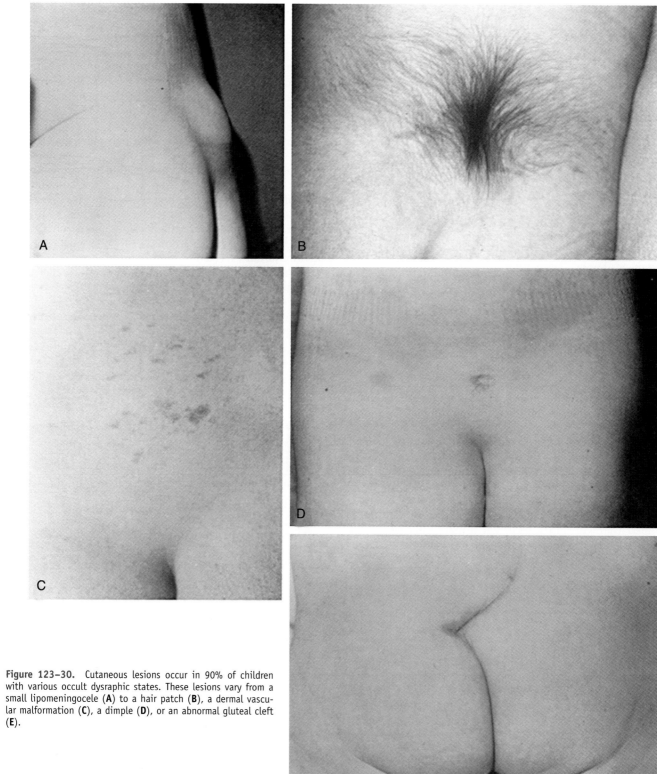

Figure 123–30. Cutaneous lesions occur in 90% of children with various occult dysraphic states. These lesions vary from a small lipomeningocele (**A**) to a hair patch (**B**), a dermal vascular malformation (**C**), a dimple (**D**), or an abnormal gluteal cleft (**E**).

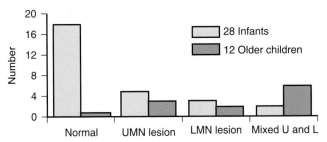

Figure 123–31. Most newborns with an occult spinal dysraphism have normal lower urinary tract function, whereas older children tend to have both upper motor neuron (UMN) and lower motor neuron (LMN) lesions.

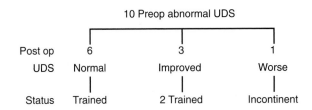

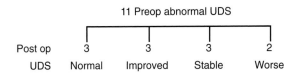

Figure 123–32. The potential for recoverable function is greatest in infants (6 of 10, 60%) and less so in older children (3 of 11, 27%). The risk of damage to neural tissue at the time of exploration to those with normal function is small (2 of 19, 11%). UDS, urodynamic study.

nerve roots by an expanding lipoma or lipomeningocele (Yamada et al, 1983), **(2) tension on the cord from tethering secondary to differential growth rates in the bony vertebrae and neural elements while the lower end of the cord is held in place by the lipoma or by a thickened filum terminale** (Dubrowitz et al, 1965), **or (3) fixation of the split lumbosacral cord by an intravertebral bony spicule or fibrous band** (Pang, 1992; Pang et al, 1992; Andar et al, 1997). The overt stretching that invariably occurs when there is a forcible flexion and/or extension of the spinal cord with normal movement leads to changes in oxidation/reduction of cytochrome oxidase, most notably in the lumbosacral spinal neurons when there is no intraspinal pathology (Yamada et al, 2004; Henderson et al, 2005). Under normal circumstances, the conus medullaris ends just below the L2 vertebra at birth and recedes upward to T12 by adulthood (Barson, 1970). When the cord does not "rise" or is fixed in place because of one of these lesions, ischemic injury may ensue (Yamada et al, 1981, 2004). Correcting the lesion in infancy has resulted not only in stabilization but also in improvement in the neurologic picture in many instances (Koyangi et al, 1997, Cornette et al, 1998; Proctor et al, 2000) (Fig. 123–32). Sixty percent of infants with abnormal urodynamic findings preoperatively revert to normal postoperatively, with improvement noted in 30%; 10% become worse with time. In older children there is a less dramatic change after surgery, with only 27% becoming normal, 27% improving, 27% stabilizing, but 19% actually becoming worse with time (see Fig. 123–32) (Keating et al, 1988; Satar et al, 1997). Older children with an overactive detrusor tend to improve, whereas those with acontractile bladders do not (Hellstrom et al, 1986; Kondo et al, 1986; Flanigan et al, 1989). Finally, 5% to 27% of children operated on in early childhood develop secondary tethering when observed for several years, suggesting that early surgery has both beneficial and sustaining effects in patients with this condition (Pierre-Kahn et al, 1997; Satar et al, 1997; Proctor et al, 2000).

As a result of these findings, it is apparent that urodynamic testing may be the only way to document that an occult spinal dysraphism is actually affecting lower spinal cord function (Keating et al, 1988; Khoury et al, 1990; Pierre-Khan et al, 1997; Sarica et al, 2003). The serial use of electromyography of the external urethral sphincter using a needle electrode to monitor individual motor unit action potentials provides a precise mechanism for measuring changes in innervation that may occur over time. Some investigators have shown that pos-

terior tibial somatosensory evoked potentials are an even more sensitive indicator of tethering and should be an integral part of the urodynamic evaluation (Roy et al, 1986). The implication of these findings lies in the fact that **early detection and early intervention can both reverse the progression of the lesion, which does not happen in the older child** (Yamada et al, 1983; Tami et al, 1987; Kaplan et al, 1988), and offers a degree of protection from subsequent tethering (Pierre-Kahn et al, 1997; Satar et al, 1997; Proctor et al, 2000), which seems to be a frequent occurrence when the lesion is not dealt with expeditiously in infancy (Chapman, 1982; Seeds and Jones, 1986).

Recommendations

In addition to MRI studies (Tracey and Hanigan, 1990), urodynamic testing including EMG of the external urethral sphincter should be performed in every child who has a questionable cutaneous or bony abnormality of the lower spine, especially if there is a radiologic abnormality of the spinal cord (Packer et al, 1986; Campobasso et al, 1988; Hall et al, 1988; Meyrat et al, 2003). This test provides the most accurate measure of sacral spinal cord function at diagnosis and provides a basis for comparison with subsequent studies when the children are either operated on or carefully observed. **In children younger than 3 months of age, the vertebral bones have not ossified; thus a window of opportunity exists for ultrasound to be a useful screening tool in visualizing the spinal canal** (Fig. 123–33) (Raghavendra et al, 1983; Scheible et al, 1983). **At this age there is good correlation between the**

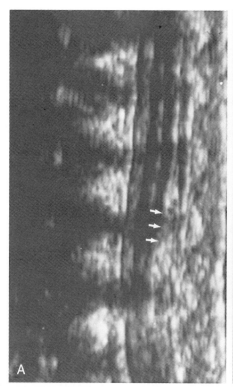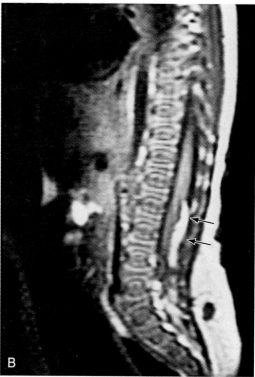

Figure 123–33. A, During the first few months of life, ultrasound can clearly demonstrate intravertebral anatomy because the posterior arches have not completely ossified. Note that the spinal cord along with its central canal is displaced anteriorly *(white arrows)* beginning at L3 because of an intradural lipoma. **B,** The MR image is juxtaposed to confirm the ultrasound findings. The longitudinal white intraspinal mass *(black arrows)* is the lipoma; the longitudinal gray mass is the spinal cord.

ultrasound imaging and MRI findings; however, the latter provides for a better definition of the spinal cord lesion. Consequently, ultrasound should not be used as the definitive imaging modality (Hughes et al, 2003).

In the past, these conditions were usually treated only by removal of the superficial skin lesions, without delving further into the spinal canal to remove or repair the entire abnormality. Currently, most neurosurgeons advocate laminectomy and removal of the intraspinal process as completely as possible without injuring the nerve roots or cord, in order to release the tether and prevent further injury with subsequent growth (Linder et al, 1982; Kondo et al, 1986; Kaplan et al, 1988; Foster et al, 1990; Atala et al, 1992; Pierre-Kahn et al, 1997; Proctor et al, 2000; Jindal and Mahapatra, 2000; Nogueira et al, 2004).

Sacral Agenesis

Sacral agenesis has been defined as the absence of part or all of two or more lower vertebral bodies. The cause of this condition is still uncertain, but teratogenic factors may play a role, because insulin-dependent diabetic mothers have a 1% chance of giving birth to a child with this disorder. Conversely, 16% or more of children with sacral agenesis have a mother affected by insulin dependent diabetes mellitus (Passarge and Lenz, 1966; Guzman et al, 1983; Wilmshurst et al, 1999). Often the mothers have only gestational insulin-dependent diabetes. The disease has been reproduced in chicks by exposing embryos to insulin (Landauer, 1945; White and Klauber, 1976). Maternal insulin-antibody complexes have been noted to cross the placenta, and their concentration in the fetal circulation is directly correlated with macrosomia (Menon et al,

1990). It is possible that a similar cause-and-effect phenomenon occurs in sacral agenesis. There is evidence that a deletion of the seventh chromosome (7q36) leading to the absence of a transcription factor may be responsible for this anomaly (Papapetrou et al, 1999). In addition, maternal drug exposure (i.e., minoxidil) has been reported to cause sacral agenesis (Rojansky et al 2002).

In familial cases of sacral agenesis associated with the Currarino syndrome (presacral mass, sacral agenesis and anorectal malformation), deletions in chromosome 7 (7q) resulting in *HLXB9* genetic mutations have been found (Ross et al, 1998). A mutation in *HLXB9*, a homeodomain gene of a 403 amino acid protein that appears to be responsible for neural plate infolding, has been identified in 20 of 21 patients with familial and in 2 of 7 sporadic cases of Currarino syndrome (Hagan et al, 2000; Kochling et al, 2001). Heterozygote carriers within these families have also been identified (Lynch et al, 2000). Thus, sacral agenesis may represent one point on a spectrum of abnormalities that encompass sacral meningoceles and anorectal malformations (Bernbeck et al, 2004).

Diagnosis

The presentation is bimodal, with more than three fourths of the disorders being detected in early infancy and the remainder discovered between 4 and 5 years of age (Wilmshurst et al, 1999). With the increased use of prenatal ultrasound, it is being diagnosed with increased frequency before birth. Sacral vertebral bony ossification begins at 15 weeks, so it is possible to detect the lesion after 18 weeks of gestation on an ultrasound examination and then to confirm it by fetal MRI (De Biasio et al, 2003). When not detected prenatally or at birth, the diagnosis is often delayed until failed

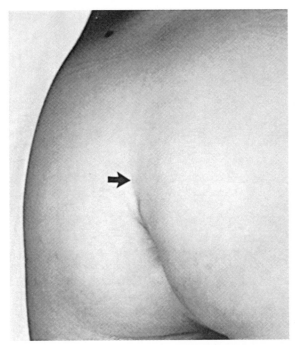

Figure 123–34. Characteristically, in sacral agenesis the gluteal crease is short and is seen only inferiorly *(below arrow)* because of the flattened buttocks.

attempts at toilet training bring the child to the attention of a physician. Sensation, including that in the perianal dermatomes, is usually intact, and lower extremity function is normal (Koff and DeRidder, 1977; Jakobson et al, 1985; Capitanucci et al, 1997). Because these children have normal sensation and little or no orthopedic deformity in the lower extremities (although high arched feet or claw or hammer toes may be present), the underlying lesion is often overlooked. In fact, 20% escape detection until the age of 3 or 4 years (Guzman et al, 1983). The only clue, besides a high index of suspicion, is flattened buttocks and a low, short gluteal cleft (Bauer, 1990) (Fig. 123–34). Palpation of the coccyx is used to detect the absent vertebrae (White and Klauber, 1976). The diagnosis is most easily confirmed with a lateral film of the lower spine, because this area is often obscured by the overlying gas pattern on an anteroposterior projection (White and Klauber, 1976; Guzman et al, 1983) (Fig. 123–35). MRI has been used to visualize the spinal cord in these cases; its imaging reveals a sharp cutoff of the conus at T12 as a consistent finding (Pang, 1993; Diel et al, 2001) (Fig. 123–36).

KEY POINTS: SACRAL AGENESIS

- Sacral agenesis has been defined as the absence of part or all of two or more lower vertebral bodies.

- On urodynamic evaluation, an almost equal number of individuals manifest either an upper or a lower motor neuron lesion (35% vs. 40%, respectively); 25% have no sign of denervation at all.

- Management depends on the specific type of neurourologic dysfunction seen on urodynamic testing.

Findings

On urodynamic evaluation, an almost equal number of individuals manifest either an upper or a lower motor neuron lesion (35% vs. 40%, respectively); 25% have no sign of denervation at all (Guzman et al, 1983; Boemers et al, 1994). Upper motor neuron lesions are characterized by an overactive detrusor, exaggerated sacral reflexes, absence of voluntary control over sphincter function, DSD, and no EMG evidence of denervation potentials in the sphincter (White and Klauber, 1976; Koff and DeRidder, 1977; Guzman et al, 1983; Capitanucci et al, 1997). The bladder tends to be thick-walled (or trabeculated) with a closed bladder neck on VCUG or ultrasonography. A lower motor neuron lesion is noted when an acontractile detrusor and partial or complete denervation of the external urethral sphincter with diminished or absent sacral reflexes are seen. In these instances the bladder is usually small and smooth walled with an open bladder neck (Wilmshurst et al, 1999). The presence or absence of the bulbocavernosus reflex is an indicator (but not a foolproof one) of an upper or a lower motor neuron lesion, respectively (Schlussel et al, 1994). The number of affected vertebrae does not seem to correlate with the type of motor neuron lesion present (Boemers et al, 1994) (Fig. 123–37). The injury appears to be stable and rarely shows signs of progressive denervation as the child grows. Sacral sensation is relatively spared, even in the presence of extensive sacral motor deficits (Boemers et al, 1994; Schlussel et al, 1994). Urinary tract infection may be detected in 75% of children over time, with vesicoureteral reflux diagnosed in 37%. Reflux is most likely in those with an upper (75%) (irrespective of whether or not they have synergy or dyssynergy) versus a lower (40%) motor neuron lesion (Schlussel et al, 1994; Wilmshurst et al, 1999).

Recommendations

Because most children who are diagnosed with this condition have a neurologic deficit, urodynamic testing is mandatory at the time of diagnosis. **Renal ultrasonography and nuclear or conventional cystography should be included as part of the evaluation process, especially if the child has a history of urinary tract infection or findings of an upper motor neuron lesion on urodynamic testing.** Additional imaging studies may be required based on the child's history and findings from baseline studies.

Management depends on the specific type of neurourologic dysfunction seen on urodynamic testing. Anticholinergic agents should be given to children with upper motor neuron findings of detrusor overactivity, whereas CIC and α-sympathomimetic medications may have to be given to individuals with lower motor neuron deficits who cannot empty their bladders or stay dry between catheterizations. When anticholinergic medication is ineffective in controlling the overactive detrusor, augmentation cystoplasty may be required to attain an adequate organ for urinary storage. Failure of α-sympathomimetic agents may require either endoscopic injection of bulking agents or even artificial urinary sphincter implantation to increase bladder outlet resistance. The bowels manifest a similar picture of dysfunction and need as much characterization and treatment as the lower urinary tract. Anorectal manometry has identified

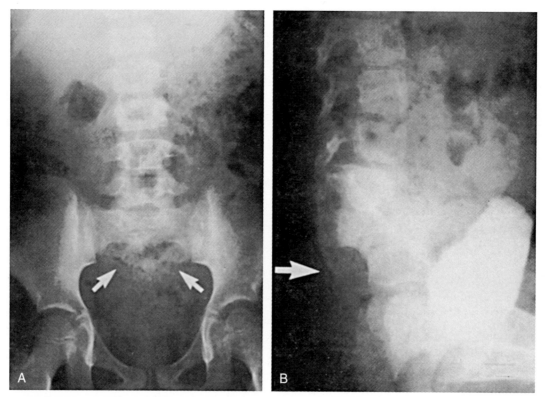

Figure 123–35. The diagnosis of partial or complete sacral agenesis *(arrows)* is easily confirmed on an anteroposterior (**A**) or lateral (**B**) radiograph of the spine if bowel gas obscures the sacral area. (From Bauer SB: Urodynamic evaluation and neuromuscular dysfunction. In Kelalis PP, King LR, Belman AB [eds]: Clinical Pediatric Urology, 2nd ed. Philadelphia, WB Saunders, 1985, vol 1, pp 283-310.)

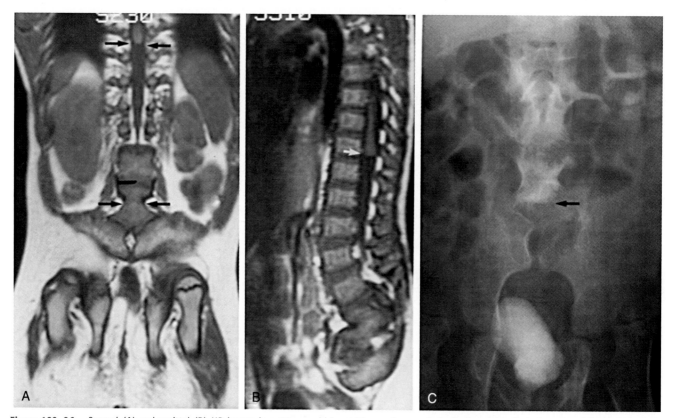

Figure 123–36. Coronal (**A**) and sagittal (**B**) MR images in a 10-year-old boy with sacral agenesis beginning at L5. Note the squared lower limit of the cord adjacent to T11 (**A**, *upper arrows;* **B**, *white arrow*) and the two sacroiliac joints (**A**, *lower arrows*), which are in the midline because of absence of the sacrum. **C**, An anteroposterior radiograph from an excretory urogram shows no vertebral bodies below L4 *(arrow)*.

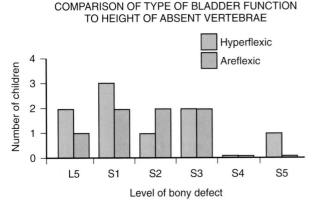

COMPARISON OF TYPE OF BLADDER FUNCTION TO HEIGHT OF ABSENT VERTEBRAE

Figure 123–37. Bladder contractility is unrelated to the number of absent vertebrae. (From Bauer SB: Urodynamic evaluation and neuromuscular dysfunction. In Kelalis PP, King LR, Belman AB [eds]: Clinical Pediatric Urology, 2nd ed. Philadelphia, WB Saunders, 1985, vol 1, pp 283-310.)

Table 123–6. Wingspread Classification of Anorectal Malformations

Female	Male
High	High
Anorectal agenesis	Anorectal agenesis
With rectovaginal fistula	With rectourethral (prostatic)
Without fistula	fistula
Rectal atresia	Without fistula
Intermediate	Rectal atresia
Rectovestibular fistula	Intermediate
Rectovaginal fistula	Rectovestibular urethral fistula
Anal agenesis without fistula	Anal agenesis without fistula
Low	Low
Anovestibular fistula	Anocutaneous fistula
Anocutaneous fistula	Anal stenosis
Anal stenosis	Rare malformation
Cloacal malformation	
Rare malformation	

abnormalities in the internal anal sphincter and in voluntary anal sphincter squeeze pressure, leading to weakness of the muscle and concomitant fecal incontinence (Morera and Nurko, 2003). It is important to identify these individuals as early as possible so that they can become continent and out of diapers at an appropriate age, thus avoiding the social stigma of fecal or urinary incontinence.

Associated Conditions—Imperforate Anus

Imperforate anus is a condition that can occur alone or as part of a constellation of anomalies that have been called the VATER or VACTERL syndrome (Barry and Auldist, 1974). This mnemonic denotes all the organs that can possibly be affected (Vertebral; Anal; Cardiac; Tracheo-Esophageal fistula; Renal; Limb). The incidence of anorectal malformations varies between 1 in 4000 to 1 in 5000 live births (Templeton and O'Neill, 1986). There is a male predominance of 1.5:1. The majority of female patients have low lesions, whereas males tend to have high ones (Santulli et al, 1971). Several classification systems have been devised, but the most commonly used one is the Wingspread Workshop on Anorectal Malformations (Table 123–6) (Shaul and Harrison, 1997). This format attempts to divide the lesions into high, intermediate, or low, depending on whether the rectum ends above, at, or below the levator ani muscle, respectively. The relative incidence for the various levels of the defect is 36% high, 14% intermediate, 47% low, and 1% a cloacal lesion. Imperforate anus may be part of a spectrum of hindgut abnormalities that include sacral agenesis and even a presacral mass or meningocele recently labeled as Currarino syndrome (Currarino et al, 1981; Hagan et al, 2000), which has genetic implications (Ross et al, 1998).

The Currarino triad is caused by an autosomal dominant defect linked to 7q36 region (Lynch et al, 1995). It can be complete when all three components are anomalous or incomplete when only two are present, but in either case a sacral bony defect is generally present (Samuel et al, 2000). Of 15 affected individuals from five families with the Currarino triad one family had 8 affected members. Linkage analysis in this family revealed that the 7q36 region was in close proximity to the *HLXB9* gene, which has also been implicated as the major gene for sacral agenesis (Emans et al, 2005).

Associated Findings

A fistulous communication with the lower urinary tract is a common occurrence, related in part to the sex of the child and the extent of the lesion: 87% of male and 79% of female babies with a high or intermediate lesion have a connection, whereas 7% of male and 10% of female children with a low lesion have such a communication (Templeton and O'Neill, 1986; Holschneider et al, 1994). Urinary tract abnormalities have been noted in 26% to 52% of affected children, with renal agenesis (primarily left-sided), and vesicoureteral reflux as the most common associated finding (Parrott, 1985). Again, the highest incidence of an abnormality is in those children with a high (70%) versus a low (infra-levator) (35%) lesion (Shaul and Harrison, 1997; Emir and Soylet 1998), with boys more prone than girls to having an anomaly (50% vs. 29%) (Metts et al, 1997). Spinal bony abnormalities range in incidence from 30% to 44%, but patients with a high lesion are more likely to be affected (48% to 54%) than those with a low lesion (15% to 27%) (Carson et al, 1984; Tsakayannis and Shamberger, 1995; Long et al, 1996). Spinal cord abnormalities including a tethered cord, thickened or fatty filum terminale, and a lipoma have been noted in 18% to 50% of patients, with the incidence varying proportionally in relation to the height of the rectal lesion (Shaul and Harrison, 1997). Not all patients with a spinal cord abnormality have a bony defect, so intraspinal imaging is mandatory to ensure the presence of a normal spinal cord especially in cases of high lesions (Rivosecchi et al, 1995). On occasion, an abnormal spinal cord can be found in patients even without one of these commonly associated other anomalies. Neurogenic bladder dysfunction is a frequent finding (Kakizaki et al, 1994) and usually manifests as incontinence, but its occurrence is rare when no spinal cord malformation exists (Hulthen de Medina et al, 2004) (Fig. 123–38). It often manifests when the child is older and the parents have difficulty with toilet training. It is not certain whether the dysfunction is caused by a spinal cord defect or by trauma to the nerves supplying the lower urinary tract or the pelvic floor musculature occasioned during surgery to repair the spinal cord or rectal defect (Parrott and Woodard, 1979). With the advent of the Peña posterior sagittal midline approach, the latter etiology is less likely (Peña, 1986; Boemers et al, 1994). Despite careful dissection techniques, 37% still have long-term problems with fecal incontinence (Peña and Hong, 2000).

Evaluation

Initial evaluation in the newborn period should include a careful inspection of the perineum looking for a fistulous site from the bowel, an examination of the upper and lower extremities, and an assessment of the bony spine and spinal cord (Carson et al, 1984; Mosiello et al, 2003). A prone cross-table lateral image with the child held in that position for 3 minutes and a radiopaque marker placed on the perineum will help delineate the distance from the end of the rectum to the skin in order to classify the extent of the rectal defect. Gas, meconium, or a gram-negative infection in the urine strongly suggests a rectal/urinary tract fistula, which then necessitates a divided colostomy very early in the postnatal period. Once the child is stable clinically, radiologic investigation of the urinary tract is begun, first with renal ultrasonography and then with VCUG, to define the presence of an abnormality and discover any clues for possible neurogenic bladder dysfunction. Vertebral bony anomalies, especially sacral level lesions, often signify an underlying spinal cord abnormality (Boemers et al, 1996). Thus, any bony abnormality warrants ultrasonography of the spine if the child is younger than 3 months of age because the vertebral bodies have not ossified, and a spinal MRI to rule out any abnormal intraspinal process (see Fig. 123–38) (Barnes et al, 1986; Tunell et al, 1987; Emir and Soylet 1998; Karrer et al, 1988; Mosiello et al, 2003). Urodynamic studies including sphincter electromyography are reserved for those children with either a bony abnormality of the spine, a spinal cord defect, or the telltale signs of dysfunction on VCUG or renal ultrasonography (Taskinen et al, 2002; Mosiello et al, 2003). These studies should be conducted early in infancy before the child has had any definitive surgery for the imperforate anus and again after a pull-through operation has been performed on the rectum, to determine, respectively, the true incidence of neurogenic bladder dysfunction and any changes that might have occurred as a result of the surgery. The presence of an abnormality on urodynamic testing in early infancy may warrant either intervention at that time to correct a spinal cord defect or watchful waiting to determine whether the lesion is progressive. Urodynamic studies are repeated subsequently or performed for the first time if secondary urinary or fecal incontinence ensues (Taskinen et al, 2002).

The most common finding on urodynamic testing is an upper motor neuron lesion with an overactive detrusor and/or bladder/urethral sphincter dyssynergy (Boemers et al, 1994; Taskinen et al, 2002), but a lower motor neuron lesion with an acontractile detrusor and a denervated sphincter may be seen as well (see Fig. 123–38) (Greenfield and Fera, 1991; Taskinen et al, 2002). EMG assessment of the perianal mus-

culature at this time helps determine the exact location of the future anus. In addition, it can provide precise information about the innervation to the levator ani muscle and its competence to function as a sphincter. The posterior midline approach espoused by Peña (1986) minimizes the chances of injuring the pelvic nerves that innervate the pelvic floor muscles and therefore reduces the risk of an iatrogenic cause for neurogenic bladder dysfunction.

CENTRAL NERVOUS SYSTEM INSULTS
Cerebral Palsy

Etiology

Cerebral palsy is a nonprogressive injury of the brain occurring in the perinatal period that produces either a neuromuscular disability, a specific symptom complex, or cerebral dysfunction (Kuban and Leviton, 1994). Its incidence is approximately 1.5 per 1000 births, but the incidence is increasing as smaller and younger premature infants survive in intensive care units (Kuban and Leviton, 1994). The condition is usually caused by a perinatal infection (e.g., sepsis, meningoencephalitis) or by a period of anoxia (or hypoxia) that affects the CNS (Nelson and Ellenberg, 1986; Naeye et al, 1989). It most commonly appears in infants who were premature, weighed less than 2 kg at birth, had intraventricular hemorrhage, and received mechanical ventilation for a prolonged time in the postnatal period and in premature infants weighing more than 2 kg who experienced a neonatal seizure (Kim et al, 1999). Maternal urinary infection in the later stages of pregnancy increases the risk of having an affected child by four to five times (Polivka et al, 1997).

Diagnosis

Affected children have delayed gross motor development, abnormal fine motor performance, altered muscle tone, abnormal stress gait, and exaggerated deep tendon reflexes. These findings can vary substantially, from obvious to very subtle when no discernible lesion is present, unless a careful neurologic examination is performed. These abnormalities may not manifest in the postnatal period, but they do become evident over time, because myelination of axons and maturation of neurons in the basal ganglia are required before spasticity, dystonia, and athetosis become apparent (Kyllerman et al, 1982). The lesions are classified according to which extremities are involved (monoplegia, hemiplegia, diplegia, and quadriplegia) and what kind of neurologic dysfunction is present (spastic, hypotonic, dystonic, athetotic, or a combination thereof). Among the more overtly affected individuals, spastic diplegia is the most common of the five types of dysfunction that characterize this disease, accounting for almost two thirds of the cases (Kuban and Leviton, 1994).

Findings

Most children with cerebral palsy develop total urinary control. Incontinence is a feature in some, but the exact incidence has never been truly determined (McNeal et al, 1983; Decter et al, 1987). In a recent survey of questionnaires sent to over 600 families with an affected child aged 4 to 18 years,

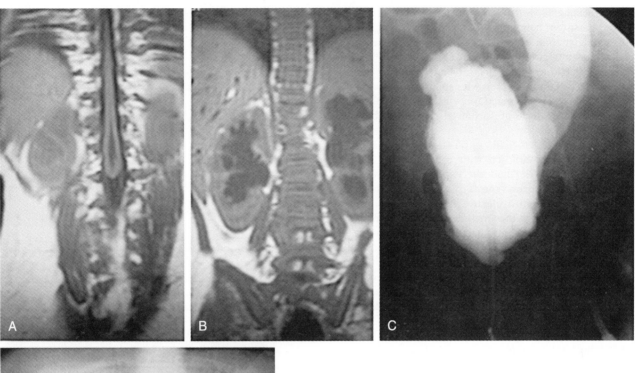

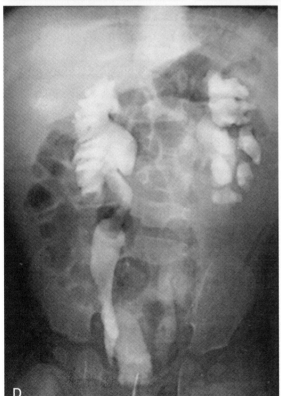

Figure 123–38. A and **B,** A 1-year-old girl with an imperforate anus and bony vertebral abnormalities has a tethered cord and bilateral hydronephrosis on MRI. **C,** Voiding cystourethrogram reveals significant trabeculation and reflux on the left. **D,** Excretory urogram demonstrates bilateral hydronephrosis secondary to the reflux on the left and a ureterovesical junction obstruction on the right. Subsequent urodynamic study revealed poor detrusor compliance and dyssynergy.

23.5% had persistent urinary incontinence (Roijen et al, 2001). When urinary continence was achieved, its development was delayed when compared with normal children of similar age. With further analysis of the data, 80% of children with spastic diplegia, 54% with tetraplegia, and 38% with low intellectual capacity attained continence. The presence of incontinence is often related to the extent of the physical impairment, because the handicap prevents the child from getting to the bathroom on time, causing an episode of wetting (Murphy et al, 1995). A number of children have such a severe degree of mental retardation that they are not trainable. They either do not recognize the need to void or cannot relate this fact to caregivers early enough to be toileted successfully (Roijen et al, 2001). The majority, however, have sufficient intelligence to learn basic societal protocols with patient and persistent handling. When continence is achieved (usually at a later than expected age), diurnal continence is attained first with nocturnal continence occurring within the subsequent year (Roijen et al, 2001). Therefore, urodynamic evaluation is reserved for children who appear to be trainable and do not seem to be hampered too much by their physical impairment but who have not achieved continence by late childhood or early puberty.

In one review (Decter et al, 1987), urodynamic studies were performed in 57 children with cerebral palsy (Table 123–7). **Forty-nine (86%) had the expected picture of a partial upper motor neuron type of dysfunction,** with exaggerated sacral reflexes, an overactive detrusor and/or DSD (Fig. 123–39), even though they manifested voluntary control over voiding. Six (11%) of the 57 had evidence of both upper and lower motor neuron denervation with an acontractile detrusor or abnormal motor unit potentials on sphincter EMG assessment (Table 123–8). Most of the children who exhibited these latter findings were found to have an episode of cyanosis in the perinatal period when their records were analyzed on a retrospective basis (Table 123–9). Therefore, a lower motor neuron lesion may be seen in addition to the expected upper motor neuron dysfunction. Similar findings have been noted by others (Mayo, 1992; Reid and Borzyskowski, 1993).

In two more recent **reviews of 65 children with cerebral palsy undergoing urodynamic studies** (Bross et al, 2004; Karaman et al, 2005) **abnormal bladder and urethral sphincter function was found in almost all.** In the first study involving 29 (Bross et al, 2004), 23 had incontinence and/or urinary tract infection whereas 6 were asymptomatic; urodynamic studies demonstrated poor compliance in 21 of the 23 symptomatic and 2 of the 6 asymptomatic children, an overactive detrusor in all symptomatic and 5 of 6 asymptomatic children, and high leak point pressure in 16 of 23 and 4 of 6 symptomatic and asymptomatic children, respectively. VCUG revealed bladder trabeculation in 58% and reflux in 9% of symptomatic, and trabeculation in 50% but no reflux in the asymptomatic, children. In the other study (Karaman et al, 2005), 66% had dysfunctional voiding symptoms, including 47.2% with day-time incontinence and 44.4% with difficulty urinating. Neurogenic detrusor overactivity was present in 47.2%, and dyssynergy between the bladder and sphincter was noted in 11%. In a meta-analysis of all published reports of urodynamic findings in children with cerebral palsy, detrusor overactivity was seen in 80%, dyssynergy between the bladder and sphincter in 5%, and normal function in only 12%

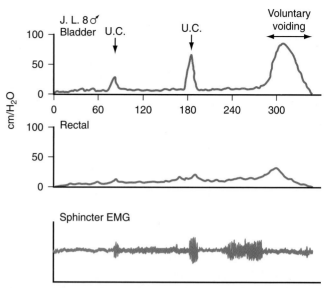

Figure 123–39. Electromyogram of an 8-year-old boy with spastic diplegia shows a typical partial upper motor neuron type bladder with uninhibited contractions (U.C.) associated with increased sphincter activity but normal voiding dynamics at capacity. Wetting is caused by these contractions when they are unaccompanied by the heightened sphincter activity.

Table 123–8. Urodynamic Findings in Cerebral Palsy*

Type of Lesion	No. of Patients
Upper motor neuron	
Uninhibited contractions	35
Detrusor sphincter dyssynergy	7
Hyperactive sacral reflexes	6
No voluntary control	3
Small-capacity bladder	2
Hypertonia	2
Lower motor neuron	
Excessive polyphasia	5
↑ Amplitude + ↑ duration potentials	4

*Some patients had more than one finding.
Adapted from Decter RM, Bauer SB, Khoshbin S, et al: Urodynamic assessment of children with cerebral palsy. J Urol 1987;138:1110.

Table 123–9. Perinatal Risk Factors in Cerebral Palsy

Factor	UMN (No. of Patients)	LMN (No. of Patients)
Prematurity	10	1
Respiratory distress/arrest/apnea	9	2
Neonatal seizures	5	—
Infection	5	—
Traumatic birth	5	—
Congenital hydrocephalus	3	—
Placenta previa/abruption	2	2
Hypoglycemia ± seizures	2	—
Intracranial hemorrhage	2	—
Cyanosis at birth	1	3
No specific factor noted	15	—

UMN, upper motor neuron lesion; LMN, lower motor neuron lesion.
Adapted from Decter RM, Bauer SB, Khoshbin S, et al: Urodynamic assessment of children with cerebral palsy. J Urol 1987;138:1110.

Table 123–7. Lower Urinary Tract Function in Cerebral Palsy

Type	Number	%
Upper motor neuron lesion	49	86
Mixed upper + lower motor neuron lesion	5	9.5
Incomplete lower motor neuron lesion	1	1.5
No urodynamic lesion	2	3

Adapted from Decter RM, Bauer SB, Khoshbin SJ, et al: Urodynamic assessment of children with cerebral palsy. J Urol 1987;138:1110.

(Decter et al, 1987; Mayo et al, 1990; Reid et al, 1993; Bross et al, 2004; Karaman et al, 2005). From these reports it is apparent that urodynamic studies can be very revealing in all children, whether or not they have urinary symptoms (Bross et al, 2004) but are especially useful if frequent toileting or initial anticholinergic treatment fails to improve incontinence, the child develops urinary infection, or renal ultrasonography reveals hydronephrosis. Upper urinary tract imaging is usually normal even in children with upper motor neuron lesions (Brodak et al, 1994).

KEY POINTS: CEREBRAL PALSY

- Cerebral palsy is a nonprogressive injury of the brain occurring in the perinatal period that produces either a neuromuscular disability, a specific symptom complex, or cerebral dysfunction.

- Affected children have delayed gross motor development, abnormal fine motor performance, altered muscle tone, abnormal stress gait, and exaggerated deep tendon reflexes.

- Most children with cerebral palsy develop total urinary control.

- The presence of incontinence is often related to the extent of the physical impairment; abnormal bladder and urethral sphincter function was found in almost all.

- Treatment usually centers on abolishing the overactive detrusor using anticholinergic medication, but residual urine must be monitored closely to ensure complete evacuation with each void.

Recommendations

Treatment usually centers on abolishing the overactive detrusor using anticholinergic medication, but residual urine must be monitored closely to ensure complete evacuation with each void. CIC may be required for those who cannot empty their bladder. Selective dorsal rhizotomy has improved bladder capacity, reduced the detrusor overactivity, and increased compliance, thus rendering the patient more continent, in a selected group of children who failed to respond to less invasive measures (Houle et al, 1998). The risk of neurourologic deterioration from this procedure is extremely low with less than 5% developing incontinence if careful mapping of dorsal nerve roots are identified (Huang 1997; Steinbok and Schrag, 1998; Liu et al, 1999). Upper and lower urinary tract imaging is not recommended unless urinary tract infection has occurred (Reid and Borzyskowski, 1993).

Traumatic Injuries to the Spine

Diagnosis

Despite increased exposure to and the potential for traumatic spinal cord injuries, **such injuries are rarely encountered in children. The incidence in Sweden is 2.6 cases per million children per year** (Augutis and Levi, 2003). **The incidence tends to increase geometrically with age** (Anderson and Schutt, 1980) (Fig. 123–40). When an injury does occur, it is more likely to happen in a male than a female child, and it is usually the result of a motor vehicle or bicycle accident (24% to 52%), a fall from a high place, a gunshot wound, or a diving or sports incident (Cass et al, 1984; Hadley et al, 1988; Decter and Bauer, 1993; Brown et al, 2001; Augutis and Levi 2003; Cirak et al, 2004). The type of causative injuries varies with age, with infants more prone to an injury from a motor vehicle accident (71%), toddlers and children those secondary to a fall (48% and 34%, respectively) and adolescents having a sports-related event (29%) (Cirak et al, 2004). An injury may also occur iatrogenically after surgery to correct scoliosis, kyphosis, or other intraspinal processes or congenital aortic anomalies or after ligation of a patent ductus arteriosus (Cass et al, 1984; Batista et al, 1995). Newborns are particularly prone to a hyperextension injury during a high forceps delivery (Adams et al, 1988; Lanska et al, 1990). Among younger children, girls are affected as often as boys (Ruge et al, 1988).

Pathogenesis

Spinal cord injuries in children are intrinsically different from those in adults because of a variety of factors, including the mechanism of injury and the difference in configuration of the cord in children compared with adults. In addition, the horizontal versus vertical orientation of the facet joints in vertebral bodies that predisposes to anteroposterior subluxation in children, the delayed supportive effect of the paraspinous musculature and ligaments, and the relative heaviness of the head, which causes a fulcrum of maximal flexion of the upper cervical region in infants and young children, all contribute to a high degree of hypermobility that places the child's spinal cord at risk for ischemic necrosis (Decter and Bauer, 1993).

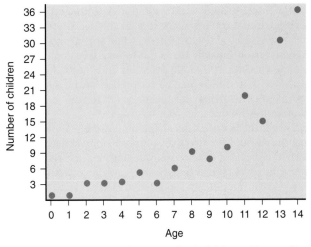

Figure 123–40. Increasing frequency of spinal injury with age. (From Anderson JM, Schutt AH: Spinal injury in children: A review of 156 cases seen from 1958 through 1980. Mayo Clin Proc 1980;55:499-504.)

SECTION XVII

KEY POINTS: TRAUMATIC INJURIES TO THE SPINE

■ The incidence in Sweden is 2.6 cases per million children per year. The incidence increases geometrically with age.

■ Spinal cord injuries in children are intrinsically different from those in adults because of a variety of factors, including the mechanism of injury and the difference in configuration of the cord in children compared with adults.

■ Patients with an upper thoracic or cervical lesion are likely to exhibit autonomic dysreflexia with a spontaneous discharge of α_1-stimulants during bladder filling and with contractions of the detrusor.

■ Monitoring of blood pressure and availability of α-antagonists are mandatory during VCUG or urodynamic studies

■ Upper spinal cord injuries produce an upper motor neuron type lesion with an overactive detrusor and detrusor-sphincter dyssynergia. The potential danger from this outflow obstruction is obvious.

Findings

The lower urinary tract dysfunction that ensues is not likely to be an isolated event but is usually associated with loss of sensation and paralysis of the lower limbs. Radiologic investigation of the spine may not reveal any bony abnormality, although momentary subluxation of osseous structures resulting from the elasticity of the vertebral ligaments can result in a neurologic injury (Pollack et al, 1988). This condition has been seen only in children (usually younger than 8 years old) and has been labeled spinal cord injury without radiologic abnormality (SCIWORA) (Pang and Wilberger, 1982; Pang and Pollack, 1989). Overall, SCIWORA can account for up to 38% of spinal cord injuries in children (Brown et al, 2001). Myelography and computed tomography show swelling of the cord below the level of the lesion (Adams et al, 1988; Lanska et al, 1990). **Often, what appears to be a permanent lesion initially turns out to be a transient phenomenon with time.** Although sensation and motor function in the lower extremities may be restored relatively quickly, the dysfunction involving the bladder and rectum may persist considerably longer.

During the acute phase of the injury, the bladder is often acontractile and the urethral sphincter nonreactive, although normal-appearing bioelectric potentials can be recorded on sphincter EMG (spinal shock). Over a variable period of time, detrusor contractility and sphincter reactivity return as spinal cord edema subsides. With this return of function, an overactive detrusor and bladder-sphincter dyssynergy develop if the lateral reticulospinal cord pathways to and from the brain stem have been disrupted. When the lesion affects the cauda equina, there is probably little to no return of bladder or sphincter function. Sacral sensation and peripheral reflexes

are not good indicators of ultimate lower urinary tract function (Shenot et al, 1998). Over time, the predominant urodynamic pattern in patients with a thoracic-level lesion is an overactive detrusor with DSD, high voiding pressures, eventual hydronephrosis, and vesicoureteral reflux. Often children exhibit a highly compliant bladder for a portion of bladder filling but then have C fiber–mediated, small, ineffective rhythmic contractions of the detrusor with simultaneous waxing and waning of external urethral sphincter activity. Some urinary leakage may occur with these contractions, but in general the bladder does not empty with them. **Patients with an upper thoracic or cervical lesion are likely to exhibit autonomic dysreflexia with a spontaneous discharge of α_1-stimulants during bladder filling and with contractions of the detrusor. Monitoring of blood pressure and availability of α-antagonists are mandatory during VCUG or urodynamic studies** (Perkash, 1997; Vaidyanathan et al, 1998b).

Management

If urinary retention occurs immediately after the injury, an indwelling Foley catheter is passed into the bladder and left in place for as short a time as possible, until the patient is stable and aseptic intermittent catheterization can be started safely on a regular basis (Guttmann and Frankel, 1966; Barkin et al, 1983). There is no difference in the incidence of urinary infection or in the development of stones in patients using sterile versus clean catheterization techniques to empty the bladder (Prieto-Fingerhut et al, 1997; VanHala et al, 1997). Rates of infection range as high as 60% to 80% (Biering-Sorensen et al, 1999), and stone formation occurs in 1.5% to 3% within the first 5 years after the trauma (McKinley et al, 1999; Donnellan and Bolton, 1999). When the child starts to void again, the timing of catheterization can be regulated so that it is used as a means of measuring the residual urine after a spontaneous void. Residual urine volumes of 25 mL or less are considered safe enough to allow reducing the frequency or even stopping the catheterization program (Barkin et al, 1983). After 4 to 6 weeks, if there is no improvement in lower urinary tract function, urodynamic studies are conducted to determine whether the condition is the result of spinal shock or to actual nerve root or spinal cord injury. An acontractile detrusor is not uncommon under these circumstances (Iwatsubo et al, 1985). On the other hand, EMG recording of the sphincter often reveals normal motor units without fibrillation potentials but absent sacral reflexes and a nonrelaxing sphincter with bladder filling, a sign that transient spinal shock has occurred (Iwatsubo et al, 1985). The outcome of this situation is guarded but good, because most cases resolve completely as edema of the cord in response to the injury subsides, leaving no permanent damage (Iwatsubo et al, 1985; Fanciullacci et al, 1988).

If and when bladder function returns and emptying is incomplete, it has been shown in the rat (Xiaa et al, 1999) that peripheral L7 dermatome stimulation initiates a micturition reflex without DSD; whether this becomes a reliable treatment in humans remains to be seen. Incomplete emptying may be enhanced by the judicious use of α–sympatholytic agents (Al-Ali et al, 1999). **The goal is balanced voiding at pressures lower than 40 cm H_2O,** which reduces the 30% risk for urinary tract deterioration seen in poorly managed patients (Giannantoni et al, 1998; Kim et al, 1998). If this cannot be achieved, then CIC is continued. Anticholinergics, either orally or intravesically (Vaidyanathan et al, 1998a; Wein, 1998), or capsaicin (an inhibitor of C-fiber stimulation [Wiart et al, 1998]) have been added and are effective in reducing an overactive detrusor, but at the cost of significant side effects. Alternative treatments that have been effective to ensure complete emptying at low pressure include external urethral sphincterotomy (Kim et al, 1998), urethral stent placement (Chancellor et al, 1999), or injection of botulinum A toxin (Botox) into the external sphincter (Schurch et al, 1997; Schurch et al, 2000: Kuo 2003; Tai et al, 2005). In some cases, a continent catheterizable abdominal urinary stoma may be created to facilitate self-catheterization in patients with low cervical or upper thoracic lesions who cannot easily catheterize themselves, in order to minimize the embarrassment of periodic genital organ exposure when care providers need to repeatedly catheterize the bladder (Sylora et al, 1997).

Recommendations

Most permanent traumatic injuries involve either the upper thoracic or cervical spinal cord but some affect the cauda equina region. The sacral cord injury most likely produces a lower motor neuron deficit of the striated sphincter that usually leads to low pressure bladder emptying with little risk of upper urinary tract deterioration. However, it probably necessitates medical and/or surgical therapy to achieve continence. On the other hand, upper spinal cord injuries produce an upper motor neuron type lesion with an overactive detrusor and detrusor-sphincter dyssynergia. The potential danger from this outflow obstruction is obvious (Donnelly et al, 1972). Substantial residual urine volumes, high-pressure reflux, urinary infections, and their sequelae are the leading causes of long-term morbidity and mortality in patients with spinal cord injury (Giannantoni et al, 1998). Even patients who voluntarily urinate and are continent or who involuntarily but spontaneously void to completion are not immune to urinary tract changes (Decter and Bauer, 1993). Urodynamic studies are imperative to identify which patients are at risk (Barkin et al, 1983). These studies should be performed within 2 to 3 months after the injury, again 6 to 9 months later, and possibly at 2 years after the trauma to determine the stability of lower urinary tract function, the need for continued CIC, and whether adjuvant drug or surgical therapy should be added (or continued) to achieve good long-term success. When these measures are employed judiciously, effective management can be achieved (Pannek et al, 1997). Renal ultrasonography early in the course and VCUG if signs of bladder outlet obstruction are present on urodynamic testing or if recurrent urinary infection ensues are also recommended. Radionuclide cystography is indicated if the patient has repeated urinary tract infection or develops hydronephrosis (Phillips et al, 1997). Because stone formation can be insidious, periodic imaging of the kidneys and bladder is necessary. Early identification and proper management may prevent the signs and effects of outlet obstruction before they become apparent on radiographic examination of the urinary tract (Pearman, 1976; Ogawa et al, 1988; Watanabe, et al, 1996).

SUGGESTED READINGS

Abrams P, Cardozo L, Fall M, et al: The standardisation of terminology in lower urinary tract function. Neurourol Urodyn 2002;21:167-178.

Abrams P, Cardozo L, Fall M, et al: The standardisation of terminology in lower urinary tract function: Report from the Standardisation Sub-committee of the International Continence Society. Urology 2003;61:37-49.

Anderson FM: Occult spinal dysraphism: A series of 73 cases. Pediatrics 1975;55:826.

Anderson JM, Schutt AH: Spinal injury in children: A review of 156 cases seen from 1950 through 1978. Mayo Clin Proc 1980;55:499.

Augutis M, Levi R: Pediatric spinal cord injury in Sweden: Incidence, etiology and outcome. Spinal Cord 2003;41:328.

Barbalais GA, Klauber GT, Blaivas JG: Critical evaluation of the Credé maneuver: A urodynamic study of 207 patients. J Urol 1983;130:720.

Barnes PD, Lester PD, Yamanashi WS, Prince JR: MRI in infants and children with spinal dysraphism. Am J Radiol 1986;147:339.

Barry JE, Auldist AW: The Vater syndrome. Am J Dis Child 1974;128:769.

Bates CP, Whiteside CG, Turner-Warwick RT: Synchronous cine/pressure/flow/cysto-urethrography with special reference to stress and urge incontinence. Br J Urol 1970;42:714.

Bauer SB, Colodny AH, Retik AB: The management of vesico-ureteral reflux in children with myelodysplasia. J Urol 1982;128:102.

Bauer SB, Hallet M, Khoshbin S, et al: The predictive value of urodynamic evaluation in the newborn with myelodysplasia. JAMA 1984;152:650.

Bauer SB, Labib KB, Dieppa RA, et al: Urodynamic evaluation in a boy with myelodysplasia and incontinence. Urology 1977;10:354.

Bauer SB, Reda EF, Colodny AH, Retik AB: Detrusor instability: A delayed complication in association with the artificial sphincter. J Urol 1986; 135:1212.

Blaivas JG, Labib KB, Bauer SB, Retik AB: A new approach to electromyography of the external urethral sphincter. J Urol 1977a;117:773.

Blaivas JG, Labib KB, Bauer SB, Retik AB: Changing concepts in the urodynamic evaluation of children. J Urol 1977b;117:777.

Bloom DA, Knechtel JM, McGuire EJ: Urethral dilation improves bladder compliance in children with myelomeningocele and high leak point pressures. J Urol 1990;144:430.

Boemers TM, van Gool JD, de Jong TP, Bax KM: Urodynamic evaluation of children with caudal regression syndrome (caudal dysplasia sequence). J Urol 1994;151:1038.

Boemers TM, de Jong TP, van Gool JD, et al: Urologic problems in anorectal malformations: II. Functional urologic sequelae. J Pediatr Surg 1996;31:634.

Botto, LD, Lisi, A, Robert-Gnansia E, Erickson, JD: International Retrospective Cohort Study of Neural Tube Defects in Relation to Folic Acid Recommendations: Are the recommendations working? Obstet Gynecol Surv 2005;60:563-565.

Bruner JP, Tulipan N, Paschall RL, et al: Fetal surgery for myelomeningocele and the incidence of shunt dependent hydrocephalus. JAMA 1999;282: 1819-1825.

Cass AS, Bloom BA, Luxenberg M: Sexual function in adults with myelomeningocele. J Urol 1986;136:425.

Cass AS, Luxenberg M, Johnson CF, Gleich P: Management of the neurogenic bladder in 413 children. J Urol 1984;132:521.

Chin-Peuckert L, Rennick JE, Jednak R, et al: Should warm infusion solution be used for urodynamic studies in children? J Urol 2004;172:1657-1661.

Cohen RA, Rushton HG, Belman AB, et al: Renal scarring and vesicoureteral reflux in children with myelodysplasia. J Urol 1990;144:541.

Currarino G, Coln D, Votteler T: Triad of anorectal, sacral, and presacral anomalies. AJR Am J Roentgenol 1981;137:395-398.

Dator DP, Hatchett L, Dyro EM, et al: Urodynamic dysfunction in walking myelodysplastic children. J Urol 1992;148:362-365.

Decter RM, Bauer SB, Khoshbin S, et al: Urodynamic assessment of children with cerebral palsy. J Urol 1987;138:1110.

Decter RM, Bauer SB: Urologic management of spinal cord injury in children. Urol Clin North Am 1993;20:475.

Diokno AC, Koff SA, Bender LF: Periurethral striated muscle activity in neurogenic bladder dysfunction. J Urol 1974;112:743.

Donnelly J, Hackler RH, Bunts RC: Present urologic status of the World War II paraplegic: 25-year follow-up comparison with status of the 20-year Korean War paraplegic and 5-year Vietnam paraplegic. J Urol 1972;108: 558.

Edelstein RA, Bauer SB, Kelly MD, et al: The long-term urologic response of neonates with myelodysplasia treated proactively with intermittent catheterization and anticholinergic therapy. J Urol 1995;154:1500.

Emir H, Soylet Y: Neurovesical dysfunction in patients with anorectal malformations. Eur J Pediatr Surg 1998;8:95.

Geranoitis E, Koff SA, Enrile B: Prophylactic use of clean intermittent catheterization in treatment of infants and young children with myelomeningocele and neurogenic bladder dysfunction. J Urol 1988; 139:85.

Giannantoni A, Scivoletti G, DiStasi SM, et al: Clean intermittent catheterization and prevention of renal disease in spinal cord injured patients. Spinal Cord 1998;36:29-32.

Goldwasser B, Barrett DM, Webster GD, Kramer SA: Cystometric properties of ileum and right colon after bladder augmentation, substitution and replacement. J Urol 1987;138:1007.

Guttmann L, Frankel H: The value of intermittent catheterization in the early management of traumatic paraplegia and tetraplegia. Paraplegia 1966; 4:63.

Guzman L, Bauer SB, Hallet M, et al: The evaluation and management of children with sacral agenesis. Urology 1983;23:506.

Hagan DM, Ross AJ, Strachan T, et al: Mutation analysis and embryonic expression of the HLXB9 Currarino syndrome gene. Am J Hum Genet 2000;66:1504.

Hellstrom WJ, Edwards MS, Kogan BA: Urologic aspects of the tethered cord syndrome. J Urol 1986;135:317.

Herndon CDA, Rink RC, Shaw MBK, et al: The Indiana experience with artificial urinary sphincters in children and young adults. J Urol 2003;169:650-654.

Holzbeierlein J, Pope JC, Adams MC, et al: The urodynamic profile of myelodysplasia in childhood with spinal canal closure during gestation. J Urol 2000;164:1336.

Hopps CV, Kropp KA: Preservation of renal function in children with myelomeningocele managed with basic newborn evaluation and close followup. J Urol 2003;169:305.

Hulthen de Medina V, Mellstam L, Amark P, et al: Neurovesical dysfunction in children after surgery for high or intermediate anorectal malformations. Acta Pediatr 2004;93:43.

Jeffs RD, Jones P, Schillinger JF: Surgical correction of vesico-ureteral reflux in children with neurogenic bladder. J Urol 1976;115:449.

Joyner BD, McLorie GA, Khoury AE: Sexuality and reproductive issues in children with myelomeningocele. Eur J Pediatr Surg 1998;8:29-34.

Kaefer M, Pabby A, Kelly M, et al: Improved bladder function after prophylactic treatment of the high risk neurogenic bladder in newborns with myelomeningocele. J Urol 1999;162:1068-1071.

Kaefer M, Rosen A, Darbey M, et al: Pressure at residual volume: A useful adjunct to standard fill cystometry. J Urol 1997a;158:1268-1271.

Kaefer M, Zurakowski D, Bauer SB, et al: Estimating normal bladder capacity in children. J Urol 1997b;158:2261-2264.

Kaplan WE, McLone DG, Richards I: The urologic manifestations of the tethered spinal cord. J Urol 1988;140:1285.

Kass EJ, Koff SA, Lapides J: Fate of vesico-ureteral reflux in children with neuropathic bladders managed by intermittent catheterization. J Urol 1981;125:63.

Keating MA, Rink RC, Bauer SB, et al: Neuro-urologic implications of changing approach in management of occult spinal lesions. J Urol 1988;140:1299.

Kroovand RL, Bell W, Hart LJ, Benfeld KY: The effect of back closure on detrusor function in neonates with myelodysplasia. J Urol 1990;144:423.

Lais A, Kasabian NG, Dyro FM, et al: Neurosurgical implications of continuous neuro-urological surveillance of children with myelodysplasia. J Urol 1993;150:1879-1883.

Landau EH, Churchill BM, Jayanthi VR, et al: The sensitivity of pressure specific bladder volume versus total bladder capacity as a measure of bladder storage dysfunction. J Urol 1994;152:1578.

Lapides J, Diokno AC, Silber SJ, Lowe BS: Clean intermittent self-catheterization in the treatment of urinary tract disease. J Urol 1972;107:458.

Laurence KM: A declining incidence of neural tube defects in UK. Z Kinderchir 1989;44(Suppl 1):51.

Laurence KM, James M, Miller MH, et al: Double-blind randomized controlled trial of folate treatment before conception to prevent recurrence of neural tube defects. BMJ 1981;282:1509.

Levesque PE, Bauer SB, Atala A, et al: Ten-year experience with artificial urinary sphincter in children. J Urol 1996;156:625.

Loening-Baucke V, Deach L, Wolraich M: Biofeedback training for patients with myelomeningocele and fecal incontinence. Dev Med Child Neurol 1988;30:781.

Mayo ME: Detrusor hyperreflexia: The effect of posture and pelvic floor activity. J Urol 1978;119:635.

Mayo ME: Lower urinary tract dysfunction in cerebral palsy. J Urol 1992; 147:419.

McGuire EJ, Woodside JR, Borden TA, Weiss RM: The prognostic value of urodynamic testing in myelodysplastic patients. J Urol 1981;126:205.

McNeal DM, Hawtrey CE, Wolraich ML, Mapel JR: Symptomatic neurogenic bladder in a cerebral-palsied population. Dev Med Child Neurol 1983; 25:612.

Mitchell ME, Piser JA: Intestinocystoplasty and total bladder replacement in children and young adults: Follow-up of 129 cases. J Urol 1987;138:1140.

Mitrofanoff P: Cystometric continente trans-appendiculaire dans le traitement de vessies neurologiques. Chir Pediatr 1980;21:297.

Montie PR, Lara RC, Dutra MA, DeCarvalho JR: New techniques for construction of efferent conduits based on the Mitrofanoff principle. Urology 1997;49:112.

Palmer LS, Richards I, Kaplan WE: Age related bladder capacity and bladder capacity growth in children with myelomeningocele. J Urol 1997;158:1261-1264.

Pang D: Split cord malformation: II. Clinical syndrome. Neurosurgery 1992;31:481-500.

Pang D, Dias M, Ahab-Barmada M: Split cord malformation: I. A unified theory of embryogenesis for double spinal cord malformations. Neurosurgery 1992;31:451-481.

Park JM, Bauer SB, Freeman MR, Peters CA: Oxybutynin chloride inhibits proliferation and suppresses gene expression in bladder smooth muscle cells. J Urol 1999;162:1110-1114.

Passarge E, Lenz K: Syndrome of caudal regression in infants of diabetic mothers: Observations of further cases. Pediatrics 1966;37:672.

Pierre-Kahn A, Zeral M, Renier D, et al: Congenital lumbosacral lipomas. Childs Nerv Syst 1997;13:298-334.

Perez LM, Khoury J, Webster GD: The value of urodynamic studies in infants less than one year old with congenital spinal dysraphism. J Urol 1992;148:584.

Pontari MA, Keating M, Kelly MD, et al: Retained sacral function in children with high level myelodysplasia. J Urol 1995;154:775.

Proctor M, Bauer SB, Scott MR: The effect of surgery for the split spinal cord malformation on neurologic and urologic function. Pediatr Neurosurg 2000;32:13-19.

Reid CJD, Borzyskowski M: Lower urinary tract dysfunction in cerebral palsy. Arch Dis Child 1993;68:739.

Roijen LE, Postema K, Limbeek VJ, et al: Development of bladder control in children and adolescents with cerebral palsy. Dev Med Child Neurol 2001;43:103.

Ross AJ, Ruiz-Perez V, Wang Y, et al: A homeobox gene, HLXB9, is the major locus for dominantly inherited sacral agenesis. Nat Genet 1998;20:358.

Salle JLP, Amarante FA, Silveira ML, et al: Urethral lengthening with anterior bladder wall flap for urinary incontinence: A new approach. J Urol 1994; 152:803.

Satar N, Bauer SB, Scott RM, et al: Late effects of early surgery on lipoma and lipomeningocele in children less than two years old. J Urol 1997;157:1434-1437.

Schulte-Baukloh H, Michael T, Schobert J, et al: Efficacy of botulinum A toxin in children with detrusor hyperreflexia due to myelomeningocele: Preliminary results. Urology 2002;59:325-328.

Schurch B, Hodler J, Rodic B: Botulism A toxin as a treatment of detrusor-sphincter dyssynergia in patients with spinal cord injury: MRI controlled transperineal injections. J Neurol Neurosurg Psychiatry 1997;63:474-476.

Schurch B, Strohrer M, Kramer G, et al: Botulinum-A toxin for treating detrusor hyperreflexia in spinal cord injured patients: A new alternative to anticholinergic drugs? J Urol 2000;164:692-697.

Sidi AA, Dykstra DD, Gonzalez R: The value of urodynamic testing in the management of neonates with myelodysplasia: A prospective study. J Urol 1986;135:90.

Spindel MR, Bauer SB, Dyro FM, et al: The changing neuro-urologic lesion in myelodysplasia. JAMA 1987;258:1630.

Stein SC, Feldman JG, Freidlander M, et al: Is myelomeningocele a disappearing disease? Pediatrics 1982;69:511.

Tarcan T, Bauer S, Olmedo E, et al: Long-term follow-up of newborns with myelodysplasia and normal urodynamic findings: Is it necessary? J Urol 2001;165:564-567.

Teichman JMH, Scherz HC, Kim KD, et al: An alternative approach to myelodysplasia management: Aggressive observation and prompt intervention. J Urol 1994;152:807.

Venes JL, Stevens SA: Surgical pathology in tethered cord secondary to meningomyelocele repair. Concepts Pediatr Neurosurg 1983;4:165.

Watanabe T, Rivas DA, Chancellor MB: Urodynamics of spinal cord injury. Urol Clin North Am 1996;23:459.

Weerasinghe N, Malone PS: The value of video-urodynamics in the investigation of neurologically normal children who wet. Br J Urol 1993;71:539.

Wein AJ: Pharmacologic options for the overactive bladder. Urology 1998;51(2A Suppl):43-47.

Wilmshurst JM, Kelly R, Borzyskowski M: Presentation and outcome of sacral agenesis: 20 years' experience. Dev Med Child Neurol 1999;41:806-812.

Woodhouse CRJ: The sexual and reproductive consequences of congenital genitourinary anomalies. J Urol 1994;152:645.

Wu H-Y, Baskin LS, Kogan BA: Neurogenic bladder dysfunction due to myelomeningocele: Neonatal versus childhood treatment. J Urol 1997; 157:2295-2297.

Yalla SV, Sharma GV, Barsamian EM: Micturitional static urethral pressure profile method of recording urethral pressure profiles during voiding and implications. J Urol 1980;124:649.

Yamada S, Won DJ, Yamada SM: Pathophysiology of tethered cord syndrome: Correlation with symptomatology. Neurosurg Focus 2004;16:E6.

Yeung CK, Godley ML, Duffy PG, Ransley PG: Natural filling cystometry in infants and children. Br J Urol 1995;76:531.

Zerin JM, Lebowitz RL, Bauer SB: Descent of the bladder neck: A urographic finding in denervation of the urethral sphincter in children with myelodysplasia. Radiology 1990;174:833-836.

Zermann DH, Lindner H, Huschke T, Schubert J: Diagnostic value of natural fill cystometry in neurogenic bladder in children. Eur Urol 1997;32:223-228.

124 Urinary Tract Reconstruction in Children

MARK C. ADAMS, MD • DAVID B. JOSEPH, MD

The goal of this chapter is to review techniques for lower urinary tract reconstruction in pediatric patients and the principles that guide their use. In general, such intervention is taken to reestablish or to construct anew a system that protects renal function, avoids significant infection, and eventually provides for urinary continence. Those, in simplistic terms, are functions of a "normal" urinary tract.

The scope of the chapter is large. Many specific techniques are presented in detail, particularly those used primarily in the pediatric population. When techniques have been used more extensively in adults, descriptions are brief with focus on adaptations for and results of use in children. Urinary diversion, both temporary and permanent with bowel, is discussed elsewhere in the text. Augmentation cystoplasty is reviewed in detail from preoperative evaluation and surgical techniques to long-term results and newer alternatives. In few areas of urology have intestinal segments been used more extensively than for bladder augmentation in pediatric patients. This experience with augmentation cystoplasty established the

groundwork for later work with continent urinary diversions and orthotopic neobladders.

Complex patients with bladder dysfunction may have bladder neck and external sphincteric problems as well. This chapter covers techniques to increase native outflow resistance in the pediatric population. Certain techniques, such as Young-Dees-Leadbetter bladder neck repair, are presented in other pediatric sections of this text. Others (i.e., sling, collagen injection, and artificial urinary sphincter) have been used more extensively in adults; again, in that setting, this chapter focuses on adaptations of those procedures for children. **Perhaps the most important contribution affecting lower urinary tract reconstruction was the introduction of clean intermittent catheterization by Lapides and colleagues** (1972, 1976). Because many pediatric patients with bladder and sphincteric dysfunction will not void adequately after reconstruction, a reliable means for easy catheterization without discomfort is an important part of their care. The work of Mitrofanoff (1980) stimulated interest in continent abdominal wall stomas within pediatric urology, and several effective techniques have since been developed. That experience serves as a nice lead into a discussion of continent urinary diversion in children as construction of an effective efferent limb that provides continence and a reliable means for catheterization is often the most challenging aspect of such diversion. "Pure" continent urinary reservoirs, such as Indiana and Kock pouches, are occasionally performed in children, and that experience is reviewed. More frequently in children, some of the patient's native urinary tract is used in the reconstruction. This is done to maintain as much urothelium-lined tissue in the urinary tract as possible, to minimize the amount of needed bowel, and, potentially at least, to minimize the morbidity to the patient. The result then is a spectrum of repairs between bladder augmentation and continent urinary diversion but rarely a continent urinary reservoir in the classic sense.

Several decades ago, many such reconstructions were performed after previous, permanent urinary diversion with use of bowel (Hendren, 1998). Today, however, few children are initially treated with permanent diversion. **Most reconstructive procedures are now undertaken primarily to correct a problem in the native urinary tract (hydronephrosis, infection, incontinence) unresponsive to medical management or after temporary diversion. Children with bladder and sphincteric dysfunction are among the most complex seen** in pediatric urology; among others, patients with diagnoses such as exstrophy, persistent cloaca and urogenital sinus, posterior urethral valves, bilateral single ectopic ureters, and prune-belly syndrome may be involved. **For most pediatric urologists, patients with myelomeningocele make up the majority of patients requiring this type of surgical intervention.** Consequently, many of the results discussed herein focus on the neurogenic population.

Many children with anomalies affecting the bladder and outlet are managed so that surgical intervention is not necessary, and a primary goal of pediatric urologists is to minimize the number of children requiring many of these techniques. Once conservative, medical therapy fails, surgical reconstruction remains an important and effective tool. When reconstruction is considered, it is imperative that the patient be thoroughly evaluated. Each child is unique, and the particular pathophysiologic changes must be understood so that surgical techniques available may be used thoughtfully to optimize results while minimizing morbidity. **The most important factor influencing the outcome of urinary tract reconstruction in children is the commitment of the patient and family to achieving good care.** Determining that commitment may at times be difficult, but its importance should not be underestimated.

THE "FUNCTIONAL" URINARY TRACT

The renal pelves and ureters should empty effortlessly into the bladder without any increase in pressure or element of obstruction. The normal ureterovesical junction prevents vesicoureteral reflux. Bladder physiology can be characterized as two different dynamic phases, passive and active. During the passive storage phase, the bladder functions as a reservoir, allowing an appropriate volume of urine to be stored without leakage while maintaining low pressure. In the active voiding phase, the bladder contracts for elimination of urine.

Basic Bladder Function

Passive: Storage

Appropriate urinary storage requires a reservoir that is compliant and of age-appropriate capacity. Age-based capacity may be estimated by formulas proposed by Koff (1988)

$$\text{volume (mL)} = 30(\text{age in years} + 2)$$

or by Kaefer and associates (1997c) for children younger than 2 years

$$\text{volume (mL)} = 32(2 \times \text{age in years} + 2)$$

and for children older than 2 years

$$\text{volume (mL)} = 30(\text{age in years} \div 2 + 6)$$

Compliance is defined as the change in bladder volume divided by the change in pressure. Normally, the bladder is considered a highly compliant vesicle in that it will accommodate an increasing volume of urine without a corresponding increase in intravesical pressure. Multiple factors contribute to this property. Initially, the bladder is in a collapsed state that allows the storage of urine at low pressure by simple unfolding. As it expands, detrusor properties of elas-

ticity and viscoelasticity take effect. Elasticity allows the detrusor muscle to stretch without an increase in tension until it reaches a critical volume. This volume should be greater than the expected bladder capacity. The viscoelastic bladder property allows a subtle continuous pressure change that occurs with bladder filling. It is associated with a small rise in pressure as the bladder stretches, balanced by a corresponding rapid pressure decay (Zinner et al, 1976; Wagg and Fry, 1999). With slow natural bladder filling, there should be no net change in bladder pressure until capacity is reached. This viscoelastic bladder property is also defined as stress relaxation and can be overcome when the rate of bladder filling exceeds normal parameters, resulting in a pattern consistent with poor compliance (Mundy, 1984; Finkbeiner, 1999). This artifact of testing is often noted when urodynamic assessment is performed at an excessive filling rate for the child's age or size (Joseph, 1992). These properties of elasticity and viscoelasticity will eventually be overcome in every child, and at that point, the bladder pressure rapidly rises. **Favorable dynamics for appropriate urine storage include a thin bladder wall with an appropriate composition of muscle and collagen allowing expression of normal elastic and viscoelastic properties.** Factors adversely affecting normal compliance include detrusor hypertrophy, fibrosis, outlet obstruction, and recurrent urinary tract infections (Mundy, 1984; Joseph, 1994).

Continence during urinary storage requires a closed bladder neck at times supported by a contracted external urinary sphincter. Fixed obstruction, neurogenic dysfunction, and chronic inflammation can affect any or all of these passive parameters, resulting in resting bladder hostility and clinical manifestations of poor compliance, upper tract deterioration, and incontinence (Brading, 1997).

Active: Voiding

Under normal conditions, the active phase of voiding requires the bladder to contract after descent of the bladder neck (Morrison, 1997). Reflexive opening of the bladder neck and sequential relaxation of the external urinary sphincter allow low-pressure balanced voiding and complete elimination of urine. Again, obstruction, neurogenic dysfunction, and chronic infection can cause physiologic changes preventing coordinated function of the detrusor, bladder neck, and external sphincter, defined as dyssynergy (Mundy et al, 1985). A poorly functioning external sphincter from denervation fibrosis may also prevent appropriate relaxation, causing elevated voiding pressure against a fixed outlet. Finally, detrusor pathophysiologic changes may prevent a sustained, coordinated bladder contraction and full elimination of all urine.

Dysfunction

Upper Tracts

It is critical to understand the dynamics of the entire urinary tract before any major reconstructive procedure. Careful evaluation is imperative. In the presence of hydronephrosis, upper tract obstruction must be excluded. With severe and long-standing bladder problems, particularly those involving poor bladder compliance and emptying, upper tract obstruction is often secondary to the bladder abnormality. Nuclear renography with a catheter in the bladder to keep the bladder empty and at low pressure may be useful to rule out a primary upper tract problem. Antegrade perfusion studies with fluoroscopy and pressure measurement are occasionally necessary. Certainly, if upper tract obstruction is present, it should be corrected at the time of bladder-sphincter reconstruction.

Much like obstruction, vesicoureteral reflux in the presence of a bladder abnormality may be primary or secondary. Differentiation between the two may be difficult. On occasion, the history is helpful. If reflux was not present initially in a patient with neurogenic dysfunction but developed later, it is typically secondary to bladder hostility. Most reflux in patients with neurogenic dysfunction requiring bladder augmentation is likely to be secondary in nature; reflux in patients with other problems (exstrophy, prune-belly syndrome, or posterior urethral valves) may be either primary or a fixed secondary problem if it persists until the time that bladder reconstruction is necessary. Previous work has suggested that reflux truly secondary to bladder dysfunction may not need surgical correction if the bladder is adequately managed. In those reports, neurogenic bladder patients requiring augmentation did not undergo reimplantation for secondary reflux, and virtually all of the low-grade reflux resolved with augmentation alone (Nasrallah and Aliabadi, 1991; Morioka et al, 1998; Lopez Pereira et al, 2001; Soylet et al, 2004). It is interesting to speculate whether reflux is even a significant problem if a large, compliant bladder is achieved (Soylet et al, 2004). Bacteria may ascend without reflux after reconstruction (Gonzalez and Reinberg, 1987). Experience with certain forms of continent diversion has not shown an increased risk of pyelonephritis in the absence of any antireflux mechanism if the reservoir is adequate (Helal et al, 1993; Pantuck et al, 2000). Although we agree that most low-grade secondary reflux is likely to resolve with adequate treatment of the bladder alone, our preference is to correct reflux present at the time of bladder reconstruction, unless it is low grade or clearly secondary, because the morbidity is low. After bladder reconstruction, many patients have chronic bacteriuria, particularly those who catheterize to empty, and the absence of reflux, at least theoretically, may decrease the likelihood of ascent to the kidney. Caution must be taken when the treatment of chronically dilated and scarred ureters is considered. Correction of reflux in that setting is certainly appropriate, but one must be careful not to trade reflux for more problematic obstruction. Overaggressive tapering or tunneling of such ureters may be fraught with complications.

Dysfunction in the upper urinary tract is usually manifested by hydronephrosis, pyelonephritis, or impairment of renal function. When such problems are present in patients with lower tract dysfunction, thoughtful evaluation and treatment are necessary. All problems should be addressed at reconstructive surgery to provide the best result for the patient.

Bladder Dysfunction

Bladder dysfunction is a composite of physiologic abnormalities, and it is helpful to assess each component of passive and active bladder function independently. **Elevated passive filling pressure becomes clinically pathogenic when a pressure higher than 40 cm H_2O is chronically reached** (McGuire et al, 1981; Wang et al, 1988; Weston et al, 1989). Pressures at this level sustained for a time impair ureteral drainage, which may result in pyelocalyceal changes, hydroureteronephrosis, and decreased glomerular filtration rate. In addition, persistent elevation in filling pressure can result in acquired vesicoureteral reflux (Sidi et al, 1986a; Cohen et al, 1990).

Pharmacologic management can play a role in decreasing filling pressure, particularly when hyperreflexic detrusor contractions are present. A combination of medications and intermittent catheterization has a positive impact, particularly in children with neurogenic dysfunction (Rink and Mitchell, 1984). Bladders that are poorly compliant because of irradiation or chronic inflammatory processes are not as likely to respond in a positive fashion to this form of therapy. When compliance is unaffected by medical management, augmentation cystoplasty will be required to improve the storage characteristics. It is an unfortunate consequence that the likelihood of detrusor contractions resulting in effective emptying is significantly diminished. With rare exceptions, intermittent catheterization should be taught to and accepted by the patient and caretaker before urinary reconstruction is contemplated.

One of the most important contributions in the care of children with bladder dysfunction came with the acceptance of clean intermittent catheterization described by Lapides and colleagues (1972, 1976) **based on the work of Guttmann and Frankel** (1966). The effective use of clean intermittent catheterization has allowed the application of augmentation and lower tract reconstruction to groups of patients who had not previously been candidates. The principle of intermittent catheterization allows the reconstructive surgeon to aggressively correct storage problems by providing an adequate reservoir and good outflow resistance. Good spontaneous voiding, although a goal, is not imperative since catheterization can be used for emptying. Intermittent catheterization can maintain a physiologic state of complete emptying on a regular basis.

Urinary incontinence is a prominent sign of bladder dysfunction. Continence is based on outflow resistance generated by the bladder neck and external urinary sphincter. Outflow resistance must remain greater than resting bladder pressure during storage throughout normal daily activity. When outflow resistance is diminished because of an abnormal bladder neck and external urinary sphincter, incontinence often will occur. Pharmacologic management with α-adrenergic agents can enhance outflow resistance when needed, but operative reconstruction is more commonly required in that setting.

When incontinence occurs during the filling phase because of poor outlet resistance, it is essential to evaluate not only the bladder neck and external urinary sphincter but detrusor characteristics. Clinical experience has shown that once appropriate resistance is achieved at the bladder neck through operative intervention, adverse detrusor characteristics may become unmasked and result in high-pressure urinary storage or uninhibited contractions not previously documented (Bauer et al, 1986; Churchill et al, 1987). For that reason, provocative urodynamic assessment with occlusion of the bladder neck is important before any bladder neck reconstruction in an attempt to identify children who will be at risk.

Normal synergistic voiding occurs when the bladder neck descends, relaxes, and opens followed by relaxation of the external urinary sphincter and subsequent detrusor contraction. The cascade results in low-pressure voiding.

Dysfunctional voiding during this active bladder phase occurs from discoordinated activity of the bladder neck, external urinary sphincter, and detrusor and can result in urinary incontinence. In addition, when neurogenic dysfunction leads to detrusor-sphincter dyssynergy, high-pressure voiding results during a period of time, having a negative impact on the bladder and upper urinary tract (Mundy et al, 1982; Bauer et al, 1984a). A similar clinical situation occurs with a fixed, fibrotic external sphincter. Initial treatment usually involves pharmacologic management and mechanical elimination of urine from the bladder through clean intermittent catheterization in an attempt to bypass the abnormal voiding mechanics.

Other Considerations

Renal function should be assessed in any patient undergoing bladder reconstruction, particularly if hydronephrosis or severe renal scarring is present. **Demos (1962) and Koch and McDougal (1985) have demonstrated that urinary solutes, particularly chloride, are absorbed from urine in contact with the mucosa of small and large bowel.** For patients with normal renal function, the kidneys are able to handle the reabsorbed load of chloride and acid without obvious difficulty. Patients with decreased renal function, however, may develop significant metabolic acidosis secondary to such reabsorption. If acidosis exists preoperatively, it will invariably worsen if urine is stored in small or large intestinal segments (Mitchell and Pizer, 1987). The first component of renal function to deteriorate after obstruction or infection is typically concentrating ability. Patients with compromised function may generate enormous volumes of urine. **The bladder volume achieved through bladder reconstruction must accommodate the patient's urinary output for an acceptable time, usually about 4 hours.** Patients with renal failure or other medical problems may conversely develop oliguria. Low urinary output may affect an augmented bladder or bowel reservoir as there is greater potential for collection and inspissation of mucus. There is also less urine for dilution and buffering of gastric secretions if stomach is used.

Abnormal function of other organ systems also influences the risk of bladder reconstruction with use of intestinal segments. Reabsorption of ammonia by large or small intestinal segments in contact with urine may be dangerous for patients with hepatic failure (McDougal, 1992a). Some medications excreted in urine may be reabsorbed by bowel mucosa (Savauagen and Dixey, 1969). Therefore, liver function tests and arterial blood gas studies may be appropriate for some patients. Careful history should be taken of the patient's preoperative bowel function; this is particularly true of adult patients who may have acquired, or secondary, gastrointestinal problems. Obviously, short-gut syndrome is a concern among patients with cloacal exstrophy, prior bowel resections, or a history of significant irradiation. A history of chronic diarrhea or fecal incontinence preoperatively should signal concern about use of the ileocecal valve in urinary reconstruction.

A critical factor to consider is the commitment of the patient and family. Urinary incontinence, at times, protects some patients from infection and upper tract deterioration. Effective storage can put the patient at risk for such problems if emptying is not accomplished on a regular basis. All must be aware of the responsibility that goes along with bladder reconstruction and urinary continence.

The timing of appropriate surgical intervention may vary dramatically among patients. It is sometimes necessary to perform early reconstruction when the upper tracts and renal function are threatened. This situation most often occurs in the presence of high outflow resistance and poor bladder compliance. More commonly, intervention may be undertaken later to achieve urinary continence. The age at which urinary incontinence becomes socially unacceptable varies among patients and families.

When appropriate, it is beneficial for the patient and family to wait for bladder reconstruction until all needs of the patient are identified. With intervention because of infection or hydronephrosis, this is not always possible. When reconstruction is undertaken to achieve continence, it is most efficient to identify all reconstructive issues and to address them with one operation. Good urodynamic assessment is usually necessary to determine whether a procedure to increase outflow resistance is necessary in addition to bladder augmentation or replacement. Introduction of intermittent catheterization preoperatively is mandatory in that it allows the patient to demonstrate the ability and desire to do so on a regular basis. It is also helpful in determining whether a continent abdominal wall stoma may help improve the reliability of catheterization and increase the patient's independence. Likewise, particularly in the neurogenic population, it is advantageous to identify the patient who may also benefit from an antegrade colonic enema. It is certainly better for the patient and surgeon to address all of these issues at one operative sitting rather than with sequential procedures.

EVALUATION OF THE PATIENT

Each patient should have upper tract imaging before bladder reconstruction. Most patients with significant bladder problems will have had routine ultrasonography as part of their surveillance. **If hydronephrosis is present, obstruction and vesicoureteral reflux should be sought with a functional renal study and voiding cystography.** Nuclear renography with a catheter in the bladder is usually adequate to rule out a primary upper tract obstruction. Reflux should be excluded with a voiding study, although that study may be done as part of videourodynamics. In the presence of any hydronephrosis, each patient should have determinations of serum electrolytes, blood urea nitrogen, and serum creatinine. For patients with elevation of the serum creatinine or significant hydronephrosis, a 24-hour urine collection for both creatinine clearance and urine volume should be obtained.

Urodynamics

Bladder Dynamics: Capacity and Compliance

Urodynamic assessment of the lower urinary tract plays an essential role in considering bladder reconstruction. It can provide reproducible results in infants and children but requires meticulous attention to detail (Joseph, 1994). Several mechanical factors may adversely influence urodynamics data, creating artifacts that can have a negative impact on the validity of the evaluation if they are not recognized. Testing is typically performed with transurethral catheter placement in this population of patients. The size of the catheter can lead to the appearance of elevated leak or voiding pressure and the inability to empty well, particularly in infants and young boys (Decter and Harpser, 1992). Suprapubic catheter placement circumvents this problem but is not practical in most cases. The testing medium and infusion rate can influence the results. Carbon dioxide is not as reliable as fluid infusion, particularly in evaluation of bladder compliance and capacity. The most common fluids used for testing are saline and iodinated contrast medium, both of which provide reproducible results (Joseph, 1993). Use of testing media at body temperature is also appropriate (Joseph, 1996). End filling pressure, and therefore bladder compliance, can be dramatically affected by simply changing the filling rate (Joseph, 1992). Bauer (1979) has suggested that cystometrography be performed at a fill rate of no more than 10% of the predicted bladder capacity per minute.

Sphincter Dynamics: Outflow Resistance

The bladder neck and external urinary sphincter work in synergy, but only one is required to maintain urinary continence. Often, neurogenic dysfunction leads to abnormalities of both the bladder neck and external urinary sphincter, resulting in diminished outlet resistance during storage or dyssynergic function with voiding. Monitoring of external urinary sphincter electrical activity is required to evaluate coordinated voiding and dyssynergic detrusor-sphincter activity. Perineal surface electrodes, abdominal wall sensors, anal plugs, vaginal monitors, electrical wires, and concentric needle electrodes have all been used for electromyography (Joseph, 1996). In children with neurogenic dysfunction, a concentric needle electrode or dual needle electrodes placed through a 25-gauge needle increase accuracy in measuring sphincter activity (Blaivas et al, 1977; Joseph, 1996).

The functional length of the external urinary sphincter also plays a role in outflow resistance, and its measurement can be undertaken with urethral pressure profilometry. Unfortunately, the short length and small diameter of the pediatric urethra make this study technically more difficult to perform than in the adult as the mechanical pulling device is not practical for pediatric use. To assess urethral pressure profile, a constant infusion of testing medium at a rate of 2 mL/min with use of a continuous Harvard pump is required (Joseph, 1996) to eliminate pressure wave artifacts noted with the standard roller ball infusion pumps. Hand withdrawal of the catheter is done while every 5 mm is marked on the recording strip. With practice, reliable measurements can be obtained. There is limited value in comparing specific urethral pressure profile results for a patient against a standard uroflow nomogram; however, a preoperative urethral pressure profile for a given patient provides baseline information that can be beneficial in assessing the intraoperative and postoperative functional urethral length.

Some surgeons use leak point pressure to evaluate outflow resistance, that bladder pressure causing leakage per urethra. It can be determined during passive filling and Valsalva maneuver. Fluoroscopy can be informative during those events. The leak point pressure may be artifactually elevated by the urodynamics catheter in a small male urethra (Decter and Harpser, 1992). Much work remains to determine how well such measurable parameters correlate.

Bladder Emptying

The patient's ability to empty the bladder before reconstruction should be assessed carefully. Useful parameters related to bladder emptying include synergistic relaxation of the external sphincter on electromyography, urinary flow rates, and measurements of postvoid residual urine. Neurologically normal patients who are able to empty the bladder well preoperatively are much more likely to do so after reconstruction than are patients who have neurogenic dysfunction or those who are unable to empty well preoperatively. **No test ensures that a patient will be able to void spontaneously and empty well after bladder augmentation or other reconstruction.** Therefore, all patients must be prepared to perform clean intermittent catheterization postoperatively. The native urethra should be examined for the ease of catheterization. Ideally, the patient should learn clean intermittent catheterization and practice it preoperatively until the patient, family, and surgeon are comfortable that catheterization can and will be done reliably. Physical and psychosocial limitations of the patient must be considered in regard to the ability to self-catheterize and to perform self-care. **Failure to catheterize and empty reliably after bladder reconstruction may result in upper tract deterioration, urinary tract infection, or bladder perforation despite a technically perfect operation.** Most patients who may catheterize per native urethra or an abdominal wall stoma will overwhelmingly prefer the latter (Horowitz et al, 1995).

PREPARATION OF THE PATIENT

Bladder and sphincter reconstructive procedures remain some of the most challenging in urology. The general status of patients should be optimized so that they have the best chance to achieve a good result with the least risk of morbidity. Each patient's general nutritional and hydration status should be determined and corrected, if necessary, before surgery. Coexisting medical problems, particularly cardiac and pulmonary, should be well managed preoperatively.

Bowel Preparation

Each patient undergoes preoperative bowel preparation to minimize the potential risk of surgery if the use of any bowel is contemplated. Even when ureterocystoplasty or other alternatives are planned, intraoperative findings may dictate the need for use of a bowel segment. A clear liquid diet for 2 days before bowel preparation aids in clearing solid stool. The patient should then undergo full mechanical bowel preparation the day before surgery. Historically, such bowel preparations have been done in the hospital; however, recent trends find this changing to an outpatient setting. Major reconstructive procedures often require many hours of operative time with large fluid shifts. It is critical that the patient be well hydrated at the time of surgery. There should be a low threshold for the use of intravenous fluids during the preoperative day. The use of oral antibiotics in bowel preparation, once dogma, is now a matter of personal preference. Special attention must be paid to the bowel preparation of patients with neurogenic dysfunction. Most of these patients have chronic constipation. Good bowel cleansing is difficult in such patients and should be done aggressively. Several days of oral cathartics and a clear liquid diet at home may be helpful.

Theoretically, gastric contents are sterile, and parenteral antibiotics and a routine bowel preparation are not necessary before gastrocystoplasty. Nonetheless, it is safest to follow the preceding guidelines for all patients because intraoperative considerations may preclude the use of stomach or ureter and necessitate ileocystoplasty or colocystoplasty.

Urine Culture

All patients should have a urine culture performed several days before bladder reconstruction. The bladder should not be opened with infected urine, which will spill intraperitoneally. Any patient with a positive preoperative urine culture should undergo treatment with either oral or intravesical antibiotics and have a second culture documenting sterile urine before the procedure. Many pediatric patients undergoing augmentation cystoplasty have spina bifida and a ventriculoperitoneal shunt. With a negative urine culture and good bowel preparation, the incidence of shunt infection or problems should be low (Yerkes et al, 2001).

Cystoscopy

Preoperative cystoscopy may be the final step in evaluating the native bladder, outflow, or ureteral orifices in pediatric patients. Endoscopy should be performed immediately before bladder reconstruction under the same anesthetic. In adult patients with interstitial cystitis or irritative bladder symptoms requiring augmentation cystoplasty, cystoscopy should be performed well before augmentation to rule out urothelial carcinoma in situ. Bladder biopsy and cytologic examination of the urine may be helpful in excluding tumor. On the basis of history, an occasional patient may warrant endoscopic or radiographic gastrointestinal evaluation.

KEY POINTS: EVALUATION AND PREPARATION

- ■ Evaluation for renal function, upper tract obstruction, and vesicoureteral reflux should be performed if hydronephrosis is present, although most such changes are secondary to the bladder dysfunction.

- ■ Careful urodynamic evaluation is critical to understand all of the problems that may contribute to the dysfunction.

- ■ The patient is likely to require clean intermittent catheterization after reconstruction and must be capable of doing so on a reliable basis.

- ■ Commitment of the patient and family is essential.

- ■ Basic preoperative preparation includes sterile urine and thorough bowel cleansing.

ANTIREFLUX

Ureteral reimplantation into a native bladder, whether the ureter is dilated or not, is a standard procedure familiar to all pediatric urologists and reconstructive surgeons. The long-term success rate is good, and complications are rare. Such reimplantation is certainly preferable and usually possible during lower tract reconstruction.

Transureteroureterostomy and Single Ureteral Reimplantation

On occasion, the urinary bladder is so small that it is inadequate for bilateral reimplantation, and alternatives must be considered. It is preferable to reimplant both ureters separately, although **if the native urinary bladder is small and adequate for only a single ureteral tunnel, transureteroureterostomy and a single reimplant may be helpful** (Fig. 124–1). Typically, the better ureter should be implanted into the bladder, draining the other across into it. The crossing ureter should be mobilized to swing gently across the abdomen to the recipient side in a smooth course without tension. It should be carefully mobilized with all of its adventitia and as much periureteral tissue as possible to preserve blood supply. Care must be taken not to angulate the crossing ureter immediately beneath the inferior mesenteric artery. The crossing ureter is widely anastomosed to the posteromedial aspect of the recipient ureter. The recipient is not mobilized or brought medially to meet the end of the other

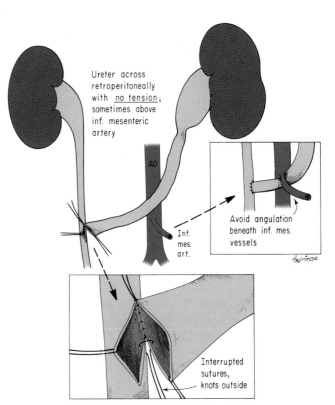

Figure 124–1. Technique for transureteroureterostomy. AO, aorta; Inf. mes. art., inferior mesenteric artery. (Courtesy of W. Hardy Hendren.)

ureter. Transureteroureterostomy, when it is fashioned appropriately, is successful and carries minimal risk for leakage or obstruction (Hodges et al, 1963; Hendren and Hensle, 1980; Noble et al, 1997; Mure et al, 2000). A history of previous calculi remains a relative contraindication to transureteroureterostomy.

The manner in which the bladder is opened may optimize its use for a single reimplant. Rather than incision of the bladder in the anterior midline, a wide, anterior U-shaped incision based cephalad can be made. This potentially elongates the bladder as a posterior plate that can be brought to one side or the other to meet a single ureter. Incision of the bladder in this way may also be useful in placing a continent catheterizable stoma to the umbilicus when the native bladder otherwise will not reach that far. For ureteral reimplantation after such an incision, a psoas hitch of the bladder fixes the bladder in position for a long, straight ureteral tunnel.

Psoas Hitch

Fixation of the bladder to the psoas muscle allows precise control of both the length and direction of a ureteral reimplant. Securing the bladder in this manner helps the bladder reach a short ureter or development of a long tunnel when necessary. A psoas hitch should prevent any angulation of the ureter with bladder filling. Such angulation may be particularly problematic or obstructive with a dilated and scarred ureter. The bladder should be secured to the psoas muscle and fascia with nonabsorbable sutures. Those sutures must not enter the bladder lumen or stones will occur. Broad, shallow purchases of the psoas muscle and fascia should be used to hold long term without trapping the sciatic nerve. The hitching sutures should not be tied so tightly that they cut through either bladder or psoas muscle. The contralateral bladder pedicle may be divided to increase bladder mobility and the length of the hitch on occasion. In general, the ureteral reimplantation should be performed before the bladder psoas hitch (Fig. 124–2).

Antireflux with Intestinal Segments

Necessity of ureteral reimplantation into an intestinal segment may occasionally determine the segment to be used for bladder augmentation or replacement. Long experience with ureterosigmoidostomy and colon conduit diversion has established an effective means of antireflux into a colonic segment. A flap valve mechanism can be constructed by tunneling the ureter beneath a taenia. Important principles learned from ureterosigmoidostomy include a direct mucosa-to-mucosa anastomosis and a submucosal tunnel of adequate length. This technique, familiar to most urologists, has provided favorable long-term results since the 1950s (Nesbit, 1949; Goodwin et al, 1953; Leadbetter and Clarke, 1954) and is based on the initial work of Coffey (1911). Implantation may be done from inside the reservoir with the intestinal segment open or from without after the intestinal segment has been completely reconfigured and closed.

If a gastric segment is used for bladder augmentation or replacement, ureters may be reimplanted into the stomach in a manner remarkably similar to that used in the native bladder. It is easy to form a submucosal tunnel with good muscle backing. The same principles for choosing the length of tunnel relative to the width of the ureter are used as with bladder. Construction of an effective antireflux mechanism into an ileal segment is more difficult. The split-nipple technique described by Griffith may prevent reflux at least at low reservoir pressure (Turner-Warwick and Ashken, 1967; Patil et al, 1976; Stone and MacDermott, 1989; Sagalowsky, 1995). A short longitudinal incision is made in the distal ureter and the ureteral wall turned back on itself. The nipple should be at least twice as long as the width of the ureter. The cuff is stabilized by suturing the ureter to itself. The adventitia of the ureter immediately proximal to the cuff is then approximated to the full thickness of the ileal wall at the hiatus so that the cuff protrudes into the lumen. Le Duc and associates (1987) described a technique in which the ureter is brought through a hiatus in the ileal wall. From that hiatus, the ileal mucosa is incised and the edges are mobilized to construct a trough for the ureter. The spatulated ureter is laid into the trough and approximated to the mucosa at the distal end. The ileal mucosa is sutured to the lateral edges of the ureter and should eventually grow over it. Long-term results with these two techniques have been conflicting but generally have not proved as reliable as a tunneled ureterocolonic anastomosis in preventing reflux (Patil et al, 1976; Le Duc et al, 1987; Rowland, 1996; Bihrle, 1997), with one exception (Lugagne et al, 1997). It is also possible to construct an antirefluxing, serosa-lined tunnel between two limbs of ileum as described by Abol-Enein and Ghoneim (1999).

Reinforced nipple valves of ileum have been used extensively for antireflux with the Kock pouch (Skinner et al, 1989). After several modifications by Skinner, good long-term results have been achieved. His technique requires a relatively long segment of ileum and use of permanent staples. Attempts have been made to secure the nipple long term without staples or mesh (Hanna and Bloiso, 1987; Gosalbez and Gousse, 1998; Tsuchiya et al, 2004). Maintenance of the intussuscepted cuff is the key to a successful result. The same forces that compress the nipple to achieve continence tend to evert or destabilize it. An ileal nipple valve may be particularly useful with short, dilated ureters; an isoperistaltic segment of ileum may be left with the nipple to replace a short ureter. Likewise, the antireflux mechanism is based on the ileal segment and not the ureter. Consequently, a very dilated ureter may be anastomosed to the ileum without tapering. In some neobladders, an isoperistaltic limb of ileum is positioned between the reservoir and ureters to discourage reflux, at least at low pressures (Studer and Zingg, 1997).

KEY POINTS: ANTIREFLUX

- Ureteral reimplantation into native bladder is preferable when necessary; the initial bladder incision may facilitate such a procedure.

- An antireflux mechanism can be constructed with any bowel segment but is most challenging with ileum.

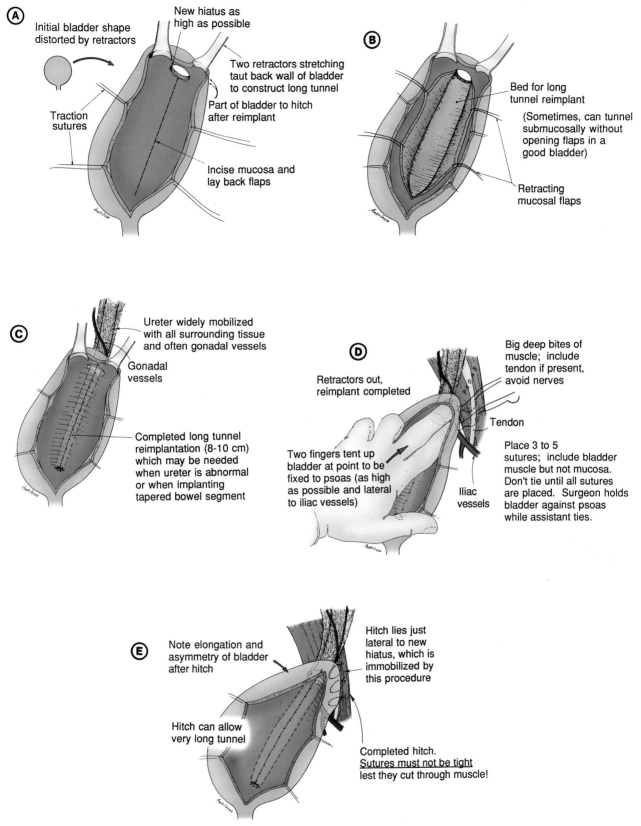

(A)
Initial bladder shape distorted by retractors
Traction sutures
New hiatus as high as possible
Two retractors stretching taut back wall of bladder to construct long tunnel
Part of bladder to hitch after reimplant
Incise mucosa and lay back flaps

(B)
Bed for long tunnel reimplant
(Sometimes, can tunnel submucosally without opening flaps in a good bladder)
Retracting mucosal flaps

(C)
Ureter widely mobilized with all surrounding tissue and often gonadal vessels
Gonadal vessels
Completed long tunnel reimplantation (8-10 cm) which may be needed when ureter is abnormal or when implanting tapered bowel segment

(D)
Retractors out, reimplant completed
Two fingers tent up bladder at point to be fixed to psoas (as high as possible and lateral to iliac vessels)
Iliac vessels
Big deep bites of muscle; include tendon if present, avoid nerves
Tendon
Place 3 to 5 sutures; include bladder muscle but not mucosa. Don't tie until all sutures are placed. Surgeon holds bladder against psoas while assistant ties.

(E)
Note elongation and asymmetry of bladder after hitch
Hitch can allow very long tunnel
Hitch lies just lateral to new hiatus, which is immobilized by this procedure
Completed hitch. Sutures must not be tight lest they cut through muscle!

Figure 124–2. Technique for psoas hitch, which allows the construction of a long reimplantation tunnel and prevents angulation of the ureter or tapered bowel segment when the bladder fills. Monofilament nonabsorbable suture material is used to fix the bladder to psoas muscle. Care must be taken to avoid entering the bladder, which might cause stone formation on a suture. (Courtesy of W. Hardy Hendren.)

BLADDER NECK RECONSTRUCTION

One of the greatest technical challenges facing the surgeon in bladder reconstruction is providing adequate outflow resistance. The bladder neck may be incompetent due to neurogenic dysfunction secondary to spinal dysraphism. Other underlying pathologic conditions, such as exstrophy, bilateral ectopic ureters, and ureteroceles, are unique problems that must be considered in addressing outlet resistance. Many operative techniques have been described for bladder neck reconstruction, indicating that no single option is best for all patients (Kryger et al, 2000; Cole et al, 2003). **It cannot be overstated that preoperative evaluation and thorough knowledge of the patient's specific physiologic limitations are required.**

The capability for a sustained bladder contraction to result in complete emptying by voiding or the absence of hyperreflexic contractions may influence the technique selected for gaining outlet resistance. Any operative technique that increases outlet resistance may do so at the expense of detrusor contractility. For reasons not clearly defined, increasing outlet resistance can change the behavior of the detrusor into a noncompliant hostile environment (Bauer et al, 1986; Burbige et al, 1987; Churchill et al, 1987). Provocative cystometry may identify only some patients at risk, and close postoperative observation is mandatory (Kronner et al, 1998b).

A spectrum of techniques are available for repair; these encompass tightening of the bladder neck, construction of a flap valve mechanism, placement of artificial or autologous bulking agents, and the artificial urinary sphincter. **The selected option should be individualized to the patient's pathologic process, needs, and personal goals.**

An important consideration is the patient's ability to empty well before reconstruction and the likelihood that the patient can afterward. Some of these repairs may prohibit spontaneous voiding. In many patients, particularly patients with neurogenic dysfunction also requiring bladder augmentation, voiding cannot be expected, and the major concern is providing adequate outflow resistance. For those with other diagnoses, especially if augmentation cystoplasty is not necessary, spontaneous voiding remains a key goal.

The following discussion covers a variety of operative techniques used to achieve urinary continence through bladder neck and external urinary sphincter reconstruction. Most of the results are based on experience in individuals with spinal dysraphism, but the techniques may be used with other pathogenic conditions. All techniques have a learning curve, which necessitates careful analysis of results and forthright reporting. An evidence-based review of operative bladder neck procedures found assessment of results to be limited by several factors, including the lack of a true, consistent definition of "success" and "continence," consideration of patients with and without concomitant bladder augmentation, and evaluation of small populations of patients with mixed pathologic conditions (Joseph et al, 2003).

Young-Dees-Leadbetter Repair

The Young-Dees-Leadbetter bladder neck reconstruction is one of the most recognized operative techniques to increase outlet resistance. The original Young procedure has evolved and remains of primary consideration in reconstruction of the exstrophic bladder neck (Ferrer et al, 2001). It has been used in patients with many diagnoses.

Technique

Young's initial description (1919) of excising a portion of the bladder neck and significantly tightening the bladder neck over a silver probe was modified by Dees (1949), who extended the length of excised tissue through the trigone. Leadbetter (1964) followed by elevating the ureters off the trigone, placing them in a more cephalad position on the bladder floor. This allowed tubularization of the trigone and further enhanced lengthening of the urethra. A detailed description and illustrations are found in Chapter 119.

Results

Reports of success with the Young-Dees-Leadbetter bladder neck reconstruction in children with neurogenic sphincter dysfunction are limited, not only in the number of patients but in overall improvement. Tanagho (1981) and Leadbetter (1985) independently reviewed their long-term results and showed minimal success in individuals with neurogenic dysfunction. They speculated that the lack of success was due to a lack of muscle tone and activity in the wrapped muscle related to the underlying neurogenic problem. Many patients in the early series did not undergo bladder augmentation, possibly compromising the continence achieved. Contrary to the results reported in exstrophy patients, the majority of individuals with neurogenic deficiency of the bladder neck will require bladder augmentation and intermittent catheterization. Sidi and colleagues (1987b) documented a 4-hour continence interval in 7 of 11 patients after such repair, although 10 required catheterization and 9 required augmentation. Five of the seven needed reoperation to achieve continence. This small series represents one of the more recent long-term results of the Young-Dees-Leadbetter reconstruction in children with neurogenic dysfunction as it has largely fallen out of favor. In an attempt to enhance the Young-Dees-Leadbetter procedure, Mitchell and Rink (1983) described the addition of external support and compression achieved through the placement of a silicone sheath around the reconstructed bladder neck. This was somewhat done to establish a plane for future placement of an artificial sphincter cuff, if necessary. In place, it seemed to improve the function of the repair by either improving coaptation or by maintaining the proximal repair in a better anatomic position. Unfortunately, most of the thicker Silastic sheaths eventually eroded and disrupted the repairs (Kropp et al, 1993). Quimby and colleagues (1996) used a thinner Silastic sheath without the same risk of erosion. They also wrapped omentum between the repair and Silastic wrap. The authors reported better results of ultimate continence and thought that placement of an artificial sphincter cuff was much easier when needed.

Donnahoo and coworkers (1999) reviewed one of the largest series of the repair used in treatment of neurogenic incontinence (38 children, 25 of whom were girls). A primary repair was performed in 24 children, a secondary procedure in 6, and a primary repair in conjunction with a silicone sheath in 8. Partial continence was achieved after the initial repair in 26 children (68%). All children with the silicone sheath were initially continent, but erosion occurred in five. More critically, 35 (92%) of the children required augmentation cystoplasty to become continent. The authors found that although continence could be achieved with this technique, it was at the expense of augmentation cystoplasty and multiple procedures. Their results are similar to those reported by Cole and associates (2003).

Fascial Sling

Sling procedures were developed in an attempt to increase resistance at the bladder neck. Both artificial and natural tissue have been used with similar technique. Resultant coaptation and elevation of the bladder neck should cause approximation of opposing epithelial surfaces and increased outlet resistance that is greater than the resting bladder pressure and the pressure achieved during stressful activity or Valsalva behavior. With sling coaptation, the bladder neck remains fixed, and although a strong detrusor contraction can establish a voiding pressure leading to urine flow, it rarely allows adequate bladder emptying in the face of anatomic or neurologic problems. The majority of pediatric patients who undergo a sling procedure must be prepared for intermittent catheterization. The resistance achieved with bladder neck slings can potentially be overcome by hyperreflexic bladder contractions or elevated pressure due to diminished bladder compliance. Therefore, simultaneous bladder augmentation has again been reported in 55% to 100% of patients who achieve urinary continence after a sling procedure (Bauer et al, 1989; Elder, 1990; Decter, 1993; Kakizaki et al, 1995; Perez et al, 1996a; Dik et al, 1999, 2003; Walker et al, 2000; Bugg and Joseph, 2003; Cole et al, 2003; Godbole et al, 2003). Alternatives to fascia, such as an expanded fluorocarbon polymer (Gore-Tex), have been used in a similar fashion, although early continence has not been maintained (Godbole and Mackinnon, 2004). Good early results have been noted with some biodegradable scaffolds (Colvert et al, 2002).

Technique

The bladder neck is exposed by clearing fatty tissue overlying the bladder neck and the lateral endopelvic fascia. An incision is made within the endopelvic fascia for approximately 2 cm. The junction between the bladder neck and proximal urethra can be identified by placing a transurethral catheter into the bladder and gently pulling down on the catheter to lodge the balloon at the bladder neck. By blunt dissection, a plane between the posterior bladder neck and vagina in girls or rectal wall in boys is developed. The proper plane may be more easily developed from the cul-de-sac by dissecting behind the bladder and ureters from above (Lottmann et al, 1999; Badiola et al, 2000). If the landmarks are not easily defined, as in a secondary repair, the dissection becomes difficult. It may be appropriate to open the bladder to help prevent inadvertent dissection into the urethra or posterior structures. Dik and colleagues (2003) proposed a transvaginal approach, eliminating the need to open the bladder or to dissect between the bladder neck and anterior vagina.

When fascial tissue is used, the technique is based on that described by McGuire and Lytton (1978) for stress urinary incontinence. Rectus abdominis fascia 1 cm in width and an appropriate length is harvested. This fascia can be taken either in vertical or horizontal fashion, depending on the initial skin incision. Fascia from other sites has been used in a similar fashion but requires a second incision. Cadaveric tissue or biodegradable scaffolds may also be used (Colvert et al, 2002). All are generally secured to the anterior rectus fascia on either side. Autologous fascial tissue has been used, combining the benefits of a compressive wrap and suspension of the proximal urethra and bladder neck. Several variations of fascial placement and configuration have been described (Woodside and Borden, 1982; McGuire et al, 1986; Elder, 1990; Perez et al, 1996a; Bugg and Joseph, 2003; Dik et al, 2003). When fascial slings and wraps are used for neurogenic sphincter incontinence, there is not as much concern for making a wrap or sling that is too tight because most patients are preferentially managed with clean intermittent catheterization.

Results

Fascial slings have been used more extensively and with better results in girls with neurogenic sphincter incompetence, although some success has recently been reported in boys. Overall long-term success with fascial slings in the neurogenic population has varied greatly from 40% to 100% (Kryger et al, 2000). A variation thought to contribute to a higher success includes a circumferential fascial wrap around the bladder neck. A circumferential wrap may equalize the compressive pressure over a greater surface area of bladder neck and posterior urethra (Walker et al, 1995). With the wrap, simultaneous suspension has also been used (Bugg and Joseph, 2003). Success rates have varied so much that it is difficult to determine whether any modification of the sling accounts for an increase in continence. Most patients who have undergone a fascial sling or wrap have also had simultaneous bladder augmentation. **Success of the sling, as with most repairs, appears to be improved with augmentation cystoplasty in this population of patients.** Perez and associates (1996a) reviewed the outcome of sling cystourethropexy in 39 children, 15 of whom were boys. One of four techniques was performed. When postoperative continence was evaluated on the basis of age, sex, underlying diagnosis, preoperative urodynamics, surgical technique, and enterocystoplasty, only concomitant enterocystoplasty was predictive of a successful outcome.

Contrary to the Silastic sheath, fascial sling erosion rarely occurs. Gormley and coworkers (1994) reported a revision rate with fascial slings of 15%. Placement of a fascial sling does not eliminate the possibility of later placement of an artificial urinary sphincter (Decter, 1993; Barthold et al, 1999). It is not unreasonable to consider placement of a fascial sling in a child with a marginally competent bladder neck and posterior urethra if the child is undergoing augmentation cystoplasty and already requires intermittent catheterization.

Bladder Neck Bulking Agents

Vorstman and colleagues (1985) reported one of the initial descriptions of injection therapy with a bulking agent into the bladder neck of incontinent children. The initial enthusiasm for use of polytetrafluoroethylene was quickly tempered because of concern about migration of particles to regional and distant sites including pelvic nodes, lungs, brain, kidney, and spleen found in animal models (Malizia et al, 1984). The technique remains of interest, and several alternatives to polytetrafluoroethylene have been assessed, including glutaraldehyde cross-linked collagen (Leonard et al, 1990a). One concern regarding the use of bovine collagen is the potential for reaction in latex-sensitive children with spina bifida since the product is not latex free (Kryger et al, 2000). In an attempt to achieve an ideal substance for injection, investigation is ongoing with autologous cartilage cells harvested from a separate site and then grown in an alginate matrix for endoscopic implantation (Bent et al, 2000). Preliminary results show a positive effect in adult women with stress incontinence. Whether this or other materials will be an appropriate alternative for neurogenic sphincter incontinence in children is yet to be seen.

In an attempt to alleviate the risks with injection of a foreign biologic product, alternatives to collagen and bovine have been investigated. Polydimethylsiloxane is one such agent. It is composed of sterile solid textured silicone particles, with an average size of 200 µg, suspended in a biologic hydrogen carrier. The large size of the particles should virtually eliminate lymphatic and distant migration (Beisang and Ersek, 1992; Guys et al, 1999; Halachmi et al, 2004).

Technique

Endoscopic exposure is used to localize the proximal urethra and bladder neck. Injection can be done directly through the working channel of the endoscope, often one with an offset lens system. Ideal placement of the material is in a subepithelial space, mobilizing the epithelium toward the lumen of the bladder neck. When it is completed in a circumferential fashion, adequate epithelial coaptation may occur that effectively raises outlet resistance. Alternatively, periurethral injection in women with a long needle placed from the perineum or through a suprapubic approach has been used. Evidence is lacking whether the exact approach affects success, but accurate placement is important and transurethral injection generally preferred.

Results

The durability and success of bladder neck and proximal urethral injection remain in doubt for the pediatric population, particularly those with neurogenic dysfunction. True continence, as defined by a 4-hour dry period between voidings or catheterization, has been reported to be at most 64% and has ranged as low as 5% (Leonard et al, 1990a; Capozza et al, 1995; Bomalaski et al, 1996; Perez et al, 1996b; Sundaram et al, 1997; Silveri et al, 1998; Guys et al, 2001; Godbole et al, 2003; Halachmi et al, 2004). Several factors play a role in the outcome, one of which is a history of any previous operative bladder neck repair. Success is enhanced by elevation of the epithelium of the bladder neck, which may be compromised by scarring from previous operative procedures. **The concept of a minimally invasive operation used to enhance a marginal result gained from a more formal bladder neck repair is enticing; unfortunately, the data are lacking to show that bladder neck injection is of lasting value in that setting.**

Sundaram and colleagues (1997) reported on the efficacy and durability of glutaraldehyde cross-linked bovine collagen in 20 children, 12 of whom had neurogenic sphincter dysfunction. More than half of the children required two or three independent injections. Success was achieved in only one patient (5%), who was considered dry; five had some improve-

ment, and 10 had either no change or transient improvement of only 2 to 90 days. In their hands, collagen therapy only delayed the ultimate need for bladder neck reconstruction. Submucosal bladder neck injection of bovine dermal collagen was used by Perez and coworkers (1996b) in 32 patients. Continence was achieved after a single injection in only 20% of the children with neurogenic dysfunction. Complications were limited to febrile urinary infections, one episode of urinary retention, and worsening incontinence in two patients. The authors concluded that even though their success was limited, the low morbidity and ease of placement justified submucosal injection in selected children.

Guys and associates (1999) treated 33 children with polydimethylsiloxane, 24 of whom had neurogenic bladder neck and sphincter incontinence. One third of the children achieved continence for more than 4 hours, and one fourth were continent for approximately 2 hours with minimal pad use. Poor results were reported in approximately 40%. Their results were not affected by previous operative procedures on the bladder neck or by detrusor hyperreflexia. Success was noted to be gender biased; 47% of girls were somewhat continent compared with only 10% of boys.

Godbole and associates (2003) and Halachmi and colleagues (2004) independently came to the conclusion that regardless of the material injected (polytetrafluoroethylene, collagen, or polydimethylsiloxane), short-term success is not long lasting. Further study is required to determine whether the same finding will be present with the use of a dextranomer–hyaluronic acid copolymer.

The cost of the bulking agents can be excessive, and there does not appear to be any financial benefit over a formal repair (Kryger et al, 2000). **At present, bulking agents play a limited role for increasing outlet resistance and should be reserved for a select group of patients. The exact criteria that define that group have not been established.** Patients with marginal native outflow resistance are probably better candidates than are those with minimal preoperative function.

Artificial Urinary Sphincter

The artificial urinary sphincter has been recognized as a device that can result in prompt continence in select children while preserving their ability to void spontaneously. The artificial urinary sphincter was introduced by Scott in 1974. The general concept and design of the initial model have been retained; however, improvements and enhancements have evolved that have positive impact on the long-term success of the artificial urinary sphincter. The current 800 model includes a seamless, pressurized balloon reservoir, nonkink tubing, and changes in the cuff that facilitate its placement and effectiveness with coaptation of the bladder neck and proximal urethra (Light and Reynolds, 1992; Barrett et al, 1993). Alternatives to the AS800 model have also been explored (Vilar et al, 2004).

Technique

Placement of the cuff should be at the level of the bladder neck in all female patients and prepubertal boys (Fig. 124–3). It is also the most desirable and effective location in pubertal boys and adult men with neurogenic sphincter incompetence. The bulbar urethra can be used as an alternative site in adult men

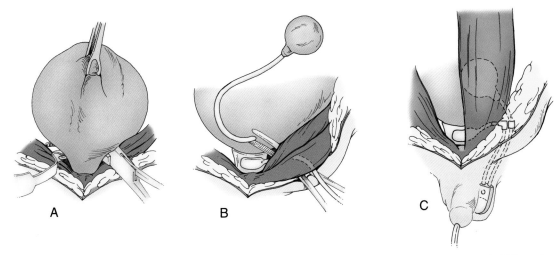

Figure 124–3. Artificial urinary sphincter placement in children. **A,** The cuff is placed around the bladder neck in prepubertal children. Dissection may be facilitated by palpation of a urethral catheter and balloon or by a posterior approach. If dissection is difficult, the bladder can be opened. **B,** The reservoir is placed beneath the rectus muscle. **C,** A tunnel is then made into the scrotum or labia for positioning of the pump on the same side as the reservoir. Tubing connections are made ventral to the rectus fascia, and the device is initially left deactivated.

with mature spongiosum. Levesque and associates (1996) have indicated that age is not a factor in placement of the cuff around the bladder neck. They found that children do not outgrow the artificial urinary sphincter as they progress through puberty and that replacement of the cuff is not routinely necessary. The artificial urinary sphincter cuff can be positioned around intestinal segments used in total urinary reconstruction but is more susceptible to erosion there. Several authors have described the successful placement of the cuff around a bowel segment, particularly when omentum is interposed between the cuff and the segment (Burbige et al, 1987; Weston et al, 1991; Light et al, 1995).

Placement of an artificial sphincter in children is the same as that described for adults. Development of the proper plane for the cuff is virtually identical to that described for a fascial sling. The cuff should be sized snugly, but not tightly, around the bladder neck. Obviously, a sterile environment is critical in considering placement of the artificial urinary sphincter to avoid infection. For that reason, preoperative antibiotics are a necessity, and confirmation of sterile urine is required. With those precautions, there is freedom to open the bladder in dissecting around the bladder neck. This will often facilitate the dissection and ensure proper placement. The AS800 model has a locking mechanism in the pump that permits the artificial urinary sphincter to be deactivated and activated without a second operative procedure. Experience has shown that leaving the unit deactivated with the cuff deflated after placement allows formation of a pseudocapsule around the cuff and decreases the risk of erosion (Furlow, 1981; Sidi et al, 1984). The noncycled artificial urinary sphincter occasionally may provide enough resistance for continence, eliminating the disadvantages of activation (Herndon et al, 2004a).

Results

There are substantial short- and long-term data regarding continence after placement of the artificial urinary sphincter, with the largest series presented by Herndon and associates (2003). **In investigation of continence, it must be placed in context of the cost experienced by the patient defined by mechanical malfunctions resulting in secondary operative procedures and more catastrophic complications, such as device infection and erosion.** Dramatic improvement regarding the need for secondary procedures has occurred with the technical refinements in the device. Ten- to 15-year long-term follow-up of the artificial urinary sphincter in children has been reported (Levesque et al, 1996; Kryger et al, 1999, 2001; Castera et al, 2001; Hafez et al, 2002; Herndon et al, 2003). All groups report an impressive continence rate of 80% and a functioning sphincter in 95% of patients. These reports are consistent with older series in children reporting continence rates of 75% to 90% and a functioning sphincter in 85% to 97% (Nurse and Mundy, 1988; Gonzalez et al, 1989a; Bosco et al, 1991; O'Flynn and Thomas, 1991; Aprikian et al, 1992; Singh and Thomas, 1996; Simeoni et al, 1996). Herndon and colleagues (2003) presented the most comprehensive long-term data. They achieved overall continence in 86% of 142 patients with an average follow-up of 10 years. Age at implementation does not appear to affect continence (Kryger et al, 2001).

Whereas the artificial urinary sphincter is one of the few surgically created continence mechanisms that does not negatively affect spontaneous voiding, intermittent catheterization remains an important adjunct in approximately 75% of children with neurogenic sphincter incompetence and can be performed successfully through the cuff (Diokno and Sonda, 1981; Gonzalez et al, 1995; Levesque et al, 1996; Kryger, 1999, 2001; Castera et al, 2001; Hafez et al, 2002; Herndon et al, 2003). As boys approach puberty, spontaneous voiding may become progressively inadequate. It has been speculated that growth of the prostate causes an increase in native outlet resistance. Kaefer and associates (1997a) evaluated increases in cuff size to facilitate spontaneous voiding in boys. In their limited series, they did not find that up-sizing restored the ability to void spontaneously. Jumper and colleagues (1990) reported on prostatic development and sexual function in pubertal boys with spinal dysraphism who had been treated with the artificial urinary sphincter. They found that the artificial sphincter did not alter sexual development, prostatic growth, or morphologic features.

Herndon and associates (2003) reported device malfunction in 64% with the pre-AS800 model and 30% with the AS800. Sphincter erosion was similar for the pre-AS800 and AS800, occurring at 19% and 16%, respectively, in their experience. Fastidious attention to detail and sterile technique diminish the risk of infection but do not eliminate it. When infection occurs without erosion, the unit can be removed and later replaced (Nurse and Mundy, 1988). Infections are minimized by sterilization of the urine preoperatively, meticulous cleaning of the wound site, preoperative bowel preparation, perioperative parenteral antibiotics, and copious antibiotic wound irrigation. Newer cuff design and a 6-week delay in activation of the device help formation of a thickened pseudocapsule that substantially decreases bladder neck and proximal urethral erosion. Kryger and associates (1999) indicated that erosion can be virtually eliminated when the cuff is placed as the primary treatment for bladder neck incompetence. They and others (Aliabadi and Gonzalez, 1990; Gonzalez et al, 1995; Simeoni et al, 1996; Levesque et al, 1996; Castera et al, 2001; Hafez et al, 2002; Herndon et al, 2003) noted that the risk of erosion substantially increases after previous failed repairs. Identification of the correct plane between the bladder neck and vagina in female patients or rectum in male patients preserves the vascularity of the bladder neck and proximal urethra and may decrease the rate of erosion (Aliabadi and Gonzalez, 1990). Initial exposure through a posterior bladder approach as described by Lottmann and coworkers (1999) may be helpful. Shankar and colleagues (2001) suggested that there is an advantage to exposure of the bladder neck with a transperitoneal approach by decreasing the potential of bleeding from the prostatic venous plexus and improving visualization of the rectal wall.

Levesque and associates (1996) evaluated the long-term outcome of the artificial urinary sphincter on the basis of date of insertion and location of the placement. Before 1985, the artificial urinary sphincter had been inserted in 36 children. Between 1985 and 1990, an additional 18 children underwent placement. In the original group, 24 of the 36 sphincters were in place and 22 functional; 12 had required at least one revision. The mean survival of the device was 12.5 years. Success rates at 5 and 10 years were 75% and 72%, respectively. In the group implanted after 1985, 78% retained a functioning sphincter. The overall continence rate in both groups was 59%; sphincter survival probability at 10 years was approximately 70%. There was no difference found between failure rates in males and females with the exception that female patients who had previously undergone bladder neck surgery were more likely to suffer an erosion. The ability to void independently without the use of intermittent catheterization was retained in 36 children (67%). Those findings are supported by contemporary series (Kryger, 1999, 2001; Levesque et al, 1996; Castera et al, 2001; Hafez et al, 2002; Herndon et al, 2003).

Upper urinary tract changes including hydronephrosis have been reported to occur in up to 15% of children after placement of the artificial urinary sphincter (Light and Pietro, 1986; Churchill et al, 1987; Gonzalez et al, 1995; Levesque et al, 1996; Kryger et al, 1999). In extreme cases, renal insufficiency has

resulted. **It is now recognized that occlusion of the bladder neck in children with neurogenic sphincter incompetence can result in the unmasking or development of detrusor hostility manifested by a decrease in bladder compliance or increase in detrusor hyperreflexia** (Bauer et al, 1986). **Careful preoperative urodynamic assessment helps identify only some of the children who are at risk** (Kronner et al, 1998b). When hostile bladder characteristics are found preoperatively, anticholinergic medications can be beneficial for hyperreflexic contractions, but augmentation cystoplasty is usually required for diminished compliance. Churchill and associates (1987) showed that favorable parameters can be maintained after placement of the artificial urinary sphincter; however, close observation is still recommended in any child undergoing bladder neck reconstruction to identify any early deterioration in bladder dynamics before upper tract changes.

Some children undergoing sphincter placement need bladder augmentation as well, and the timing of the two procedures may be questioned because of the concern for artificial urinary sphincter infection. Light and colleagues (1995) reported a 50% infection rate with simultaneous augmentation compared with 9.5% when the procedures were staged. On the contrary, a contemporary review by Miller and coworkers (1998) found that infection necessitating removal of the device occurred in only 2 of 29 such patients (7%). This low rate is similar to that noted by others (Strawbridge et al, 1989; Gonzalez et al, 1989b). Several reports have evaluated various factors and found that the intestinal segment selected for augmentation appeared to be the only parameter affecting results; gastric augmentation was the least offensive regarding infection (Ganesan et al, 1993; Miller et al, 1998; Holmes et al, 2001). Gonzalez and associates (2002) reported an alternative technique using a seromuscular colocystoplasty and simultaneous placement of the artificial urinary sphincter. They achieved continence in 89% without the need for additional procedures and no deterioration of the upper urinary tract.

The AS800 is the subject of most reviews when the artificial urinary sphincter is discussed, but alternative devices have been reported. Lima and colleagues (1996) reported on the combined use of enterocystoplasty and a "new type" of artificial urinary sphincter. The new device is a one-piece adjustable cuff connected to an inflatable port. The injection port is placed subcutaneously and made available for percutaneous access to adjust the fluid valve and pressure of the cuff needed to achieve continence. It is too early to determine whether this will be an acceptable alternative.

The ultimate benefits of the artificial urinary sphincter lie in its ability to achieve a high rate of continence while maintaining the potential for spontaneous voiding. For practical purposes, when intermittent catheterization is required along with augmentation cystoplasty, use of native tissue for continence eliminates the long-term concern for infection or erosion and the risk of mechanical failure.

Urethral Lengthening

Young's original description of bladder neck reconstruction (1919) consisted of two components—excision of a segment of anterior urethral bladder neck tissue and narrowing of the adjacent remaining posterior portion. This, however, ultimately led to failure because the tubularized segment remained unsupported within the bladder. Refinements by Dees (1949) and Leadbetter (1964) maximized good muscle tone at the bladder neck and extension of the urethral tube through the trigone.

With similar principles, Tanagho (1981) described a cephalad-based anterior detrusor wall tube. Closure of the tubularized bladder neck formed circularly oriented muscle fibers that Tanagho described as a sphincter mechanism. However, he cautioned against the use of this technique in the neurogenic population. Because of potential breakdown of that tubularized bladder neck and poor results, other techniques have been developed on the basis of the concept of a flap valve mechanism for urinary retention. Kropp and Angwafo (1986) described urethral lengthening and construction of a flap valve for neurogenic bladder neck and sphincter dysfunction. The technique is based on an anterior detrusor wall tube that is kept in continuity with the urethra, tubularized, and implanted into a submucosal tunnel within the trigone. Conceptually, this is effective; however, difficulty with catheterization is a common problem and significant concern.

Technique

A Foley catheter is placed intravesically and the bladder filled to capacity. The bladder is exposed through either a midline or low transverse abdominal incision. The bladder neck is then identified with application of gentle catheter traction. A 6 × 2-cm rectangular flap based on the bladder neck and urethra is then isolated. Stay sutures are placed, and the flap is mobilized in continuity with the proximal urethra. The detrusor musculature at the bladder neck is then divided, separating the bladder and urethra, or the muscle may be left intact at the 5- and 7-o'clock positions. The anterior vaginal wall is exposed in girls; the seminal vesicles are exposed in boys. The rectangular strip based on the urethra is tubularized posteriorly around the urethral catheter with a continuous absorbable suture. The distal portion of the tubularized strip should be approximated in an interrupted fashion to facilitate excision of excessive tissue without jeopardizing the suture line. A capacious submucosal tunnel through the trigone is then developed posteriorly for the proximal neourethra (Fig. 124–4). A wide tunnel is required to prevent kinking at the level of the bladder neck, which will impede catheterization. It is important to eliminate dead space at the entrance of the urethra into the bladder, and this can be accomplished by placement of lateral anchoring sutures in the region of the bladder neck. The detrusor tube must be pulled straight through the tunnel without curve or deviation to facilitate catheterization. Waters and colleagues (1997) and Kropp (1999) have not found it necessary to reimplant all ureters in a cephalic location; they now typically reimplant only refluxing ureters (Kropp, 1999). When the bladder is closed, the lateral wings in the region of the bladder neck are approximated and incorporate adventitia of the tubularized urethra. This enhances a watertight closure and is continued for 2 to 3 cm anteriorly, often up to the area of augmentation. The tubularized neourethra should be long enough to reach the true lumen of the bladder, where it is exposed to pressure as an effective flap valve.

Because of the difficulties with catheterization, modifications of the Kropp bladder neck procedure have been described. Belman and Kaplan (1989) suggested a simplified approach. They harvested a rectangular strip from the anterior bladder wall similar to that described by Kropp. The lateral and posterior muscles at the bladder wall are not incised, however, and the proximal urethra and bladder are not separated. The flap is tubularized over an 8 French catheter. The epithelium on the floor of the bladder is incised, contrary to the tunnel made by Kropp. The tube is placed within the trough with the proximal meatus secured on the floor of the bladder. The epithelial edges of the trough are then secured to the lateral aspect of the tube. As in the initial description, the suture line for tubularization of the urethra is posterior against trigonal muscle. Closure of the bladder begins with reapproximation of the lateral walls of the bladder to the tube until the bladder edges meet. The remaining portion of the bladder is covered by an augmentation. Regardless of any modification to the Kropp bladder neck procedure, catheterization potentially remains problematic, and therefore the patient should be prepared for a catheterizable abdominal-vesicle channel.

Results

Snodgrass (1997) examined the results in 23 children, 22 of whom had neurogenic sphincter incompetence, and noted continence in more than 90% of the children. The most common complication was difficult catheterization, particularly in boys. Less than half of the boys in Snodgrass' series catheterize through the native urethra; the majority do so through an abdominal wall stoma. Postoperative vesico-ureteral reflux was identified in 9 of 18 children, and Snodgrass speculated that this was due to lateral retraction of the ureters. The recommendation was made to leave the posterior bladder wall open and flat in receiving the augmentation to prevent this distortion. Kropp (1999) has not had as much problem with catheterizations in his patients and likewise has achieved a high rate of continence without a high incidence of new reflux.

Some patients with an effective flap valve mechanism constructed by urethral lengthening will virtually never leak per urethra. This potentially puts them at risk for upper tract deterioration or bladder rupture, particularly if they do not or cannot catheterize reliably. Snodgrass (1997) thought that his modification was beneficial in that it resulted in a shorter intravesical tunnel for the neourethra, allowing leakage per urethra with overfilling.

Pippi-Salle Procedure

In an attempt to maximize the benefits of the Kropp technique and to decrease problems with catheterization, Salle (1994) reported an anterior bladder onlay flap. With this technique, the posterior wall of the neourethra is intact, theoretically providing less potential hang-up during catheterization. Modifications have been made since the first report to improve flap viability, to minimize fistula formation, and to extend the indications for the procedure beyond that of the neurogenic bladder (Salle et al, 1997).

Technique

An anterior, full-thickness bladder wall flap 5 × 1 cm is mobilized to the bladder neck with 0.1 cm of its epithelial edges

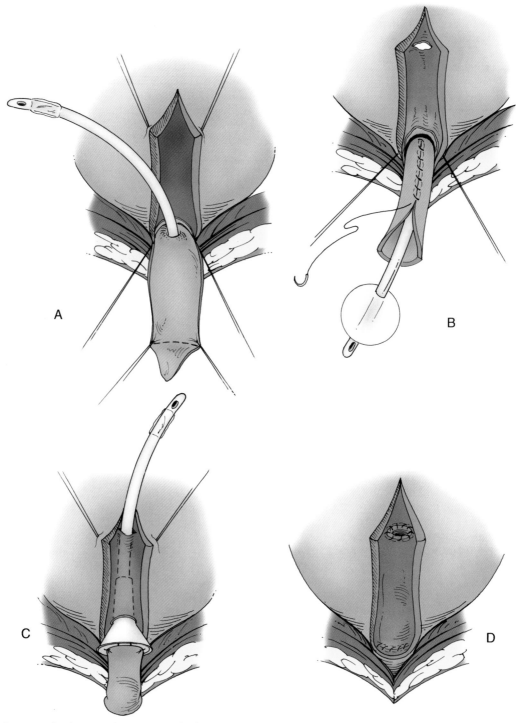

Figure 124–4. Kropp anterior detrusor tube. **A,** An anterior flap of bladder (2 cm in width by 5 to 6 cm in length) is developed in continuity with the urethra. **B,** The anterior flap is tubularized over a catheter. A tunnel beneath the mucosa of the trigone is made between the ureteral orifices for the length of the tube. **C,** The tubularized flap is brought through the tunnel. **D,** The detrusor tube is secured to the floor of the trigone with interrupted absorbable suture in a straight course.

excised to avoid overlapping suture lines. Two parallel incisions down to the level of the muscle are made in the mucosa of the trigone from the native bladder neck. The anterior flap is secured to the midline strip of trigone mucosa to form a tube of lengthened urethra with absorbable suture. The muscle on either side of the posterior epithelial strip may be

incised superficially to provide an edge to which the muscle of the anterior flap may be approximated with a second layer of suture in an effort to avoid fistula (Fig. 124–5). The more lateral mucosa of the trigone is mobilized and closed over the midline urethra. Distally, the muscle of the bladder neck is wrapped fairly tightly around the urethra with closure. More

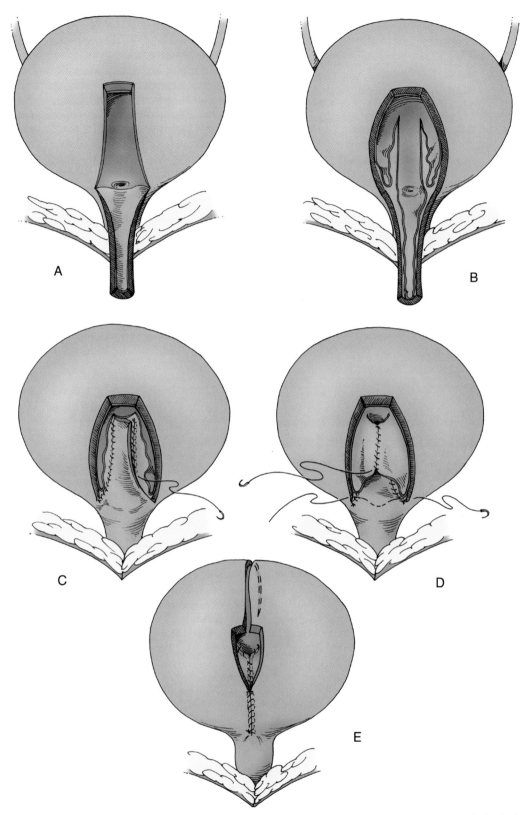

Figure 124–5. Pippi-Salle anterior detrusor tube onlay. **A,** An anterior detrusor tube (1 cm by 4 to 5 cm) is mobilized to the level of the bladder neck. **B,** A central strip on the floor of the bladder is developed by incision of the epithelium on either side. **C,** The anterior detrusor flap is secured to the strip in a two-layer fashion, approximating the epithelium with the first layer and muscle with the second. **D,** The lateral mucosa of the trigone is mobilized and secured over the lengthened urethra. Distally, the bladder is closed to itself and should incorporate a portion of the anterior detrusor flap to ensure a water-tight seal. **E,** After distal closure, the remaining portion of the bladder is left open if augmentation cystoplasty is necessary.

proximally, the lengthened urethra should extend well into the lumen of the bladder.

Results

Initial complications of this procedure included persistent incontinence, urethrovesical fistula, and partial necrosis of the intravesical neourethra. Widening the base of the urethra at the level of the bladder neck may decrease these problems. Children who have previously undergone bladder surgery can have a secondary Salle repair if the anterior bladder flap is lateralized slightly to avoid any old midline suture line and increased potential for scarring or necrosis.

Salle and coworkers (1997) found that continence was achieved in 12 of 17 patients (70%) for more than 4 hours. Catheterization difficulties occurred in only 3 of 17 children, one of whom subsequently underwent an appendicovesicostomy. Fistula formation at the base of the flap between the proximal, intravesical urethra and bladder occurred in two children and resulted in recurrent incontinence. This problem appears to be diminished by making a wider base to the flap and generously trimming the epithelial edges. Jawaheer and Rangecroft (1999) reported a diurnal continence rate of 61% for 3 hours or longer with the Salle procedure. However, only 44% of their patients were dry through the night. Less trouble with catheterization has occurred relative to the Kropp technique, and it rarely remains a problem. Continence rates have not been quite as high in most series (Rink et al, 1994; Mouriquand et al, 1995; Cole et al, 2003).

Bladder Neck Division

The ultimate procedure to increase bladder outlet resistance is to divide the bladder neck so that it is no longer in continuity with the urethra. It must be accompanied by construction of a continent abdominal wall stoma and should be performed only in patients who will reliably catheterize. If effective, it prevents any leakage or pop-off per urethra and potentially increases the risk for upper tract deterioration or bladder rupture if emptying is not performed. Division is seldom performed as a primary procedure but may be considered if the previously mentioned repairs fail.

Such a procedure effectively moves the reconstructive effort into the realm of continent urinary diversion. The bladder neck is abandoned from a physiologic standpoint, although the bladder may be used as part of the reservoir. Effective division of the bladder neck is not a simple procedure. The bladder must be aggressively mobilized away from the urethra after complete division of the bladder neck. The bladder should be closed distally in several layers. Omentum has generally been interposed. Without these steps, fistulization and leakage per urethra can occur.

AUGMENTATION CYSTOPLASTY

The initial approach to the patient for augmentation cystoplasty is similar regardless of the bowel segment to be used. Cystoscopy should be performed preoperatively to identify any unsuspected anatomic abnormalities that may affect the surgery or postoperative care. If other bladder procedures, such as ureteral reimplantation, are to be performed, the bladder is left full after cystoscopy. If only augmentation is

---

KEY POINTS: BLADDER NECK RECONSTRUCTION

- Any bladder neck repair other than placement of an artificial urinary sphincter, particularly in combination with augmentation cystoplasty, is likely to make spontaneous voiding inadequate.

- Young-Dees-Leadbetter bladder neck repair in the spina bifida population may have variable success related to the underlying neurogenic dysfunction.

- Fascial slings have been used more extensively and with better results in girls than in boys with neurogenic sphincter incompetence, although those results have varied greatly.

- Experience does not yet suggest that injection of bladder neck bulking agents has a lasting effect on severe neurogenic sphincter incompetence.

- A functioning, well-positioned artificial urinary sphincter device generally provides good outflow resistance and is best suited for patients who can empty adequately with spontaneous voiding.

- Urethral lengthening procedures construct an effective flap value mechanism for continence that disrupts any chance of spontaneous voiding and may make catheterization per urethra difficult.

- The success of all bladder neck repairs in the neurogenic population is improved when the repair is associated with bladder augmentation.

- Any bladder neck repair may unmask or result in new bladder hostility; careful follow-up is mandatory.

---

indicated, the bladder is emptied to allow easy access to the peritoneal cavity.

As a general rule, a midline incision is preferred for intestinal cystoplasty, although these procedures can be performed through a lower transverse incision if there has been no previous abdominal surgery. Laparoscopic assistance with mobilization of the intestine may allow augmentation through a smaller, lower incision (Hedican et al, 1999). Associated bladder procedures should be performed before the peritoneal cavity is opened to minimize third-space fluid loss. For gastrocystoplasty, the incision needs to extend from the pubis to xiphoid to allow more cephalad exposure.

Management of the Native Bladder

In the past, it had been recommended that the majority of the "diseased" bladder be excised in preparation for augmentation. This meant removal of the supratrigonal bladder, leaving only a small cuff of higher bladder for anastomosis to the intestinal segment. Despite the cuff, a relatively small area is left for anastomosis to the bowel segment; most of the bowel is approximated to itself. **Most surgeons now preserve the native bladder as long as it is widely opened to prevent a** narrow-mouthed anastomosis, which can result in the augmentation segment's behaving like a diverticulum (Fig. 124–6). A sagittal incision to bivalve the bladder is generally useful (Fig. 124–7). The incision is carried from a point several centimeters cephalad to the bladder neck anteriorly to a position just above the trigone posteriorly. Such an incision allows a technically easier anastomosis to the bowel segment and leaves the native bladder to add to the overall capacity. A greater circumference for the anastomosis can be provided, if needed, by opening the bladder in a stellate fashion with a second transverse incision into the two bladder halves. There have been reports of severe penile or perineal pain in sensate boys after augmentation with preservation of the native bladder (Phelps and Malone, 2004). Although four such patients required secondary excision of the bladder, similar problems have not been frequent enough to warrant routine excision at the time of augmentation.

Management of Intestinal Segments

Hinman (1988) and Koff (1988) have thoroughly demonstrated the advantages of opening a bowel segment on its antimesenteric border, which allows detubularization and reconfiguration of that intestinal segment. **Reconfiguration into a spherical shape provides multiple advantages, including maximization of the volume achieved for any given surface area, blunting of bowel contractions, and improvement of overall capacity and compliance.** All intact, tubular

intestinal segments have been noted to generate pressures of 60 to 100 cm H_2O with contractions, including ileum (Kock, 1969; Light and Engleman, 1985; Fowler 1988; Camey et al, 1991). Detubularization lowered the maximal contractile pressure from 63 to 42 cm H_2O in the right colon and 81 to 28 cm H_2O with use of ileum (Goldwasser et al, 1987). Furthermore, a shorter intestinal segment can be used to achieve the same capacity than when it is left in tubular form. **Detubularization and reconfiguration should always be performed during augmentation cystoplasty.**

Mathematical models based on the length and width of the bowel segment used may predict the volume needed but are cumbersome (Rink and Mitchell, 1990). Depending on the volume needed, 20 to 40 cm of ileum or approximately 20 cm of colon is generally used for cystoplasty. This somewhat depends on the volume of the native bladder being augmented. If the cystoplasty is being done on a bladder of moderate volume that generates high pressure by uninhibited contractions, less bowel is necessary than for one that is tiny in capacity. Unless it is otherwise contraindicated, the surgeon should err by making the bladder too large rather than too small. Appreciation of the patient's urinary volumes also should influence the size of the bladder required. Patients with upper tract damage, particularly to concentrating ability, may make huge volumes of urine and require a larger capacity.

Ileocystoplasty

Goodwin and associates (1959) were among the first to demonstrate the numerous ways of anastomosing a patch of ileum to the native bladder. Virtually all surgeons recognize that ileum should be detubularized and reconfigured to achieve the most spherical shape possible.

Technique

A segment of ileum at least 15 to 20 cm proximal to the ileocecal valve should be selected. The distal portion of terminal

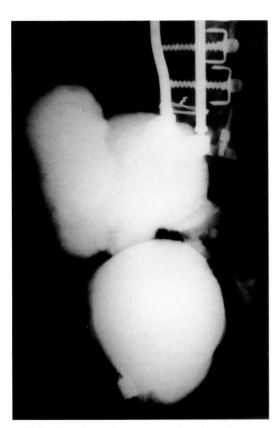

Figure 124–6. Cystogram after augmentation demonstrates a narrow anastomosis of the bowel segment to bladder. The segment behaves like a diverticulum.

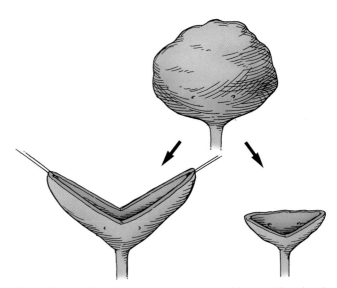

Figure 124–7. The native bladder can be managed by supratrigonal excision of the diseased bladder. More typically, the bladder is opened widely in a sagittal plane (left).

ileum is unique from a physiologic standpoint and should be avoided. The isolated segment should be 20 to 40 cm in length, depending on the patient's size, native bladder capacity, and desired final capacity. With short ureters, an extra tail of isoperistaltic ileum can be useful to reach the foreshortened ureters. This requires construction of an ileal nipple valve to prevent reflux as in the Kock or hemi-Kock pouch. This type of construction may require up to 60 cm of small intestine. **The segment to be used should have an adequate mesentery to reach the native bladder without tension.**

After selection of the appropriate segment, the mesentery is cleared from the bowel at either end for a short distance to make a window. The bowel is divided at these ends, and a hand-sewn ileoileostomy or stapled anastomosis is performed. The harvested ileal segment is irrigated clear with 0.25%

neomycin solution and opened on its antimesenteric border (Fig. 124–8A). **The ileum is folded in a U shape most commonly, although longer segments can be folded further into an S or W configuration.** The ileum is anastomosed to itself with running absorbable sutures (Fig. 124–8B). The suture line should approximate the full thickness of ileum to ileum while inverting the mucosa. If the bladder was not opened previously, it is incised in a sagittal plane. The anastomosis of the ileum to native bladder is easily done when it is started posteriorly. The anastomosis may be done in a one- or two-layer fashion, always with absorbable suture (Fig. 124–8C). Permanent sutures should never be used for any cystoplasty because they serve as a nidus for stone formation.

A suprapubic tube is brought out through the native bladder when possible and secured. The anterior aspect of the

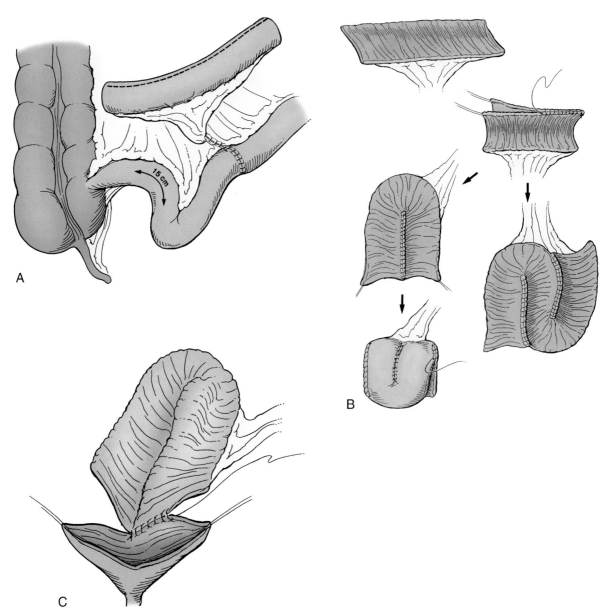

Figure 124–8. A, Ileocystoplasty. A 20- to 40-cm segment of ileum at least 15 cm from the ileocecal valve is removed and opened on its antimesenteric border. Ileoileostomy reconstitutes the bowel. **B,** The opened ileal segment should be reconfigured. This can be done in a U, S, or W configuration. It can be further folded as a cup patch. **C,** The reconfigured ileal segment is anastomosed widely to the native bladder.

anastomosis is then completed. The mesenteric window at the bowel anastomosis is closed to prevent an internal hernia. A drain is placed near the bladder and brought out of the pelvis through a separate stab incision. It should be removed promptly if it is not draining urine, particularly in neurogenic patients with a ventriculoperitoneal shunt. The wound is thoroughly irrigated, and the abdomen is closed in layers.

Cecocystoplasty and Ileocecocystoplasty

Couvelaire described the use of the cecum for augmentation cystoplasty in 1950, and numerous reports of simple cecocystoplasty have appeared since then. Presently, cecocystoplasty is an uncommon operative procedure and is not discussed because it has largely been replaced by various forms of ileocecocystoplasty. With this technique, the cecum is opened, reconfigured, and used to augment the bladder alone, leaving a segment of ileum to reach the ureters or for construction of a continent abdominal wall stoma based on imbrication of the ileocecal valve and proximal ileum. Conversely, the ileal segment can be opened and used as a patch on the cecal segment before augmentation cystoplasty. Many modifications of the technique exist, but all start with mobilization of the cecum and right colon by incision of the peritoneum along the white line of Toldt up to the hepatic flexure. Approximately 15 to 30 cm of the terminal ileum is used. The length of the ileal segment depends on the technique employed. As with all intestinal cystoplasties, before division of the bowel segment, it should be noted that it will reach the bladder without tension (Fig. 124–9A).

Technique

The isolated ileocecal segment is irrigated clear with neomycin solution and opened on its antimesenteric border through the ileocecal valve for its entire length. In the typical ileocecal augmentation, the ileal and cecal segments are of equivalent length such that the borders of the open segment can be anastomosed and then folded on themselves to form a cup cysto-

plasty (Fig. 124–9B). The anastomosis of the reconfigured segments is done in either a one- or two-layer closure with absorbable suture. The opening should be left large enough to provide a wide anastomosis to the bivalved bladder. **If more volume is necessary, the ileal segment can be significantly longer, allowing it to be folded before anastomosis to the cecum.** The Mainz ileocecocystoplasty uses an ileal segment twice the length of the cecal segment. The opened edge of the cecal portion is anastomosed to the first portion of the ileal segment. The first and second portions of the ileal segment are next approximated. The compound ileocecal patch is then anastomosed to the bladder (Fig. 124–10). The mesenteric window is closed, and a suprapubic tube is placed through the native bladder and secured through the abdominal wall.

Appendix. One potential advantage of ileocecocystoplasty is the presence of the appendix. Particularly in children, the appendix is useful in construction of a reliable continent abdominal wall stoma. The appendix may be removed with a small cuff of cecal wall and tunneled into the native bladder or a taenia of the cecal segment to provide a continence mechanism. Likewise, it may be left in situ and the base safely tunneled beneath a taenia. If the appendix is not to be used, an appendectomy is performed with standard ileocecocystoplasty.

Ileocecal Valve. The ileocecal segment has been used extensively in the adult population undergoing reconstruction and bladder replacement. It has been used less frequently in children because the majority of patients undergoing augmentation cystoplasty do so for neurovesical dysfunction. Those patients generally have neurapraxic bowel dysfunction as well. Removal of the ileocecal valve in such children can result in intractable diarrhea (Gonzalez and Cabral, 1987; King, 1987). Use of the ileocecal valve in such patients should be avoided unless other advantages of the segment outweigh the risk of diarrhea and fecal incontinence.

There are potential advantages to the use of the ileocecal segment. Antireflux tunnels can easily be performed into the taenia of the cecum when necessary. Again, for the short ureter, a tail of ileum can be left intact to bridge the gap and

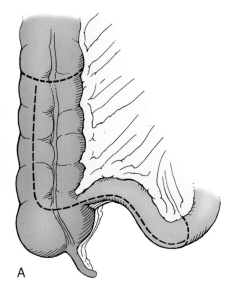
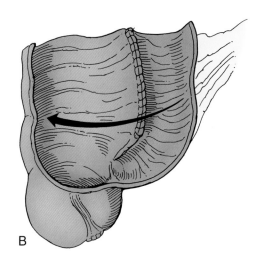

Figure 124–9. Ileocecocystoplasty. **A,** An ileocecal segment is selected. The length of segment chosen depends on the technique employed. After removal, it is opened on the antimesenteric border *(dashed lines).* **B,** The opened ileal and cecal segments are anastomosed to form a cup in the standard ileocecal cystoplasty.

A

B

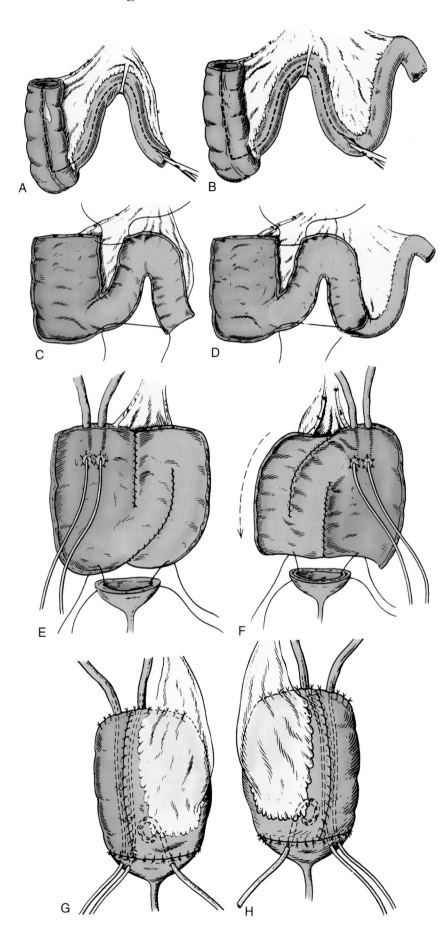

Figure 124–10. The Mainz ileocecocystoplasty. **A** and **B,** The ileal segment is twice the length of the cecal segment. **C** and **D,** It is opened on the antimesenteric border. **E** and **F,** The ureters can be reimplanted into the opened cecal segment if necessary. **G** and **H,** The ileocecal segment is anastomosed to the native bladder. (From Thuroff JW, et al: In King LR, Stone AR, Webster GD, eds: Bladder Reconstruction and Continent Urinary Diversion. Chicago, Year Book, 1987.)

the imbricated ileocecal valve used for antireflux. The same imbrication technique can be used to construct a continent abdominal wall stoma as with the appendix. Cain and associates (Cain and Husmann, 1994; Cain et al, 1999) have proposed use of the ileocecal segment for augmentation with the plicated ileal segment brought to the abdominal wall as a catheterizable stoma as in the Indiana pouch.

Sigmoid Cystoplasty

Use of the sigmoid colon for augmentation cystoplasty was first reported by Lemoine in 1912 (Charghi et al, 1967) and continues to be used commonly. **Because of the strong unit contractions of the sigmoid, it is imperative to detubularize and reconfigure the segment to provide maximal compliance and disruption of contractions.**

Technique

Fifteen to 20 cm of sigmoid colon is identified and mobilized. The mesentery is transilluminated to identify the vascular arcade to the segment. After identification of this blood supply, the surgeon must ensure that the segment can reach

the bladder without tension. If so, the bowel segment is divided between clamps and a colocolostomy performed (Fig. 124–11A). The remainder of the abdominal cavity is carefully packed to prevent contamination from the open sigmoid segment. Detubularization and reconfiguration are done in a fashion determined by the surgeon's preference. The sigmoid patch is anastomosed to the bivalved bladder in a manner similar to that previously described for ileocystoplasty. Again, a large suprapubic tube is brought out through the native bladder and secured to the bladder and skin exit sites. Drains are placed as previously noted.

Reconfiguration of Sigmoid. Sigmoid colon segments are generally reconfigured in one of two ways. Mitchell (1986) suggested closing the two ends and then opening the segment longitudinally opposite its blood supply. The segment easily fits on the bivalved bladder in either the sagittal or coronal plane (Fig. 124–11B). More radical reconfiguration, and perhaps breakup of unit contractions, may be achieved by folding the sigmoid segment in a U shape similar to that described for ileocystoplasty (Sidi et al, 1987a) (Fig. 124–11C). A slightly longer segment of sigmoid may be necessary for effective reconfiguration in this manner.

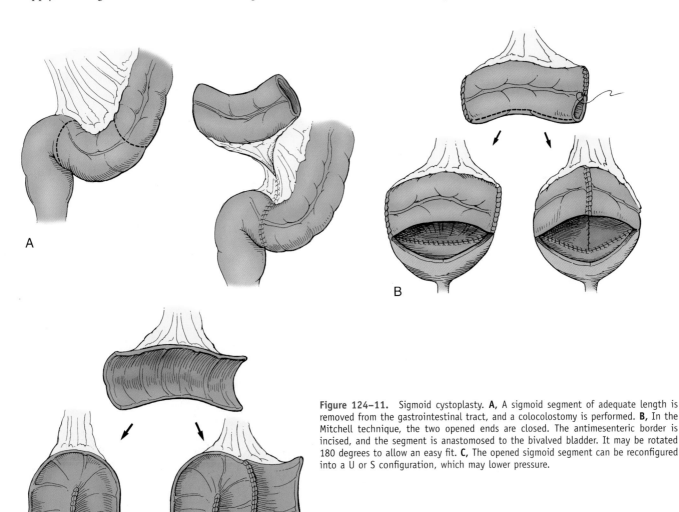

Figure 124–11. Sigmoid cystoplasty. **A,** A sigmoid segment of adequate length is removed from the gastrointestinal tract, and a colocolostomy is performed. **B,** In the Mitchell technique, the two opened ends are closed. The antimesenteric border is incised, and the segment is anastomosed to the bivalved bladder. It may be rotated 180 degrees to allow an easy fit. **C,** The opened sigmoid segment can be reconfigured into a U or S configuration, which may lower pressure.

Gastrocystoplasty

Two basic techniques exist for use of stomach in bladder augmentation.

Technique with Use of Antrum

Leong and Ong (1972) described the use of the entire gastric antrum with a small rim of body for bladder replacement. With their technique, the left gastroepiploic artery is always used as a vascular pedicle. If the right gastroepiploic artery is dominant and the left vessel ends high of the greater curvature, a strip of body along the greater curvature from the left gastroepiploic artery to the antrum is maintained and pro-

vides adequate blood supply (Leong, 1988). Continuity of the upper gastrointestinal tract is restored by a Billroth I gastro-duodenostomy.

Technique with Use of Body

A gastric wedge based on the midportion of the greater curvature may be used (Adams et al, 1988) (Fig. 124–12A). **The gastric segment used in this technique is made up mainly of body and consequently has a higher concentration of acid-producing cells. The right or left gastroepiploic artery may be used as a vascular pedicle to this segment.** The right artery is commonly dominant and thus more frequently used. The

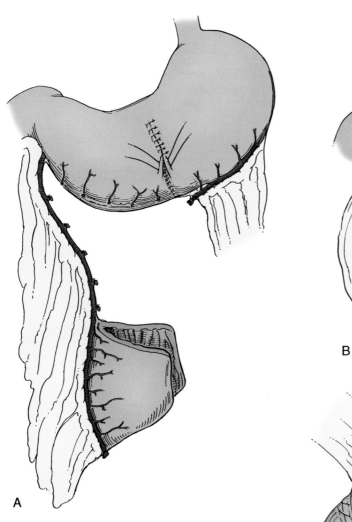

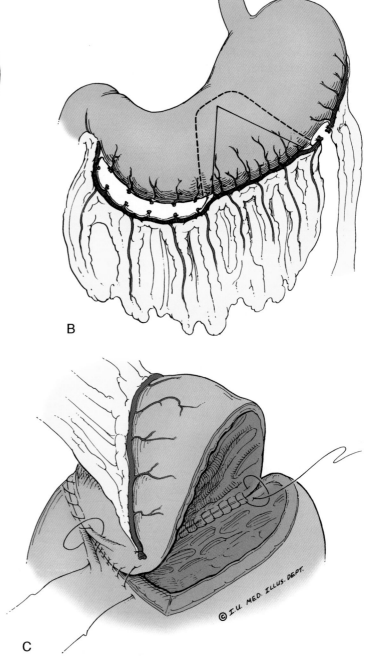

Figure 124–12. Gastrocystoplasty with use of the body. **A,** Gastric segment of body is mobilized on the right gastroepiploic artery. The left vessel may also be used; neither vessel as a pedicle should be free-floating through the peritoneum. **B,** Longer gastric segment along greater curvature with wider apex provides more surface area for augmentation. **C,** The gastric segment is anastomosed to the bivalved bladder with the mucosa inverted.

wedge-shaped segment of stomach includes both the anterior and posterior wall. The segment used may be 10 to 20 cm along the greater curvature, depending on the patient's age and size as well as the needed volume (Fig. 124–12*B*). The incision into the stomach is stopped just short of the lesser curvature to avoid injury to branches of the vagus nerve controlling the gastric outlet. Branches of the left gastric artery just cephalad to the apex of this incision are suture ligated in situ before incision to avoid significant bleeding. Parallel atraumatic bowel clamps are placed on either side of the gastric incisions to avoid excessive bleeding or spillage of gastric contents. Alternatively, the stomach may be incised by use of a gastrointestinal stapling device that places a double row of staples on each side of the incision (Mitchell et al, 1992). The staple lines, however, must eventually be excised. The native stomach is closed in two layers with permanent sutures on the outer seromuscular layer.

Branches of the gastroepiploic artery to the antrum on the right or to the high corpus on the left are divided to provide mobilization of the gastroepiploic pedicle. For the eventual pedicle to be long enough to reach the bladder, the appropriate segment may be higher on the greater curvature if the right vessel is used as a pedicle or lower if it is based on the left. The vascular pedicle, with omentum, should not be free-floating through the abdomen. The segment and pedicle may be passed through windows in the transverse mesocolon and mesentery of the distal ileum and carefully secured to the posterior peritoneum. Despite careful consideration for an adequate pedicle length, on occasion the gastric segment initially may not reach the bladder without tension. Either gastroepiploic artery may be mobilized closer to its origin for further length. The first few branches from the gastroepiploic artery to the isolated gastric segment may also be divided. Because of the rich submucosal arterial plexus in the stomach, devascularization of the isolated segment does not result. Rarely, it may be necessary to approximate some of the isolated gastric segment to itself in one corner. The gastric segment should be approximated to the native bladder with one or two layers of absorbable sutures, with care taken to invert the mucosa (Fig. 124–12*C*).

Raz and colleagues (1993) and Lockhart and associates (1993) have described the use of a much longer, more narrow segment of stomach based along the greater curvature. Use of this segment, which includes both body and antrum, somewhat narrows the lumen of the stomach along its entire length except at the fundus and pylorus. Raz and colleagues have isolated this segment with a gastrointestinal stapler so that the native stomach is never open. The segment used in both of these series is similar to that first described by Sinaiko (1956), the first surgeon to use stomach in bladder replacement. **Postoperative bladder and gastric drainage is no different from that described for intestinal cystoplasty.** H$_2$ blockers are often given in the early postoperative period to promote healing (Rink et al, 2000).

Postoperative Management

Early Management

Care of patients after cystoplasty is similar regardless of the gastrointestinal segment used in the procedure. **All patients are maintained on nasogastric decompression until bowel function recovers, including patients after gastrocystoplasty. Attention to fluid and electrolyte management is important because third-space losses may be significant after extensive reconstructive surgery.**

Continuous drainage of the bladder is achieved by suprapubic cystostomy. Mucus production from small or large bowel may be excessive and can potentially occlude the drainage catheter. **The suprapubic tube should be irrigated at least three times daily and whenever drainage is slowed by mucus.** Extravesical drains may be removed after several days, if drainage of urine is not apparent. The drains are generally removed more promptly in patients with a ventriculoperitoneal shunt to avoid potential infection. Some surgeons prefer a cystogram before discharge of the patient; others wait approximately 3 weeks for the study before clamping the suprapubic tube. All patients begin on clean intermittent catheterization every 2 to 3 hours during the day and one or two times at night after bladder healing is documented. The suprapubic tube is removed after catheterization is successfully under way and well tolerated. The duration between catheterizations is gradually increased during several weeks but should not exceed 4 to 5 hours during the day. Patients without neurologic impairment may eventually attempt to void spontaneously. All must check postvoid residual volumes and continue catheterizations if the residuals are significant.

Late Management

Routine radiographic surveillance of the upper urinary tract is indicated at 6 weeks, 6 months, and 1 year after augmentation cystoplasty. Most such surveillance may be done with ultrasonography. Serum electrolyte, blood urea nitrogen, and creatinine determinations along with urine cultures are performed several times in the first year after surgery. Not all positive urine cultures need to be treated in patients on clean intermittent catheterization. Certainly, symptomatic cystitis or infections involving urea-splitting organisms should be cleared. Evaluation by ultrasonography and serum chemistries is then appropriate once a year. Eventually, yearly endoscopy for tumor surveillance may be performed. No consensus exists about the initiation or frequency of cystoscopic examination; however, we generally begin such surveillance approximately 5 years after augmentation. There is no experience demonstrating that routine endoscopy is cost-effective or successful in this population.

Results and Complications of Augmentation Cystoplasty

The effect of cystoplasty on the patient should be considered in two main categories. One must first consider the effect of removal of a relatively small portion of the gastrointestinal tract for use in urinary reconstruction. **Any more than rare development of gastrointestinal problems would be prohibitive, even if results were perfect from the standpoint of the urinary bladder.** Second, the effect of augmentation cystoplasty on the urinary bladder must be reviewed. The primary goal of augmentation is to provide a compliant urinary reservoir. **Therefore, the main consideration after augmentation is the storage pressure and capacity that are achieved. Any** other effect on the urinary bladder is a side effect or complication that exists because bowel is not a perfect physiologic substitute for native bladder.

Gastrointestinal Effects

Postoperative bowel obstruction is uncommon after augmentation cystoplasty, occurring in approximately 3% of patients after augmentation (Gearhart et al, 1986; King, 1987; Mitchell and Pizer, 1987; Hollensbe et al, 1992; Rink et al, 1995a). **The rate of obstruction is equivalent to that noted after conduit diversion or continent urinary diversion** (McDougal, 1992b). Delicate handling of tissues, closure of mesenteric windows, and elimination of sites of internal herniation help avoid obstruction. Occasional series have suggested differing rates of bowel obstruction, depending on the segment used. These differences have not been consistent in most series and therefore are not likely to be significant; the incidence of bowel obstruction is low regardless of the gastrointestinal segment used and should not influence the choice of a particular segment for enterocystoplasty.

Reports of chronic diarrhea after bladder augmentation alone have been rare. Diarrhea can occur after removal of large segments of ileum from the gastrointestinal tract, although the lengths of the segments typically used for augmentation are rarely problematic unless other problems coexist. Much longer segments required for continent urinary diversion may increase the risk. The use of a typical colonic segment for augmentation only rarely results in a change in bowel function. **Removal of a segment from the gastrointestinal tract including the ileocecal valve is more likely to cause diarrhea.** Some children with neurogenic impairment depend on controlled constipation for fecal continence. Removal of the ileocecal valve from the gastrointestinal tract may significantly decrease bowel transit time. Loss of the valve can also allow bacterial backflow into the ileum, and the organisms may interfere with fat and vitamin B_{12} metabolism. Studies have noted chronic diarrhea in 10% to 23% of patients with neurogenic dysfunction after displacement of the ileocecal valve (King, 1987; Roth et al, 1995), although the risk may be lower for carefully selected patients (Husmann and Cain, 1999).

Ileum is the sole site of vitamin B_{12} absorption. **Removal of the distal ileum from the gastrointestinal tract may therefore result in vitamin B_{12} deficiency and megaloblastic anemia. Certainly, the terminal 15 to 20 cm of ileum should not be used for augmentation, although problems may arise even if that segment is preserved** (Steiner and Morton, 1991; Racioppi et al, 1999). Again, the risk is greater if longer segments of ileum are used as with continent diversion. Thirty-five percent of patients observed for 5 years after a Kock pouch were found to be deficient in vitamin B_{12} in one series (Akerlund et al, 1989). In general, the length of ileum used for augmentation is less than half of that used for a Kock pouch, so that vitamin B_{12} deficiency seems unlikely after routine bladder augmentation. Canning and associates (1989) evaluated 26 patients after bladder augmentation or replacement and found no patients with either fat malabsorption or vitamin B_{12} deficiency. Only three patients, however, were observed longer than 3 years, and longer observation is necessary because existing body vitamin B_{12} storage may last considerably longer (Stein et al, 1997a). Eventually, determination

of vitamin B_{12} levels or routine injections of the vitamin may be appropriate after ileocystoplasty.

Early satiety may occur after gastrocystoplasty but usually resolves with time. Disorders of gastric emptying should be extremely rare, particularly when gastric body is used.

Bladder Compliance after Augmentation

An early lesson of past clinical experience with augmentation cystoplasty is the value of detubularization and reconfiguration of the bowel segment (Hinman, 1988; Koff, 1988). **Bowel in its native, tubular form continues to display peristalsis or mass contraction. The tubular form does not maximize the volume achieved for the surface area of bowel used.** Hinman (1988) demonstrated with a mathematical model that the maximum volume achieved for a given surface area occurs when a sphere is formed. No finished cystoplasty is a perfect sphere but should approach it as nearly as possible.

Some surgeons with extensive experience in augmentation cystoplasty and continent diversion have concluded that ileum is superior to other segments in terms of compliance after augmentation, although controlled experimental examination of similarly sized and used bowel or gastric segments is lacking (Goldwasser and Webster, 1986; Rink and McLaughlin, 1994; Studer and Zingg, 1997). On the contrary, one report has suggested superior results with colon compared with ileum (Shekarriz et al, 2000) when a longer colonic segment reconfigured into a U shape was used. Good results have been achieved with all segments in most cases, and it is more important to use a bowel segment well than to choose a particular bowel segment for every patient.

Most problems with pressure after augmentation cystoplasty occur from uninhibited contractions, apparently in the bowel segment. It is extremely rare not to achieve an adequate capacity or flat tonus limb unless a technical error has occurred with use of the bowel segment. On occasion, a small, scarred pelvis may prevent adequate expansion of the augmented bladder. When pressure contractions occur in the bladder after augmentation, they are often noted in a rhythmic or sinusoidal pattern occasionally with increasing amplitude (Fig. 124–13). Contractions that begin at low amplitude later in filling and progress only near capacity may be of no clinical significance at all. Early contractions of higher pressure may occasionally result in persistent incontinence, delayed perforation, hydronephrosis, or vesicoureteral reflux. If patients have such clinical problems after augmentation, repeated urodynamic testing is necessary. One cannot assume the bladder is compliant after augmentation. Rhythmic contractions have been noted postoperatively with all bowel segments, although ileum seems the least likely to demonstrate remarkable urodynamic abnormalities and stomach the most.

After bladder augmentation or replacement, some urodynamic evaluation has suggested that colonic segments, whether cecum or sigmoid, still generate more pressure than ileum despite detubularization (Berglund et al, 1987; Jakobsen et al, 1987; Thuroff et al, 1987; Lytton and Green, 1989; Studer and Zingg, 1997). Some work has suggested that pressure contractions from the colon decrease with time (Hedlund et al, 1984; Sidi et al, 1986b). Nonetheless, Goldwasser's review of enterocystoplasty demonstrated contractions above 15 cm H_2O in 42% of patients after ileocystoplasty versus 60% of those after colocystoplasty (Goldwasser et al,

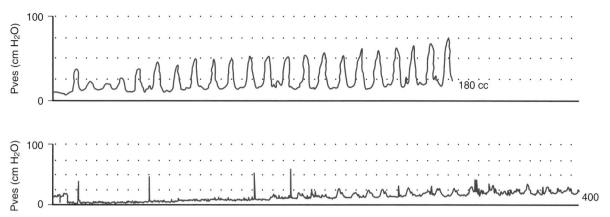

Figure 124–13. Rhythmic, sinusoidal contractions (above) may occur after bladder augmentation, in this case with stomach. Contractions of significant amplitude early in filling occasionally require secondary augmentation. After secondary augmentation with ileum (below), urodynamics show that contractions still occur but are much lower in pressure and occur later in filling.

1987). Significant contractions, defined as those above 40 cm H_2O at a volume of less than 200 mL, were not noted in any of the ileal augmentations but persisted in 10% of colocystoplasties. Their work agreed with that of Berglund and colleagues (1987) and Studer and Zingg (1997) in suggesting that ileal reservoirs have lower basal pressures and less motor activity. None of these studies critically controlled for the size of the bowel segment or the technique in which it was used.

Rhythmic contractions after gastrocystoplasty have been noted in up to 62% of patients (Adams et al, 1988; Atala et al, 1993a; Gosalbez et al, 1993a; Roth et al, 2000). The segment of stomach initially described for augmentation with the body was much smaller than segments of ileum or colon commonly used for cystoplasty. Use of a slightly larger gastric segment that is longer along the greater curvature results in improved urodynamics after augmentation with less prominent contractions (Adams et al, 1995; Kurzrock et al, 1998; Koraitim et al, 1999; DeFoor et al, 2003b). Leong (1988) has suggested that an antral segment of stomach is less likely to demonstrate such contractions.

In perhaps the largest experience with pediatric bladder augmentation, Hollensbe and associates at Indiana University found that approximately 5% of several hundred patients had significant uninhibited contractions after augmentation cystoplasty causing clinical problems (Hollensbe et al, 1992). Pope and Rink (1999) found that 6% of more than 300 patients required secondary augmentation of a previously augmented bladder for similar problems in long-term follow-up. These secondary augmentations represent true failures of the primary cystoplasty, not from any side effect or complication but from failure to achieve the objective, capacity and compliance. In that series, sigmoid colon followed by stomach and then ileum were more likely to require reaugmentation. A colonic segment closed at the ends and not generally reconfigured otherwise was typically used in that experience. Other studies have suggested that stomach is more likely than colon to require secondary intervention (El-Ghoneimi et al, 1998).

Metabolic Complications

Chloride Absorption and Acidosis. The first recognized metabolic complication related to storage of urine within

intestinal segments was the occasional development of hyperchloremic metabolic acidosis after ureterosigmoidostomy (Ferris and Odel, 1950). Patients with this metabolic derangement were noted to have fatigue, weakness, anorexia, and polydipsia. **Koch and McDougal** (1985) **demonstrated the mechanisms by which acid is absorbed from urine in contact with intestinal mucosa.** Resorption in the form of ammonium results in chronic acid loading. Patients with normal renal function are generally able to handle the resorbed load of chloride and acid without frank acidosis. **In 1987, Mitchell and Piser noted that essentially every patient after augmentation with an intestinal segment had an increase in serum chloride and a decrease in serum bicarbonate level, although full acidosis was rare if renal function was normal.** Similar trends of increased serum chloride and decreased bicarbonate have been noted with ileal conduits (Malek et al, 1971) and continent urinary reservoirs (Allen et al, 1985; McDougal, 1986; Ashken, 1987; Thuroff et al, 1987; Boyd et al, 1989). More severe acidosis and electrolyte disturbances requiring treatment have been reported despite normal renal function (Schmidt et al, 1973; Whitmore and Gittis, 1983). Such derangements may be debilitating to the patient if they are not recognized and treated; death of patients has been reported (Heidler et al, 1979). **Hall and colleagues noted that there is an increase in the urinary acid load with wasting of bone buffers even in the absence of frank acidosis** (Hall et al, 1991). Such wasting may result in bone demineralization and could potentially cause retarded growth in children after augmentation cystoplasty (Abes et al, 2003; Hafez et al, 2003; Vajda et al, 2003). Patients with acidosis should receive bicarbonate therapy. Whether all patients with intestine in the lower urinary tract might benefit from supplemental bicarbonate is controversial. Nurse and Mundy (1989) have suggested that arterial blood gas values may be more sensitive than serum bicarbonate or chloride levels for detecting acidosis. Stein and associates (1998) thought that measurements of arterial blood gas for base deficit allowed early treatment of acidosis and avoidance of bone demineralization. In severe cases of acidosis, chloride transport can be blocked with chlorpromazine and nicotinic acid.

Although jejunum is rarely used for bladder reconstruction, storage of urine in this segment results in a unique

metabolic pattern of hyponatremic, hypochloremic, and hyperkalemic metabolic acidosis. The problem is often associated with significant hypovolemia.

Gastric mucosa is a barrier to chloride and acid resorption and, in fact, secretes hydrochloric acid (Piser et al, 1987). This difference was the primary factor in the initial consideration of stomach for use in the urinary tract. This secretory nature was shown to be of benefit in azotemic animals during acid loading (Piser et al, 1987; Kennedy et al, 1988). **Serum chloride does decrease and serum bicarbonate increases slightly after gastrocystoplasty, whether antrum or body is used in patients with normal and impaired renal function** (Adams et al, 1988; Ganesan et al, 1991; Kurzrock et al, 1998). In 21 patients with renal insufficiency, serum bicarbonate improved in all patients except one after gastrocystoplasty, and many patients requiring oral bicarbonate therapy before cystoplasty did not do so after gastrocystoplasty (Ganesan et al, 1991). A similar benefit has been noted in a smaller group of patients with renal failure (Sheldon and Gilbert, 1991).

Patient Growth. Delayed or slowed growth in some children after intestinal cystoplasty has previously been recognized (Wagstaff et al, 1991, 1992; Mundy and Nurse, 1992). A delay in linear growth was noted in 20% of almost 200 pediatric patients without any gross biochemical abnormalities. However, no control patients were included in the series, and body habitus and growth are difficult to measure and predict in children with myelodysplasia. Such patients make up the majority in most series of augmentation cystoplasty. More recently, Gros and colleagues (2000) at the Johns Hopkins Hospital evaluated growth in exstrophy patients. Patients requiring augmentation were matched retrospectively with a similar group not requiring bladder augmentation. Hydronephrosis was not mentioned in the patients but was unlikely with a diagnosis of exstrophy. Only one patient was noted to have acidosis in either group. Other factors that might affect growth, such as urinary tract infection, were not controlled. Of 17 patients with adequate measurements before and after augmentation cystoplasty, 14, or 82%, had a decline in percentile height postoperatively. The decline corresponded to a 1.5-inch decrease in expected height. The pattern of growth was significantly different between patients with and without augmentation in the series. That series is small, and no evaluation of familial growth patterns or ultimate height was possible; however, the findings are worrisome, particularly since Feng and coworkers (2002) noted similar differences in exstrophy patients. In the absence of any serum abnormalities, the exact mechanism of delayed growth was not evident, although it seems likely to be related to chloride absorption and subclinical acidosis (Koch and McDougal, 1988; Bushinsky, 1989; Hochstetler et al, 1997). Three recent series did show effect of bowel cystoplasty on bone mineral density in some patients (Abes et al, 2003; Hafez et al, 2003; Vajda et al, 2003), although Mingin and associates (2002) noted no such changes clinically. Better analysis of subtle metabolic alterations after enterocystoplasty may establish better understanding of the effect on growth, minimize changes, or aid in early treatment to avoid the complication (Brkovic et al, 2004).

Alkalosis. The secretory nature of gastric mucosa may at times be detrimental to the patient and can result in two unique complications of gastrocystoplasty. Severe episodes of hypokalemic, hypochloremic metabolic alkalosis that followed acute gastrointestinal illnesses have been noted in 5 of 37 patients after gastrocystoplasty (Hollensbe et al, 1992). The episodes were significant enough to require hospitalization in all cases and were recurrent in two patients. Three of the five patients suffering the complication had renal insufficiency and would not have been good candidates for augmentation with other segments because of acidosis. Ganesan and associates (1991) noted similar episodes of alkalosis in 5 of 21 patients with renal insufficiency after gastrocystoplasty. **Those patients with the primary indication for consideration of gastrocystoplasty may be the ones at greatest risk for this unusual complication.** It has been proposed that the alkalosis results from ongoing chloride loss from the gastric segment in the bladder in the face of decreased oral intake. McDougal (1992a) suggested that the decreased ability to excrete bicarbonate from an impaired kidney may compound the problem. Gosalbez and associates (1993b) demonstrated persistently increased fractional excretion of chloride despite profound hypochloremia, suggesting that inappropriate gastric secretion is likely to be the primary mediator. One patient in their series eventually required resection of three quarters of the gastric segment in the bladder because of recurrent problems with alkalosis, and several required therapy with H_2 blockers or H^+-K^+ ion pump inhibitors.

All patients and families should be made aware of this potential problem as it has been reported to occur intermittently in between 3% and 24% of patients. A composite reservoir of stomach and ileum or colon may provide a more metabolically neutral reservoir (McLaughlin et al, 1995; Austin et al, 1997, 1999, 2001), although they have typically been constructed in only complex patients or circumstances. Duel and associates (1996) have used stomach and colon together to advantage in a staged fashion for oncology patients; patients initially diverted with a colon conduit after cystectomy had a composite reservoir constructed later after cure from tumor was ensured.

Hematuria-Dysuria Syndrome

Acid secretion by gastric mucosa may result in another unique problem after gastrocystoplasty, the hematuria-dysuria syndrome. Mitchell's group has characterized this syndrome well (Nguyen et al, 1993; Plaire et al, 1999). **Virtually all patients after gastrocystoplasty with normal sensation have occasional hematuria or dysuria with voiding or catheterization beyond that which is expected with other intestinal segments** (Leonard et al, 1999). **All patients should be warned of this potential problem, although these symptoms are intermittent and mild in most patients and do not require treatment.** The problem has led one group to recommend avoiding gastrocystoplasty in patients with bladder exstrophy (El-Ghoneimi et al, 1998). The dysuria is certainly not as problematic in patients with neurogenic dysfunction. In the experience of Nguyen and colleagues (1993), 36% of patients have developed signs or symptoms of the hematuria-dysuria syndrome after gastrocystoplasty; 14% of patients have required treatment with medications, including 9% on a regular basis. They believe that patients who are incontinent or have decreased renal function are at increased risk. Others have noted a similar requirement for short-term and chronic medical therapy (Hollensbe et al, 1992; Adams et al, 1995). In the authors' experience and that of Nguyen and colleagues, the symptoms of the hematuria-dysuria syndrome do respond well to H$_2$ blockers and hydrogen ion pump blockers. Bladder irrigation with baking soda may also be effective. It has been demonstrated that urine pH may decrease remarkably after meals following gastrocystoplasty (Bogaert et al, 1995). The signs and symptoms of the hematuria-dysuria syndrome are most likely secondary to acid irritation. Recent work has suggested that *Helicobacter pylori* may play a role in this complication as it may in acid complications in the native stomach (Celayir et al, 1999). Such problems can occur but are less frequent after antral cystoplasty where there is a smaller load of parietal cells (Ngan et al, 1993).

Acid in the urine may also cause external irritation. Leong first noted glanular excoriation after gastrocystoplasty in a patient with voiding symptoms (Ngan et al, 1993). Similar meatal irritation has been noted in other patients after gastrocystoplasty; most have had significant dysuria. Nguyen and associates (1993) noted skin excoriation in 8 of 57 patients after gastrocystoplasty; all 8 patients had some element of urinary incontinence. **It is imperative to achieve reliable urinary continence in patients undergoing gastrocystoplasty because urine leakage may result in the exposure of the skin to gastric secretions and in gastric secretions that are poorly diluted and buffered.** Such dilution is important; Reinberg and coworkers (1992) reported a perforation of a gastric segment in a defunctionalized bladder after gastrocystoplasty. They then evaluated the influence of urine on gastrocystoplasties in dogs (Castro-Diaz et al, 1992). The animals developed marked inflammation of the gastric segment and native bladder after construction of a dry gastrocystoplasty; three of nine dogs developed ulceration and perforation. Use of H$_2$ blockers resulted in some protection for the animals; however, such a clinical situation should certainly be avoided. Rare perforations and ulcerations have been noted clinically without defunctionalization (El-Ghoneimi et al, 1998; Mingin et al, 1999b).

Mucus

Intestinal segments continue to produce mucus after placement in the urinary tract. The proteinaceous material can potentially impede bladder drainage during voiding or clean intermittent catheterization, particularly in pediatric patients in whom the use of small-caliber catheters is necessary. Mucus may serve as a nidus for infection or stone formation when it remains in the bladder for long periods. Mucus production often increases after cystoplasty in the presence of cystitis. Kulb and associates (1986) have shown experimentally in dogs that colonic segments produce more mucus than ileum does and that gastric segments produce the least amount. This has been noted clinically as well. Most patients do not require any routine bladder irrigations for mucus after gastrocystoplasty. Villous atrophy in the ileum has been documented after long-term placement in the urinary tract. It has been suggested that such atrophy may result in decreased mucus production (Gearhart, 1987), although laboratory demonstration of any decrease in production with time has not been evident (Murray et al, 1987). Hendren and Hendren (1990) noted a decrease in mucus production from colonic segments over years; however, others have not been impressed with such changes (Rink et al, 1995a). Glandular atrophy in colonic

mucosa has not been noted histologically (Mansson et al, 1984). **Routine use of daily bladder irrigations to prevent mucus buildup may minimize complications of enterocystoplasty, such as urinary tract infection and calculi** (Hensle et al, 2004).

Urinary Tract Infection

Bacteriuria is common after intestinal cystoplasty, particularly among patients requiring intermittent catheterization (Gearhart et al, 1986; Hendren and Hendren, 1990; King, 1991). Recent experience with bowel neobladders has demonstrated that patients who are able to spontaneously void to completion frequently maintain sterile urine. **It appears that the use of clean intermittent catheterization is a prominent factor in the development of bacteriuria in patients after augmentation cystoplasty.** Bacteriuria has been noted even when patients are maintained on daily oral antibiotics or antibiotic irrigation (Gearhart et al, 1986; Casale et al, 1999). In Hirst's (1991) experience, persistent or recurrent bacteriuria occurred in 50% of patients augmented with sigmoid colon versus 25% of those after ileocystoplasty. Hollensbe and coworkers (1992) noted bacteriuria much more commonly in patients requiring clean intermittent catheterization regardless of the segment considered. The incidence of symptomatic cystitis after cystoplasty probably depends on the length of follow-up and the diligence with which symptoms are sought. All patients and families should be told to expect some signs or symptoms of cystitis. Recurrent episodes of symptomatic cystitis requiring treatment occurred in 23% of patients after ileocystoplasty, 17% after sigmoid cystoplasty, 13% after cecocystoplasty, and 8% after gastrocystoplasty at Indiana University (Hollensbe et al, 1992). Febrile urinary tract infections occurred in 13% of those 231 patients after augmentation. The same trend among different bowel segments was noted for febrile infections, although there was no statistically significant difference among the various segments. **The incidence of pyelonephritis after augmentation cystoplasty, as long as upper tract problems are corrected, is similar to that noted for conduit diversion, whether refluxing or not** (McDougal, 1992b). Recurrent infections resulting in deterioration of renal function in the absence of other problems have been rare after effective augmentation. Infections may occasionally be more problematic in an immunocompromised patient (Alfrey et al, 1997).

Not every episode of asymptomatic bacteriuria requires treatment in patients performing clean intermittent catheterization. Bacteriuria should be treated for significant symptoms, such as incontinence or suprapubic pain, and maybe for hematuria, foul-smelling urine, or remarkably increased mucus production. **Bacteriuria should be treated if the urine culture demonstrates growth of a urea-splitting organism that may lead to stone formation.** To minimize infection, patients requiring clean intermittent catheterization must perform it on a regular basis to avoid increased reservoir pressures and work to empty the bladder completely. This process may require periodic irrigation of mucus as well as patience with the catheter in place. Special care must be taken by patients catheterizing through a continent abdominal wall stoma. Such patients may have more difficulty completely emptying the bladder from a nondependent stoma. Most can do so with effort (Ludlow et al, 1995). Although catheterization is not routinely a sterile technique, proper clean technique should be emphasized.

Calculi

Another long-term complication of augmentation cystoplasty is bladder calculus. In the early 1990s, several series reported calculi in 18% of patients after augmentation cystoplasty (Hendren and Hendren, 1990; Hirst, 1991). Blyth and associates (1992) noted calculus formation in 30% of such patients; they found that patients catheterizing through an abdominal wall stoma have the highest risk, probably because of incomplete emptying. Palmer and colleagues (1993) noted urolithiasis in 52% of patients after augmentation cystoplasty. Rink and associates (1995a) noted only an 8% rate of bladder stone formation in 231 patients with long-term follow-up after enterocystoplasty; the reasons for these remarkable differences are not clear. **The majority of bladder stones in this population of patients are struvite in composition, and bacteriuria has been thought to be an important risk factor.** Any infection with a urea-splitting organism should therefore be treated aggressively. All patients requiring clean intermittent catheterization, particularly those who have already formed stones, should make every effort to empty the bladder completely with each catheterization. If stones are found in patients voiding spontaneously after augmentation, the adequacy of emptying should be reevaluated. The association of urinary stasis with stone formation is well established. Routine bladder irrigations to avoid buildup of inspissated mucus may remove a nidus for stone formation. The group at Indiana and others have stressed irrigations and asked patients and families to routinely irrigate the bladder several times a day after augmentation (Rink et al, 1995a; Hensle et al, 2004). Compliance with such irrigations may lower the frequency of stone formation.

Stones have been noted after the use of all intestinal segments, with no significant difference noted between small and large intestine. Struvite stones are less likely after gastrocystoplasty (Kaefer et al, 1998; Kronner et al, 1998a), probably because of decreased mucus production and acid that minimizes bacteriuria. Uric acid calculi have rarely been noted in the bladder after gastrocystoplasty (Kaefer et al, 1998). Clearly, any foreign body will serve as a nidus for stone formation; the use of permanent suture or staples in the urinary tract should be avoided during enterocystoplasty. Khoury and associates (1997) looked for metabolic problems in patients after augmentation and noted low urinary citrate levels in patients with and without stones. They thought that poor emptying and mucus buildup were more significant factors.

Tumor Formation

A well-recognized complication of ureterosigmoidostomy has been the development of tumors, primarily adenocarcinoma, at the ureterocolonic anastomotic site. In Husmann and Spence's (1990) review of reported tumors after ureterosigmoidostomy, the latency for development of such tumors averaged 26 years and ranged from 3 to 53 years. Adenocarcinomas were the prominent tumors that developed, but benign polyps and other types of carcinoma were also found. Eraklis and Folkman (1978) estimated that the risk for development of such tumors is increased by 7000-fold over that of age-matched controls after ureterosigmoidostomy. The exact basis

for the increased risk is unknown; however, N-nitroso compounds thought to originate from a mixture of urine and feces may be carcinogenic. These compounds have been noted in the urine of patients with conduit diversion and augmentation (Treiger and Marshall, 1991). Husmann and Spence (1990) suggested that those compounds are more likely to be enhancing agents rather than a lone cause of tumor development. It has been proposed that inflammatory reaction at the anastomotic site may induce growth factor production, which in turn increases cellular proliferation.

Filmer and Spencer (1990) **identified 14 patients who have developed adenocarcinoma in an augmented bladder, and several more have been reported since then.** Nine of those tumors occurred after ileocystoplasty and five after colocystoplasty. **Experimental work in the rat demonstrated hyperplastic growth in the augmented bladder with use of all intestinal segments; no segment showed any particular increased risk** (Klee et al, 1990; Buson et al, 1993; Spencer et al, 1993; Little et al, 1994). The applicability of such findings to humans is uncertain. The long latency noted for tumor development after ureterosigmoidostomy suggests that short-term follow-up after augmentation cystoplasty is not adequate to evaluate tumor formation. **Patients undergoing augmentation cystoplasty should be made aware of a potential increased risk for tumor development. Yearly surveillance of the augmented bladder with endoscopy should eventually be performed; the latency period until such procedures are necessary is not well defined** (Vajda et al, 2002). The earliest reported tumor after augmentation was found only 4 years after cystoplasty (Carr and Herschorn, 1997). Transitional cell carcinoma, hyperplasia, and dysplasia have also been noted near the anastomosis in humans (Gregoire et al, 1993; Barrington et al, 1997; Soergel et al, 2004). Urine cytology or flow cytometry may ultimately become useful in surveillance.

Delayed Spontaneous Bladder Perforation

Perhaps the most disturbing complication of augmentation cystoplasty is delayed bladder perforation. Patients presenting with spontaneous perforation after augmentation cystoplasty are generally quite ill with abdominal pain, distention, and fever. Sepsis has been common. Nausea, decreased urine output, and shoulder pain from diaphragmatic irritation have also been noted. Perforations have been found in evaluation of asymptomatic pelvic masses (Pope et al, 1999). **Patients with neurogenic dysfunction often have impaired lower abdominal sensation and present later in the course of the illness; severe sepsis and death have occurred.** Patients with perforation after gastrocystoplasty often present promptly because of acid irritation. **A high index of suspicion for perforation is necessary. Contrast cystography is diagnostic in most cases** (Braverman and Lebowitz, 1991; Rosen and Light, 1991; Bauer et al, 1992) (Fig. 124–14). Thorough technique is important to identify as many true positives as possible with cystography (Braverman and Lebowitz, 1991). Some reports of perforations have noted a significant false-negative rate on cystography (Rushton et al, 1988; Sheiner and Kaplan, 1988; Pope et al, 1999) and suggested that ultrasonography and computed tomography improve diagnostic accuracy. They recommended that one of those studies be done in any child thought to have a perforation if the initial cystogram is normal.

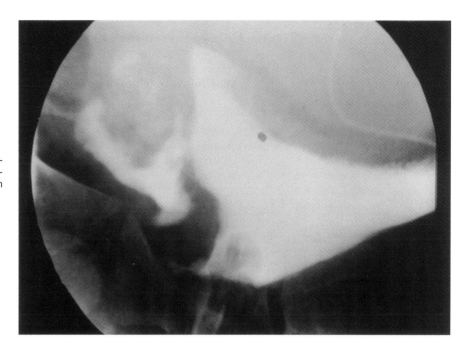

Figure 124–14. After complete filling, a sagittal view on the cystogram demonstrates a spontaneous bladder perforation on the post-drain view.

Etiology. **The etiology of delayed perforations within a bowel segment is unknown.** It has been suggested that perforation might be secondary to traumatic catheterization in some cases (Elder et al, 1988; Rushton et al, 1988). Perforation of a bladder not previously augmented has been recognized after clean intermittent catheterization (Reisman and Preminger, 1989). It seems unlikely that catheterization trauma is the lone cause in most patients. The location of the perforations has been variable among patients and even in a single patient with multiple perforations. Perforations have occurred after augmentation in patients who did not catheterize at all. Others have suggested that trauma to the bowel because of fixed adhesions resulting in shearing forces with emptying and filling may result in perforation (Elder et al, 1988). Chronic, transmural infection of the bladder wall has also been proposed as a cause. **Histologic examination of bowel segments adjacent to areas of perforation has noted necrosis, vascular congestion, hemorrhage, and hemosiderin deposition compatible with chronic bowel wall ischemia** (Crane et al, 1991). **Chronic overdistention of the bladder might result in such ischemia.** Decreased perfusion in dog bowel used for augmentation can be induced experimentally with high intravesical pressure (Essig et al, 1991). Those changes were noted more prominently at the antimesenteric border of the bowel. Chronic ischemia may thus play a significant role in at least some delayed bladder perforations. Anderson and Rickwood (1991) have reported perforations occurring in bladders with significant uninhibited contractions after augmentation, as have others (Pope et al, 1998). **High outflow resistance may maintain bladder pressure rather than allow urine leakage and venting of the pressure, potentially increasing ischemia.** Hyperreflexia alone is not likely to be a solitary cause of perforation; the complication was essentially never recognized in the era before bowel detubularization and reconfiguration when persistent pressure contractions were more common after augmentation cystoplasty. **Once bowel is reconfigured, however, it may be more susceptible to ischemia if high**

pressure does persist. Failure to perform clean intermittent catheterization on a regular basis when needed to empty may exacerbate such issues (DeFoor et al, 2003a).

The majority of patients suffering perforations after augmentation cystoplasty have had myelodysplasia. The incidence of perforation has been lower in series of patients with other diagnoses requiring bladder reconstruction (Hendren and Hendren, 1990). The role of neurogenic dysfunction in the etiology of these perforations is unclear. No matter what the etiology, there is likely to be some field effect on the entire segment. Once a patient has suffered a spontaneous perforation, the chance of recurrence is significant (Hollensbe et al, 1992). One third of patients with ruptures in one series had a recurrence (Pope et al, 1999). Consideration must eventually be given to removal of the original segment and replacement by another after repeated perforation.

Incidence. This problem has been noted with increasing frequency after augmentation cystoplasty and may involve all segments. Early postoperative leaks from the bowel-to-bowel or bowel-to-bladder anastomoses after augmentation cystoplasty are rare and represent a technical error or problem with early healing. **Delayed perforations more commonly occur within the bowel segment itself and represent a problem with long-term storage of urine within an intestinal segment.** There may be no particular increased risk of one intestinal segment over another. At Indiana University, perforations were noted in 32 of 330 patients undergoing cystoplasty (Pope et al, 1999) an average of 4.3 years after augmentation. Analysis of this experience suggested that the use of sigmoid colon was the only significantly increased risk. Several other large series of patients with sigmoid cystoplasty have noted a low incidence of delayed perforation (Sidi et al, 1987a; Hendren and Hendren, 1990; Shekarriz et al, 2000). At Children's Hospital Boston, the incidence of perforation after augmentation was highest in ileum (9.3%) and less frequent in ileocecal, sigmoid, and gastric segments (Bauer et al, 1992).

With inconsistent differences across multiple large series, it is unlikely that any given enteric segment is at significantly increased risk for perforation and that likely multiple factors influence the risk for the complication. Pope, Rink, and the Indiana group (1999) still believe strongly from their experience that sigmoid colon has a greater risk for perforation based on a four-time higher rate than ileum there. Some other experienced surgeons think the same (Ransley, 1998).

Treatment. **The standard treatment of spontaneous perforation of the augmented bladder is surgical repair, as it is for intraperitoneal rupture of the bladder after trauma.** There are reported series of conservative management for suspected perforation (Slaton and Kropp, 1994). Conservative management including catheter drainage, antibiotics, and serial abdominal examinations was successful in 87% of the patients, although only 2 of the 13 patients with suspected ruptures had x-ray documentation unequivocally identifying a perforation. Even patients who do well with conservative management during the acute episode often require eventual surgical intervention (Pope et al, 1999). Such management may be a consideration in a stable patient with sterile urine. The surgeon should certainly have a low threshold for surgical exploration and repair. The majority of patients with perforations have myelodysplasia and present late in the course of the disease because of impaired sensation. Increasing sepsis and death of the patient may result from a delay in diagnosis or treatment.

Pregnancy

Good success has been reported for female patients after bladder augmentation, bladder neck repair, or continent urinary diversion in terms of continence and upper tract preservation. Little note has been made of fertility issues. **Limited information exists regarding the outcome of pregnancy in women who have undergone augmentation cystoplasty, as many of these patients are just reaching childbearing age.** Older women undergoing bladder replacement for oncologic reasons often are rendered infertile by the nature of the disease and treatment.

Three major issues are raised in the context of pregnancy and bladder reconstruction: how the expanding uterus will affect the pedicle of the reconstruction; how to manage bacteriuria during pregnancy; and whether cesarean section is needed in all or some of these patients and, when it is performed, how to manage the pedicle of the augmentation patch.

Experience during pregnancy related to the pedicle of a prior bladder augmentation is limited. Hatch and colleagues (1991) and Schumacher and coworkers (1997) have noted that the mesenteric pedicle to bladder augmentations did not appear to be stretched at the time of cesarean section. In those cases, the pedicle was not located near the exposed anterior uterus but deflected laterally. Schilling and colleagues (1996) recognized a difference between urinary diversion and augmentation. With diversion, the pedicle of the intestinal segment extended cranially and laterally away from the uterus, whereas the pedicle covered the uterus after bladder augmentation. Neither process prevented the rise of the uterus during pregnancy. Those authors speculated that the mesentery underwent changes that enabled deflection or stretch without

any adverse effect on circulation. Loss of the augmentation due to mechanical effect on the pedicle from the enlarging uterus has not been reported. Pregnancy itself has not had a reported detrimental effect on the augmentation. Successful pregnancy with spontaneous vaginal delivery has been observed in a few cases with bladder augmentations (Quenneville et al, 2003) and other forms of urinary reconstruction, such as ureterosigmoidostomy and ileal conduit urinary diversion (Pedlow, 1961; Asif and Uehling, 1969). Schumacher and coworkers (1997) reviewed their experience with pregnancy and delivery in patients who had undergone continent catheterizable ileocecal diversion and found no major complications. It is likely that this would also be true for other forms of reconstruction. (Wren et al, 2003). Urgency and late difficulty with catheterization have been noted with Kock continent ileostomies (Ojerskog et al, 1988) and could occur with continent urinary diversion.

Urinary tract infections may be problematic in women who have undergone urinary reconstruction including bladder augmentation. Ureteral dilation, increased residual urine, and diminished tone to the upper tract may all be important risk factors (Hill et al, 1990; Hatch et al, 1991). On the basis of those experiences, prophylactic nonteratogenic antibiotics may be appropriate, particularly once symptomatic infection has occurred. Placement of an indwelling stent might benefit some patients. Uterine prolapse has been noted to occur at a higher rate with pregnancy, particularly in exstrophy patients (Kennedy et al, 1993). Because of such concerns, Stein and associates (1994) suggested fixation of the uterus during reconstructive surgery.

The need for cesarean section is probably not universal for all women with bladder reconstructions. Adequate progression of spontaneous vaginal delivery, however, may require flaccid, distensible pelvic tissues, which may not be present after extensive pelvic surgery. It is unknown if tissues fixed from previous operative repairs can undergo the trauma of delivery and resume the same level of function as before the pregnancy. Our bias would be that women having undergone extensive bladder neck repair would benefit from cesarean delivery, particularly if the progression toward spontaneous vaginal delivery is slowed or difficult at all. Although there are reports of spontaneous vaginal delivery in the presence of an artificial urinary sphincter (Creagh et al, 1995), the presence of such a prosthetic device raises a concern for erosion with a long, difficult delivery.

If cesarean section is required or selected, it is imperative to protect the augmentation and its pedicle. The anterior uterus can typically be exposed atraumatically, although some time and patience may be required to protect the bladder. Such exposure may be more difficult if multiple abdominal stomas are present. The reconstructive urologist familiar with the patient and her anatomy should be present during cesarean section to maximize safety.

Choice of Segment

The use of bowel for augmentation of the bladder was first described experimentally by Tizzoni and Foggi in 1888 and in humans by Mikulicz in 1898 (Orr et al, 1958). Extraordinary advances have been made in the use of the bowel in urinary tract reconstruction since then. Bladder augmentation is used for patients with bladder dysfunction related to a small-capacity, noncompliant reservoir. **Enterocystoplasty improves bladder capacity and compliance in most cases when medical management fails.** It is obvious from the preceding discussion that there is no one single bowel segment that is perfect for augmentation in all patients. All gastrointestinal segments have been used and continue to be used with good results. Unremitting medical problems or complications requiring surgical intervention are relatively rare after augmentation cystoplasty. No one bowel segment has a clear advantage over another when all such problems are considered. Diagnosis, anatomy, and physiology may suggest that one bowel segment is preferable for a particular patient. Each surgeon interested in augmentation cystoplasty should be familiar with the advantages and disadvantages of each segment in different settings.

In many routine cases, any gastrointestinal segment may be chosen for cystoplasty purely on the basis of the personal preference and familiarity of the surgeon. The surgeon's experience and confidence in using a segment are important. **The authors believe that no one bowel segment is the best choice in all patients and that optimal results are achieved when the bowel segment is chosen on the basis of the needs of the particular patient. The segment must then be used correctly.** We prefer ileum if there is no clear advantage to or reason for use of another segment. We reserve stomach for children with renal insufficiency and acidosis, short-gut syndrome, and heavy irradiation. We do continue to use sigmoid cystoplasty in select patients without reservation; clearly, good results can be expected with any segment if it is used properly.

Alternatives to Gastrointestinal Cystoplasty

Largely because of the complications and side effects just reviewed, alternative methods that can achieve a large-capacity, compliant reservoir remain attractive. Efforts have covered the spectrum from synthetic materials and autologous grafts to construction of a bladder diverticulum (autoaugmentation) and to various forms of neural stimulation. **Some of these alternatives appear to hold promise, but none has stood the test of time for true comparison to intestinal cystoplasty.**

An ideal tissue for increasing capacity and improving compliance would have transitional epithelium to be relatively impermeable and avoid metabolic changes. The lining would also not produce mucus and carry no increased potential for tumor development. The ability to augment the bladder without violation of the peritoneal cavity would also decrease potential morbidity. Two such alternative procedures are ureterocystoplasty and autoaugmentation. With ureterocystoplasty, there is good muscle backing of transitional epithelium; collagen eventually backs the transitional mucosa of an autoaugmentation.

Ureterocystoplasty

It has been noted for years that in patients with posterior urethral valves, unilateral reflux may behave like a "pop-off" valve to lower intravesical pressures and protect the contralateral upper tract (Hoover and Duckett, 1982; Rittenberg

et al, 1988; Kaefer et al, 1995). In many of these patients, the refluxing ureter is massively dilated, draining a poorly functioning or nonfunctioning kidney. **It was a logical extension to use this ureteral tissue to augment the bladder.**

Technique. Ureterocystoplasty may be performed through a midline, intraperitoneal incision. This incision provides access to the intestine should mobilization of the ureter for augmentation be unsatisfactory. **Bellinger (1993), Dewan and colleagues (1994a), and Reinberg and colleagues (1995) have shown that ureterocystoplasty can be done through two incisions, remaining completely extraperitoneal.** The general technique is the same. A standard nephrectomy is performed with great care to preserve the renal pelvic and upper ureteral blood supply. All adventitia and periureteral tissue is swept from the peritoneum toward the ureter during mobilization to protect the ureteral blood supply. Proximally, this blood supply typically arises medially. As the ureter enters the true pelvis, the blood supply arises posterior and laterally. After mobilization of the ureter into the pelvis, the bladder is opened in the sagittal plane. Posteriorly, this incision has typically been carried off-center directly into and through the ureteral orifice of the ureter used for cystoplasty. The ureter is *not* detached from the bladder but is opened longitudinally along its entire length, with care taken to avoid its main blood supply (Fig. 124–15). The incision in the bladder and distal ureter should avoid branches of the superior vesical artery that serves as an important blood supply to the mobilized ureter. The ureter is folded on itself, and the ureter-to-ureter and ureter-to-bladder anastomosis is performed with running absorbable suture. A suprapubic tube is left indwelling through the native bladder for 3 weeks during healing. After cystography documents the absence of leakage, clean intermittent catheterization is started. Patients, particularly those without neurogenic dysfunction, may attempt to void spontaneously. It is our impression that children are more likely to void adequately after ureterocystoplasty than after intestinal cystoplasty, although all must prove that they can empty appropriately by checking postvoid residuals.

Alternatively, the bladder incision can be stopped approximately 2 cm from the orifice and a similar length of distal ureter left in situ and intact without incision. The resulting small loop of intact ureter does not cause clinical problems or adversely affect the end volume in a significant manner (Adams et al, 1998). This modification of technique is easier and may be safer in that it avoids potential injury to the blood supply of the mobilized ureter near the ureterovesical junction.

Results. Early reports suggested that ureterocystoplasty could be achieved after nephrectomy by bivalving the bladder through the vesicoureteral junction and laying in the open ureter (Mitchell et al, 1992; Bellinger, 1993). Later reports modified and improved the procedure by noting that with meticulous care, the vascularity to the entire renal pelvis could be preserved, allowing more tissue for cystoplasty (Churchill et al, 1993; Landau et al, 1994; McKenna and Bauer, 1995; Reinberg et al, 1995). As with intestinal cystoplasty, folding the ureter into a more spherical configuration maximizes the volume that can be achieved. If a massively dilated ureter drains a functioning kidney, the distal ureter alone may be used for augmentation; the proximal ureter is either

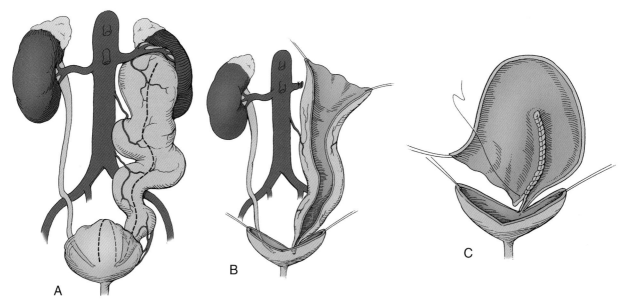

Figure 124–15. Ureterocystoplasty. **A,** After nephrectomy, the bladder is bivalved, with the posterior aspect of the incision carried off the midline to enter the ureteral orifice. The ureter is not detached from the bladder. **B,** The ureter is opened opposite its main blood supply. **C,** The ureter is reconfigured as in intestinal cystoplasty before anastomosis to the bladder.

reimplanted into the bladder or anastomosed to the contralateral ureter (Bellinger, 1993).

Numerous series have reported good results after augmentation with use of ureter, some with follow-up as long as 8 years. The upper tracts have remained stable or improved in virtually all patients. Complications have been uncommon, with only a rare early extravasation of urine reported (Churchill et al, 1993). Landau and colleagues (1994) compared age-matched and diagnosis-matched children having ureterocystoplasty or ileocystoplasty. **The total mean bladder capacity was 470 mL in the ureterocystoplasty group and 381 mL in the ileocystoplasty group. Bladder volumes at 30 cm H_2O were 413 mL and 380 mL after ureterocystoplasty and ileocystoplasty, respectively.** Ureter effectively enhanced both volume and compliance. There was one failure in the group that occurred in a child in whom the distal ureter did not provide enough volume. Work has shown that one dilated ureter typically is enough for cystoplasty (Zubieta et al, 1999).

The main disadvantage to ureterocystoplasty is the limited population of patients with a nonfunctioning kidney draining into a megaureter. McKenna and Bauer (1995) have reported the use of a normal-sized ureter. The ultimate success of ureterocystoplasty with normal ureter requires further follow-up, particularly since Gonzalez (1999) has stated that one quarter of his patients with posterior urethral valves have failed ureterocystoplasty with a dilated ureter because of their huge urinary volume. Husmann and colleagues (2004) noted even worse results if the ureter used was less than 1.5 cm in diameter. Atala and colleagues (1994) presented an experimental technique to slowly dilate a normal ureter for later use. Work continues to develop such a technique that is clinically applicable for patients (Stifelman et al, 1998; Desai et al, 2003).

Autoaugmentation

Techniques and Results. Cartwright and Snow (1989a, 1989b) described an ingenious method to improve bladder compliance and capacity with use of native urothelial tissue. In their procedure, known as autoaugmentation, they excised the detrusor muscle over the dome of the bladder, leaving the mucosa intact to protrude as a wide-mouth diverticulum. Initially, they made a midline incision through the bladder muscle (Fig. 124–16A). With the bladder distended with saline so that mucosa bulged from the incision, the muscle was then mobilized and excised laterally in each direction (Fig. 124–16B). The lateral edges of the detrusor muscle were then secured to the psoas muscle bilaterally to prevent collapse of the diverticulum (Fig. 124–16C). Their early experience noted improved compliance in most and increased capacity in some patients (Cartwright and Snow, 1989a).

This procedure has since been modified by a number of surgeons, each providing a different name for the procedure, depending on whether the detrusor muscle is simply incised or excised to make the diverticulum. In an effort to determine if incision or excision provided superior results, Johnson and colleagues (1994) performed 16 vesicomyotomies and 16 vesicomyectomies in rabbits after previously reducing the bladder capacity. Functional bladder capacity in the animals increased by 43.5%, and there was no statistical difference between the two techniques. They then performed vesicomyotomies (incision) in 12 patients with neurogenic bladder dysfunction and demonstrated a mean increase in capacity of 40% and a mean decrease in leak point pressure of 33% (Stothers et al, 1994). They concluded that detrusor excision offered no advantage over incision. All patients demonstrated some increase in capacity (15% to 70%), and no patient in early follow-up clinically deteriorated and required enterocystoplasty.

Detrusorectomy, leaving a small cap of muscle at the dome through which a suprapubic tube can be placed, has been proposed by Landa and Moorehead (1994). **They have been concerned that although these procedures usually improve compliance, increase in volume is "modest at best," a**

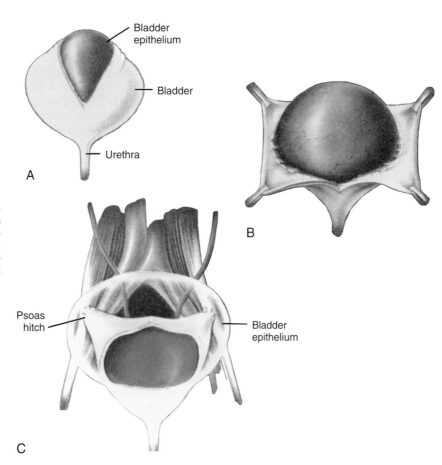

Figure 124–16. Autoaugmentation. **A,** The detrusor is incised. **B,** Detrusor is stripped and excised from mucosa. **C,** The detrusor muscle is anchored bilaterally so that the mucosa bulges with bladder filling. (From Cartwright PC, Snow BW: Bladder autoaugmentation: Early clinical experience. J Urol 1989;142: 505.)

concern shared by others (Snow and Cartwright, 1996; Cartwright and Snow, 1998). In a report of 12 detrusorectomies, five patients were considered to have excellent results, two had acceptable results, and one was lost to follow-up. There were four failures (one hydronephrosis, two persistent incontinence, one worsening renal insufficiency), of which three have undergone gastrocystoplasty or ileocystoplasty (Landa and Moorehead, 1994). In a combined series at those two institutions, only 52% of patients had a good result with autoaugmentation; 20% had a poor outcome (Snow and Cartwright, 1996). Reoperative enterocystoplasty was not hampered by the prior detrusorectomy. The urothelial diverticulum at the time of augmentation cystoplasty was noted to be thick and fibrous, similar to a leather bag.

There are obvious advantages to autoaugmentation and its variants. Native urothelial tissue is used. It is an extraperitoneal procedure, which shortens operative time and avoids the risks of intestinal surgery and adhesions. Autoaugmentation is compatible with clean intermittent catheterization and does not seem to complicate subsequent intestinal cystoplasty when it is necessary.

Complications from the procedures are generally uncommon. Perforation, a major concern after intestinal cystoplasty, has not been reported. Inadvertent opening of the mucosa during the procedure can make subsequent mobilization more difficult and may promote prolonged postoperative extravasation. Such extravasation usually stops with bladder drainage (Landa and Moorehead, 1994; Stothers et al, 1994). Prolonged drainage, however, may result in compromised results from

collapse of the diverticulum. If concomitant ureteral reimplantation or bladder neck surgery is necessary, various authors have recommended that it be done first and the bladder then closed before detrusorectomy (Stothers et al, 1994).

Ehrlich and Gershman (1993) first reported laparoscopic myotomy (incision). A laparoscopic approach uses a smaller incision and perhaps shortens postoperative hospitalization; it may make effective fixation of the detrusor muscle in an open fashion to allow good bulging more difficult. It remains to be seen whether autoaugmentation provides effective long-term results for pediatric patients and whether it can be done as well laparoscopically.

Concerns. **The main disadvantage of autoaugmentation is a limited increase in bladder capacity such that adequate preoperative volume may be the most important predictor of success** (Landa and Moorehead, 1994). If the maximum capacity and the volume of urine held at 40 cm H_2O are similar, the patient may be better served by immediate intestinal cystoplasty. It is of note that some patients have demonstrated clinical improvement after these procedures without a significant change in urodynamics. The reason for the improvement in that setting is unknown.

In most series of autoaugmentation, no matter what the technique, it has been noted in occasional patients or concern has existed at the time of the initial procedure that adequate expansion was not achieved. In most such cases, it was elected to proceed with enterocystoplasty immediately at the time

(Landa and Moorehead, 1994). These patients are not included in the failure rate of autoaugmentation. The patient and surgeon must be prepared for such an event on occasion. Stohrer's group (1999) as well as Leng and associates (1999) reported good results with the technique among patients with hyperreflexia. Even if adequate expansion is achieved initially, there is concern that any improvement may not persist long term (Dewan et al, 1994b). In animals, the surface area of the autoaugmentation site was noted to decrease approximately 50% at 12 weeks. Progressive thickening and contracture of the site have been noted because of collagenous infiltrate (Johnson et al, 1994). Milam (2000) has noted that almost half of his adult patients with hyperreflexia who had a good early result after autoaugmentation have failed with longer follow-up. Similar delayed failures have been noted in pediatric patients (Lindley et al, 2003) including one series with very poor results (MacNeily et al, 2003).

At this point, autoaugmentation should probably be considered only in patients who have reasonable capacity but poor compliance due to uninhibited contractions. **If a significant increase in capacity is needed, autoaugmentation is unlikely to be as definitive as other techniques.**

Seromuscular Enterocystoplasty

Based on concerns about collagen deposition and contraction around autoaugmentation, efforts have been made to cover the bulging urothelium with demucosalized enteric segments. The use of enteric segments without bowel mucosa within the bladder is not new. As far back as the 1950s, seromuscular augmentation cystoplasty was performed with the serosal side of the bowel turned to the bladder lumen (Shoemaker and Marucci, 1955; Shoemaker et al, 1957). Urothelium soon covered the serosa. Gonzalez's group experienced good results with reversed seromuscular cystoplasty in rats, as did others with rabbits (Celayir et al, 1995), but contracture of the patch occurred in larger animals (De Badiola et al, 1991; Long et al, 1992). Others left the exposed submucosa facing the bladder lumen and noted re-epithelialization with urothelium in animals (Oesch, 1988; Salle et al, 1990). Despite the re-epithelialization, patch contracture occurred (Salle et al, 1990). Several recent series have re-evaluated demucosalized augmentation in humans after taking care to preserve the submucosa. Better results have been noted (Lima et al, 1998, 2004; de Badiola et al, 1999; Dayanc et al, 1999), although regrowth of metaplastic enteric mucosa was found in the second study. Early placement of a silicone balloon or mold may help prevent contracture (Lima et al, 2004).

Techniques and Results. To avoid contracture, a combination of autoaugmentation after detrusorectomy and coverage with a demucosalized enteric segment has now been used. This has been done to potentially preserve the advantages of both procedures. In a similar fashion, the combination has been undertaken with both colon and stomach. Buson and colleagues (1994) used reconfigured, demucosalized sigmoid colon placed over the urothelium (seromuscular colocystoplasty lined with urothelium). They and others noted that the intestinal submucosa should be preserved to avoid contracture (Buson et al, 1994; Vates et al, 1997) (Fig. 124–17). This procedure has been performed clinically with early reports of good results in most patients (Gonzalez et al,

1994). Postoperative bladder capacity increased an average of 2.4-fold (139 to 335 mL) in 14 of 16 patients, and end filling pressure decreased from an average of 51.6 to 27.7 cm H_2O. Two patients failed and required ileocystoplasty; their urodynamic data were excluded. Two other patients developed an hourglass deformity (Gonzales et al, 1994). Endoscopic biopsy findings of the segments have been interesting. Of 10 biopsies in the series, one noted urothelium with islands of colonic mucosa; two others found only colon mucosa. Removal of all of the enteric mucosa is important when sigmoid is used to prevent mucoceles or overgrowth of intestinal mucosa (Gonzalez et al, 1994; Lutz and Frey, 1994). Dewan and associates (1997) thought that preservation of the submucosa eventually promoted regrowth of bowel mucosa. The interaction of the two different tissues will be interesting to follow. The long-term effects on the urothelium by the seromuscular segment and vice versa are unknown. Work has shown that persistent transitional lining will protect from metabolic problems and mucus production (Denes et al, 1997).

Dewan and Byard (1993) and Close and associates (2004) alternatively used demucosalized stomach to cover an autoaugmentation, first in sheep and then in patients. Early results showed improved bladder function both clinically and by urodynamics (Dewan and Stefanek, 1994; Horowitz and Mitchell, 1993; Horowitz et al, 1994; Robinson et al, 1994), although long-term results are not as encouraging (Carr et al, 1999). These procedures are technically more demanding than simple augmentation or autoaugmentation and are associated with more blood loss and a longer operative time (Gonzalez et al, 1994; Horowitz et al, 1994). Increased bleeding is particularly true when stomach is used. These urothelium-lined, seromuscular augmentations are theoretically attractive. Thus far, the failure and reoperation rate after such procedures remains higher than that noted for standard enterocystoplasty (Vates et al, 1997; Carr et al, 1999; Shekarriz et al, 2000). The best results have been reported with colon (Shekarriz et al, 2000). Those results may be partially attributed to the learning curve with a new, complex procedure. Longer follow-up and more experience are necessary to determine whether the complication rate will decrease with experience or increase because of problems with the combination.

Bladder Regeneration

Other efforts to find alternatives to intestinal cystoplasty in the 1950s included the use of alloplastic materials for bladder substitution (Gleeson and Griffith, 1992). Early research efforts met with limited success. Further work with biodegradable, collagen-rich tissues to serve as a scaffold for bladder regeneration has also been reported (Kelami, 1971; Fishman et al, 1987; Kambic et al, 1992; Kropp et al, 1995; Zhang et al, 2004). Atala and coworkers have applied bioengineering techniques to culture and combine various bladder cells in tissue culture for regeneration (Atala et al, 1992, 1993b; Cilento et al, 1994; Oberpenning et al, 1997; Yoo et al, 1998; Fauza et al, 1998; Lai et al, 2002; Zhang et al, 2004). Early efforts are exciting but preliminary. Clinical applicability in the human with a diseased bladder requires more study. It should be determined in a diseased bladder model whether regenerated tissue is functionally normal or assumes the characteristics of the abnormal native bladder. Because enterocystoplasty is not a perfect physiologic substitute for the native

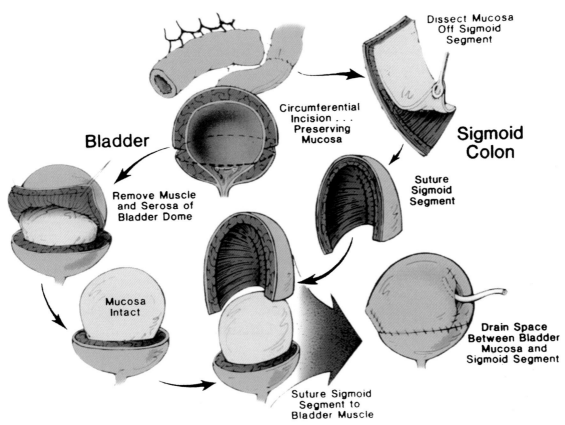

Figure 124–17. Seromuscular enterocystoplasty with use of sigmoid colon. Detrusor incision is performed as in autoaugmentation; however, the bulging mucosa is covered with a demucosalized segment of sigmoid colon. (From Buson H, Manivel JC, Dayanc M, et al: Seromuscular colocystoplasty lined with urothelium: Experimental study. Urology 1994;44:745.)

bladder, these continued efforts are certainly warranted and should be encouraged.

A Decreasing Necessity?

Although augmentation cystoplasty works well for most patients who require it, and work on alternatives to bowel cystoplasty may lower morbidity for the patient, a primary goal for every pediatric urologist is to minimize the number of patients needing cystoplasty. Newer medical regimens and neuromodulation may prove effective for some patients who presently do not respond to conservative measures (Aslan and Kogan, 2002). No matter what the diagnosis, earlier and more aggressive treatment of bladder dysfunction may minimize the insult to the bladder and maximize recovery as well as ultimate bladder function. Early urodynamic evaluation of boys with posterior urethral valves may identify treatable bladder problems and improve the prognosis from the standpoint of the kidneys and bladder (Misseri et al, 2002). Grady and colleagues (2003) have suggested that complete primary repair of bladder exstrophy results in early bladder cycling that improves eventual bladder function and decreases the likelihood of augmentation cystoplasty.

With perhaps the most compelling evidence to date, Kaefer and associates (1999b) found that only 17% of patients with hostile neurogenic bladder dysfunction treated immediately

on diagnosis required augmentation cystoplasty compared with 41% of similar patients treated expectantly. Although the series included no collaborative urodynamic data and might be subject to lag time bias, the authors thought that there was a significant difference in the outcomes for the two groups. Because there are no prospective, randomized trials evaluating early evaluation and treatment of pediatric bladder dysfunction, recommendations that expectant treatment may lower the necessity for augmentation cystoplasty (Bauer, 2003; Mitchell, 2003) remain a personal bias rather than a scientific fact. Critical, prospective evaluation of such treatment is needed and will, it is hoped, demonstrate how to manage these patients successfully so that they will not need augmentation cystoplasty. It is likely that such improvements will minimize the need for cystoplasty but not completely remove it.

CONTINENT URINARY DIVERSION

The frequency with which continent urinary diversion is performed in children depends on one's definition of continent diversion. In adults, total bladder replacement is not uncommon after cystectomy for transitional cell carcinoma. This has led to extensive experience with continent urinary diversion and orthotopic neobladders that allow spontaneous voiding. Tumors resulting in cystectomy among children are much less common. It is in that setting, and the occasional child in

KEY POINTS: AUGMENTATION CYSTOPLASTY

- No matter the gastrointestinal segment used, that segment should be reconfigured and widely anastomosed to the native bladder to maximize capacity and compliance.

- Failures to achieve adequate compliance are rare (~5%) and are usually related to rhythmic pressure contractions.

- Gastrointestinal effects are rare, although chronic diarrhea may occur if the ileocecal segment is used in the neurogenic population.

- Ammonium resorption from urine in contact with intestinal mucosa can cause chronic metabolic acidosis, particularly among patients with renal insufficiency.

- Acid secretion after gastrocystoplasty results in two unique potential complications: hematuria-dysuria syndrome and acute metabolic alkalosis.

- Bacteriuria is common after cystoplasty and does not always require treatment.

- Bladder calculi, usually struvite, occur in 10% to 30% of patients after augmentation cystoplasty but may be minimized by routine irrigations for mucus.

- Adenocarcinoma in the intestinal segment has been reported as early as 4 years after augmentation cystoplasty but, thus far, has not occurred with the frequency noted after ureterosigmoidostomy.

- Delayed spontaneous perforation of the bowel segment can be expected in 5% of patients after augmentation. It has occurred most frequently in colonic segments used in the neurogenic population.

- Ureterocystoplasty avoids the complications associated with bowel segments but may not provide adequate volume if the ureter is not remarkably dilated.

- Autoaugmentation, no matter what the technique, seldom adds significant capacity and may not always improve compliance long term.

- More experience and longer follow-up with seromuscular enterocystoplasty are needed to determine its appropriate role.

- Care for the underlying bladder dysfunction should be improved to lower the need for augmentation cystoplasty.

infrequently. Neurogenic or anatomic problems at the outlet prevent spontaneous voiding in many cases. Even among patients having undergone cystectomy for tumors, irradiation can interfere with voiding. On occasion, a child with neurogenic dysfunction may be a candidate for orthotopic bladder substitution (Stein et al, 2000). It is not clear how many of those patients with neurogenic dysfunction can be expected to void adequately.

More frequently in children, series of continent diversion have included patients undergoing a mix of the techniques discussed in this chapter. Some authors have defined combinations of bladder augmentation, continent abdominal wall stoma, and some procedure at the outlet as continent diversions (Kaefer et al, 1997b). Division and closure of the bladder neck to prevent incontinence per native urethra has typically meant inclusion. Certainly, maximal use of the native urinary tract is beneficial to the child. Much like urinary undiversion, these procedures typically have been performed in complex patients with multiple problems that must be addressed, often after numerous previous surgeries.

Considerations

The amount of bowel used in continent urinary diversion may vary according to the patient. Total bladder replacement requires much more intestine than simple augmentation. Typically, a 40-cm segment of small bowel is used for an ileal reservoir in a Kock pouch compared with the 20 cm often used for augmentation. Likewise, the entire right colon with the hepatic flexure may be used in an Indiana pouch with or without a patch of small intestine, whereas only 15 to 20 cm of colon is needed for colocystoplasty. Because of the potential morbidity associated with use of a larger intestinal segment, the native bladder is often incorporated in children if it provides any significant volume. To do so, however, may require repair of the outlet if outflow resistance is low. Otherwise, incontinence per native urethra will result.

Imbrication of the ileocecal valve and terminal ileum has proved to be a simple and reliable means for construction of an effective efferent limb in continent diversion among adults and children. Despite reports to the contrary in select patients (Husmann and Cain, 1999), concern about fecal incontinence secondary to use of the ileocecal valve persists for patients with neurogenic dysfunction. The flap valve continence mechanism provides numerous alternatives for those surgeons with such concerns in continent diversion. The good results achieved with the appendix or tapered intestinal segments has led to their increased use in recent years.

Whereas maintenance of the native urethra for catheterization is ideal, it may not be appropriate or possible in all individuals. As indicated previously, reconstructive bladder neck procedures are often subject to difficulty with catheterization. **Children with neurogenic sphincter incompetence may have associated neurologic limitations that prevent easy access to the native urethra. This is particularly true for the wheelchair-bound child. For children without neurologic deficits, normal sensation in the native urethra can prevent compliance with a routine catheterization schedule because of discomfort. For these reasons, a continent catheterizable stoma provides an adequate and sometimes a more reliably useful alternative.**

whom the bladder is congenitally absent or so small as to be virtually useless, that a pure continent urinary diversion in the classic sense of an Indiana or Kock pouch might be performed. Very good results with continent diversion in children have been achieved, equivalent to those reported in adults. Orthotopic neobladders in children are performed

CONTINENCE MECHANISMS AND CATHETERIZABLE SEGMENTS

Ureterosigmoidostomy and Its Variants

Ureterosigmoidostomy can be an effective form of continent urinary diversion in some patients. Its major advantage is the potential for spontaneous emptying by evacuation of urine with stool. The significant complications of hyperchloremic acidosis, infection, hydronephrosis, and the development of colonic malignant neoplasms have led to disfavor and disuse, particularly in the United States. **Although good results with standard ureterosigmoidostomy have been reported in some children, the procedure is rarely performed as originally described. The morbidity of acidosis and upper tract changes may increase with time, making those complications particularly worrisome for children with a long life expectancy. The significant risk of adenocarcinoma commits the patients to a lifetime of close surveillance for an avoidable tumor.** It is unlikely that ureterosigmoidostomy, as classically described, will regain acceptance for children.

Several modifications of ureterosigmoidostomy have been described in an attempt to decrease the significant complication rate. **The most basic of the modifications is the sigma rectum or the Mainz II pouch.** The colon is incised along the antimesenteric border for 6 cm both proximal and distal to the rectosigmoid junction. The ureters are implanted in an antirefluxing fashion, and that portion of colon is then reconfigured and closed. This is done to potentially make a rectosigmoid reservoir of lower pressure to protect the upper tracts. The Mainz II pouch has been used in children primarily with bladder exstrophy (Stein et al, 1997a). Continence in appropriately selected patients is good, although acidosis is still a significant problem because of exposure of the entire colon to urine (Fisch et al, 1996; Mingin et al, 1999a; Gerharz et al, 1999). The potential for development of adenocarcinoma still exists with this technique. Long-term follow-up is necessary to determine if the reconfiguration of the sigmoid in the area of ureteral implantation is truly effective for protection of the upper tracts. Stricture at the ureterocolonic anastomosis has been the most common complication in relatively short follow-up (Fisch et al, 1996).

In an effort to control the amount of colon to which urine is exposed, Kock and associates (1988a, 1988b) described a colorectal valve to confine urine to the distal segment. The intussuscepted nipple valve is stabilized with permanent staples. The distal rectal segment is opened and patched with ileum to lower pressure. With short-term follow-up, the valve is effective in that Kock noted no necessity for sodium bicarbonate or potassium citrate therapy (Kock et al, 1988b), a finding duplicated by others (Mahran et al, 1999). An increased risk for tumor development probably still exists with this modification as the ureterocolic anastomoses are still exposed to an admixture of stool and urine, and long-term follow-up of its use in children is needed to see if it is truly less morbid in terms of infection and upper tract deterioration. Urodynamic evaluation has revealed low pressure in the rectal reservoir (Kock et al, 1988b).

If placement of a colorectal valve avoids most complications of metabolic acidosis from ureterosigmoidostomy and construction of a reservoir with lower pressure better protects the upper tracts, the last remaining major concern about ureterosigmoidostomy is tumor development. The concern is significant; of 94 children observed in Boston after ureterosigmoidostomy, adenocarcinoma developed in 7, of whom 4 died of the tumor (Rink and Retik, 1991). Kock and colleagues (1988b) followed by Skinner and associates (1989) used a hemi-Kock pouch to augment the distal rectal segment. A colorectal valve was made to isolate urine to the distal colonic reservoir. The afferent nipple valve kept stool away from the ureteroileal anastomoses, perhaps lowering the risk for tumor development. Simoneau and Skinner (1995) reported their results with the procedure in 15 patients, including 4 children. Their complication rate, both early and late, was relatively high. This is not surprising, considering the relatively complex nature of the procedure. They did think that the pediatric patients were better suited for the procedure. Rink and Retik (1991) suggested that the rectum could be augmented with a nonrefluxing ileocecal conduit in a similar fashion.

Before any variant of ureterosigmoidostomy is considered, competence of the anal sphincter must be ensured. Tests used to assess sphincter integrity include manometry, electromyography, and practical evaluation of the ability to retain an oatmeal enema in the upright position for a time without soilage. Incontinence of a mixture of stool and urine results in foul soilage and must be avoided. Consequently, most patients with neurogenic dysfunction, who are incapable of fecal continence in the presence of diarrhea, are not candidates for these procedures. Procedures that separate the fecal and urinary streams within the rectal sphincter have been described but have not been widely used among children.

Nipple Valves

The greatest experience with nipple valves used to achieve urinary continence has been with the Kock pouch. Skinner and associates (1989) made a series of modifications to aid in maintenance of the efferent nipple. Even with experience and these modifications, a failure rate of 15% or higher can be expected (Benson and Olsson, 1998) (Fig. 124–18). Several authors have reported a reoperative rate of approximately 33% with the Kock pouch, most frequently related to the efferent nipple (deKernion et al, 1985; Waters et al, 1997). Equivalent results with the nipple valve and a Kock pouch have been achieved in children (Hanna and Bloiso, 1987; Skinner et al, 1988; Kaefer et al, 1997b; Abd-El-Gawad et al, 1999). The last report noted a significant incidence of hyperchloremic acidosis and new hydronephrosis, although those complications were likely due to the complex nature of the patients rather than the particular continent diversion used.

Intussuscepted nipple valves have also been used with colonic and ileocolonic reservoirs, particularly the Mainz I pouch. Again, evolution of the nipple valve in the Mainz pouch occurred over time (Thuroff et al, 1986, 1988; Hohenfellner et al, 1990; Stein et al, 1995). Most recently, the intussuscepted ileum is fixed with staples, passed through the intact ileocecal valve, and fixed again. Much as with the Kock pouch, the incidence of incontinence decreased with experience and modifications. The Mainz I pouch has been used in

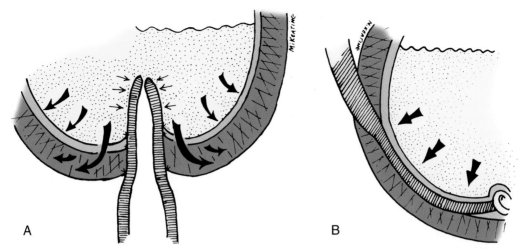

Figure 124–18. Continence mechanisms. **A,** The same pressures that create continence tend to efface nipple valves. **B,** This is not true of flap valves, which have been more reliable in pediatric reconstruction.

children with good results and low rates of incontinence with the latest modifications (Stein et al, 1995, 1997a, 2000; Steiner et al, 1998). Maintenance of normal upper tracts has been good, and metabolic problems are rare (Stein et al, 1997b). In fact, improvement of preexisting hydronephrosis has been more common than worsening. For the past several years, the group in Mainz has used a flap valve mechanism and the appendix for a continent catheterizable stoma with less incontinence (Stein et al, 1995; Gerharz et al, 1997).

Flap Valves and the Mitrofanoff Principle

Mitrofanoff (1980) described a continence mechanism with use of the appendix and ureter to make a flap valve. He recognized that any tubular structure could be implanted

effectively into a low-pressure reservoir. This continence mechanism circumvents many of the secondary potential complications associated with harvesting of the ileocecal valve or use of other gastrointestinal segments.

The foundation for the success of the Mitrofanoff principle is based on construction of a submucosal tunnel for a supple, small-diameter conduit. As the reservoir fills, the rise in intravesical pressure is transmitted through the epithelium and to the implanted conduit, coapting its lumen (Fig. 124–19). **The appendix is an ideal natural tubular structure that can be safely removed from the gastrointestinal tract without significant morbidity. The small caliber of the appendix facilitates construction of a short functional tunnel with the bladder wall. Experience has shown that continence can be achieved with only a 2-cm appendiceal tunnel** (Kaefer and Retik, 1997). Whether in a continent urinary reservoir or native bladder, the appendix has been

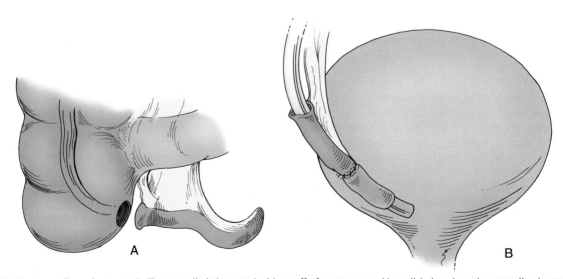

Figure 124–19. Appendicovesicostomy. **A,** The appendix is harvested with a cuff of cecum on a wide pedicle based on the appendiceal artery. A flap of cecum can be harvested in continuity with the appendix and tubularized to increase the length. **B,** The distal appendix is tunneled into the bladder to provide continence after the end is amputated. The proximal end of the appendix, the cecal cuff, is brought to the umbilicus or right lower quadrant as a catheterizable stoma.

used as an efferent limb with very good results (Jayanthi et al, 1995; Mollard et al, 1997; Kaefer et al, 1997b; Cain et al, 1999). The appendix has been particularly useful in children as it is relatively longer and the abdominal wall generally thinner. The flap valve is probably the most reliable of all of the surgically constructed continence mechanisms. This is good in terms of continence when the patient is catheterized reliably. Many patients with good flap valves will virtually never leak per stoma. This potentially puts them at greater risk for upper tract deterioration or spontaneous rupture of the bladder or reservoir if catheterization is not performed.

If the appendix is used in situ as a continence mechanism in a continent urinary reservoir, the reservoir by necessity will include the right colon. Duckett and Snyder (1986, 1987) used the right colon and appendix with good results and called it the Penn pouch. The mesoappendix, in most cases, allows mobilization of the appendix for use in the native bladder or virtually any reservoir.

Technique

Appropriate preoperative planning is required to position the skin incision to allow adequate mobilization of the appendix to the bladder. In most children, this can be achieved by making a low midline or a transverse incision. On occasion, the cecum may be high in the abdomen. Mobilization of the ascending colon along the line of Toldt may be required to gain mobilization of the appendix and its mesentery. Cadeddu and Docimo (1999) have used laparoscopy to aid in mobilization of the ascending colon and cecum. Once the cecum has been mobilized, the base of the appendix is amputated, leaving a small cuff of cecum with the appendix. Use of the cuff at the stoma may decrease the risk of stenosis. The cecum is closed in a fashion similar to an open appendectomy. If the length of the appendix is marginal, a greater portion of the cecum can be harvested, which effectively increases the functional length of the appendix (Cromie et al, 1991). A portion may be tubularized with the appendix (Bruce and McRoberts, 1998).

After harvesting, a location is selected for implantation of the appendix into the bladder. The location is based on the length of the appendix, the mobility of the bladder, and the location for the appendiceal stoma. Typically, the distal end of the appendix is tunneled into a posterolateral position within the bladder (see Fig. 124–19).

The base of the appendix is brought to the abdominal wall in a location chosen preoperatively to suit the patient. If a patient wears a supportive brace, stomal positioning must take this into account. The appendix should be brought up to reach the skin without tension, and care must be taken not to twist the pedicle or to occlude it as it passes through the abdominal wall fascia. The base of the appendix can often be hidden within the umbilicus, which allows elimination of a small but obvious abdominal stoma. Because of the small circular diameter of the appendiceal base, stomal stenosis is common, and techniques have been described to prevent this problem. Various flaps have been described as a method for avoiding stomal stenosis (Keating et al, 1993; Kajbafzadeh, et al, 1995; Kaefer and Retik, 1997). **For prevention of kinking and problems with catheterization, it is advisable to maintain as short a conduit as possible.** Securing the appendix and bladder wall to the peritoneum beneath the fascia will help

diminish the problem of conduit kinking with reservoir filling. The importance of meticulous operative detail in securing the Mitrofanoff limb cannot be overemphasized.

When appendix or any catheterizable stoma is used, it is advisable to repeatedly catheterize the channel after each step in reconstruction to confirm easy passage. If the catheter does not pass easily into the reservoir, the preceding step needs to be revised. Problems with catheterization by the surgeon during the operative procedure usually result in more difficulty for the patient afterward. It is also beneficial to catheterize at variable reservoir volumes to confirm proper fixation of the reservoir and the absence of any kinking. A 6 to 10 French Silastic stent is typically left for 10 to 14 days within the efferent catheterizable channel during the healing process. It is advisable for the surgeon to personally catheterize the efferent limb before allowing the patient or other family members to do so. Catheterization should be repeated at least every 4 hours during the day for reservoir drainage, maintenance of patency, and minimalization of the risk of stomal stenosis.

The appendix may not be available for use in all patients because of previous appendectomy, its location or length, congenital absence, involvement with adhesions, or its use for continence enemas. Histologic abnormalities of the appendix have been reported to occur in as many as 30% of patients (Liebovitch et al, 1992) and to increase with age. They rarely are of enough clinical significance to preclude use (Mulvihill et al, 1983).

Results

Several papers have reviewed large series of patients after appendicovesicostomy (Kaefer et al, 1997b; Cain et al, 1999, Harris et al, 2000). The populations of patients have been typical of most pediatric groups, the majority having neurogenic dysfunction. Inability to use the appendix, other than because it was needed in situ for antegrade continence enemas, has been rare. The results, in terms of continence, have been superb, usually above 95% (Gerharz et al, 1997, 1998; Kaefer and Retik, 1997; Mor et al, 1997; Suzer et al, 1997; Gosalbez et al, 1998; Cain et al, 1999; Castellan et al, 1999; Liard et al, 2001). **Incontinence is a rare event with the Mitrofanoff principle and may result from inadequate length of the flap valve mechanism or persistently elevated reservoir pressure.** Urodynamic evaluation is required to evaluate the cause of the incontinence. Whereas injection of collagen or other biomaterials is a possible treatment for inadequate outflow resistance, a more formal approach with takedown and revision of the leaking Mitrofanoff valve is usually required (Kaefer and Retik, 1997). **The most common complication has been stomal stenosis, which has generally occurred in 10% to 20% of patients.** Such stenosis resulting in difficult catheterization may occur early in the postoperative course and require formal revision (Harris et al, 2000). Another recognized complication has been appendiceal perforation. Stricture and necrosis, particularly of cecal extensions of the appendix, have occurred rarely. Abdominal stomas may be associated with a higher risk of reservoir calculi because of the potential for incomplete emptying.

Follow-up in the recent series has averaged approximately 4 years. Patients from Mitrofanoff's early experience (1980) should now have follow-up of more than 20 years, suggesting that the appendix may provide a durable alternative for pediatric patients with a long life expectancy, a finding also noted by others (Cain et al, 1999; Harris et al, 2000; Liard et al, 2001).

Alternatives

When the appendix is unavailable for use, other tubular structures can provide a similar mechanism for catheterization and continence. Mitrofanoff (1980) described a similar technique with ureter (Kaefer et al, 1997b). Care must be taken to preserve the distal blood supply to prevent ischemia. Refluxing ureters have even been used after extravesical reimplantation (Ashcraft and Dennis, 1986; Duel et al, 1996; Kaefer et al, 1997b). Stomal stenosis seems to be more problematic with use of the ureter compared with the appendix, possibly owing to compromised blood supply. In addition, distention of the ureter due to catheter passage has caused discomfort in some individuals (Duckett and Lofti, 1993).

Woodhouse and MacNeily (1994) as well as others have used the fallopian tube, which can accommodate catheterization. Stenosis appears to be a significant problem with the fallopian tube. In addition, the effect on fertility should be considered when there is a normal ipsilateral gonad. Bihrle and associates (1991) fashioned a gastric tube mobilized on the gastroepiploic artery for implantation in continent reservoirs. Acid irritation of the skin was a problem in some patients. They then used a tapered segment of ileum as well (Adams et al, 1992). By narrowing the segment longitudinally along the mesenteric border with permanent staples in series, they were able to construct a uniform tube of adequate length that was easy to catheterize and provided good continence rates. Others (Hasan et al, 1994; Woodhouse and MacNeily, 1994) have had similar good results. It is ideal for such tubes to be long enough to reach from the reservoir to skin without tension; however, they should then be kept as short and straight as possible to facilitate easy catheterization. Any long and free catheterizable channel within the abdomen can potentially kink and result in difficult catheterization or perforation.

Monti has been credited with a novel modification of the tapered intestinal segment that can be reimplanted according to the Mitrofanoff principle (Monti et al, 1997). **Recognition should also be directed to another report of this procedure by Yang** (Yang, 1993). A very short (1 to 2 cm) segment of small bowel is opened longitudinally along the antimesenteric border and then closed transversely (Fig. 124–20). By this reconfiguration, the initial circumference of the segment is converted to the length, and the original length to the circumference of the reconfigured tube. A uniform tube is made with a small mesentery toward the center. The two ends are devoid of mesentery, making them easy to tunnel into bladder and bring through the abdominal wall. If the first incision is made directly at the antimesenteric border, both limbs are of equal length. By making the incision well around one side, one limb may be made much longer than the other. Experience has shown that one need not achieve a long tunnel in the bladder or reservoir to achieve continence with such a small tube, and the longer limb has typically been used to reach the skin through a thick abdominal wall.

Very good results have been achieved with the Yang-Monti tube as a catheterizable stoma, and it is certainly an efficient use of bowel. Some surgeons have suggested that it may be easier to catheterize than an ileal segment tapered longitudinally because circular mucosal folds are redirected longitudinally in the direction of catheter passage. Flap valves constructed with ileum may have a lower rate of stomal stenosis than those made with appendix (Kaefer et al, 1999a). The one potential disadvantage of the Yang-Monti tube is that it remains relatively short and may not reach the skin without tension in obese patients. Despite extensive use of skin flaps, such tension may lead to stomal stenosis. Two separate reconfigured tubes can be anastomosed together for better length (Kaefer and Retik, 1997). Casale (1999) has used an initial segment that is twice as long, partially split in the middle, and then opened in a spiral fashion on opposite sides to make a longer strip that can be tubularized in continuity. Narayanaswamy and colleagues (2001) noted difficulty with catheterizations through Yang-Monti channels in 28% of a large series of patients due to "pouch-like dilatation." Such a problem has been avoidable in most series.

Ileocecal Valve

Use of the ileocecal valve as a continence mechanism began with Gilchrist (1950) and was popularized by the Indiana group (Rowland et al, 1985; Bihrle, 1997). Various modifications exist. In general, a short segment of terminal ileum, whether imbricated or tailored, is used as an efferent limb. This segment should be kept as short and straight as possible to facilitate easy intermittent catheterization. Continence is based on the imbricated ileocecal valve, not the length of the efferent limb. The imbrication is usually secured with interrupted, permanent sutures, involving the very distal ileum and ileocecal valve, and the imbrication is carried well onto the cecum. The reservoir itself is constructed from reconfigured right colon up through the hepatic flexure, with or without a patch of ileum. Standard ureterocolonic anastomoses are done beneath the taenia to prevent reflux. Staplers using absorbable staples have been used for reconfiguration of the reservoir (Kirsch et al, 1996) and may shorten the operative time for reconstruction.

The Indiana pouch has been used in children with excellent results, as it has in adults. Besides the appendix, this continence mechanism is perhaps the simplest and has the shortest learning curve to achieve reliable results. Continence rates as high as 95% have been reported with preservation of normal upper tracts (Rowland et al, 1985; Lockhart et al, 1990; Rink and Bihrle, 1990; Hensle and Ring, 1991; Rowland, 1995; Kaefer et al, 1997b). Rare reports have noted higher rates of incontinence (Canning, 1998). Husmann and Cain (1999) have used the cecal segment for bladder augmentation and the efferent limb to construct a continent catheterizable stoma with equally good results. They noted a low incidence of detrimental effect on gastrointestinal function in a select group of patients with neurogenic dysfunction.

Hydraulic Valves

Benchekroun (1982, 1989) developed an interesting hydraulic valve as a continence mechanism that was modified by Guzman and coworkers (1989). Urine from the reservoir and any pressure generated there is allowed to enter a sleeve of ileum around the catheterizable channel. Compression of the

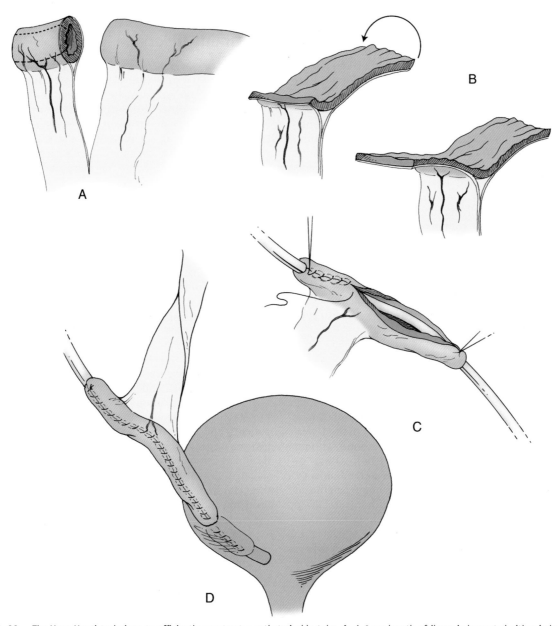

Figure 124–20. The Yang-Monti technique to efficiently construct a catheterizable tube. **A,** A 2-cm length of ileum is harvested either independently or next to a segment for augmentation cystoplasty. The segment is opened horizontally and tubularized in a longitudinal fashion. **B,** If the segment is opened directly on the antimesenteric border, two equal-length limbs result with a central mesenteric pedicle. Initial incision may be made to one side to form a shorter limb for implantation in the bladder and a longer one to be brought through the abdominal wall. **C,** The reconfigured ileal segment is tubularized over a 12 French catheter in a two-layer technique with absorbable sutures. **D,** A continent catheterizable stoma is constructed.

inner tube theoretically provides continence, and early results were encouraging. Initial continence rates approached 75% and then 90% with a single revision (Benchekroun et al, 1989). Others have not been able to duplicate those results (Sanda et al, 1988; Leonard et al, 1990b), and the valve has largely been abandoned.

Koff and associates (1989) added hydraulic compression to the terminal ileum of an Indiana pouch by anastomosing a segment of tubular ileum to the cecum and then wrapping it around the efferent limb. The procedure has not gained popularity, probably because of the excellent success of the standard Indiana pouch.

Continent Vesicostomy

Yachia (1997) described construction of a bladder tube fashioned from a wide flap of the anterior bladder wall. No attempt was made to produce continence at the level of the bladder. The continence mechanism was fashioned by weaving the bladder tube through the rectus muscle to produce compression and continence. Continence in the small, short-term series was reported at 100% but has not been duplicated.

Hanna and colleagues (1999) described a continence mechanism based on either a flap of bladder or intestinal tissue fashioned after prior enterocystoplasty. A rectangular flap in continuity with the bladder is tubularized over a 14 to 16 French catheter. The bladder is plicated around the proximal 3 cm of the tube with nonabsorbable suture to make a type of nipple similar to gastric fundoplication. No significant morbidity has been identified in a limited series of five children, and all children have remained dry on intermittent catheterization. Macedo and Srougi (2000) described a similar continence mechanism made at the time of initial augmentation. They achieved acceptable continence in eight of their first nine patients. Their technique is potentially appealing for patients requiring augmentation and having no appendix because of the simplicity; however, continence is based on a type of nipple valve that historically has been difficult to keep fixed. The same forces that create continence tend to efface the continence mechanism.

Casale (1991) has described a form of continent vesicostomy in which the continence mechanism is based on a flap valve made from a tubularized strip of bladder mucosa. It is particularly suitable when the bladder is compliant and of large capacity. An anterior detrusor strip is also used to construct a catheterizable limb.

Technique

Parallel incisions 3 cm apart are made into the anterior bladder and used to form a long rectangular flap. The abdominal wall should be measured to ensure that the strip is long enough to reach the skin without tension. The full-thickness strip is tubularized down to the bladder, typically in two layers. The muscle portion is left broad to come around without tension and provide good blood supply. The mucosa may be trimmed in width before tubularization to avoid redundancy. A strip of mucosa within the bladder, 2 to 3 cm in length and 1.5 cm in width, is incised in a direct line with the mobilized bladder tube. The edges of this strip are mobilized until it can be tubularized along its entire length. It may be beneficial to mobilize only one edge over to the other side, which allows one to avoid overlapping suture lines. Casale (1991) originally incised the mucosa transversely at the end of the intravesical strip to be tubularized; Rink and associates (1995b) then suggested that it could be left intact (Fig. 124–21). The bladder mucosa from either side of the tube is then mobilized and closed to make a flap valve. More extensive mobilization of the side opposite that mobilized for the inner tube allows closure without overlapping suture lines, which may help avoid fistula formation and incontinence. A soft stent is usually left through the tube for 3 weeks during healing to prevent stenosis. It does tend to close if it is not catheterized regularly and may be even more susceptible than other catheterizable channels to stomal stenosis (Cain et al, 2002; Thomas et al, 2005).

Results

Continence rates have been good, as with most flap valve mechanisms (Cain et al, 1999, 2002). Stomal stenosis remains a significant problem, 45% in the experience at Indiana University (Cain et al, 2002). Skin flaps and avoidance of tension to reach the skin may minimize this risk but not remove it. Advantages include avoidance of an intraperitoneal procedure and bowel anastomosis; the appendix can be reserved for use with enemas. It does use some bladder and decreases capacity, which may not be appropriate for some patients.

Results with Pediatric Continent Diversion

Continent urinary reservoirs have been performed in children with very good results, equivalent to those achieved for adults. Construction of an adequate reservoir and an antireflux mechanism has generally been straightforward. For review of issues concerning compliance of the reservoir or mechanisms by which reflux can be prevented, the reader may review earlier parts of this chapter or the chapter on continent urinary diversion in adults. The most challenging aspect of continent diversion remains construction of an efferent limb that provides reliable continence and easy catheterization. The continence mechanism most familiar to pediatric urologists is the flap valve. The appendix is simple to use, suitable for most children, and associated with very good continence rates. If the appendix is not present or is to be used for antegrade colonic enemas, tapered intestinal segments provide a nice alternative. Nipple valves are the most complex continence mechanism and therefore have a longer learning curve. Continence rates of approximately 85% can be expected with stapled nipple valves (Kaefer et al, 1997b; Benson and Olsson, 1998), even with extensive experience. With use of the other efferent limbs, continence rates above 90% and approaching 95% have routinely been reported in children (Duckett and Snyder, 1986; Hensle and Ring, 1991; Kaefer et al, 1997b; Surer et al, 2003). Those continence rates have been achieved with preservation of the upper tracts. With proper selection of patients and appropriately performed continent diversion, hydronephrosis in children is rare postoperatively. Particularly if catheterization is not performed reliably, new hydronephrosis can occur (Abd-El-Gawad et al, 1999). There is no evidence that children suffer more hydronephrosis after continent diversion compared with conduit diversion (Stein et al, 2000).

Children undergoing continent diversion have a long life expectancy. The incidence of complications after continent diversion will probably increase with longer follow-up. Those patients will be subject to the same complications discussed at length for bladder augmentation. All of those complications, including infection, hydronephrosis, calculi, spontaneous perforation, and tumor, have been reported after continent diversion, in adults if not in children. These are largely a function of the use of intestine as a urinary reservoir. Because more intestine is usually required in continent diversion than in bladder augmentation, the incidence of complications may ultimately be higher than with simple augmentation as follow-up increases. Certainly, serum changes of increased chloride, decreased bicarbonate, and acidosis have been noted in some patients after continent diversion (Allen et al, 1985; Ashken, 1987; Thuroff et al, 1987; Boyd et al, 1989; McDougal, 1992a). Spontaneous perforation has occurred in up to 1.5% of patients (Mansson et al, 1997).

The most common complication in pediatric continent diversion thus far has been stomal stenosis. Such stenosis occurs more commonly at the umbilicus and when appendix is used compared with tapered ileal segments (Fichtner et al, 1997; Kaefer et al, 1999a). Various skin flaps may be placed into the terminal end of the appendix or intestinal segment to lower the rate of stenosis but do not eliminate it (Kajbafzadeh et al, 1995). Bladder calculi have also been common problems (Surer et al, 2003).

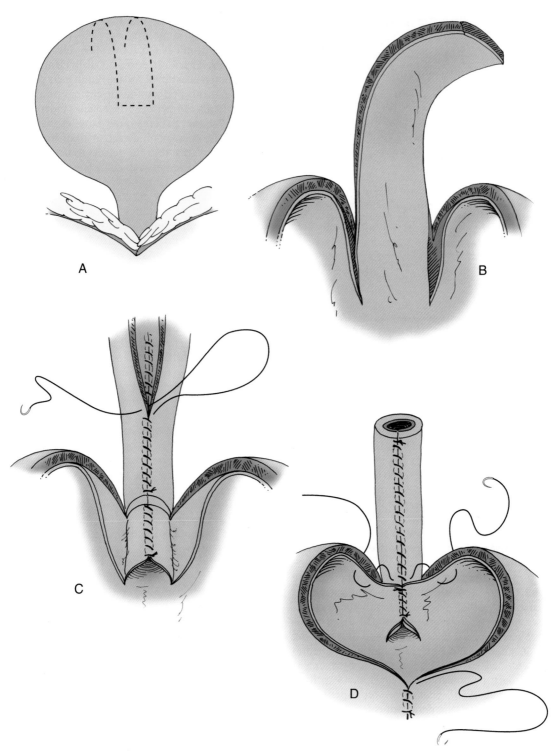

Figure 124–21. Casale continent catheterizable stoma. **A,** Parallel incisions are made in the bladder dome, forming a full-thickness bladder strip. **B,** The epithelium of the bladder is then incised for an additional 2.5 cm. The edges of the epithelium are mobilized, allowing tubularization. **C,** The epithelium is tubularized from the bladder out to the tip of the strip with an absorbable suture. The muscle of the bladder strip is then tubularized with an absorbable suture. **D,** The lateral edges of the epithelium within the bladder are reapproximated over the tubularized bladder segment with absorbable suture. The bladder is then closed with absorbable suture, incorporating the bladder tube with the initial sutures to prevent kinking.

ANTEGRADE CONTINENCE ENEMAS

Fecal incontinence may be more socially debilitating to patients than urinary incontinence. In a sense, it has been easier to work surgically on urinary incontinence because urologists and their patients have intermittent catheterization to reliably empty. Unfortunately, that has not been the case with constipation and fecal incontinence, particularly among patients with neurogenic dysfunction. **Malone and colleagues (1990) have described use of the appendix for antegrade continence enemas (MACE) to control constipation and achieve fecal continence in patients with complex gastrointestinal disorders refractory to conservative management.** These enemas, usually performed once a day, provide a thorough cleansing in a short time. Patients, particularly those with neurogenic dysfunction, often will not stool again until their next enema (Curry et al, 1999). Cecostomy tubes, cecostomy buttons, and tapered intestinal segments tunneled into the cecum have been used for the enemas when the appendix is not suitable or is unavailable. Antegrade continence enemas as originally described by Malone have been used extensively in the neurogenic population (Koyle et al, 1995; Rink et al, 1999; Curry et al, 1999). Enemas are often performed with plain tap water. Metabolic derangements are unusual, although water treated in a softener should be avoided as it can cause hypernatremia (Yerkes et al, 2000).

Average irrigating volumes in most series have approached 400 mL but occasionally reach 900 mL. The transit time for the enema after insertion varies among patients but averages 25 minutes and ranges from 15 minutes to an hour (Rink et al, 1999). Smaller volumes and less transit time may be required for left colon antegrade enemas (Churchill et al, 2003). Additives to the irrigant may decrease the transit time in some patients (Kajbafzadeh and Chubak, 2000). The enemas are begun daily as soon as bowel function returns after reconstructive surgery. The initial volume used is low and typically increased every 2 or 3 days until adequate decompres-

sion is achieved. Fecal continence until the next enema has been consistent for most patients with neurogenic dysfunction and ranges from 67% to above 90% (Hensle et al, 1998; Rink et al, 1999; Herndon et al, 2004b). Hensle and colleagues (1998) noted occasional soilage requiring a pad in one quarter of their patients performing the enemas routinely. The majority of patients can perform the enemas independently. Almost universally, the patients and families have continued to perform the enemas on a regular basis in these series, good evidence that they find the results to be worth any time and effort involved (Yerkes et al, 2003; Herndon et al, 2004b). Rare patients may have severe colonic spasms with flushing that preclude use (Bau et al, 2000). They occasionally respond better to multiple flushings with smaller volumes. The most common complication, as with use of the appendix as a catheterizable stoma elsewhere, has been stomal stenosis, although stenosis may not occur as commonly as when the appendix is moved to the bladder (Kaefer et al, 2000). Some children require catheterization of the appendix twice a day to avoid contracture or a cicatrix at the skin level. Perforation of the appendix has been noted with catheterization, as has false passage parallel to the appendix. Subsequent intraperitoneal injection of the enema fluid has resulted in peritonitis. Such patients require antibiotics and close observation. They do not routinely require reoperation (Brock, 2000). Kokoska and associates (2004) reported two cases of cecal volvulus among 164 patients using these enemas.

The appendix can be used easily in situ (Fig. 124–22). Windows in the mesoappendix may be made and permanent Lembert sutures used to approximate the cecal wall in each window. This effectively wraps the cecum around the base of the appendix to prevent spillage. Alternatively, one taenia leading to the appendix may be incised longitudinally and reapproximated in the windows of the mesoappendix. Others have made no attempt to construct a continence mechanism at the appendicocecal junction, particularly surgeons

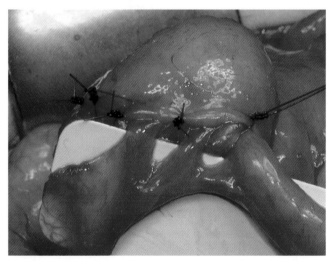

Figure 124–22. The appendix used in situ for antegrade continence enema or urinary continent catheterizable stoma. The appendix and its mesentery are mobilized without detachment from the cecum. Windows are carefully made in the mesentery between vessels to the proximal appendix. The taeniae from either side of the cecum are approximated in those windows with permanent sutures to ensure continence of the stoma. The distal end of the appendix is brought to the abdominal wall for catheterization.

performing antegrade continence enemas laparoscopically (Cadeddu and Docimo, 1999). Most MACE procedures are performed by urologists at the time of a major reconstructive procedure involving the bladder. Their long experience with construction of continent catheterizable stomas for the urinary bladder has taught them the principles to ensure a good result. Our preference is to provide some continence mechanism at the base of the appendix in that setting to avoid any spillage (Donohoe et al, 2004).

URINARY UNDIVERSION

The role and frequency of urinary undiversion have changed dramatically during the past several decades. Before the acceptance of clean intermittent catheterization (Lapides et al, 1976), many children were not candidates for complex reconstructive procedures because of an inability to empty afterward. Many were initially treated with permanent urinary diversions with use of an intestinal segment with high expectations. Over time, it became clear that such diversions had significant complications including infection, stones, and nephropathy (Smith, 1972; Richie et al, 1974; Shapiro et al, 1975; Middleton and Hendren, 1976; Pitts and Muecke, 1979). With the recognition of those complications and the routine use of clean intermittent catheterization, urinary undiversion became a relatively common procedure for the reconstructive surgeon (Hendren, 1974, 1987, 1990; Perlmutter, 1980). Fewer patients now require diversion. Better anesthetic and perioperative surgical care has allowed safe definitive repair of primary problems in younger infants. The occasional diversion presently done in extreme cases is usually temporary rather than permanent with use of bowel. Consequently, undiversion now is infrequent and typically involves closure of some urinary stoma rather than takedown of an intestinal segment.

Permanent diversions in children are now typically confined to cancer patients with a poor prognosis and short life expectancy. When their outcome is better than expected, they may still be candidates for undiversion or a change to continent urinary diversion. The Boston group has favored initial temporary diversion with a transverse colon conduit to avoid irradiated bowel. Once cure is ensured, the conduit can be converted to a continent reservoir by augmenting the colonic segment with stomach to provide an adequate reservoir and by providing a continent catheterizable efferent limb (Duel et al, 1996).

The key to urinary undiversion is understanding the original pathologic process that led to diversion. This may be relatively easy if the surgeon involved has cared for the patient throughout his or her course. If the original diversion was done by someone else years previously, such understanding may be difficult and require thorough investigation. Accurate understanding of the underlying disease may be made more difficult because of defunctionalization of the remaining urinary tract. It is important to review the patient's original history and studies to understand the pathophysiologic changes before any intervention. For example, failure of the urinary bladder in a patient with neurogenic dysfunction to respond adequately to anticholinergic medication and intermittent catheterization before vesicostomy diversion might well predict that it will not do so after vesicostomy closure.

Special nuances in the current evaluation may also be necessary. Urodynamic evaluation of a bladder diverted for several years with a vesicostomy will virtually always show a small capacity. A repeated study after several days of bladder cycling or occlusion of the vesicostomy may be more predictive of bladder function. The bladder may respond to bladder cycling quickly (Bauer et al, 1986; McGuire, 1996). Temporary occlusion of a vesicostomy with a gastrostomy button may be informative (de Badiola et al, 1995). Occlusion of the vesicostomy during urodynamics may be necessary to achieve good bladder filling and to accurately define the adequacy of outflow resistance. Such parameters must be evaluated before undiversion and may have changed since the time of diversion, particularly in patients with neurogenic dysfunction. Antegrade perfusion studies may be helpful and necessary in evaluation of the upper tract previously diverted by ureterostomy or pyelostomy.

Correction of Original and New Pathologic Processes

It is essential that all pathophysiologic change is appreciated, whether it is original or new. Failure to do so can result in recurrent clinical problems for the patient (i.e., renal insufficiency, hydronephrosis, infection, and incontinence) in the face of a technically perfect operation. Once the reconstructive surgeon well understands those problems, the reconstructive options available at undiversion must be evaluated. Considerations include the length, dilation, and scarring of the ureters; the volume, compliance, and fibrosis of the native bladder; and the function of the outlet in terms of resistance for continence and synergistic relaxation for emptying. More global problems, such as renal insufficiency and neurogenic dysfunction, may influence the choices of technique as well. In patients with an existing permanent diversion involving an intestinal segment, the quality, length, and volume of that segment should be considered to determine how it might best be used in reconstruction. An existing ileal conduit might be used as an ileal ureter, as a segment for bladder augmentation, or for tapering as a continent stoma, depending on the needs of the patient.

For examples that illustrate the potentially complex nature of many undiversion cases, we refer the reader to Dr. Hendren's chapter on undiversion in prior editions of this text (Hendren, 1998). No one has more experience, and his cases demonstrate the total command of all surgical alternatives that is required to manage these patients well. The illustrated cases there are typical of the types of patients that historically underwent undiversion.

Results

Hendren (1998) reported a 26-year experience with urinary undiversion in 216 patients. Two thirds of the patients had permanent diversions, often of long duration. He noted that many of the patients had impaired renal function, either from their underlying problems or as morbidity related to the diversion. More than 10% of the patients required renal transplantation after undiversion, and even more are likely to require such in the future. With successful relief of obstruction, prevention of reflux, and provision of a compliant bladder, undiversion prolonged the time to renal failure in some patients and may have avoided it altogether in others. Undiversion may protect renal function rather than contribute to any decline if it is properly selected and performed.

In that series, management of the bladder was relatively straightforward and effective with bladder augmentation as necessary. Inadequate outflow resistance was usually treated with Young-Dees-Leadbetter bladder neck repair. Most complications were related to the ureters; 23 patients required reoperation for persistent reflux; 10 did so for partial obstruction of the ureter. Those reoperation rates are indicative of the difficulty one faces in dealing with short, dilated, and scarred ureters that may be present after urinary diversion (Hendren, 1998). Others have had similar good success (Gonzalez et al, 1986; Mitchell and Rink, 1987) with undiversion.

The success of many of the techniques necessary for urinary undiversion should be similar to the success of those done in primary reconstruction. In other words, the good results of ileocystoplasty or appendicovesicostomy should be equivalent whether they are done as part of a urinary undiversion or not. As noted in Hendren's cases and series, many problems may be present and multiple techniques might be required for a given patient. **The key to achieving a good result in urinary undiversion is to understand all of the patient's problems and to correct each. The most difficult measure of complex undiversion, and the one most prone to complication, relates to the short, dilated, and chronically scarred ureter that may be the residual of the original problem or previous surgical procedures including diversion.**

In occasional cases of urinary undiversion, conversion to a continent urinary reservoir is appropriate. This is true of cases in which the native bladder is congenitally absent, removed, or heavily irradiated. In those rare cases, the volume and quality of the patient's native tissue may be so poor that inclusion in the reconstruction is not warranted. **In the majority of cases of urinary undiversion, reconstruction of the native urinary tract is preferable to continent diversion.** Such reconstruction can minimize the morbidity to the patient.

KEY POINTS: URINARY UNDIVERSION

- Most undiversion now involves takedown of a urinary stoma rather than an intestinal diversion.

- It is key to understand the patient's underlying pathophysiologic process as well as any problems related to diversion.

- Chronically scarred and shortened ureters may be a challenge in these patients.

SUMMARY

Every effort should be made to treat pediatric bladder dysfunction, no matter what the etiology, early and aggressively to minimize the number of patients requiring reconstructive surgery for bladder and sphincter dysfunction. Some such surgery will still be necessary, and the patients must be carefully evaluated so that all problems are identified and can be addressed. The surgeon should then be flexible and prepared to use the bowel segments and techniques that best fit each patient. **Whereas a given surgeon's result with any technique may improve with experience and confidence, each patient's unique problems and anatomy may make some choices better than others. Forcing one procedure to fit every patient should be avoided.**

Preoperative evaluation should identify upper tract obstruction or vesicoureteral reflux. Such problems should be corrected at the time of surgery. It is imperative to provide the patient with an adequate bladder or reservoir, one capable of holding at low pressure a urinary volume that will be produced between voidings or catheterizations. This can be accomplished by either augmentation or construction of a continent reservoir with use of any gastrointestinal segment. Each has its own set of advantages and disadvantages that should be considered. If adequate outflow resistance is lacking, it should be created at the bladder neck to prevent incontinence. Any patient undergoing reconstructive surgery for bladder or sphincter dysfunction must be prepared to perform and be capable of performing intermittent catheterization on a reliable basis; many will require it routinely. This is particularly true of those patients with neurogenic dysfunction.

As much of the patient's native urinary tract as possible should be preserved in pediatric urologic reconstruction. The urothelial lining avoids much of the morbidity associated with intestinal segments. If necessary, however, virtually any portion of the lower urinary tract may be reconstructed or replaced with intestine. Unfortunately, occasional complications do occur when intestinal segments are used in that manner. They are not perfect physiologic substitutes. The most important factor in avoiding problems with such complex pediatric patients is the motivation of the patient and family to achieve a successful outcome. Assessment of that commitment is critical.

SUGGESTED READINGS

Cain MP, Casale AJ, King SJ, Rink RC: Appendicovesicostomy and newer alternatives for the Mitrofanoff procedure: Results in the last 100 patients at Riley Children's Hospital. J Urol 1999;162:1749-1752.

Filmer RB, Spencer JR: Malignancies in bladder augmentations and intestinal conduits. J Urol 1990;143:671.

Hendren WH: Urinary tract refunctionalization after long-term diversion: A 20 year experience with 177 patients. Ann Surg 1990;212:478-495.

Herndon CD, Rink RC, Shaw MB, et al: The Indiana experience with artificial urinary sphincters in children and young adults. J Urol 2003;169:650-654.

Husmann DA, Snodgrass WT, Koyle MA, et al: Ureterocystoplasty: Indications for a successful augmentation. J Urol 2004;171:376-380.

Koch MO, McDougal WS: The pathophysiology of hyperchloremic metabolic acidosis after urinary diversion through intestinal segments. Surgery 1985;98:561-570.

Kropp KA, Angwafo FF: Urethral lengthening and reimplantation for neurogenic incontinence in children. J Urol 1986;135:533.

Kryger JV, Gonzalez R, Spencer Barthold J: Surgical management of urinary incontinence in children with neurogenic sphincteric incompetence. J Urol 2000;163:256-263.

Lapides J, Diokno AC, Gould FR, Lowe BS: Further observations on self-catheterization. J Urol 1976;116:169-171.

Liard A, Seguier-Lipszyc E, Mathiot A, Mitrofanoff P: The Mitrofanoff procedure: 20 years later. J Urol 2001;165:2394-2398.

McGuire EJ, Woodside JR, Borden TA, Weiss RM: Prognostic value of urodynamic testing in myelodysplastic patients. J Urol 1981;126:205-209.

Rink RC, Hollensbe D, Adams MC: Complications of augmentation in children and comparison of gastrointestinal segments. AUA Update Series 1995;14:122-128.

125 Hypospadias

JOSEPH G. BORER, MD • ALAN B. RETIK, MD

Hypospadias is a relatively common congenital defect of the male external genitalia. It is present in approximately 1 in 250 male newborns. Hypospadias may be an isolated defect or a phenotypical component of a more complex condition such as an intersex state. There are a multitude of techniques at the disposal of the experienced surgeon faced with reconstruction of hypospadias. Dr. John W. Duckett, Jr., defined *hypospadiology* as "the in-depth study of the art and science of the surgical correction of hypospadias" (Duckett, 1981b, 1995). This chapter provides a detailed account of all aspects of care regarding the individual with hypospadias.

Definition

Hypospadias, in boys, is defined as an association of three anomalies of the penis: (1) an abnormal ventral opening of the urethral meatus that may be located anywhere from the ventral aspect of the glans penis to the perineum, (2) an abnormal ventral curvature of the penis (chordee), and (3) an abnormal distribution of foreskin with a "hood" present dorsally and deficient foreskin ventrally (Fig. 125–1) (Mouriquand et al, 1995). The second and third characteristics are not present in all cases.

Diagnosis

Hypospadias is typically diagnosed at newborn physical examination. This is not always the case for boys with milder forms of hypospadias or a nonretractile prepuce (Boisen et al, 2005) or for those with the megameatus intact prepuce (MIP) variant (Duckett and Keating, 1989; Hatch et al, 1989). These boys may escape diagnosis until the foreskin is fully retracted or circumcision is performed (Fig. 125–2). **Although uncommon, simple apparently isolated hypospadias may be the only visible indication of a significant underlying abnormality** (Aarskog, 1971).

Classification Schemes

Many different classification systems have been proposed, as reviewed by Sorensen (1953) and summarized more recently (Sheldon and Duckett, 1987). **Culp, in 1959, was perhaps the first to classify the level of hypospadias after any necessary treatment of penile curvature (orthoplasty) and to realize the importance of this method. In 1973, Barcat more formally proposed designating the location of the hypospadiac meatus, and thus the true extent of the urethral defect requiring repair, after orthoplasty.** Both categorical designations and specific anatomic description of the meatal level are helpful to the discussion of hypospadias as it pertains to diagnostic classification and management (Fig. 125–3).

In all commonly used classification systems, glanular, coronal, and subcoronal (anterior/distal) defects constitute the great majority (50% to 70%) of hypospadias (Sheldon and Duckett, 1987; Sauvage et al, 1993; Borer et al, 2001). Duckett (1998) has reported overall rates of approximately 50%, 30%, and 20% for distal, middle, and posterior/proximal hypospadias, respectively.

KEY POINTS: DEFINITION, DIAGNOSIS, CLASSIFICATION SCHEMES

- *Hypospadias* is defined as an ectopic urethral meatus on the ventral aspect of the penis, scrotum, or perineum with or without ventral penile curvature.

- Apparent isolated hypospadias may be associated with a significant underlying abnormality.

- Classification of the level of hypospadias is most accurately performed after correction of penile curvature.

DEVELOPMENT
Embryology

Glenister (1954) performed serial sectioning of 37 human fetuses (21 male, 12 female, and 4 in the indifferent stage) to evaluate embryologic development of the urethral plate and urethra. **Based on a thorough review of the subject, Glenis-**

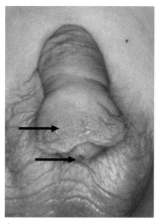 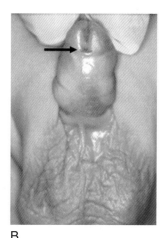

A B

Figure 125–1. Appearance of mild hypospadias. **A,** Dorsal "hood" foreskin *(upper arrow)* and distal glanular groove *(lower arrow)*. **B,** Ventral view of same patient showing paucity of ventral foreskin and proximally placed urethral meatus *(arrow)*.

ter believed the origin of the urethral plate to be an outgrowth from the walls of the cloaca and urogenital sinus. According to Glenister, development of the urethra begins at the 10-mm stage (at approximately the 4th week of development) (Stephens et al, 1996) when the urethral plate is recognizable as a thickening of the anterior wall of the endodermal cloaca. **A *urethral groove* is established by the development of the urethral folds on the ventrum of the phallic portion of the urogenital sinus on either side of the urethral plate.** These folds are covered by surface epithelium, and it is suggested that the groove between them be called the *primary* urethral groove (Glenister, 1954). A *secondary* urethral groove develops at the 35-mm stage (at approximately the 8th week) (Stephens et al, 1996) as a result of disintegration of the roof of the primary groove. Continuation of this process eventually establishes the *definitive* urethral groove.

In the male fetus, at the 50-mm stage (at approximately the 11th week of development) (Stephens et al, 1996) when the interstitial (Leydig) cells of the testis increase in number, size, and function, the urethral folds begin to fuse ventrally in the midline to form the urethra (Glenister, 1954). Via a similar process, the proximal portion of the glanular urethra forms shortly thereafter and is thus derived from the urethral plate (endodermal origin). **The distal portion of the glanular urethra is formed by lamellar ingrowth of the surface epithelium (ectodermal origin) that grows toward the distal extent of the urethral plate, becoming stratified squamous epithelium at the completion of development. This classical "ectodermal ingrowth theory" for development of the distal glanular urethra has recently been challenged by the "endodermal differentiation theory"** (Kurzrock et al, 1999).

The *endodermal differentiation theory* described by **Kurzrock and colleagues (1999) is based on the results of** immunohistochemical staining for different cytokeratins in 36 serially sectioned human fetal phallic specimens of gestational ages 5 to 22 weeks. **According to these investigators the urethral plate extends to the tip of the phallus and maintains patency and continuity throughout urethral development; therefore, the epithelium of the entire urethra originates from the urogenital sinus (endoderm).** Sections of the distal glanular urethra showed no evidence of ectodermal tissue ingrowth. **Kurzrock and colleagues (1999) provided further support for the endodermal differentiation theory using**

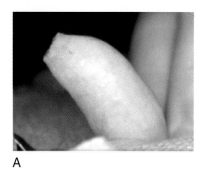 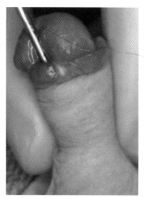 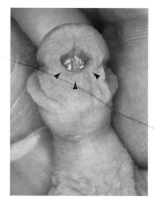

A B C

Figure 125–2. Megameatus intact prepuce (MIP) variant of hypospadias. **A,** Normal appearance of foreskin on lateral view. **B,** Sound passed within gaping hypospadiac meatus. **C.** Typical appearance of meatus *(arrowheads)* after newborn circumcision in a patient with the MIP variant.

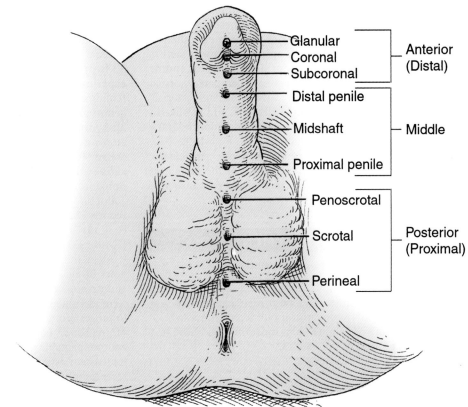

Figure 125–3. Levels of hypospadias based on the position of the meatus after orthoplasty, within three major categories.

tissue recombinant grafting techniques, which suggest that under the correct cellular signaling conditions endodermally derived epithelium (urethral plate) differentiates into the stratified squamous epithelial phenotype present in the fully developed distal glanular urethra.

Yamada and colleagues (2003) have described cellular and molecular mechanisms of external genitalia development. Petiot and coworkers (2005) have reported that mice lacking the IIIb isoform of fibroblast growth factor receptor 2 (Fgfr2) exhibit severe hypospadias. These authors also showed that blocking the androgen receptor leads to loss of *Fgfr2-IIIb* and *Fgf10* expression in the urethra and hypospadias and believe that this represents the first example of integration of input from systemically circulating androgens by a locally expressed growth factor pathway in the developing genitourinary system.

With regard to preputial development, Hunter (1935) noted that at the 40-mm stage preputial tissue did not uniformly surround the phallus in the form of a circle; rather, it was present in an oblique orientation, radiating out on either side of the phallus from the point of the urethral opening, with the urethral opening placed "well back" on the ventral surface of the phallus at this stage of development. According to Hunter, at this early stage of development the preputial tissue appears as a "hood" dorsally and gradually becomes less well marked ventrally as it approaches the urethral meatus. Complete preputial covering of the glans occurs at approximately the 130-mm stage (20th week) of development (Stephens et al, 1996).

Neurovascular Anatomy

Using immunohistochemical localization and three-dimensional computer reconstructive techniques, Baskin and colleagues (1998) studied neural and vascular anatomic features of 10 normal and one hypospadiac fetal penis. These investigators showed that **the nerves that innervate the penis originate proximally as two well-defined bundles under the pubic rami superior and slightly lateral to the urethra. This was similar for both the hypospadiac and normal fetal penises compared.** As the two crural bodies converge into the corpora cavernosa, the nerves diverge, spreading around the corpora cavernosa to the junction with the urethral spongiosum. **Nervous tissue fans out in this manner from the 11- and 1-o'clock positions all along the penis and does not remain confined to two well-defined bundles.** The absence of neuronal structures at the 12-o'clock position along the entire shaft of the penis was also noted (Baskin et al, 1998). Yucel and Baskin (2003) have expanded our understanding of proximal neuroanatomy via characterization of the path of perineal nerves from their pudendal nerve origin to their terminal distribution on the ventral aspect of the penis and corpus spongiosum.

On further comparison of normal and hypospadiac fetal penile anatomy using immunostaining techniques, Baskin and colleagues (1998) noted that the most striking difference detected was that of relative vascularity. **There was extensive vascularity of the distal urethral spongiosum and glans in the hypospadiac compared with that of the normal penises** examined. **These researchers proposed implications for hypospadias repair in that an incision of these sites (distal urethral spongiosum and glans) rich in large endothelial-lined sinuses results in release of epithelial growth factors that encourage tissue repair without significant scar and/or stricture formation.** Several authors have compared normal and hypospadiac preputial skin with vascular (arterial) systems categorized as single, double, H-type, and net-like in appearance at transillumination (Perovic and Radojicic, 2003; Yucel et al, 2004a). All contributors to the knowledge base of normal and hypospadiac penile anatomy, particularly neural and vascular, stress the importance of the awareness of such factors for safe and efficacious penile reconstructive procedures.

KEY POINTS: DEVELOPMENT

- Urethral folds fuse ventrally in the midline in the 11th week of gestation, forming the urethra.

- The endodermal differentiation theory suggests that endodermally derived epithelium differentiates into stratified squamous epithelium for formation of the glanular portion of the urethra.

- The rich vascular supply of the corpus spongiosum has implications for hypospadias repair.

ETIOLOGY
Hypospadias

A detailed report by Sorensen (1953) and more recent reviews by Sweet and colleagues (1974) and Baskin (2000) suggest a multifactorial etiology of hypospadias, fitting a polygenic model. Responsible etiologic factors may include one or more of an environmental or other endocrine disruptor; an endocrinopathy, enzymatic or local tissue abnormality; and/or a manifestation of arrested development.

The characteristic defects of hypospadias may result from one or more of the following: (1) abnormal androgen production by the fetal testis, (2) limited androgen sensitivity in the target tissues of the developing external genitalia, or (3) premature cessation of androgenic stimulation secondary to premature involution of Leydig cells of the fetal testis (Devine and Horton, 1977). **Other possible causes include insufficient testosterone and/or dihydrotestosterone synthesis (presumably defective or deficient 5α-reductase enzyme activity) and/or defective androgen receptor quality and/or quantity. Several entities in the spectrum of androgen resistance (androgen insensitivity syndromes) have been elucidated at the clinical and molecular level** (Griffin and Wilson, 1987; Griffin, 1992).

Several endocrinopathic/enzymatic factors have been identified in both humans and animal models of hypospadias. Experimentally, the importance of steroid hormone synthesis in normal development of genitalia has been reinforced. Genotypic male rats experience peak activity of 3β-hydroxysteroid dehydrogenase enzyme in the testis at the time of urethral fold fusion (Goldman and Bongiovanni, 1967). Greene

and colleagues (1938) showed that administration of estrogens antenatally reproducibly causes feminization in male rats. The same **investigators produced profound congenital adrenal hyperplasia experimentally with the use of a 3β-hydroxysteroid dehydrogenase enzyme inhibitor. The experimental gonadal males had severe hypospadias** (Goldman and Bongiovanni, 1967). **It has been observed that genotypic male infants born with a severe form of 3β-hydroxysteroid dehydrogenase enzyme (microsomal enzyme essential in biosynthesis of nearly every biologically active steroid hormone) deficiency have incomplete masculine development and hypospadias** (Goldman and Bongiovanni, 1967). Additional evidence, in humans, of an endocrinopathic etiology is provided in several detailed reports (Allen and Griffin, 1984; Aaronson et al, 1997; Albers et al, 1997) including monozygotic twin studies (Roberts and Lloyd, 1973; Fredell et al, 1998).

Allen and Griffin (1984) evaluated 15 boys younger than 4 years of age with "advanced degrees" of hypospadias for an endocrinopathy. Six different endocrine-related abnormalities were identified in 11 boys. One child each had been exposed to progesterone given to the mother during the first trimester of pregnancy, had an abnormal karyotype, and had a unilateral nonpalpable gonad. One patient with a family history of Reifenstein's syndrome (partial androgen resistance) had low receptor numbers, and 3 boys with normal receptor levels exhibited a poor genital response to exogenous testosterone (perhaps due to abnormal receptor function or dihydrotestosterone production). On the contrary, Holmes and coworkers (2004) studied 48 boys with hypospadias and 20 controls and found that defects in the enzymatic steps from cholesterol to androstenedione are unlikely in boys with any degree of hypospadias without associated genital defects.

With regard to endocrine disruptors, Aarskog (1979) retrospectively studied a personal series of 130 hypospadiac patients with special reference to pathogenetic mechanisms that might have interfered with fetal testicular differentiation and/or function. In 11 patients there was a history of maternal progestin intake early in pregnancy, either for treatment of threatened abortion or in combination with estrogen for pregnancy testing. **When the position of the urethral meatus was compared with the week of gestation at which progestin therapy was begun, a positive correlation was noted for more proximal hypospadias in mothers treated in the first month of pregnancy** (Fig. 125–4).

The implication of a role for maternal progestin exposure in development of hypospadias has been both supported (Goldman and Bongiovanni, 1967) and discounted (Mau, 1981). Alternatively, Paulozzi (2000) has suggested that the real risk factor for hypospadias in these patients is related to that responsible for threatening the loss of pregnancy rather than the progestin itself. However, this would not explain hypospadias development in offspring of those exposed to a combination of progestin and estrogen during pregnancy testing. **Further support of an endocrine disruptor etiology for hypospadias may be provided by markedly increased rates of hypospadias in male offspring conceived by in-vitro fertilization (progesterone given early for pregnancy support)** (Macnab and Zouves, 1991; Silver et al, 1999). Hussain and coworkers (2002) noted a 10-fold increase in hypospadias in their neonatal intensive care unit population

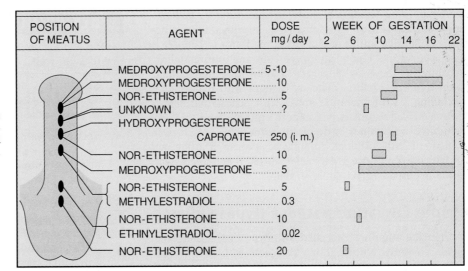

Figure 125-4. Hypospadias associated with maternal (gestational) treatment with progestins. (Reprinted from Aarskog D: Maternal progestins as a possible cause of hypospadias. N Engl J Med 1979;300:75-78.)

from 1987 to 2000. Hypospadias was significantly more common in infants who had uniformly poor intrauterine growth originating in early gestation, suggesting that common environmental factor(s) that have an impact on both conditions may be involved. Advanced maternal age (35 to 40 years) has been associated with hypospadias (odds ratio of 1.85) (Reefhuis and Honein, 2004). Although a possible causative role for environmental factors and endocrine disruptors in hypospadias is of significant concern, this is not yet clear (Paulozzi, 1999; Myers, 2000; Landrigan et al, 2003; Vrijheid et al, 2003; Silver, 2004).

The hypothesis of an "arrest of development" as noted by **Mettauer** (1842) and **Van Hook** (1896) **would seem the most plausible explanation for hypospadias. Although this theory does not identify a possible specific cause(s) of the arrested development, it would account for the concomitant occurrence of all three typical characteristics of hypospadias, including penile curvature, hypospadiac meatus, and deficient foreskin.** Complete straightening of the phallus does not occur until approximately the same time as the completion of urethral closure and just before completion of preputial formation. In addition, the dorsal "hood" appearance of the prepuce described by Hunter (1935) in the early stages of development is an exact description of the observed appearance of the preputial defect typically associated with hypospadias. This "hood" appearance is present at a time during development when the meatus is still hypospadiac in location.

Baskin (2000) has proposed that future areas of study, such as endocrine disrupters, mesenchymal-epithelial interactions, and mechanisms of penile growth, may hold the key to explaining the etiology of hypospadias (Yucel et al, 2004b). Recently, this group has shown that disruption of the fibroblast growth factor (FGF)-10 gene results in hypospadias (Baskin et al, 2000). FGF-10 is known to be important in growth, development, and wound healing. Morgan and coworkers (2003) have shown that mutations in the *Hoxa13* gene and loss of function leads to hypospadias occurring as a result of the combined loss of Fgf8 and Bmp7 expression in the urethral plate epithelium. These authors also noted that mice mutant for *Hoxa13* also exhibit changes in androgen receptor expression.

Penile Curvature (Chordee)

According to E. D. Smith (1997), Galen (130-199 AD) was the first to use the term "hypospadias" as well as to emphasize the major significance of penile curvature. Although there were references to penile curvature in the 1500s (Ambrose Paré) and 1700s (Pierre Dionis) (Smith, 1997), there was apparently no understanding of its cause(s) until an attempt at such by Mettauer in 1842. Mettauer implicated subcutaneous structures proximal to the meatus and described a "skin tethering" etiology for penile curvature (Smith, 1997). This concept was ignored for more than 100 years until championed by D. R. Smith in 1955. According to Smith, the major cause of curvature was skin and correction of curvature depended on freeing attachments of the ventral skin and corpora cavernosa distal to the urethral meatus (Smith, 1955). Creevy, in 1958, acknowledged D. R. Smith's thoughts regarding the significance of skin and proposed his own hypothesis regarding the etiology of penile curvature, implicating the tissue now commonly referred to as the urethral plate, stating that the urethral plate is shorter than the corresponding segment of penis and "so produces the characteristic ventral bowing."

In the past decade, **study of penile development via examination of fetal specimens has led to the understanding that penile curvature is a part of the early stages of normal penile development** (Glenister, 1954; Kaplan and Lamm, 1975). It follows that interruption of development (e.g., termination of pregnancy) or other detrimental effect on fetal development during this stage(s) could result in fixation of penile development at a time when curvature is present and, thus, be observed in the newborn carried to term. These observations support the "arrest of development" hypothesis for etiology of hypospadias as proposed by Mettauer (1842) and Van Hook (1896). **Currently, three major theories are proposed for the cause of penile curvature. These include (1) abnormal development of the urethral plate; (2) abnormal, fibrotic mesenchymal tissue at the urethral meatus; and (3) corporal disproportion or differential growth of normal dorsal corpora cavernosal tissue and abnormal corporal tissue ventrally** (Kaplan and Lamm, 1975; Bellinger, 1981; Duckett et al, 1996).

A report by Snodgrass and colleagues (2000) challenges most of the historical tenets that typically vilified the urethral plate as the sole source or a contributing factor in chordee or penile curvature. Using light microscopy and routine staining techniques, these investigators showed that subepithelial biopsy of the urethral plate in 17 boys with hypospadias, including 5 with curvature and 4 with penoscrotal defects, revealed well-vascularized smooth muscle and collagen without fibrous bands or dysplastic tissue. These results were consistent with histologic findings at autopsy in a boy with proximal hypospadias (Marshall et al, 1978) and a fetus with distal hypospadias (Baskin et al, 1998).

Penile Curvature without Hypospadias

Although commonly associated with hypospadias, congenital penile curvature (chordee) may also occur with an orthotopically positioned urethral meatus. Devine and Horton (1973) described three classes of chordee or penile curvature without hypospadias. In class I, the most severe defect, there is a very thin "mucous membrane" urethra and deficiency of corpus spongiosum from the site at which curvature begins and continuing to the level of the glans. According to these authors, dense fibrous tissue lying beneath the urethra is the cause of curvature in these cases. In class II, the urethra is surrounded by normal corpus spongiosum with abnormal Buck's and dartos fascia present. In class III, only the dartos fascia is abnormal.

Several authors have described this entity in similar terms of classification and treatment (Cendron and Melin, 1981; Hurwitz, 1986; Devine et al, 1991; Caldamone and Diamond, 1999). A report from **Donnahoo and colleagues (1998) evenly divided the etiology of congenital penile curvature without hypospadias in a series of 87 patients into three categories: (1) skin tethering, (2) fibrotic dartos and Buck's fasciae, or (3) corporal disproportion.** According to these authors, a congenitally short urethra was a rare cause of isolated curvature.

Dorsal or lateral curvature of the penis, both with and without hypospadias, has also been described (Udall, 1980; Redman, 1983; Spiro et al, 1992; Adams et al, 1999). Methods used for treatment of congenital penile curvature are discussed later in this chapter.

EPIDEMIOLOGY
Prevalence: General Population

In a comprehensive review, Sorensen (1953) credited Rennes in 1831 with reporting a prevalence for hypospadias of 1 in 300 "recruits" and also reported the same figure for live male births in Denmark. In 1896, Van Hook (1896) quoted Orth's figure for hypospadias prevalence of 1 in 300 live births; and in a postmortem series of 12,280 children in 1947, Campbell reported a prevalence of 1 in 1,100 boys. **In the frequently quoted Rochester, Minnesota, community-wide case-control study of hypospadias, Sweet and colleagues (1974) reported their 30-year experience and reviewed the epidemiology of hypospadias. During the inclusive period 1940 to 1970, there were 113 cases of hypospadias in 13,776 (1 in 122) live male births.** Of note, 87% of defects were coronal or

---

KEY POINTS: ETIOLOGY

- Several investigators suggest a multifactorial etiology of hypospadias fitting a polygenic model.

- Insufficient testosterone, insufficient dihydrotestosterone, or androgen receptor defect may be responsible for hypospadias in some cases.

- Ventral curvature of the penis is normal in early fetal development, and this fact supports an arrest of development etiology for penile curvature with or without hypospadias.

- The three leading theories for etiology of penile curvature are abnormal development of the urethral plate; abnormal, fibrotic mesenchymal tissue at the urethral meatus; and corporal disproportion or differential corporal growth.

---

glanular. In this review of the literature from five different countries, Sweden had the lowest reported prevalence of (1 in 1,250) live male births. **In 1997, two independent and well-established surveillance systems in the United States, the Metropolitan Atlanta Congenital Defects Program (MACDP) and the nationwide Birth Defects Monitoring Program (BDMP), reported near doubling of hypospadias rates in the most recent compared with immediately preceding decades** (Paulozzi et al, 1997). As measured by the BDMP, hypospadias rates increased from 2.02 per 1000 male births in 1970 to 3.97 per 1000 male births in 1993. In other words, approximately one boy in every 250 live male births had hypospadias. **The rate of severe hypospadias increased threefold to fivefold from 0.11 per 1000 male births in 1968 to between 0.27 and 0.55 per 1000 male births per year from 1990 to 1993 as recorded by the MACDP** (Paulozzi et al, 1997). The rising trend may simply reflect a more frequent or early diagnosis of mild forms of hypospadias over time or an increasing tendency to report the disorder to congenital anomaly registries. However, the results suggest that the ratio of minor to severe cases is decreasing, not increasing, as one would expect if the change in hypospadias rates was secondary to more frequent reporting of minor forms (Dolk, 1998). In a recent report of a cohort of 1072 Danish boys the prevalence of hypospadias in newborns was 1.03% (Boisen et al, 2005). This prevalence rose to 4.64% at 3 years of age on full reduction of the foreskin. All boys diagnosed at 3 years of age had a glanular defect.

Prevalence: Other

Pertinent familial aspects include the finding of hypospadias in 6% to 8% of fathers of affected boys and 14% of male siblings of the index patient with hypospadias (Sweet et al, 1974; Bauer et al, 1979, 1981; Sorber et al, 1997). **Roberts and Lloyd (1973) noted an 8.5-fold higher rate of hypospadias in one of monozygotic male twins compared with singleton live male births. They suggested that this strong association of monozygotic twinning and hypospadias may be due to an inability of a single placenta and reduced human chorionic gonadotropin (hCG) levels to meet the requirements of two**

developing male fetuses. In an evaluation of monozygotic male twins discordant for hypospadias, Fredell and colleagues (1998) found that 16 boys with hypospadias, from 18 such pairs, had a statistically significant lower birth weight than their unaffected twin and a more pronounced difference in birth weight than that found in unaffected monozygotic twin males. This would seem to further support an endocrinopathic etiology, namely, the mismatch in the "supply and demand" of hCG (of placenta and fetuses, respectively) hypothesis suggested by Roberts and Lloyd (1973) as an explanation.

KEY POINTS: EPIDEMIOLOGY

■ In the United States, hypospadias rates increased from 2 cases per 1000 male births in 1970 to approximately 4 cases per 1000 (1 in 250) male births in 1993.

■ The prevalence of hypospadias recorded at birth may underestimate the true prevalence because some patients are not diagnosed until later in life when the foreskin is retracted.

■ There is a 8.5-fold increase in hypospadias in one of monozygotic twin males compared with singleton gestation males.

ASSOCIATED FINDINGS
Genetic Associations

Aarskog (1970) was one of the first to perform cytogenetic analysis in patients with hypospadias. He found a normal karyotype in all cases of glanular hypospadias **and noted that an abnormal karyotype tended to occur among patients with the most severe degrees of hypospadias, especially those with associated cryptorchidism. Yamaguchi and colleagues (1991) studied 110 consecutive patients who had cryptorchidism and/or hypospadias.** Seven of the patients (6.4%) were found to have chromosomal anomalies. **The prevalence of chromosomal abnormalities in patients with cryptorchidism only was 4/83 (4.8%), in patients with hypospadias only the prevalence was 1/18 (5.6%), and in concomitant cases the incidence was 2/9 (22.2%).**

Cryptorchidism/Inguinal Hernia

Associated abnormalities include cryptorchidism (7% to 9%) and inguinal hernia and/or hydrocele (9% to 16%) (Sweet et al, 1974; Khuri et al, 1981; Sorber et al, 1997; Wu et al, 2002). **Wu and coworkers (2002) found that the prevalence of inguinal hernia was similar in anterior, mid, and posterior hypospadias at approximately 12% but cryptorchidism was predominant in boys with posterior defects.** Boys with concomitant occurrence of hypospadias and cryptorchidism even in the setting of unambiguous genitalia should alert the urologist to evaluate for the possible presence of an intersex state.

Syndromes

According to the authoritative, encyclopedic reference *Smith's Recognizable Patterns of Human Malformation,* there are approximately 49 recognized syndromes in which hypospadias is either a "frequent" (15) or an "occasional" (34) associated finding (Table 125–1) (Jones, 1997). **Interestingly, of the 49 syndromes in which hypospadias is an associated finding, 38 (78%) also have associated micropenis, cryptorchidism, and/or a scrotal abnormality. This would seem to further support an endocrinopathic cause of hypospadias.** The issue of intersexuality is not specifically discussed in this reference (Jones, 1997).

Intersex States

In general terms, any divergence from the orderly sequence of events involved in normal sexual differentiation culminating in anything less than completely normal phenotype and/or function per respective gender may be considered a disorder of sexual differentiation or an intersex state. Perhaps taken to the extreme, Jost regarded all hypospadias as a form of male pseudohermaphroditism (Aarskog, 1971). **A high index of suspicion for an intersex state should accompany presumed males with any degree of hypospadias and cryptorchidism** (Rajfer and Walsh, 1976; Borer et al, 1995; Albers et al, 1997; Smith and Wacksman, 1997; Kaefer et al, 1999). In 1976, Rajfer and Walsh reported the incidence of intersexuality in children with cryptorchidism, hypospadias, and otherwise nonambiguous genitalia to be 27%.

In a detailed evaluation of hypospadias level and exact status of concomitant cryptorchidism, Kaefer and colleagues (1999) evaluated 79 presumed males presenting with an undescended testis(es) and hypospadias. Intersex conditions were identified with nearly equal frequency in the 44 cases (30%) of unilateral and 35 cases (32%) of bilateral cryptorchidism. **In the unilateral cryptorchid testis group, patients with a nonpalpable testis were at least threefold more likely to have an intersex condition than those with a palpable undescended testis (50% vs. 15%). In the bilateral cryptorchid group, patients with one or more nonpalpable testes were also nearly threefold as likely to have an intersex condition compared with those with bilateral palpable undescended gonads (47% vs. 16%).** Meatal position was graded as anterior in 33% of cases, mid in 25%, and posterior in 41%, with the more posterior location conferring a significantly greater likelihood of intersexuality (anterior 2 of 26, mid 1 of 20, and posterior 21 of 33) (Kaefer et al, 1999).

KEY POINTS: ASSOCIATED FINDINGS

■ Approximately 15% of individuals with hypospadias and a palpable undescended gonad will have an intersex condition.

■ Approximately 50% of individuals with hypospadias and a unilateral nonpalpable gonad will have an intersex condition.

■ A chromosomal abnormality will be present in approximately 22% of individuals with hypospadias and cryptorchidism.

Table 125-1. Syndromes with Hypospadias as a Feature

Syndrome (S.)	Relative or Approximate % of Cases with Hypospadias	Other Notable Findings of the Genitalia
Aniridia-Wilms' tumor association	Frequent	Cryptorchidism
Deletion 4p S.	Frequent	Cryptorchidism
Deletion 11q S.	50%	Cryptorchidism
Deletion 13q S.	Frequent	Cryptorchidism
Fetal trimethadione S. (tridione S.)	Frequent	Ambiguous genitalia
Fraser S. (cryptophthalmos S.)	Frequent	Cryptorchidism
Fryns S.	86%	Cryptorchidism, bifid scrotum
Opitz S. (hypertelorism-hypospadias S., Opitz-Frias S., Opitz oculo-genito-laryngeal S.)	Frequent	Cryptorchidism, bifid scrotum
Rapp-Hodgkin ectodermal dysplasia S. (hypohidrotic ectodermal dysplasia, autosomal dominant type)	Frequent	
Rieger S.	Frequent	
Schinzel-Giedion S.	100%	Micropenis, hypoplastic scrotum
Smith-Lemli-Opitz S.	70%	Micropenis, hypoplastic/bifid scrotum
Triploidy S. and diploid/triploid mixoploidy S.	Frequent	Micropenis, cryptorchidism
X-linked α-thalassemia/mental retardation (ATR-X) S.	Frequent	Micropenis, hypoplastic scrotum
Brachmann-de Lange S. (Cornelia de Lange S., de Lange S.)	33%	Cryptorchidism (73%)
Beckwith-Wiedemann S. (exomphalos-macroglossia-gigantism S.)	Occasional	Cryptorchidism
Craniofrontonasal dysplasia	Occasional	
Dubowitz S.	Occasional	
Duplication 4p S. (trisomy for the short arm of chromosome 4, trisomy 4p S.)	Occasional	Micropenis, cryptorchidism
Duplication 9p S. (trisomy 9p S.)	Occasional	Micropenis, cryptorchidism
Escobar S.	Occasional	Cryptorchidism
Duplication 10q S.	Occasional	Cryptorchidism, streak gonads
Fanconi pancytopenia S.	20%	Micropenis, cryptorchidism
Fetal hydantoin S. (fetal Dilantin S.)	Occasional	Cryptorchidism, micropenis, ambiguous genitalia
Fetal rubella effects (fetal rubella S.)	Occasional	Cryptorchidism
Fetal valproate S.	Occasional	
FG S.	Occasional	Cryptorchidism (36%)
Hay-Wells S. of ectodermal dysplasia (ankyloblepharon-ectodermal dysplasia-clefting S., AEC S.)	Occasional	Micropenis
Hydrolethalus S.	Occasional	
Johanson-Blizzard S.	Occasional	Micropenis, cryptorchidism
Killian/Teschler-Nicola S. (Pallister mosaic S., tetrasomy 12p)	Occasional	
Lenz-Majewski hyperostosis S.	Occasional	Cryptorchidism
Peters'-plus S.	Occasional	Cryptorchidism
Levy-Hollister S. (lacrimo-auriculo-dento-digital S., LADD S.)	Occasional (coronal)	
Marden-Walker S.	Occasional	Micropenis, cryptorchidism
Multiple lentigines S. (LEOPARD S.)	Occasional	Cryptorchidism, hypogonadism
Oto-palato-digital S., type II	Occasional	Cryptorchidism
Restrictive dermopathy	Occasional	
Roberts-SC phocomelia (pseudothalidomide S., hypomelia-hypotrichosis-facial hemangioma S.)	Occasional	Cryptorchidism
Russell-Silver S. (Silver S.)	Occasional	Seminoma
Shprintzen S. (velo-cardio-facial S.)	Occasional	Cryptorchidism
Simpson-Golabi-Behmel S.	Occasional	Cryptorchidism
Townes-Brocks S.	Occasional	
Trisomy 13 S. (D1 trisomy S.)	<50%	Cryptorchidism (>50%)
Trisomy 18 S.	<10%	Cryptorchidism (≥50%), bifid scrotum (<10%)
XXY S., Klinefelter S.	Occasional	Micropenis, cryptorchidism
XXXY S. and XXXXY S.	Occasional	Micropenis (80%), cryptorchidism (28%)
XYY S.	Occasional	Micropenis, cryptorchidism
Zellweger S. (cerebro-hepato-renal S.)	Occasional	Cryptorchidism

Adapted with permission from Jones KL: Smith's Recognizable Patterns of Human Malformation, 5th ed. Philadelphia, WB Saunders, 1997, p 835.

SPECIAL CONSIDERATIONS: PREOPERATIVE
Indications

According to Cecil (1932), the only reason for operating on any hypospadiac patient was to correct deformities that interfered with the function of urination and procreation. There is no question that **more severe degrees of hypospadias require** **repair to provide the ability to micturate in a standing position, achieve sexual intercourse, and effectively inseminate.** However, questions regarding the need for repair of anterior hypospadias are noted throughout history. Early on, unsatisfactory results of anterior hypospadias repair were responsible for the sentiment that the balanitic type of hypospadias was best treated by "masterly neglect" (Cabot, 1936). This sentiment has changed, in part, because of both superior results of current techniques and caregiver concern regarding cosmesis. As Backus and De Felice (1960) stated, "The cosmetic considerations are definitely secondary and usually of more concern to the parents than the patient. However, this does not constitute a valid excuse to dismiss them entirely."

Few have studied the natural history of untreated distal hypospadias. One such report by Fichtner and colleagues (1995) examined the meatal location of 500 adult men admitted for transurethral treatment of either prostatic or bladder disease. A meatus located in the distal third of the glans was considered to be in "normal" position and was noted in only 55% of the 500 men examined. Sixty-five (13%) of the men had either glanular (49), coronal (15), or subcoronal (1) hypospadias. Of the 16 men with a coronal or subcoronal defect, only 6 were aware of the abnormality, all reported no difficulties with sexual intercourse or voiding in a standing position without downward deflection of the stream, and all 15 heterosexuals had fathered children. These data led Fichtner and colleagues to narrow their indications for repair of anterior hypospadias. There are no long-term patient satisfaction data in men with hypospadias comparing those who have undergone repair with those who have not.

Intersex Evaluation

Although not indicated for isolated anterior and middle hypospadias, the necessity for an intersex evaluation in the setting of concomitant hypospadias and cryptorchidism has been discussed. The idea that evaluation for an endocrine abnormality and/or intersex state should be undertaken in those with posterior hypospadias, regardless of gonadal position or palpability, is controversial but supported in the literature, because significant, identifiable, and treatable abnormalities are common (Allen and Griffin, 1984; Aaronson et al, 1997; Albers et al, 1997). It has been suggested that for patients with severe, apparently isolated hypospadias, a standardized set of diagnostic evaluations including ultrasonography, genitography, and chromosomal, gonadal (histology), biochemical, and molecular testing should be performed as a minimum (Rajfer and Walsh, 1976; Albers et al, 1997). Not all authors support routine karyotyping in patients with hypospadias and cryptorchidism even with the finding of abnormality in 8 of 48 (17%) patients (McAleer and Kaplan, 2001). We would argue in support of karyotyping in patients with severe hypospadias, particularly in those with associated cryptorchidism, because of the potential significant impact on the child and family, for fertility, genetic counseling, and therapeutic implications.

Radiologic Evaluation

In general, the literature does not support routine imaging of the urinary tract with either ultrasonography (Cerasaro et al, 1986; Davenport and MacKinnon, 1988) or intravenous urography (McArdle and Lebowitz, 1975; Cerasaro et al, 1986) for evaluation of children with isolated hypospadias, particularly when the hypospadiac meatus is middle or anterior in location. Retrograde injection of radiographic contrast material into the presumed urethral meatus (genitogram) is an essential component of the intersex evaluation when such an evaluation is deemed appropriate. Preoperative evaluation may include voiding cystourethrography (VCUG) or cystourethroscopy in patients with a scrotal or perineal defect to evaluate the frequent presence and extent of a prostatic utricle (Retik, 1996).

Hormonal Manipulation

There is considerable controversy surrounding the use of hormonal stimulation or supplementation for the purpose of penile enlargement before hypospadias repair. Topics of debate include agent, route, dose, dosing schedule, and timing of treatment to be employed.

Androgen Stimulation

Koff and Jayanthi (1999) presented evidence that supports the use of hCG before repair of proximal hypospadias. hCG was started 6 to 8 weeks preoperatively with 250 and 500 IU hCG injected twice weekly in boys younger than 1 year and 1 to 5 years old, respectively. An increase in penile size and length was noted in 12 boys aged 8 to 14 months. Observations included a decrease in hypospadias and chordee severity in all patients, increased vascularity and thickness of proximal corpus spongiosum, and allowance for more simple repairs in 3 of the 12 boys receiving hCG preoperatively. Shima and colleagues (1986) noted impaired gonadotropin and testosterone response to luteinizing hormone-releasing hormone (LHRH) and hCG stimulation (100 µg of LHRH and 4000 units of hCG for a 1.6 m^2 average *adult* body surface area) in prepubertal boys 2 to 8 years old with hypospadias, but neither penile nor meatal response to stimulation was discussed.

Androgen Supplementation/Replacement

Various preparations including testosterone ointment, applied to the glans penis for 2 weeks before surgery, have been used to stimulate penile growth (Perovic and Vukadinovic, 1994). Citing variable absorption and inconsistent results with the use of topical testosterone, Gearhart and Jeffs (1987) administered testosterone enanthate intramuscularly (2 mg/kg), 5 and 2 weeks before reconstructive penile surgery. The authors noted a 50% increase in penile size and an increase in available skin and local vascularity in all patients. A near doubling (from 3 to 5 cm) of the mean transverse length of the inner prepuce was also noted in some. In addition, Gearhart and Jeffs reported minimal side effects and return of plasma testosterone levels to within the normal range for age within 6 months after therapy. Others have employed variations in the total dose and schedule of testosterone enanthate administration, using 25 mg intramuscularly once weekly for a total of either two (Belman, 1997) or three injections (Stock et al, 1995). Chalapathi and coworkers (2003) administered testosterone either topically or intramuscularly to patients with hypospadias. They concluded that intramuscular testosterone enanthate (2 mg/kg weekly for 3 consecutive weeks) was superior because absorption via the topical route may be unpredictable.

Monfort and Lucas (1982) have employed a 4-week period of local penile stimulation with daily application of dihydrotestosterone (DHT) cream before hypospadias or epispadias repair. The authors reported a mean increase in penile circumference and length by 50% of pretreatment measurements, without any lasting side effects or gonadotropin level perturbation or effects in the pubertal or postpubertal period.

Timing of Hormonal Manipulation

Hormonal manipulation, at any age, is not without risk. Caution must be exercised with regard to neonatal administration of hCG, in that evidence obtained from an experimental rat micropenis model supports delaying hormonal therapy until the pubertal period (McMahon et al, 1995). However, in their study of boys with congenital hypogonadotropic hypogonadism and micropenis, **Bin-Abbas and colleagues (1999) concluded that one or two short courses of testosterone therapy in infancy and childhood (puberty) augmented adult penile size into the normal range.** These results refute the theoretical concern, and experimental evidence, that testosterone treatment in infancy or childhood impairs penile growth in adolescence and compromises adult penile length. **The conclusion that prepubertal exogenous testosterone administration does *not* adversely affect ultimate penile growth has been supported by the study of men with true precocious puberty or congenital adrenal hyperplasia** (Sutherland et al, 1996) **and by the study of growth and androgen receptor status of testosterone-stimulated human fetal penile tissue in vitro** (Baskin et al, 1997).

KEY POINTS: SPECIAL CONSIDERATIONS: PREOPERATIVE

■ Intramuscular injection of testosterone enanthate, either 25 mg/dose or 2 mg/kg/dose, given for a total of two or three doses before hypospadias repair is a reliable means of obtaining penile growth in the appropriate patient.

■ Prepubertal exogenous testosterone administration does not appear to impair ultimate penile growth.

HISTORICAL ASPECTS OF HYPOSPADIAS REPAIR

Hauben (1984) credits Heliodor and Antyl (1st, 2nd, and 3rd centuries AD) as the first to describe hypospadias and its surgical correction. Perhaps no surgical concern in history has inspired such widespread and varied opinion with regard to management as has hypospadias. From the earliest recorded description of hypospadias to the present, several hundred surgical approaches and/or variations on a theme have been described. Early contributors to the field of hypospadiology and a brief description of their contribution are listed in the chapter on this subject in the 8th edition of this textbook (Retik and Borer, 2002). Several comprehensive accounts of historical aspects (Murphy, 1972; Hauben, 1984; Smith, 1997; Hodgson, 1999) and early technical reviews (Cecil, 1932; Young and Benjamin, 1948; Creevy, 1958; Backus and De Felice, 1960) regarding hypospadias are available.

KEY POINT: HISTORICAL ASPECTS OF HYPOSPADIAS REPAIR

■ Several hundred surgical approaches or modifications of existing techniques have been described for the repair of hypospadias.

GENERAL PRINCIPLES OF HYPOSPADIAS REPAIR

Regardless of the technique employed for repair of hypospadias and its associated defects, attention to penile curvature and its correction (orthoplasty), urethroplasty, meatoplasty and glanuloplasty, and, finally, skin coverage are universal concerns.

Orthoplasty

Assessment of Penile Curvature

Preoperatively, the degree of penile curvature may be assessed in the infant or young boy who has an erection at the time of examination. A photograph taken at home during an erection in the adolescent/adult may also be very helpful in assessing penile curvature with or without hypospadias. **Intraoperative assessment of penile curvature by either artificial or pharmacologic methods is a critical step in hypospadias repair and is typically performed after degloving of the penile shaft skin. A subjective impression or an objective (protractor) measurement** (Bologna et al, 1999) **of the observed curvature helps guide management.**

Artificial Erection. Gittes and McLaughlin (1974) were the first to describe artificial erection as an aid to the evaluation of penile curvature. This technique has gained wide acceptance (Horton and Devine, 1977) and is depicted in Figure 125–5A. Injection of normal saline with a "butterfly" needle into the corpora directly is performed by insertion of the needle through the lateral aspect of one or the other corpora cavernosa. Alternatively, the needle may be passed through the glans to eliminate the possibility of hematoma formation beneath Buck's fascia. The degree of curvature may vary with force of injection and/or the method used to impede saline outflow.

Pharmacologic Erection. Intracorporal injection of the arterial vasodilator prostaglandin E_1 has been used for pharmacologic induction of erection during hypospadias repair (Perovic et al, 1997; Kogan, 2000). **Proponents of a pharmacologically induced erection argue that the physiologic erection allows for a more accurate and continued assessment of penile curvature before, during, and after its correction.** It would seem wise to defer use of the pharmacologic method if underlying neurologic pathology and/or injury is either known or suspected.

Management of Penile Curvature with or without Hypospadias

Aside from simple release of skin tethering for correction of mild curvature, **penile curvature may be addressed with procedures that are carried out on either the dorsal, ventral, or lateral aspects of the penis. The site for orthoplasty and the specific technique employed are dictated by the direction and severity of curvature and/or penile size.** Except where indicated per technique description, orthoplasty techniques may be performed on any surface of the penis. **Occasionally, repair of severe ventral curvature without hypospadias may require concomitant (interposition) urethroplasty.**

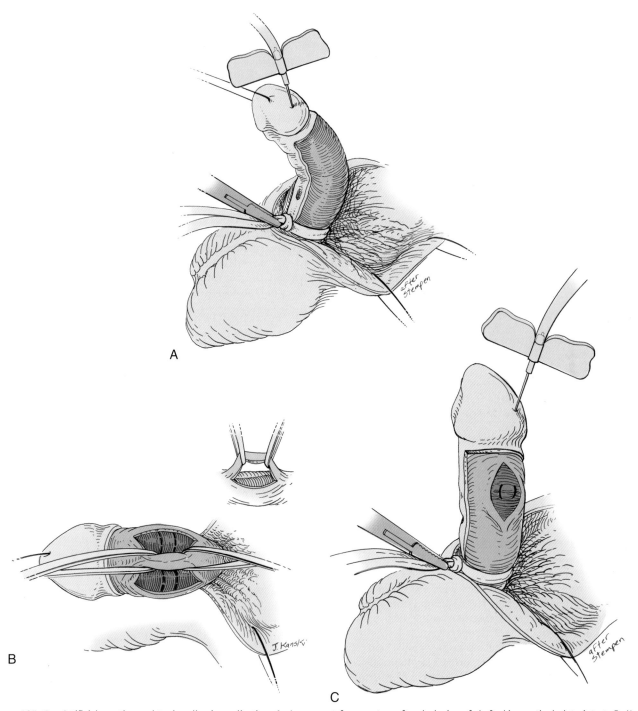

Figure 125–5. Artificial erection and tunica albuginea plication. **A,** Assessment for curvature after degloving of shaft skin, urethral plate intact. **B,** Neurovascular bundles isolated and elevated. Proposed parallel lines of incision bilaterally are opposite point of maximal curvature. **C,** Outer edges of incisions have been approximated, and both the intervening strip of tunica albuginea and the knots are buried. (Modified from Baskin LS, Duckett JW: Dorsal tunica albuginea plication [TAP] for hypospadias curvature. J Urol 1994;151:1668.)

Skin Release/Transfer. Penile skin may be the sole source or a contributor to penile curvature (Smith, 1955) or torsion (Culp, 1966). In 1968, Allen and Spence observed this association with distal hypospadias, when on making a circumcising incision proximal to a coronal hypospadiac meatus they noted that freeing of penile shaft skin from the underlying urethra permitted penile straightening. As part of the repair, preputial skin was transposed ventrally. King (1970) recog-

nized the utility of this concept and incorporated it into tubularized urethroplasty and later summarized the concept of "cutaneous chordee" (King, 1981). As summarized by Smith (1955), others have employed ventrally transposed, pedicled preputial skin as an aid to correction of penile curvature in two-stage correction of severe hypospadias. A similar technique has been described for correction of minor penile curvature without hypospadias (Allen and Roehrborn, 1993).

Plicating/Heineke-Mikulicz Techniques. Nesbit (1965) described removing "vertical elliptical segments" of tunica albuginea (transversely oriented) from the disproportionately longer, convex aspect of the penis to correct curvature. Another method for correcting the disparity in tunica albuginea length consists of lengthening the shorter concave surface by using the Heineke-Mikulicz principle (Udall, 1980). Several transverse incisions in the tunica are closed longitudinally to achieve lengthening of the concave aspect of the penis (Saalfeld et al, 1973). The Nesbit and Heineke-Mikulicz principle can be used simultaneously on opposing aspects of the curvature (Udall, 1980). Either the Nesbit technique or simple dorsal plicating sutures may be used to repair the "glans tilt" deformity. Cross-hatched incisions of the corpora cavernosa followed by simple plicating sutures has been described as a successful orthoplasty technique (Perovic et al, 1998). Placing multiple parallel plicating sutures in the midline opposite the site of maximal curvature is a recently reported technique that has become the preferred technique for the treatment of penile curvature by the reporting authors (Baskin and Lue, 1998). This technique does not require mobilization of the neurovascular bundle. Longitudinal incision of the tunica albuginea in the dorsal midline appears to be an advantageous adjunct to suture placement alone (Soygur et al, 2004).

Tunica Albuginea Plication. Initially described by Baskin and Duckett (1994a), the tunica albuginea plication has become a popular technique for correction of penile curvature (Klevmark et al, 1994). After degloving the penile shaft of its skin, the neurovascular bundles are dissected free from the surface of the corpora cavernosa bilaterally (see Fig. 125–5). Parallel lines of incision approximately 1.0 cm in length and 0.5 to 1.0 cm apart are marked bilaterally on the anterolateral surface of the tunica albuginea, directly opposite the point of maximal penile curvature. The tunica albuginea is incised at these sites with a fine knife. A tourniquet placed at the base of the penis decreases blood loss and optimizes visualization during this procedure. After incision, the outer edges of the parallel incisions are approximated with 4-0 polydioxanone suture with simple interrupted technique and inversion of the knot. This technique buries the intervening strip of tunica albuginea and shortens the disproportionately long corporal surface, thus correcting the opposing penile curvature. Chertin and coworkers (2004) reported acceptable efficacy at a median follow-up of 6 years. Twenty-eight of 83 patients had an erection test during repeat hypospadias repair or fistula repair: 22 had a straight penis, and 6 required repeat plication for a satisfactory cosmetic outcome.

Corporal Rotation. Corporal rotation, achieved via a ventral, midline longitudinal incision alone, was described by Koff and Eakins in 1984 for correction of ventral penile curvature in a hypospadiac patient. Medial rotation and suture fixation of the dorsal aspect of the corpora cavernosa has been described for management of severe curvature. This may be performed with (Snow, 1989) or without (Kass, 1993) simultaneous longitudinal incision of the corporal septum in the ventral midline. Decter (1999) has described a similar technique for correction of ventral curvature in severe hypospadias in which, after urethral plate division, the septum between the corpora cavernosa is partially split with a ventral midline incision. This incision and freeing of the neurovascular bundles on the dorsal aspect of the corpora cavernosa facilitate medial rotation of the dorsal aspect of the corpora. Nonabsorbable sutures are placed in the area of maximal convex curvature from the dorsolateral aspect of one corpus cavernosum across the midline to the other side such that the corpora are rotated toward the dorsal midline. **The corporal rotation technique allows one-stage reconstruction while achieving and/or maintaining maximal penile length.**

Dermal Graft. The dermal graft has been used extensively for repair of significant penile curvature (Devine and Horton, 1975; Hendren and Keating, 1988; Hendren and Caesar, 1992; Horton et al, 1993; Pope et al, 1996; Lindgren et al, 1998). **This orthoplasty technique is ideal for the short phallus with severe ventral penile curvature in which techniques applied to the dorsal aspect of the penis may be inadequate to correct the curvature or further shorten the penis.** After assessing the degree of curvature, the dermal graft is harvested from a non–hair-bearing donor site typically in the groin (Fig. 125–6). The donor site is marked in an elliptical shape at a length slightly longer than the ventral defect to be created by transverse linear corporotomy. The graft is sharply dissected, defatted, and placed in saline. **A transverse incision is made at the site of maximal curvature (concavity), and the dermal graft is anastomosed to the edges of the corporal defect** with a running simple suture of 6-0 polyglactin.

Small Intestinal Submucosa. Small intestinal submucosa (SIS) is an acellular collagen-based material derived from porcine small intestine used as an interposition graft for severe penile curvature. Single-layer SIS appears to have advantage over multilayer SIS most likely secondary to the ability of one-layer SIS to regenerate and/or revascularize (Kropp et al, 2002; Soergel et al, 2003; Weiser et al, 2003). **The best results appear to be obtained when one-layer SIS is used for management of severe ventral penile curvature at the first stage of a two-stage repair for severe hypospadias.**

Tunica Vaginalis Graft. Perlmutter and colleagues (1985) described use of a tunica vaginalis free graft as a ventral corporal patch orthoplasty technique for repair of severe curvature in 11 boys with chordee and hypospadias. Only one patient had "some degree" of ventral angulation on follow-up ranging from 2 to 37 months. Others have reported a 91% success rate at 33 months mean follow-up for correction of curvature with a tunica vaginalis patch graft as the first stage (orthoplasty) of a two-stage repair of severe hypospadias (Stewart et al, 1995). Ritchey and Ribbeck (2003) stressed the need for long-term follow up after initial success.

Total Penile Disassembly. A radical approach, penile disassembly and corporoplasty, has been described by Perovic and colleagues (1998). According to the authors, the total penile disassembly technique is ideal for correction of (1) glans tilt, (2) ventral curvature without hypospadias, and (3) curvature with hypospadias. They also report that the total penile disassembly technique corrects curvature without the need for placement of an interposition corporal graft, thus minimizing the work of straightening the penis and lengthening the urethra in those with associated hypospadias.

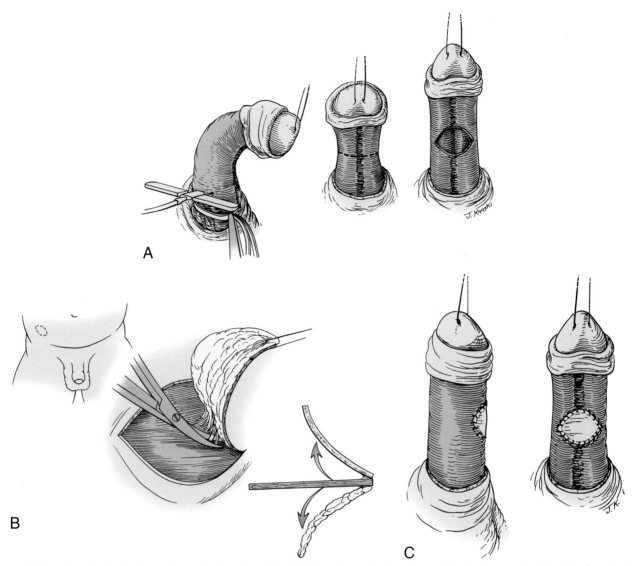

Figure 125–6. Dermal graft. **A,** Degree of curvature is noted with artificial erection and a transverse incision has been made at the site of maximal curvature. **B,** Isolation of elliptical dermal graft from non–hair-bearing donor site. Graft is then defatted. **C,** Dermal graft sutured to the edges of the defect. (Reprinted from Retik AB: Proximal hypospadias. In Marshall FF [ed]: Textbook of Operative Urology. Philadelphia, WB Saunders, 1996.)

Urethroplasty

Neourethral Formation

Several basic principles and techniques govern successful urethroplasty during hypospadias repair. Among these is the term *tissue transfer,* which implies the movement of tissue(s) for the purpose of reconstruction. Techniques for urethroplasty typically employ use of either immediately adjacent tissue, local tissue flaps, and/or free grafts of genital or extragenital tissue.

Immediately Adjacent Tissue. The neourethra may be formed via reconfiguration of tissue immediately juxtaposed to the hypospadiac meatus and/or along the path of proposed urethroplasty. This, in fact, may be the least risky and least technically challenging of all forms of urethroplasty. An example would be simple tubularization of the urethral plate.

Local Tissue Flaps. Although immediately adjacent tissue is moved to some degree when incorporated into urethroplasty, in other techniques, specific local penile or other genital tissue may be transferred to the penile ventrum to be employed in the urethroplasty or another component of hypospadias repair. **The term *flap* implies that the tissue used is excised and transferred with the vasculature preserved or surgically reestablished at the recipient site** (Jordan, 1999a, 1999b). Tissue flaps may be classified by their vascularity such that a *random* flap does not have a defined cutaneous vascular territory, and **the term *axial* flap implies the presence of specific, defined vasculature in the base of the flap.** With regard to elevation technique, another means of flap classification, the vascular and cutaneous continuity of the flap remains intact in a *peninsula* flap, whereas **the term *island* flap implies maintenance of vascular and division of cutaneous continuity** (Jordan, 1999a).

Local tissue flaps used for urethral reconstruction must be thin, nonhirsute, and reliably tailored. These flaps are properly termed *fasciocutaneous* flaps, and the extended fascial system is called the dartos fascia (Jordan, 1999a). **The vessels of the fasciocutaneous flap are preserved within the fascia, which provides a conduit for smaller arteries and veins. Axial blood supply and drainage is typically provided by branches of the deep and superficial external pudendal vessels, which are medial branches of the femoral vessels** (Hinman, 1991; Standoli, 1988; Jordan, 1999a).

Local or Extragenital Free Grafts. The term *graft* implies that tissue has been excised from one location and transferred to a graft host bed, where a new blood supply develops by a process called "take" (Jordan, 1999a). As with all free grafts, a well-vascularized recipient site is crucial for optimal graft survival. **The initial phase of take, called *imbibition,* relies on diffusion of nutrient material from the adjacent graft host bed into the graft and requires approximately 48 hours. This is followed by the second phase of take, *inosculation,* which is the formation of new and permanent vascularization of the graft, also requiring approximately 48 hours** (Jordan, 1999a).

Neourethral Coverage (Second Layer)

Subcutaneous (Dartos) Flap. Second layer coverage of the neourethra with the use of various vascularized flaps has significantly decreased urethrocutaneous fistula as a complication of hypospadias repair (Smith, 1973; Belman, 1988; Retik et al, 1988; Churchill et al, 1996). As previously described by Retik and colleagues (1988, 1994b), the dorsal prepuce is unfolded and the underlying dartos layer is sharply dissected to the base of the penis and then incised longitudinally in the midline (Fig. 125–7). One side of the flap or, alternatively, a dartos flap raised from the lateral penile shaft skin is then brought around to the ventral aspect of the penis and secured over the neourethra with simple, interrupted, fine absorbable suture. Glans wings must be incised deeply to accommodate this additional tissue cover of the neourethra.

Tunica Vaginalis. Tunica vaginalis tissue may be used as an alternative for second layer coverage of the neourethra (Fig. 125–8) (Snow, 1986; Kirkali, 1990; Snow et al, 1995). Before tunica vaginalis coverage the inferolateral border of the neourethral mesentery may be advanced over the edges of the neourethra as a buttress. The testis to be used as the donor of tunica vaginalis is delivered into the operative field and isolated from its scrotal attachments. The tunica vaginalis is incised, and an appropriate width of flap is isolated from the testis and widely mobilized on its own vascular pedicle. The tunica vaginalis flap is then secured over the neourethra by placement of simple interrupted sutures, and the testis is replaced in the scrotum.

Corpus Spongiosum. Paraurethral (spongiosal) tissue approximation in the midline as a second cover of the initial suture line was initially described by van Horn and Kass (1995) as an adjunct to distal hypospadias repair. In a recent cohort repaired with this technique, the complication rate was 1.7% for distal and 7.7% for midshaft hypospadias repair (Kass and Chung, 2000). Similarly, Yerkes and colleagues (2000a) described mobilization of distal spongiosum lateral to the open urethra along with the urethral plate away from the corpora cavernosa, subsequently wrapping it around various types of urethroplasty for distal hypospadias to prevent fistula formation. In 25 patients with more than 1-year follow-up, there were no urethrocutaneous fistulas. The distal wrap of

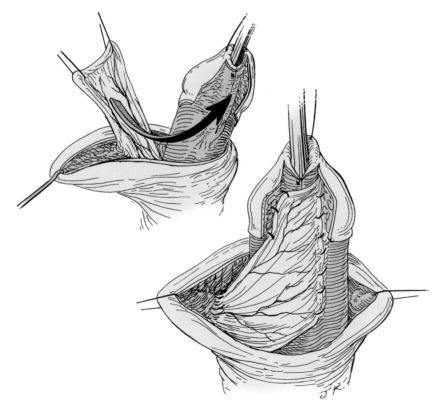

Figure 125–7. Second-layer coverage of neourethra with subcutaneous (dartos) tissue flap harvested from lateral or dorsal penile shaft and repositioned ventrally over the neourethra.

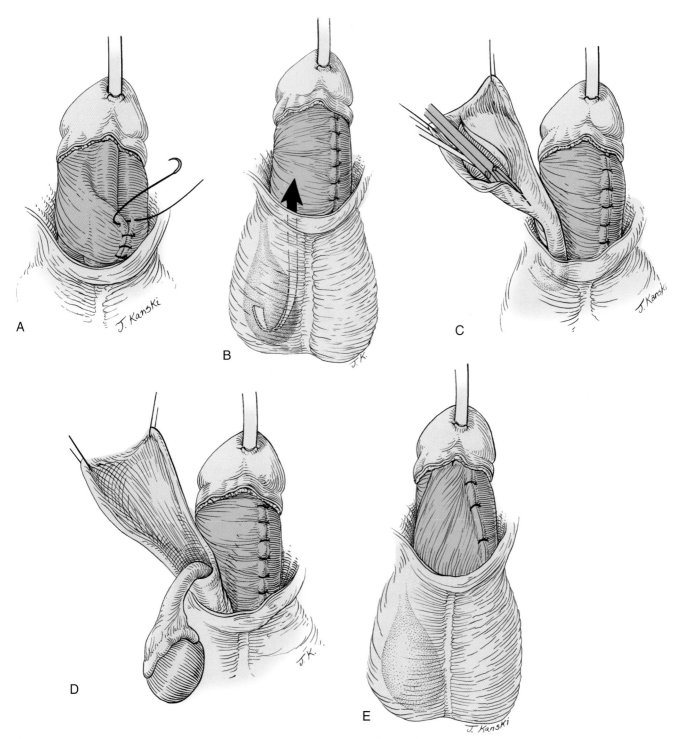

Figure 125–8. Tunica vaginalis neourethral coverage (performed over mesentery of onlay island flap repair in this case). **A,** Lateral border of onlay or tube pedicle may be advanced as a second layer of neourethral coverage. **B,** Testis to be delivered for harvest of tunica vaginalis as supplemental or sole source for second layer coverage. **C,** Harvest of tunica vaginalis. **D,** Isolation of flap graft from testis and distal spermatic cord. **E,** Tunica vaginalis graft has been secured over the neourethra. (Reprinted from Retik AB: Proximal hypospadias. In Marshall FF [ed]: Textbook of Operative Urology. Philadelphia, WB Saunders, 1996.)

corpus spongiosum appears to avoid fistula formation without causing residual or recurrent curvature.

Meatoplasty and Glanuloplasty

These two components of hypospadias repair are discussed together because successful completion of one is dependent on that of the other. Although nuances of glanuloplasty and meatoplasty are typically discussed per specific hypospadias repair, some principles may have more broad application. In 1977, Devine and Horton (1977) described the V-flap glanuloplasty as an adjunct to tubularized skin graft urethroplasty. This technique involves extensive dissection of the glans penis with development of a midline anteriorly based flap of glans epithelium. Underlying subepithelial tissue is removed from the glans flap, and the flap is fixed to the tunica of the corpora cavernosa, consistently fashioning a widely patent, complication-free meatus. A double-faced preputial flap transposed ventrally has been described for enhancement of the glans and meatus for the small and deformed glans (Perovic et al, 2003). Others have incorporated a glanular W-shaped flap meatoplasty with urethroplasty (Sensöz et al, 1997).

Penile Shaft Skin Coverage

Various techniques have been employed for the purpose of completing hypospadias with adequate skin coverage of the penis. These techniques have included those describing **ventral transfer of preputial skin either with a buttonhole through the skin for through-passage of the glans penis** (Ombredanne, 1932; Nesbit, 1941), **or midline longitudinal split of the prepuce or dorsal penile skin followed by lateral transfer of the skin on either side of the penis for ventral coverage** (Thiersch, 1869; Byars, 1951; Mustarde, 1965). The transverse outer preputial island flap has also been described (Galifer and Kalfa, 2003).

KEY POINTS: GENERAL PRINCIPLES OF HYPOSPADIAS REPAIR

- Assessment for presence and severity of penile curvature is an important component of successful hypospadias repair.

- Placement of plicating sutures in the dorsal midline of the penis will reliably correct mild to moderate ventral penile curvature.

- A dermal graft of elliptical shape harvested from non–hair-bearing skin is perhaps the most reliable means of correcting severe ventral penile curvature.

SPECIAL CONSIDERATIONS: PERIOPERATIVE
Timing (Age at Repair)

In 1975, an ad hoc committee of the American Academy of Pediatrics, composed of urologists and pediatricians, concluded that the optimal time for surgery, from a psychologi-

cal perspective, was during the fourth or fifth year of life (Kelalis et al, 1975). Then, in 1979, Lepore and Kesler reported a prospective study of boys undergoing hypospadias repair between 2 and 6 years of age. They noted a distinctive pattern of postoperative behavior characterized by anger, aggression, and negative interactions as compared with children undergoing other types of surgery. This and other studies that followed (Manley and Epstein, 1981; Schultz et al, 1983) prompted a more recent review of the subject by the American Academy of Pediatrics (Kass et al, 1996). In this report, **as a result of a combination of factors including an improved understanding of the psychological implications of genital surgery in children, improvement in the technical aspects of surgery for hypospadias, and advances in pediatric anesthesia, it was suggested that "the best time for surgery for hypospadias is between 6 and 12 months of age."** Albeit a different population, Hensle and colleagues (2001) reported a significantly higher complication rate for hypospadias repair in 42 men 18 to 47 years old. This included a 38% complication rate in 8 patients without previous hypospadias surgery, further supporting the benefit of repair at a younger age.

Anesthesia/Analgesia

General anesthesia, typically with endotracheal intubation, has been the mainstay of anesthetic technique for hypospadias repair. General anesthesia provides uninterrupted performance of the repair without concern for patient movement or sensation of pain. Adjunctive analgesia in the form of long-acting injectable agents, delivered via a caudal route or as a dorsal penile nerve block, has proven safe and efficacious. **A popular agent for adjunctive analgesia is bupivacaine (0.25%) without epinephrine administered as either a caudal or dorsal penile nerve block.** Bupivacaine given in this manner at the beginning of hypospadias repair will allow time for onset of action during the planning and preliminary stages of the repair. Newer concepts regarding perioperative analgesic administration have been reported by Chhibber and colleagues (1997). Patients undergoing outpatient hypospadias repair were randomly assigned to receive a penile block with the same total dose of bupivacaine at the completion of surgery, before the incision or before and at the completion of surgery. **A statistically significant improvement in postoperative pain control was noted for those patients who received a penile block both at the beginning and completion of hypospadias repair, compared with the other groups** (Chhibber et al, 1997). Similarly, caudal injection of bupivacaine provided significantly better pain management when given both at the start and at the end of surgery when compared with administration at the start of surgery alone (Samuel et al, 2002).

Antibiotics

One intravenous dose of a broad-spectrum antibiotic may be indicated for those in whom the urethra is catheterized intraoperatively. Cephalexin given 1 day after surgery to 2 days after urethral catheter removal has been shown to significantly decrease the rate of complicated (febrile) urinary tract infection compared with boys not receiving prophylaxis (Meir and Livne, 2004). Preferential use of perioperative antibiotics has been described by others (Winslow and Devine, 1996).

Hemostasis

Based on the hypothesis that some complications such as urethrocutaneous fistula and repair breakdown are, in part, a result of ischemic tissue necrosis, use of electrocautery should be limited during hypospadias repair (Zaontz, 1990). **The current of monopolar electrocautery is dispersed to the remote grounding site, generally along the vessels, and in this way may irreparably damage tissue microvasculature** (Jordan, 1999a). Others employing electrocautery may prefer the bipolar variant and the use of fine-point neurologic forceps (Winslow and Devine, 1996). We favor injection of a vasoconstrictive agent (epinephrine diluted 1:200,000 with lidocaine) deep to proposed glanular incision, as well as intermittent use of a tourniquet at the base of the penis during urethroplasty. Other options for effective temporary hemostasis without permanent tissue devitalization include intermittent compression with gauze soaked in iced saline and/or epinephrine solution.

Optical Magnification

Wacksman (1987) reported that a microscope compared favorably with previous results with loupe magnification and allowed use of small sutures with great accuracy. Shapiro (1989) compared the results of hypospadias repair using 3.5× magnification (loupes) and the Zeiss reconstruction microscope. Shapiro did not show any significant difference in outcome, and his prediction that the microscope would be used more often in the repair of hypospadias in the future does not appear to have come to fruition.

Suture/Suture Technique

Stay sutures are used whenever possible to limit tissue handling. Delicate forceps with fine teeth may limit crushing of tissues when handling is necessary. Typically, a subcuticular technique is employed during longitudinal closure of the neourethra when performing a tubularization technique. **Perhaps, the most important aspect of closure of the neourethra is exact suture placement such that the edge of the epithelial surface is inverted and the raw surfaces of the subepithelial tissue are approximated.** Healing then provides a "watertight" anastomotic suture line that, at least theoretically, would decrease the risk of urethrocutaneous fistula formation. However, Hakim and associates (1996) reported that the technique, either subcuticular or full thickness, did not affect results provided the suture used was of polyglactin composition. In contrast, Ulman and colleagues (1997) have documented a statistically significant lower fistula rate (4.9% vs. 16.6%) for subcuticular compared with full-thickness technique. **Disandro and Palmer** (1996) **reported a fourfold increase in urethral stricture rate after hypospadias repair with polydioxanone suture (PDS) compared with chromic or polyglycolic acid suture.**

Laser Techniques

Although its use in hypospadias repair is not popularized as yet, Scherr and Poppas (1998) have published an exhaustive review of current laser technology. Kirsch and colleagues (1997) have updated their experience with the use of laser-tissue welding for urethral surgery, as either an adjunct to suturing in 25 patients or as the primary means of tissue approximation in 11 patients. Preoperative diagnoses included hypospadias, urethral stricture, urethral diverticulum, and urethral fistulas. With follow-up ranging from 3 months to 3 years, no strictures or diverticula developed. Overall, 5 patients developed fistulas between 2 weeks and 6 months postoperatively. In the initial experience (Kirsch et al, 1996b), the overall complication rate using laser soldering was 19%, with one half of the complications occurring in reoperative repairs. The fistula rate was 14% overall and 6% for primary cases (Kirsch et al, 1996b).

Neourethral Intubation

Another source of controversy in hypospadias repair is the use or omission of postoperative urethral catheterization. Stressing the importance of a watertight urethroplasty, Rabinowitz (1987) performed Mathieu hypospadias repair without urethral catheter drainage or urinary diversion in 59 boys, achieving excellent cosmetic and functional results with few complications. **In one multicenter report combining the experience of 4 institutions** (Hakim et al, 1996), **excellent results were obtained in 96.7% of 336 patients repaired with the Mathieu technique** as modified by Rabinowitz (1987). Complications occurred in 11 patients and consisted of urethrocutaneous fistula, meatal retraction, and meatal stenosis in 9, 1, and 1 patient, respectively. **Results were not affected by urethral catheterization status.** In a prospective, randomized study, McCormack and colleagues (1993) found no difference in outcome after comparing 19 boys with urinary diversion and indwelling urethral catheter versus 16 boys without, all of whom underwent Mathieu hypospadias repair. Further experience with limited use of a urethral catheter in over 200 patients undergoing Mathieu hypospadias repair was reported by Retik and colleagues (1994b), who noted a complication rate of 0.98% and no urethrocutaneous fistulas.

Others report rates of urethrocutaneous fistula formation and meatal stenosis twofold greater in those with a urethral catheter versus those diverted suprapubically after hypospadias repair (Demirbilek and Atayurt, 1997). **Based on these results and those for the more extensively studied Mathieu repair, there does not appear to be an advantage to or necessity for use of a urethral catheter after some hypospadias repairs.** This may be true for some of the more recently described techniques as well (Steckler and Zaontz, 1997). However, **El-Sherbiny** (2003) **reported significantly less dysuria, urinary extravasation, urinary retention, and fistula formation in toilet-trained boys whose urethra was stented (continuous bladder drainage) compared with unstented after tubularized incised plated hypospadias repair.**

Dressing

Several different dressing techniques have been described (Cromie and Bellinger, 1981). In 1982, De Sy and Oosterlinck described a soft, pliable foam dressing, the "silicone foam elastomer," as a significant improvement in postoperative penile dressing. After mixture of elastomer and catalyst, the sterile foam is molded around the penis. This dressing appears to be well tolerated and easily removed in 4 to 6 days. This silicone foam elastomer has been used in conjunction with pantaloon spica cast postoperative immobilization after free graft hypospadias repair (Cilento et al, 1997). **In two recent prospective randomized trials, it has been shown that there is little or no advantage to the application of a dressing to the operated hypospadias** (Van Savage et al, 2000; McLorie et al, 2001). Randomized patients received either transparent film dressing, elastic wrap dressing, or no dressing. Antibiotic ointment was used to coat the penis in those receiving no dressing. **Method of postoperative care (dressing vs. no dressing) did not impact surgical success rate or wound healing. In general, a regimen of no dressing (antibiotic ointment only) appears to result in increased patient comfort and decreased burden for the caregiver.**

Postoperative Penile Erection, Bladder Spasm

Sengezer and coworkers (2002) have shown that patient-controlled epidural analgesia provides effective pain control and prevents penile erection in adults after hypospadias repair. Stock and Kaplan (1995) reported use of ketoconazole as a reliable method for preventing postoperative penile erections after penile surgery in 8 patients ranging in age from 14 to 42 years. **Ketoconazole reduces adrenal and testicular androgen production through the inhibition of 17,20-desmolase, thereby preventing the conversion of cholesterol to testosterone. Hepatotoxicity is a recognized side effect of ketoconazole.** The authors recommended obtaining liver function tests before starting therapy, on the third day of therapy, and after completion. Amyl nitrite has also been used to prevent penile erections (Horton and Horton, 1988). Judicious use of anticholinergic medication has been described for postoperative bladder spasm in stented patients (Horton and Horton, 1988; Minevich et al, 1999). Follow-up schedule and length of follow-up are specific to surgeon preference but in general should be at least 6 months to 1 year for successful repairs (Caldamone and Diamond, 1999).

INTRAOPERATIVE ALGORITHM

At surgery, the decision-making process for determining an appropriate repair for a given defect begins with a general assessment of native meatal location, penile size and curvature, and characteristics of ventral, proximal shaft skin (Fig. 125–9). Occasionally, it may be necessary to longitudinally incise ventral, deficient skin and urethral tissue proximal to the hypospadiac meatus to incorporate healthy, well-developed tissue at the proximal extent of the repair (Fig. 125–10). Some are proponents (Yang et al, 2000) and others are critics (Elbakry, 2001b) of preservation of this thin distal urethra.

KEY POINTS: SPECIAL CONSIDERATIONS: PERIOPERATIVE

- Bipolar electrocautery is a safer alternative to monopolar electrocautery.

- When appropriate, judicious use of a vasoactive agent that provides hemostasis without permanent tissue damage is preferable to electrocautery.

- Optical magnification of 2.5× to 3.5× is the norm for hypospadias repair, although some surgeons prefer the operating microscope with up to 10× magnification.

- For most distal repairs there is no clear advantage to the use of a temporary indwelling urethral catheter in the immediate postoperative period.

The penile shaft is degloved of its skin with care taken to preserve the urethral plate in all but the most severe (scrotal and perineal) defects. The assessment and management of penile curvature follows. **In general, both the level of the hypospadiac meatus and the severity of penile curvature dictate appropriate repair options. Distal, middle, and some proximal defects are usually amenable to repair by preservation of the urethral plate, dorsal orthoplasty procedure as needed, and then one of several appropriate urethroplasty techniques** (Sozubir and Snodgrass, 2003).

The use of well-vascularized local tissue is preferred for urethroplasty. Most distal defects are typically repaired with one of several advancement techniques. In instances where simple advancement is not sufficient or appropriate, defects may be managed with various tubularization or flap techniques. Defects with a deep glanular groove and a phallus (including urethral plate) with sufficient width are perhaps amenable to a simple tubularization technique. When the glanular groove is shallow and/or the urethral plate narrow, midline longitudinal incision of the urethral plate may allow neourethral tubularization free of tension.

Various perimeatal-based flap techniques using ventral, proximal shaft skin may also be employed in the setting of a shallow glanular groove and narrow urethral plate provided the proximal extent of the flap does not include hair-bearing skin. Perimeatal-based flaps may not be favored secondary to inferior meatal cosmesis and poor flap vascularity relative to other repairs. An onlay technique may be preferred in the setting of a small penis that is inadequate in width for tubularization alone or with midline longitudinal incision of the urethral plate, or in the specific case of a conical (convex ventral) glans with a shallow groove. **Thus far, preferable technical options assume either absent, mild, or moderate penile curvature (amenable to dorsal orthoplasty techniques) and allow one to preserve the urethral plate and incorporate it into the neourethra.**

For more proximal defects, with mild to moderate curvature, dorsal orthoplasty techniques may be sufficient, allowing one to preserve the urethral plate and perform one of several tubularization or flap urethroplasty techniques. **In some proximal hypospadias, associated curvature is severe and**

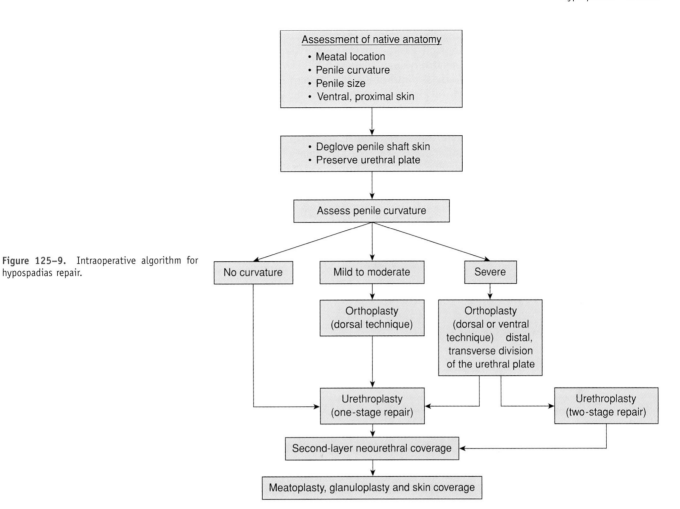

Figure 125–9. Intraoperative algorithm for hypospadias repair.

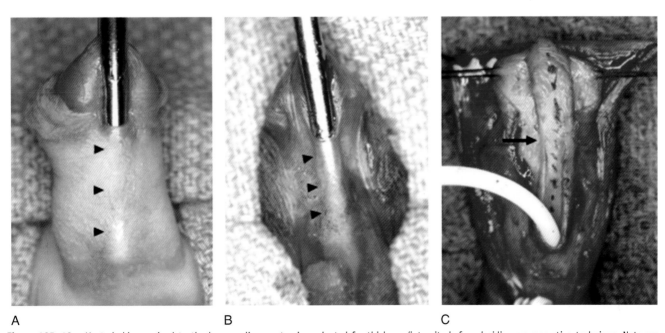

A   B   C

Figure 125–10. Ventral skin proximal to the hypospadiac meatus is evaluated for thickness/integrity before deciding on reparative technique. Note urethral sound passed into meatus. **A,** Thick, healthy skin overlying urethra *(arrowheads)* proximal to hypospadiac meatus. **B,** Thin, near-transparent skin and urethra *(arrowheads)* proximal to meatus before, and **C,** same patient as in **B** after midline incision proximally from site of the native meatus *(arrow)* to the point of encountering healthy tissue in preparation for urethroplasty. Note catheter within neomeatus. The urethral plate has been outlined with incisions and marked in the midline with a longitudinal *dotted line* (see Fig. 125–12*C* to *G*).

the urethral plate may have a tethering effect on the penis and thus, may at least in part be responsible for the curvature. In this setting, with or without a relatively small penis, it may be necessary to divide the urethral plate in some cases, followed by dissection of the urethral plate proximally off of the ventral aspect of the corpora cavernosa to the level of the meatus. Curvature, if persistent, may then be corrected with placement of a ventral interposition graft before urethroplasty performed via tubularization of either pedicled local skin, a free graft of local or extragenital tissue, or, alternatively, a two-stage repair (Hensle et al, 2002; Snodgrass and Lorenzo, 2002b; Hayashi et al, 2003).

KEY POINTS: INTRAOPERATIVE ALORITHM

- The level of the hypospadias, degree of penile curvature, and tissue availability and quality dictate repair options.

- Distal hypospadias is typically amenable to advancement or tubularization techniques.

- Middle hypospadias is typically amenable to tubularization or vascularized flap techniques.

- Proximal defects are treated with tubularization, vascularized flap, two-stage techniques, or the incorporation of extragenital skin for repair.

PRIMARY HYPOSPADIAS REPAIR

There is no single, universally applicable technique for hypospadias repair. Several well-established techniques exist for the repair of all hypospadias defects with which the surgeon is presented. A discussion of various currently popular techniques for respective hypospadias level follows. Techniques listed and discussed are intended to be neither exhaustive nor exclusive per level of hypospadias. Generalizations are presented with the expectation of overlap and/or exclusion of technique applicability for a given defect based on surgeon preference and case-specific anatomy. Included in the discussion are specifics of technique, as performed by the current authors, for several of the most commonly performed repairs.

Distal Hypospadias Procedures

Advancement Techniques

Glanular and some coronal hypospadias defects are amenable to the meatoplasty and glanuloplasty (MAGPI) technique (Fig. 125–11), with excellent functional and cosmetic results provided there is adequate urethral mobility and no penile curvature (Duckett, 1981a; Duckett and Snyder, 1992; Park et al, 1995). The MAGPI technique is performed by first making a circumferential incision 5 mm proximal and parallel to the corona of the glans. If present, the typical transverse glanular tissue "bridge" in the urethral plate that separates the hypospadiac meatus and distal glanular groove is incised longitudinally. The incised tissue edges are

then approximated transversely in Heineke-Mikulicz fashion. This step obliterates the tissue bridge and advances the meatus slightly. The ventral edge of meatus is pulled distally with the aid of a stay suture placed in the midline, and the medial edges of the glans are then trimmed before midline approximation in two layers. Approximation of the glans and skin with simple, interrupted, fine absorbable suture completes the repair. Excision of a flap of tissue from the midline of the glans may allow placement of the urethra more deeply in the glans, decrease the risk of meatal stenosis, and improve cosmesis (Taneli et al, 2004).

Another successful technique for the repair of glanular and coronal defects is a modification of the MAGPI technique described by Arap and colleagues (1984). According to these authors, incorporation of urethroplasty (distal tubularization) with meatal advancement and glanuloplasty enables treatment of the more severe cases of distal hypospadias. Proponents of other modifications on the theme of **distal urethral advancement and glanuloplasty** have reported long-term results of 95% or greater success rates and low reoperation rates of 2% (Harrison and Grobbelaar, 1997) and 5% (Caione et al, 1997).

Distal urethral **circumferential dissection and advancement** was first described by Beck in 1898 for repair of distal hypospadias. Atala (2002) has described a similar technique. Taken to the extreme, the principle of urethral advancement may gain 2.0 to 2.5 cm of urethral length in children, with mobilization of the urethra to the bulbar level using the **bulbar elongation anastomotic meatoplasty (BEAM)** procedure for hypospadiac urethroplasty. According to Turner Warwick and colleagues (1997), this degree of mobilization is necessary to prevent the formation of penile curvature.

Tubularization Techniques

Thiersch (1869) **and Duplay (1880) were the initial descriptors of the simple urethral plate tubularization technique that has come to be known as the Thiersch-Duplay urethroplasty.** Several techniques, including that described by King (1970, 1981), employ tubularization of the urethral plate for repair of distal hypospadias. The **glans approximation procedure (GAP)** described by Zaontz (1989) is an ideal repair for glanular and coronal defects with a deep glanular groove. This technique has excellent functional and cosmetic results. **A recent study involving over 500 repairs with the combined use of the Heineke-Mikulicz meatoplasty and the GAP reported a complication and reoperation rate of only 2.1% for the entire group** (Stock and Hanna, 1997). **Glanuloplasty and in-situ tubularization** of the urethral plate has been touted as an excellent technique for distal and midshaft hypospadias (van Horn and Kass, 1995). In a recent cohort of patients repaired with this technique, the complication rate decreased to 1.7% for distal and 7.7% for midshaft hypospadias repair (Kass and Chung, 2000).

A modification of the Thiersch-Duplay (Thiersch, 1869; Duplay, 1880) **technique has been described by Snodgrass (1994). The tubularized incised plate (TIP) urethroplasty combines modifications of the previously described techniques of urethral plate incision** (Rich et al, 1989) **and tubularization** (Thiersch, 1869; Duplay, 1880). **The concept of a urethral plate "relaxing incision" as an adjunct to hypospadias repair to allow tension-free neourethral tubularization**

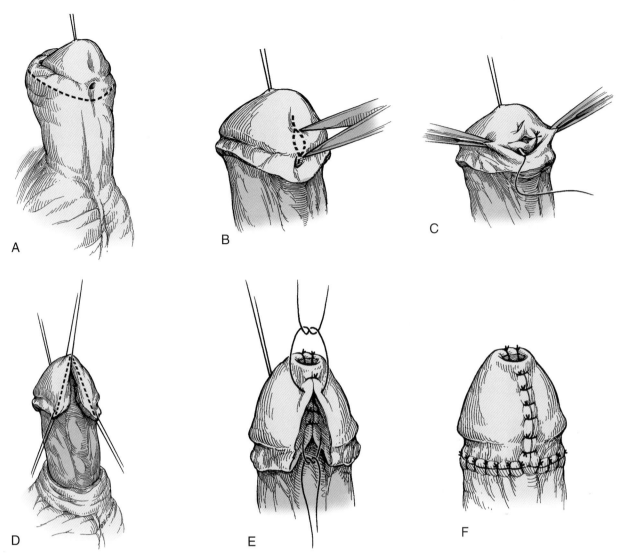

Figure 125–11. Meatoplasty and glanuloplasty (MAGPI). **A,** Circumferential subcoronal incision is marked. **B,** Longitudinal incision. **C,** Transverse approximation (Heineke-Mikulicz procedure) of transverse glanular "bridge" in urethral plate. **D,** Ventral edge of meatus is pulled distally, and medial glans "trimming" incisions are marked. **E,** Deep suture approximation of the glans. **F,** Superficial approximation of the glans and skin. (Reprinted from Duckett JW: Hypospadias. In Walsh PC, Retik AB, Vaughan ED Jr, Wein AJ [eds]: Campbell's Urology, 7th ed. Philadelphia, WB Saunders, 1998, vol 2, pp 2093-2119.)

was also described simultaneously by **Perovic and Vukadinovic** (1994). Since the initial description in 1994 for use in distal hypospadias repair, additional experience using the TIP urethroplasty technique for distal and more proximal defects has been reported by several authors (Snodgrass et al, 1996, 1998; Ross and Kay, 1997; Steckler and Zaontz, 1997; Retik and Borer, 1998; Decter and Franzoni, 1999). Complication rates of 1% to 5% have been reported for primary hypospadias repair with the TIP urethroplasty technique. Excellent results have also been reported for TIP urethroplasty use in reoperative and complex hypospadias repair (Snodgrass et al, 1996; Borer et al, 2001; Borer and Retik, 2002; Snodgrass and Lorenzo, 2002a).

Modifications to the TIP urethroplasty technique have been previously described (Retik and Borer, 1998; Borer and Retik, 1999) and are summarized here (Fig. 125–12). After stay suture placement in the glans, the urethral plate is outlined at a width of 7 to 9 mm, depending on the size of the phallus.

Dilute epinephrine is injected deep to the proposed sites of incision, and parallel longitudinal incisions demarcating the urethral plate are made from the tip of the glans to the hypospadiac meatus. A transverse incision across the skin overlying the urethra completes the U-shaped incision outlining the urethral plate. A circumferential incision 5 to 7 mm proximal to the coronal margin is extended from each longitudinal incision, followed by degloving of the penile shaft skin. Orthoplasty is performed as needed.

The *first* critical point in the TIP urethroplasty involves a longitudinal midline incision of the urethral plate from the level of the hypospadiac meatus to the tip of the penis, as necessary. The depth of the urethral plate incision depends primarily on the configuration of the glans and the glanular groove. With the aid of a tourniquet, the urethral plate is then tubularized over a 6-Fr Silastic catheter with a running subcuticular fine polyglactin suture. The *second* critical point involves fashioning a wide meatus. Second layer coverage of

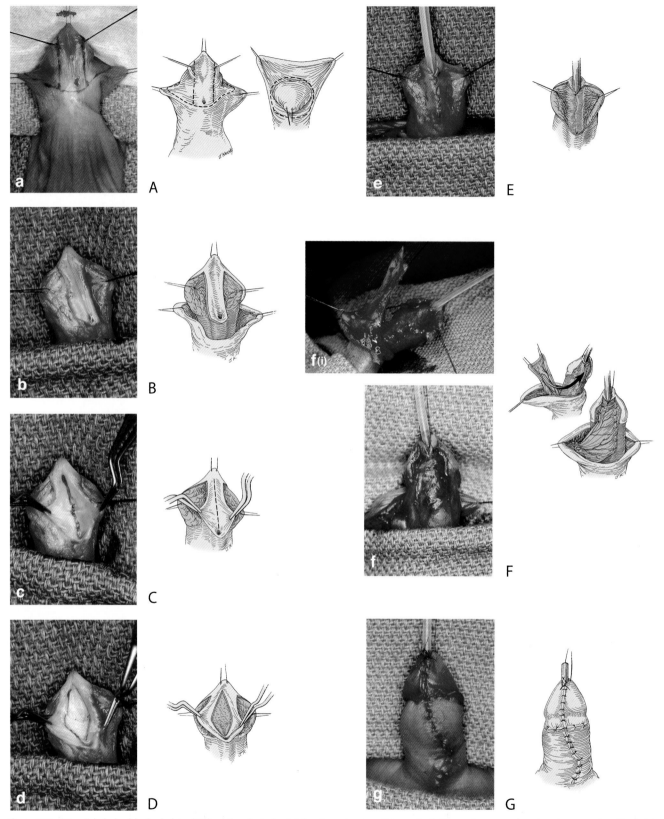

Figure 125–12. Tubularized incised plate (TIP) urethroplasty in distal, primary hypospadias repair. **A,** Stay sutures are placed, and proposed urethral plate demarcating and circumferential incisions are marked. **B,** Parallel longitudinal and circumferential incisions have been made. **C,** Proposed longitudinal line of incision in the midline of the urethral plate. **D,** Urethral plate has been incised. **E,** Urethral plate tubularized over a 6-Fr Silastic catheter with care not to close the distal extent (meatus) of the incised urethral plate too tightly. **F,** Subcutaneous (dartos) tissue flap is harvested from lateral or dorsal penile shaft and repositioned over the neourethra as a second layer of coverage. **G,** Glans penis has been approximated in two layers, redundant skin excised, and indwelling bladder catheter secured. (Reprinted from Retik AB, Borer JG: Primary and reoperative hypospadias repair with the Snodgrass technique. World J Urol 1998;16:186.)

the neurethra with a well-vascularized subcutaneous (dartos) tissue flap, harvested from the dorsal preputial and shaft skin, is the *third* critical aspect of the TIP urethroplasty. The glans wings are then approximated without tension in two layers, the indwelling Silastic urethral catheter is secured to the glans penis, and skin coverage completes the repair. The TIP urethroplasty technique is performed similarly for previously circumcised boys and for more proximal defects (see Fig. 125–10C) and results in a normal-appearing penis with a "slit-like," vertically oriented meatus. Modification of the meatoplasty component of the repair has been suggested to decrease the meatal stenosis rate (Jayanthi, 2003). Others recommend midline longitudinal incision of the urethral plate as the first step in this technique also to reduce the meatal stenosis rate as discussed by Zaontz in editorial comments (Nguyen et al, 2004).

Flap Techniques

Among the more commonly used local tissue flap techniques for coronal and subcoronal defects is the **Mathieu, perimeatal-based flap** technique (Mathieu, 1932). In 1994, Retik and colleagues reported a series of 204 perimeatal-based repairs performed with the addition of dorsal dartos flap coverage of the neourethra and a complication rate of 0.98%. In a recent multicenter report combining the experience of four institutions, an excellent functional and cosmetic result was obtained in 96.7% of 336 patients repaired with a modified Mathieu technique (Hakim et al, 1996). Urethrocutaneous fistula was the most common complication and occurred in only 9 patients.

The *Mathieu* hypospadias repair (Fig. 125–13) starts with measuring the length of the defect from the urethral meatus to the glans tip. An equal distance from the meatus is measured on the proximal penile shaft skin. With the aid of calipers, the urethral plate and perimeatal-based flap are then marked at appropriate widths. Typically, a width of 7.5 mm is measured for the proximal flap. This width is tapered to 5.5 mm at the distal extent of the glans, and longitudinal lines outlining the urethral plate are then drawn. A line is marked beginning at either lateral margin of the previously marked urethral plate and carried around the dorsal aspect of the penis 5 to 7 mm proximal to the corona of the glans. Injection of dilute epinephrine is followed by skin and glanular incisions. Glans wings are incised deeply, the penile shaft skin is degloved, and the penis is evaluated for curvature.

After a straight penis is either appreciated or achieved with an orthoplasty technique, the premeasured segment of penile skin proximal to the meatus is mobilized off of the urethra in a proximal to distal direction with the aid of skin hooks, fine stay sutures, and tenotomy scissors. This tissue is folded over at the meatus (perimeatal-based flap), and bilateral, longitudinal, running subcuticular sutures approximate this flap to the lateral aspects of the urethral plate, thereby creating the neourethra. Tubularization is performed over a 6-Fr Silastic catheter using fine polyglactin suture. The meatus is matured at the glans tip with simple, interrupted, fine absorbable suture, and second-layer neourethral coverage is performed with dorsal dartos tissue. The glans wings are then approximated without tension in two layers, and skin coverage is completed. Many believe that the Mathieu hypospadias repair provides less than optimal meatal cosmesis. A V-shaped

modification at the ventral apex of the meatus appears to provide significant benefit (Boddy and Samuel, 2000).

The **Barcat balanic groove** technique is similar to the Mathieu repair but includes dissection of the urethral plate distal to the meatus and advancement of the approximated (now tubularized) flaps to the tip of the glans (Barcat, 1973; Redman, 1987; Koff et al, 1994; Barthold et al, 1996). **Perimeatal-based flap repairs such as the Mathieu and initial and modified Barcat balanic groove procedures incorporate the use of tissue flaps with blood supply that may be compromised** (Keating and Duckett, 1995). **In addition, these repairs require ventral penile shaft skin of sufficient length without incorporation of proximal hair-bearing skin.** Often this results in a skin defect that requires complex rotational skin flaps for coverage and a horizontally oriented abnormal-appearing urethral meatus. A technique described initially by **Bevan** (1917) and later by **Mustarde** (1965) represents a combination of a perimeatal-based, ventral skin flap that is then tubularized and passed through a glans channel to achieve a meatus at the penile tip.

Others

The **MIP** (see Fig. 125–2), **a variant of distal hypospadias so named by Duckett and Keating** (1989), **was simultaneously described by Hatch and colleagues** (1989). A repair specific to this hypospadias variant, **the "pyramid" procedure,** has also been described (Duckett and Keating, 1989). Other techniques, including the MAGPI, Thiersch-Duplay urethroplasty, and Mathieu, have been used to successfully repair this particular defect (Hatch et al, 1989; Hill et al, 1993; Nonomura et al, 1998). **The split prepuce in-situ onlay technique** (Rushton and Belman, 1998) has been reported for use in distal and middle hypospadias and is discussed in detail in a later section.

Middle Hypospadias Procedures

Numerous successful procedures with acceptable complication rates have been described for the repair of middle hypospadias with mild to moderate penile curvature. Popular techniques include the **TIP urethroplasty** (Snodgrass, et al, 1996; Retik and Borer, 1998; Borer et al, 2001) and the **Mathieu, perimeatal-based flap** (Mathieu, 1932), both of which have been described for repair of distal hypospadias. Although primary utility may be in repair of coronal and subcoronal defects, the Mathieu technique may also be employed for repair of distal penile shaft hypospadias.

Onlay Techniques

Among the most commonly used techniques for repair of middle hypospadias is the onlay island flap (OIF) technique (Elder et al, 1987). **Since its introduction for the repair of subcoronal and midshaft hypospadias, use of the OIF technique has expanded both in frequency and indication to include more proximal defects.** In 1994, Baskin and colleagues (1994) reported use of the OIF in 374 patients, or 33% of the total hypospadias repairs during a 5-year period. Complications requiring reoperation occurred in 32 (8.6%) of the patients. Twenty-three (6%) of the patients developed a urethrocutaneous fistula.

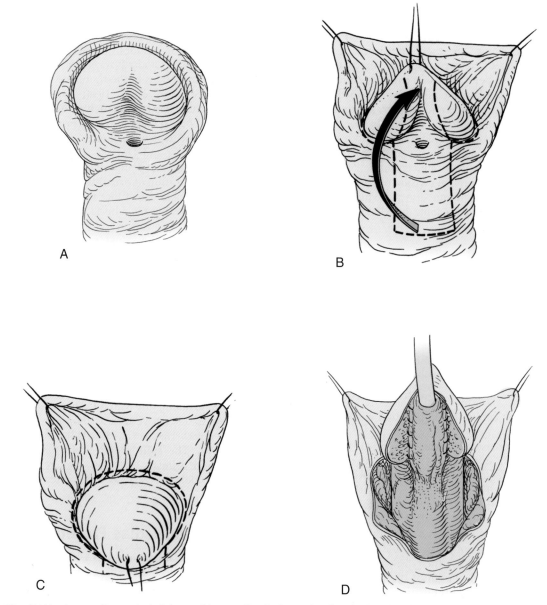

Figure 125–13. Mathieu hypospadias repair. **A,** Subcoronal hypospadias. **B,** Appropriate flap size is outlined proximal to urethral meatus. **C,** Proposed circumferential incision. **D,** Proximal flap has been elevated from penile ventrum and sutured to the urethral plate with running subcuticular technique.

The OIF repair (Fig. 125–14) begins by placing a traction suture in the glans penis and fine stay sutures at the corners of the prepuce. The urethral plate is measured to a width of approximately 6 mm, and proposed parallel longitudinal incisions outlining the urethral plate are marked from the hypospadiac meatus to the glans tip. A near-circumferential incision that preserves the urethral plate is also marked on the distal penile shaft. Dilute epinephrine solution is injected to facilitate hemostasis, and the skin incisions are then made with a fine knife. **After correction of penile curvature if necessary, the length of the defect from the urethral meatus to the glans tip is measured. This is the length required of the rectangular preputial onlay to be harvested for repair. We**

typically use a width of 9 to 10 mm for the onlay flap when used for repair in infants. The preputial skin is marked, incised, and then dissected with its pedicle from the outer preputial layer and dorsal penile shaft skin. Dissection of the pedicle to the base of the penis minimizes torque on the penis and tension on the repair.

The rectangular preputial OIF is held with a fine stay suture in each corner and is passed around the penis to the ventrum. Care is taken to ensure that the flap reaches the site of anastomosis without tension on its pedicle. Tubularization is performed over a 6-Fr Silastic catheter and is begun with a full-thickness running 6-0 or 7-0 polyglactin suture that approximates the previous proximal edge of the onlay flap

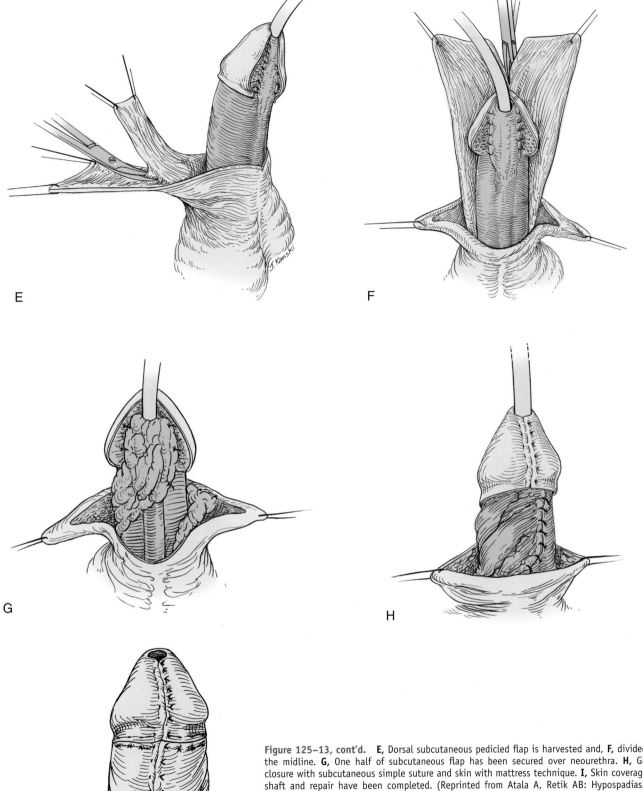

E

F

G

H

I

Figure 125–13, cont'd. **E,** Dorsal subcutaneous pedicled flap is harvested and, **F,** divided in the midline. **G,** One half of subcutaneous flap has been secured over neourethra. **H,** Glans closure with subcutaneous simple suture and skin with mattress technique. **I,** Skin coverage of shaft and repair have been completed. (Reprinted from Atala A, Retik AB: Hypospadias. In Libertino JA [ed]: Reconstructive Urologic Surgery, 3rd ed. St. Louis, Mosby–Year Book, 1998, p 467.)

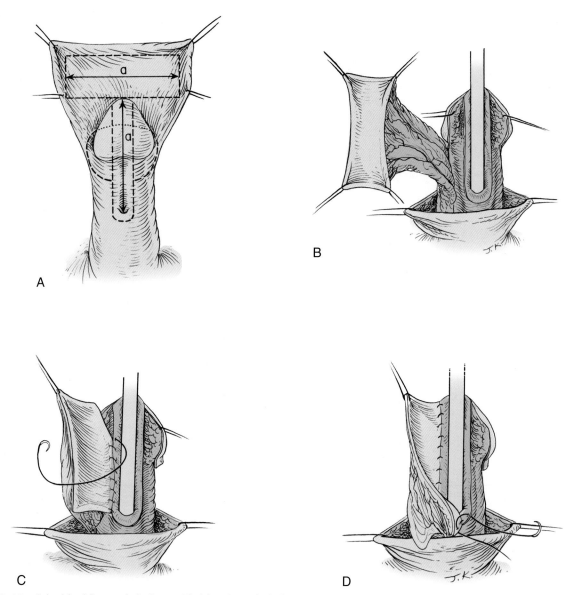

Figure 125–14. Onlay island flap repair. **A,** Proposed incisions for urethral plate and preputial skin onlay. **B,** Pedicled preputial skin onlay with stay sutures. **C,** Initial full-thickness suture approximation of onlay flap and urethral plate. **D,** Approximation at proximal extent. *Continued*

(now oriented longitudinally) with the edge of urethral plate ipsilateral to the side of flap transfer. A full-thickness running suture is also used for the transverse proximal anastomosis, and the remainder of the tubularization is performed with a running subcuticular technique. **The inferolateral border of the pedicle is advanced over the lines of anastomosis, and a tunica vaginalis flap may be employed for second-layer coverage.** Maturation of the urethral meatus, securing of the Silastic catheter, glans approximation, and skin closure are then performed.

Rushton and Belman (1998) have reported excellent results with the **split prepuce in-situ onlay** (Fig. 125–15) modification of the OIF technique. In this modification, it is **preservation of the whole blood supply to one half of the prepuce (onlay segment harvested in longitudinal orientation and transferred ventrally) used for coronal to midshaft hypospa-**dias repair that the authors believe is responsible for the low 4% urethrocutaneous fistula and 5% reoperative rates. In further contrast to the standard OIF repair (onlay segment harvested in transverse orientation) (Elder et al, 1987), **the split prepuce island onlay does not require separate mobilization of both inner preputial and skin vascular supplies. The outer epithelial layer is simply excised, simplifying the repair and optimizing blood supply to the onlay flap.** The authors suggest that this technique would be applicable for more proximal repairs as well (Rushton and Belman, 1998). Yerkes and colleagues (2000b) have also reported excellent preliminary results with this technique. Another variation of the onlay, the **double-onlay preputial flap,** as described by Gonzalez and colleagues (1996), primarily for the repair of proximal hypospadias has also been employed for repair of midshaft hypospadias (Barroso et al, 2000).

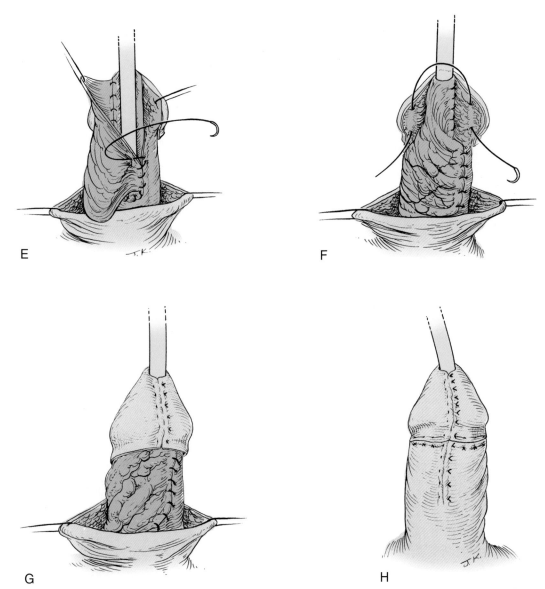

Figure 125–14, cont'd. **E,** Completion of anastomosis with running subcuticular technique. **F,** Inferolateral border of onlay pedicle has been advanced as a second layer coverage of proximal and longitudinal suture lines. **G,** Approximated glans. **H,** Completed repair. (Reprinted from Atala A, Retik AB: Hypospadias. In Libertino JA [ed]: Reconstructive Urologic Surgery, 3rd ed. St. Louis, Mosby–Year Book, 1998, p 467.)

Tubularization Techniques

Other popular and successful techniques include the tubularization technique described by King (1970) (whose initial description of the technique involved a patient with midshaft hypospadias) and the TIP urethroplasty. As stated in the discussion of anterior hypospadias repair, the TIP urethroplasty has become a popular technique for primary and reoperative repair of middle as well as anterior hypospadias (Snodgrass et al, 1996; Retik and Borer, 1998; Borer et al, 2001a).

Proximal Hypospadias Procedures

Proximal hypospadias defects represent the most challenging and complex manifestations of this entity and may be successfully treated with one of several one- or two-stage repairs. Arguments for either one- or two-stage repair of proximal hypospadias continue to be discussed with as much passion as any aspect of hypospadiology (Gershbaum et al, 2002; Hensle et al, 2002; Shukla et al, 2004).

One-Stage Repairs

Onlay Techniques. The *onlay island flap,* **initially described for distal and midshaft repairs** (Elder et al, 1987), **has been increasingly employed for repair of more severe hypospadias** (Hollowell et al, 1990; Dewan et al, 1991; Mollard et al, 1991; Gearhart and Borland, 1992; Baskin et al, 1994; Perovic and Vukadinovic, 1994). Baskin and colleagues (1994) reported the repair of penoscrotal and perineal hypospadias defects in 33 and 5 patients, respectively, with excellent results.

Recently, a variation of the onlay principle, the *onlay-tube/onlay urethroplasty* technique, which is composed of a **central tubularized and distal and proximal onlay compo-**

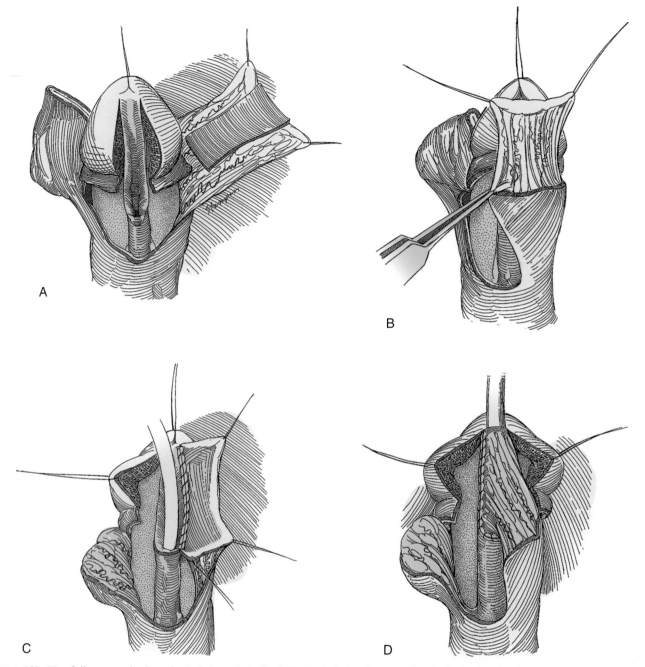

Figure 125–15. Split prepuce in-situ onlay technique. **A,** Penile shaft skin is degloved, prepuce is split in the dorsal midline, and the urethral plate is outlined. The one half of split prepuce used for the island flap is isolated by de-epithelializing adjacent inner prepuce. **B,** Outer skin of preputial onlay is de-epithelialized. **C,** The onlay flap is sutured to the urethral plate beginning with a running 7-0 polyglactin suture and, **D,** completed with subcuticular technique.

Continued

nents, has been described. This repair, based on the same strip of penile shaft and preputial skin (harvested in longitudinal orientation) (Perovic and Vukadinovic, 1994) or preputial skin alone (harvested transversely) (Flack and Walker, 1995), has been described in four patients each with "severe" and perineal hypospadias. Other modifications of this onlay-tube combination have been reported (Kocvara and Dvoracek, 1997).

The **double-onlay preputial flap,** as described by Gonzalez and colleagues (1996) combines the principles of the OIF and

the double face preputial flap. The preputial onlay segment is harvested transversely and transposed ventrally with a "buttonhole" in the vascular pedicle. **This repair preserves the urethral plate, as do other onlay techniques, but obviates the need for separation of the inner and outer preputial layers and the need for separate skin coverage of the onlay segment used for urethroplasty.** Use in proximal hypospadias included 11 patients with penoscrotal and 1 with a perineal meatus. According to the authors, there were no problems with vascular supply to the flaps or ventral bulkiness. Complications

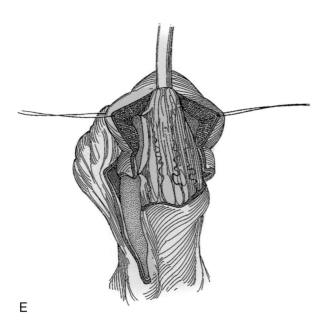

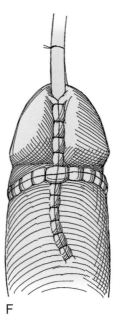

Figure 125–15, cont'd. **E,** Edges of the vascular pedicle are secured lateral to neourethral suture lines as second-layer coverage. **F,** The repair is completed with skin coverage and securing of an 8-Fr intravesical stent to the glans. (Reprinted from Rushton HG, Belman AB: The split prepuce in situ onlay hypospadias repair. J Urol 1998;160:1134-1136.)

requiring reoperation occurred in 4 patients with penoscrotal hypospadias (Gonzalez et al, 1996). Barroso and colleagues (2000) updated this experience and have now performed the double-onlay preputial flap in a total of 47 patients. Complications requiring reoperation occurred in 12 patients (25%). In 8 (17%) boys a fistula developed, of whom 6 had perineal and 2 had penoscrotal hypospadias. Successful closure was achieved with one procedure in 6 patients and required an additional fistula repair in 1 patient. Diverticulum, meatal recession, and persistent penile curvature requiring repeat dorsal plication occurred in 4 (9%), 2 (4%), and 2 (4%) patients, respectively. Revision for a bulky ventral skin strip was required in one boy (2%) (Barroso et al, 2000).

Tubularization Techniques. Credit for the first description of preputial skin use for a tubularized, pedicled flap neourethra goes to Weller Van Hook, who, in 1896, described use of a pedicled preputial flap for creation of a tubularized neourethra in a patient with proximal hypospadias. Several others have described similar techniques (Wehrbein, 1943; Hodgson, 1970; Toksu, 1970; Duckett, 1980; Harris, 1984).

In 1969, Hamilton described urethroplasty with a **longitudinally oriented preputial island flap.** A similar technique has been described by Chen and colleagues (1993). In 1971, Asopa and coworkers (1971) described use of preputial skin for formation of a tubularized neourethra transferred to the ventrum for hypospadias repair as a single unit with the inner prepuce as the tubularized neourethra and the attached outer prepuce for skin cover. Yavuzer and colleagues (1998) described a similar technique for repair of midshaft or proximal hypospadias in 26 patients, with a success rate of 92.3%.

The **transverse preputial island flap (TPIF)** employs preputial skin for formation of a tubularized neourethra transferred to the ventrum for hypospadias repair as separate components of the repair; the inner prepuce with its vascular pedicle for the neourethra is separated from and followed by transfer of the longitudinally split outer prepuce as skin cover. The TPIF described, named, and popularized by Duckett (1980) is often referred to as the "Duckett tube" and is perhaps the most frequently performed one-stage tubularized repair for proximal hypospadias.

The TPIF technique (Fig. 125–16) begins with placement of fine traction sutures in the glans and prepuce. A ventral midline longitudinal incision is marked from the urethral meatus to the distal circumcising incision. The urethral meatus is marked circumferentially for planned incision as well. The skin is incised, the penile shaft is degloved, and the penis is assessed for curvature. **Curvature that persists after release of skin and tethering subcutaneous tissues may require division of the urethral plate. Curvature is then reassessed and, if necessary, corrected with a ventral orthoplasty technique. After orthoplasty, a transversely oriented rectangle of preputial skin is marked at a length equal to the distance from the urethral meatus to the glans tip and approximately 15 mm in width.** Once dissected from the outer layer of prepuce and dorsal penile skin, the pedicled inner prepuce is tubularized over a 6-Fr Silastic catheter to form the neourethra. The anastomosis is performed in a running, subcuticular first layer closure with fine polyglactin suture and a second layer with inverting Lembert technique using the same material. The last 0.5 to 1.0 cm of the anastomosis is closed with a simple interrupted technique to allow future tailoring of the distal neourethral length.

The neourethra is transferred to the penile ventrum on a tension-free pedicle and oriented such that the sutured line of anastomosis is facing the ventral surface of the corpora cavernosa after anastomosis. The dorsal aspect of the native meatus, before anastomosis with the neourethra, is fixed with simple interrupted sutures to the ventrum of the corpora cavernosa to stabilize the anastomosis. Additionally, a small

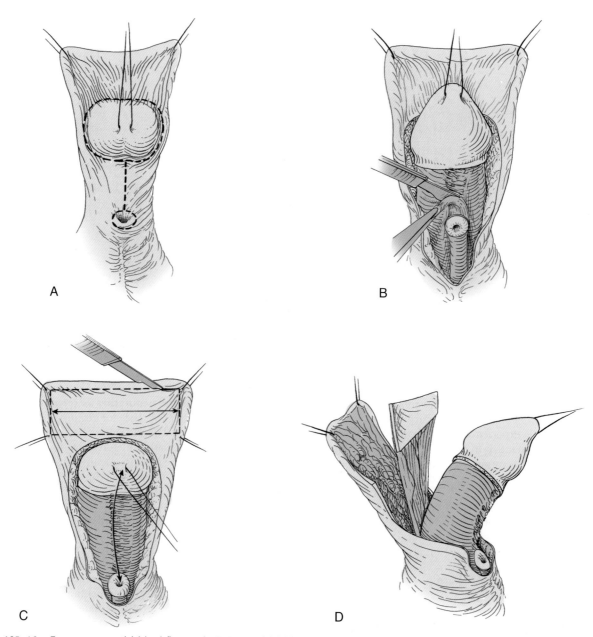

Figure 125–16. Transverse preputial island flap repair. **A,** Proposed initial incisions for proximal shaft/penoscrotal hypospadias. **B,** Release of tethering urethral plate and "dropping" of meatus proximally. **C,** Incision of preputial skin of appropriate dimensions for length of defect and width for desired luminal diameter. **D,** Harvested transverse preputial island flap.

Continued

circular incision is marked in the glans penis at the proposed site for the neomeatus. **A wide channel is fashioned, initially with tenotomy scissors and finally to a No. 16 to No. 18 urethral sound caliber, to accommodate passage of the distal neourethra. A core of glans tissue is excised to achieve sufficient channel caliber. Alternatively, the glans may be deeply incised in the midline to allow advancement of the neourethra and proper placement of the meatus.** The proximal anastomosis is performed first with two separate sutures and a running, locking full-thickness technique. The distal extent of the neourethra is then passed through the glans channel, and the meatus is trimmed, if necessary, to appropriate length and fixed to the glans with fine polyglactin

simple interrupted suture. **The inferolateral border of the pedicle is advanced over the neourethra and then covered by a tunica vaginalis flap.** Securing of the Silastic catheter and skin closure complete the repair. Patel and coworkers (2005) have recommended transfer of the preputial flap and proximal anastomosis before tubularization as a means of decreasing stricture and diverticulum rate.

In a comparison of techniques for the repair of proximal hypospadias, Wiener and colleagues (1997) reported similar results in overall complication rate (31% vs. 36%) and fistula rate (14% vs. 17%) for the OIF when compared with the TPIF. Baskin and colleagues reported similar fistula rates for the OIF and TPIF, 10% vs. 15%, respectively, and postulated that the

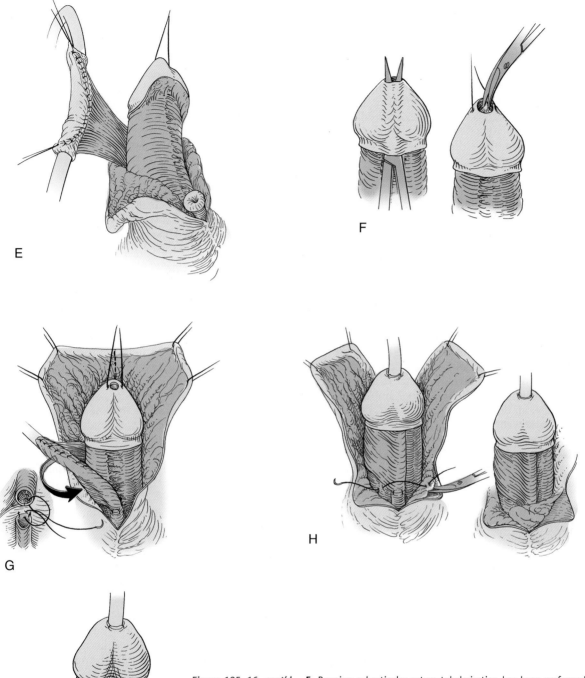

Figure 125–16, cont'd. **E,** Running subcuticular suture tubularization has been performed over a Silastic catheter to be followed by a second-layer running Lembert suture. **F,** Generous glans channel is fashioned for neourethral passage. A core of glans tissue is excised to achieve sufficient caliber. **G,** Native urethral meatus is fixed to corpora cavernosa before performing proximal anastomosis with the neourethra. **H,** Dartos tissue coverage of anastomosis. **I,** Maturation of neourethral meatus and penile shaft skin coverage have been completed. (Reprinted from Atala A, Retik AB: Hypospadias. In Libertino JA [ed]: Reconstructive Urologic Surgery, 3rd ed. St. Louis, Mosby–Year Book, 1998, p 467.)

lower fistula rate for the OIF may be due to improved healing of the repair with preservation of the spongiosa-supported urethral plate (Baskin et al, 1994).

Others

A modification of the TPIF incorporates tubularization of proximal nonhirsute interscrotal tissue as an adjunct to the TPIF (Glassberg, 1987). Tubularization of the nonhirsute interscrotal tissue has been described previously as an adjunct to distal skin graft urethroplasty (Devine and Horton, 1977). In some cases, where anatomy necessitates division of the urethral plate, the current authors have performed a similar modification with incorporation of a longitudinal midline incision and tubularization of the urethral plate, proximally, with repair of the remaining distal defect using the TPIF technique. These modifications, in effect, decrease the length of defect requiring repair with the TPIF technique.

A one-stage urethroplasty with the "parameatal foreskin flap" technique described for repair of proximal hypospadias with or without penoscrotal transposition has been promoted as having universal applicability and is depicted in Figure 125–17 (Koyanagi et al, 1994). This technique has also been referred to as the meatal based "manta-wing flap" and has similarities to the "clergyman's stole" (strip of prepuce in continuity with longitudinal, ventral penile skin strips) technique described by Russell in 1900. Complication rates range from 20% to 50% for this procedure (Koyanagi et al, 1994; Glassberg et al, 1998; Hayashi et al, 2001; DeFoor and Wacksman, 2003). Modifications described by Hayashi and coworkers (2001) include preservation of all dartos (pedicle) tissue that provides vascular support with buttonhole transfer to the ventrum and elimination of longitudinal incision in the distal extent of the preputial collar. Radical bulbar dissection is a rapid adjunctive technique applicable to all proximal hypospadias (Baker et al, 2000). According to the authors, benefits realized by this technique include release of proximal tethering of the scrotum and subcutaneous fibrous bands resulting in correction of curvature in some and at times decreased severity of the hypospadias requiring repair.

Two-Stage Repairs

Because the majority of hypospadias can be repaired with a one-stage procedure, the use of two-stage techniques for repair of posterior hypospadias is controversial. In the setting of scrotal or perineal hypospadias, severe curvature, and a small penis, we prefer to perform a two-stage repair as described by Retik and colleagues (1994a, 1996). In a series of 58 repairs performed with this two-stage technique, a urethrocutaneous fistula developed in 3 patients (5.2%) postoperatively.

At the *first stage*, orthoplasty is performed and the prepuce is repositioned ventrally (Fig. 125–18). Depending on the severity of penile curvature, resection of ventral tethering tissue and division of the urethral plate, with dropping of the urethral meatus proximally, may not be sufficient for correction. Orthoplasty may be performed with one of several techniques. We prefer to use an interposition dermal graft inlay after transverse incision of the corpora cavernosa directly at the apex of maximal concave curvature. When flat, the glans penis is deeply incised in the ventral midline distally to the point of the eventual neomeatus. For those with a deep glanular groove, longitudinal incisions may be placed lateral to the groove, bilaterally. Another option would be to leave the glans intact, cover the ventral shaft with approximation of prepuce to the subcoronal circumcising incision, and perform TIP urethroplasty for the distal aspect of the neourethra at the second stage of the repair.

A midline longitudinal incision is made in the preputial and dorsal distal penile shaft skin. Each half is brought around its respective lateral aspect of the penis and anastomosed with fine, interrupted absorbable suture to the penile ventrum beginning at the distal apex of the glans incision. Identical suture is placed with simple interrupted full-thickness technique to approximate the transferred skin in the ventral midline. Simple interrupted sutures approximate transferred skin and native meatus proximally. In some cases, it may take all of the preputial skin to cover the ventral aspect of the liberated and straightened shaft. This step prepares well-vascularized tissue to be used for neourethral formation (tubularization) at the second stage.

The *second stage* is performed 6 months or more after completion of the first stage. The primary goal of the second stage of the procedure is to create a neourethra that bridges the defect between the hypospadiac meatus and the tip of the penis. Tubularization of local skin in Thiersch-Duplay fashion is the preferred technique. Tissue to be used for neourethral construction is marked on the ventral aspect of the penis at a width of approximately 15 mm, centered on the midline. Once incised, the lateral edges of this tissue are dissected only minimally toward the midline so as preserve the vascular supply to the neourethra. Second-layer neourethral coverage is either with local subcutaneous tissues or a tunica vaginalis flap. Subcutaneous tissues and penile skin are approximated in the ventral midline with "pullout" running sutures of 4-0 nylon. Urinary diversion is with either urethral and/or suprapubic catheter for 7 to 10 days postoperatively. Others have described modification of the two-stage technique (Gershbaum et al, 2002; Cheng et al, 2003).

Free Graft for Neourethral Formation

Various techniques incorporating the use of free skin, bladder, or buccal mucosa graft alone or in combination have also been described for the repair of proximal hypospadias. These include graft of non–hair-bearing skin (genital or extragenital) (Hendren and Horton, 1988; Hendren and Keating, 1988), bladder mucosa (Hendren and Reda, 1986; Baskin and Duckett, 1994b), and buccal mucosa (Bürger et al, 1992; Dessanti et al, 1992; Baskin and Duckett 1994b, 1995), which may be used alone or in combination (Ransley et al, 1987; Retik, 1996).

The use of skin for urethroplasty was first described by Nové-Josserand in 1897 and later in 1914. In 1941, Humby used tubularized skin as a free graft for primary hypospadias repair in 12 patients, and in 1961 Devine and Horton popularized use of the tubularized skin graft with their description of a preputial, free graft tubularized neourethra in 1961. Bracka (1995a, 1995b) has continued to be a proponent of the skin graft tube as the second stage of a universally applicable two-stage technique for hypospadias repair.

The use of bladder mucosa was first reported by Memmelaar in 1947 and later by others (Marshall and Spellman, 1955; Hendren and Reda, 1986) for primary repair

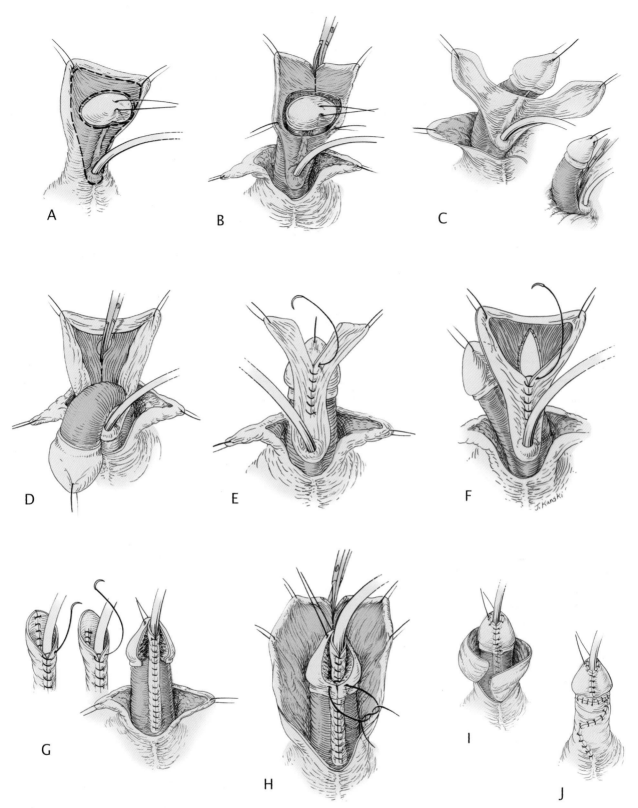

Figure 125–17. Koyanagi repair. **A,** Proposed incisions are marked. The first is a distal circumferential incision 5 mm proximal and parallel to the corona of the glans and includes division of the urethral plate. The second encompasses the perimeter of the tissue to be tubularized as the neourethra. Note stay sutures placed in the glans and dorsal hood foreskin. **B,** Both the distal circumferential and perimeter incisions have been made and the proximal shaft skin has been degloved. Incision of the dorsal midline longitudinal marking is in progress. **C,** The latter incision creates two "wings" that are brought around either side of the penile shaft to the ventrum. *Inset* depicts freeing of proximal urethral plate and urethra. Fibrotic corpus spongiosum is excised, and curvature is assessed and treated as needed. **D,** Alternatively, the "neourethral" epithelial and subcutaneous tissue collar is left intact and passed to the ventrum via a "buttonhole" in the dartos fascia (Hayashi et al, 2001). **E,** Dorsal running suture line in progress for tubularization of the neourethra. **F,** Closure of dorsal wall with Hayashi modification. **G,** Ventral suture is placed in similar fashion to complete tubularization of the neourethra. In the penis with a deep glanular groove glans, wings are formed and the neourethra is matured at the glans tip with simple interrupted sutures. Alternatively, with a shallow groove, the neourethra may be passed to the tip through a glans tunnel (see Fig. 125–16F). Consider tunica vaginalis second layer coverage (see Fig. 125–8). **H,** The glans is approximated in the ventral midline in several layers to cover and support the distal neourethra. **I,** Dorsal penile shaft skin has been incised longitudinally in the midline creating Byar's skin flaps for skin coverage. **J,** Skin flaps are approximated to the coronal cuff and in the midline as shown here, or as a Z-plasty.

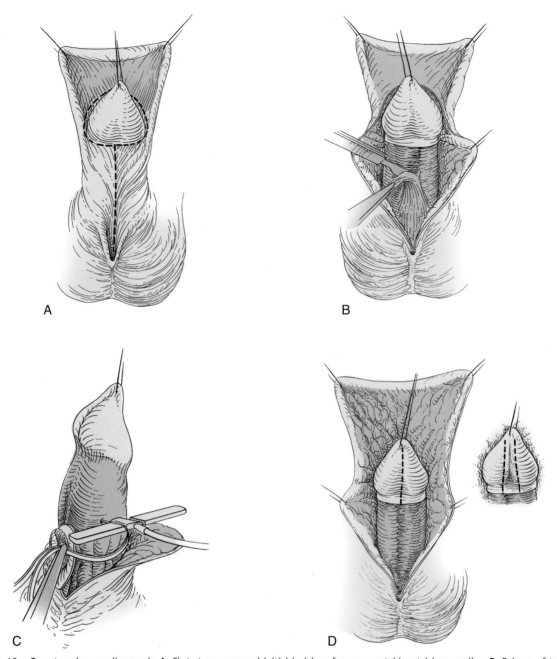

Figure 125–18. Two-stage hypospadias repair. **A,** First stage: proposed initial incisions for penoscrotal/scrotal hypospadias. **B,** Release of tethering ure-thral plate and "dropping" of meatus proximally. **C,** Curvature is assessed with artificial erection. **D,** Either midline incision or longitudinal incisions on either side of a deep glanular groove are placed in the glans. *Continued*

of severe hypospadias in cases with a paucity of local tissue. However, protruding mucosa at the neomeatus resulted in a significant reoperation rate for revision at that site. Unlike bladder mucosa, which tends to shrink and requires a greater size of tissue at harvest relative to the defect to be repaired, buccal mucosa may be harvested in a 1:1 ratio (Bürger et al, 1992; Dessanti et al, 1992; Baskin and Duckett, 1994b, Baskin and Duckett, 1995). **This characteristic of buccal mucosa is secondary to a lamina propria rich with vascularity. As with all free grafts, a well-vascularized graft host bed is a necessity for successful take via the processes of imbibition and inosculation.**

Bladder mucosa **is harvested by distending the bladder with saline and dissecting the detrusor muscle off of the underlying mucosa** (Fig. 125–19). A rectangular donor site is marked to a size 10% greater than the size of the defect to be repaired. **As part of a composite repair, tubularized skin or buccal mucosa may be added to the distal extent of the tubu-larized bladder mucosa graft to decrease the risk of meatal complications. The length of bladder mucosa graft har-vested should equal that of the defect when used in a com-posite repair.** The two grafts are approximated with two running sutures of 6-0 or 7-0 polyglactin. The composite graft is then tubularized over a Silastic catheter using a running,

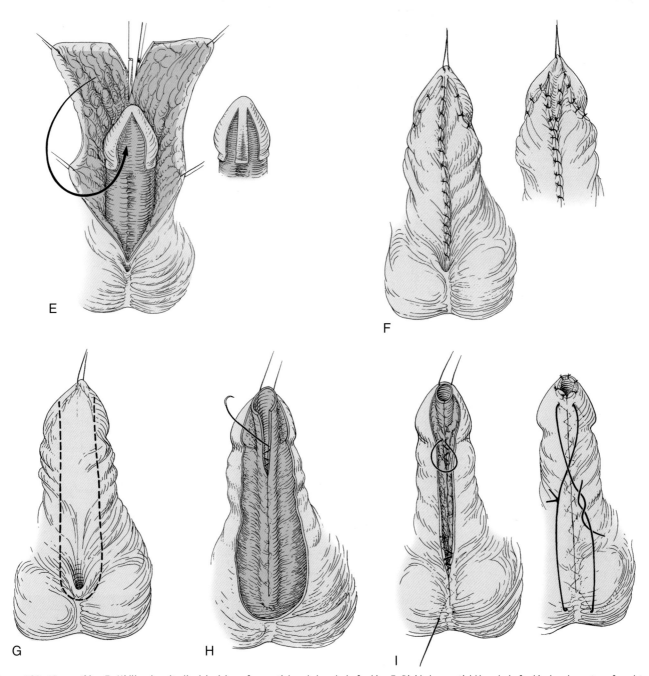

Figure 125–18, cont'd. **E,** Midline longitudinal incision of preputial and dorsal shaft skin. **F,** Divided preputial/dorsal shaft skin has been transferred to the penile ventrum. **G,** Second stage: line of incision for Thiersch-Duplay tubularization. **H,** Running subcuticular closure of neourethra. **I,** The meatus is secured to the glans, the subcutaneous tissues approximated, and the skin closed with nylon suture, the ends of which are tied to each other. (Reprinted from Retik AB: Proximal hypospadias. In Marshall FF [ed]: Textbook of Operative Urology. Philadelphia, WB Saunders, 1996.)

locking technique. The proximal anastomosis is performed with two running, locking sutures of fine polyglactin, and the neomeatus is matured with simple, interrupted, fine absorbable suture. **A second layer of neourethral coverage is provided either by a dorsal subcutaneous flap or by tunica vaginalis.** The bladder is drained with a suprapubic catheter, and the repair is stented for 7 to 10 days postoperatively with a Silastic catheter. **Immobilization of the patient in the early postoperative period is crucial to graft survival.**

The technique for use of *buccal mucosa* in hypospadias repair begins with general anesthetic induction and *naso-*

tracheal intubation. A self-retaining retractor is then placed in the oral cavity; and **with care taken to avoid Stensen's duct, an appropriate-sized graft is marked on the mucosa of the cheek and/or lip** (see Fig. 125–19). **Epinephrine (diluted 1:200,000 in 0.5% lidocaine) is injected submucosally, fine stay sutures are placed in the corners of the graft, and the graft is harvested with sharp dissection superficial to the buccinator muscle.** Buccal mucosal edges at the harvest site are approximated with 5-0 chromic catgut suture in a running simple fashion. The graft is defatted on a sterile cardboard scaffold and then tubularized in a manner similar to that for

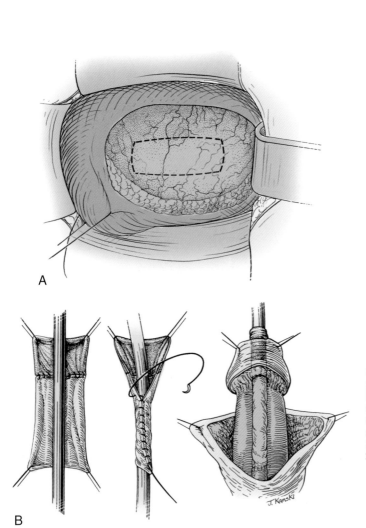

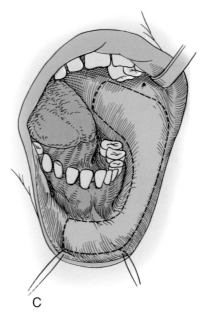

Figure 125–19. Bladder and buccal mucosa hypospadias repair. **A,** Proposed site of bladder mucosa harvest on anterior wall of saline-filled bladder after dissection of detrusor muscle. **B,** Buccal mucosa harvest site is marked with care taken to avoid Stensen's duct. **C,** Tubularization of bladder or buccal mucosa in combination with a full-thickness penile skin graft distally. (Reprinted from Retik AB: Proximal hypospadias. In Marshall FF [ed]: Textbook of Operative Urology. Philadelphia, WB Saunders, 1996.)

bladder mucosa. Proximal and meatal anastomoses and second-layer neourethral and skin coverage/closure are performed similarly as well. The repair is stented for 7 to 10 days postoperatively. Improved results are noted when buccal mucosa is used in an onlay fashion compared with a tubularized technique (Duckett et al, 1995; Ahmed and Gough, 1997). Long-term outcome of buccal mucosa has shown efficacy for this technique (Hensle et al, 2002; Dessanti et al, 2003; Fichtner et al, 2004).

COMPLICATIONS

Complications of hypospadias repair include bleeding/hematoma, meatal stenosis, urethrocutaneous fistula, urethral stricture, urethral diverticulum, wound infection, impaired healing, and breakdown of the repair (Duckett et al, 1980; Horton and Horton, 1988; Retik et al, 1988; Keating and Duckett, 1995). When reoperation is indicated, complications such as meatal stenosis, urethrocutaneous fistula, and urethral stricture can be repaired rather expeditiously, with appropriate timing. However, more serious complications involving

KEY POINTS: PRIMARY HYPOSPADIAS REPAIR

- The tubularized incised plate (TIP) urethroplasty is a popular technique that combines midline, longitudinal urethral plate incision and tubularization.

- The onlay island flap technique is ideal for middle hypospadias defects. This technique requires an intact urethral plate and correction of mild to moderate penile curvature, when indicated, with a dorsal plication technique.

- Some proximal defects with severe penile curvature may require division of the urethral plate and repair with a transverse preputial island flap (TPIF) technique.

- For the patient with proximal hypospadias, severe penile curvature, and a small penis, a two-stage approach to repair may be an excellent alternative.

either partial or complete breakdown of the hypospadias repair may require a major reconstructive effort. At times, this involves the task of performing a complete repair in the presence of less than optimal tissues and conditions. **In general, unless immediate reexploration is indicated for bleeding, infection, or débridement, reoperation for complications should not be performed less than 6 months after previous repair.**

Bleeding and Hematoma

Bleeding is the most common complication of hypospadias repair. This may require simple addition of a compressive dressing due to persistent oozing. At other times, significant postoperative bleeding may require exploration to identify and treat the source. Hematoma may form as a result of persistent bleeding and if large may require wound exploration and hematoma evacuation. Consequences of hematoma formation range from simple temporary cosmetic issues to wound or repair breakdown (Elbakry et al, 1998). **Patients with excessive bleeding and/or hematoma formation, particularly those requiring reoperation, should undergo evaluation for bleeding diathesis/dyscrasias** (Horton and Horton, 1988).

Meatal Stenosis

The complication of meatal stenosis is perhaps most commonly due to technical issues at the time of repair, such as fashioning of the urethral meatus with too narrow a lumen or performance of glanuloplasty too tightly. Urethral (meatal) dilation or meatotomy may be sufficient for the mildest forms of meatal stenosis. However, a more complex distal urethral stricture also involving the meatus may require a more extensive flap procedure (De Sy, 1984).

Urethrocutaneous Fistula

The suspicion of a urethrocutaneous fistula is often reported by a parent or caregiver. This can be confirmed on physical examination with or without voiding, or with retrograde injection of dye such as methylene blue either alone or with glycerin (Horton and Horton, 1988; Retik et al, 1988). Fistula may result from, or be associated with, distal stricture or meatal stenosis. Other risk factors include failure to invert all epithelial edges at urethroplasty, devitalization of tissue, or failure to add appropriate second-layer urethroplasty coverage. The latter of these, **second layer coverage of the neourethra, has been shown to significantly reduce the fistula rate as reported by several authors** (Smith, 1973; Belman, 1988; Retik et al, 1988; Churchill et al, 1996). Repair of urethrocutaneous fistula is optimized by the same principle (Davis, 1940; Cecil, 1946; Goldstein and Hensle, 1981; Retik et al, 1988; Elbakry, 2001a; Waterman et al, 2002; Landau et al, 2003; Richter et al, 2003; Santangelo et al, 2003). **At times, larger or multiple fistulas may require incision of the intact skin bridges and delayed repeat hypospadias repair.**

Infection

Infection is an uncommon complication of hypospadias repair. When suspected, culture, incision and drainage, and débridement when indicated are incorporated with appropriate antibiotic therapy. Severe infection may lead to breakdown of the entire repair.

Urethral Diverticulum

Although infrequent, urethral diverticulum formation may follow hypospadias repair. **Similar to urethrocutaneous fistula, urethral diverticula may be associated with distal stricture or meatal stenosis.** Zaontz and colleagues (1989) have described repair of this entity with circumferential skin incision, penile shaft skin degloving, diverticula excision, and urethral closure, followed by "pants over vest" subcutaneous tissue coverage of the repair, with excellent results. A similar technique has been described by others (Radojicic et al, 2004). For more extensive lesions, Aigen and colleagues (1987) described repair similar to that for megalourethra.

Balanitis Xerotica Obliterans

Balanitis xerotica obliterans (BXO) is a chronic inflammatory process of unknown etiology. BXO can arise spontaneously or may follow minor trauma or penile surgery such as circumcision or hypospadias repair or may complicate these surgeries (Gargollo et al, 2005). Kumar and Harris (1999) reported 8 patients with histologically proven BXO. Seven of the patients presented with difficult micturition, and meatal stenosis or neourethral stricture, at varying periods from 1 to 8 years after primary hypospadias repair. These authors recommended use of bladder or buccal mucosal free grafts for repair of such cases, to improve on an alarming 50% complication rate with the use of skin grafts for urethroplasty. Venn and Mundy (1998) have described similar techniques for repair in this difficult setting.

Recurrent Penile Curvature

Late-onset, recurrent curvature has been described as a complication of orthoplasty alone or in conjunction with hypospadias repair. Farkas (1967) reported that a second operation (and sometimes more) was required in approximately 50% of cases of hypospadias and initial severe curvature. In a more contemporary report, **late-onset curvature in 22 patients with initial proximal penile or penoscrotal hypospadias and successful orthoplasty was believed to be due equally to either extensive fibrosis of the reconstructed urethra, corporeal disproportion, or both** (Vandersteen and Husmann, 1998). Soergel and coworkers (2003) and others have recommended against the use of four-layer small intestinal submucosa because of a high rate of recurrent penile curvature.

Urethral Stricture

Urethral stricture other than meatal stenosis may be a complication of proximal hypospadias repair. The proximal anastomotic site of a tubularized repair such as the TPIF appears to be particularly at risk. **This type of stricture may be successfully treated with less invasive means such as endoscopic cold knife urethrotomy** (Scherz et al, 1988). Hsiao and coworkers (2003) reported a success rate of only 50% in 20 patients who underwent direct vision internal urethrotomy for urethral stricture after hypospadias repair. The authors suggested that the 50% success rate should not deter the surgeon from a single attempt to treat a stricture with this technique. We would reserve this for a short, film-like stricture. **A more extensive stricture may warrant patch with free graft or, preferably, vascularized flap urethroplasty with either of these two techniques achieving greater success when used as an onlay versus a tubularized segment.** In a thorough review of anterior urethral stricture repair techniques, Wessells and McAninch (1998) reported near-identical overall success rates of approximately 85% for both free graft and pedicled skin flap methods. However, these authors noted that many of the reports reviewed did not specifically state the site of repair.

Others have discussed the usefulness of mucosal grafts for treatment of urethral stricture disease (Baskin and Duckett, 1994b; Ahmed and Gough, 1997). In 1989, a two-stage mesh-graft urethroplasty using split-thickness skin was described for application in the absence of available pedicled flap tissue or an appropriate graft bed (Wessells and McAninch, 1998; Schreiter and Noll, 1989). The mesh-graft technique would be useful in those instances when all other options have failed.

Intraurethral Hair Growth

Intraurethral hair growth is an uncommon complication of hypospadias repair and occurs when hair-bearing skin is incorporated into the repair either as transferred skin or tubularization of proximal penile or scrotal skin. Crain and coworkers (2003) have described laser hair ablation for management of this complication.

Repair Breakdown

Repair breakdown may occur secondary to devascularization of local tissues or flaps used in urethroplasty or other components of hypospadias repair. **Breakdown may also result from urethroplasty and/or approximation of the glans (glanuloplasty) under tension. Breakdown of the repair may also result from devitalized tissue due to excessive use of electrocautery, unidentified vascular pedicle injury during repair, or hematoma formation** (Elbakry et al, 1998). Regardless of the etiology, repair breakdown may require débridement of devascularized, necrotic tissue before repair (Horton and Horton, 1988).

Hypospadias Cripples

Horton and Devine (1970) **used the term** *hypospadias cripple* **to describe the patient who has undergone multiple, unsuccessful hypospadias repair attempts, with significant resultant penile deformity. These patients represent perhaps the most perplexing of hypospadias repair complications in that they require extensive repair amid scarred and devitalized tissue** (Gershbaum et al, 2002; Amukele et al, 2003). Options for the repair of the hypospadias cripple are discussed in the next section.

KEY POINTS: COMPLICATIONS

- Bleeding/persistent oozing from the repair site is the most common complication of hypospadias repair.

- A well-vascularized second layer of tissue coverage placed over the neourethral suture line is perhaps the single most important step in decreasing the risk of urethrocutaneous fistula.

- Clinically significant stricture of the neourethral may occur at the meatus (meatal stenosis) or at the proximal anastomotic site of the repair—such as with use of the TPIF technique.

REOPERATIVE HYPOSPADIAS REPAIR
General Principles

In general, attempts at reoperative hypospadias surgery should not be undertaken less than 6 months after the previous failure. Certainly, no attempt at repair should be entertained until all edema, infection, and/or inflammation has resolved and healing is complete. Radiographic imaging with **retrograde urethrogram and/or voiding cystourethrogram for complete urethral visualization may be necessary in complex reoperative hypospadias** cases as an important aspect of preparation for definitive repair. Inspection of available tissue to determine whether adequate local tissue exists, versus the need for an extragenital tissue graft, will significantly impact and dictate repair options. This decision-making process is critical to achieving a successful result.

Specific Techniques
Immediately Adjacent or Local Tissue Flap

When possible, the use of immediately adjacent or local pedicled, well-vascularized tissue is preferred for reoperative hypospadias surgery. This may be in the form of a simple tubularization procedure or a modification such as the TIP urethroplasty. The TIP urethroplasty technique is performed similarly for previously operated patients as for primary repair (see Fig. 125–12). The use of TIP urethroplasty in reoperative hypospadias repair was reported in a multicenter experience (Snodgrass et al, 1996). **Based, in part, on a 95% success rate for primary hypospadias repair, we have employed TIP urethroplasty for reoperative hypospadias. Results are similar to that for primary repair when all components of the TIP technique, as described for primary repair, are incorporated** (Borer et al, 2001; Borer and Retik, 2002). Several institutions have reported excellent success rates with TIP urethroplasty in reoperative hypospadias (Shanberg et al, 2001; Yang et al, 2001; Elbakry 2002; Borer and Retik, 2002; El-Sherbiny et al, 2004; Nguyen and Snodgrass, 2004). Complications consisted mostly of urethrocutaneous fistulas and complication rates had a narrow range among these institutions, with rates ranging from 15% of patients to 28% of patients.

For reoperative hypospadias repair, advantages of the TIP urethroplasty include use of local, usually supple tissue with well-established vascularity for urethroplasty and skin

coverage, as well as a cosmetically superior result. The TIP urethroplasty technique is ideal for repair after failed Mathieu, OIF, and tubularization procedures because, theoretically, the native vascularity of the urethral plate has not been altered. **The absence of preputial skin in reoperative cases makes TIP urethroplasty an ideal option because additional skin flaps are not necessary for urethroplasty or for skin coverage because mobilized ventral penile shaft skin is usually sufficient for the latter.**

Based on issues of tissue availability, it has been our experience that the OIF is rarely a feasible option in reoperative hypospadias repair. However, this impression regarding the use of the OIF in reoperative repair is not universal. **In a recent report of reoperative repair using Mathieu and OIF techniques, secondary complications occurred in 24% and 14% of reoperative surgeries performed with these techniques, respectively** (Simmons et al, 1999). Emir and Erol (2003) reported a 25% complication rate in 55 patients who underwent reoperation with the Mathieu technique. With similar concerns regarding skin coverage and a complication rate of 30% in reoperative cases (Koff et al, 1994), we would not recommend the modified Barcat technique as a viable alternative in such cases. The Duckett tube has been used in reoperative hypospadias with a complication rate of 24% (5 of 21 patients), including distal fistula, proximal diverticula, and stenosis of the meatus and proximal anastomosis (Soutis et al, 2003). Johanssen (1953) described a useful two-stage technique for repair of severe urethral stricture after hypospadias repair.

Joseph and Perez (1999) have reported the use of the **tunica vaginalis flap** as an onlay salvage procedure after multiple previously failed hypospadias repairs in 10 boys and 1 adult male. **This option for reoperative hypospadias has fallen into disfavor because of a complication rate of 60% for both meatal stenosis and urethral stricture.** A tubularized technique with tunica vaginalis tissue was previously described in several patients (Snow and Cartwright, 1992).

Free Graft with Local or Extragenital Tissue

Horton and Devine (1970) described the use of a tubularized free skin graft urethroplasty in patients with multiple, previously failed hypospadias repairs. This nonhirsute skin graft may be from a genital or extragenital source. **Similarly, and perhaps for use in more severe reoperative cases, free graft bladder mucosa** (Baskin and Duckett, 1994b), **buccal mucosa ("dry" or "wet," onlay or tubularized)** (Baskin and Duckett, 1994b; Duckett et al, 1995; Ahmed and Gough, 1997; Caldamone et al, 1998), **or a combination of the above may be used** (Ransley et al, 1987; Retik, 1996).

It appears that for the skin-deficient hypospadias requiring reoperation, buccal mucosa has become the preferred material for reconstruction (Bracka, 2002). Buccal mucosa as a "dry" onlay (first stage of a planned two-stage repair) followed by tubularization at the second-stage repair for reoperative hypospadias is becoming an attractive alternative. Snodgrass and Elmore (2004) reported 25 patients who underwent stage 1 of the repair with complete graft take in 22 (88%) cases. Three had focal scarring or graft contracture successfully "patched" before tubularization (stage 2). At publication, 20 patients had undergone stage 2 with fistula in 1 of 18 when

dartos or tunica vaginalis second-layer coverage was used, with partial glans dehiscence in 4 boys. Fichtner and coworkers (2004) reported a complication rate of 24% (12 of 49 patients) using buccal mucosa strictly as an onlay method. In the 49 cases with available follow-up after 5 years, 9 of the 12 complications occurred within the first postoperative year including two graft contractures. Hensle and coworkers (2002) reported use of buccal mucosa as either a tube graft in 12 patients or as an onlay graft in 35 patients requiring complex urethroplasty. The overall complication rate was 32% with rates of 50% for free tube grafts and 20% for onlay grafts. Major complications of graft contracture or slough were seen in 6 patients, 4 when buccal mucosa was used as a tube and 4 in the authors' early experience (first 10 cases) (Hensle et al, 2002). Buccal mucosa has also been used in adult reoperation urethroplasty for multiple indications (Andrich and Mundy, 2001). Free graft of bladder mucosa has also been used for successful repair in complex reoperative cases (Mollard et al, 1989).

Split-thickness mesh skin graft as first stage, followed by tubularization as second stage, may be a last resort for the hypospadias cripple in whom multiple previous attempts at repair have failed (Schreiter and Noll, 1989). Ehrlich and Alter (1996) have described the use of split-thickness skin graft and tunica vaginalis flaps for reoperative hypospadias. With the use of a two-stage procedure, 10 patients with failed hypospadias repair(s) were treated by a varied combination of split-thickness mesh graft urethroplasty and tunica vaginalis flap. A tunica vaginalis flap was placed as a bed for the mesh graft in 3 patients. Tunica vaginalis flaps were also used as an intermediate layer during stage 2 of the repair. No strictures or fistulas occurred in 8 patients. Two patients await second stage of repair after successful placement of the mesh graft. The combination of split-thickness mesh graft urethroplasty and a tunica vaginalis flap appears to achieve success in the difficult patient with complex hypospadias subsequent to multiple failed repairs.

It is predicted that tissue engineered constructs for urethral replacement may have a major impact on reoperative hypospadias repair in the future (Atala et al, 1999). Intestinal free flap urethroplasty has also been described for use in reoperative hypospadias (Bales et al, 2002).

KEY POINTS: REOPERATIVE HYPOSPADIAS REPAIR

- As a general rule, reoperation for failed hypospadias repair should not be attempted less than 6 months after failure.

- Provided sufficient penile tissue of appropriate quality is available, several techniques applicable to primary repair may also be used for reoperation.

- Multiple previous failures of hypospadias repair in a patient may be best treated with a 2-stage technique that, at times, incorporates extragenital skin or buccal mucosa.

LONG-TERM FOLLOW-UP
Gender Identity Issues

Sandberg and colleagues (1995) studied gender-role behavior of middle childhood boys (175 boys aged 6 to 10 years of age) with hypospadias. Parents completed standardized questionnaires regarding their son's behavior. Both questionnaires, the Child Behavior and Attitude Questionnaire and the Child Game Participation Questionnaire, may help to differentiate between gender-typical boys and boys with gender-identity disorders. **Hypospadias subjects did not show consistent differences from a community control group, and the severity of hypospadias was unrelated to gender-role behavior.** A greater number of hospitalizations were associated with increased gender-atypical behavior, but overall **it was concluded that hypospadias and possible associated "hypoandrogenization" did not interfere with development of gender-typical masculine behavior.**

Eberle and colleagues (1993) reported "satisfactory" results in two thirds of the 42 patients after childhood posterior hypospadias repair available for long-term follow-up. However, there were 13 patients who at follow-up still presented with complex sexual ambiguity. In 6 of these patients, androgen receptor defects were detected by means of biochemical as well as molecular-biologic investigations. **These authors emphasized the importance of androgen metabolism for male sexual development and underline the necessity of careful evaluation in children with posterior hypospadias.**

Patient Satisfaction
Cosmesis

Mureau and colleagues (1995a, 1995b) studied children and adolescents and men with previous hypospadias repair. **Although many of the children and adolescents (39%) desired functional and/or cosmetic penile improvement, they were reluctant to seek advice for these and other issues and, therefore, should be observed through adolescence** (Mureau et al, 1995a). Similarly, adult hypospadias patients reported a more negative genital appraisal than comparison subjects and 37% desired functional or cosmetic penile improvement (Mureau et al, 1995b).

Psychosexual Issues

Mureau and colleagues (1995a) studied psychosexual adjustment of children and adolescents. Relative to "comparison" subjects, 116 boys aged 9 to 18 years had a more negative genital appraisal, and anticipated more ridicule by a partner because of penile appearance than comparison subjects, but sexual adjustment did not differ. The surgical procedures, the number of operations, or the age at final surgery did not significantly impact outcome. Mureau and colleagues (1995b, 1997) also evaluated psychosexual adjustment, sexual functioning, and genital appraisal in adult (≥18 years of age) hypospadias patients. A total of 73 hypospadias patients and 50 comparison subjects received a semi-structured interview. **More hypospadias patients (32.8%) than comparison subjects (12.8%) had been inhibited in seeking sexual contacts. The severity of hypospadias negatively affected genital appraisal. Patient age**

at final operation positively correlated with sociosexual development. The majority of patients experienced a normal adult sex life but were reluctant to seek advice for problems. Several authors have reviewed this subject (Woodhouse, 1994; Bracka, 1999; Mieusset and Soulie, 2005).

Functional Issues
Uroflow

Several authors have evaluated uroflowmetry parameters both in normal boys (Szabo and Fegyverneki, 1995; Gutierrez Segura, 1997) and in boys after hypospadias repair (Svensson and Berg, 1983; Garibay et al, 1995; Jayanthi et al, 1995; Malyon et al, 1997). **At some centers, this noninvasive study is a postoperative evaluation routine and has been of value in identifying asymptomatic urethral stricture in some patients** (Garibay et al, 1995). Jayanthi and colleagues included uroflowmetry data after TPIF hypospadias repair and after stricture and/or fistula repair and concluded that the neourethra was functionally equivalent to a normal urethra in most boys after the aforementioned repairs (Jayanthi et al, 1995). TIP urethroplasty has been evaluated by uroflowmetry. Hammouda and coworkers (2003) studied 48 boys and found that 33 had normal peak flow rate and 15 had low peak flow rate 6 months after repair. Of 21 patients with a mean follow-up of 1.8 years after TIP urethroplasty, flow rates were normal (>25th percentile) in 14 and equivocally obstructed in 4 and obstructed (<5th percentile) in 3 (Marte et al, 2001).

Sexual Function and Fertility

Several authors have reported relatively normal adult sexual function and fertility (Berg et al, 1981; Svensson and Berg, 1983; Woodhouse, 1994; Mureau et al, 1995b; Bracka 1999). Selection bias may influence these results because those with a less than optimal outcome or outlook may not wish to divulge such information and, therefore, may not be represented in these reports. Bubanj and coworkers (2004) concluded that sexual function of patients who underwent surgery for hypospadias in general is not affected. However, a difference in certain aspects of sexual behavior was noted in that patients with hypospadias were significantly less sexually active and had a smaller total number of sexual partners compared with control subjects and control subjects were significantly more completely satisfied with their sexual life. An extensive review of these issues is available (Mieusset and Soulie, 2005).

KEY POINTS: LONG-TERM FOLLOW-UP

■ Careful evaluation for underlying errors in androgen metabolism may have significant consequences and, when treatable, significant positive impact on long-term outcome in some individuals with severe hypospadias.

■ Several authors have reported relatively normal adult sexual function and fertility.

■ Noninvasive uroflow evaluation may help identify clinically silent, but significant urethral stricture. It may be the trend in uroflow velocity over time in an individual patient that is most helpful.

CURRENT TRENDS

It is clear that preservation of the urethral plate, if at all possible, has become a priority in current hypospadias repair. This, in part, explains the popularity and increasing indications for use of several tubularization and onlay techniques with the goal being completion of repair in a single-stage whenever possible. For cases of hypospadias with severe curvature it is clear that the use of small intestinal submucosa as an interposition graft is gaining in popularity (Kropp et al, 2002).

For a relatively wide range of hypospadias, the TIP urethroplasty has gained popularity, becoming the technique of choice for both primary and reoperative middle and anterior hypospadias repair at our institution (Borer et al, 2001) and touted as the ideal repair for distal hypospadias by others (Decter and Franzoni, 1999). **As the use of TIP urethroplasty for reoperative repair increases, perhaps the need for extragenital tissue use in this setting will decrease.**

Many, including its originators, have favored the OIF technique for a wide and increasing range of hypospadias. In 1994, Baskin and colleagues reported use of the OIF in 374 or 33% of the total hypospadias repairs during a 5-year period. This represented an increase from 10% of the total repairs over an immediately preceding 5-year period. The decreased fistula rate relative to the TPIF was believed to be due to improved healing of the repair with preservation of the spongiosa-supported urethral plate. **The current preference for onlay versus tubularized techniques, whenever possible, was predicted by Hodgson** (1993).

A variation of the OIF, the split prepuce in-situ onlay technique described by Rushton and Belman (1998), **has achieved excellent early results and has become the preferred technique for anterior hypospadias repair at some institutions** (Yerkes et al, 2000b). The OIF and several modifications are gaining popularity for repair of more proximal defects, complementing proven success over an already wide range of hypospadias. **This trend is supported by a comparison of results for proximal hypospadias repair using free grafts as an onlay versus a tube, with significantly higher proximal stricture rates for the latter** (Powell et al, 2000). **Transition away from the use of free grafts, toward increased use of pedicled, vascularized flaps has also been reported** (Winslow and Devine, 1996). It appears that for the skin deficient hypospadias requiring reoperation, buccal mucosa has become the preferred material for reconstruction (Bracka, 2002).

FUTURE CONCEPTS

To this point, detailed principles and techniques for treatment of hypospadias have been discussed. With regard to hypospadias repair, tissue used for urethroplasty is typically obtained from genital skin, extragenital skin, or mucosal grafts from either bladder or buccal origin. **Although, at times, the only viable option for repair, the use of extragenital donor tissue may increase the morbidity of the procedure and/or length of hospital stay for the patient. Ideally, a readily available and biocompatible alternative source of tissue would be helpful in this setting.**

Atala and colleagues (1999) have explored the use of a human cadaveric, bladder submucosal, collagen-based inert matrix as a potential substitute for use in hypospadias repair. In this preliminary report, four patients with failed previous repair(s), underwent urethroplasty with the collagen-based inert matrix material in an onlay fashion. Length of tissue used ranged from 5 to 15 cm, and all repairs were covered with a tunica vaginalis flap. One patient developed a urethrocutaneous fistula that was repaired using standard techniques. Postoperative urethrography and endoscopy showed a normal-appearing urethra in all patients. Although a preliminary report, the human cadaveric, bladder submucosal, collagen-based inert matrix material may have a specific role for use in more complex reoperative cases with insufficient local tissue. Ideally, this type of urethral tissue substitute would obviate the need for use of extragenital skin in the future. Novel methods of human skin transplantation may also improve the management of complex hypospadias in the future (Stern et al, 2004).

KEY POINT: FUTURE CONCEPTS

- Tissue-engineered constructs for urethral replacement may have a major impact on hypospadias repair in the future.

SUMMARY

Innovative concepts and techniques continue to emerge in the field of hypospadiology, and with time may herald improvements to even the most basic of principles necessary for successful hypospadias repair. Hypospadiologists must be cognizant of the general principles of repair, be well versed in several appropriate techniques for all levels of hypospadias, and, most importantly, be dedicated to meticulous and uncompromising surgical technique and patient care as they strive for perfection in this ever-flourishing field (Duckett, 1981b, 1995).

SUGGESTED READINGS

Aaronson IA, Cakmak MA, Key LL: Defects of the testosterone biosynthetic pathway in boys with hypospadias. J Urol 1997;157:1884-1888.

Albers N, Ulrichs C, Gluer S, et al: Etiologic classification of severe hypospadias: Implications for prognosis and management [see comments]. J Pediatr 1997;131:386-392.

Allen TD, Griffin JE: Endocrine studies in patients with advanced hypospadias. J Urol 1984;131:310-314.

KEY POINTS: CURRENT TRENDS

- When possible, single-stage repair with preservation of an intact urethral plate is the ideal approach to surgical management of hypospadias.

- Two-stage repair of hypospadias is optimal for the most severe hypospadias defects or for reoperation after multiple previous failures.

Amukele SA, Lee GW, Stock JA, et al: 20-year experience with iatrogenic penile injury. J Urol 2003;170:1691-1694.

Atala A, Guzman L, Retik AB: A novel inert collagen matrix for hypospadias repair. J Urol 1999;162:1148-1151.

Baskin LS, Duckett JW, Ueoka K, et al: Changing concepts of hypospadias curvature lead to more onlay island flap procedures. J Urol 1994;151:191-196.

Belman AB: De-epithelialized skin flap coverage in hypospadias repair. J Urol 1988;140:1273-1276.

Boisen K, Chellakooty M, Schmidt I, et al: Hypospadias in a cohort of 1072 Danish newborn boys: Prevalence and relationship to placental weight, anthropometrical measurements at birth, and reproductive hormone levels at 3 months of age. J Clin Endocrinol Metab 2005;90:4041-4046.

Borer JG, Bauer SB, Peters CA, et al: Tubularized incised plate urethroplasty: Expanded use in primary and repeat surgery for hypospadias. J Urol 2001;165:581-585.

Bracka A: A versatile two-stage hypospadias repair. Br J Plast Surg 1995b; 48:345-352.

Bracka A: Hypospadias repair: The two-stage alternative [see comments]. Br J Urol 1995a;76(Suppl 3):31-41.

Bracka A: Two-stage urethroplasty revisited. In Snodgrass W (ed): Dialogues in Pediatric Urology. Pearl River, NJ, William J. Miller Associates, 2002. vol 25, pp 7-8.

Bracka A: Sexuality after hypospadias repair. BJU Int 1999;83(Suppl 3):29-33.

Byars LT: Technique of consistently satisfactory repair of hypospadias. Surg Gynecol Obstet 1955;100:184-190.

Chalapathi G, Rao KL, Chowdhary SK, et al: Testosterone therapy in microphallic hypospadias: Topical or parenteral? J Pediatr Surg 2003;38: 221-223.

Chhibber AK, Perkins FM, Rabinowitz R, et al: Penile block timing for postoperative analgesia of hypospadias repair in children. J Urol 1997;158:1156-1159.

Dessanti A, Iannuccelli M, Ginesu G, et al: Reconstruction of hypospadias and epispadias with buccal mucosa free graft as primary surgery: More than 10 years of experience. J Urol 2003;170:1600-1602.

Duckett JW: Transverse preputial island flap technique for repair of severe hypospadias. Urol Clin North Am 1980;7:423-430.

Duckett JW, Kaplan GW, Woodard JR, et al: Panel: Complications of hypospadias repair. Urol Clin North Am 1980;7:443-454.

Duckett JW, Snyder HM: Meatal advancement and glanuloplasty hypospadias repair after 1,000 cases: Avoidance of meatal stenosis and regression. J Urol 1992;147:665-669.

Duplay LS: Sur le traitement chirurgical de l'hypospadias et de l'epispadias. Arch Gen Med 1880;5:257-276.

Erickson JD: Epidemiology of hypospadias. Adv Exp Med Biol 2004;545:25-29.

Griffin JE: Androgen resistance—the clinical and molecular spectrum. N Engl J Med 1992;326:611-618.

Hakim S, Merguerian PA, Rabinowitz R, et al: Outcome analysis of the modified Mathieu hypospadias repair: Comparison of stented and unstented repairs. J Urol 1996;156:836-838.

Hayashi Y, Kojima Y, Nakane A, et al: A strategy for repairing moderately severe hypospadias using onlay urethroplasty versus onlay-tube-onlay urethroplasty. Urology 2003;61:1019-1022; discussion 1022.

Hensle TW, Kearney MC, Bingham JB: Buccal mucosa grafts for hypospadias surgery: Long-term results. J Urol 2002;168:1734-1736; discussion 1736-1737.

Hensle TW, Tennenbaum SY, Reiley EA, et al: Hypospadias repair in adults: Adventures and misadventures. J Urol 2001;165:77-79.

Hauben DJ: The history of hypospadias. Acta Chir Plast 1984;26:196-199.

Hendren WH, Keating MA: Use of dermal graft and free urethral graft in penile reconstruction. J Urol 1988;140:1265-1269.

Jordan GH: Techniques of tissue handling and transfer. J Urol 1999b;162: 1213-1217.

Kaefer M, Diamond DA, Hendren WH, et al: The incidence of intersexuality in children with cryptorchidism and hypospadias: Stratification based on gonadal palpability and meatal position. J Urol 1999;162:1003-1006; discussion 1006-1007.

Kass E, Kogan SJ, Manley C et al: Timing of elective surgery on the genitalia of male children with particular reference to the risks, benefits, and psychological effects of surgery and anesthesia. American Academy of Pediatrics. Pediatrics 1996;97:590-594.

Kropp BP, Cheng EY, Pope JC, et al: Use of small intestinal submucosa for corporal body grafting in cases of severe penile curvature. J Urol 2002;168: 1742-1745; discussion 1745.

Landrigan P, Garg A, Droller DB: Assessing the effects of endocrine disruptors in the National Children's Study. Environ Health Perspect 2003; 111:1678-1682.

Manzoni G, Bracka A, Palminteri E, et al: Hypospadias surgery: When, what and by whom? BJU Int 2004;94:1188-1195.

Mieusset R, Soulie M: Hypospadias: Psychosocial, sexual, and reproductive consequences in adult life. J Androl 2005;26:163-168.

Morgan EA, Nguyen SB, Scott V, et al: Loss of Bmp7 and Fgf8 signaling in Hoxa13-mutant mice causes hypospadias. Development 2003;130:3095-3109.

Mureau MA, Slijper FM, Slob AK, et al: Psychosocial functioning of children, adolescents, and adults following hypospadias surgery: a comparative study. J Pediatr Psychol 1997;22:371-387.

Murphy LJT: The urethra. In Murphy LJT (ed): The History of Urology. Springfield, IL, Charles C Thomas, 1972, pp 453-481.

Patel RP, Shukla AR, Austin JC, et al: Modified tubularized transverse preputial island flap repair for severe proximal hypospadias. BJU Int 2005;95:901-904.

Paulozzi LJ, Erickson JD, Jackson RJ: Hypospadias trends in two US surveillance systems. Pediatrics 1997;100:831-834.

Petiot A, Perriton CL, Dickson C, et al: Development of the mammalian urethra is controlled by Fgfr2-IIIb. Development 2005;132:2441-2450.

Rajfer J, Walsh PC: The incidence of intersexuality in patients with hypospadias and cryptorchidism. J Urol 1976;116:769-770.

Retik AB, Borer JG: Hypospadias. In Walsh PC, Retik AB, Vaughan ED Jr, Wein AJ (eds): Campbell's Urology, 8th ed. Philadelphia, WB Saunders, 2002, vol 3, pp 2284-2333.

Retik AB, Keating M, Mandell J: Complications of hypospadias repair. Urol Clin North Am 1988;15:223-236.

Silver RI: Endocrine abnormalities in boys with hypospadias. Adv Exp Med Biol 2004;545:45-72.

Snodgrass W: Snodgrass technique for hypospadias repair. BJU Int 2005;95:683-693.

Snodgrass W, Elmore J: Initial experience with staged buccal graft (Bracka) hypospadias reoperations. J Urol 2004;172:1720-1724; discussion 1724.

Snodgrass W, Koyle M, Manzoni G, et al: Tubularized incised plate hypospadias repair: Results of a multicenter experience. J Urol 1996;156:839-841.

Snodgrass W, Lorenzo A: Tubularized incised-plate urethroplasty for proximal hypospadias. BJU Int 2002;89:90-93.

Soergel TM, Cain MP, Kaefer M, et al: Complications of small intestinal submucosa for corporal body grafting for proximal hypospadias. J Urol 2003;170:1577-1578; 1578-1579.

Sozubir S, Snodgrass W: A new algorithm for primary hypospadias repair based on tip urethroplasty. J Pediatr Surg 2003;38:1157-1161.

Smith ED: The history of hypospadias. Pediatr Surg Int 1997;12:81-85.

Sweet RA, Schrott HG, Kurland R, et al: Study of the incidence of hypospadias in Rochester, Minnesota, 1940-1970, and a case-control comparison of possible etiologic factors. Mayo Clin Proc 1974;49:52-58.

Thomas DF: Hypospadiology: Science and surgery. BJU Int 2004;93:470-473.

Woodhouse CR: The sexual and reproductive consequences of congenital genitourinary anomalies. J Urol 1994;152:645-651.

Yamada G, Satoh Y, Baskin LS, et al: Cellular and molecular mechanisms of development of the external genitalia. Differentiation 2003;71:445-460.

Yucel S, Liu W, Cordero D, et al: Anatomical studies of the fibroblast growth factor-10 mutant, Sonic Hedge Hog mutant and androgen receptor mutant mouse genital tubercle. Adv Exp Med Biol 2004b;545:123-148.

Zaontz MR: The GAP (glans approximation procedure) for glanular/coronal hypospadias. J Urol 1989;141:359-361.

Abnormalities of the Genitalia in Boys and Their Surgical Management

JACK S. ELDER, MD

Neonatal genital anomalies are common and may result from a disorder of sexual differentiation, genital differentiation, or genital growth. Many genital anomalies are associated with developmental abnormalities of other organ systems. **Although most genital deformities are recognized at birth, they may occasionally be detected in utero** (Vijayaraghavan et al, 2002; Pinette et al, 2003). For example, Cheikhelard and colleagues (2000) reported that in 43 cases in which a genital abnormality was identified by sonography at a mean gestational age of 29 weeks, the diagnosis was accurate in 34 (79%).

Recognition of normal embryology is essential to understanding the pathogenesis of genital anomalies. **In the male embryo, differentiation of the external genitalia occurs between weeks 9 and 13 of gestation and requires production of testosterone by the testes as well as conversion of testosterone to dihydrotestosterone under the enzymatic influence of 5α-reductase in the genital anlagen. Under the influence of dihydrotestosterone, the genital tubercle differentiates into the glans penis, the genital folds become the shaft of the penis, and the genital swellings migrate inferomedially, fusing in the midline to become the scrotum. In the female, because of the absence of testosterone and dihydrotestosterone, the genital tubercle develops passively into the clitoris, the genital folds become the labia minora, and the genital swellings become the labia majora.** The same changes may also occur in males with an abnormality in fetal testosterone production, a 5α-reductase deficiency, or an androgen receptor defect.

NORMAL GENITALIA AND ASSOCIATION WITH OTHER ABNORMALITIES

Fetal penile length increases significantly with gestational age, from a mean value of 6 mm at 16 weeks to 26.4 mm at 38 weeks (Johnson and Maxwell, 2000; Zalel et al, 2001). **In a normal, full-term male neonate, the penis is 3.5 ± 0.7 cm in stretched length and 1.1 ± 0.2 cm in diameter** (Table 126–1). At birth, the inhibitory effect of maternal estrogens on the fetal pituitary disappears; this change in the hormonal milieu causes a rebound surge in gonadotropins, which results in an early, transient surge in testosterone production by the Leydig cells that stimulates penile growth during the first 3 months of life. During the remainder of childhood, the penis grows much more slowly. In the mature male, stretched penile length ranges from 10 to 16.5 cm. Male adolescents often have concerns about penile size, and reference to published tables is generally reassuring (Lee and Reiter, 2002).

Normally, the penis has a fully developed foreskin and a median raphe on the shaft. However, in 10% of males, the raphe deviates, usually to the left side (Ben-Ari et al, 1985). Deviation of the raphe may be associated with penile torsion or chordee without hypospadias or may be an insignificant finding. However, in the newborn boy with deviation of the raphe, careful inspection of the glans is important. Congenital ventral or lateral curvature of the penis affects approximately 0.6% of male neonates (Yachia et al, 1993). A urethral deformity such as hypospadias or epispadias occurs in approximately 1 of every 250 males. At puberty, the penis and testes show predictable changes that are classified as Tanner stages (Table 126–2).

Congenital anomalies of the genitalia are often associated with abnormalities of other organ systems or are part of recognized syndromes (Table 126–3). **As many as 50% of children with congenital anorectal malformations also have an associated urologic malformation,** and the external genitalia are frequently involved. For example, in one series of boys with high imperforate anus, 29% had an abnormality of the external genitalia, including hypospadias, penile duplication,

Table 126–1. Stretched Penile Length (cm) in Normal Male Subjects

Age	Mean ± SD	Mean − 2.5 SD
Newborn, 30 wk gestation	2.5 ± 0.4	1.5
Newborn, 34 wk gestation	3.0 ± 0.4	2.0
0–5 mo	3.9 ± 0.8	1.9
6–12 mo	4.3 ± 0.8	2.3
1–2 yr	4.7 ± 0.8	2.6
2–3 yr	5.1 ± 0.9	2.9
3–4 yr	5.5 ± 0.9	3.3
4–5 yr	5.7 ± 0.9	3.5
5–6 yr	6.0 ± 0.9	3.8
6–7 yr	6.1 ± 0.9	3.9
7–8 yr	6.2 ± 1.0	3.7
8–9 yr	6.3 ± 1.0	3.8
9–10 yr	6.3 ± 1.0	3.8
10–11 yr	6.4 ± 1.1	3.7
Adult	13.3 ± 1.6	9.3

Data from Feldman KW, Smith DW: Fetal phallic growth and penile standards for newborn male infants. J Pediatr 1975;86:895; Schonfeld WA, Beebe GW: Normal growth and variation in the male genitalia from birth to maturity. J Urol 1987;30:554; Tuladhar R, Davis PG, Batch J, Doyle LW: Establishment of a normal range of penile length in preterm infants. J Paediatr Child Heath 1998;34:471.

Table 126–2. Tanner Classification of Sex Maturity Stages in Boys

Stage	Pubic Hair	Penis	Testes
1	None	Preadolescent	Preadolescent
2	Scanty, long	Slight enlargement; slightly pigmented	Enlarged scrotum, pink, texture altered
3	Darker, starts to curl, small amount	Longer	Larger
4	Resembles adult type but less in quantity; coarse, curly	Larger; glans and breadth increase in size	Larger, scrotum dark
5	Adult distribution, spread to medial surface of thighs	Adult size	Adult size

Modified from Tanner JM: Growth at Adolescence, 2nd ed. Oxford, England, Blackwell Scientific Publications, 1962.

Table 126–3. Male Genital Anomalies that Commonly Occur in Various Syndromes (Microphallus, Hypospadias, Ambiguous Genitalia, and Bifid Scrotum)

Anencephaly
Aniridia–Wilms' tumor association (WAGR syndrome)
Bladder exstrophy
Borjeson-Forssman-Lehman syndrome (microcephaly, mental retardation, large ears)
Carpenter's syndrome (acrocephaly, polydactyly and syndactyly of feet, congenital heart disease)
CHARGE association (*c*oloboma, *h*eart malformation, *a*tresia choanae, *r*etarded growth and development, *g*enital anomalies, *e*ar anomalies and/or deafness)
Cloacal syndrome
Fraser's syndrome (cryptophthalmos, mental retardation, ear anomalies)
Johanson-Blizzard syndrome (hypoplastic alae nasi, hypothyroidism, mental retardation, pancreatic insufficiency, deafness)
Meckel-Gruber syndrome (occipital encephalomeningocele, micrognathia, polydactyly, cystic renal dysplasia)
Noonan syndrome (webbed neck, pectus excavatum, pulmonic stenosis, short stature)
Opitz syndrome (hypertelorism, hypospadias, mild to moderate mental retardation)
Pallister-Hall syndrome (hypothalamic hamartoblastoma, hypopituitarism, imperforate anus)
Popliteal pterygium syndrome (popliteal web, cleft palate, lower lip pits)
Prader-Willi syndrome (hypotonia, obesity, small hands and feet, mild to moderate mental retardation)
Rapp-Hodgkin ectodermal dysplasia syndrome (hypohidrosis, oral clefts, dysplastic nails)
Rieger syndrome (iris dysplasia, hypodontia)
Robinow syndrome ("fetal face syndrome"; flat facial profile, hypertelorism, short forearms, thoracic hemivertebrae)
Schinzel-Giedian syndrome (growth deficiency, mental retardation, widely patent fontanelles, short forearms and legs, renal anomalies)
Smith-Lemli-Opitz syndrome (ptosis of eyelids, syndactyly of second and third toes, microcephaly, failure to thrive with short stature, mental retardation)
Triploidy syndrome
Trisomy 4p, 9p, 18, 20p, 21, 22, 9p, 10q, 11p, or 15q deficiency
XXY, XXXXY

From Jones KL: Smith's Recognizable Patterns of Human Malformation, 5th ed. Philadelphia, WB Saunders, 1997.

MALE GENITAL ANOMALIES
Penile Anomalies

Phimosis

At birth, there is normally a physiologic phimosis or inability to retract the foreskin because natural adhesions exist between the prepuce and the glans. During the first 3 to 4 years of life, as the penis grows, epithelial debris (smegma) accumulates under the prepuce, gradually separating the foreskin from the glans. Intermittent penile erections cause the foreskin to become completely retractable. **By 3 years of age, 90% of foreskins can be retracted, and less than 1% of males have phimosis by 17 years of age** (Oster, 1968).

Early forceful retraction of the foreskin generally is not recommended because recurrent adhesions between the de-epithelialized glans and foreskin may occur, and a cicatrix may form at the tip of the foreskin, causing secondary phimosis. However, **in boys older than 4 or 5 years and in those who**

micropenis, or scrotal deformity, whereas hypospadias was the primary genital abnormality in those with low imperforate anus (Hoekstra et al, 1983). Among boys with esophageal atresia or tracheoesophageal fistula, genital anomalies are also common, including hypospadias (6%), penile agenesis, penoscrotal transposition, scrotal malformation, and scrotal agenesis (1.5% each) (Berkhoff et al, 1989). Consequently, involvement of the urologist in the initial evaluation and long-term management of these patients is important. A guide to the early diagnosis and management of genital anomalies has been published by the American Academy of Pediatrics (AAP) Committee on Genetics and Sections on Endocrinology and Urology (2000).

develop balanitis or balanoposthitis, application of a topical corticosteroid cream (e.g., 0.1% triamcinolone) to the foreskin three or four times daily for 6 weeks loosens the phimotic ring in 70% to 80% of cases and usually allows the foreskin to be retracted manually (Yang et al, 2005). This effect is durable, but if phimosis recurs, another course of steroid cream is generally effective (Lund et al, 2005). In older boys with phimosis, balanitis xerotica obliterans is common, affecting approximately 40% (Kiss et al, 2005). Topical corticosteroids are beneficial even if the foreskin is involved with balanitis xerotica obliterans (Kiss et al, 2001). Formal lysis of adhesions is rarely indicated. In uncircumcised boys older than 7 or 8 years with phimosis that is resistant to topical corticosteroids and in boys with phimosis that causes ballooning of the foreskin or recurrent balanitis, strong consideration should be given to circumcision. An alternative to circumcision is preputioplasty (Dean et al, 2000), which can be performed under local anesthesia (Dessanti et al, 2005).

Circumcision

In pediatrics, few topics generate as much controversy as whether the newborn boy should undergo a circumcision, perhaps because it is the most common surgical procedure in the United States and because it is usually performed for cosmetic reasons. There are several recent reviews of the issues (Christakis et al, 2000; Alanis and Lucidi, 2004; Hutcheson, 2004). Although some have alleged that neonatal circumcision can lead to sexual dysfunction, long-term studies have not supported this view (Fink et al, 2002; Bleustein et al, 2005). A hospital-based study demonstrated that 61% of male neonates in the United States undergo circumcision and that the incidence is increasing (Nelson et al, 2005).

In support of circumcision is the prevention of penile cancer, urinary tract infection (UTI), sexually transmitted disease including human immunodeficiency virus (HIV) infection, and phimosis as well as lessening of the risk of balanitis.

Carcinoma of the penis develops almost exclusively in men who were not circumcised at birth. Schoen and coworkers (2000b) reported that of 89 men in a large health maintenance organization with invasive penile cancer, only 2 (2%) had been circumcised at birth. Furthermore, of 116 men with penile carcinoma in situ, 16 (14%) had had a neonatal circumcision. **Phimosis is a significant risk factor** (Tsen et al, 2001). On the other hand, although carcinoma of the penis develops primarily in uncircumcised men, in Scandinavian countries, where few men are circumcised and genital hygiene is excellent, the incidence of penile cancer is low.

Uncircumcised newborns and infants are predisposed to UTI (Singh-Grewal et al, 2005). In a study of 100 neonates with UTI, Ginsburg and McCracken (1982) found that only 3 (5%) of the 62 boys who developed a UTI were circumcised. Subsequently, Wiswell and colleagues (1985) studied more than 2500 male infants and found that 41 had symptomatic UTIs; of these, 88% were uncircumcised. In that study, uncircumcised boys were almost 20 times more likely than circumcised neonates to develop a UTI. Other studies of larger groups of infants have confirmed these reports (Wiswell, 2000; Zorc et al, 2005) and have demonstrated that neonatal circumcision is less costly than treating UTIs in uncircumcised boys (Schoen et al, 2000a). The increased risk

seems to affect boys at least through 5 years of age (Craig et al, 1996), and the incidence of epididymitis is reduced (Bennett et al, 1998). The increased risk of UTIs can be attributed to colonization of the prepuce by urinary pathogens (Gunsar et al, 2004; Bonacorsi et al, 2005). It has been calculated that it takes 111 neonatal circumcisions to prevent one UTI (Singh-Grewal et al, 2005).

Whether circumcision reduces the risk of sexually transmitted diseases has been controversial. An increased risk has been attributed to minor frenular injuries acquired during intercourse and to the larger surface area of the penis in uncircumcised men. In some studies, however, an increased incidence of sexually transmitted diseases in uncircumcised men has been attributed to demographic factors. Nevertheless, Lavreys and associates (1999) studied 746 men who were seronegative for HIV-1 infection and found that uncircumcised men were four times more likely to become HIV-1 positive and 2.5 times more likely to develop genital ulcers compared with circumcised men. However, there was not an increased incidence of genital warts in uncircumcised men. Currently, three clinical trials in South Africa, Kenya, and Uganda are studying whether circumcision reduces this rate of HIV infection. Preliminary unpublished results of the South African study demonstrated that circumcision reduced the risk of HIV infection by 70% (Schoofs et al, 2005), and reportedly this trial has been stopped.

In 1989, the AAP concluded, "Newborn circumcision has potential medical benefits and advantages as well as disadvantages and risks. When circumcision is being considered, the benefits and risks should be explained to the parents and informed consent obtained" (AAP Task Force on Circumcision, 1989). **More recently, the AAP again updated its policy statement** (AAP Task Force on Circumcision, 1999; Lannon et al, 2000). **Its position was essentially unchanged, with the exception that it emphasized the importance of local anesthesia for the procedure. The AAP does not endorse routine circumcision.**

When neonatal circumcision is performed, local anesthesia is recommended. Available options include the topical application of a cream containing eutectic mixture of local anesthetic (EMLA; lidocaine and prilocaine), a dorsal penile nerve block, and a penile ring block (Hardwick-Smith et al, 1998). Randomized controlled trials have demonstrated that a dorsal penile nerve block is more effective than EMLA cream (Howard et al, 1999; Taddio et al, 2000). In addition, the prilocaine in EMLA cream poses a risk for methemoglobinemia (Couper, 2000), although the risk is low. Consequently, a dorsal penile nerve block or ring block at the base of the penis with 1% lidocaine is preferred. Circumcision can be performed under local anesthesia even in older boys. For example, Jayanthi and colleagues (1999) reported a series of 287 infants aged 3 days to 9 months (20% older than 3 months) who underwent office circumcision with local anesthesia. At that time, the mean cost (excluding professional fees) was $196 for office circumcision, compared with $1805 for circumcision under general anesthesia.

Circumcision should not be performed in neonates with hypospadias, chordee without hypospadias, dorsal hood deformity, webbed penis, or small penis (Fig. 126–1). **In addition, many neonates with a large hydrocele or hernia are more likely to develop secondary phimosis and a buried**

penis if circumcision is performed (see Fig. 126–1). In a report by Williams and associates (2000), 8% of boys referred for initial circumcision had an "inconspicuous penis" (see later discussion), as did 63% of boys referred for circumcision revision.

KEY POINTS: CIRCUMCISION

- The AAP does not endorse routine circumcision.

- Potential benefits of circumcision are the reduced risk of UTI in an infant and the prevention of carcinoma of the penis, balanitis, phimosis, and possibly sexually transmitted disease.

- By 3 years of age, in uncircumcised boys, 90% can retract the foreskin.

- In boys with phimosis, topical application of corticosteroid cream loosens the phimotic ring in 70% to 80%; the cream does not cause separation of preputial adhesions.

- Circumcision should not be performed in neonates with hypospadias, chordee without hypospadias, dorsal hood deformity, webbed or hidden penis, or micropenis.

- In neonatal circumcision, the AAP recommends use of local anesthetic.

- The complication rate of neonatal circumcision is 0.2% to 3%. Early complications include bleeding, wound infection, penile adhesions, skin bridge, removal of excessive or insufficient skin, secondary phimosis, and penile injury. The most common late complication is meatal stenosis.

Circumcision Complications. The complication rate for newborn circumcision is 0.2% to 3% (Christakis et al, 2000; Ben Chaim et al, 2005). Minor complications include early problems such as bleeding, wound infection, penile adhesions, and removal of too much or too little skin; secondary phimosis with a trapped or hidden penis (see later discussion); and injury to the glans, urethra, or penile shaft by inadvertent excision or by a thermal injury (Baskin et al, 1996). The most common late complication is meatal stenosis.

Post-circumcision bleeding usually results from oozing from the frenulum or occasionally from a large arterial or venous vessel on the penile shaft. Bleeding can usually be controlled with compression, but cautery with a silver nitrate stick or ophthalmic cautery is occasionally necessary. Application of silver nitrate over the urethra should be avoided in most cases. On occasion, hemorrhage must be controlled with a suture.

Wound infection is rare and usually prevented by application of antibiotic ointment to the circumcision wound. Another potential complication is severe penile vasoconstriction secondary to inadvertent injection of concentrated epinephrine instead of lidocaine. Treatment of this unusual problem is either local infiltration with 0.4 mg of phentolamine or insertion of a caudal catheter to induce a sympathetic block (Adams et al, 2000).

Many of the other problems with healing can be managed in the office if the baby is seen 2 or 3 weeks after the circumcision. **Filmy penile adhesions after circumcision are common and have been reported to be present in 71% of infants, 30% of 1- to 5-year-olds, and 2% of those older than 9 years** (Van Howe, 1997; Ponsky et al, 2000). Typically, epithelial debris accumulates and helps separate the adhesion.

If too much penile shaft skin is removed, application of an antibiotic ointment and adherent gauze to the open wound usually yields a satisfactory result. Typically, most of the skin grows back and bridges the epithelial defect. **Immediate skin grafting is rarely necessary** and may result in a disfigured penis and graft site. In addition, suturing the skin edges together to bridge the gap is not recommended because the penile shaft may end up with insufficient skin. If too much skin is left, revision of circumcision may need to be considered. In some babies, the penis retracts into the suprapubic fat pad or scrotum. This situation is most common if the baby had a large hydrocele or hernia or was born with a webbed penis. A cicatricial scar may result, producing a trapped penis, which can cause urinary retention or UTI in the most severe cases. If this situation is recognized early, the cicatrix may be opened bluntly in the office. Alternatively, application of a topical corticosteroid cream may loosen the scar tissue (Palmer et al, 2005). If the problem is not corrected satisfactorily, correction of hidden penis under anesthesia is necessary when the child is older (Fig. 126–2) (see later).

The most serious circumcision complications are urethral injury and removal of part of the glans or part or all of the penile shaft. **Partial glans removal has been reported to occur with a Mogen clamp; in these cases, the excised tissue should be preserved and immediately sutured back to the penis** (Sherman et al, 1996). A microscopic repair is unnecessary. When repair is performed within 8 hours after the injury, the penis heals nicely in most cases.

In extremely rare cases, penile necrosis can result from thermal injury. For example, a thermal injury can occur if a metal clamp is applied to the foreskin and the cautery is used to excise the foreskin; if the cautery comes into contact with the metal clamp, an electrical-thermal injury to the shaft can result. Thermal injury to the penis also can result from inappropriate use of the yttrium-aluminum-garnet (YAG) contact laser in performing a circumcision. **The optimal therapy for an ablative penile injury is unresolved at this time. One option is to reassign the baby to a female gender and perform bilateral orchiectomy** (Bradley et al, 1998). Unfortunately, these children may grow up with a male identity, presumably from androgen imprinting in utero and shortly after birth (Reiner, 1996; Diamond and Sigmundson, 1997; Diamond, 1999). On the other hand, current efforts for penile reconstruction in such cases have suboptimal cosmetic and functional results. These patients should be referred immediately to a tertiary center with a team approach that includes specialists from pediatric urology, endocrinology, plastic surgery, child psychiatry, and ethics for definitive management.

In some cases, dense skin bridges form between the penile shaft and glans; these never come apart and need to be excised

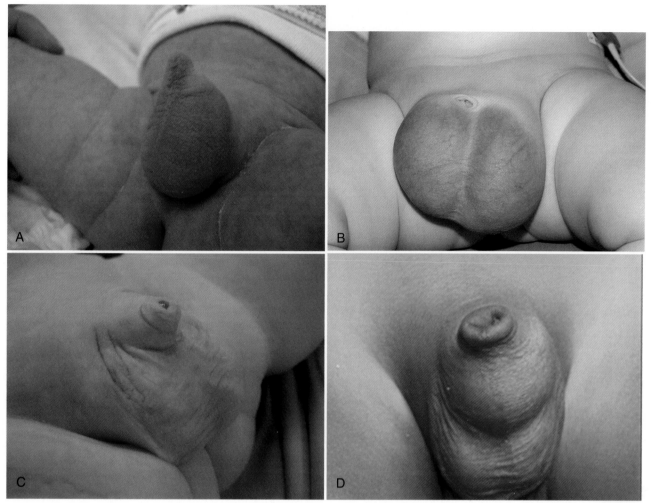

Figure 126–1. Examples of inconspicuous penis in uncircumcised boys; all have normal size penis. Newborn circumcision should be avoided in these cases. **A,** Hidden penis. **B,** Hidden penis secondary to bilateral large hydroceles. **C,** Webbed penis. **D,** Megaprepuce.

(Fig. 126–3). This procedure often can be performed in the office under local anesthesia, but if the adhesions are extensive, excision under general anesthesia is necessary.

Meatal Stenosis. **Meatal stenosis is a condition that almost always is acquired after neonatal circumcision.** One theory is that after disruption of the normal adhesions between the prepuce and glans and removal of the foreskin, a significant inflammatory reaction occurs, causing severe meatal inflammation and cicatrix formation, which results in a narrow meatus, a membranous web across the ventral aspect of the meatus, or an eccentric healing process that produces a prominent lip of ventral meatal tissue.

Another cause of meatal stenosis is balanitis xerotica obliterans, which can cause urinary retention. After meatoplasty, topical application of corticosteroid cream may be effective in reducing the risk of recurrent meatal stenosis.

Symptoms of meatal stenosis vary with the appearance. **In most cases, meatal stenosis does not become apparent until after the child is toilet trained. If the meatus is pinpoint, the boy voids with a forceful, fine stream that has a great casting distance. Some boys have a dorsally deflected stream or a** prolonged voiding time. Dysuria, frequency, terminal hematuria, and incontinence are symptoms that may lead to discovery of meatal stenosis **but generally are not attributable to this abnormality. In other boys with meatal stenosis, deflection of the urinary stream is the only sign.**

In a boy with suspected meatal stenosis, the meatus can be calibrated with a bougie or assessed with infant sounds. The majority of boys up to 3 years of age have a meatus that is 10 French; from 4 to 10 years, it is 12 French; and in older boys, the majority have a meatus that is 14 French (Litvak et al, 1976). Not infrequently, an asymptomatic boy with suspected meatal stenosis actually has a compliant meatus of normal caliber. If the meatus is diminished in size or if the child has abnormal voiding symptoms, a renal and bladder ultrasound examination may be indicated. If the child has a history of UTIs, voiding cystourethrography should be done also. However, **meatal stenosis rarely causes obstructive changes in the urinary tract.**

In many cases, meatoplasty can be accomplished in the physician's office with use of EMLA cream for local anesthesia (Cartwright et al, 1996). In addition, 1% lidocaine with

SECTION XVII

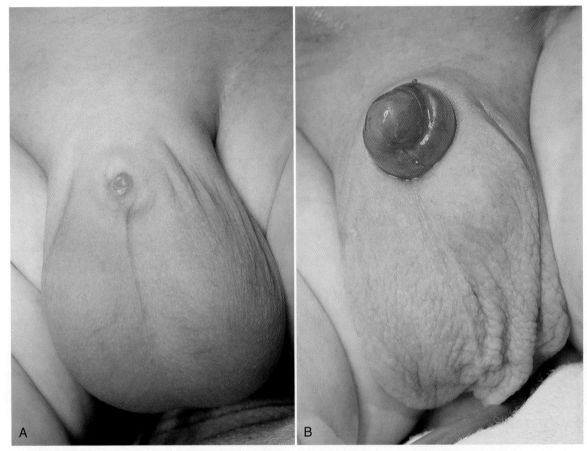

Figure 126–2. **A,** Trapped (concealed) penis resulting from circumcision. **B,** The same patient after revision of circumcision.

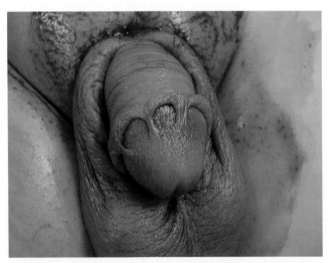

Figure 126–3. Penile skin bridges after newborn circumcision. These need to be excised.

1:100,000 epinephrine may be infiltrated in the ventral web with a 26-gauge needle for local anesthesia and vasoconstriction. A ventral incision is made toward the frenulum and long enough to provide a meatus of normal caliber, which can be checked with the bougie. The urethral mucosa is sutured to the glans with fine chromic catgut sutures. If the procedure is performed under general anesthesia, the bladder may be filled with saline and compressed manually to be certain that the stream is straight. Cystoscopy is unnecessary unless the child has obstructive symptoms and has not had voiding cystourethrography.

When meatal stenosis is congenital, it occurs primarily in neonates with coronal or subcoronal hypospadias. Obstruction in these cases is unusual, but UTI occasionally occurs or catheterization is necessary during hospitalization, and urgent meatoplasty may need to be performed.

Penile Cysts

The most common cystic lesion of the penis is accumulation of epithelial debris, or smegma, under the unretractable foreskin. In general, the foreskin should not be retracted because it will eventually retract by itself.

Congenital epidermal cysts occasionally form along the median penile raphe on the penile shaft or on the glans. Epidermal inclusion cysts may form after circumcision, hypospadias repair, or other forms of penile surgery and result when islands of epithelium are left behind in the subcutaneous tissue. These cystic lesions should be treated with simple excision.

Inconspicuous Penis

The term *inconspicuous penis* refers to a penis that appears to be small (Bergeson et al, 1993). **Several entities are included in this term, including webbed penis, concealed penis, and trapped penis, in which the penis is normal in size** (see Fig. 126–1), **and micropenis, in which the penis is abnormally small**. When an infant has an inconspicuous penis, prompt evaluation is necessary for proper treatment, and the family must be informed as to whether the penis is or is not normal. The stretched penile length should be measured from the pubic symphysis to the tip of the glans. In addition, the diameter of the penile shaft may be measured by palpation.

Webbed Penis. **Webbed penis is a condition in which the scrotal skin extends onto the ventrum of the penis** (see Fig. 126–1C). When this condition is congenital, the penis, the urethra, and the remainder of the scrotum typically are normal and the deformity represents an abnormality of the attachment between the penis and the scrotum. This condition may also be iatrogenic after circumcision or other penile surgery, in which case it results from excessive removal of ventral penile skin.

Although the webbed penis is usually asymptomatic, the cosmetic appearance is often unacceptable. On occasion, this condition may be corrected by incision of the web transversely, separation of the penis from the scrotum, and closure of the skin vertically. In other cases, a circumferential incision is made 1.5 cm proximal to the coronal sulcus, Byars' preputial skin flaps are transferred to the ventral surface of the penis, and the redundant foreskin is excised. The scrotum may be anchored to the base of the penis to prevent recurrence of the webbed appearance. **In rare cases, the distal urethra is hypoplastic, necessitating urethral reconstruction.**

Concealed (Buried or Hidden) Penis. **A concealed penis is a normally developed penis that is camouflaged by the suprapubic fat pad; this anomaly may be congenital, or it may occur iatrogenically after circumcision.** In infants and young children, the congenital condition has been thought to result from inelasticity of the dartos fascia (which normally allows the penile skin to slide freely on the deep layers of the shaft); extension of the penis is restricted because the penile skin is not anchored to the deep fascia (Fig. 126–4). In older children and obese adolescents, the abundant fat on the abdominal wall may hide the penile shaft.

On inspection, the contour of the penile shaft and the glans cannot be seen. However, careful palpation allows one to determine that the penile shaft actually is concealed and normal in size and is not a microphallus or a penis that has undergone circumcision injury. The clinician should determine whether the glans can be exposed simply by retracting the skin covering the glans. If so, it remains the surgeon's judgment whether correction is warranted.

Numerous techniques have been described to correct the concealed penis (Maizels et al, 1986; Casale et al, 1999; Elder, 2001; Frenkl et al, 2004; Gillett et al, 2005). The indications for this type of surgery and the timing of reconstruction are controversial. In moderately severe cases, the dysgenic bands of tissue, which are located primarily on the dorsal surface of the shaft of the penis, must be removed. The prepuce should be unfurled and used for ventral skin coverage. In addition, the subcutaneous tissue on the dorsal aspect of the penis

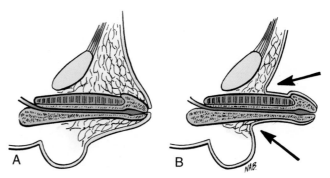

Figure 126–4. Concealed penis (**A**), which may be visualized by retraction of the skin lateral to the penile shaft (**B**).

should be fixed to the pubic fascia, and the subcutaneous tissue of the scrotum should be fixed to the ventral aspect of the base of the penile shaft with nonabsorbable suture. In addition, penoscrotal Z-plasty and lateral penile shaft Z-plasty often are necessary. In the most severe cases, the suspensory ligament of the penis must be divided, the suprapubic fat excised, and the spermatic cords protected. Liposuction has been reported to be helpful in severe cases (Maizels et al, 1986; Shenoy et al, 2000). However, this technique should be reserved for adolescent boys because prepubertal boys may lose their fat pad with somatic growth. In some cases, an island pedicle of ventral preputial skin or a skin graft may be used to cover the penis and aid in reconstruction.

Trapped Penis. **Trapped penis is an acquired form of inconspicuous penis; the term refers to a phallus that has become embedded in the suprapubic fat pad after circumcision. This deformity may occur after neonatal circumcision in a baby who has significant scrotal swelling due to a hydrocele or hernia or after routine circumcision in a baby with a webbed penis.** In some neonates, the penile shaft seems to retract naturally into the scrotum, and if circumcision is performed in this situation, the skin at the base of the penis may form a cicatrix over the retracted phallus (see Fig. 126–2). In its most severe form, this complication can predispose the child to UTIs and may cause urinary retention. In one series, secondary phimosis occurred in 2.9% of newborn circumcisions (Blalock et al, 2003). These patients were managed with forceful dilation of the cicatrix with a fine hemostat in the office. We have found that application of topical steroids for 6 weeks is effective and avoids a subsequent operative procedure in two thirds of infants (Palmer et al, 2005). If topical steroid application is ineffective, correction under general anesthesia is necessary, although the anesthetic risk is higher in the first few months of life. Elective repair of the trapped penis at 6 months is preferred. The surgical technique is similar to that for concealed penis.

Micropenis

Micropenis is a normally formed penis that is at least 2.5 standard deviations (SD) below the mean in size (Aaronson, 1994) (Fig. 126–5A). Typically, the ratio of the length of the penile shaft to its circumference is normal. In a few cases, the corpora cavernosa are severely hypoplastic. The scrotum is usually fused but often diminutive. The testes are usually small and frequently undescended.

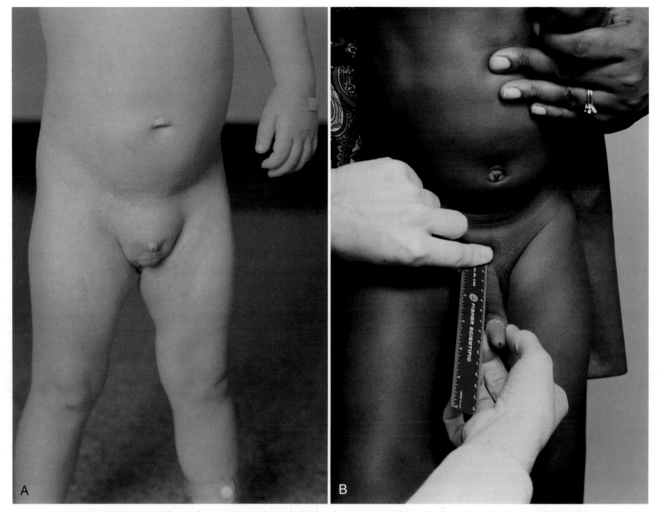

Figure 126–5. **A,** Micropenis secondary to hypopituitarism in an 8-year-old boy. **B,** Measuring stretched penile length.

Assessment of length is made by measuring the penis from its attachment to the pubic symphysis to the tip of the glans (Fig. 126–5*B*). In an obese infant or child, one must be careful to depress the suprapubic fat pad completely to obtain an accurate measurement. Stretched penile length is used because it correlates more closely with erectile length than does the relaxed length of the penis. The measurements should be compared with standards for penile length (see Table 126–1). **In general, the penis of a full-term newborn should be at least 1.9 cm long. A webbed or concealed penis often resembles micropenis, but examination shows a normal penile shaft.**

Knowledge of the endocrinologic regulation of penile development allows an understanding of how micropenis occurs. Differentiation of the male external genitalia is complete by the 12th week of gestation and requires a normal testis producing testosterone, stimulated by maternal human chorionic gonadotropin (hCG). During the second and third trimesters, growth of the penis occurs under the direction of fetal androgen, which is controlled by the secretion of fetal luteinizing hormone (LH). An abnormality in the production or use of testosterone results not only in a small penis but usually in hypospadias also, whereas a true micropenis often seems to be a consequence of a deficiency of gonadotropic

hormones. **Therefore, micropenis results from a hormonal abnormality that occurs after 14 weeks of gestation.**

There are numerous causes of micropenis (Table 126–4), including isolated gonadotropin defects without involvement of other organ systems and generalized endocrinopathies that may be associated with central nervous system defects. **The most common causes of micropenis are hypogonadotropic hypogonadism, hypergonadotropic hypogonadism (primary testicular failure), and idiopathic** (Lee et al, 1980b). In addition, micropenis is often associated with major chromosomal defects, including Klinefelter's syndrome (47,XXY); other X polysomy syndromes; and translocations, deletions, and trisomy involving chromosomes 8, 13, and 18 (Aaronson, 1994).

The most common cause of micropenis is failure of the hypothalamus to produce an adequate amount of gonadotropin-releasing hormone (GnRH). This condition, termed hypogonadotropic hypogonadism, may result from hypothalamic dysfunction, as in Kallmann's syndrome (genital-olfactory dysplasia), Prader-Willi syndrome, Laurence-Moon-Biedl syndrome (Walsh et al, 1978; Danish et al, 1980), **and the CHARGE association** (Ragan et al, 1999). In other cases, there is an associated growth hormone

Table 126-4. Etiology of Micropenis

Deficient testosterone secretion
  Hypogonadotropic hypogonadism
    Isolated, including Kallmann's syndrome
    Associated with other pituitary hormone deficiencies (e.g.,
      CHARGE association)
    Prader-Willi syndrome
    Laurence-Moon syndrome
    Bardet-Biedl syndrome
    Rud's syndrome
  Primary hypogonadism
    Anorchia
    Klinefelter's syndrome and poly X syndrome
    Gonadal dysgenesis (incomplete)
    Luteinizing hormone receptor defects (incomplete)
    Genetic defects in testosterone steroidogenesis (incomplete)
    Noonan's syndrome
    Down syndrome
    Robinow's syndrome
    Bardet-Biedl syndrome
    Laurence-Moon syndrome
Defects in testosterone action
  Growth hormone/insulin-like growth factor 1 deficiency
  Androgen receptor defects (incomplete)
  5α-reductase deficiency (incomplete)
  Fetal hydantoin syndrome
Development anomalies
  Aphallia
  Cloacal exstrophy
Idiopathic
Associated with other congenital malformations

Modified from Bin-Abbas B, Conte FA, Grumbach MM, Kaplan SL: Congenital hypogonadotropic hypogonadism and micropenis: Effect of testosterone treatment on adult penile size—why sex reversal in not indicated. J Pediatr 1999;134:579.

deficiency or neonatal hypoglycemia secondary to congenital hypopituitarism. Other major causes include congenital pituitary aplasia and midline brain defects, such as agenesis of the corpus callosum and occipital encephalocele.

Another cause of micropenis is primary testicular failure. Micropenis secondary to hypergonadotropic hypogonadism may result from gonadal dysgenesis or rudimentary testes syndrome, and it also occurs in Robinow's syndrome (Lee et al, 1980b). Failure of serum testosterone concentration to rise appropriately after stimulation by hCG has been the test most frequently used to identify this subgroup. However, in patients with Kallmann's syndrome and undescended testes, the serum testosterone level may not increase after hCG administration. Rarely, a patient with partial androgen insensitivity syndrome has micropenis; more commonly, the patient has sexual ambiguity.

Some patients have an idiopathic form of micropenis and a normal hypothalamic-pituitary-testicular axis as demonstrated by endocrine studies. In these cases, micropenis may result from improper timing or delayed onset of gonadotropin stimulation in the fetus (Lee et al, 1980a).

A karyotype should be performed in boys with micropenis. Consultation is usually obtained from the pediatric endocrinology service to help determine the cause of the micropenis and to assess whether other abnormalities are also present. Several issues need to be addressed, the most important of which is the growth potential of the penis. In addition, the endocrine abnormality needs to be defined. Testicular function may be assessed by measuring serum testosterone

levels before and after hCG stimulation. Primary testicular failure produces an absent response and elevated basal concentrations of LH and follicle-stimulating hormone (FSH). In some cases, a GnRH stimulation test is done also. Anterior pituitary screening tests include serial measurements of serum glucose, sodium, potassium, and serum cortisol concentrations and thyroid function tests. The endocrine evaluation of patients with micropenis is not standardized. Magnetic resonance imaging of the head should be done to determine the anatomic integrity of the hypothalamus and the anterior pituitary gland as well as the midline structures of the midbrain.

Before extensive evaluation of the hypothalamic-pituitary-testicular axis, **androgen therapy should be administered to determine the end-organ response. In general, intramuscular testosterone enanthate, 25 mg per month for 3 months, is given. Although prolonged treatment might advance skeletal maturation, short courses of treatment do not affect height.** Transdermal testosterone also has been used in these patients (Choi et al, 1993). Levy and Husmann (1996) proposed the use of growth hormone alone to stimulate penile development in boys with micropenis and isolated growth hormone deficiency; in a series of eight patients, seven had an adult stretched penile length in the normal range, but the average was 1.73 SD below the mean. In contrast, with use of a combination of growth hormone and testosterone in five boys with multiple pituitary hormone deficiencies, Bin-Abbas and coworkers (1999) reported that the mean stretched adult penile length was only 0.56 SD below the mean.

If androgen treatment in a neonate with a micropenis is used to increase the size of the penis so that it falls within the normal range, what will happen at puberty? The answer is not known with certainty. In a mouse model of hypogonadotropic hypogonadal micropenis, there was evidence that significant prepubertal exposure of the penis to androgens reduced the ultimate growth response to androgens (Husmann and Cain, 1994; McMahon et al, 1995). However, more recently, Bin-Abbas and coworkers (1999) described eight boys with micropenis who were treated with androgens both at birth and at puberty. The final penile stretched length averaged 10.3 cm and was in the normal range in all cases. Until longer term studies are available, exogenous stimulation at birth and at puberty with testosterone enanthate seems most reasonable (Tietjen et al, 1998).

If the penis does not respond to testosterone, the question of whether to recommend gender reassignment is controversial. In the past, gender reassignment was recommended, but this position has more recently come under criticism, in large part because of the lack of long-term data regarding the risks and benefits of reassigning these patients to a female gender (Calikoglu, 1999; Diamond, 1999). Husmann (2004) described 20 adult men born with micropenis who had a suboptimal response to testosterone therapy and were raised as males. At adulthood, 90% had a micropenis, and all had a male gender identity; five were undergoing psychiatric counseling for fear of rejection, and eight had not been sexually active.

In an important long-term retrospective study, Reilly and Woodhouse (1989) described 20 patients with a primary diagnosis of micropenis in infancy. Almost all had received androgen therapy during childhood. None of the adults had a penis within the "normal" range of size. Parents of patients in the prepubertal group considered their children to be normal boys and thought that the penile appearance was satisfactory but expressed concern about the size of the penis and wondered whether sexual function in adulthood would be a problem. All of the boys stood to urinate. Of the 12 patients in the adult group, 9 had a normal male appearance; 3 appeared eunuchoid despite regular testosterone therapy. All had a strong male identity, although half had experienced teasing because of their genital appearance; 9 of the 12 patients were sexually active. In a study of 22 adult men born with micropenis, Lee and Houk (2004) had similar findings. Wisniewski and Migeon (2002) reported that their patients had a male gender identity but were generally dissatisfied with their genital appearance and function. These studies demonstrate that **although ultimate penile size may not fall within what is considered a normal range, men born with micropenis have a male gender identity, and the majority can have satisfactory sexual function.**

KEY POINTS: MICROPENIS

■ Micropenis is a normally formed penis that is at least 2.5 SD below the mean in size (i.e., less than 1.9 cm in a term newborn).

■ A micropenis can be confused with a webbed or hidden penis.

■ Micropenis most commonly occurs secondary to failure of the hypothalamus to produce an adequate amount of GnRH (hypogonadotropic hypogonadism). Consider Kallmann's, Prader-Willi, Laurence-Moon-Biedl, and CHARGE syndromes. It may result from primary testicular failure (gonadal dysgenesis, rudimentary testes, Robinow's syndrome).

■ Evaluation includes karyotype; determination of serum LH and FSH concentrations; measurement of testosterone levels before and after hCG stimulation; serum studies of anterior pituitary function; magnetic resonance imaging of the head to assess the hypothalamus, anterior pituitary, and midbrain; and assessment of penile growth after androgen stimulation.

■ In adulthood, most men born with micropenis have male gender identity and satisfactory sexual function, even if penile size is less than what is considered in the normal range.

■ Gender reassignment is controversial.

Penile Torsion

Penile torsion is a rotational defect of the penile shaft (Fig. 126–6). Almost always, the shaft is rotated in a counterclockwise direction (i.e., to the left side). In most cases, penile size is normal and the condition is unrecognized until circumcision is performed or until the foreskin is retracted. Penile torsion may also be associated with hypospadias or a dorsal hood deformity without a urethral abnormality. In most cases

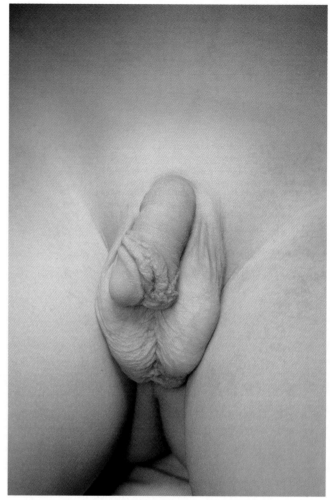

Figure 126–6.   Example of penile torsion.

of penile torsion, the median raphe spirals obliquely around the shaft. In general, the defect has primarily cosmetic significance, and correction is unnecessary if the rotation is less than 60 to 90 degrees from the midline.

Although the glans may be directed more than 90 degrees from the midline, the orientation of the corporal bodies and the corpus spongiosum at the base of the penis is normal. In mild forms of penile torsion, the penile skin may be degloved and simply reoriented so that the median raphe is restored to its normal position. However, in boys with penile torsion of 90 degrees or more, simple rearrangement of the skin on the shaft of the penis is insufficient. Instead, the base of the penis must be mobilized so that dysgenic bands of tissue can be identified and incised. If the penis still remains rotated, correction may be accomplished by placing a nonabsorbable suture through the lateral aspect of the base of the corpora cavernosa on the side opposite the direction of the abnormal rotation (i.e., on the right corporal body) and fixing it to the pubic symphysis dorsal to the penile shaft (Elder, 2001).

Lateral or Dorsal Curvature of the Penis

Lateral penile curvature is usually caused by overgrowth or hypoplasia of one corporal body. Lateral penile curvature is usually congenital; however, it is often unrecognized until later in childhood because the penis is normal when flaccid and the disparity in corporal size becomes apparent only during an erection. Surgical repair of this lesion involves degloving the penis and performing a modified Nesbit procedure, in which ellipses of tunica albuginea are excised from the site of maximum curvature to allow straightening of the penis.

Another deformity is congenital dorsal penile curvature. Many of these boys have a slender phallus more than 2 SD above the mean (unstretched length) (Adams et al, 1999). Some also have hypospadias. Repair is performed by excision of ellipses from the ventral corporal bodies.

The intraoperative technique of artificial erection with use of a normal saline solution is critical to the procedure's success. During correction, one must be careful to avoid injury to the neurovascular bundles (Baskin and Lue, 1998; Baskin et al, 2000).

Paraphimosis

Paraphimosis develops when the tip of the foreskin retracts proximal to the coronal sulcus and becomes fixed in position. Severe edema of the foreskin occurs within several hours, depending on the tightness of the tip of the foreskin. In most cases, manual compression of the glans with placement of distal traction on the edematous foreskin allows reduction of the paraphimotic ring. Other treatments that have been effective include application of an iced glove for 5 minutes, application of granulated sugar for 1 to 2 hours, and placement of multiple punctures in the edematous skin (Mackway-Jones and Teece, 2004).

Priapism

Priapism is a persistent penile erection at least 4 hours in duration that continues beyond, or is unrelated to, sexual stimulation. Typically, only the corpora cavernosa are affected (Montague et al, 2003). There are three subtypes.

1. **Ischemic (veno-occlusive, low-flow) priapism** is characterized by little or no cavernous blood flow, and cavernous blood gases are hypoxic, hypercapnic, and acidotic. The corpora are rigid and tender to palpation.
2. **Nonischemic (arterial, high-flow) priapism** is caused by unregulated cavernous arterial inflow. Typically, the penis is neither fully rigid nor painful. There is often a history of antecedent trauma resulting in a cavernous artery–corpora cavernosa fistula.
3. **Stuttering (intermittent) priapism** is a recurrent form of ischemic priapism with painful erections with intervening periods of detumescence.

The most common cause of priapism in children is sickle cell disease, which is characterized by predominance of sickle hemoglobin (Hb SS). **As many as 27.5% of children with sickle cell disease develop priapism** (Mantadakis et al, 1999). The priapism is generally related to a low-flow state, secondary to sickling of red blood cells within the sinusoids of the corpora cavernosa during normal erection, resulting in venous stasis. This situation results in decreased local oxygen tension and pH, which potentiates further stasis and sickling (Bruno et al, 2001). Priapism typically occurs during sleep, when mild hypoventilatory acidosis depresses oxygen tension and pH in the corpora. The pain that is experienced is a sign of ischemia. On examination, there is typically significant corporal engorgement with sparing of the glans penis. If there is spon-

giosal involvement, voiding may be impaired. Evaluation includes complete blood count and serum chemistry. If sickle cell status is unknown, hemoglobin electrophoresis should be performed. In some cases, corporal aspiration is performed to distinguish between a high-flow and low-flow state. Typically, the PO_2 is below 30 mm Hg, PCO_2 is above 60 mm Hg, and pH is less than 7.25 (Montague et al, 2003). Cavernous blood gases in patients with nonischemic priapism typically are similar to arterial blood.

In the past, priapism secondary to sickle cell disease was managed primarily by medical therapy, including exchange transfusion, hydration with hypotonic intravenous fluid, alkalinization, pain management with morphine, and oxygen. The American Urological Association guidelines on priapism also recommended concurrent intracavernous treatment beginning with corporal aspiration and irrigation (Montague et al, 2003). Typically, a 19- or 21-gauge butterfly needle is inserted. In many patients, general anesthesia or intravenous sedation will be necessary. Intracavernous irrigation with a sympathomimetic agent, such as phenylephrine, is performed in conjunction with a local anesthetic. In adolescents, the phenylephrine should be diluted with normal saline to a concentration of 100 to 500 µg/mL, and 1-mL injections should be made every 3 to 5 minutes for up to 1 hour. In prepubertal children, a lower concentration of phenylephrine solution and a smaller volume should be used. It is important to use phenylephrine promptly after diagnosis; if priapism has been present longer than 48 hours, ischemia and acidosis impair the intracavernous smooth muscle response to sympathomimetics (Montague et al, 2003). If irrigation and medical therapy are unsuccessful, a corporoglanular shunt should be considered. This shunt can be performed either with a large biopsy needle (Winter shunt) or a scalpel inserted through the glans or with excision of a piece of the tunica albuginea at the tip of the corpus cavernosum. For stuttering priapism, administration of an oral α-adrenergic agent (pseudoephedrine) once or twice daily is first-line therapy. If this treatment is unsuccessful, an oral β agonist (terbutaline) is recommended; a GnRH analog plus flutamide is recommended as third-line therapy (Maples and Hagemann, 2004). In a long-term follow-up study of 15 adults treated for sickle cell disease as children, satisfactory erectile function was inversely related to the patient's age at onset of priapism and duration of priapism (Chakrabarty et al, 1996).

In children, ischemic priapism is also associated with numerous factors including leukemia and sildenafil ingestion (Cantrell, 2004), and it is often idiopathic. Initial treatment with corporal aspiration and irrigation with a phenylephrine solution is appropriate.

Nonischemic (high-flow) priapism most commonly follows perineal trauma, such as a straddle injury, that results in laceration of the cavernous artery. Other causes include Fabry's disease and sickle cell anemia (Volkmer et al, 2001). In these cases, corporal irrigation is diagnostic only, not therapeutic. In addition, injection of sympathomimetic agents may have significant systemic adverse effects. Typically, the aspirated blood is bright red, and the aspirate is similar to arterial blood. Color Doppler ultrasonography often will demonstrate the fistula. Spontaneous resolution may occur. If not, angiographic embolization is indicated (Volkmer et al, 2001; Montague et al, 2003; Kuefer et al, 2005).

KEY POINTS: PRIAPISM

- Priapism can be ischemic (veno-occlusive, low flow), nonischemic (arterial, high flow), and stuttering (intermittent).

- The most common cause in children is sickle cell disease (ischemic).

- Treatment of a child with priapism secondary to sickle cell disease includes corporal aspiration and irrigation with a sympathomimetic agent with local anesthetic, exchange transfusion, hydration with intravenous fluids, alkalinization, pain management with morphine, and oxygen.

- Nonischemic priapism most commonly follows perineal trauma with corporal fistula formation. Angiographic embolization is necessary if spontaneous resolution does not occur.

- In a child with stuttering priapism, administration of an oral α-adrenergic agent (pseudoephedrine) is first-line therapy, an oral β agonist (terbutaline) is second-line therapy, and a GnRH analog plus flutamide is third-line therapy.

Genital Lymphedema

Lymphedema of the genitalia is a disfiguring disorder characterized by impaired lymphatic drainage that causes progressive penile or scrotal swelling. Lymphedema may be congenital or acquired. Congenital lymphedema is expressed at various ages and may be sporadic (85%) or inherited (15%) (McDougal, 2003). If it is inherited as an autosomal dominant trait, it is termed Milroy's disease. If it occurs at puberty and is sporadic, it is termed lymphedema praecox; whereas if it is inherited (autosomal dominant with variable penetrance) and occurring at puberty, it is termed Meige's disease. Approximately 80% with congenital lymphedema demonstrate onset of the disease at puberty (McDougal, 2003). The lymphedema may involve the penis, scrotum, or both. Congenital lymphedema has been associated with Turner's, Noonan's, Klinefelter's, and intestinal lymphangiectasia syndromes. Many with congenital lymphedema also have lower extremity involvement.

Initial management involves observation. If lymphedema remains significant or progresses, surgical therapy is necessary. The goal of surgical treatment is to remove all involved tissue. On the penile shaft, the penis is degloved and all tissue between Buck's fascia and the skin as well as redundant penile skin must be excised. If the patient is uncircumcised, the prepuce may be unfurled to provide coverage of the penile shaft (Shenoy et al, 2001). If the scrotum is involved, most of the scrotal skin must be excised, with the exception of the posterior skin, and the spermatic cords and testes should be preserved (Ross et al, 1998). **The penis may be covered with local skin flaps, and the scrotal contents may be covered with uninvolved posterior skin flaps** (Bolt et al, 1998; Ross et al, 1998). **If inadequate healthy skin is available, the penis and scrotum must be covered with split-thickness skin flaps**

(McDougal, 2003). After definitive surgical therapy, lymphedema in adjacent areas may recur.

Megaprepuce

Megaprepuce refers to a severely redundant inner foreskin covering a normal glans penis (see Fig. 126–1D). The foreskin cannot be retracted. Typically, during voiding, there is tremendous penoscrotal swelling; significant discomfort or even UTI may be present, and the urine trapped in the foreskin is often malodorous. Manual decompression of the swelling typically relieves the discomfort. Correction of this problem involves degloving of the penis and excision of the redundant skin (Shenoy and Rance, 1999; Summerton et al, 2000). Ideally, the penile shaft should be covered with the dorsal penile skin, which should be anchored to Buck's fascia in each quadrant.

Chordee without Hypospadias

A variant of hypospadias is chordee without hypospadias. In this anomaly, there is a dorsal hood and a variable degree of chordee, and the urethra is at the tip of the glans (Fig. 126–7). In most cases, there is deficiency of the ventral skin and the urethra is normal. In these boys, the deformity can generally be corrected by degloving of the penis and development of Byars' flaps. In more severe cases, simple dorsal plication, Nesbit dorsal excision, or corporal rotation is necessary. In the most severe cases, the urethra is short and an interposition island flap of dorsal foreskin must be performed. Intraoperative erection with injectable normal saline is necessary to be certain that complete chordee correction has been performed. The principles of chordee correction are identical to those in which hypospadias is present and are described in detail in Chapter 125.

Aphallia

Penile agenesis results from failure of development of the genital tubercle. The disorder is rare and has an estimated incidence of 1 in 10,000,000 to 30,000,000 births; approximately 80 cases have been reported. In these cases, the

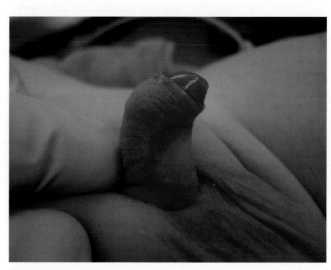

Figure 126–7. Chordee without hypospadias, side view. Note dorsal hood deformity of foreskin. Urethral meatus is at tip of glans.

karyotype almost always is 46,XY, and the usual appearance is that of a well-developed scrotum with descended testes and an absent penile shaft (Fig. 126–8). The anus is usually displaced anteriorly. The urethra often opens at the anal verge adjacent to a small skin tag; in other cases, it opens into the rectum.

Associated malformations are common and include cryptorchidism, vesicoureteral reflux, horseshoe kidney, renal agenesis, imperforate anus, and musculoskeletal and cardiopulmonary abnormalities (Skoog and Belman, 1989; Evans et al, 1999). The connection between the genitourinary and gastrointestinal tract is variable. Skoog and Belman (1989) reviewed 60 reports of aphallia and found that the more proximal the urethral meatus, the higher the incidence of other anomalies and the greater the likelihood of neonatal death. At least 60% of patients had a postsphincteric meatus located on a peculiar appendage at the anal verge (Fig. 126–8*B*). There were an average of 1.2 associated anomalies, and the mortality rate was 13%. Among the 28% of patients who had a presphincteric urethral communication (prostatorectal fistula), the mortality rate was 36%. In the 12% with a vesicorectal fistula and urethral atresia, there were an average of four anomalies per patient, and mortality rate was 100%.

Children with this lesion should be evaluated immediately with a karyotype and other appropriate studies to determine whether there are associated malformations of the urinary tract or other organ systems. Magnetic resonance imaging may be beneficial in determining the severity of the defect (Lapointe et al, 2001). **Prompt gender assignment is important. Some of these patients have a male gender identity despite reconstruction as a female, presumably because of in utero or postnatal sex steroid imprinting** (Diamond, 1999). **Consequently, the recommendation to perform gender reassignment should be made carefully and only after full evaluation by an ambiguous genitalia assessment team** that

includes a pediatric urologist, endocrinologist, and psychiatrist. As a male, the patient would potentially be fertile, but currently there is an inability to construct a cosmetically acceptable phallus that would allow normal urinary, sexual, and reproductive function. The issues are similar to those under consideration in many genetic males born with cloacal exstrophy. Gender reassignment involves orchiectomy and feminizing genitoplasty in the newborn period. At a later age, construction of a neovagina is necessary. Urinary tract reconstruction with simultaneous construction of an intestinal neovagina through a posterior sagittal and abdominal approach in patients with penile agenesis has been described (Hendren, 1997).

Diphallia

Duplication of the penis is a rare anomaly and has a range of appearances from a small accessory penis to complete duplication (Gyftopoulos et al, 2002). In some cases, each phallus has only one corporal body and urethra, whereas others seem to be a variant of twinning, with each phallus having two corpora cavernosa and a urethra. The penes are usually unequal in size and lie side by side. Associated anomalies are common, including hypospadias, bifid scrotum, duplication of the bladder, renal agenesis or ectopia, and diastasis of the pubic symphysis (Maruyama et al, 1999). Anal and cardiac anomalies are also common. Evaluation should include imaging of the entire urinary tract. Magnetic resonance imaging can also be done to assess penile development (Lapointe et al, 2001). Treatment must be individualized to attain a satisfactory functional and cosmetic result.

Congenital Urethral Fistula

A rare anomaly is the congenital urethral fistula, in which **the urethra and meatus are normal and a urethrocutaneous**

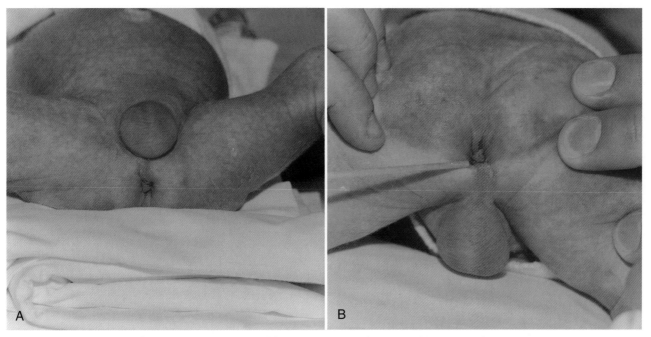

Figure 126–8. **A,** Neonate with aphallia. **B,** Urethral meatus at skin tag on anal verge.

fistula is present, typically coronal or subcoronal. This abnormality is usually an isolated deformity, but it may be associated with imperforate anus or ventral chordee (Ritchey et al, 1994). In a series of 14 boys with a congenital fistula, 4 had distal hypospadias and 2 had chordee (Caldamone et al, 1999). The cause of congenital urethral fistula is unknown but probably involves a focal defect in the urethral plate that prevents fusion of the urethral folds. Some patients have undergone circumcision before diagnosis (Caldamone et al, 1999), raising the possibility that the fistula may have been iatrogenic rather than congenital in some of these cases. Treatment usually consists of one of two techniques: the fistula can be circumscribed and then closed in multiple layers, similar to a urethrocutaneous fistula after hypospadias repair; or if the glans bridge is thin, the ventral glans can be opened through the distal urethra, and the distal urethra is then closed by a Thiersch-Duplay tubularization or tubularization and incision of the urethral plate technique.

Parameatal Urethral Cysts

The parameatal urethral cyst is another rare anomaly. Shiraki (1975) suggested that these cysts may result from occlusion of paraurethral ducts or in other cases from faulty preputial separation from the glans along the coronal sulcus. The cyst wall may consist of transitional and squamous as well as columnar epithelium. Treatment is simple excision under anesthesia, with care taken not to cause meatal stenosis.

Scrotal Anomalies

Penoscrotal Transposition (Scrotal Engulfment)

Penoscrotal transposition may be partial or complete (Fig. 126–9). Its less severe forms have been termed bifid scrotum, doughnut scrotum, prepenile scrotum, and shawl scrotum. Presumably, this anomaly results from incomplete or failed inferomedial migration of the labioscrotal swellings. Frequently, the condition occurs in conjunction with perineal, scrotal, or penoscrotal hypospadias with chordee (Pinke et al, 2001). It has also been associated with caudal regression (Lage et al, 1987), Aarskog syndrome (Shinkawa et al, 1983), and sex

chromosome abnormalities (Yamaguchi et al, 1989). When there is complete penoscrotal transposition and a normal scrotum, as many as 75% of patients have a significant urinary tract abnormality (MacKenzie et al, 1994), and renal sonography and voiding cystourethrography should be performed.

When scrotal engulfment is associated with severe hypospadias, hypospadias repair is often accomplished by a transverse preputial island flap in conjunction with Thiersch-Duplay tubularization of the proximal urethra. To minimize the possibility of devascularization of the preputial flap, correction of the scrotal engulfment is usually done as a second-stage procedure 6 months later (Elder and Duckett, 1990; Germiyanoglu et al, 1994). If the penis is normal, scrotoplasty can be accomplished when the child is 6 to 12 months of age.

Scrotoplasty is begun by circumscribing the superior aspects of each half of the vertical aspect of the scrotum and extending these incisions laterally to include at least half of the scrotum (Fig. 126–10). The medial aspects of the incision are joined on the ventral aspect of the penis, and the incision is carried down the midline along the median raphe for 4 or 5 cm. Before the incision is made, it is helpful to infiltrate the skin with 1% lidocaine with 1:100,000 epinephrine to diminish bleeding. Traction sutures are placed on the superior aspect of the scrotal flaps, and these are dissected out in the areolar layer. Deeper dissection may result in cutting of the tunica vaginalis and may injure the spermatic cord. The scrotal wings are rotated medially under the penis and sutured together in the midline in an everted manner. During this dissection, moderate oozing from the areolar tissue frequently occurs, and it may be necessary to leave a small dependent Penrose drain in place for 24 to 48 hours. In many cases, the bare area on either side of the penis can be closed. However,

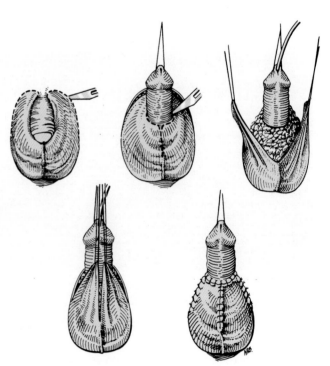

Figure 126–10. Repair of penoscrotal transposition (see discussion in text).

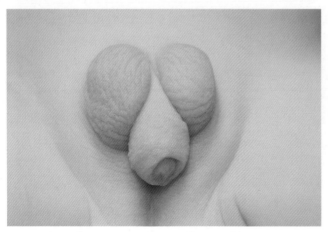

Figure 126–9. Penoscrotal transposition.

in more severe cases of penoscrotal transposition, dorsal interposition flaps may be necessary, allowing caudal advancement of the skin of the abdominal wall (Pinke et al, 2001). Scrotoplasty can usually be accomplished as an outpatient procedure.

An alternative technique is to identify the correct position for the penis and make a buttonhole by excising a plug of epidermis, dermis, and suprapubic fat. The penis is then degloved, and the penile shaft is brought through the buttonhole. The penile shaft skin remains behind, is split down the ventrum, and is mobilized superiorly to the penile shaft. A window of the dartos pedicle is made, and the penile shaft is brought through this window. The degloved penis is then resurfaced with shaft skin. In a report of 15 patients who underwent this technique, all had an excellent cosmetic result (Kolligian et al, 2000).

Ectopic Scrotum

Ectopic scrotum, the anomalous position of one hemiscrotum along the inguinal canal, is a rare condition. Most commonly, it is suprainguinal (Fig. 126–11), although it may also be infrainguinal or perineal (Elder and Jeffs, 1982). This

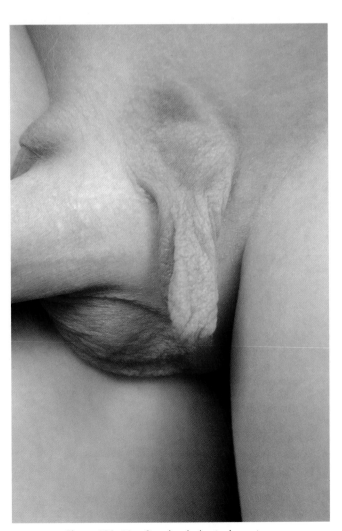

Figure 126–11. Suprainguinal ectopic scrotum.

anomaly has been associated with cryptorchidism, inguinal hernia, and exstrophy as well as with the popliteal pterygium syndrome (Cunningham et al, 1989). In one review, 70% of boys with a suprainguinal ectopic scrotum exhibited ipsilateral upper urinary tract anomalies, including renal agenesis, renal dysplasia, and ectopic ureter (Elder and Jeffs, 1982). Another study indicated that an associated perineal lipoma was found in 83% of these children; 68% of those with a lipoma had no associated anomalies, whereas 100% of those without a lipoma had associated genital or renal malformations (Sule et al, 1994). Consequently, children with this anomaly should undergo upper urinary tract imaging. Because the embryology of the gubernaculum and that of the scrotum are intimately related chronologically and anatomically, it seems likely that the ectopic scrotum results from a defect in gubernacular formation that prevents migration of the labioscrotal swellings (Hoar et al, 1998). Scrotoplasty and orchiopexy may be performed at 6 to 12 months of age or earlier if other surgical procedures are necessary.

Bifid Scrotum

Bifid scrotum refers to the deformity in which the labioscrotal folds are completely separated. Almost always, this anomaly is associated with proximal hypospadias.

Scrotal Hypoplasia

Scrotal hypoplasia, the underdevelopment of one or both sides of the scrotum, **occurs most commonly in boys with an undescended testis** and frequently is noted in infants with genital ambiguity. The deformity probably results from lack of gubernacular swelling of the labioscrotal folds.

Vascular Lesions of the Genitalia

Vascular lesions of the genitalia are uncommon, and there is disagreement about their classification, etiology, and treatment. **These deformities include hemangiomas and vascular malformations. A hemangioma is on the skin and often is present at birth. It may show significant growth in the postnatal period followed by slow involution. Vascular malformations, on the other hand, are present at birth in the subcutaneous tissues and tend to persist or to enlarge. They may expand secondary to trauma, sepsis, or hormonal changes** (Ramos et al, 1999). **Vascular malformations can be subdivided into either slow-flow (capillary, lymphatic, venous) or fast-flow (arterial, arteriovenous) types.**

Congenital hemangiomas are common and affect the genitalia in approximately 1% of all hemangiomas (Alter et al, 1993). **Strawberry hemangiomas, the most common type, result from proliferation of immature capillary vessels.** These are also categorized as cutaneous hemangiomas because they occur on the skin. Although the lesions may undergo a period of rapid growth lasting 3 to 6 months, gradual involution is common, and most lesions require no treatment (Casale and Menashe, 1989). If ulceration develops, intervention is necessary to prevent complications from bleeding. The most popular form of therapy is short-term oral steroid therapy. In some cases, surgical excision is necessary. Treatment with a pulsed dye laser (585-nm wavelength) allows selective photothermolysis and destruction of superficial blood vessels (Ward et al, 1998).

Subcutaneous hemangiomas, also referred to as cavernous hemangiomas, are much less common than the cutaneous variety (Sule et al, 1993; Ferrer and McKenna, 1995) and are probably more appropriately classified as a vascular malformation. They may be detected at birth or later in life. **In contrast to cutaneous hemangiomas, which tend to involute, cavernous hemangiomas tend to enlarge gradually.** Physical examination reveals a "bag of worms" sensation similar to that of a varicocele, although the lesions tend to be firm and do not decompress when the patient is recumbent. Because examination does not disclose the extent of the lesion, ultrasonography with color Doppler study, computed tomographic scanning, or magnetic resonance imaging is advised to delineate the size of the hemangioma (Aizenstein et al, 1996). Definitive treatment by en bloc resection is advised, and preoperative angioembolization may help reduce the size of the mass and the risk of bleeding.

Klippel-Trénaunay-Weber syndrome is a triad of cutaneous vascular malformation, most commonly nevus flammeus, in combination with soft tissue and bone hypertrophy. The anomaly is present at birth and typically involves a lower extremity but often may involve the trunk or face. The vascular lesions have a propensity to bleed. In a review of 214 patients from a single institution, Husmann and colleagues (2005) **found that 30% had genitourinary cutaneous or visceral involvement. Of the 48 (22%) who had cutaneous genital involvement, 29% developed intractable bleeding. Excision of the hemangiomas was associated with significant blood loss.**

Vascular malformations may also affect the penis. Although these lesions are congenital, they usually are not diagnosed until the teenage years or young adulthood and are characterized as a faint blue patch or a soft blue mass. If the lesion affects the glans penis, the neodymium:YAG laser may yield a better result than surgical excision (Ramos et al, 1999).

Miscellaneous Genital Anomalies

Cysts of the median raphe can occur on the perineum, scrotum, or shaft of the penis (Little et al, 1992). The lesions probably result from epithelial rests that become buried during the urethral infolding process. Excision is recommended unless the cysts are small and asymptomatic.

Juvenile xanthogranulomas appear as one or more lesions of rapid onset; they measure 2 to 20 mm in diameter and are orange, gold, or brown. These lesions can affect the penis (Hautmann and Bachor, 1993) or scrotum (Goulding and Traylor, 1983). As many as 20% are present at birth. The lesion is often self-limited, and a period of 1 year of expectant waiting is advised to avoid potentially unnecessary ablative genital surgery.

Meconium peritonitis causes genital manifestations on occasion, among them meconium hydrocele (Ring et al, 1989) and congenital rupture of the scrotum, termed **scrotoschisis** (Salle et al, 1992; Chun and St-Vil, 1997). When an unusual inflammatory condition of the scrotum is detected, the clinician should suspect meconium peritonitis and proceed with the appropriate evaluation.

SUGGESTED READINGS

Aaronson IA: Micropenis: Medical and surgical implications. J Urol 1994;152:4-14.

American Academy of Pediatrics, Task Force on Circumcision: Circumcision policy statement. Pediatrics 1999;103:686-693.

Baskin LS, Canning DA, Snyder HM, Duckett JW: Treating complications of circumcision. Pediatr Emerg Care 1996;12:62-68.

Baskin LS, Erol A, Li YW, Liu WH: Anatomy of the neurovascular bundle: Is safe mobilization possible? J Urol 2000;164:977-980.

Bergeson PS, Hopkin RJ, Bailey RB Jr, et al: The inconspicuous penis. Pediatrics 1993;92:794-799.

Casale AJ, Beck SD, Cain MP, et al: Concealed penis in childhood: A spectrum of etiology and treatment. J Urol 1999;162:1165-1168.

Elder JS: Circumcision, urethral prolapse, penile torsion, buried penis, webbed penis and megalourethra. In Frank JD, Gearhart JP, Snyder HM III, eds: Operative Pediatric Urology, 2nd ed. London, Churchill Livingstone, 2001:273-285.

Husmann DA: The androgen insensitive micropenis: Long-term follow-up into adulthood. J Pediatr Endocrinol Metab 2004;17:1037-1041.

Lee PA, Houk CP: Outcome studies among men with micropenis. J Pediatr Endocrinol Metab 2004;17:1043-1053.

Lee PA, Mazur T, Danish R, et al: Micropenis: I. Criteria, etiologies and classification. Johns Hopkins Med J 1980;146:156-163.

McDougal WS: Lymphedema of the external genitalia. J Urol 2003;170:711-716.

Montague DK, Jarow J, Broderick GA, et al: American Urological Association guideline on the management of priapism. J Urol 2003;170:1318-1324.

Palmer JS, Elder JS, Palmer LS: The use of betamethasone to manage the trapped penis following newborn circumcision. J Urol 2005;174:1577-1578.

Ross JH, Kay R, Yetman RJ, Angermeier K: Primary lymphedema of the genitalia in children and adolescents. J Urol 1998;160:1485-1489.

Skoog SJ, Belman AB: Aphallia: Its classification and management. J Urol 1989;141:589-592.

Walsh PC, Wilson JD, Allen TD, et al: Clinical and endocrinological evaluation of patients with congenital microphallus. J Urol 1978;120:90-95.

127 Abnormalities of the Testes and Scrotum and their Surgical Management

FRANCIS X. SCHNECK, MD • MARK F. BELLINGER, MD

TESTICULAR EMBRYOLOGY AND NORMAL DESCENT

The embryologic origin of testicular development begins early in fetal life. Although chromosomal sex is determined at the time of fusion of the gametes by the presence or absence of the Y chromosome, male sexual differentiation does not begin until **testicular differentiation is initiated in the seventh week of gestation by the *SRY* gene. During male sexual differentiation, hormones produced by the fetal testes initiate and sustain normal male development, whereas absence of testicular hormones results in female sexual differentiation.** Normal male sexual differentiation involves gonadal development, stabilization of the wolffian (mesonephric) ducts with simultaneous regression of müllerian (paramesonephric) duct structures, and testicular descent into the scrotum. **The hormones that control embryonic male sexual differentiation include the testicular androgens, produced by Leydig cells, and müllerian inhibiting substance (MIS), produced by Sertoli cells. Androgens (testosterone, dihydrotestosterone [DHT]) mediate differentiation of the paired wolffian ducts into the seminal vesicles, epididymis, vas deferens, and ejaculatory ducts.** Masculinization of the external genitalia is under similar influence of the testicular androgens.

At 4 to 6 weeks' gestation, the genital ridges organize, followed by migration of primordial germ cells (Wylie, 1993).

Primordial germ cells, located along the caudal wall of the embryonic yolk sac near the allantoic stalk, begin migration by amoeboid movement to the genital ridges via the dorsal mesentery. At this stage, the gonadal primordium is indifferent and arises from a thickening of the coelomic epithelium between the root of the mesentery and the mesonephros. The segmented mesonephros extends along the posterior abdominal wall as a ridge from the lower cervical to the lumbar region. The coelomic epithelium develops epithelial cords (germinal cords) into the underlying mesenchyme to form the genital ridges. Chemotactic factors are produced by the thickened coelomic epithelium and attract the primordial germ cells.

Cells other than germ cells, including Sertoli cells, are derived from cells that migrated from the mesonephros. **By 7 weeks, primitive Sertoli cells have developed. Germ cells differentiate into gonocytes on entering the testicular cords to become fetal spermatogonia by 15 weeks of gestation.** Gonocytes and Sertoli cells form testicular cords within the testis and canalize to form seminiferous tubules; however, a lumen will not be present within the tubule until puberty. By the eighth week of gestation, Leydig cells have differentiated around the testicular cords in the gonadal mesenchyme between the seminiferous tubules (Huhtaniemi, 1994). The testicular cords are separated from the coelomic epithelium by a well-vascularized connective tissue layer that later becomes the tunica albuginea. The rete testis forms at the ends of the testicular cords and converges at the hilus of the testis to connect to the efferent ductules that differentiate from the mesonephric tubules. The gonadal ridge rounds off into an oval organ.

During the eighth week, the fetal testis begins to secrete testosterone and MIS independent of pituitary hormonal regulation. This signals stabilization and differentiation of the wolffian ducts and external genitalia. Fetal Leydig cells secrete testosterone, a paracrine hormone, which is converted by intercellular 5α-reductase in target tissues to DHT. DHT is responsible for inducing differentiation of the wolffian duct into the epididymis and vas deferens. Testosterone synthesis plus secretion is regulated by maternal human chorionic gonadotropin (hCG) and peaks at 12 to 14 weeks of gestation. MIS is secreted by Sertoli cells and causes degeneration of the müllerian structures after the eighth week of gestation (Lee and Donahue, 1993). MIS expression is detectable by week 7 and is limited to Sertoli cells only. MIS induces degeneration of basement membrane integrity of the epithelial and mesenchymal müllerian cells within the genital ridge (Catlin et al, 1993). The gene for MIS maps to chromosome 19p13.3 (Cohen-Haguenauer et al, 1987).

The gubernaculum appears at the seventh week of embryologic development as a condensation of mesenchymal tissue within the subserous fascia on either side of the vertebral column that extends from the gonad to the fascia between the developing external and internal oblique muscles. The cranial aspect of the gubernaculum envelops the cauda epididymis and lower pole tunica albuginea of the testis and extends caudally into the inguinal canal, where it maintains a firm attachment. This distal attachment has been shown experimentally to be important in normal development of the processus vaginalis (Clarnette et al, 1996). Mechanical disruption of the gubernaculum resulted in lack of development of the processus vaginalis, but proximal gubernaculectomy had no effect on development of the processus vaginalis when the testis descended into the scrotum. In dissections of fetuses less than 23 weeks' gestation, before descent of the testis, Heyns (1987) demonstrated that the gubernaculum does not extend beyond the external inguinal ring. Controversy regarding the caudal extent of gubernaculum attachment during development is especially relevant when considering the theoretical mechanisms of gubernacular function during testicular descent. Many investigators have observed that the gubernaculum itself does not extend into the scrotum during fetal development (Heyns, 1987). The gubernaculum is not firmly attached to the scrotum but is in continuity with the scrotum by the mesenchymatous tissue that fills the scrotum.

Before descent, the testis lies atop the gubernaculum, which resembles a cylindrical, Wharton's jelly–like structure covered by peritoneum on all sides except posteriorly along the mesorchium, which is retroperitoneal. Histologically, the gubernaculum is composed of undifferentiated spindle-shaped cells with a large amount of extracellular material containing glycosaminoglycans. Just before testicular descent, the gubernaculum undergoes a significant increase in length and rapid enlargement in gubernacular mass as a result of increased water uptake. The glycosaminoglycan fraction within the gubernaculum is probably responsible for the increase in water in the extracellular matrix (Heyns et al, 1990). Backhouse (1964) suggested that this increased water may serve to dilate the inguinal canal to facilitate testicular passage. Gubernacular swelling coincides with lengthening of the testicular vasculature and vas deferens. The bulbous lower end of the gubernaculum loses its firm attachments to the inguinal canal after the testis descends through the canal. Therefore, it has been observed that **the gubernaculum has an important role in fixation of the testis to the inguinal canal before descent, but its role in descent of the testis through the canal and into the scrotum is less obvious and requires further analysis.**

As the cranial portion of the mesonephros involutes, a mesenchymatous ridge persists between the gonad and diaphragm and becomes part of the cranial gonadal mesentery (Backhouse, 1982b). Backhouse (1982a) considered this embryologic structure, the cranial suspensory ligament (CSL),

to have an insignificant role in the mechanism of testicular descent, an observation that has been clinically correlated. The testes, like the ovaries, are initially located near the developing kidney, between the CSL and gubernaculum. The CSL in the male regresses while the gubernaculum proliferates during the transabdominal and transinguinal phases of descent. Evidence suggests that androgens mediate regression of the CSL and possibly the transinguinal phase of descent, although normal positioning of the ovaries in 46,XX individuals with prenatal androgen exposure demonstrates that regression of the CSL alone is insufficient to cause gonadal descent (Scott, 1987).

This is also the stage when the inguinal canal develops. Its role is to convey the testes to the developing scrotum. The developing trilaminar anterior abdominal wall musculature is present at 6 weeks' gestation. During the eighth week, the inguinal canal begins development as a caudal evagination of the abdominal wall that forms in conjunction with caudal elongation of the processus vaginalis. The processus vaginalis develops as a herniation of peritoneum at the deep inguinal ring and lies on the anterior aspect of the gubernaculum. The processus encounters the three layers of the abdominal wall via the large hiatus of the transversus abdominis muscle. The first layer is the transversalis fascia, which lies just deep to the transversus abdominis muscle at the deep inguinal ring. This eventration embryologically becomes the internal spermatic fascia of the spermatic cord. The next layer encountered, the internal oblique muscle, becomes the cremasteric muscle of the spermatic cord, although there is debate regarding the origin of this layer (Backhouse, 1964). The cremasteric muscle extends along the developing processus vaginalis. The last layer is the external oblique muscle, which becomes the external spermatic fascia. The anatomic boundaries of the inguinal canal are the deep (internal) inguinal ring superiorly and the superficial (external) inguinal ring inferomedially. The canal itself is filled by mesenchyme, through which the genital branch of the genitofemoral nerve (GFN) and ilioinguinal nerve pass (Backhouse, 1982a).

The external genitalia develop between the 8th and 16th weeks of gestation. Differentiation is induced by DHT, the active androgen converted from testosterone by 5α-reductase. The genital swellings contain undifferentiated mesenchyme and differentiate under androgenic stimulation into the scrotum. The testes at this time are intra-abdominal and develop never more than 1.3 mm from the internal ring (Hutson and Donahoe, 1986). **The testes lie dormant within the abdomen until about the 23rd week of gestation, during which time the processus vaginalis continues its elongation into the scrotum.** The testis, epididymis, and gubernaculum have been observed to descend en mass through the inguinal canal posterior to the patent processus vaginalis. Transinguinal transit of the testes is a rapid process that probably occurs within a period of several days (Scorer and Farrington, 1971; Backhouse, 1982a; Heyns, 1987; Sampaio and Favorito, 1998). Heyns (1987) found that 75% of testes passed through the inguinal canal between 24 and 28 weeks of gestation and only 2.6% of testes were present within the inguinal canal during the period of descent. His postmortem dissections of spontaneously aborted human fetuses showed that **testicular descent had occurred in 10% at 24 weeks' gestation, in 50% at 27 weeks, in 75% at 28 weeks, and in 80% at 34 weeks to**

birth (Heyns, 1987). This coincides with a 72% descent rate reported in fetuses that weighed less than 1200 g or had a crown-rump length greater than 270 mm (Heyns, 1987). Sampaio and Favorito (1998) observed, similarly, that before 23 weeks of gestation the majority of testes remained intra-abdominal, yet by 30 weeks all testes were descended into the scrotum. Complete descent from the external ring to the bottom of the scrotum may take more than 3 to 4 weeks (Curling, 1843; Scorer and Farrington, 1971). Sampaio and Favorito (1998) reported that transinguinal migration occurred between 21 and 25 weeks after conception. In addition, testes remained undescended in fetuses that weighed less than 990 g or had a crown-rump length of 245 mm or less, whereas all testes were descended in fetuses that weighed more than 1220 g or had a crown-rump length greater than 275 mm. **These data support epidemiologic findings in newborn boys with cryptorchidism and suggest that fetal and birth weights are a significant determinant of descent in males after 30 weeks' gestation.**

KEY POINTS: TESTICULAR EMBRYOLOGY AND NORMAL DESCENT

■ Sex determination is the process of testis formation, whereas sexual differentiation is the subsequent process that results in the male phenotype.

■ The *SRY* gene, located in a 35-kb region on the short arm of the Y chromosome, appears to be primarily responsible for male sexual differentiation.

■ Testicular differentiation is initiated by the *SRY* gene in the seventh week of gestation.

■ By 7 weeks primitive Sertoli cells have developed, and by the 8th week Leydig cells have differentiated.

■ Germ cells differentiate into gonocytes on entering the testicular cords at 7 weeks and become fetal spermatogonia by 15 weeks of gestation.

■ The gubernaculum appears in the seventh week and extends from the gonad to the fascia between the developing external and internal oblique muscles.

■ Testosterone and MIS, produced by the fetal testes in the eighth week, initiate and sustain normal male development independent of pituitary hormonal regulation.

■ Testicular descent occurs in 10% at 24 weeks' gestation, in 50% at 27 weeks, in 75% at 28 weeks, and in 80% at 34 weeks to birth.

THE UNDESCENDED TESTIS
Definition

The cause of cryptorchidism is multifactorial. An undescended testis can be located anywhere between the abdominal cavity and just outside the anatomic scrotum. Less commonly, the testis can also migrate to ectopic positions outside the scrotum, not along the normal path of descent. *Cryptorchidism* is a term that has been used interchangeably with the term *undescended testis*. Both terms refer to an abnormally positioned testis, but cryptorchidism literally means "hidden testis." Therefore, an undescended testis may be a more appropriate term because most testes that are not within the scrotum at birth are detectable by palpation. To fully appreciate the diversity of this congenital disorder, one must concede that it is not a single disease process with a common pathogenesis but a group of commonly recognized clinical abnormalities with multiple causes. Evidence for this is that cryptorchid testes exhibit wide variation in phenotypic expression. Differences in the resting anatomic position of the testis, unilateral versus bilateral maldescent, paratesticular structural anomalies, intrinsic structural and hormonal abnormalities of the testis, and association with other congenital conditions (e.g., hypospadias) represent common variations of cryptorchidism. With respect to the comparative developmental and pathophysiologic origins of cryptorchidism, categorization of testes that are retractile, ectopic, absent, or have ascended to an abnormal location late in childhood is also clinically debated. A large body of research and clinical observations have begun to answer important etiologic questions, but to date the exact mechanism of what is perhaps the most common congenital abnormality at birth in male children is unknown.

Incidence

Isolated cryptorchidism is one of the most common congenital anomalies found at birth and affects upward of 3% of full-term male newborns (Scorer and Farrington, 1971; Cryptorchidism, 1992; Berkowitz et al, 1993; Thong et al, 1998). Unilateral cryptorchidism is more common than bilateral cryptorchidism, which occurs in 1.6% to 1.9% of boys. Testicular descent into the scrotum is usually complete by the second trimester; however, a significantly higher rate of cryptorchidism in premature boys suggests that the process of descent may not be complete until close to term. Scorer and Farrington (1971) reported a 30.3% incidence of undescended testes in premature infants. Many other studies have confirmed similar results in preterm male infants less than 37 weeks' gestation and weighing less than 2500 g. Several large series have identified groups of newborns at risk for cryptorchidism in order to characterize the natural history and factors that affect postnatal descent. These studies found that undescended testes are significantly more prevalent in preterm, small-for-gestational-age, low-birth-weight, and twin neonates. The Cryptorchidism Study Group prospectively examined more than 7400 consecutive normal boys at birth and showed that the rate of cryptorchidism was 7.7%, 2.5%, and 1.41% at 3 months of age for babies weighing, respectively, less than 2000 g, between 2000 and 2499 g, and 2500 g or more (Cryptorchidism, 1992).

Berkowitz and colleagues (1993) reported that the rate of cryptorchidism in 6935 newborn boys declined from 3.7% at birth to 1.0% by 3 months of age and remained essentially constant by 1 year of age. **Approximately 70% to 77% of cryptorchid testes will spontaneously descend, usually by 3 months of age.** Wenzler et al (2004) reported that only 6.9% of cryptorchid testes descended spontaneously beyond 6 months of age. Factors that predict complete spontaneous descent by 3 months of age include low birth weight, bilateral cryptorchidism, normal scrotal anatomy, and testis that are positioned lower along the normal path of descent; boys with a small or poorly rugated scrotum and those with hypospadias are more likely to be cryptorchid at 3 months (Cryptorchidism, 1992). Other factors that may help determine late testicular descent include black or Hispanic ethnicity; a family history of cryptorchidism, low birth weight, and preterm birth delivery; and cola consumption during pregnancy (Berkowitz and Lapinski, 1996). By 1 year of age, the incidence of cryptorchidism declines to about 1% and remains constant throughout adulthood.

Epidemiology

Establishing epidemiologic factors that affect the risk for undescended testes is made more difficult by the complex interactions among anatomy, heredity, the hormonal milieu, and socioeconomic and environmental conditions. Nevertheless, risk factors for the presence of an undescended testis at birth and by 1 year of age need to be considered. As described earlier, cryptorchidism is more common in premature and low-birth-weight male newborns, including boys born prematurely because of maternal, fetal, and unknown causes, intrauterine growth retardation, and twin gestation. **However, more accurate analysis of data leads to the conclusion that birth weight alone is the principal determinant of cryptorchidism at birth and at 1 year of life, independent of the length of gestation** (Hjertkvist et al, 1989; Mayr et al, 1999). Jones and associates (1998) found that gestational age was not an independent risk factor after adjusting for birth weight, as did Weidner and coworkers (1999), who found that the risk for cryptorchidism and hypospadias both increased with decreasing birth weight, independent of gestational age.

A study of 1002 Malaysian male newborns found that premature infants with an undescended testis were more likely than term newborns with an undescended testis to demonstrate complete testicular descent (Thong et al, 1998). This finding implicates factors that result in low birth weight, such as intrauterine growth retardation and poor placental function, to be a more important risk factor for testicular maldescent. Neonates with congenital malformations, who often have low birth weight, are at increased risk for cryptorchidism. Other studies examining maternal causes of cryptorchidism have discovered a number of possible risk factors. Important factors common to all reports include preeclampsia, breech presentation of the fetus, delivery by cesarean section or complicated delivery, and a family history of cryptorchidism (Hjertkvist et al, 1989; Mori et al, 1992; Berkowitz and Lapinski, 1996; Jones et al, 1998; Akre et al, 1999; Mayr et al, 1999). This again implicates factors that may disrupt uteroplacental function and affect fetal viability and development. Few studies have examined ethnicity; however, Asian descent may be a relative risk factor for the development of cryptorchidism (Berkowitz and Lapinski, 1996). Investigators have postulated a possible common genetic, hormonal, or environmental cause for cryptorchidism and hypospadias. The simultaneous presence of hypospadias and cryptorchidism has been shown to occur more commonly than would be predicted (Weidner et al, 1999). Czeizel and associates (1981) reported

that the incidence of undescended testes was 1.5% to 4.0% in the fathers and 6.2% in the brothers of index patients with cryptorchidism, thus supporting a multifactorial pattern of inheritance. A recent study found almost 23% of index patients with cryptorchidism to have a positive family history in other family members (parents, brothers, uncles, cousins, great cousins, and grandfathers) versus 7.5% in control families (Elert et al, 2003). **The familial cluster (risk for an undescended testis in a newborn male if a family member is already affected) is 3.6-fold overall, 6.9-fold if a brother is affected, and 4.6-fold if the father is affected.** To date, the precise molecular and genetic mechanisms underlying cryptorchidism in humans remain unknown.

Classification

Normal testicular descent is defined as a testis that remains stationary within the dependent portion of the scrotum. Therefore, cryptorchidism is a developmental defect in which the testis fails to descend completely into the scrotum. Although this is a useful general definition, there is considerable anatomic variation among cryptorchid testes. In addition, classification by anatomic position alone no doubt underestimates the variable anatomy, physiology, etiology, and natural history of an undescended testis and skews many published studies. Anatomic variation in testicular size and consistency, epididymal and vasal anomalies, and an associated patent processus vaginalis or inguinal hernia should be taken into account. These factors reflect the dimorphic nature of male sexual differentiation and suggest that multiple causes may be responsible for the variations in phenotypic expression. Consideration of the normal embryologic sequence of testicular descent helps in understanding the possible ectopic positions that the testis may attain when it fails to descend to an orthotopic intrascrotal position.

It is sometimes difficult to accurately classify the position, integrity, and presence of an undescended testis. Body habitus, testicular position, and compliance of the child during the examination can significantly complicate the clinical evaluation and result in diagnostic error. Classification systems can be useful in determining management and predicting outcome. Although a number of classification systems have been devised, Kaplan (1993) proposed the most popular system, which categorizes cryptorchid testes as either *palpable* or *nonpalpable*. Excluding atrophic or vanishing testes, palpable testes have descended beyond the abdomen (internal ring), whereas nonpalpable testes are intra-abdominal. The subjective nature of the physical examination confounds the accurate classification of testicular position; more accurate assessment occurs at the time of surgery. **Cryptorchid testicular position is most simply described at the time of exploration as intra-abdominal, intracanalicular, extracanalicular (suprapubic or infrapubic), or ectopic.**

Approximately 80% of undescended testes are clinically palpable and 20% are nonpalpable. Looking more closely at children with nonpalpable testes, Cisek et al (1998) reported that 18% of these testes could be palpated during physical examination under anesthesia and 12.6% of viable testes discovered at exploration were distal to the inguinal canal and simply missed on physical examination. Between a third and two thirds of children with a nonpalpable testis will be monorchid.

An *intra-abdominal testis* is usually located just inside the internal ring, commonly within a few centimeters, although intra-abdominal testes have been observed anywhere along a line between the lower pole of the kidney and the internal ring. Testes may also lie at a high annular position at the internal ring. These testes have been referred to as "peeping" because they can move between the abdominal cavity and inguinal canal. Rarely, a testis is found in ectopic intra-abdominal positions such as in the perihepatic and perisplenic regions. An intracanalicular testis is occasionally difficult to palpate and by definition lies within the inguinal canal, between the internal and external ring. An emergent or suprapubic testis lies just beyond the external ring, above the level of pubic symphysis, and an infrapubic testis lies just below the pubic symphysis, often just outside the anatomic scrotum in the retroscrotal space. The testis may also be located in an ectopic position. An ectopic testis completes normal transinguinal migration but is misdirected outside the normal path of descent below the external ring. **The most common ectopic location is within a superficial pouch between the external oblique fascia and Scarpa's fascia, a structure that has been termed the Denis-Browne pouch. Other abnormal locations include transverse scrotal, femoral, perineal, and prepenile ectopia.** Theories of descent do not include adequate data, either observational or experimental, to explain testicular ectopia, and presently the mechanism of pathologic descent is unknown. Studies of human fetuses by both Backhouse in 1982 and Heyns in 1987 did not support the finding of multiple distal attachments of the gubernaculum, originally credited to Lockwood in 1888 to account for testicular ectopia (Backhouse 1982b; Heyns 1987).

The terms "nonpalpable testis" and "retractile testis" are ubiquitous. These terms deserve further definition and incorporation into this discussion because they may confound accurate classification of cryptorchidism. **The term "nonpalpable testis" implies that the testis cannot be detected on physical examination and therefore is either intra-abdominal, absent (vanishing), atrophic, or missed on physical examination.** A vanishing or absent testis is usually encountered during exploration for a nonpalpable testis. The anatomic hallmark of a vanishing testis is blind-ending spermatic vessels that are found just proximal to the internal inguinal ring. An atrophic testis is a smaller than normal testis that may be cryptorchid. These testes can be encountered anywhere along the course of normal descent from within the abdomen to the scrotum.

A "retractile testis" withdraws spontaneously out of the scrotum toward the inguinal canal by an active cremasteric reflex but can easily be brought down into a dependent position within the scrotum and remains there after traction has been released. This condition is considered a variant of normal; however, the risk of ascent may be as great as 50% in children with a "significantly" retractile testis. A retractile testis can be found anywhere along the course of descent, but it is usually palpable in the groin on initial examination. Retractile testes are most commonly encountered between the ages of 3 and 7 years. The retractability of the testes is caused by an overactive cremasteric reflex. A cremasteric reflex, initiated by stroking the skin of the inner aspect of the thigh, is present in about 50% of boys younger than 30 months and in most boys older than 30 months (Caesar and Kaplan, 1994).

If a testis can be milked down to the bottom of the scrotum, it is probably retractile and does not require therapy (Wyllie, 1984). However, there is debate regarding whether retractile testes are a subtle variant of their undescended counterpart. A retractile testis is not truly cryptorchid, although an uncommon phenomenon of delayed spontaneous testicular ascent has perhaps been falsely ascribed to a retractile testis. In cases of ascent, boys previously documented to have normally descended testes are found later in childhood to be cryptorchid. **Ascent probably represents an undescended testis that is almost completely descended.** Rabinowitz and Hulbert (1997) observed that the cause of this condition is a missed diagnosis at a younger age. The testis is usually located in a superficial inguinal pouch and is diagnosed as undescended with somatic growth. **Therefore, children with retractile testes should be monitored regularly (yearly), at least up to puberty, until the testes are no longer retractile and remain intrascrotal.** This phenomenon was noted by Scorer and Farrington (1971) and other investigators, who reported a higher incidence of cryptorchidism in 5-year-old boys than in younger children. Recently, Barthold and Gonzalez (2003) reported that cryptorchidism may be acquired in a significantly greater number of cases, in large part because of retractile testes. Based on the reviewed published literature, they noted higher than anticipated cumulative orchidopexy rates of 2% to 4%, with the mean age at surgery reported to be 7 years in the majority of series. The most common testicular position was observed to be distal to the external inguinal ring, and in about half the cases the processus vaginalis was patent (Barthold and Gonzalez, 2003). Although Puri and Nixon reported that children with retractile testes have normal testicular volume and a normal fertility rate in adulthood, testicular development has been reported to be abnormal in both retractile testes and ascending testes, with histology similar to that of undescended testes (Puri and Nixon, 1977; Ito et al, 1986; Saito and Kumamoto, 1989; Han et al, 1999). The abnormally low total germ cell counts were comparable to primary undescended testes, thus suggesting a similar pathophysiology (Rusnack et al, 2002).

KEY POINTS: GENERAL

- Cryptorchidism affects 3% of full-term male newborns. Approximately 70% to 77% of cryptorchid testes will spontaneously descend, usually by 3 months of age.

- Birth weight may be the principal determinant of cryptorchidism at birth and at 1 year of life, independent of the length of gestation.

- Eighty percent of undescended testes are palpable and 20% are nonpalpable. The most common location for an ectopic undescended testis is within the superficial pouch.

- Children with retractile testes require annual follow-up until puberty or the testis is no longer retractile.

- The germ cell histology of ascended testes is abnormal and comparable to that of primary undescended testes.

Testicular Maldescent

Theories of Descent and Maldescent

The past 2 centuries have given rise to theories of testicular descent and maldescent that remain controversial because they are mired in myth, misconceptions, and misinterpretation of previous data. As yet, there is no universally agreed on theory of descent, but important pieces of the puzzle have been postulated from careful anatomic and embryologic observations. Testicular descent and maldescent are now being explored on a molecular level, but most of our current understanding is based on observation. John Hunter, an English anatomist, published the first important and highly accurate description of testicular descent in 1762. He is credited with describing and naming the gubernaculum, which is derived from the Latin word meaning *helm* or *rudder*. Hunter also recognized the importance of this structure with regard to testicular descent but was cautious in postulating its function (Backhouse, 1982b). Since that time, many theories have been proposed that involve the effect of intra-abdominal pressure, gravity, cremasteric muscle contraction, endocrine factors, and structures unique to the male fetus—but none more important than the gubernaculum. The popular theories of descent are presented in this section to underscore the diversity and complexity of this condition.

For normal spermatogenesis to occur, it is necessary for the testes to descend into the scrotum, a specialized, low-temperature environment that maintains a temperature 2° F to 3° F lower than core body temperature. Under normal embryologic conditions in humans, the fetal testis begins its multistaged descent into the scrotum from its position of origin, the abdominal cavity. Gier and Marion (1969) proposed three phases of testicular descent in the human fetus: (1) nephric displacement by degeneration of the mesonephros at 7 to 8 weeks' gestation, (2) transabdominal passage of the testis from the metanephros to the inguinal ring by 21 weeks, and (3) inguinal transit of the testis from the peritoneal cavity to a position along the processus vaginalis at 28 weeks. Hutson and Hasthorpe (2005) proposed a schema in which testicular descent occurs in two phases: transabdominal and inguinoscrotal. Transabdominal descent is generally dependent on hormonal control by MIS, whereas the inguinoscrotal phase of descent is mediated by androgen. Anatomically, the transabdominal phase is viewed as a combination of CSL regression under the regulation of androgen and gubernacular swelling controlled by both androgen and MIS. Conceptually, however, testicular descent is best illustrated in three phases: (1) transabdominal, (2) transinguinal, and (3) extracanalicular migration (descent from the external ring to the scrotum).

To briefly review, transabdominal descent of the testis toward the internal ring results from differential growth of the lumbar vertebral column and pelvis. The testis is adjacent to the kidney by the 8th week of gestation, and further migration does not begin until about the 23rd week. The intra-abdominal position of the testis before transinguinal descent is just inside the internal ring. The rapid transinguinal phase of descent requires the testis to travel through the inguinal canal alongside and posterior to the processus vaginalis into the scrotum. The final phase of descent, from the external ring to the scrotum, occurs after 28 weeks; in most cases testicular descent is complete between the 30th and 32nd week. Many investigators agree with this basic outline and time course, but controversy exists regarding the mechanism of descent after 23 weeks of gestation until the testis is intrascrotal because most theories are extrapolated from static observation of fetal human dissections. Animal models have not provided a satisfactory comparison to human testicular descent. Most theories of testicular descent are concentrated on development of the gubernaculum, processus vaginalis, inguinal canal, spermatic vessels, and scrotum because the analogous structures in the female fetus are substantially different and the gubernaculum truly has no analog in the female (Heyns and Hutson, 1995).

Endocrine Factors

A normal hypothalamic-pituitary-gonadal axis is usually a prerequisite for testicular descent to occur (Toppari and Kaleva, 1999). Defects may occur in gonadotropin production, androgen biosynthesis, or androgen action. The primary hormones that regulate the testes are luteinizing hormone (LH) and follicle-stimulating hormone (FSH). Both hormones are secreted by basophilic cells in the anterior pituitary. The primary site of action of FSH is on the epithelium of the seminiferous tubule. Gonadotropin regulation is under the control of luteinizing hormone–releasing hormone (LHRH) stimulation from the hypothalamus, which interacts with high-affinity cell surface receptor sites on the plasma membrane of pituitary gonadotrophs. Plasma FSH levels are often elevated in patients with testicular pathology, including those with cryptorchidism. FSH stimulates Sertoli cells and therefore has an important role in spermatogenesis. Plasma FSH levels usually correlate inversely with spermatogenesis, and therefore FSH is considered the most clinically useful endocrine marker in the evaluation of infertile men. However, in children, circulating FSH, LH, and testosterone levels may not accurately reflect testicular development or the presence of testicular pathology.

Androgens. The androgens testosterone and DHT are necessary for testicular descent to occur. They may act either directly or indirectly, such as in the neuroendocrine modulation of the GFN and release of calcitonin gene–related peptide (CGRP), as proposed by Hutson and associates in 1994. Clinical examples supporting this theory include patients with androgen insensitivity syndrome (AIS) and hypogonadotropic hypogonadism who have bilateral cryptorchidism. In the majority of humans with AIS, the testes are located in close proximity to the inguinal canal, thus indicating that transabdominal descent has not been effected (Ahmed et al, 2000). The testes were palpable in the labioscrotal folds or the inguinal region in 77% and 41% of cases of complete AIS and partial AIS, respectively. In addition, transabdominal descent occurs normally in mice with androgen insensitivity (Hutson and Donahoe, 1986). Prenatal exposure to the anti-androgen agent flutamide did not interfere with transabdominal descent in rats (Shono et al, 1994).

From these data it can be surmised that androgens do not mediate the first phase of testicular descent. However, androgens appear to be important for the inguinal-scrotal phase of testicular descent. Failure of gubernacular involution has been observed in humans with AIS (Hutson and Donahoe, 1986).

Delayed gubernacular migration and regression have been described in animal models of gonadotropin deficiency associated with low testosterone concentrations and in AIS. Additional support for androgen action is the presence of androgen binding by the gubernaculum in rodent models. Evidence indicating that androgens mediate CSL regression includes (1) persistence of the CSL in humans with AIS and (2) persistence of the CSL in animal models with prenatal anti-androgen exposure (Hutson and Donahoe, 1986; Shono et al, 1994). **Therefore, impaired androgen biosynthesis or action can impede the second phase of testicular descent.**

Analysis of the androgen receptor in DNA samples obtained from 21 boys with isolated unilateral or bilateral cryptorchidism identified no abnormalities (Wiener et al, 1998). However, exon 1 was not evaluated, and it contains a polymorphic CAG trinucleotide repeat expansion. Longer repeats are associated with decreased androgen action, manifested as an increased incidence of oligozoospermia or azoospermia in otherwise normal men (Tut et al, 1997; Dowsing et al, 1999). Undervirilized 46,XY patients have been found to have longer CAG repeats, which suggests that this locus functions as a modifier locus (Lim et al, 2000). Therefore, variations in the trinucleotide repeat in exon 1 of the androgen receptor may have a role in cryptorchidism.

In utero testosterone deficiency can be caused by decreased LH, by impaired function of gonadotropin-releasing hormone (GnRH) or LH receptors, or by loss-of-function mutations in the proteins involved in testosterone biosynthesis. Complete loss-of-function mutations are associated with sex reversal in 46,XY fetuses and with variable testicular location. The spectrum of testicular location includes an intra-abdominal position to the labia majora. Experimental evidence links gonadotropin deficiency and cryptorchidism. Although a small penis is a common clinical finding in boys with gonadotropin deficiency, cryptorchidism does occur (Van Dop et al, 1987). Hypogonadotropic hypogonadism as a result of mutation in the *KAL*, *DAX1*, or GnRH receptor (*GNRHR*) genes is a monogenic disorder associated with gonadotropin deficiency in which cryptorchidism has been described as one of the clinical features (Habiby et al, 1996; Pralong et al, 1999). Because anosmia occurs infrequently in the majority of patients with cryptorchidism, *KAL* mutations are probably an extremely rare cause of isolated cryptorchidism. Deletion of the GnRH gene in GnRH[hpg] mice often results in intra-abdominal testes (Mason et al, 1986). Mutations in the *GNRHR* gene are associated with autosomal recessive hypogonadotropic hypogonadism (de Roux et al, 1997; Layman et al, 1998). Abnormalities of the LH receptor show a theoretical possibility of affecting testicular descent. Two variants of the LHβ gene have been described that show an increased clearance rate from serum, although their relationship to cryptorchidism has not been evaluated (Furui et al, 1994; Suganuma et al, 1996). A mutation in the LHβ gene has been shown to impair the ability of LH to bind to its receptor and is associated with impaired steroidogenesis and infertility in heterozygotic carriers; it results in delayed puberty, oligospermia, and Leydig cell hypoplasia (Weiss et al, 1992). Cryptorchidism has been described in association with Leydig cell hypoplasia, an autosomal recessive disorder characterized by impaired Leydig cell differentiation secondary to loss-of-function mutations in the LH receptor gene (*LHR*)

(Martinez-Mora et al, 1991; Kremer et al, 1995; Wu et al, 1998).

Errors in testosterone biosynthesis have also been associated with cryptorchidism. The specific enzyme genes include 17α-hydroxylase/17,20-lyase (*CYP17*), 3β-hydroxysteroid dehydrogenase type 2 (*HSD3B2*), and 17β-hydroxysteroid dehydrogenase type 3 (*HSD17B3*). Children with complete **CYP17 deficiency** are usually assigned female gender at birth and are initially evaluated in adolescence for delayed puberty. Affected 46,XY individuals can have intra-abdominal testes or genital ambiguity with undescended testes (Biason et al, 1991; Lin et al, 1991; Geller et al, 1997). **3β-Hydroxysteroid dehydrogenase type 2 deficiency** is a rare cause of congenital adrenal hyperplasia in which the affected 46,XY fetus is undervirilized because of mutations in *HSD3B2* (Kenny et al, 1971; Rheaume et al, 1992). Whereas hypospadias is typical, testicular position is variable (Rheaume et al, 1994). Affected 46,XY individuals with **17β-hydroxysteroid dehydrogenase type 3 deficiency** have a female phenotype or ambiguous genitalia at birth, with undescended testes (Gross et al, 1986). Testicular conversion of androstenedione to testosterone is affected, and these individuals are often initially seen in adolescence with virilization and primary amenorrhea (Geissler et al, 1994; Andersson et al, 1996; Park et al, 1996). The clinical spectrum of 5α-reductase type 2 (*SRD5A2*) deficiency ranges from the female phenotype to hypospadias. Testicular position is variable and ranges from intra-abdominal to labial-scrotal (Imperato-McGinley et al, 1991; Nordenskjold and Ivarsson, 1998).

Müllerian Inhibiting Substance. MIS is secreted by the fetal Sertoli cells and is responsible for regression of the müllerian ducts. MIS has also been implicated in effecting testicular descent. MIS levels normally surge in the first year of life, peak at 4 to 12 months, and subsequently decline with age. **Yamanaka and colleagues (1991) reported that patients with cryptorchidism do not demonstrate a surge in the first year of life and that mean MIS serum concentrations in cryptorchid boys are significantly lower than in controls.** There was also a significant reduction in mean MIS levels in children with bilateral cryptorchidism when compared with those with unilateral undescended testes. However, the authors concede that the difference in MIS levels may have resulted from secondary intrinsic Sertoli cell dysfunction rather than being a consequence of cryptorchidism.

MIS has been further investigated as a factor mediating testicular descent because cryptorchidism is a common feature of persistent müllerian duct syndrome (PMDS) (Hutson and Donahoe, 1986). PMDS is characterized by normal male differentiation with failure of regression of müllerian duct derivatives secondary to mutations in the MIS or MIS II receptor gene (Knebelmann et al, 1991; Josso et al, 1993; Imbeaud et al, 1996). However, it is more likely that anatomic obstruction is the cause of cryptorchidism associated with PMDS because the testes are tethered to the intra-abdominal müllerian duct derivatives. Therefore, the weight of evidence suggests that MIS does not play a significant role in the regulation of testicular descent, based on the following: (1) normal testicular descent occurs in MIS-deficient knockout mice (Behringer et al, 1994), (2) normal testicular descent occurs in fetal rabbits immunized against bovine MIS (Tran et al,

1986), (3) ovarian descent is not observed in transgenic female mice overexpressing MIS (Behringer et al, 1994), and (4) the majority of patients with intra-abdominal testes do not have retained müllerian derivatives.

Estrogen. Estrogens have been postulated to impair testicular descent. Prenatal treatment with diethylstilbestrol (DES), a nonsteroidal synthetic estrogen, is associated with urogenital abnormalities in both male and female fetuses. Undescended testes is one of the abnormalities observed in 46,XY fetuses (Stillman, 1982). Animal studies on mice confirmed that prenatal estrogen exposure disrupts the transabdominal phase of testicular descent (McLachlan et al, 1975; Shono et al, 1994). Estrogens are thought to impair gubernacular development and to cause persistence of müllerian duct derivatives. Testicular position was noted to be similar in INSL3 (insulin-like 3) knockout animals and in DES-exposed normal animals. To determine the relationship between prenatal estrogen exposure and INSL3 expression, experimental evidence determined that prenatal DES exposure was associated with decreased testicular INSL3 expression in mice. However, no change in steroidogenic factor 1 (SF1) expression was noted in DES-treated animals (Emmen et al, 2000a). SF1 has been shown to play an essential role in transcriptional activation of the INSL3 gene promoter. In a different animal model, testicular expression of SF1 was decreased by prenatal DES exposure (Majdic et al, 1997). Prenatal testosterone treatment does not correct cryptorchidism induced by prenatal estrogen exposure, thus indicating independent mechanisms of action (Hutson and Watts, 1990).

Skakkebaek and colleagues maintained that the frequency of cryptorchidism and poor semen quality is increasing and speculated that this was occurring because of greater exposure to endocrine disruptors in the environment (Toppari and Skakkebaek, 1998). Evidence cited against their hypothesis included the absence of differences in maternal estrogen concentrations during pregnancy in woman who had sons with cryptorchidism and controls (Key et al, 1996). However, because the maternal circulation is far removed from local fetal hormone concentrations, maternal estrogen concentrations may not be valid measures of fetal estrogen exposure.

Descendin. Conflicting views on the role of androgen stimulation and gubernacular development resulted in the concept of an androgen-independent factor, descendin, a gubernacular-specific growth factor. Hosie and associates (1999) demonstrated direct androgen stimulation of the human gubernaculum testis via specific intranuclear hormone receptor binding, thus implicating its role in gubernacular swelling through an increase in glycosaminoglycans. The quality and quantity of androgen receptors would therefore theoretically influence the extent of transinguinal testicular descent. However, evidence suggests that gubernacular development is not completely androgen dependent. In dogs, fetal orchiectomy prevented gubernacular swelling and regression but was not completely rectified by testosterone supplementation (Baumans et al, 1982; Baumans et al, 1983). Gubernacular regression was not completely prevented by fetal supplementation of testosterone, and some descent of the remaining epididymis occurred. In contrast, dogs orchidectomized neonatally and supplemented with an autotransplant of testicular tissue demonstrated normal gubernacular devel-

opment and epididymal descent. Cryptorchidism induced by the antiandrogen flutamide was also shown to specifically inhibit only gubernacular regression (McMahon et al, 1995). Furthermore, normal gubernacular development was observed to occur in the presence of complete testicular feminization (Hutson and Donahoe, 1986). **Indirect evidence that growth of the gubernaculum during descent is not the result of androgen stimulation supports the existence of an androgen-independent factor** (Heyns and Pape, 1991). Testicular descent was examined in a fetal porcine model, and it was demonstrated that during the first phase of testicular descent, a bioactive, low-molecular-weight factor is present that stimulates gubernacular cell growth (Fentener van Vlissingen et al, 1988). This paracrine factor, descendin, is believed to be secreted from the testis in an androgen-independent fashion and to be responsible for changes in the first phase of gubernaculum development, which is characterized by rapid cell proliferation (outgrowth) and concomitant synthesis of sulfated glycosaminoglycans, hyaluronic acid, and collagen (Fentener van Vlissingen et al, 1989).

Gubernaculum

The singular importance of the gubernaculum in testicular descent cannot be underestimated; however, its exact physiologic mechanism has the subject of considerable debate and study. There are many theories regarding the function of the gubernaculum, including the gubernaculum as a guide into the scrotum, the gubernaculum as a wedge that swells and dilates the inguinal passage of the testis, and various theories espousing gubernacular contraction, involution, traction, and stationary fixation in combination with differential somatic growth. Heyns (1987) defined the primary differences between the countervailing theories of gubernaculum-mediated testicular descent in relation to three points: (1) the cranial and caudal attachments, (2) the type of cell forming its "active" constituent, and (3) gubernacular morphogenesis relative to inguinal-scrotal development during testicular descent. All evidence implicates the gubernaculum as the major factor responsible for testicular descent.

Research from many species has simultaneously advanced and muddled our understanding of testicular descent; nonetheless, several key mechanistic properties of the gubernaculum have been established. The earliest theories were based on preconceived notions of testicular descent and suggested that the testis was pulled into the scrotum by the gubernaculum. However, substantial evidence indicates that there is no firm attachment of the gubernaculum to the scrotum (Wensing, 1968; Scorer and Farrington, 1971; Heyns, 1987; Wensing, 1988; Hutson et al, 1997). **Consequently, the testis cannot be pulled *into* the scrotum.** The gubernaculum is anchored near the future inguinal canal and stabilizes the testis near the groin while the kidney migrates to a cranial position. The processus vaginalis allows the previously intra-abdominal testis to migrate from the abdominal cavity (Heyns and Hutson, 1995). Once the testis has passed through the inguinal canal and descent is complete, the bulb of the gubernaculum is resorbed (Backhouse, 1966). Clinical and experimental data indicate that hormones, transcription factors, and possibly neural factors influence development. At present, it appears that testicular descent is a complex event mediated by both hormonal and mechanical factors.

The hormone INSL3 has been implicated in mediating testicular descent through gubernacular development. Produced by the fetal testis, specifically the Leydig cells, INSL3 is related to insulin and relaxin and is believed to mediate transabdominal descent. Targeting of transgenic mice for *INSL3* gene knockout resulted in bilateral cryptorchidism (Nef and Parada, 1999; Zimmermann et al, 1999). The mice were found to have small, undifferentiated gubernacula and intraabdominal testes. Emmen et al (2000b) then demonstrated gubernacular outgrowth to be dependent on both androgen and INSL3. INSL3 binds specifically to LGR8, a leucine-rich G protein–coupled receptor (Kumagai et al, 2002). Further evidence supporting the essential relationship of INSL3 and LGR8 was demonstrated in mice with mutations in the receptor *LGR8* gene and transgenic mice deficient for the *LGR8* gene overexpressing INSL3. In both experimental models, bilateral intra-abdominal testes developed similar to the INSL–/– phenotype (Overbeek et al, 2001; Bogatcheva et al, 2003; Tomiyama et al, 2003). Though a tantalizing cause-and-effect relationship that might have explained the admittedly small subset of patients with cryptorchidism who have bilateral intra-abdominal testes, analysis of published studies indicates that mutations in either of these two genes account for only a minority of cases of cryptorchidism in the human population and thus support a multifactorial etiology for the most common manifestation of this disease (Tomboc et al, 2000; Klonisch et al, 2004; Bogatcheva and Agoulnik, 2005).

Genitofemoral Nerve and Calcitonin Gene–Related Peptide

Lewis first presented evidence in 1948 that transecting the GFN in neonatal rats resulted in cryptorchidism. Hutson repeated this study and presented data proposing that the GFN induced testicular descent and gubernacular differentiation. Transection of the GFN in rats resulted in the testes remaining in the abdomen and prevented gubernacular migration (Beasley and Hutson, 1987; Fallat et al, 1992). The concept that the GFN acts as a "second messenger" is based on evidence that androgens increase the number of GFN cell bodies and promote gubernacular migration, mediated by CGRP (Hutson and Beasley, 1987). CGRP has been identified as a neurotransmitter in the GFN and its nerve branches (Larkins et al, 1991). Gubernacula in vivo showed rhythmic contractility and demonstrated a high degree of motility during testicular descent (Park and Hutson, 1991). This theory is supported by evidence that the androgen receptor is present in the lumbar spinal cord near the cremasteric nucleus before the onset of maximal androgenic action (Cain et al, 1994).

GFN morphology has been shown to be altered by a reduction in motor neuron number and neural diameter in association with flutamide-induced cryptorchidism (Husmann et al, 1994). Prenatal androgen blockade with flutamide has been shown to inhibit masculinization of the GFN with a significant reduction in its CGRP content (Goh et al, 1994). These findings support the hypothesis that androgens directly regulate the development and morphology of the sexually dimorphic GFN during testicular descent and that CGRP acts as a second messenger. However, a number of studies present evidence to the contrary, including the observation that CGRP release is increased by androgen withdrawal and that the cremasteric nucleus may not be androgen dependent (Popper and Micevych, 1989; Barthold et al, 1994). CGRP also fails to induce murine testicular descent (Houle and Gagne, 1995). Additionally, CGRP is a neuromuscular transmitter that has been demonstrated to act on the muscular component of the rodent's developing gubernaculum, which is primarily cremasteric muscle (Husmann and Levy, 1995). The human gubernaculum lacks a muscular component; this fact most likely excludes CGRP from playing a significant role in human testicular descent (Heyns, 1987).

Epididymis

The theoretical association uniting normal testicular descent to epididymal function is based on the observation that epididymal abnormalities often accompany cryptorchidism. The difficulty arises in that it is unknown whether epididymal anomalies are the cause or the result of the undescended testis. The concept that normal testicular descent depends on the epididymis is challenged by the demonstration that either elimination of the epididymis or epididymal agenesis does not impede testicular descent (Frey and Rajfer, 1982; Baikie and Hutson, 1990). Many of the theories related to epididymal anomalies link the causative theories of cryptorchidism, and it stands to reason that the same factors are responsible for both cryptorchidism and fusion anomalies of the epididymis (Merksz, 1998). Most theories suggest that fetal androgen deficiency plays an important role in this association.

Embryologically, the epididymis is in direct contact with the gubernaculum and precedes the testis into the scrotum. It has been suggested that abnormal embryologic attachment of the cranial gubernaculum may account for abnormalities noted in the mode of descent of adjacent paratesticular structures (Abe et al, 1996). Epididymal anomalies are encountered in patients with undescended testes (including ectopic testes), hernias, and hydroceles. Epididymal abnormalities were found to be more common in boys with undescended testes (41%) than in boys with ectopic testes (25.9%) (Kucukaydin et al, 1998). One large series of 652 cases of cryptorchidism reported that epididymal and vasal anomalies occurred with an overall frequency of 36% (Mollaeian et al, 1994). **Koff and Scaletscky (1990) reported similar findings but found a much higher incidence of complex epididymal abnormalities in those with cryptorchidism, approaching 90%.** Thirty-nine percent of ectopic testes displayed more severe epididymal abnormalities, whereas 33% showed only an elongated epididymis and 29% were normal. The higher the arrest of testicular descent, the more grossly abnormal the associated ductal system (Gill et al, 1989). Epididymal anomalies associated with cryptorchidism also include a significantly higher incidence of patent processus vaginalis. Barthold and Redman (1996) reported that epididymal anomalies were more frequently found in association with undescended than with descended testes (72% versus 34%, respectively), with a greater frequency depending on the extent of patency of the processus vaginalis. A closed, partially closed, or open processus vaginalis was associated with an abnormal epididymis in 14%, 36%, and 69% of cases, respectively.

Elder (1992a), by comparing epididymal abnormalities in descended testes, concluded that most epididymal abnormalities probably do not contribute to testicular maldescent.

Excluding intra-abdominal testes, 50% of boys with a hydrocele or hernia had an epididymal abnormality if the processus was patent and communicated with the testis, as compared with only 10% if no communication was present. In children with an undescended testis, 71% had an epididymal abnormality if there was a patent processus versus 16% without a patent processus.

Epididymal abnormalities range from minor structural findings, such as elongation, to more complex anatomic aberrations in fusion, to complete disjunction, to an absent structure altogether. **Perhaps the most salient point concerning this association as it relates to future fertility is that despite early surgical treatment of children with cryptorchidism to preserve normal germ cell development, fusion anomalies commonly exist that must ultimately affect sperm maturation and transport** (Mollaeian et al, 1994). In addition, biopsy of testes with severe anomalies in ductal fusion showed preservation of germ cells in 69% and diminished germ cells in 31% (Gill et al, 1989). Therefore, prognostic indicators of future fertility should consider the epididymal anomalies detected at the time of surgery because such anomalies might coexist with excellent testis histology.

Intra-abdominal Pressure

Conditions that result in cryptorchidism hypothetically associated with decreased intra-abdominal pressure include prune-belly syndrome, cloacal exstrophy, omphalocele, gastroschisis, and a number of syndromes characterized by both cryptorchidism and congenital abdominal wall muscular defects or agenesis (Levard and Laberge, 1997; Koivusalo et al, 1998). Abdominal pressure probably has an ancillary role in migration of the testis from the abdominal cavity to the inguinal canal, but thereafter it plays a more significant role in transinguinal descent into the scrotum (Quinlan et al, 1988; Attah and Hutson, 1993; Hutson et al, 1997). The patent processus vaginalis probably works in conjunction with intra-abdominal pressure, which is transmitted to the testis during transinguinal migration. Androgens may also play a role in conjunction with abdominal pressure at this stage of development to deliver the testis into the scrotum (Frey et al, 1983; Frey and Rajfer, 1984; Hadziselimovic et al, 1987a). Frey demonstrated experimentally that in the presence of androgen, a silicone prosthesis will descend from the abdominal cavity into the scrotum but that such descent occurs less frequently when androgen is removed (Frey et al, 1983; Frey and Rajfer, 1984).

Histopathology

Normal germ cell development during childhood is a continuous process that is completed at puberty (Hadziselimovic et al, 1987b). The concept that a testis was more likely to be histologically abnormal the longer it remains cryptorchid was proposed by Cooper in 1929. Undescended testes demonstrate more pronounced impairment in germ cell development the higher the testes are located, although newborns with intra-abdominal testes have a normal number of germ cells (Hadziselimovic et al, 1987b). **The histopathologic hallmarks associated with cryptorchidism are evident between 1 and 2 years of age and include decreased numbers of Leydig cells, degeneration of Sertoli cells, delayed disappearance of**

***

KEY POINTS: DESCENT PATHOPHYSIOLOGY

- Testicular descent is normally complete between the 30th and 32nd week of gestation.

- A normal hypothalamic-pituitary-gonadal axis is usually necessary for testicular descent.

- Testosterone and DHT are necessary for the inguinal-scrotal phase of descent.

- In utero testosterone deficiency can be caused by decreased LH, by impaired function of GnRH or LH receptors, or by loss-of-function mutations in the proteins involved in testosterone biosynthesis.

- Up to 90% of cases of cryptorchidism have associated epididymal anomalies.

***

gonocytes, delayed appearance of adult dark (Ad) spermatogonia, failure of primary spermatocytes to develop, and reduced total germ cell counts (Huff et al, 1987; Rune et al, 1992; Huff et al, 1993). A decrease in cryptorchid testis volume by 6 months of age has been reported (Cendron et al, 1993). The earliest postnatal histologic abnormality in cryptorchid testes was hypoplasia of the Leydig cells, which was observed from the first month of life (Huff et al, 1991). Mininberg and colleagues (1982) reported peritubular fibrosis by 1 year of age in undescended testes. Huff and associates (1989) documented significantly defective maturation of gonocytes in bilateral testicular biopsy specimens from unilaterally cryptorchid boys aged 1 to 13 years, as well as decreased numbers of germ cells from the first year of life. Specifically, transformation of gonocytes to Ad spermatogonia, which is normally complete at 6 months of age, and transformation of Ad spermatogonia to primary spermatocytes, which is normally initiated at 3 years of age, were delayed or defective, or both. The total germ cell count was similar to that of normal controls until the seventh month of age, at which time secondary degeneration of untransformed gonocytes led to a decrease in the total germ cell count (Huff et al, 1991). Numbers of Leydig cells were also abnormally decreased.

Similar pathology as described above was observed in the contralateral descended testis, though to a lesser extent, which supports the theory of hypogonadotropic hypogonadism as the possible cause of the decreased fertility seen in males with unilateral cryptorchidism (Huff et al, 1989; Huff et al, 1993). McAleer and coworkers (1995) reported similar abnormalities in the undescended and descended testes of boys with unilateral cryptorchidism; no significant differences in the fertility index were seen in children before 1 year of age, but there were significant differences in all other age groups. A continuous process of Sertoli cell degeneration is also evident from 1 year of age in undescended testis. It is not related to age but depends on testicular position (Rune et al, 1992). Sertoli cell degeneration may help account for the reduction in germ cell number.

These reports all demonstrate early histopathologic evidence of abnormal spermatogenesis in boys well before 2 years of age that is probably related, in part, to deficient hormonal stimulation. Other parameters that provide evidence of testicular injury include the physical examination and the appearance of the testis at the time of orchiopexy. Concentrations of circulating gonadotropins and gonadal hormones correlate with testicular dysfunction in adults; however, because of the relative quiescence of the pituitary during infancy and early childhood, these hormones do not provide an accurate and direct measurement of testicular maturation and pathology in young boys. Barthold et al (2004) were unable to identify any significant differences in hormone levels (testosterone, estradiol, LH, FSH, inhibin B, sex hormone–binding globulin, and leptin) between controls and boys with nonsyndromic cryptorchidism during activation of the pituitary-testicular axis in early infancy, thus suggesting that impairment of this process is uncommon.

Consequences of Cryptorchidism

Infertility

An important consideration in the assessment of future fertility is recognizing the implications of predicting outcomes based on testis histopathology obtained during orchidopexy in childhood, spermiograms obtained in adulthood, and paternity rates. Impairment of germ cell maturation is a well-recognized consequence of cryptorchidism. A tenet of treatment is that early surgical repositioning of the testis into the scrotum before the onset of histopathologic changes reduces the risk for subfertility. However, increasing evidence suggests that orchiopexy may not significantly reduce this risk. Initial reports focused on the histologic changes that were seen in undescended testes after 1 year of age as a rationale for early surgical treatment to preserve spermatogenic function. McAleer and coworkers (1995) reported that no significant difference in the fertility index was seen in patients 1 year or younger when comparing undescended with descended testes but that fertility index differences were significantly abnormal in all other age groups. However, fertility index measurements were significantly decreased from normal expected values in all age groups with unilateral cryptorchidism, which suggests that potential fertility may be significantly impaired regardless of patient age at the time of surgery. One study conducted after orchiopexy noted severe changes in histomorphologic characteristics of the testicular tissue if surgery was performed after 5 years of age (Tzvetkova and Tzvetkov, 1996). Cortes et al (2001) reported a decrease in germ cells from 18 months, with the frequency increasing with age. In addition, sperm counts were reported to be normal in approximately 20% of men with a history of bilateral cryptorchidism and 80% of men with unilateral cryptorchidism. A later study by this same group concluded that infertility was probable in a third of patients despite orchiopexy; however, the median age at surgery was nearly 13 years and 11 years for bilateral and unilateral cryptorchidism, respectively (Cortes et al, 2003). With respect to histopathologic damage, Gracia et al (1995) failed to show any correlation between the tubular fertility index or tubular diameter and the time of surgery or testicular location in 1342 boys (2000 testes).

Grasso and associates (1991) assessed the fertility of 91 patients with unilateral cryptorchidism who underwent postpubertal orchiopexy and found that 83.5% of patients were azoospermic or oligospermic, with or without asthenospermia. Another study concluded that in postpubertal males with unilateral cryptorchidism, the undescended testis should be removed because of the risk for future malignancy, because the majority of such testes cannot contribute to fertility (only 1 in 52 orchiectomy specimens showed normal spermatogenesis), and because of the risk for torsion (Rogers et al, 1998). Two patients (4%) had carcinoma in situ of the testicle. Fifteen percent of men treated for unilateral cryptorchidism between 4 and 14 years of age were found to be azoospermic, and an additional 30% were oligospermic (sperm count less than $20 \times 10^6/mL$). Untreated men with unilateral cryptorchidism had very similar spermiograms. No untreated, bilaterally cryptorchid patient had normal fertility, whereas a quarter of those who were treated achieved normal fertility (Chilvers et al, 1986). Experimental evidence has demonstrated that early orchiopexy can reverse the histologic changes in cryptorchid testes (Lugg et al, 1996). These data provide support to the value of orchiopexy in the treatment of cryptorchidism.

Attempts have been made to correlate future fertility to testis histopathology at the time of orchidopexy. Hadziselimovic and colleagues (1987c) showed a positive correlation between the number of germ cells in prepubertal testes and the sperm count after puberty. Cortes and Thorup (1991) evaluated boys with bilateral undescended testes by biopsy at the time of orchidopexy and found histology to positively correlate with sperm density and with testes volume in adulthood and negatively correlate with serum FSH; only 11 of 91 patients had a sperm density of 20 million/mL or greater, 41% had normal serum FSH, and 32% had a bilateral testicular volume of 15 mL or greater. Others have demonstrated that patients with bilateral undescended testes had uniformly poor results on semen analysis as young men, with sperm densities of less than 20 million/mL in 75% of patients, whereas men with unilateral cryptorchidism had varied histologic findings, with sperm densities of less than 20 million in 57% of men with testis biopsies that initially showed severe histopathology (Rusnack et al, 2003). **It needs to be kept in mind when interpreting these data that in the era in which these biopsies were performed, much older children (most just prepubertal) were being treated, with a median age at orchidopexy years beyond the current treatment recommendations of orchidopexy at 6 months of age.**

Histopathologic studies in younger cohorts of patients have provided evidence of abnormal germ cell maturation correlating with spermiograms in adulthood. **Biopsy findings from children with unilateral cryptorchidism typically demonstrate reduced total germ cell counts as a result of failure of the two prepubertal steps involved in maturation and proliferation of germ cells: (1) transformation of the fetal stem cell pool (gonocytes) into the adult stem cell pool (Ad spermatogonia) at 2 to 3 months of age and (2) transformation of Ad spermatogonia into primary spermatocytes (meiosis) at 4 to 5 years (Huff et al, 2001a).** These investigators also found similar, but less severe histopathologic changes in the *contralateral* descended testis. Other studies have supported these observations. Prepubertal (median age of 3.5 years at orchidopexy) and postpubertal testicular biopsy specimens have demonstrated varying degrees of germinal hypoplasia that correlate with histopathologic changes and spermiograms in men with infertility (Nistal et al, 2000). Hadziselimovic and Herzog found a negative association between age and germ cell count by 6 months of age in children undergoing orchidopexy. Surprisingly, a third of boys younger than 6 months with a normal germ cell count had an abnormal sperm cell count 20 years later, and although testis histology was abnormal in all boys *older* than 6 months at orchidopexy, the total sperm count was no different between groups (Hadziselimovic and Herzog, 2001). When the specific stage of germ cell maturation was examined, **transformation of gonocytes into Ad spermatogonia between 2 and 3 months of age appeared to be critical for male fertility**, not the total number of germ cells. The risk for later infertility, defined as less than 40 million sperm per ejaculate, was as high as 90% in the absence of transformation.

This important phase in spermatogenesis, which is probably androgen dependent and associated with blunting of the normal surges in gonadotropins and testosterone, has prompted investigators to treat children with GnRH in the hope of improving their fertility index. Postoperative treatment with the GnRH analog buserelin after successful orchidopexy resulted in significant improvement in the fertility index in adulthood, although these patients were treated preoperatively with hCG (Hadziselimovic and Herzog, 1997). Seventy-five percent of boys with severely reduced germ cell counts treated with another GnRH analog (nafarelin) after orchidopexy and bilateral testicular biopsy demonstrated improvement in total germ cell counts on follow-up biopsies within 5 months of completing hormonal therapy (Huff et al, 2001b). Neoadjuvant GnRH therapy in prepubescent boys with cryptorchidism may also have a positive effect on future fertility, with the highest fertility indices reported with therapy before 2 years of age (Schwentner et al, 2005).

Lee (1993) postulated that paternity would be a better index for verification than the sperm count because it is known that men with subnormal sperm counts can have normal paternity rates. **When compared with a control group, paternity was significantly compromised in men with previous bilateral, but not unilateral cryptorchidism (53% versus 75%, respectively)** (Lee et al, 1995). It was also demonstrated that paternity was not correlated with age at orchidopexy. In more recent studies, up to 90% of men with unilateral undescended testes demonstrated paternity, whereas only 33% to 65% of men with bilateral undescended testes fathered children (Cendron et al, 1989; Lee and Coughlin, 2001). Higher FSH and LH levels and lower sperm counts and inhibin B levels were shown to correlate inversely, both in formerly unilaterally cryptorchid men versus controls and in the subset of men who reported unsuccessful attempts at paternity versus those reporting paternity; LH, testosterone, and other results of semen analysis did not differ (Lee et al, 1998; Lee and Coughlin, 2001). Therefore, increased FSH and a low sperm count may be weighed as risk factors for infertility in formerly cryptorchid men. Other risk factors include the placement of a parenchymal testicular suture at the time of orchiopexy (Bellinger et al, 1989; Coughlin et al, 1998). Monorchidism resulting from either absence/atrophy or removal of a testis during childhood does not appear to diminish the paternity rate when compared with unilateral cryptorchid men corrected during childhood or the normal general male population (Lee and Coughlin, 2002).

Neoplasia

It is a well-established fact that children born with undescended testes are at increased risk for testicular malignancy. Testis tumors usually develop during puberty and thereafter, although there are reports of tumor development before 10 years of age. Approximately 10% of testicular tumors arise from an undescended testis (Whitaker, 1970; Abratt et al, 1992). The incidence of a testicular tumor in the general population is 1 in 100,000, and the incidence of a germ cell tumor in men formally cryptorchid is 1 in 2550; therefore, the relative risk (RR) is approximately 40 times greater (Farrer et al, 1985). It is controversial whether orchiopexy affects the natural history of development of a testicular tumor, although emerging evidence supports the claim that prepubescent orchiopexy may lessen the risk. An indication for orchiopexy is to permit a more thorough examination of the testis, which would theoretically allow for earlier detection of malignant degeneration.

Uncorrected cryptorchidism is now rarely seen in the West, but 14% of adult patients from New Delhi, India, with primary germ cell tumors of the testis were found to have cryptorchidism (Raina et al, 1995). The United Kingdom Testicular Cancer Study Group (Aetiology, 1994; Social, 1994) found a significant association of testicular cancer with undescended testis and inguinal hernia. However, the risk associated with an undescended testis was eliminated in men who underwent orchiopexy before 10 years of age, and therefore it was concluded that the trend to perform orchiopexy at younger ages may reduce the associated risk for testicular malignancy. The study also found that the increased risk for tumor formation was associated with early age at puberty and low amounts of exercise. These findings may be related to the effects of exposure to endogenous hormones and may partly contribute to the increasing rates of testicular cancer observed in the past few decades (Social, 1994).

Moller and associates (1996) reported on a large cohort of men in Denmark and found the RR for testicular cancer in men with treated or persisting cryptorchidism to be 3.6 (95% confidence interval [CI], 1.8 to 6.9), but no increase in risk was observed in men who reported a history of undescended testes that underwent spontaneous descent. This study also provided evidence that the RR for cancer in men who were treated for cryptorchidism increased with age at treatment. Testicular atrophy was associated with both testicular cancer and cryptorchidism. Contrary to the previous study, inguinal hernia was not associated with testicular cancer in the absence of cryptorchidism or testicular atrophy. Another study demonstrated that the incidence of undescended testes was statistically significantly higher in both black and mixed-race patients than in white patients with testis tumors (Abratt et al, 1992). However, a study bias probably accounts for this finding because the orchiopexy rate was 71% in mixed-race patients, 87% in whites, and zero in blacks. In addition, the mean age at initial evaluation was 40 years for black patients, 32 years for those of mixed race, and 33 years for whites. Black patients also had abdominal or inguinal tumors rather than scrotal tumors. **These studies provide evidence to support the contention that early orchiopexy may protect against the development of malignancy.** Although the study by Prener and coworkers (1996) found the risk for testicular cancer to be increased in men with a history of cryptorchidism (RR, 5.2; 95% CI, 2.1% to 13.0%), there was no observed decrease in risk associated with treatment in early childhood.

The location of the undescended testis also affects the RR for tumor development. The higher the position of the undescended testis, the greater the risk for development of a malignancy (Martin and Menck, 1975; Martin, 1982). Almost half the tumors that develop from undescended testes occur in testes located abdominally, sixfold higher than for inguinal testes (Campbell, 1942). **The most common tumor that develops from a cryptorchid testis is seminoma** (Martin, 1979; Batata et al, 1980; Abratt et al, 1992). Of 125 patients treated with a history of cryptorchidism and testicular germ cell tumor, pure seminoma was found in 54, embryonal carcinoma in 35, teratocarcinoma in 33, and pure choriocarcinoma in 3 (Batata et al, 1980).

The cause of the increased risk for malignant degeneration of an undescended testis is at this time theoretical. Theories have included exposure of the testis to increased temperature, but most compelling is the idea of an intrinsic pathologic process affecting both testes. This theory is supported by evidence of an increased risk for tumor formation in normally descended contralateral testes (Johnson et al, 1968; Batata et al, 1980; Martin, 1982). One study found that the RR for testicular cancer in the contralateral, normally descended testis in unilaterally cryptorchid men was increased to 3.6 (Prener et al, 1996). The risk for development of a tumor in the contralateral testis is 15% in men with bilaterally undescended testes when the other testis is already involved with tumor (Gilbert and Hamilton, 1970).

In 1972, Skakkebaek reported finding carcinoma in situ in the testis of an infertile man with an undescended testis in whom a germ cell tumor developed 16 months later. Since that time, it has been estimated that **the prevalence of carcinoma in situ is 1.7% in patients with cryptorchidism.** Carcinoma in situ is more commonly detected in abdominal testes than in testes that have undergone further descent (Ford et al, 1985). These findings bring into question the extent to which testicular biopsies taken during childhood orchiopexy can exclude the development of a tumor in adult life. Premalignant changes could not be demonstrated in biopsies of cryptorchid testis before adulthood (Muffly et al, 1984). In addition, no evidence of histologic premalignant changes occurring before the onset of puberty was observed in men in whom testicular malignancies later developed (Parkinson et al, 1994). Therefore, routine testicular biopsy during childhood orchiopexy appears to have no predictive value for the development of later malignant degeneration.

Hernia

A patent processus vaginalis is found in more than 90% of patients with an undescended testis (Scorer and Farrington, 1971; Grosfeld, 1989; Elder, 1992a). The processus normally closes between the period after complete testicular descent and the first month after birth. A higher incidence of epididymal anomalies is associated with a patent processus vaginalis, thus supporting the theory that androgenic stimulation may be required for closure of the processus (Barthold and Redman, 1996). The clinical significance of a patent processus vaginalis is that it has been shown to affect the efficacy of hor-

monal treatment of cryptorchidism. This issue was investigated in children with cryptorchidism who received hCG and later underwent inguinal herniorrhaphy. The incidence of testicular descent was 49.5% in patients with a nonpatent (normal) processus vaginalis and zero in testes associated with a patent processus vaginalis (Varela Cives et al, 1996). Adamsen and colleagues (1989) unexpectedly found a hernia or hydrocele at surgery in 77% of cases after failed hCG treatment of cryptorchidism.

Testicular Torsion

The increased susceptibility of the testis to undergo torsion is the result of a developmental anatomic abnormality between the testis and its mesentery. The mechanism is believed to be related to a greater relative broadness of the testicle than its mesentery (Scorer and Farrington, 1971). This may explain the phenomenon of torsion of an undescended testis associated with a testicular tumor. Riegler (1972) found that 64% of adults with torsion in an undescended testis had an associated germ cell tumor. Intravaginal spermatic cord torsion and testicular infarction were reported in an infant with bilateral cryptorchidism who was receiving hCG treatment (Sawchuk et al, 1993). Although torsion of an undescended testis is rare, it should be considered in any child with abdominal or groin pain and an empty ipsilateral hemiscrotum.

KEY POINTS: ADVERSE CONSEQUENCES

- Two critical prepubertal steps in germ cell maturation and proliferation are defective in patients with cryptorchidism: (1) transformation of the fetal stem cell pool (gonocytes) into the adult stem cell pool (Ad spermatogonia) at 2 to 3 months of age and (2) transformation of Ad spermatogonia into primary spermatocytes (meiosis) at 4 to 5 years.

- Hypoplasia of the Leydig cells, observed from the first month of life, is the earliest postnatal histologic abnormality in cryptorchid testes.

- There are no accurate hormonal markers that provide either a direct or an indirect measurement of testicular function or impairment in infants or prepubertal boys with cryptorchidism.

- Paternity has been found to be significantly compromised in men with previous bilateral, but not unilateral cryptorchidism.

- Monorchidism does not appear to diminish the paternity rate.

- The prevalence of carcinoma in situ is 1.7% in patients with cryptorchidism; the most common tumor that develops from an undescended testis is seminoma.

- It is yet inconclusive whether orchidopexy performed at an early age will protect against the development of malignancy.

Workup

When a child is referred for an undescended testis, the testis is palpable in approximately 80% and the remainder are nonpalpable. Most nonpalpable testes are intra-abdominal. However, a nonpalpable testis does not exclude an intracanalicular or absent testis. Approximately 20% of nonpalpable testes are absent and 30% are atrophic. Determination of whether the testis is present on physical examination is critically important because it guides further workup and treatment. Many times children are found to have retractile testes, and frequently only follow-up examination is required to document a normally palpable state without retraction of the testis. Furthermore, up to 25% of children with cryptorchidism have bilaterally undescended testes. The workup begins with a thorough history that includes the following:

- Preterm and maternal history, including the use of gestational steroids
- Perinatal history, including documentation of a scrotal examination at birth
- The child's medical and previous surgical history
- Family history of cryptorchidism or syndromes

The physical examination ideally requires a relaxed child observed first in the supine position. Examination of the child in general should include any other birth defects that might suggest a syndromic association. The genital examination includes inspection for any penile malformations, including hypospadias, micropenis, or ambiguous genitalia. It should be noted whether the scrotum is asymmetric or underdeveloped. The examination also includes inspection of the inguinal canal and common sites of testicular ectopia for any masses. If only one testis is descended, this gonad should be carefully examined for size, turgor, any palpable paratesticular anomalies, and the presence of a hernia or hydrocele. In the case of a unilaterally nonpalpable testis, contralateral testicular hypertrophy of the normally descended testis has been suggested to represent absence of the ipsilateral testis. Huff et al (1992) found that the mean volume of the contralateral descended testis of boys with an absent testis was greater than that of boys with an intra-abdominal testis at all ages, but this was not a reliable criterion for differentiating the two conditions. It has also been suggested, based on spermiograms, that compensatory hypertrophy of one testis does not prevent testicular insufficiency in adulthood (Laron et al, 1980). The child may be placed in one of several positions to assist in locating the undescended testis, including a sitting or squatting position. Examination for the undescended testis is best performed with warm hands and soapy water on the fingertips to reduce skin friction. The examiner's fingers are swept down from just above the internal ring along the inguinal canal into the scrotum. The clinician should feel either a testis moving back under the fingertips against the direction of palpation or a "pop" as the testis springs back into its cryptorchid position. Ectopic areas of testicular descent should also be carefully examined.

The overall accuracy of radiologic testing for an undescended testis is 44% (Hrebinko and Bellinger, 1993). The purpose of testing is usually to determine the location or presence of the undescended testis. However, because surgical exploration is necessary in either case, imaging becomes a fruitless and expensive endeavor that in most situations does not influence the decision to operate, the surgical approach, or the viability or salvageability of the cryptorchid testis. Many modalities have been used, including ultrasound, computed tomography, magnetic resonance imaging, testicular angiography and venography, pneumoperitoneography, and herniography. Many of these techniques are invasive, require anesthesia, are technically difficult to perform, or are associated with a significant rate of false-negative results.

The workup for bilateral nonpalpable testes merits special consideration because it may represent a life-threatening situation if it is associated with either hypospadias or ambiguous genitalia. The diagnosis of bilateral anorchia should be considered if a male karyotype is confirmed. Endocrinologic evaluation is necessary and may help determine whether one or both testes are present. Childhood is a quiescent phase in testicular activity, and the hCG stimulation test is widely used to evaluate testicular function. The hCG stimulation test can be performed to induce testosterone production and would confirm the presence of at least one testis. However, there may be a false-negative response if the Leydig cells are unresponsive to exogenous hCG. If basal gonadotropin levels, FSH in particular, are increased in a prepubescent boy, further endocrine workup is unnecessary because it probably represents bilateral anorchia (Jarow et al, 1986). If gonadotropin levels are normal in a boy with bilateral nonpalpable testes, an hCG stimulation test can be performed to further establish the diagnosis. Although there are many, but no standard test method of hCG stimulation, a conventional regimen is 5000 U hCG divided into six injections over a period of 3 weeks, with DHT, FSH, and LH levels rechecked within 24 hours of last dose. **However, all boys with nonpalpable testes and normal serum gonadotropin levels must undergo surgical exploration regardless of the results of the hCG stimulation test.** MIS and inhibin B are also specific testicular markers, and measurement of these markers may be of benefit in determining whether testicular tissue is present. Inhibin B, a testicular peptide regulating FSH secretion, is a marker of Sertoli cell function and spermatogenesis in adults and probably regulates FSH secretion in early childhood (Byrd et al, 1998). In contrast to the other hormones of the hypothalamic-pituitary-gonadal axis, it is secreted in detectable amounts during childhood and may predict prepubertal testicular function (Raivio and Dunkel, 1999; Kubini et al, 2000).

Management of Cryptorchidism

Tenets of Treatment

Important tenets for the treatment of a child with an undescended testis include the following:

- **Proper identification of the anatomy, position, and viability of the undescended testis**
- **Identification of any potential coexisting syndromic abnormalities**
- **Placement of the testis within the scrotum in timely fashion to prevent further testicular impairment in either fertility potential or endocrinologic function**
- **Attainment of permanent fixation of the testis with a normal scrotal position that allows for easy palpation**
- **No further testicular damage resulting from the treatment**

Definitive treatment of an undescended testis should take place between 6 and 12 months of age. Because spontaneous descent occurs in most boys by 3 months of age and uncommonly thereafter, earlier intervention should be considered in order to theoretically prevent the complications of cryptorchidism that may be manifested before 1 year of age. The approach and timing should be predicated on the anatomic position and whether both testes are undescended. For instance, there may be a theoretical advantage to bringing down a solitary undescended testis before 1 year of age if the contralateral testis is absent or intra-abdominal. Every effort should be made to preserve any testicular tissue at an early age, especially in children with unilateral or bilateral intra-abdominal testes. This recommendation is based on the poor paternity rates in men with a history of bilateral cryptorchidism. Orchiectomy is typically reserved for postpubescent males with a contralateral normally descended testis when the cryptorchid testis is either anatomically or morphologically abnormal or too far from the scrotum to allow for tension-free placement without compromising the vascular integrity of the testis. Extraordinary means are occasionally necessary to preserve a solitary testis or bilateral intra-abdominal testes, especially when the initial clinical evaluation is delayed.

Hormonal Therapy

Two types of medical treatment of an undescended testis can be provided: exogenous hCG and exogenous GnRH or LHRH. The mechanism of action in both cases increases serum testosterone production by stimulation at different levels of the hypothalamic-pituitary-gonadal cascade. This therapy is based on experimental observations that descent is mediated by androgen and involves testicular synthesis of the active metabolite in high local concentrations (Rajfer and Walsh, 1977). hCG stimulates Leydig cells directly to produce testosterone, whereas GnRH stimulates the pituitary to release LH and thereby promote testicular production of testosterone. Serum testosterone levels during therapy for cryptorchidism in prepubertal boys are much higher with hCG than with GnRH (Rajfer et al, 1986).

Patient selection has been found to be critical in achieving good results. Successful results are more commonly reported in older groups of children and in testes that were retractile or below the external inguinal ring—that is, **the lower the pretreatment position, the better the success rate** (Rajfer et al, 1986; De Muinck Keizer-Schrama et al, 1987; Pyorala et al, 1995; Fedder and Boesen, 1998). A retrospective evaluation of boys treated with LHRH revealed a previous scrotal position of the testes in 43% of those with successful treatment but in only 17% of those with failed treatment (De Muinck Keizer-Schrama et al, 1987). Similar results were reported by Fedder and Boesen (1998), who found a 56% success rate in boys in whom both testes were documented to be descended by 1 week after birth. These findings certainly help explain the earlier studies that reported high success rates with hormonal therapy. In most of these cases, surgical exploration revealed an anatomic anomaly that most likely caused testicular ascent. Regular reexamination of children treated with hormonal therapy is indicated because re-ascent has been reported in up to 25% of patients. Hormonal treatment is not indicated in patients with previously operated testes or prior surgery that would result in inguinal scar tissue formation, in those with

ectopic testes, or in those with an inguinal hernia. Presently, however, only hCG is available for patient use in the United States.

The use of hCG for the treatment of cryptorchidism has been both widespread and debated since the 1930s. hCG is structurally analogous to LH and is a potent stimulator of Leydig cells. Reported therapeutic success rates have varied considerably, from 14% to 59% (Ehrlich et al, 1969; Job et al, 1982; Adamsen et al, 1989). Treatment regimens have also varied greatly, and the most effective treatment was demonstrated to be a total dose of at least 10,000 IU to achieve maximal stimulation of the Leydig cells and avoid the complications associated with doses exceeding 15,000 IU (Job et al, 1982). A typical treatment schedule is 1500 IU/m^2 given by intramuscular injection twice a week for 4 weeks. A downside of hCG treatment is that it must be given parenterally on a frequent basis. FSH appears to influence spontaneous descent of the testis and to induce LH receptors; however, efficacy studies of combination treatment with hCG have shown mixed results and such treatment cannot be recommended at this time (Saggese et al, 1989; Hoorweg-Nijman et al, 1994).

Side effects of hormonal treatment include increased rugation and pigmentation of the scrotum. Rarely, there is an increase in size of the penis and the development of pubic hair, which regresses after cessation of therapy. A significant increase in weight increment velocity was seen in 7- to 9-year-olds treated with a dose of 10,000 IU (Adamsen et al, 1989). A number of studies have evaluated the controversial issue of adverse histologic effects on the testis after hCG treatment. Although hCG induced a significant increase in the volume density of both interstitial tissue and blood vessels in normally descended and undescended testes, there appeared to be no permanent damage (Kaleva et al, 1996). However, hCG withdrawal was implicated as the mechanism of increased germ cell apoptosis in the hormonal treatment of cryptorchidism (Heiskanen et al, 1996). hCG should also be avoided in immunosuppressed patients because of a transient decrease in the absolute number of total peripheral blood lymphocytes, total T cells, helper-inducer T cells, and CD8+ subsets during therapy. In addition, the percentage of CD8+ cells and the lymphocyte response to the mitogen concanavalin A decreased significantly with hCG treatment and returned to normal after hCG withdrawal (Maghnie et al, 1991).

Exogenous GnRH was developed as a therapy for cryptorchidism because of the less than ideal results of exogenous hCG. It has the advantage of nasal spray administration, and an effective dose for stimulating LH is 1.2 mg/day for 4 weeks (Rajfer et al, 1986). The results of previous trials may have been falsely optimistic because of the inclusion of patients with retractile testes; reported success rates ranged from 32% to 73% (Illig et al, 1977; Hadziselimovic et al, 1982; Witjes et al, 1990). Rajfer and associates (1986) found that testicular descent into the scrotum occurred in 19% of patients treated with GnRH and in 6% of those treated with hCG. In addition, there appears to be a difference in the success rate in patients with unilateral versus bilateral cryptorchidism. One multicenter study demonstrated the effect of LHRH in cryptorchid boys and found a therapeutic gain in 8.1% of those with bilaterally undescended testes and no effect in those with unilateral undescended testis (Olsen et al, 1992). A success rate of 9% for LHRH nasal spray and 8% for placebo was reported in 252 prepubertal boys with 301 undescended testes (De Muinck Keizer-Schrama et al, 1987). Hormonal evaluation revealed no abnormalities in cryptorchid boys when compared with control subjects. These results confirmed similar findings reported by Pyorlala and coworkers (1995), who performed a meta-analysis of 33 studies from 1958 to 1990 in which the results of treatment with LHRH and hCG were assessed in 3282 boys with cryptorchidism. Analysis of randomized, controlled trials showed that LHRH was not significantly more effective than hCG (21% versus 19%). The low success rate with GnRH has been demonstrated to not be caused by defective LH secretion by the hypothalamus or testosterone secretion by the testes (Rajfer et al, 1986). **In summary, the overall efficacy of hormonal treatment is less than 20% for cryptorchid testes and is significantly dependent on pretreatment testicular location. Therefore, surgery remains the gold standard for the management of undescended testes.**

Surgical Treatment

It is very useful to examine the child after induction of general and regional anesthesia to reaffirm testicular position or attempt to establish testicular position in the case of a previously nonpalpable testis. With anesthesia, the anterior abdominal musculature relaxes, thereby offering the surgeon the opportunity to perform a more thorough physical examination in the occasional case in which the initial examination was complicated by body habitus, uncooperative behavior, or guarding. In general, success rates for orchiopexy are directly related to the anatomic position of the testis. A 1995 analysis of surgical therapy for undescended testes by Docimo revealed a success rate of 92% for testes below the external ring, 89% for inguinal testes, 84% for microvascular orchiopexy, 81% for standard abdominal orchiopexy, 77% for staged Fowler-Stephens orchiopexy, and 67% for standard Fowler-Stephens orchiopexy.

Standard Orchiopexy. The key steps in this procedure are (1) complete mobilization of the testis and spermatic cord, (2) repair of the patent processus vaginalis by high ligation of the hernia sac, (3) skeletonization of the spermatic cord without sacrificing vascular integrity to achieve tension-free placement of the testis within the dependent position of the scrotum, and (4) creation of a superficial pouch within the hemiscrotum to receive the testis.

A transverse inguinal skin incision is made in the midinguinal canal, usually in a skin crease in children younger than 1 year (Fig. 127–1). The dermis is opened with electrocautery, and subcutaneous tissue and Scarpa's fascia are opened sharply. The skin and subcutaneous tissue are quite elastic in younger children and allow for a tremendous degree of mobility by retractor positioning for viewing the entire length of the inguinal canal. Therefore, a large incision is usually unnecessary. One should be careful to observe that the testis is in the superficial inguinal pouch and that it lies between Scarpa's fascia and the external oblique fascia. Sharp dissection cleans the surface of the external oblique fascia of prefascial fat, and gentle spreading over Poupart's ligament defines the full lateral extent of the external oblique fascia. This maneuver is helpful to maintain anatomic orientation when defining the area directly over the inguinal canal.

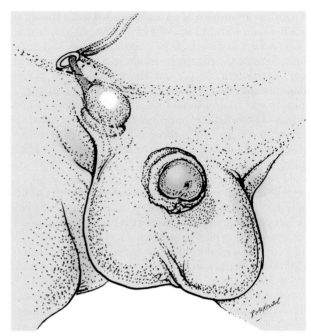

Figure 127–1. A transverse skin incision is made in an inguinal skin crease.

The testis will be lying within its tunics either in the inguinal canal or just outside it in most cases. If the testis is intracanalicular, the external oblique fascia is opened with a small superficial incision that is carried through the external ring, with care taken to preserve the ilioinguinal nerve (Fig. 127–2A). The tunics overlying the testis are grasped and the distal gubernacular attachments are sharply dissected to free the testis up into the wound. The cremasteric muscular fibers and any anomalous fibrous attachments from the superficial peripheral fascia are then dissected sharply away from the testis and spermatic cord (Fig. 127–2B). Once the spermatic cord is freely mobilized to the internal ring from the cremasteric attachments in the inguinal canal, the tunica vaginalis is opened over the testis. This is a good time to carefully inspect the anatomy and integrity of the paratesticular structures and measure the testis.

Complete mobilization of the spermatic cord is essential to achieve adequate cord length for tension-free placement of the testis in the scrotum. Such mobilization should not be done at the risk of devitalizing the vascular supply to the testis or damaging the paratesticular structures, including the vas deferens. The key steps in this part of the operation include (1) complete transection of the fused fibers between the cremasteric muscle and the internal oblique muscle; (2) complete separation of the patent processus vaginalis from the elements of the spermatic cord (Fig. 127–3), with mobilization of the hernia sac/peritoneum to a position at least just inside the internal ring (Fig. 127–4); and (3) dissection of the internal spermatic fascia from the cord structures (Fig. 127–5). In most cases, division of the processus vaginalis and cremasteric muscle attachments provides adequate cord length to allow for placement of the testis in the scrotum. It is also helpful to separate the vas deferens from the vascular elements at the level of the internal ring because these structures diverge at this

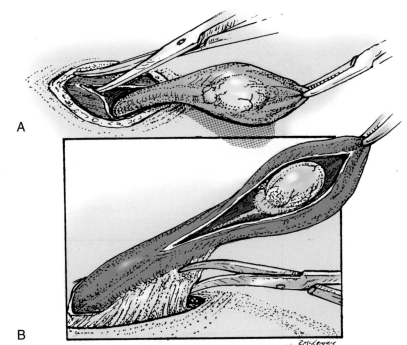

Figure 127-2. **A,** The external ring is opened. **B,** Cremasteric fibers are dissected from the cord.

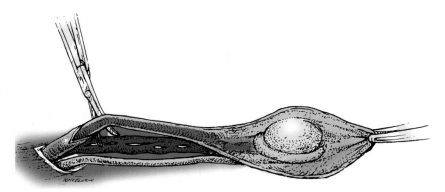

Figure 127-3. Dissection to separate the processus vaginalis from the cord structures.

level. If additional cord length is needed at this point, retroperitoneal dissection is necessary. A Ragnell retractor placed within the internal ring allows adequate visualization of the spermatic vessels cephalad for gentle blunt mobilization with either a cotton-tipped applicator, sponge, or Kittner dissector. The external oblique should be opened above the level of the internal ring, and the internal oblique muscle can be divided 1 to 2 cm from the superior lateral margin of the internal ring.

Experimental evidence has documented that transparenchymal suture fixation causes testicular damage by inducing an inflammatory reaction regardless of suture size and material. **In comparison, dartos-fixed testes demonstrated complete circumferential adherence, with only 5% of the animals in the dartos pouch group showing an inflammatory response and normal spermatogenesis in 94%** (Bellinger et al, 1989; Dixon et al, 1993). Based on these studies, transparenchymal sutures should be avoided, with only two exceptional circumstances: (1) for a tethered testis when its position is tenuous after complete mobilization of the spermatic cord and short-term external fixation to a nylon

button is required and (2) for testicular fixation of the ipsilateral and contralateral testes because of clinical torsion of the spermatic cord. A significant variation of the technique, however, is to completely avoid deep transparenchymal placement of the sutures by superficial placement just under the tunica albuginea. The sutures used in these cases are fine, permanent monofilament suture, such as 5-0 or 6-0 Prolene, on a noncutting needle. It is important to be familiar with the intragonadal vascular anatomy in such cases, especially when ligation of the spermatic vessels is being contemplated. The collateral arterial circulation through the deferential artery, which communicates with the internal spermatic arterial system both in the spermatic cord and at the lower pole of the testis, was found to be compromised in all testes with placement of a traction suture (Jarow, 1991).

The testis can be adequately and permanently secured in the scrotum by placement of the testis within a superficial dartos pouch. The dartos pouch has a long and proven record of success. Placement of the testis within a dartos pouch results in complete circumferential adherence of the tunica albuginea to the scrotal skin. A transverse midscrotal superficial skin

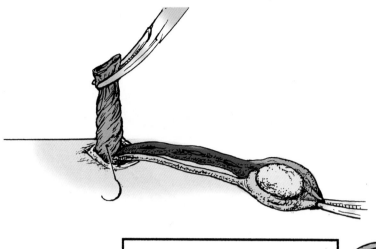

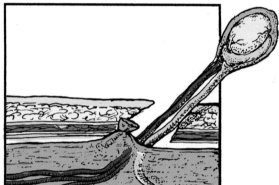

A

B

Figure 127–4. A, High ligation of the processus vaginalis at the internal inguinal ring. **B,** The ligated processus and the cord structures.

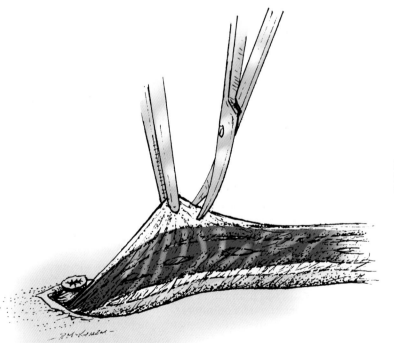

Figure 127–5. Separation of the internal spermatic fascia from the cord structures after ligation of the processus vaginalis.

incision is made within a rugal skin fold, and a mosquito hemostat is then used to develop a tissue plane just under the scrotal skin of the ipsilateral hemiscrotum (Fig. 127–6). The scrotal pocket should be developed from the median raphe and the lateral scrotal margin, with creation of the space inferiorly to encourage preferential fixation of the testis as dependently in the scrotum as possible. After the testis and cord are completely mobilized and the tunica vaginalis is opened and everted over the testis, a hemostat is passed just over the pubic symphysis from the inguinal incision through the tough dartos fascia into the scrotum (Fig. 127–7A). It is important to pass the hemostat into the medial aspect of the scrotum to avoid lateral placement or migration of the testis. The most direct path to the scrotum allows for the most dependent placement of the testis. A second hemostat is back-passed from the scrotum into the inguinal incision; the most dependent tunica vaginalis or remnant of gubernaculum is grasped, and the testis is passed into the scrotum, with care taken to avoid torsion of the spermatic cord (Fig. 127–7B and C).

The dartos fascial window is closed with fine absorbable suture, with the option of placing this suture through the redundant tunica vaginalis well above the level of the testis to indirectly secure the cord at this position. The testis is then placed within the dartos pouch and the scrotal skin closed with fine interrupted absorbable sutures such as 4-0 chromic vertical mattress sutures. The external oblique fascia is closed with running or interrupted absorbable suture with re-creation of the external ring, although not to such a degree that it impinges on the spermatic cord or the cord is redirected and kept from the most direct path to the scrotum. Subcutaneous tissue and skin are closed in the usual fashion. We prefer interrupted subcuticular closure of the skin with fine absorbable suture and collodion placed as a dressing.

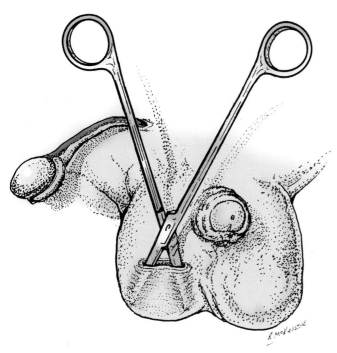

Figure 127–6. Formation of a dartos pouch.

Techniques for High Undescended Testes. Occasionally, greater mobilization of the proximal spermatic cord structures does not provide adequate length to allow for tension-free placement of the testis within the scrotum. Greater cord length can be obtained by mobilizing the spermatic vessels medially. The spermatic vessels are usually the limiting factor in these circumstances. The Prentiss maneuver was described in 1960 and is occasionally helpful in adding length to the spermatic vessels by positioning the spermatic vessels medially and thereby choosing the hypotenuse of the triangle, or the most direct course to the scrotum, created by the natural course of the vessels laterally through the internal ring (Prentiss et al, 1960). It is performed by incising the floor of the inguinal canal through the external ring and dividing the inferior epigastric vessels. The internal ring and transversalis fascia are then closed lateral to the cord. In addition, thorough retroperitoneal dissection, especially of the lateral attachments, is carried out in conjunction with this procedure.

A high inguinal approach or Jones incision is an open surgical alternative for a high canalicular or intra-abdominal testis (Jones and Bagley, 1979). This procedure shares similar indications and surgical principles with laparoscopic orchidopexy and was the popular surgical approach before the advent of laparoscopic management of an intra-abdominal testis. Principles include preservation of the spermatic vessels, high retroperitoneal mobilization of the spermatic vessels, and passage of the testis directly through the abdominal wall at the pubic tubercle (Prentiss maneuver). The procedure may also be performed in combination with laparoscopy to help locate the testis and aid in dissection. A transverse incision is made medial to the anterior superior iliac spine and carried down to the external oblique fascia just superior to the internal ring. Once the fascia is incised, a muscle-splitting technique is performed to expose the retroperitoneum and mobilize the peritoneum medially. The internal ring and processus vaginalis, if present, are identified and the peritoneum opened at this level to deliver the testis into the field. After ligating the hernia sac, the spermatic vessels are dissected from the lateral spermatic fascia as far cranial as possible, and a Prentiss maneuver is performed by passing the testis under the floor of the inguinal canal to an exit site just above the pubic tubercle. If there is tension on the testis after delivery into the subdartos pouch, an external nylon fixation button helps maintain a dependent scrotal position.

If anatomic conditions prevent adequate spermatic vessel length from being achieved during primary orchidopexy or if, under unusual circumstances, a two-stage procedure is undertaken with planned preservation of the spermatic vessels, a staged orchiopexy can be performed as described by Persky and Albert in 1971. The testis is anchored to the external ring or pubic symphysis after maximal mobilization in the first stage, and a second procedure is performed 6 to 12 months later. Wrapping of the cord and testis in a Silastic sheath may reduce adhesion formation and render the second-stage procedure less difficult (Corkery, 1975; Steinhardt et al, 1985).

Fowler-Stephens Orchiopexy. Ligation of the testicular vessels occasionally becomes a necessary consideration, especially in the management of a high inguinal or intra-abdominal testis. The testicular artery and veins often limit the distal mobility of these testes. The surgical complexity of this con-

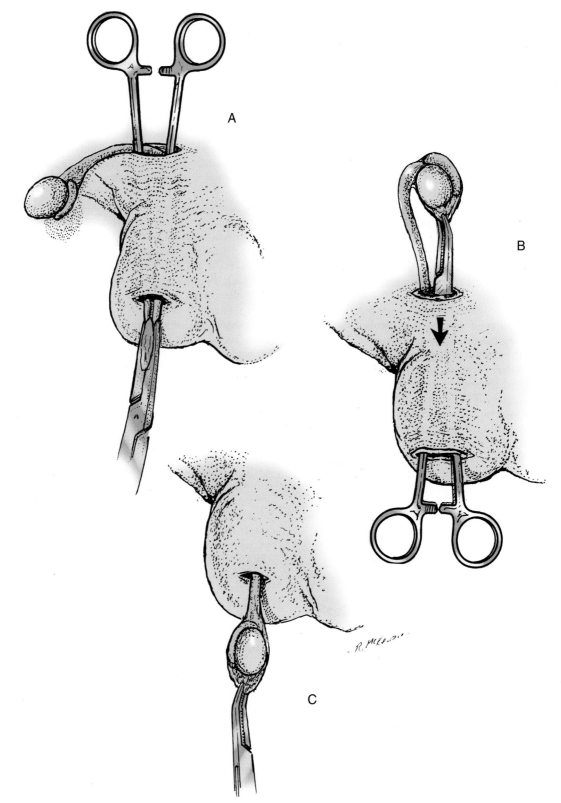

Figure 127–7. A, Formation of a passage to the scrotum. **B** and **C,** Passage of the testis into the scrotal pouch.

dition was recognized well before the 20th century. Bevan's 1899 attempt at remedying this conundrum resulted in a procedure that included division of the testicular artery. The results of this technique were poor and produced testicular atrophy. It was not until 1959 that Fowler and Stephens studied the vascular anatomy of the testis and devised a means to repair a high undescended testis and preserve its blood supply via collateral circulation. The testis has three sources of arterial blood supply: the testicular artery (primary), the deferential artery of the vas deferens, and the cremasteric arteries (Fowler and Stephens, 1959). **When the spermatic vessels are divided, blood supply to the testis is dependent on collateral circulation from the deferential artery, a branch of the inferior vesical artery, and the cremasteric system, a branch of the inferior epigastric artery.**

The technique described by Fowler and Stephens was originally a one-stage procedure, but it may also be performed in two stages. If a one-stage repair is to be performed, it is critical early in the dissection that a wide pedicle of peritoneum be preserved with the vas deferens to maintain collateral blood flow. It is also important to remember that the testis is technically a retroperitoneal organ, as is its blood supply and that of the vas deferens. A high transverse inguinal incision is made that can be extended laterally in a cranial direction. The external oblique fascia is opened in the direction of its fibers, and the contents of the inguinal canal are examined. If a hernia sac is present, it is carefully dissected up to the level of the internal ring and opened. More commonly, there is no canal or sac, and therefore the anterior abdominal muscles are opened to expose the peritoneum, which is then opened.

After the testis is identified, it is gently mobilized up into the incision without transecting any structures proximal to the testis. Careful inspection is then required to identify the primary and collateral vessels to the testis, as well as the course of the vas deferens. Anatomic variations in the vascular supply to the testis are especially common in patients with a long, looping vas. It has been reported that this most important requirement for successful Fowler-Stephens orchiopexy is present in less than a third of boys with true intra-abdominal testes (Bloom et al, 1994). Children with a long, looping vas that extends down the inguinal canal are the ideal candidates for a one-stage repair. True intra-abdominal testes lie at least 1 cm from the internal ring and have shortened spermatic vessels. If a long, looping vas is present, it is carefully mobilized up from the inguinal canal and protected. Once it has been determined that the testis will not traverse the distance to the scrotum, the spermatic vessels are divided.

The Fowler-Stephens test is a method of testing the collateral blood supply to the testis. It is performed by temporarily occluding the testicular artery with a vascular clamp for 5 minutes and inspecting the testis for color, as well as making a small incision in the tunica albuginea of the testis to document arterial bleeding. Care must be taken to distinguish the tunica blood supply, which tends to be preserved despite testicular arterial occlusion, from the true blood supply to the testicular parenchyma. If the blood supply is at this point considered tenuous, a two-stage repair should be performed to allow for development of the collateral circulation.

If the testis appears viable, the testicular artery is ligated and divided high above the testis. The testis is then mobilized on a wide swath of peritoneum with the vas deferens. An incision is made in the lateral peritoneal reflection, and the peritoneum medial to the testis is left undisturbed. Care is taken to not injure the ureter during dissection of the deep vasal pedicle. If a long, looping vas is present, the loop is straightened by dividing the peritoneum in the center to extend the length of the pedicle. The course of the vasal pedicle should be as medial as possible to choose the shortest distance to the scrotum, which may require direct placement of the testis and pedicle through a neohiatus in the abdominal wall over the symphysis pubis or medial to the inferior epigastric vessels via the Prentiss maneuver. From this point forward the procedure is carried out as a standard orchiopexy with creation of a dartos pouch.

The anticipated advantage of a two-stage orchiopexy with spermatic vessel ligation is twofold: (1) to allow for development of collateral blood supply to compensate for division of the main blood supply to the testis and (2) to allow for greater mobility of the testis to place it within the scrotum (Elder, 1989; Elder, 1992b). The two-stage orchiopexy is typically performed by ligating the spermatic vessels in situ as close to the origin as possible and then returning after 6 months or longer to complete the vasal-peritoneal pedicle mobilization with the standard Fowler-Stephens technique. Koff and Sethi (1996) reported excellent results with a technique of low spermatic vessel ligation and demonstrated that high ligation of the spermatic vessels does not need to be performed to preserve testicular viability.

Laparoscopic Management of an Undescended Testis

Laparoscopy has attained its greatest degree of general acceptance, both diagnostically and therapeutically, in the realm of pediatric urology for the management of a nonpalpable testis. Since the earliest reported cases over a quarter of a century ago, there are now several thousand cases in the literature documenting the impact that laparoscopy has made in the management of a nonpalpable testis. The principles of surgery for a nonpalpable testis are equal to, if not enhanced by a laparoscopic approach; exposure, lighting, and magnification remain critical to this pediatric procedure. **However, the advantages of laparoscopy over a conventional "open" surgical approach to a nonpalpable testis include accurate anatomic assessment of testicular position and viability and, when necessary, optimal accessibility to the crux of the surgical problem.**

Diagnostic Laparoscopy for a Nonpalpable Testis

A nonpalpable testis accounts for approximately one fifth of children with an undescended testis. Diagnostic laparoscopy is commonly used for the assessment of a nonpalpable testis, with the accuracy of testicular localization reported to be greater than 95% (Moore et al, 1994; Tennenbaum et al, 1994). Numerous reports attest to radiographic and less invasive means of determining whether a testis is present within the abdomen, but a surgical procedure cannot be avoided in the evaluation and treatment of a nonpalpable testis. Radiographic imaging studies carry unacceptable false-negative and false-positive rates (Hrebinko and Bellinger, 1993; Siemer et al, 2000). Elder reported that inguinal ultrasound, perhaps the most common test ordered to evaluate boys with a non-palpable testis, rarely localizes a true nonpalpable testis and in only 18% of cases correctly identified testes located in the inguinal canal (Elder, 2002). Magnetic resonance imaging has been shown to be an effective method of detection in 37% of cases (Bakr and Kotb, 1998). As important, radiographic testing is also not adequately sensitive enough to determine the *quality* of the testis when compared with direct visualization. This includes assessing whether the testis is dysmorphic or hypoplastic or whether epididymal or vasal nonunion anomalies coexist that would ultimately have an impact on the type of surgical procedure performed. Any technique, whether radiographic or surgical, must be highly accurate because the fate of a missed intra-abdominal testis is potentially serious with respect to preserving testicular function and can be catastrophic because of the risk for malignancy. Diagnostic laparoscopy has also been shown to be useful in the management of a previous inconclusive open exploration for a nonpalpable testis (Diamond and Caldamone, 1992; Lakhoo et al, 1996; Barqawi et al, 2003).

Diagnostic laparoscopy is the most accurate means of determining whether a testis is intra-abdominal and has been shown to be a safe procedure in experienced hands (Orlando et al, 2003). **Potential major complications** include vascular injury and bowel and bladder perforation; however, these complications become rare when an open technique is used for trocar placement. **Minor complications** are those that would not necessarily require termination or conversion of the laparoscopic procedure and include abdominal wall injury, such as hematoma, and subcutaneous insufflation.

Peters reported in 2004 that in approximately 50% of patients, diagnostic laparoscopy will assist or guide further surgical exploration. A common example is in the case of vanishing testis syndrome, which occurs in up to 47% of boys with a nonpalpable testis (Cisek et al, 1998; Van Savage, 2001; Barqawi et al, 2003; Radmayr et al, 2003). Diagnostic laparoscopy will also help in determining intra-abdominal testicular anatomy and the feasibility of a single- or two-stage orchidopexy or, if indeed the testis is abnormal, whether orchiectomy is indicated. Surgery is the only means to either bring the salvageable testis into a scrotal position or remove it if abnormal. Conversion to therapeutic laparoscopy provides options over the standard open technique when a viable testis or remnant is present. **By using an already existing port site, diagnostic laparoscopy can naturally transition to extend the operative procedure from diagnostic to therapeutic.**

Technique

The technique of diagnostic laparoscopy begins with access either blind with a Veress needle or via the preferred open technique. The open technique begins with either a semilunar supraumbilical or an infraumbilical incision that is carried down to the rectus fascia. This layer is opened and the properitoneal fat spread until the peritoneum is exposed, grasped, and brought up into the incision. This layer is opened sharply and the trocar placed usually between the obliterated umbilical arteries. The open technique lessens the risk of inadvertent trauma to the intra-abdominal structures, as well as extraperitoneal insufflation. The choice of trocar depends on the size of the laparoscope and whether the intended procedure

requires larger instruments. Usually, a 5-mm zero-degree laparoscope is available in most pediatric hospitals, but smaller-diameter systems and laparoscopes such as 3 or 2 mm via a Veress needle cannula are now in wide use. Our preference is a radially dilating disposable trocar that will accommodate up to 5-mm instruments. Pneumoperitoneum is created with CO_2 at a flow rate between 8 and 10 L/min with a pressure limit of 8 to 10 mm Hg. A 2-0 absorbable U-stitch can be placed in the rectus fascia to help maintain the pneumoperitoneum and facilitate quick closure, especially if the fasciotomy is generous. We request the anesthesiologist to not give NO_2 during induction or any portion of the procedure performed via the laparoscope to avoid bowel distention.

Intraperitoneal pelvic anatomy viewed through the laparoscope is elegantly displayed. Magnification is of added benefit in discerning delicate blood vessels and structures leading to the testis and in dissecting and preserving these same structures. The midline structure first viewed is the urinary bladder, which should be drained throughout the procedure. Just lateral and running along the anterior abdominal wall is the obliterated umbilical arteries, which serve as prominent anatomic markers for identifying the internal ring, vas deferens, and ureter. **Examining the side opposite the pathology is useful for comparing normal anatomy, especially in the case of a vanishing testis, so that the degree of atresia can be directly measured. The finding of normal internal spermatic vessels implies an intracanalicular testis, which may be normal but difficult to palpate on physical examination, and therefore surgical exploration should proceed to an inguinal incision. If the processus vaginalis is patent, the laparoscope can be advanced into the inguinal canal in most cases to again help identify the position and viability of the testis.**

Laparoscopic Assessment

There are three distinct possible findings—and courses of action—when laparoscopy is used to assess a nonpalpable testis. Findings include

1. **Blind-ending vessels above the internal ring (vanishing testis)**
2. **Cord structures entering the internal ring (viable intracanalicular testis versus an intracanalicular or scrotal atrophic testis)**
3. **Intra-abdominal testis** (Fig. 127–8)

A forth possibility is true testicular agenesis, but this more infrequent condition will be treated in a similar manner as a vanishing testis. Exploration along the course of descent is necessary to definitively determine whether the testis is absent, whether orchidopexy should be performed if the testis is present and viable, or whether excision should be performed if the testis is abnormal or consists of an atrophic remnant. An intra-abdominal vanishing testis, or the rarer possibility of testicular agenesis, also needs to be confirmed. **Examination of the contralateral testis has been helpful in predicting the fate of the nonpalpable testis; however, it is not a reliable method of definitively determining testicular presence or absence.** Hypertrophy of a normally descended testis may connote monorchia. A dysgenetic or hypoplastic testis will not usually result in contralateral testicular hypertrophy, defined as a testis greater than 2 mL or testicular length greater than 2 cm. Several groups have addressed this phenomenon and

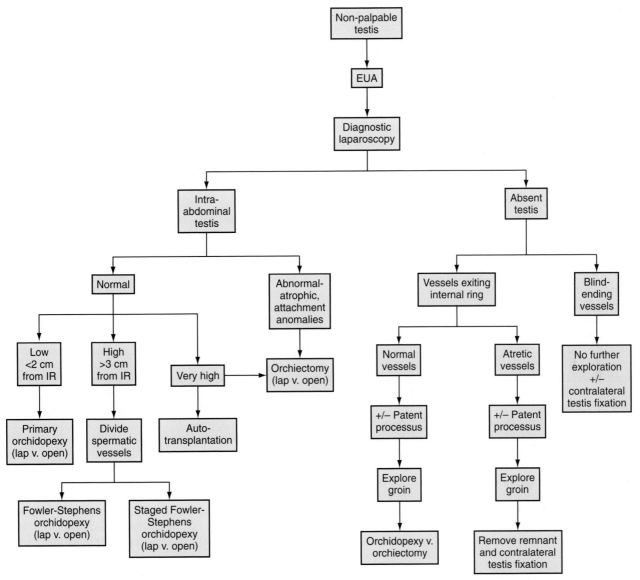

Figure 127–8. Management of a nonpalpable testis. EUA, examination under anesthesia; IR, internal ring.

noted that in particular a contralateral testis length of 2.0 cm or greater predicted monorchia in over 90% of cases (Koff, 1991; Hurwitz and Kaptein, 2001; Belman and Rushton, 2003).

Approximately 36% to 64% of children with a nonpalpable testis will be monorchid (Rappe et al, 1992; Wilson-Storey and MacKinnon, 1992; Elder, 1994; Moore et al, 1994; Perovic and Janic, 1994; Ferro et al, 1996; Baillie et al, 1998; Cisek et al, 1998). **A vanishing testis may be either an intra-abdominal or inguinal-scrotal event.** It is most commonly an in utero event caused by either torsion or a compromising vascular event. In both cases the spermatic vessels are generally hypoplastic or atretic when compared with the contralateral vessels. An intra-abdominal vanishing testis will demonstrate the classic anatomy of a blind-ending vas and spermatic vessels, usually within a few centimeters of the internal ring. No testicular tissue will be present. **When blind-ending spermatic vessels are found, no further surgical intervention is**

necessary, although consideration should be given to performing a trans-scrotal testicular fixation procedure on the normally descended contralateral testis because of the reported risk for abnormal testicular fixation (bell-clapper deformity) (Bellinger, 1985; Van Savage, 2001).

When the spermatic vessels and vasa exit the internal ring, including those that are comparatively hypoplastic, one must consider viable testicular elements within the caudad extent of descent. Therefore, inguinal-scrotal exploration should be performed and the cord remnant excised. However, this is controversial because atretic vessels are predictive of a nonviable testicular remnant. **Even though most testicular remnants or nubbins will demonstrate histologic evidence of ischemia and necrosis (fibrosis, hyalinization, calcification, and hemosiderin deposition), in up to 13% of cases viable residual testicular elements will be present** (Plotzker et al, 1992; Turek et al, 1994; Rozanski et al, 1996; Grady et al, 1998; De Luna et al, 2003). DeLuna et al (2003) reported that approximately 10% of testicular remnants contained residual tubules, 5.6% of which contained germ cells. Carcinoma in situ has not yet been reported within these specimens. It has been argued that inguinal exploration is not necessary for removal of the testicular remnant because the risk for malignant degeneration is low (Grady et al, 1998). In these circumstances, the groin can be effectively explored through a low inguinal incision and the remnant cord structures removed.

An intra-abdominal testis usually resides within a few centimeters of the internal ring. In most cases the processus vaginalis is patent and the vas deferens can exit into the inguinal canal (long looping vas deferens). An intra-abdominal testis can also be much further from the internal ring and has been reported, though rarely, in perinephric, perihepatic, or crossed ectopic locations. Careful laparoscopic inspection of the contralateral pelvic region is also important because an ectopic testis or remnant may be dissociated from the vas and vessels and identification of these structures may not be a reliable indicator of a testicular remnant (De Luna et al, 2003). **The vas deferens can demonstrate nonunion with any cryptorchid testis and therefore, when blindly ending, is not confirmative of a vanishing testis.** Accordingly, the entire abdomen should be inspected at the time of diagnostic laparoscopy if the testis is not readily apparent close to its internal ring. Thereafter, searching along the course of the spermatic vessels toward its origin at the level of the kidneys should lead to the testis. To facilitate identification of the spermatic vessels and testis, a child positioned in the supine position can be laterally rotated and placed in the Trendelenburg position so that the intestines fall away from the course of the spermatic vessels along the psoas muscle. Occasionally, the left colon or cecum may hide the testis, in which case another port can be placed in the contralateral lower abdominal quadrant for laparoscopic dissection. Every effort should be made to either locate the testis or determine its fate.

Most undescended testes discovered in infancy and located in the groin are associated with a patent processus vaginalis. Likewise, if on initial scrotal or inguinal exploration the processus is found to be patent, a nonpalpable testis will probably be present in the abdomen. Inspection of the ipsilateral internal ring during diagnostic laparoscopy is therefore important because in 91% of boys with a patent processus vaginalis the testis will be viable whereas if the processus is closed, 97% of testes will be vanished or absent (Elder, 1994). **Therefore, a patent processus vaginalis found during inguinal exploration for a nonpalpable testis requires intra-abdominal exploration; however, a negative inguinal exploration does not rule out the possibility of an intra-abdominal testis.**

Inguinal versus Laparoscopic Exploration

The choice of traditional surgical exploration versus primary laparoscopy for assessment of a nonpalpable testis is a matter of debate. Most reports are retrospective and biased toward one methodology or the other. Open surgical exploration via an inguinal incision was the procedure most commonly used before the era of laparoscopy for the management of a nonpalpable testis. Many urologists undoubtedly continue this practice because of long established merits. The argument exists that although diagnostic laparoscopy is valuable, especially when an intra-abdominal testis is confirmed, inguinal-scrotal exploration is nonetheless necessary to evaluate the cord and gonadal structures exiting the internal ring, and thus laparoscopy may have been avoided altogether (Gulanikar et al, 1996; Ferro et al, 1999; Belman and Rushton, 2001). In addition, the method of exploration, whether transinguinal or laparoscopic, will probably influence the type of procedure ultimately performed. Ferro and colleagues (1996) demonstrated that a significantly greater percentage of intra-abdominal testes were managed with Fowler-Stephens orchidopexy initially approached laparoscopically.

Kanemoto and associates (2002) combined inguinal exploration and transinguinal laparoscopy to test this strategy as an alternative. They found that an extended incision was unnecessary in the case of a blind ending vas and vessels in the peritoneum because this could be easily assessed with transinguinal laparoscopy. Laparoscopy was avoided in 73.3% of cases altogether because the testis, its remnant or testicular vessels, and the vas deferens were detected by inspecting the inguinal region. Ravasse et al (2003) reported similar results. Laparoscopy was subsequently performed in 38% of boys with a nonpalpable testis when no viable testis was demonstrated by inguinal exploration. The authors concluded that laparoscopy was critical to a change in management for only 23% of patients. Schleef and colleagues (2002) reported a variation of diagnostic laparoscopy. Laparoscopic groin exploration via a nonpatent internal ring was performed and the remnant cord structures resected when the spermatic cord appeared to be hypoplastic. In this small series, management was predicated on the laparoscopic findings, the nuance being that open groin exploration could be avoided when a vanishing testis is encountered. Belman and Rushton (2001) recommend primary scrotal exploration for a unilateral nonpalpable testis. This strategy is based on the authors' rationale that (1) a third to half of boys with a nonpalpable testis will have a vanishing testis and (2) a vanishing testis, believed to be due to perinatal testicular torsion, occurs not as an abdominal or inguinal event, but most often as a scrotal event. Laparoscopy can then be limited to those in whom scrotal exploration is negative and an intra-abdominal testis is suspected.

Other reports have generally found utility in at least 50% of patients when diagnostic laparoscopy was performed as the primary approach to a nonpalpable testis. Cisek et al (1998) reported that in 66% of cases patients benefited from a primary laparoscopic diagnosis and treatment strategy that would have otherwise resulted in compromised exposure via an inguinal exploration. Mikaelsson and associates (1999) concluded that the accuracy of diagnostic laparoscopy resulted in 51% of patients avoiding more extensive inguinal exploration or laparotomy. **Therefore, it is difficult to criticize traditional nonlaparoscopic techniques of exploration; however, laparoscopy, whether primary or adjunctive to an open exploration, offers a logical extension of surgical principles, especially if conversion to a therapeutic laparoscopic procedure is anticipated.**

Laparoscopic Orchidopexy

Laparoscopic orchidopexy is now standard in the urologists' armamentarium of management for an intra-abdominal testis. A laparoscopic approach in the management of an intra-abdominal undescended testis has advantages over standard orchidopexy performed through either an extended inguinal incision or a high inguinal incision (Jones incision). Laparoscopy accurately assesses the presence, absence, viability, and entire anatomy of an intra-abdominal testis. Success in testicular mobilization may require complete and proximal dissection of the spermatic vessels and redirecting the line of "descent" to the shortest distance to the scrotum. Laparoscopic orchidopexy allows accessibility to the entire course of the spermatic vessels to their origin, usually the limiting factor in tension-free mobilization of an intra-abdominal testis. Dissection close to the origin of the spermatic vessels is possible because the surgeon's range of motion with laparoscopic instrumentation extends across the entire abdominal cavity. Magnification of these delicate vessels aids in dissection and preservation of the main and collateral blood supply.

Jordan et al first described primary, nonstaged laparoscopic orchidopexy in 1992 and the first staged procedures in 1994. Success rates of laparoscopic orchidopexy are comparable to results published for open orchidopexy and are based on postoperative testicular position and viability. Although testicular atrophy is a well-recognized complication of orchidopexy, especially for an intra-abdominal testis, it has been more apt to occur in patients who have undergone previous surgery, presumably because of dissection around the vas deferens (Chang et al, 2001). A number of series have demonstrated laparoscopic orchidopexy to have higher success rates than historically reported for open techniques. A recent retrospective, nonrandomized multi-institutional analysis found higher success rates in the management of a nonpalpable testis (Baker et al, 2001). Success rates were dependent on the method (97.2% for "primary" laparoscopic orchidopexy, 74.1% for one-stage Fowler-Stephens orchidopexy, 87.9% for two-stage Fowler-Stephens orchidopexy), with an overall atrophy rate of 6.1%. Atrophy rates were found to be highest in the single-stage Fowler-Stephens orchidopexy at 22%, whereas atrophy occurred in only 2% of testes after a straightforward laparoscopic orchidopexy. Two-stage Fowler-Stephens orchidopexy had intermediate results of a 10% atrophy rate. Lindgren et al (1998) reported an overall 93% success rate without a case of testicular atrophy when either primary or Fowler-Stephens laparoscopic techniques were used. Chang et al (2001) reported a large single-group experience with similar success rates for all laparoscopic techniques of orchidopexy, specifically, an overall 85% success rate for one- or two-stage Fowler-Stephens procedures with a 4% failure rate as a result of atrophy. However, of the 20 one-stage Fowler-Stephens orchidopexy procedures, 85% were successfully placed in the scrotum without atrophy.

The age at which laparoscopic orchidopexy should be performed is the same as for standard orchidopexy, usually between 6 and 8 months and certainly before 1 year of age. The surgical procedure for a boy with a nonpalpable testis starts with examination under anesthesia. This will give the surgeon an excellent opportunity to examine the child, especially if it was difficult to do so in the office. In approximately 18% of boys a previously nonpalpable testis will be palpable on examination under anesthesia (Cisek et al, 1998). Attention should be especially directed to the location of a peeping or emergent testis at the internal ring or to identification of an atrophic nubbin in the scrotum. An 8 French infant feeding tube is placed per urethra to drain the bladder before and

during the entire procedure. Intraoperative antibiotics are unnecessary.

Diagnostic laparoscopy is first performed. We recommend an open technique for placement of the first trocar in a child to reduce the inherent complications associated with blind placement of a Veress needle, such as extraperitoneal emphysema or bowel injury. A small infraumbilical or supraumbilical incision is made and carried down to the rectus fascia, which is opened transversely. Properitoneal fat is spread and the peritoneum grasped, elevated, and opened sharply while being careful to avoid bowel. Either a 5-mm Hossan trocar is placed or a comparably sized disposable port such as a 5-mm radially dilating port. If necessary, a 2-0 Vicryl suture can be placed as a U-stitch into the rectus fascia, which can then be drawn upon with a cardiac slider to ensure an airtight seal around this port. Pneumoperitoneum is created with CO_2 insufflation at pressures between 8 and 10 mm H_2O and a gas flow rate of 8 to 10 L/min to create and maintain a working space. A 0-degree 5-mm laparoscope is used in most cases. The child can be placed in the Trendelenburg position or turned laterally to help mobilize the bowel away from the area of interest. The surgeon should be on the contralateral side of the patient with the assistant operating the camera. The monitor is best positioned at the foot of the table. Smaller instruments and telescopes have been developed. Pediatric telescopes of 1.9 or 3.5 mm provide excellent illumination and visual detail, and 3.5-mm reusable instruments (trocars, scissors, graspers) handle tissue well (Humke et al, 1998).

An intra-abdominal testis is usually found within 1 to 2 cm of the internal ring, which is usually patent. If the testis is immobile and beyond 2.5 cm from the internal ring, it may be prudent to perform a staged orchidopexy consisting of clipping the internal spermatic vessels and returning 6 months later to mobilize the testis on collateral vessels and the deferential artery. Attention to the distal paratesticular elements is necessary to determine whether the vas deferens exits beyond the internal ring into the inguinal canal. The first element of testicular mobilization is drawing the "gubernacular" attachment from the internal ring/inguinal canal, transecting it, and using it as a grasping point for safe testicular manipulation.

After it has been determined to proceed with laparoscopic orchidopexy, two more 3- or 5-mm ports are placed under direct laparoscopic vision. A 5-mm port is at present the smallest port size that can accommodate a clip applier if spermatic vessel transection is anticipated. It is the surgeon's preference where these ports should be placed to achieve the greatest degree of instrument freedom and avoid crossing instruments during dissection. Two port placement configurations are presented here: one configuration is to place the other two ports in the midclavicular line, usually opposing each other at the level of the umbilicus. An alternative configuration, especially useful in infants, is to place the port ipsilateral to the intra-abdominal testis higher in the abdomen, just below the subcostal margin, to move the camera port away from the working ports. The second port can then be placed in the contralateral lower abdominal quadrant. When placing these additional ports, especially in infants, there is not a great deal of room, particularly in the breadth of the abdominal cavity, and the peritoneum tends to push away from the anterior abdominal wall, thereby further restricting safe working space. It may be necessary to tent the child's skin in the opposing direction of port advancement. This maneuver should nonetheless be monitored laparoscopically.

The initial dissection begins with taking down the distal attachments sharply inside or at the internal ring while being careful to not damage the vas deferens or epididymis and assessing for vasal descent into the inguinal canal, in which case a hernia would be present. Electrocautery, when necessary, is used at low current to maintain hemostasis and avoid damage to neighboring structures. Sharp dissection begins with a peritoneal incision at the internal ring made well lateral to the spermatic vessels and carried along the abdominal sidewall or psoas muscle parallel and cranial toward the origin of the vessels. The other line of dissection is caudad to the course of the vas deferens and carried along the pelvic sidewall toward the bladder. A triangular wedge of peritoneum is preserved between the spermatic vessels and vas deferens, with the testis at the apex. It is sometimes necessary to open the window of peritoneum between these structures to gain more length. **However, if a single-stage Fowler-Stephens orchidopexy is the intended or possible procedure, the peritoneum between the spermatic vessels and vas needs to be carefully preserved to prevent disruption of the collateral vasculature.** Therefore, the isolated peritoneal sheath should be left intact until the commitment is made to bring the testis into the scrotum with the spermatic vasculature intact. This swath of peritoneum, which includes the vas and vessels, is mobilized away from the posterior retroperitoneum. An approximate indication that laparoscopic dissection is near completion is when the testis can be brought beyond the contralateral internal ring without any tension. The ipsilateral internal ring is not closed despite the presence of a hernia because it has not been demonstrated to result postoperatively in a clinical hernia.

Transfer of the testis into the scrotum has been described in many ways, but passing a curved hemostat from the subdartos pouch over the symphysis pubis into the peritoneal cavity where the laparoscope can guide its path medial to the obliterated umbilical artery is simple and effective. Others have described passing an additional port trans-scrotally into the abdomen over the symphysis for grasper access. **It is critical for the surgeon to personally monitor tension on the spermatic cord as the testis is passed into the scrotum to avoid inadvertent avulsion of the spermatic vessels. Further mobilization of the spermatic vessels may be necessary and can be performed by two methods: dissecting the peritoneum away from the spermatic vessels and carrying the dissection of the spermatic vessels more cephalad toward the kidney.** When tension is encountered that does not allow the testis to rest comfortably within the mid to dependent scrotum, incising the peritoneum overlying the spermatic vessels as cephalad as possible is helpful in improving effective spermatic cord length. Gentle traction on the testis outside the scrotum can be applied to help determine laparoscopically which elements require further mobilization or division. In either case, great care must be taken to not damage or avulse the vessels because dissection can be tedious. The subdartos pouch is created in a manner already described. Many times an external nylon fixation button is useful in maintaining testicular position securely in the scrotum when tension is present. It is usually left in place for 5 to 7 days.

Before port removal, bleeding should be assessed laparoscopically under low intra-abdominal pressure by releasing the pneumoperitoneum. On removing the ports, hemostasis should also be assessed at the port sites, as well as being sure that the umbilical closure does not include bowel or omentum.

Laparoscopic Fowler-Stephens Orchidopexy

The spermatic vessels are usually the length-limiting factor in accomplishing a tension-free orchidopexy. The decision whether to divide these vessels needs to be made early in the course of laparoscopic orchidopexy. There are no absolute criteria for when transection needs to be performed, but the obvious maxim is the further the distance that the testis is from the scrotum, the greater the likelihood that vessel transection will be necessary. As a general guideline, a testis within 2 cm of the internal ring can be brought down without vessel transection, between 2 and 4 cm is a gray area, and beyond 4 cm vessel transection needs to be seriously considered before any peritoneal dissection. Keeping in mind that staged orchidopexy carries a higher complication rate with regard to testicular atrophy, vessel transection may not be as necessary in children younger than 1 year because the critical distance of the testis to the scrotum is not significantly more than that for an intracanalicular testis. During the initial laparoscopic evaluation, it may be necessary to place more than one port to manipulate the testis for determination of its mobility, position, and anatomy. Vessel ablation with surgical clips or a harmonic scalpel can be performed via a 5-mm port placed in the contralateral lower abdominal quadrant.

The second stage of the orchidopexy is usually completed 6 months later. It can be performed in either open or laparoscopic fashion. The same principles apply as with an open second-stage procedure if performed laparoscopically. After the spermatic vessels are divided, a peritoneal incision is made wide and lateral to the distal spermatic vessels and testis. A second incision is made distal to the vas deferens. The testis is mobilized on a wide triangular swath of peritoneum while carefully preserving the vasal artery and any collateral vasculature. The remainder of the procedure is as described earlier.

Microvascular Autotransplantation

The indications for performing autotransplantation of an intra-abdominal testis must be weighed in light of the circumstances of the clinical findings; the indications are similar to those for a Fowler-Stephens orchiopexy. **An important consideration that weighs in favor of this procedure is the variability of collateral blood supply in patients with a high undescended testis, which may potentially compromise the Fowler-Stephens procedure.** The results of testicular autotransplantation have been demonstrated to be superior to the predicted results reported with division of the spermatic vessels for a high intra-abdominal testis. The success of this technique is heavily dependent on microvascular expertise, which may not be universally available and most likely accounts for why this approach has not been more widely adopted.

Silber and Kelly (1976) first reported using a microvascular anastomosis to bring extra blood supply to the testis after mobilization of a high intra-abdominal testis in a child with prune-belly syndrome. The initial series were limited to older boys whose internal spermatic artery was large enough to be anastomosed to the inferior epigastric artery, but the technique was demonstrated to be successful in boys younger than 2 years (Harrison et al, 1990). Overall success rates are in excess of 80% (Wacksman et al, 1982; Bianchi, 1984; Harrison et al, 1990; Bukowski et al, 1995c; Bukowski et al, 1995b). Bukowski and associates (1995b) reported a 96% success rate for testicular autotransplantation over a 17-year period. Diagnostic laparoscopy is used in conjunction with autotransplantation to locate and assess the viability of the testis. Laparoscopically assisted testicular autotransplantation was reported to be successful in five children, with a median operative time of 5 hours (Wacksman et al, 1996). Therefore, microvascular testicular autotransplantation may be the procedure of choice for a solitary, high intraabdominal testis rather than an open or two-stage Fowler-Stephens approach.

Before surgery, hCG or testosterone can be given to increase vascular caliber. The procedure is performed through a Gibson incision, which offers high intraperitoneal exposure. Donor vessel preparation requires 1 to 3 cm of the vessel to be dissected free of surrounding tissue for anastomosis of the spermatic vessels to the ipsilateral inferior epigastric artery and vein. The spermatic vessels are mobilized proximally and divided near their origin after the vas and its collateral vessels have been preserved and mobilized on a wide patch of peritoneum. Vascular spasm can be relieved with 1% lidocaine, and systemic anticoagulation with heparin may be established. Further preparation of the vessels and anastomoses is based on microvascular techniques. Fixation of the testis in the scrotum is performed by the dartos pouch method. Doppler ultrasound or radioactive isotope perfusion scanning can be used postoperatively to determine patency of the anastomosis.

Reoperative Orchiopexy

Reoperative orchiopexy is performed in cases of secondary cryptorchism after orchiopexy or inguinal hernia repair. Testes that are at risk for iatrogenic ascent after hernia repair many times appear to be normally descended when in fact they are retractile or represent a subtle variant of a cryptorchid testis. In this case, the testis may be ectopic and located in a low-lying position within a superficial pouch. In many cases the testis is also in a retroscrotal plane just outside the confines of the anatomic scrotum. The testis is usually located near the pubic tubercle, but depending on age and delay in treatment, it may be as high as just outside the external ring. The skin incision and initial exposure should be in a previously non-operated area to identify landmarks and approach the testis from normal to scarred tissue.

The initial dissection should be toward the lower pole of the testis. The inguinal ligament should also be identified early in the procedure. After the testis is freed, care is taken to mobilize the spermatic cord, which has probably been previously skeletonized. Dense scarring may be found between the anterior aspect of the cord and the undersurface of the external oblique fascia. To lessen the risk of injury to the spermatic vessels, dissection is performed lateral and medial to the cord in more normal tissues, and in some cases it is beneficial to leave a strip of fascia overlying the cord during the initial mobilization. It may also be necessary to mobilize the cord proximally above the internal ring to gain length in a now relatively inelastic cord. The usual surgical principles of a standard orchiopexy can then be applied, including positioning the cord more medially.

Complications of Orchiopexy

Complications of orchiopexy include testicular retraction, hematoma formation, ilioinguinal nerve injury, postoperative torsion (either iatrogenic or spontaneous), damage to the vas deferens, and testicular atrophy. Atrophy of the testis is the most devastating complication, but it is seldom seen with standard orchiopexy. Devascularization with atrophy of the testis can result from skeletonization of the cord, from overzealous electrocautery, from inadvertent torsion of the spermatic vessels during passage of the testis into the scrotum, or as a result of ligation and division of the spermatic vessels during Fowler-Stephens orchiopexy. Devascularization may also be caused by excessive axial tension on the spermatic vessels, particularly if the collaterals are poor. Some degree of postoperative hematoma is common, but a large hematoma increases the risk for infection and abscess formation. Although retraction is usually caused by inadequate retroperitoneal dissection, insufficient cord length precludes successful orchiopexy no matter how much dissection is performed. If the patent processus vaginalis is ligated within the canal and not above the internal ring, the peritoneum remains adherent to the spermatic vessels, and complete retroperitoneal mobilization of vessels is not feasible.

HERNIAS AND HYDROCELES

The differential diagnosis of acute and chronic swelling of the inguinal and scrotal area is of daily concern to urologists who deal with children. Although there has been a trend toward imaging of the groin in some circles, physical examination and a history of the clinical findings remain the hallmarks of physical diagnosis.

KEY POINTS: MANAGEMENT OF UNDESCENDED TESTES

- Radiologic testing does not have a relevant role in the assessment of undescended testes and should not influence surgical management.

- Bilateral nonpalpable testes warrant immediate assessment in the newborn period to determine the presence or absence of testes and to rule out an intersex state.

- Surgical intervention on an undescended testis should be performed between 6 and 12 months of age.

- The efficacy of hormonal treatment is less than 20% for cryptorchid testes and is significantly dependent on pretreatment testicular location.

- Nonpalpable testes account for 20% of children with an undescended testis; approximately 50% of these patients will be monorchid.

- Viable testicular elements will be present in up to 13% of testicular remnants/nubbins and should therefore be removed.

Hydrocele

As the testis descends into the scrotum from its abdominal position, it carries with it a tongue of peritoneum (the processus vaginalis). Normally, the processus is obliterated from the internal inguinal ring to the upper scrotum, with a small potential space remaining in the scrotum that partially surrounds the testis. During the normal embryologic processes that involve descent of the testis and closure and obliteration of the processus vaginalis, a number of embryologic misadventures may occur that can result in commonly seen inguinal or scrotal pathology (hydrocele, hydrocele of the cord, and communicating hydrocele).

A simple (scrotal) hydrocele is an accumulation of fluid within the tunica vaginalis. All hydroceles in infants and children result from persistence or delayed closure of the processus vaginalis. Simple hydroceles, in which the processus appears to be obliterated and fluid trapped within the tunica vaginalis of the scrotum persists, are commonly seen at birth, are frequently bilateral, and may be quite large. They transilluminate and may appear quite tense but are not painful. No fluid is evident in the groin in most cases, but occasionally a large, simple hydrocele extends toward the internal inguinal ring. Most simple scrotal hydroceles found at birth deserve long-term observation, and most resolve during the first 2 years of life. Aspiration of infant hydroceles is contraindicated because of the risk for infection, which in the case of a patent processus, would extend into the peritoneal cavity. If surgical repair of an infant hydrocele is elected, an inguinal approach should be used in case a patent processus is encountered.

Communicating Hydrocele and Inguinal Hernia

Persistence of the processus vaginalis allows peritoneal fluid to freely communicate with the scrotal limits of the processus, and a communicating hydrocele results. **The classic description of a communicating hydrocele is that of a hydrocele that vacillates in size, usually related to activity.** Most communicating hydroceles are smaller in the morning and become more prominent as the day progresses, enlarging in response to the upright position, activities that increase intra-abdominal pressure, and in many cases, fever. The scrotal swelling may be soft or tense, and it may change in consistency. In infants, the hydrocele sac may be thick or thin. Thin sacs frequently present a bluish hue through thin scrotal skin. Hydroceles easily transilluminate. Tense hydroceles may prohibit adequate palpation of the testis. Because most undescended testes are found at exploration to have an accompanying patent processus, it is important that a cryptorchid testis not be missed when assessing a child with a communicating hydrocele. Inguinal hernias represent the same anatomic defect that is seen in cases of communicating hydrocele. Small intestine, omentum, bladder, or genital contents may be found in the sac.

Communicating hydroceles may be diagnosed by history or by physical examination. If a scrotal hydrocele can be compressed and the fluid within the scrotum evacuated into the abdomen, a patent processus must be present. In many cases, however, the processus is small and it is not possible to express fluid out of the scrotum. In these cases, one must rely on the observations of the child's caretakers to determine whether a communication exists. In most cases, observation permits differentiation of simple from communicating hydroceles. On occasion, however, a hydrocele is explored because of the assumption that it communicates and is found to have an obliterated processus vaginalis.

Communicating hydroceles are by definition congenital in origin. However, it is not uncommon for a communicating hydrocele to be manifested for the first time clinically in an older child or adolescent. In our experience, many of these late-onset communicating hydroceles are found to be omental hernias in which descent of a plug of omentum through the internal inguinal ring has caused a sudden increase in the amount of fluid in the scrotum. In some of these cases, a palpable thickening in the inguinal canal may suggest the presence of entrapped omentum.

All communicating hydroceles should be explored through an inguinal incision. A small incision, 1 cm or less in length, should be made in an inguinal skin crease. The subcutaneous tissue and Scarpa's fascia are incised. The cord structures may be isolated outside the external inguinal ring in infants because of the very short oblique course of the inguinal canal; however, in most cases a short incision through the aponeurosis of the external oblique or through the external ring provides adequate access to the cord just below the internal inguinal ring. Once the cord structures have been isolated, the cremasteric fibers are spread to identify the shiny sac, which should be located on the anteromedial aspect of the cord. The sac may be isolated from the cord structures or opened on its anterior wall to allow the back wall to be dissected off the cord under direct vision. This technique is particularly appealing and offers safety to the cord structures when a very large sac is present. It is imperative that the sac be opened when the anatomy is confusing or the sac is very thickened. Failure to do so may result in disastrous consequences if bowel, bladder, or ovary is contained in the sac and not recognized.

Once the sac has been isolated from the cord structures, it should be divided distal to the internal ring. High ligation of the stump of the sac is then performed at the internal ring after the sac is twisted to strengthen it for suture ligation. If the internal ring is patulous, it may be tightened with one or two sutures, with care taken to not close it too tightly around the remaining cord structures. If the cord was pulled into the wound during the procedure, the testis should now be pulled back into the scrotum. The distal sac does not need to be completely removed. If fluid remains in the distal sac, the proximal portion of the distal hydrocele can be unroofed through the inguinal incision, or a small needle can be passed through the scrotum to aspirate the remaining fluid. If there is concern that the testis is not completely in the scrotum, a scrotal incision and orchidopexy are indicated. The external oblique, subcutaneous tissue, and dermis are then closed with absorbable sutures.

The quandary of whether to explore an asymptomatic contralateral inguinal canal in children with an inguinal hernia or communicating hydrocele has been a controversial topic since the 1950s. Several areas of concern are raised when this question is discussed, including the incidence of a contralateral patent processus vaginalis, the incidence of a clinically apparent hernia or communicating hydrocele developing after unilateral inguinal herniorrhaphy, and the potential for injury to the vas or testicular blood supply that is inherent during repair of an inguinal hernia. The incidence of a patent processus vaginalis has been confirmed at exploration to be between 48% and 63% and varies with the age of the child (Rowe et al, 1969; Holder and Ashcraft, 1980). Rowe and colleagues reviewed 1965 infants and children with a clinically unilateral hernia who underwent contralateral exploration and found a patent processus in 46%, with an incidence of 63% in those younger than 2 months and 41% in those aged 2 to 16 years. These data must be considered in light of the much lower incidence of a contralateral clinical hernia and communicating hydrocele developing after unilateral inguinal herniorrhaphy. Sparkman (1962) analyzed data from seven studies and found the average incidence to be 15.8%, similar to the finding of 14.9% in the study by Bock and Sobye (1970) and 22% in the study by McGregor and colleagues (1980). In practice, the frequency of contralateral exploration has varied according to patient age from institution to institution. Wiener and coworkers (1996) surveyed the Surgery Section of the American Academy of Pediatrics in 1996 and found that open contralateral exploration was carried out in 65% of boys up to 2 years of age and in 84% of girls up to 4 years of age.

A concern was raised by Sparkman (1962) about the morbidity associated with contralateral inguinal exploration, which causes pathologically proven vas injury in 1.6% of patients. He postulated that the true incidence of vas injury might be much higher. With the advent of small laparoscopic instrumentation, evaluation of the contralateral internal inguinal ring can be performed endoscopically, a trend that has grown significantly over the past several years (DuBois et al, 1997; Gardner et al, 1998; Yerkes et al, 1998; Van Glabeke et al, 1999; Owings and Georgeson, 2000). This technique would seem to obviate any concern about injury to the vas and vessels.

No consensus has been reached about which technique to use or the age below which evaluation of the contralateral inguinal canal should be strongly considered in patients with a clinically unilateral inguinal hernia or communicating hydrocele. However, it is important that the question of contralateral disease be addressed completely by both history and examination at the time of initial consultation. Any past or present history of contralateral inguinal or scrotal pathology should be considered an indication for contralateral evaluation at the time of herniorrhaphy. In addition, any child with a ventriculoperitoneal shunt or other source of increased intraperitoneal fluid (e.g., peritoneal dialysis) should undergo bilateral exploration.

Hydrocele of the Cord

One of the vagaries of closure of the processus vaginalis that may occur is segmental closure of the processus, which leaves a loculated hydrocele of the cord that may or may not communicate with the peritoneal cavity (communicating hydrocele of the cord). Hydrocele of the cord is usually manifested as a painless groin mass contiguous with the cord structures

and located at any position from just above the testis to the inguinal canal. The mass is mobile and transilluminates. It may vacillate in size when communication with the peritoneal cavity is present. The differential diagnosis of inguinal masses also includes sarcomas of the cord and paratesticular tissues and inguinal hernia (especially with impacted omentum). Ultrasound may be helpful in determining the diagnosis (Martin et al, 1996). Inguinal exploration of a hydrocele of the cord in most cases delineates a circumscribed, cystic mass connected to an obliterated or patent processus vaginalis. High ligation of a patent processus at the internal ring and excision or unroofing of the encysted hydrocele are curative.

Abdominoscrotal Hydrocele

An abdominoscrotal hydrocele is a rare clinical entity in which a large, bilobed hydrocele spans the internal inguinal ring; it consists of a large inguinoscrotal component and a large intra-abdominal component. It is thought that the abdominal component results from a large inguinoscrotal hydrocele that is separated from the peritoneal cavity by only a short obliterated segment at the internal ring. As fluid continues to accumulate, the hydrocele expands into the relatively low pressure of the abdominal cavity and forms the abdominal component (Gentile et al, 1998). The diagnosis is usually made on physical examination when a child with a large hydrocele has a palpable abdominal mass. Pressure on the abdominal mass generally results in an increase in size of the scrotal hydrocele. Ultrasound examination is definitive. At inguinal exploration it is important to remove all of the abdominal component, which is advanced into the wound as the proximal end of the sac is dissected. Failure to recognize the abdominal component is a cause of recurrence.

ACUTE SCROTUM

A child or adolescent with acute scrotal pain, tenderness, or swelling should be looked on as an emergency situation requiring prompt evaluation, differential diagnosis, and potentially immediate surgical exploration. Adolescent boys do not always understand the potential significance of acute scrotal conditions, and evaluation in many cases is delayed. As a result, a subacute or even chronic scrotal condition may in certain situations merit prompt evaluation and intervention.

Differential Diagnosis

The list of differential diagnoses for an acute scrotum is extensive. In all instances it is imperative to rule out torsion of the spermatic cord, a clinical diagnosis requiring emergency surgical intervention (Table 127–1).

Torsion of the Spermatic Cord (Intravaginal)

Torsion of the spermatic cord is a true surgical emergency of the highest order. Irreversible ischemic injury to the testicular parenchyma may begin as soon as 4 hours after

Table 127–1. Differential Diagnosis of Acute/Subacute Scrotum

Torsion of the spermatic cord
Torsion of the appendix testis
Torsion of the appendix epididymis
Epididymitis
Epididymo-orchitis
Inguinal hernia
Communicating hydrocele
Hydrocele
Hydrocele of the cord
Trauma/insect bite
Dermatologic lesions
Inflammatory vasculitis (Henoch-Schönlein purpura)
Idiopathic scrotal edema
Tumor
Spermatocele
Varicocele
Nonurogenital pathology (e.g., adductor tendinitis)

occlusion of the cord. Bartsch and colleagues (1980) demonstrated that although testes operated on less than 8 hours after the onset of symptoms of torsion retained normal testis size and showed just slight changes in testicular morphology, only 50% of men whose testes underwent detorsion less than 4 hours after symptoms began had normal semen analysis. It appears that the degree of torsion that occurs may have a significant influence on the potential for viability of the testis over time. The significance of this situation is magnified by the findings of Barada and coworkers (1989), who reported that patients younger than 18 years were more prone to testicular loss after acute torsion because of a median delay in medical evaluation of 20 hours after the onset of scrotal pain, an indication of the need for improved awareness of the significance of scrotal pain in adolescents.

Intravaginal torsion, or torsion of the cord within the space of the tunica vaginalis, may result from lack of normal fixation of an appropriate portion of the testis and epididymis to the fascial and muscular coverings that surround the cord within the scrotum. In effect, the normally segmental area of the free space between the parietal and visceral layers of the tunica vaginalis is expanded to surround the testis and epididymis and extends proximally up the cord for a variable distance. This creates an abnormally mobile testis that

hangs freely within the tunica space (a "bell-clapper deformity") (Fig. 127–9).

Although torsion of the cord does occur in prepubertal males, it appears that the added weight of the testis after puberty adds a physical dimension that may be more likely to allow the testis to twist on its vascular stalk. Torsion can occur in association with trauma or athletic activity, but in most cases spontaneous torsion of the cord is reported; in many cases the adolescent is awakened from sleep. It is thought that sudden contraction of the cremasteric muscle, which inserts onto the cord in a spiral configuration, is the inciting event in most cases and initiates a rotational effect on the testis as it is pulled upward. The cord may twist as many as several complete (360-degree) rotations.

The classic manifestation of acute torsion of the spermatic cord is that of an acute onset of scrotal pain, but in some instances the onset appears to be more gradual, and in some boys the degree of pain is minimized. A large number of boys with acute scrotal pain give a history of previous episodes of severe, self-limited scrotal pain and swelling. It is likely that these incidents represent previous episodes of intermittent torsion of the cord with spontaneous detorsion. Nausea and vomiting may accompany acute torsion, and some boys have pain referred to the ipsilateral lower quadrant of the abdomen. Dysuria and other bladder symptoms are usually absent.

The history is an important factor in the differential diagnosis of an acute scrotum, but the physical examination may perhaps be even more crucial in determining whether the diagnosis is torsion of the cord or otherwise (i.e., whether the patient does or does not require immediate surgical exploration). Inspection of the genitalia may prove helpful if the affected testis is riding high in the scrotum, perhaps indicating foreshortening of the spermatic cord as the result of twisting of the cord. In some cases, the affected testis has an abnormally transverse orientation, but in many cases, in particular when several hours have passed since onset, an acute hydrocele or massive scrotal edema obliterates all landmarks. **The absence of a cremasteric reflex is a good indicator of torsion of the cord.** Rabinowitz (1984) found 100% correlation between absence of a cremasteric reflex and the presence of torsion in 245 boys over a 7-year period. In some cases, assessment of this physical finding is difficult. When the patient is cooperative enough to allow examination of the affected hemiscrotum, effort should be made to assess

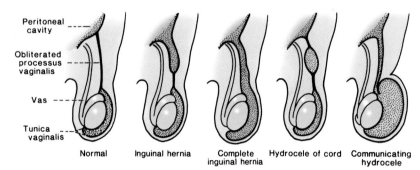

Figure 127–9. Anomalies of the inguinal canal and scrotum that may result from anomalous closure of the processus vaginalis. (From Welch KA, Randolph JG, Ravitch MM, et al [eds]: Pediatric Surgery, vol 2, 4th ed. St Louis, Year Book, 1986, p 780.)

anatomic landmarks to primarily look for an appreciation of normal structures in an attempt to identify a swollen and tender epididymis or a twisted appendix of the testis or epididymis. If torsion of the cord seems likely, manual detorsion should be attempted as part of the initial examination because the patient may be uncooperative with an extended examination because of discomfort. Classically, torsion of the cord occurs such that the anterior surface of each testis turns toward the midline as viewed from the patient's perspective (Sparks, 1971). To accomplish detorsion of the cord, a rotational effort should be made in the opposite direction. Kiesling and associates (1984) described detorsion through two planes, with rotation in a caudal-to-cranial direction and simultaneous medial-to-lateral rotation. In actuality, the examiner should try to twist or "unscrew" the testis in one direction (usually outward, toward the thigh) and then in the opposite direction if the first attempt is unsuccessful. When detorsion is successful, the testis "flips" into a different rotation and pain relief may be almost instantaneous, with the cord appearing to lengthen and the testis dropping into the scrotum. If manual detorsion does not totally correct the rotation that has occurred, prompt exploration is indicated. However, when the patient becomes almost immediately comfortable, it can be assumed that blood flow to the testis has been restored, at least to a significant degree, yet this should not be used to defer exploration.

When the diagnosis of torsion of the cord is suspected, prompt surgical exploration is warranted. Although adjunctive tests are commonly used to aid in the differential diagnosis of an acute scrotum, these tests are most appropriately performed when their purpose is to confirm the absence of torsion of the cord in cases in which surgical intervention is believed to be unnecessary. Doppler examination of the cord and testis to determine whether blood flow is present was once touted as a helpful diagnostic test, but false-positive and false-negative results have led most examiners to abandon this technique. Color Doppler ultrasound examination has become the adjunctive investigation of choice in many institutions for the evaluation of both acute and chronic scrotal conditions. Color Doppler studies allow an assessment of anatomy (e.g., presence of a hydrocele, swollen epididymis) while determining the presence or absence of blood flow to the testis. Baker and associates (2000) showed that in patients with acute scrotal swelling and an uncertain diagnosis, color Doppler examination had a diagnostic sensitivity of 88.9% and a specificity of 98.8%, with a 1% rate of false-positive results. Allen and Elder (1995), however, reported five cases in which color Doppler interpretations were inconsistent with findings at surgery. It is clear that as in most clinical situations, ultrasound imaging is inherently operator dependent.

Radionuclide imaging, originally the study of choice for assessment of an acute scrotum, is more limited because it allows evaluation of only testicular blood flow (Kogan et al, 1979). Although Levy and associates (1983) found the study to have a positive predictive value of 75%, a sensitivity of 90%, and a specificity of 89%, a false impression of blood flow may result from hyperemia of the scrotal wall. In addition, children with small scrotal sacs and testes that are not dependent may be difficult to image with radionuclide techniques. Despite these shortcomings, Paltiel and colleagues (1998) found the efficacy of color Doppler imaging and radionuclide imaging

to be equivocal in the diagnosis of torsion of the spermatic cord in boys with indeterminate clinical diagnoses. In most institutions, clinicians learn to place most trust in the imaging technique and in radiographers with the most interest, experience, and reliability in the differential diagnosis of an acute scrotum.

When surgical exploration is elected, it should be performed promptly. A median raphe scrotal incision may be used to explore both sides, or a transverse incision following the skin creases may be placed in each hemiscrotum. The separate incisions are more appropriate for dartos pouch placement of the testes. The affected side should be examined first. After the skin has been incised, a dartos pouch may be created into which the testis can later be placed; then the tunica vaginalis is entered and the testis is examined. The cord should be detorsed to reestablish blood flow to the testis. Testes with marginal viability should be placed in warm sponges and reexamined after several minutes. A necrotic testis should be removed by dividing the cord into two or three segments and doubly ligating each segment with silk suture. Testes with marginal viability may be preserved, although there has been some concern about "sympathetic orchiopathy" in the contralateral testis secondary to circulating antibodies released from the injured testis (Cosentino et al, 1982; Nagler and White, 1982). The validity of comparing animal studies with the human situation, however, has been called into question, and most urologists choose to preserve testes that seem marginally viable.

If the testis is to be preserved, it should be placed in the dartos pouch with suture fixation. It has been shown experimentally that placing sutures through the tunica albuginea of the testis can produce local injury to the testis, and therefore fixation should be performed with fine, nonreactive, nonabsorbable sutures placed so that they avoid superficial blood vessels on the surface of the testis (Bellinger et al, 1989). **When torsion of the spermatic cord is found, exploration of the contralateral hemiscrotum must be carried out. In almost all cases a bell-clapper deformity is found. The contralateral testis must be fixed to prevent subsequent torsion.**

Intermittent Torsion of the Spermatic Cord

A significant percentage of adolescents with acute torsion of the spermatic cord give a history of previous episodes of acute, self-limited scrotal pain that appear clinically to have been episodes of intermittent torsion with spontaneous detorsion (Stillwell and Kramer, 1986). It is not uncommon to be asked to evaluate an adolescent for one or more episodes of acute scrotal pain that resolved spontaneously, was severe in nature, and in many cases was associated with vomiting or even a visit to the emergency room. At the time of evaluation the physical examination will be normal. If suspicion is strong that episodes of intermittent torsion and spontaneous detorsion have occurred, our experience has been that the finding of a bell-clapper deformity at exploration can be expected. Elective scrotal exploration should be undertaken, and scrotal fixation of both testes should be performed when bell-clapper deformities are identified (Eaton et al, 2005). The purpose of prophylactic fixation of the testes is to prevent an episode of torsion that might lead to testicular atrophy.

Torsion of the Testicular and Epididymal Appendages

The appendix testis, a müllerian duct remnant, and the appendix epididymis, a wolffian remnant, are prone to torsion in adolescence, presumably as a result of hormonal stimulation, which increases their mass and makes them more likely to twist on the small vascular pedicle on which they are based.

The symptoms associated with torsion of an appendage are extremely variable, from an insidious onset of scrotal discomfort to an acute condition identical to that seen with torsion of the cord. In this sense, torsion of an appendage and epididymitis might be difficult to distinguish clinically. When seen at an early stage, an adolescent with torsion of an appendage may have localized tenderness of the upper pole of the testis or epididymis, where a tender nodule may be palpated. In some instances, the infarcted appendage is visible through the skin as a "blue dot sign" (Dresner, 1973). In cases in which the inflammatory changes are more significant, scrotal wall edema and erythema may be severe. The cremasteric reflex should be present, and the testis should be mobile. Radionuclide scans or color Doppler studies may show normal or increased flow, and ultrasound imaging may delineate the swollen appendage. Though often interpreted as "epididymitis," it is not likely to be bacterial in origin.

When the diagnosis of torsion of an appendage is confirmed clinically or by imaging, nonoperative management allows most cases to resolve spontaneously. Limitation of activity, administration of nonsteroidal anti-inflammatory agents, and observation permit most symptoms to subside as the acute changes of ischemic necrosis resolve. In an occasional clinical situation, acute exploration is performed because of suspicion of torsion of the cord, or delayed exploration is performed because of failure of spontaneous resolution of the inflammatory changes and discomfort. Simple excision of the twisted appendage in these cases is therapeutic.

Epididymitis

Inflammation or infection of the epididymis is an important part of the differential diagnosis of an acute scrotum. Epididymitis is reported to be a rare clinical diagnosis in the pediatric age group. Siegel and associates (1987) reported fewer than five cases per year at a major pediatric hospital, most documented at the time of scrotal exploration. Likitnukul and colleagues (1987) reported 35 cases in a 20-year retrospective review. The most common clinical symptoms at the initial encounter are scrotal swelling, erythema, and pain; these symptoms are found equally in boys subsequently determined to have anatomic anomalies of the urogenital system and in boys with normal anatomy. In fact, it appears that in many cases the diagnosis of epididymitis is a "wastebasket" diagnosis for patients without torsion of the spermatic cord who have swollen, painful scrotal contents. It is possible that some cases of appendage torsion, for example, are misdiagnosed as epididymitis. This results, in part, from the varied severity of

symptoms of epididymitis: from localized epididymal tenderness, to tenderness and swelling of the entire epididymis, to a massively inflamed hemiscrotum with absence of definable landmarks and increased blood flow on scrotal scintigraphy or color Doppler study.

Epididymitis is classically described as an indolent process, in contrast to the rather acute onset of torsion of the spermatic cord. In adolescents, however, clinical distinction between the two entities is frequently less easily categorized. The presence of dysuria and fever is more common in the epididymitis group, although many boys with clinical epididymitis have neither. A past history of urinary tract infections, urethritis, urethral discharge, sexual activity, urethral catheterization, or urinary tract surgery may indicate a higher likelihood for epididymitis. Epididymitis has been associated with Henoch-Schönlein purpura, presumably on a systemic inflammatory basis, and has been noted in boys treated with the antiarrhythmic agent amiodarone (Hutcheson et al, 1998). Dysfunctional voiding has also been implicated as a potential cause of epididymitis, presumably as a result of urinary reflux into the ejaculatory duct (Bukowski et al, 1995a). Physical examination may reveal localized epididymal tenderness, a swollen and tender epididymis, or a massively swollen hemiscrotum with the absence of landmarks. **The cremasteric reflex should be present in patients with epididymitis, and its absence is highly suggestive of torsion of the spermatic cord;** however, it may be difficult to demonstrate in the acutely swollen scrotum of those with epididymitis (Rabinowitz, 1984).

The presence of pyuria, bacteriuria, or a positive urine culture is important evidence that epididymitis should be high on the list of differential diagnoses, although urine cultures may be sterile in 40% to 90% of patients. Normal urinalysis results do not rule out epididymitis. The most common finding in this age group is gram-negative bacteria (Likitnukul et al, 1987; Siegel and Snyder, 1987). Our experience, in fact, would demonstrate that most boys with a clinical diagnosis of epididymitis have sterile urine (Gislason et al, 1980; Likitnukul et al, 1987; Siegel and Snyder, 1987). Conversely, there is a low incidence of clinical epididymitis in patients who require nonsterile intermittent catheterization. Thirumavalavan and Ransley (1992) found the incidence in this group to be only about one episode of epididymitis per 10 patient-years. Bennett and colleagues (1998) documented a relationship between epididymitis in boys with infected urine and the presence of an uncircumcised penis.

Scrotal imaging may be an important part of making the diagnosis of epididymitis and thus avoiding unnecessary surgery, especially in a patient with a massively swollen scrotum. Color flow Doppler and radionuclide imaging reveal increased blood flow; ultrasound may demonstrate a swollen testis or testis and epididymis, frequently with the presence of a hydrocele, which may contain echogenic debris when bacterial infection is present. In current practice, the trend toward imaging of an acute scrotum has made the finding of epididymitis at scrotal exploration less common.

Radiographic imaging of the urinary tract is commonly performed during follow-up of boys in whom epididymitis has been diagnosed. Likitnukul and coworkers (1987) found radiographic abnormalities in four of five such boys with positive urine cultures. Abnormalities included urethral stricture, ureteral ectopia into the seminal vesicle, and reflux of contrast into the seminal vesicles in two patients. In Siegel and Snyder's series (1987), 47% of prepubertal boys with epididymitis were found to have radiographic abnormalities, including ectopia of the vasa or ureter and urethral anomalies, all having the common end result of predisposing the genital duct system to reflux of urine. The younger the child with epididymitis, the more likely it is that a urinary tract infection, radiographic anomaly, or both will be found (Merlini, 1998). **Because the majority of boys with epididymitis have sterile urine and apparently radiographically normal urinary tracts, it would seem most appropriate to reserve renal and bladder ultrasonography and voiding cystourethrography for prepubertal boys with positive urine cultures.** When epididymitis is diagnosed on color Doppler study, it is expeditious to proceed with imaging of the bladder and the upper urinary tract at the same sitting.

Epididymitis in adolescents should be treated aggressively, whether in an early or advanced stage. Because all boys with acute scrotal swelling of any cause will clinically worsen when allowed to resume normal activities, limitation of activity, especially that of a strenuous nature, should be enforced. In many cases, bed rest for 1 to 3 days results in a less protracted clinical course of pain and scrotal swelling. Following this period with a more extended course of relative restriction (sports, gymnastics) continues to promote resolution of scrotal swelling and discomfort. Scrotal elevation, the use of an athletic supporter, and the application of cold or warmth to the area may prove beneficial in reducing discomfort. Prompt and aggressive parenteral antibiotic therapy should be instituted when urinary tract infection is documented or suspected. Urethral instrumentation should be avoided if at all possible. After the acute episode has subsided, prophylactic antibiotic therapy should be continued until a voiding cystourethrogram is performed. In boys with sterile urine, the same limitations in physical activity should be imposed. Oral nonsteroidal anti-inflammatory agents may promote resolution of the inflammation.

Miscellaneous Causes of Acute Scrotal Swelling

Scrotal swelling, erythema, or pain may be initiated by lesions primary to the scrotal contents, the scrotal wall or skin, or the inguinal canal. On occasion, pain thought to originate in the scrotum is found to have an extrascrotal origin.

Acute idiopathic scrotal edema is a self-limited process of unknown cause that is not usually associated with scrotal erythema (Qvist, 1956). Fever is not present, and scrotal tenderness is usually minimal, but pruritus may be significant. Although the process is considered to be idiopathic, allergic or chemical dermatitis, insect bites, trauma, and other known potential causes of scrotal inflammation may be responsible but undiagnosed. Examination should include a complete assessment of the perineum and perianal region to rule out scrotal edema secondary to a contiguous process (e.g., perirectal abscess). In most cases, the scrotal wall is thickened but the testes can be palpated. When in doubt about the cause of scrotal edema, ultrasound evaluation with color flow Doppler should be performed. No therapy is indicated.

Henoch-Schönlein purpura is a systemic vasculitis that can cause scrotal swelling secondary to involvement of the testis, epididymis, or both (Clark and Kramer, 1986). The cause of vasculitis is unknown. The purpura is a nonthrombocytopenic process that may be manifested as abdominal and joint pain, nephritis and hematuria, and skin lesions. Scrotal involvement is merely part of the systemic manifestation; it is seen in up to 35% of patients. Scrotal findings are generally diffuse and consist of swelling, erythema, and tenderness. Urinalysis may demonstrate hematuria and proteinuria. Color Doppler study or scintigraphy shows increased blood flow. Observation of the scrotal findings is a part of managing the systemic symptom complex, which is usually a self-limited process but may require steroid therapy.

Perinatal Torsion of the Spermatic Cord

Torsion of the spermatic cord may occur prenatally (months, weeks, or days before birth or during the process of labor) or in the immediate postnatal period. Although the term *perinatal torsion* has been used to group both prenatal and postnatal torsion into a single clinical diagnosis, they may in fact represent distinctly different pathophysiologic processes that should be approached very differently. The major points of contention that arise when perinatal torsion is discussed are the utility of prompt surgical exploration and the need for contralateral scrotal exploration and fixation of the testis.

Prenatal (in utero) torsion is typified by the finding at delivery of a hard, nontender testis fixed to the overlying scrotal skin. The skin is commonly discolored by the underlying hemorrhagic necrosis. This clinical scenario is pathognomonic of a resolving infarction process, the acute phase of which occurred before delivery. Pathologic examination of testes that have undergone prenatal torsion reveals that in most cases, extravaginal torsion (torsion of the cord and its tunics) has occurred. Duckett (1991) argued that the incidence of prenatal torsion is probably much higher than usually quoted. He postulated that the blind-ending spermatic cord ("vanishing testis") discovered on exploration for a nonpalpable testis is in many cases the result of antenatal torsion. This thought is corroborated by the common finding of hemosiderin in the pathologic examination of the distal sections of blind-ending spermatic cords removed surgically. Prenatal torsion may merely be a late gestational representation of the same process that if it had occurred earlier, would have produced a blind-ending spermatic cord (Duckett, 1991).

Classic teaching has held that testes found to be hard, nontender, and fixed to the skin at birth do not merit surgical exploration because of the delayed nature of the pathologic process at the time of initial evaluation. In fact, the reported salvage rate of testes presumed to have undergone torsion before birth is negligible. Despite prompt exploration, Brandt found no salvageable testes in 25 explorations, a finding confirmed by others (Brandt et al, 1992; Stone et al, 1995). However, controversy has arisen regarding the need for prompt exploration of the contralateral testis.

Contralateral scrotal exploration traditionally has not been recommended in cases of prenatal torsion because extravaginal torsion is not associated with the testicular fixation defect (bell-clapper deformity) that is recognized as the cause of intravaginal torsion. However, reports of asynchronous peri-natal torsion have made the practice of avoiding prompt sur-gical exploration of the contralateral testis controversial (Olguner et al, 2000).

The postnatal manifestation of acute scrotal swelling may present a problem for urologists who are unsure of whether the process is truly a prenatal or a postnatal event. Postnatal torsion is usually associated with swelling and tenderness of the scrotum. Fixation of the skin is not typically present. Burge (1987) described 30 infants with acute scrotal swelling, 18 of whom underwent prompt surgical exploration. Ten were found to have extravaginal torsion, 3 had intravaginal torsion, 1 had torsion of an appendix testis, 1 had torsion of an undescended testis, and 1 had a normal testis. Pinto and Noe (1987) described salvage of 2 of 10 testes explored within 6 hours of discovery. The diagnosis may be aided by color flow Doppler examination, even in small neonates (Stone et al, 1995).

Prompt exploration of suspected postnatal torsion of the spermatic cord is indicated (in conjunction with explo-ration of the contralateral testis) when the patient's general condition and anesthetic considerations allow for a safe pro-cedure. The 17% incidence of bell-clapper deformity and the 20% incidence of salvage of a solitary contralateral testis (pre-vention of anorchia) must be weighed against the risk associ-ated with general anesthesia in neonates. Tiret and colleagues (1988) reported the incidence of major anesthetic-related complications in children older than 1 year to be 0.5 per 1000, and in those younger than 1 year it was 0.7 per 1000. Mortal-ity occurred in 1 in 40,000 anesthesia procedures. Others showed that the incidence of intraoperative and postoperative complications was greatest in infants younger than 1 month (Cohen et al, 1990). Clearly, the decision to subject a neonate with suspected torsion of the spermatic cord to surgery should be carefully considered by weighing the clinical assessment of the acuity of the torsion episode, the risk to the contralateral testis, and the risk related to general anesthesia. The decision may be even more difficult when the neonate is located at a distance from a tertiary referral center that can offer skilled pediatric anesthesia because both the risk associated with neonatal transport and the time lost in transport may be crit-ical if acute postnatal torsion is to be salvaged. Clearly, if the cause of scrotal swelling appears to be related to an acute post-natal event, all efforts should be made to pursue prompt sur-gical intervention.

Exploration, when elected, should be carried out through an inguinal incision to allow for the most efficacious treat-ment of other potential or unexpected causes of scrotal swelling. **If torsion is confirmed, contralateral scrotal explo-ration with testicular fixation should be carried out** (Bellinger, 1985). The most effective and safest form of testic-ular fixation involves dartos pouch placement (Bellinger et al, 1989).

VARICOCELE

Ectatic and tortuous veins of the pampiniform plexus of the spermatic cord are found in approximately 15% of male adolescents, with a marked left-sided predominance (Steeno

et al, 1976). It was documented in the 1880s that varicoceles predominated on the left side, were rarely observed before puberty, and in some cases were associated with ipsilateral tes-ticular volume loss that appeared to be reversible in some instances after varicocele ligation (Barwell, 1885). In fact, Bennett in 1889 described improved seminal fluid after vari-cocele ablation. Varicoceles rarely become clinically evident before early adolescence. Once present, they are not thought to regress. Because varicoceles rarely have been reported to arise in older men, it seems that the population of boys with varicoceles probably represents the population of adults who will have varicoceles. Although varicoceles are commonly dis-covered for the first time in adolescence, the pathophysiology of varix formation remains a subject of conjecture. Oster (1971) surveyed 1072 schoolboys and found the incidence of varicocele to be 0% in those younger than 10 years and 16.2% in those 10 to 19 years old. Other studies have estimated the incidence between 10 and 17 years of age to be 9% to 25.8%, with an incidence in adulthood of approximately 15% (Skoog et al, 1997). However, because most adolescent varicoceles are asymptomatic and many are discovered on routine physical examination, the true incidence of adolescent varicocele is likely to be much higher than expected, especially in later adolescence. The prevalence of varicocele in adolescence, the association of varicocele with male infertility, and the improvement in semen quality that may be seen in infertile men after varicocele ligation have brought increased interest to the study of adolescent varicocele and its associated sper-matogenic dysfunction.

Pathophysiology

Approximately 90% of varicoceles are left sided. Because ret-rograde flow of blood in the internal spermatic vein is respon-sible for venous dilation and tortuosity, differences in the configuration of the right and left internal spermatic veins and their embryologic origins are thought to contribute to this marked left-sided predominance. Varicocele formation has been attributed to one of three primary factors: increased venous pressure in the left renal vein, collateral venous anas-tomoses, and incompetent valves of the internal spermatic vein.

The pathophysiology of adolescent varicocele may be mul-tifactorial, but some believe that the normal physiologic changes that occur during puberty and result in increased tes-ticular blood flow might expose underlying venous anomalies to overperfusion and cause venous ectasia to become clinically evident.

Pathology of Testicular Dysfunction

The presence of a varicocele is known to be associated with an adverse effect on spermatogenesis in a subset of men. The pathophysiology of this testicular dysfunction has been attributed to one or a combination of several mechanisms, including reflux of adrenal metabolites, hyperthermia, hypoxia, local testicular hormonal imbalance, and intrates-ticular hyperperfusion injury. The toxic effect of varicocele may be manifested as testicular growth failure, semen abnormalities, Leydig cell dysfunction, and histologic changes (tubular thickening, interstitial fibrosis, decreased

spermatogenesis, maturation arrest). Lyon and Marshall (1982) found ipsilateral volume loss in 77% of testes associated with a varicocele; this was confirmed by Steeno (1991), who documented diminished ipsilateral volume in 34.4% of boys with a grade 2 varicocele and in 81.2% of boys with a grade 3 varicocele. Because testis volume increases rapidly during adolescence, it should not be surprising that differences in testis size are most easily appreciated in teenagers. This ipsilateral growth failure is reversible in some cases after varicocele ablation.

Because the rapid increase in testis volume in adolescence is in part caused by an increase in seminiferous tubule diameter and an increase in germ cell number, it is not unexpected that testicular growth failure secondary to varicocele may be associated with a decrease in sperm count. **Semen analysis is rarely performed in adolescents, and the utility of this most important measure of varicocele effect is limited when the impact of varicocele on the adolescent testis is analyzed. As a result, testis volume, a much less precise and more end-stage manifestation of orchiopathy, is used to guide therapy.**

Leydig cell dysfunction in patients with varicocele may in part be caused by diminished intratesticular testosterone levels, but serum levels of FSH, LH, and testosterone are not predictably abnormal, and normal peripheral blood levels of these hormones cannot exclude the possibility that Leydig cell dysfunction exists (Su and Goldstein, 1995). Castro-Magana and colleagues (1990) found exaggerated LH and FSH levels in adolescents with unilateral varicocele after stimulation with GnRH and testosterone and concluded that normalization of gonadotropin and testosterone responses to GnRH stimulation occurred after varicocele ablation in boys whose testis biopsies demonstrated no histologic abnormalities. Kass et al (1993), however, measured the gonadotropin response pattern in 53 adolescents and found that an abnormal response paralleled a finding of ipsilateral testicular volume loss; they concluded that increased serum FSH and LH levels after gonadotropin stimulation may indicate an irreversible testicular parenchymal injury to both Leydig cells and germinal epithelium. Hudson and Perez-Marrero (1985) confirmed these findings by showing that an exaggerated gonadotropin response to GnRH stimulation correlated with abnormal sperm density.

Histologic evaluation of the testes in men with unilateral varicocele and infertility may show bilateral findings that include decreased spermatogenesis, maturation arrest, and tubular thickening. In addition, Leydig cell abnormalities ranging from atrophy to hyperplasia may be noted. These findings are present in both testes and are more pronounced on the side ipsilateral to the varicocele. Hadziselimovic (1986) studied bilateral testis biopsies in adolescents with unilateral varicocele. Histologic findings in the seminiferous tubules included impaired spermatogenesis and varying degrees of degenerative changes in the Sertoli cells. When changes in the Sertoli cells were not irreversible, Leydig cell atrophy was present. However, when Leydig cell hyperplasia was found, irreversible Sertoli cell damage was seen. Hadziselimovic concluded that normal testicular histology was seen in all boys younger than 13 years. Abnormal histologic findings, when present, were found in both testes but were more pronounced ipsilateral to the varicocele. Leydig cell atrophy was invariably present, with Leydig cell hyperplasia being uncommon.

Clinical Findings

Because adolescent varicocele is usually asymptomatic, many are discovered on routine physical examination performed for school entry, driver's license examination, or preseason sports participation. In large part because of dissemination of information regarding self-examination for detection of testicular cancer, an increasing number of adolescents have sought medical evaluation for self-discovered scrotal masses. Many scrotal masses of unknown origin referred from primary care physicians are found to be varicoceles. Inguinal hernia, communicating hydrocele, omental hernia, hydrocele of the cord, epididymal cyst (spermatocele), and scrotal hydrocele are common differential diagnoses for such generally painless scrotal masses in adolescents. Rarely, an adolescent seeks evaluation for a painful varicocele, usually one that is symptomatic with inguinal or scrotal aching discomfort that in many cases is relieved by assuming the supine position.

Physical examination should be carried out in a warm room with the patient in both the supine and standing positions and with and without a Valsalva maneuver. Failure to use the standing position or Valsalva maneuver may result in missing some cases of varicocele. A varicocele is a painless, compressible mass above and in some cases surrounding the testis. The classic description of the varices is the consistency of a "bag of worms" that decompresses when the patient is in the supine position. Varicoceles have been graded according to physical characteristics: grade III (large, visible through the scrotal skin), grade II (moderately sized, easily palpable without a Valsalva maneuver), and grade I (small, palpable only with a Valsalva maneuver). Bilateral varicoceles are palpable in less than 2% of males.

A crucial part of the physical examination of all boys with varicocele is an accurate assessment of testicular volume and consistency. Although assessment of testicular consistency (firmness) is extremely subjective, measurement of testis volume can be accurately and reproducibly performed with the use of either a Prader or disk orchidometer (Nagu and Takahira, 1979). In standard practice, the volume of the left testis is compared with that of the right. Behre and Nashan (1991) showed that the measurement of testis volume by ultrasound offers little practical advantage and significant expense when compared with orchidometer measurement.

Adjunctive Assessment

Assessment of subclinical varicocele by Doppler examination does not have a role in adolescent varicocele evaluation, primarily because the significance of subclinical varicocele in adolescents is unknown. Although Kass (1990) found an exaggerated response to GnRH stimulation in 43% of adolescents with grade II or III varicocele independent of the testicular volume differential, the relationship between GnRH stimulation testing and future fertility issues in adolescents remains unclear. Carillo and coauthors (1999) studied nine boys and found four with an exaggerated response to GnRH stimulation. They also measured levels of inhibin B but failed to find a correlation with varicocele size or laterality or with asymmetry in testicular volume. It appears that few pediatric urologists rely on hormonal stimulation as a basis for determination of which patients should undergo varicocele ablation.

Varicocele Ablation: Treatment Considerations

Few studies are available regarding the effect of varicocele on semen analysis in adolescents. Paduch and Niedzielski (1996) compared 36 boys without varicocele and 38 boys with varicocele and found statistically significant differences in sperm motility and viability and total sperm counts between the two groups, thus indicating that varicocele does have a noxious effect on semen parameters in adolescents. Because semen analysis in adolescent boys is not usually considered practical from a psychological and ethical point of view and because of the lack of widespread acceptance of hormonal stimulation testing, testis volume measurements have become the mainstay of assessment of whether surgical management is appropriate. **In adults and adolescents, testis size (volume) should be approximately equal bilaterally, with the differential normally not greater than 2 mL or 20% of volume (Kass, 1990).** When the testis ipsilateral to a varicocele varies by more than this differential, many examiners believe that varicocele ablation is indicated, in a large part because catch-up growth has been reported after varicocele ablation in adolescents.

Ipsilateral testis catch-up growth after varicocele ablation has been evaluated by several observers. Kass and Belman (1987) studied 20 adolescents with grade II or III varicocele and ipsilateral testicular volume loss averaging 70%. At an average interval of 3.3 years after varicocele ligation, a statistically significant increase in testis volume (50% to 104%; average, 91%) was found in 16 of the 20 patients. The remaining four patients had an increase in ipsilateral testis volume that was not statistically significant. Gershbein and associates (1999) retrospectively studied 42 patients (average age, 14.7 years) with palpable varicoceles at least 6 months after ligation (average follow-up, 22.6 months). Preoperatively, 54.8% had a small ipsilateral testis. Postoperatively, left testicular hypertrophy (testis volume at least 10% greater than that of the contralateral side) developed in 38%. Though not statistically significant, the hypertrophy was found to be more common in younger boys and those with smaller varicoceles. Further data, perhaps from a prospective multicenter study, is needed to sort out the specifics of patient age, varicocele size, and the potential for reversibility of testicular volume loss as related to GnRH stimulation and future semen parameters. Until such data are available, **it appears that an ipsilateral testis volume loss greater than 2 mL is a reasonable criterion to use as an indicator for adolescent varicocele ablation, which offers expected improvement in testis volume in the majority of those undergoing ablation.**

Treatment Alternatives

When varicocele ablation is determined to be appropriate, several therapeutic options must be considered. Because most of the available techniques for varicocele ablation have proved to have very nearly the same efficacy, it is imperative that the relative advantages and disadvantages of each technique be reviewed with particular attention to the unique circumstances posed by adolescents. Currently, it appears that multiple different techniques are applied clinically, with the choice of technique guided by the experience of the surgeon and by taking into account the age, body habitus, and peculiarities of the patient and varicocele in question.

Retroperitoneal and Laparoscopic Ligation

Retroperitoneal ligation of the internal spermatic vein, described by Palomo in 1949, remains a commonly used technique for varicocele ablation in adolescents, in part because of a relatively short operative time and quick recovery. The procedure is commonly performed with the adolescent under general anesthesia in an outpatient setting. A small (1.5-inch) muscle-splitting incision is made at the level of the anterior superior iliac spine, and the retroperitoneal space is entered, with the peritoneal envelope swept medially to identify the internal spermatic vessels. At this level, the testicular artery and a single vein or a small number of veins may be present. Ligation is performed, the wound is closed with running absorbable suture, a local anesthetic is infiltrated, and the patient is discharged soon after the procedure. Retroperitoneal ligation may be performed by mass ligation of the spermatic vessels or by an artery-sparing technique. Preservation of the artery can be difficult to accomplish in adolescents, even with the assistance of optical magnification, because of both the small size of the testicular artery and the small and rather deep dissection that is necessary with this technique. Kass and Marcol (1992) found no recurrences when the mass ligation technique was used, but an 11% incidence of persistent varicocele when testicular artery sparing was attempted.

Laparoscopic varicocele ligation is a technique that is easily mastered by surgeons familiar with laparoscopic technique and is in many ways similar to open retroperitoneal ligation of the internal spermatic vein. Mandressi et al (1996) compared open and laparoscopic techniques in adults and concluded that laparoscopic varix ligation was much more costly than open techniques because of the added equipment and operating room time, although hospitalization was briefer. The conclusion was that there was little indication to use laparoscopy. Ogura and colleagues (1994) found a similar diminution in recovery time in adults. Ulker and associates (1997) found the laparoscopic technique to be superior for preservation of the testicular artery. Today's surgeons find that any of the aforementioned techniques can be accomplished in adolescent boys as an outpatient procedure with rapid recovery.

Inguinal and Subinguinal Ligation

Inguinal ligation (opening of the external oblique aponeurosis) is performed through a small incision over the inguinal canal that follows the skin lines. The inguinal canal is opened through the external inguinal ring along the direction of the fascial fibers to gain access to the cord just below the internal ring. The cord is isolated over a Penrose drain, with the ilioinguinal nerve excluded, and is delivered into the wound. With optical magnification and the help of Doppler ultrasound, the testicular artery should be located and preserved. The veins of the cord, except those associated with the vas, are doubly ligated with 4-0 silk and divided. Attention should be paid to the lymphatic vessels, which should be preserved when possible. The inguinal approach is best avoided when a previous inguinal surgical procedure has been performed.

The subinguinal approach involves a transverse skin fold incision below the inguinal ring at about the level of the pubic tubercle, with isolation and delivery of the testis as in the inguinal approach. The inguinal canal is not opened. Because a larger number of veins will be encountered in this location, the testicular artery may be more difficult to identify. Dissection of the cord should follow the technique described for dissection within the inguinal canal. When either the inguinal or the subinguinal approach is used, a cord block or caudal block may provide adequate postoperative analgesia (Ogura et al, 1994).

When using the inguinal or subinguinal approach for varicocele ablation, several adjunctive techniques may be considered that have been reported to improve results in several series. Doppler identification of the testicular artery is an important adjunct. Goldstein and coworkers (1992) reported that delivery of the testis out of the wound allows improved access for ligation of external spermatic and gubernacular vessels, which are thought to be avenues of persistent venous drainage in some cases of persistent or recurrent varicocele. Lemack and colleagues (1998), in addition to delivering the testis for ligation of the cremasteric and gubernacular vessels, performed microsurgical ligation of the spermatic veins, a technique that has become standard in the practice of many adult fertility specialists and that seems to minimize the potential for recurrence. Intraoperative spermatic venography has been reported to improve the success of varicocele ablation in adolescents (Levitt et al, 1987; Hart et al, 1992).

Transvenous Occlusion

Interventional radiographic techniques typically involve transfemoral access to the spermatic vein for venography and embolization, with detachable balloons or steel coils used to accomplish venous occlusion. Although transvenous embolization in adults can often be carried out under local anesthesia, adolescents usually require general anesthesia and the procedures may take several hours to complete. In addition, the relatively small caliber of the adolescent venous system makes the potential for vascular complications higher in this age group.

Comparison of Techniques and Complication Rates

The potential complications of varicocelectomy of primary concern are hydrocele formation, varicocele recurrence (failure to decompress the varicocele), and testicular infarction (atrophy). Hydrocele formation is related to failure to preserve the lymphatic vessels associated with the spermatic cord. Hydrocele formation seems most common after retroperitoneal ligation, especially when a mass ligation technique is used, and it is least likely to occur after transvenous embolization. Failure to decompress a varicocele or recurrence appears to be minimized by microsurgical ligation. Table 127–2 compares the success and complication rates of the various varicocele ablation procedures.

Table 127–2. **Outcome of Varicocele Ablation Procedures**		
Technique	*Hydrocele*	*Recurrence or Failure*
Open inguinal/sublingual	3%–9%	15% average
Microscopic inguinal/ sublingual	<1%	1%–3%
Retroperitoneal mass ligation	7.2%	2%
Retroperitoneal artery sparing	<7.2%	11%
Laparoscopic	Similar to open	Similar to open
Embolization	None	10%–25%

Summary

Adolescent varicocele presents the urologist with dilemmas about the necessity, timing, and method of intervention. It is hoped that further studies will clarify some of the answers to these uncertainties.

CONGENITAL ANOMALIES OF THE VAS DEFERENS, SEMINAL VESICLES, AND EPIDIDYMIS

The closely parallel development of the müllerian and wolffian ducts and the structures that derive from them invites the formation of a wide spectrum of congenital anomalies of the lower genital and urinary tracts. Congenital anomalies of the vas deferens, seminal vesicles, epididymis, and lower urinary tract are encountered with regularity in both adult and pediatric urologic practice. It is not feasible to catalog every known congenital anomaly of the genital ducts because of the infinite number of variations that may be seen clinically. However, an appreciation of the broad categorization of the potential embryologic misadventures involved in various clinical scenarios will promote optimal evaluation and management of each case.

Agenesis of the Vas Deferens

Agenesis of the vas deferens may occur unilaterally or bilaterally. Bilateral agenesis has been closely associated with cystic fibrosis and occurs in 65% to 95% of men with the disease (Vohra and Morgentaler, 1997). The relationship between cystic fibrosis and vasal anomalies appears to be related to the cystic fibrosis transmembrane conductance regulator (*CFTR*) gene, mutations of which may result in cystic fibrosis, unilateral absence of the vas, bilateral absence of the vas, unilateral or bilateral absence of the ejaculatory duct, or unilateral or bilateral epididymal obstruction (Stuhrmann and Dork, 2000). In fact, it has been suggested that all men with idiopathic obstructive azoospermia merit genetic counseling and molecular genetic analysis of the *CFTR* gene. Bilateral agenesis of the vas results in infertility, whereas unilateral agenesis may be clinically inconsequential.

Agenesis of the vas deferens may be associated with unilateral or bilateral hypoplasia or absence of other portions of the wolffian duct derivatives. In the presence of unilateral agenesis of the vas, 75% of patients have only the caput of the epididymis present, 20% have no ipsilateral epididymis, 86% have ipsilateral agenesis of the seminal vesicle, and 20% have bilateral seminal vesicle agenesis. In bilateral vas agenesis, 68% have absence of a portion of the epididymis bilaterally, and approximately 45% have absence of the seminal vesical (Schlegel et al, 1996).

Men with vasal agenesis should be screened with renal ultrasonography. In men with bilateral vas agenesis, the incidence of renal anomalies is 14% to 21%, and in men with unilateral agenesis, it is 26% to 79%. The most common renal anomaly found is unilateral renal agenesis.

Persisting Mesonephric Duct

The term *persisting mesonephric duct* was first used by Schwarz and Stephens (1978) to describe junction of the vas and ureter. In reality, this anomaly probably represents failure of incorporation of the distal mesonephric duct into the urogenital sinus and subsequent separation of the ureteral bud from the mesonephric (wolffian) duct. In most cases the ipsilateral kidney is poorly functioning, and in many cases renal dysplasia is detected. Boys found to have a persisting mesonephric duct may initially be evaluated for urinary tract infection or epididymitis. Persisting mesonephric duct syndrome has been associated with imperforate anus (Vordermark, 1983). The focus of surgical intervention depends primarily on function of the unilateral kidney.

Epididymal Cyst (Spermatocele)

Epididymal cysts are usually asymptomatic, and in adolescents they are often found on routine physical examination, in many cases a preparticipation sports-related examination. Increased awareness of the importance of testicular self-examination in adolescents has made self-discovery an important contribution to the diagnosis of spermatocele. Patients with von Hippel-Lindau disease have an increased incidence of epididymal cysts, as do the offspring of women treated with DES (Vohra and Morgentaler, 1997).

Epididymal cysts are smooth, spherical, and in many cases located at the head of the epididymis. Although most cysts are small, on occasion a large cyst or one that has gradually enlarged is identified. The cysts transilluminate. Usually, physical examination is sufficient to differentiate an epididymal cyst from other scrotal pathology. Scrotal ultrasound has proved successful in the differential diagnosis of scrotal masses in children and adolescents (Finkelstein et al, 1986). Surgical excision of epididymal cysts may be performed if continued enlargement of the cysts or pain occurs. However, long-term observation has shown that in most cases intervention is unnecessary.

SUGGESTED READINGS

Barthold JS, Gonzalez R: The epidemiology of congenital cryptorchidism, testicular ascent and orchiopexy. J Urol 2003;170:2396-2401.

Cisek LJ, Peters CA, Atala A, et al: Current findings in diagnostic laparoscopic evaluation of the nonpalpable testis. J Urol 1998;160:1145-1149; discussion 1150.

Cortes D, Thorup JM, Visfeldt J: Cryptorchidism: Aspects of fertility and neoplasms. A study including data of 1,335 consecutive boys who underwent

KEY POINTS: HERNIAS, ACUTE SCROTUM, AND VARICOCELES

- Contralateral inguinal exploration should be considered in any child younger than 2 years with an inguinal hernia or communicating hydrocele.

- Torsion of the spermatic cord is a surgical emergency; irreversible ischemic injury to the testicular parenchyma may begin as soon as 4 hours after occlusion of the cord.

- A large number of boys with acute torsion of the spermatic cord give a history of previous episodes of severe, self-limited scrotal pain that may have represented prior episodes of intermittent testicular torsion.

- When torsion of the spermatic cord is found, exploration of the contralateral hemiscrotum with testicular fixation must be performed because of the high risk for a contralateral bell-clapper deformity.

- Prompt exploration of suspected postnatal torsion of the spermatic cord is indicated in conjunction with fixation of the contralateral testis.

- The incidence of varicoceles in adolescent men is 15%, but only a small subset are at risk for infertility.

- Varicocele-related testicular dysfunction is postulated to be due to one or a combination of several mechanisms, including reflux of adrenal metabolites, hyperthermia, hypoxia, paraendocrine imbalance, and intratesticular hyperperfusion injury.

- The histologic effects of a varicocele may be present bilaterally and include tubular thickening, interstitial fibrosis, decreased spermatogenesis, and maturation arrest, as well as Leydig cell abnormalities ranging from atrophy to hyperplasia.

- Testis volume loss greater than 2 mL or 20% is a reasonable criterion to use as an indicator for adolescent varicocele ablation.

testicular biopsy simultaneously with surgery for cryptorchidism. Horm Res 2001;55:21-27.

Docimo SG: The results of surgical therapy for cryptorchidism: A literature review and analysis. J Urol 1995;154:1148-1152.

Hadziselimovic F, Herzog B: The importance of both an early orchiopexy and germ cell maturation for fertility. Lancet 2001;358:1156-1157.

Hrebinko RL, Bellinger MF: The limited role of imaging techniques in managing children with undescended testes. J Urol 1993;150:458-460.

Huff DS, Fenig DM, Canning DA, et al: Abnormal germ cell development in cryptorchidism. Horm Res 2001;55:11-17.

Hutson JM, Hasthorpe S: Testicular descent and cryptorchidism: The state of the art in 2004. J Pediatr Surg 2005;40:297-302.

Lee PA, Coughlin MT: Fertility after bilateral cryptorchidism. Evaluation by paternity, hormone, and semen data. Horm Res 2001;55:28-32.

Skoog SJ, Roberts KP, Goldstein M, Pryor JL: The adolescent varicocele: What's new with an old problem in young patients? Pediatrics 1997;100:112-121.

128 Sexual Differentiation: Normal and Abnormal

DAVID A. DIAMOND, MD

NORMAL SEXUAL DIFFERENTIATION

ABNORMAL SEXUAL DIFFERENTIATION

EVALUATION AND MANAGEMENT OF THE NEWBORN WITH AMBIGUOUS GENITALIA

KEY POINT: NORMAL SEXUAL DIFFERENTIATION

According to the Jost paradigm, three steps must occur for sexual differentiation: establishment of chromosomal sex at fertilization, which determines development of the undifferentiated gonads into testes or ovaries, and subsequent differentiation of the internal ducts and external genitalia as a result of endocrine functions associated with the type of gonad present (Jost et al, 1973).

Disorders of sexual differentiation are among the most fascinating and complex disease processes encountered by the urologist. Indeed, since antiquity physicians have been fascinated by sexual differentiation. In the 2nd century AD, Galen suggested that sperm from the right testis was "male," that sperm from the left testis was "female," and a hermaphrodite resulted when sperm from both testes joined in fertilization. Considerable progress has been made since then. In particular, over the past 2 decades, remarkable advances in molecular biology and genetic research have provided new insight into the precise mechanisms responsible for sexual differentiation and for specific intersex disorders.

NORMAL SEXUAL DIFFERENTIATION

Under normal circumstances, sexual differentiation is a dynamic and sequential process. **According to the Jost paradigm, three steps must occur: establishment of chromosomal sex at fertilization, which determines development of the undifferentiated gonads into testes or ovaries, and subsequent differentiation of the internal ducts and external genitalia as a result of endocrine functions associated with the type of gonad present** (Jost et al, 1973). Therefore, development of the sexual phenotype represents the result of complex interactions of genetic and hormonal signals. Interference with this highly ordered process at any step can result in a disorder of sexual differentiation.

Chromosomal Sex

In 1921, Painter demonstrated cytologically that humans have X and Y chromosomes. Based on chromosomal studies of *Drosophila*, it was assumed that sex was determined by the X chromosomes possessed by the individual (Bridges, 1921). The Y chromosome was thought to impart no genetic infor-

mation until karyotyping of mammalian chromosomes, developed in the 1950s, demonstrated that the Y chromosome specified development of the testis. Specifically, reports in the late 1950s describing the karyotype 47,XXY as male with Klinefelter's syndrome and 45,XO as female with Turner's syndrome demonstrated that the presence of a Y chromosome, independent of the number of X chromosomes, resulted in the development of a male embryo, whereas in the absence of a Y chromosome the embryo developed as a female (Ford et al, 1959; Jacobs and Strong, 1959). Therefore, the Y chromosome appeared to possess a gene or genes that determined the destiny of the bipotential gonad as a testis or ovary. **In the human, the hypothetical Y-chromosomal gene was termed the testis-determining factor (TDF).**

During the following years, the search for TDF was the focus of intense research. The observation that antibodies raised in inbred female mice transplanted with male skin grafts resulted in graft rejection whereas female-to-male skin grafts were accepted in the same strain of mice led to the proposal that the histocompatibility Y or H-Y antigen was the product of TDF (Eichwald and Silmser, 1955). Assays for quantifying H-Y antigen were developed. With the use of these assays, it was discovered that the presence of a testis resulted in serologically detectable levels of H-Y antigen. This was confirmed in normal and intersex patients as well as in males of other species. **Therefore, it was believed that the H-Y gene was the TDF** (Wachtel, 1977). **This theory was considered valid for more than 10 years.**

Problems with the H-Y antigen theory developed, however. A number of women with 45,X gonadal dysgenesis were found to be H-Y antigen positive. In addition, a mouse model for the male sex reversal syndrome (XX male) was studied in which mice have two X chromosomes and testes because a fragment of Y is translocated onto one of the X chromosomes (McLaren et al, 1984). These mice were H-Y antigen negative and azoospermic. **As a result of these findings, the hypothesis that the H-Y antigen was the product of TDF was excluded.**

Further study of the Y chromosome suggested that the genetic information responsible for maleness was on the short arm of the chromosome near the centromere. This theory was supported by experiments of nature in which the short arm of the Y chromosome was lost and only the long arm remained, the result being a female phenotype.

Further progress was made by studying 46,XX males, paradoxical individuals who develop as phenotypic males in the presence of a normal female 46,XX karyotype (Magenis et al, 1982). The simplest explanation for their sex reversal would be the presence of Y chromosomal material (including TDF), owing to mosaicism or in submicroscopic cellular quantities. The application of molecular techniques to evaluate Y chromosomal sequences present in XX males, as well as deletions of the Y chromosome in XY females, led to the cloning of TDF (Lukusa et al, 1992). **Deletion maps based on the genomes of these individuals were constructed by a number of laboratories, and TDF was mapped to the most distal aspect of the Y-unique region of the short arm of the Y chromosome, adjacent to the pseudoautosomal boundary** (Fig. 128–1).

ZFY and SRY

Page and coworkers (1987) constructed a more detailed genomic map and defined a 140-kilobase (kb) interval thought to contain the TDF by aligning the Y-specific DNA present in an XX male with a Y chromosome deletion of the same region in an XY female. These investigators identified a gene encoding a protein with multiple "zinc finger" domains, characteristic of a class of proteins that bind DNA in a sequence-specific manner and regulate transcription. In addition, these sequences demonstrated evolutionary conservation. **Based on its position and structural similarity to regulatory genes, ZFY (zinc finger gene on Y chromosome) was proposed as a candidate for the TDF.**

However, in subsequent years, data were accumulated that excluded ZFY as the TDF. This included the discovery that in marsupials ZFY was located not on the sex chromosomes but on autosomes (Sinclair et al, 1988). **ZFY was excluded with certainty as a candidate for TDF when four individuals with testicular development were found to have inherited a fragment of the Y chromosome that did not include ZFY** (Palmer et al, 1989).

The renewed search for TDF led to the discovery of Y-specific sequences in XX males lacking ZFY and imposing new limits on the location of TDF to a 35-kb region adjacent to the pseudoautosomal boundary (Fig. 128–2). **Using probes from this region, Sinclair and colleagues (1990) discovered a single-copy male-specific sequence that was evolutionarily conserved. This gene was termed SRY (sex-determining region Y gene)** in humans and *Sry* in mice. Analysis of the SRY gene demonstrated there to be a highly conserved region with homology to a DNA-binding motif referred to as high-mobility group (HMG) box (Fig. 128–3). When the HMG box was used as a probe, a subfamily of closely related genes was identified. Members of this family, defined as those encoding a region with 60% or greater amino acid similarity to the SRY HMG-box motif, were called SOX (SRY-box-related) genes (Goodfellow and Lovell-Badge, 1993).

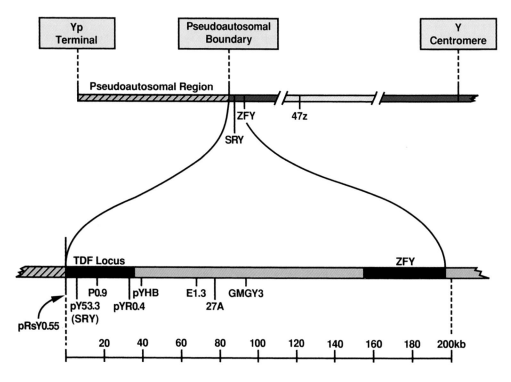

Figure 128–1. Genetic map of the short arm of the human Y chromosome. The top of the diagram shows the pseudoautosomal region of the short arm of the Y chromosome and the locus of the *SRY* and *ZFY* genes near the pseudoautosomal boundary. The lower part of the diagram represents an enlargement of the Y chromosome near the pseudoautosomal boundary and the location of the *SRY* and *ZFY* genes. (From Migeon CJ, Berkovitz GD, Brown TR: Sexual differentiation and ambiguity. In Kappy MS, Blizzard RN, Migeon CJ [eds]: Wilkins, The Diagnosis and Treatment of Endocrine Disorders in Childhood and Adolescence. Springfield, IL, Charles C Thomas, 1994, p 588.)

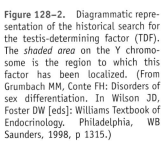

Figure 128–2. Diagrammatic representation of the historical search for the testis-determining factor (TDF). The *shaded area* on the Y chromosome is the region to which this factor has been localized. (From Grumbach MM, Conte FH: Disorders of sex differentiation. In Wilson JD, Foster DW [eds]: Williams Textbook of Endocrinology. Philadelphia, WB Saunders, 1998, p 1315.)

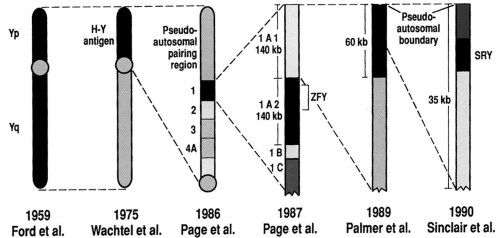

| 1959 | 1975 | 1986 | 1987 | 1989 | 1990 |
| Ford et al. | Wachtel et al. | Page et al. | Page et al. | Palmer et al. | Sinclair et al. |

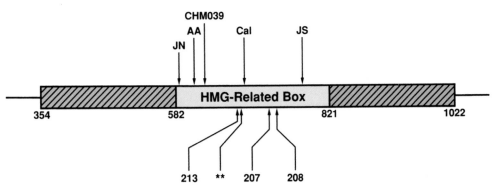

Figure 128–3. Diagram of the *SRY* (sex-determining region Y gene) locus, with the so-called high-mobility group (HMG)-related box in the center. The HMG box encodes the DNA binding region of the SRY protein. Various *arrows* represent the location of the mutations that have been identified in patients with 46,XY complete gonadal dysgenesis. (From Migeon CJ, Berkovitz GD, Brown TR: Sexual differentiation and ambiguity. In Kappy MS, Blizzard RN, Migeon CJ [eds]: Wilkins, The Diagnosis and Treatment of Endocrine Disorders in Childhood and Adolescence. Springfield, IL, Charles C Thomas, 1994, p 620.)

KEY POINTS: CHROMOSOMAL SEX

Sinclair and colleagues (1990) discovered the testis-determining factor (TDF) a single-copy male-specific sequence that was evolutionarily conserved. This gene was termed *SRY* (sex-determining region Y gene) in humans and *Sry* in mice.

Considerable evidence has accumulated that *SRY* is the TDF. In the mouse, expression of *Sry* correlates with testicular determination in the gonadal ridge (Koopman et al, 1990). *SRY* is an evolutionarily conserved gene on the Y chromosome of mammals. Chromosomal fragments related to *SRY* (i.e., the *SOX* genes) are very much conserved evolutionarily, being demonstrated in various vertebrates and marsupials. **SRY is localized to the smallest region of the Y chromosome capable of inducing testicular differentiation in humans and in mice** (Gubbay et al, 1992). In fact, Koopman and coworkers (1991) introduced into XX mouse embryos a 14-kb mouse genomic DNA fragment containing *Sry* and no other Y-linked gene sequences and demonstrated that it was capable of giving rise to normal testicular development in the transgenic mice.

The *SRY* protein functions as a transcription factor that, by binding and producing bending of the DNA, promotes protein-protein interaction and is able to activate downstream gene expression (Fig. 128–4).

An expectation for TDF was that mutations in its protein sequence would result in sex reversal. Examination of the *SRY* sequence in XY females has identified more than 20 mutations in the protein-coding sequences. All but one of these point mutations and microdeletions lie within the DNA-binding domain. Another prediction for TDF is that its presence can cause XX male sex reversal. All but one XX male with Y-specific sequences have been found to contain *SRY* (Goodfellow and Lovell-Badge, 1993). This suggests a causative role of *SRY* in these cases of XX sex reversal. **Therefore, genetic and molecular data have established that *SRY* can be equated to the TDF.** Biochemical data have provided insight into how the gene may function, but the identities of genes that interact directly with *SRY*, both upstream and downstream, are currently being pursued (Bogan and Page, 1994). However, the initial step—establishment of gonadal sex in the previously undifferentiated urogenital ridge—provides a model of a genetic switch in organogenesis. Identification of *SRY* as the testis-determining factor may potentially lead to biochemical characterization of this switch.

Other Genes Involved in Sex Determination

Genes other than *SRY* that have been found to be involved in sex determination include *WT1, SF1, SOX9, DAX1,* and *WNT4* (Fig. 128–5).

WT1. The *WT1* gene was originally isolated in cloning experiments that identified an oncogene on human chromosome 11 as being involved in the etiology of Wilms' tumor (Call et al, 1990). This gene, originally localized by examining chromosomal deletions in children with WAGR syndrome (Wilms' tumor, aniridia, genitourinary abnormalities, gonadoblastoma, and mental retardation), was found to

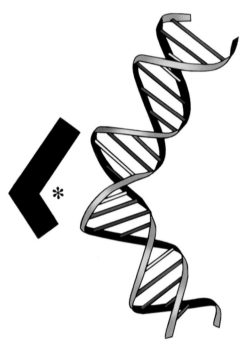

Figure 128–4. Schematic model of the L-shaped HMG box *(left)* and bent DNA site *(right).* (From Peters R, King CY, Ukiyama E, et al: An *SRY* mutation causing human sex reversal resolves a general mechanism of structure-specific DNA recognition: Application to the four-way DNA junction. Biochemistry 1995;34:4569-4576.)

be expressed primarily in the kidney and gonads of the developing human embryo (Kreidberg et al, 1993). The first reported mutations in the Denys-Drash syndrome, which includes Wilms' tumor, renal failure, and gonadal and genital abnormalities, were found to involve the WT1 protein (Pelletier et al, 1991a, 1991b). Indeed, mutations involving *WT1* have been found responsible for both the Frasier and Denys-Drash syndromes, which appear to represent a spectrum of genetically induced abnormalities involving the gonads and kidneys, due to the earlier involvement of *WT1* in the differentiation of both gonads and kidneys. Frasier syndrome is characterized by both gonadal dysgenesis and renal abnormalities that result in streak gonads and a nephrotic syndrome (MacLaughlin and Donahoe, 2004). If it occurs in the XY genotype, sex reversal results. As a result of alternative splicing of the *WT1* gene, patients with Frasier syndrome are not susceptible to Wilms' tumor whereas those with Denys-Drash are (Koziell and Grundy, 1999). In addition, with the Denys-Drash syndrome, gonads differentiate more completely than with Frasier syndrome. Research on *Wt1* in the mouse suggests that it exerts its effects upstream of *Sry* and is likely to be necessary for commitment and maintenance of gonadal tissue (Lim and Hawkins, 1998).

SF1. Experiments in the mouse have demonstrated the nuclear receptor, *SF1,* to be expressed in all steroidogenic tissue, including adrenal cortex, testis (Leydig cells), ovarian theca, granulosa cells, and corpus luteum. *SF1* appears to be a key regulator of enzymes involved in steroid production, including the sex hormones. In addition, it may well play a role in early gonadal differentiation. **SF1 appears to be a regulator of müllerian-inhibiting substance** (MIS) (Shen et al, 1994; Imbeaud et al, 1995). *Sf1* knockout mice fail to develop adrenal glands and gonads and die at birth (Lala et al, 1992).

SOX9. The *SOX9* gene was originally identified in patients with camptomelic dysplasia, a congenital disease of bone and cartilage formation that is often associated with XY sex reversal (Wagner et al, 1994). **The gene is structurally quite similar to *SRY*, with 71% similarity of the *SOX9* HMG-box amino acid sequence to that of *SRY*.** Expression of the gene in adults is greatest in the testes. *SOX9* is also a transcription factor that is thought likely to be involved in gonadal differentiation (Josso and Rey, 1996). *SOX9* is probably activated by *SRY* because both genes are expressed by fetal Sertoli cells in a

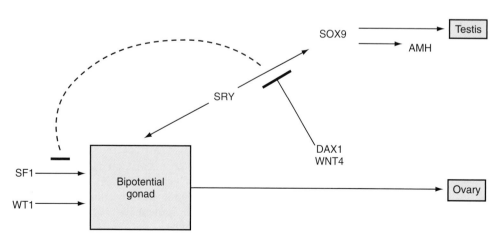

Figure 128–5. Genes determining testis or ovarian differentiation from bipotential gonad. (From Hughes IA: Intersex. BJU Int 2002;90:771.)

temporally related fashion. *SOX9* also upregulates *AMH* gene expression (MacLaughlin and Donahoe, 2004).

DAX1. The first indication that an X-specific gene was involved in human sex determination was provided in 1978 with the identification of a family with an X-linked mode of inheritance of 46,Y gonadal dysgenesis. Subsequent studies of a number of sex-reversed subjects confirmed the presence of X-chromosomal genetic duplication and a normal Y chromosome (Ogata et al, 1992). **This finding has suggested that the duplicated X chromosome causes XY sex reversal by expressing a double dose of the gene normally subject to X inactivation. Screening of XY females with a normal *SRY* gene detected such a submicroscopic duplication, a 160-kb region designated DSS** (dosage-sensitive sex reversal). Subsequent study of this region revealed a gene, *DAX1*, that was implicated in adrenal hypoplasia congenita, an inherited disorder of adrenal gland development (Guo et al, 1995). The common origin of adrenals and gonads from primordial mesenchyme and their shared steroidogenic properties support *DAX1* as the probable gene for both adrenal hypoplasia congenita and DSS.

WNT4. *WNT4* on chromosome 1p34 appears to be an additional anti-testis gene based on sex reversal in an XY female. Early inactivation of *Wnt4* in mice causes failure of the formation of müllerian duct derivatives in both sexes. A recent report supports the role of *WNT4* in development and maintenance of the female phenotype in women by regulating müllerian duct development and ovarian steroidogenesis (Biason-Lauber et al, 2004).

Gonadal Stage of Differentiation

During the first 6 weeks of embryonic development, the gonadal ridge, germ cells, internal ducts, and external genitalia are bipotential in both 46,XY and 46,XX embryos. Under the genetic influences of sex determination, the bipotential gonadal ridges differentiate into either ovaries or testes and germ cells develop into either oocytes or spermatocytes.

Primordial germ cells can be recognized in the 3rd week of gestation on the posterior wall of the secondary yoke sac. **Migration of the germ cells begins in the 5th week of gestation as a result of ameboid movements through the mesentery to the medial ventral aspect of the urogenital ridge** (Jirasek, 1998) (Fig. 128–6). This process is dependent on chemoattractants and cell adhesion molecules (Hughes, 2002). Overall, a population of 1000 to 2000 primordial germ cells reaches the gonadal blastema by the 6th week of gestation.

Transformation of the germ cells into spermatogonia and oogonia results from differentiation of the epithelial gonadal compartments referred to as testicular and ovarian "cords." *SRY* **initiates the switch that induces a cascade of genes directing the indifferent gonad toward testicular organogenesis.** The precise moment at which this occurs remains unknown. Initially, differentiation of Sertoli cells is noted as testicular cords form at 6 to 7 weeks' gestation, creating the basement membrane, or blood-testis barrier, of spermatogonia and Sertoli cells on one side and mesenchymal fibroblasts on the other. **The differentiation of Sertoli cells is associated**

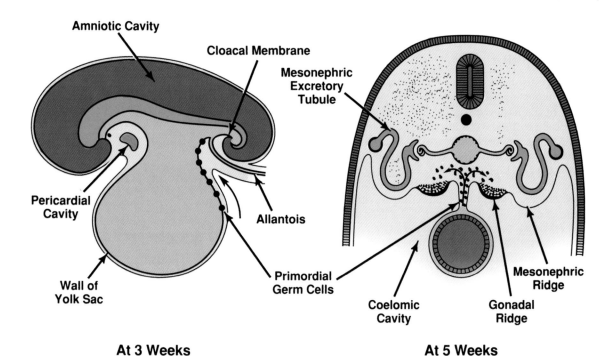

Figure 128–6. Migration of primordial germ cells. At 3 weeks, primordial germ cells are being formed and migrate along the wall of the yolk sac to reach the caudal part of the fetus. By 5 weeks, they have reached the level of the gonadal ridge. (From Migeon CJ, Berkovitz GD, Brown TR: Sexual differentiation and ambiguity. In Kappy MS, Blizzard RN, Migeon CJ [eds]: Wilkins, The Diagnosis and Treatment of Endocrine Disorders in Childhood and Adolescence. Springfield, IL, Charles C Thomas, 1994, p. 584.)

with the production of MIS, a glycoprotein encoded by a gene on the short arm of chromosome 19 (Haqq et al, 1994).

In males, a second line of primordial cells of steroidogenic mesenchyme remain among the testicular cords and represent future Leydig cells, which differentiate at 8 to 9 weeks.

In the absence of *SRY*, ovarian organogenesis results. Little is known about the genetic control of ovarian development. To date, no genes whose products direct development of the ovary have been identified. **It does appear necessary that there be duplicate copies of at least one X chromosomal locus (which presumably explains the dysgenetic ovaries in the 45,XO Turner's syndrome patients).** A potential candidate is *DAX1* on Xp-21, which, when duplicated, promotes male-to-female "sex reversal" (Lopez et al, 1998).

Unlike the testis, which functions primarily as a fetal endocrine organ, the ovary has primarily exocrine activity. **In embryonal ovaries, germ cells undergo intense mitotic proliferation (preceding the onset of meiotic prophase) and in the process exhaust their entire mitotic potential prenatally, reaching a maximum endowment of 20 million cells by 20 weeks' gestation.** The presence of two X chromosomes appears to be responsible for differentiation of the granulosa cells into the protective mantle of the granulosa layer and "rescue" of 30% of germ cells (approximately 2 million) (Byskov and Westergaard, 1998).

KEY POINT: GONADAL STATE OF DIFFERENTIATION

During the first 6 weeks of embryonic development, the gonadal ridge, germ cells, internal ducts, and external genitalia are bipotential in both 46,XY and 46,XX embryos.

Gonadal Function

The initial endocrine function of the fetal testes is the secretion of MIS by the Sertoli cells at 7 to 8 weeks' gestation. MIS, one of the two hormones necessary for male sexual differentiation, acts locally to produce müllerian regression. It is a member of the transforming growth factor-β (TGF-β) family, and the human gene has been cloned and mapped to chromosome 19 (Cate et al, 1986). Little is known about the cellular mechanism of action of MIS. Because the hallmark of MIS-mediated müllerian duct regression is the formation of a ring of connective tissue around the epithelial cells, it is likely that the mesenchyme is the primary target of MIS.

Testosterone secretion by the fetal testes is detectable shortly after the formation of Leydig cells in the interstitium at approximately 9 weeks' gestation (Siiteri and Wilson, 1974). There is a rise in serum and testicular testosterone to a peak concentration at 13 weeks and then a decline. The rate-limiting enzyme for fetal testosterone synthesis is 3β-hydroxysteroid dehydrogenase, which is concentrated approximately 50 times more highly in the fetal testes than in the ovary. Androgens are synthesized by the Leydig cells, initially autonomously, but then dependent on placental human chorionic gonadotropin (hCG) secretion. Later in gestation, with declining hCG concentrations, androgen synthesis is con-

trolled by luteinizing hormone (LH) secretion by the fetal pituitary gland. **Jost and colleagues (1973) clearly demonstrated that androgen is essential for virilization of wolffian duct structures, the urogenital sinus, and genital tubercle. Testosterone, the major androgen secreted by the testes, enters target tissues by passive diffusion.** Organs such as the wolffian duct, adjacent to the fetal testis, also take up testosterone by pinocytosis. **The local source of androgen is important for wolffian duct development, which does not occur if testosterone is supplied only via the peripheral circulation. In some cells, such as those in the urogenital sinus, testosterone is converted to dihydrotestosterone (DHT) by intracellular 5α-reductase.** Testosterone or DHT then binds to a high-affinity intracellular receptor protein, and this complex enters the nucleus, where it binds to acceptor sites on DNA, resulting in new messenger RNA and protein synthesis (Fig. 128–7). The androgen receptor has been characterized as a high-affinity receptor that mediates the action of testosterone and DHT in all androgen-dependent tissues. In disorders of the androgen receptor, such as androgen insensitivity syndrome, testosterone production is normal but the hormone is unable to reach the nucleus and interact with DNA. Various defects in the androgen receptor result in a spectrum of phenotypic abnormalities in the genetic male. Because gonadal females have androgen receptor within their tissues, exogenous androgen produces virilization.

DHT binds to the androgen receptor with greater affinity and stability than does testosterone. Therefore, in tissues equipped with 5α-reductase at the time of sexual differentiation (e.g., prostate, urogenital sinus, external genitalia), DHT is the active androgen (George and Peterson, 1988). The 5α-reductase activity has two optimal pH values in cultured genital skin fibroblasts—one at pH 5.5 and a second one near pH 8—that correspond to two distinct enzymes (Jenkins et al, 1992). The alkaline enzyme, human steroid 5α-reductase type I, was cloned first; however, the primary enzyme in the prostate is 5α-reductase type II (Andersson and Russell, 1990). A deletion in the gene coding for this enzyme has been discovered in intersex patients with 5α-reductase deficiency (Andersson et al, 1991).

The gene encoding the androgen receptor has been cloned and mapped to the X chromosome at Xq 11-12 (Lubahn et al, 1988).

KEY POINT: GONADAL FUNCTION

DHT binds to the androgen receptor with greater affinity and stability than does testosterone. Therefore, in tissues equipped with 5α-reductase at the time of sexual differentiation (e.g., prostate, urogenital sinus, external genitalia), DHT is the active androgen (George and Peterson, 1988).

Ovary

Estrogen synthesis is detectable in the female embryo just after 8 weeks of gestation. The rate-limiting enzyme is aromatase, which is higher in the fetal ovary than in the fetal testis. Estrogens are not required for normal female differentiation of the reproductive tract, but they can interfere with

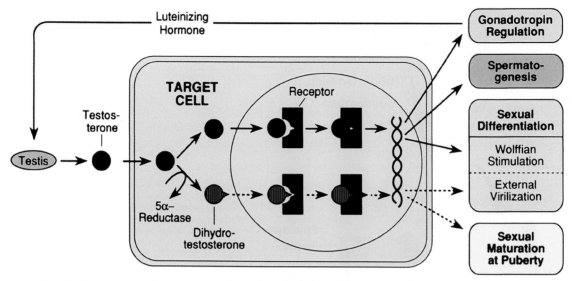

Figure 128–7. Schematic diagram of normal androgen physiology. The major actions of androgens are listed on the right. Testosterone enters androgen target tissues and either binds to the androgen receptor in cell nuclei or is converted by 5α-reductase to dihydrotestosterone (DHT). DHT binds to the same receptor but with greater affinity. Androgen actions mediated by testosterone are indicated by *solid arrows,* and those mediated by DHT are indicated by *dashed arrows.* (From Griffin JE, Wilson JD: Syndromes of androgen resistance. Hosp Pract 1987;22:99-114.)

male differentiation. Estrogen can block the effect of MIS on müllerian ducts, and prenatal estrogen treatment of mothers has been associated with male reproductive tract abnormalities (Gill et al, 1979; Vigier et al, 1989).

Phenotypic Sexual Differentiation

Before the 8th week of gestation, the urogenital tract is identical in the two sexes. Both the wolffian and the müllerian duct systems are present as anlagen of the internal accessory organs of reproduction (Fig. 128–8). In addition, at this stage, the anlagen of the external genitalia of male and female embryos are indistinguishable (Fig. 128–9).

In the male fetus, Sertoli cells produce MIS, which acts locally and unilaterally to suppress the müllerian ducts, and Leydig cells produce testosterone, which permits local development of the wolffian ducts. By 10 weeks of gestation, degeneration of the müllerian ducts is almost complete and the wolffian ducts have become more prominent (see Fig. 128–8). Adjacent to the testes, convolutions of the ducts organize to form the epididymis. The wolffian ducts of the epididymis join with the collecting portion of the testicular tubules (rete testes). Distally, the ducts join the urogenital sinus by about 30 days' gestation, where they develop into the seminal vesicles.

In the female fetus, testosterone is not secreted by the ovaries and therefore the wolffian ducts regress. Because the ovary does not produce MIS, the müllerian ducts are maintained and develop into the female internal reproductive tract. The cephalic ends are anlagen of the fallopian tubes, and the caudal ends fuse to form the uterus (see Fig. 128–8). Contact of the müllerian ducts with the urogenital sinus induces formation of the uterovaginal plate, which ultimately forms the lumen of the vagina. The relative contributions of the müllerian ducts and urogenital sinus to the formation of the vagina remain somewhat controversial; however, there is

some agreement that the proximal two thirds of the vagina is contributed by the müllerian ducts and the distal one third by the urogenital sinus.

Masculinization of the male fetus starts between 7 and 8 weeks of gestation (Fig. 128–10). **The first sign of male phenotypic differentiation is degeneration of the müllerian ducts adjacent to the testes as a result of MIS secretion by the Sertoli cells. Whereas the effects of androgen on the wolffian ducts are related to diffusion of testosterone from the adjacent gonad, masculinization of the external genitalia results from the systemic delivery of testosterone with local conversion to dihydrotestosterone.** By 10 weeks, an increase in distance between genital tubercle and anal folds can be seen. The genital tubercle thickens and elongates to become the penis, and the urethral folds fuse from posterior to anterior over the urethral groove (Fig. 128–11). Near the bladder, the urethra is surrounded by the prostate. The urogenital swellings migrate posteriorly to the genital tubercle and fuse to form the scrotum. **By 12 to 13 weeks' gestation, the genitalia of the male fetus is completed with closure of the elongated urogenital cleft.** Under the influence of androgen secreted by the fetal testes, penile growth and testicular descent occur in the third trimester (see Fig. 128–10).

In the female fetus, the absence of circulating testosterone maintains the appearance of the external genitalia at the 6-week gestational stage. The genital tubercle develops only slightly to form the clitoris. The lateral genital swellings become labia majora, and the adjacent urethral folds become the labia minora (Fig. 128–12). Between the labia minora will develop the vaginal introitus and urethral meatus.

Psychosexual Differentiation

Humans have been recognized as having sexually dimorphic behavior, which has several aspects: (1) *gender identity,* the identification of self as either male or female; (2) *gender role,*

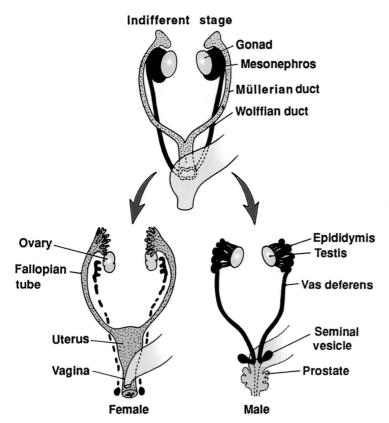

Figure 128–8. Differentiation of the wolffian and müllerian duct and urogenital sinus in the male and female. (From Wilson JD: Embryology of the genital tract. In Harrison HH, Gittes RF, Perlmutter AD, et al [eds]: Campbell's Urology, 4th ed. Philadelphia, WB Saunders, 1979, p 1473.)

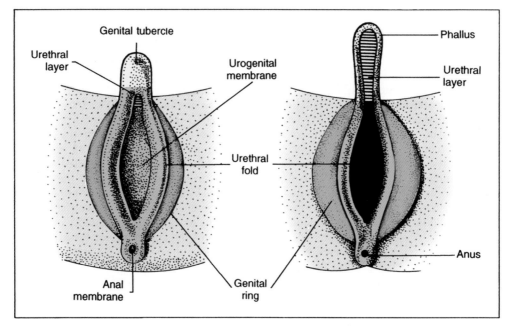

Figure 128–9. Schematic diagram of external genitalia in the undifferentiated period. (From Martinez-Mora J: Development of the genital tract. In Martinez-Mora J: Intersexual States: Disorders of Sex Differentiation. Barcelona, Ediciones Doymer, 1994, p 52.)

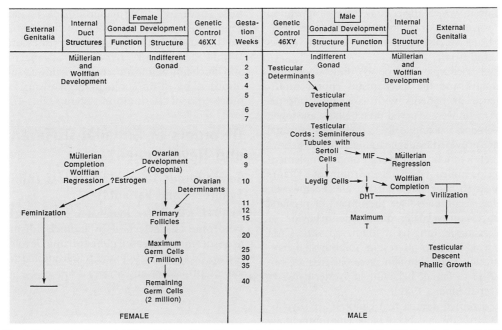

External Genitalia	Internal Duct Structures	Female Gonadal Development		Genetic Control 46XX	Gesta- tion Weeks	Genetic Control 46XY	Male Gonadal Development		Internal Duct Structure	External Genitalia
		Function	Structure				Structure	Function		
Müllerian and Wolffian Development			Indifferent Gonad		1 2 3 4 5 6 7	Testicular Determinants	Indifferent Gonad Testicular Development Testicular Cords: Seminiferous Tubules with Sertoli Cells		Müllerian and Wolffian Development	
Müllerian Completion Wolffian Regression	?Estrogen	Ovarian Development (Oogonia)	Ovarian Determinants		8 9 10	Leydig Cells→	→MIF DHT	Müllerian Regression Wolffian Completion →Virilization		
Feminization		Primary Follicles			11 12 15	Maximum T				
		Maximum Germ Cells (7 million)			20 25 30 35					Testicular Descent Phallic Growth
		Remaining Germ Cells (2 million)			40					
FEMALE						MALE				

Figure 128–10. Timetable of normal sexual differentiation. (From Diamond D: Intersex Disorders: I and II. AUA Update Series, Vol IX, Lessons 9 and 10, Houston, TX, American Urological Association Office of Education, 1990.)

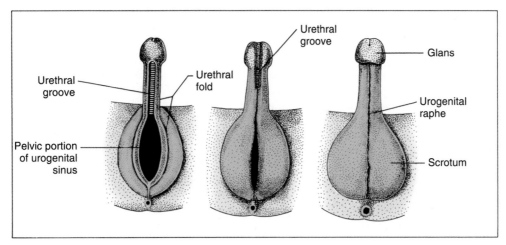

Figure 128–11. Schematic diagram of differentiation of the male external genitalia. (From Martinez-Mora J: Development of the genital tract. In Martinez-Mora J: Intersexual States: Disorders of Sex Differentiation. Barcelona, Ediciones Doymer, 1994, p 53.)

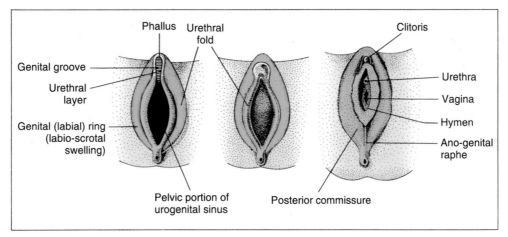

Figure 128–12. Schematic diagram of differentiation of the female external genitalia. (From Martinez-Mora J: Development of the genital tract. In Martinez-Mora J: Intersexual States: Disorders of Sex Differentiation. Barcelona, Ediciones Doymer, 1994, p 52.)

aspects of behavior in which males and females appear to differ; (3) *gender orientation*, or choice of sexual partner (heterosexual, homosexual, or bisexual); and (4) *cognitive differences* (Grumbach and Conte, 1998).

Gender identity is a complex and poorly understood phenomenon in humans, and the mechanisms appear multifactorial. Experience in patients with congenital adrenal hyperplasia (CAH) who were exposed prenatally to androgen and in patients reared in a sex opposite to their chromosomal or gonadal sex have provided evidence to indicate that gender identity is not merely a function of chromosomal complement or prenatal endocrine milieu. Postnatal environmental factors and learning appear to have an important effect. However, strong evidence has accumulated for the impact of prenatal hormonal influences on sexually dimorphic behavior or gender role. For example, long-term follow-up with CAH patients has supported a greater interest in "tomboyish behavior" than in unaffected girls, although these patterns are not abnormal in relation to female behavior in Western society (Erhardt and Meyer-Bahlberg, 1981).

The previously accepted dogma that children are psychosexually neutral at birth and capable of being environmentally oriented (the blue room/pink room theory) has been seriously challenged by those who support the concept of prenatal psychosexual differentiation (Money and Erhardt, 1972; Diamond and Sigmundson, 1997). Support for either theory in humans is based on the assessment of a limited number of affected patients. An improved understanding of the "nature versus nurture" controversy will probably prove important in the optimal management of patients with intersex disorders. However, our increased awareness of physiologically normal patients with genuine "gender dysphoria" has illustrated the complexity of this process.

KEY POINT: PSYCHOSEXUAL DIFFERENTIATION

The previously accepted dogma that children are psychosexually neutral at birth and capable of being environmentally oriented (the blue room/pink room theory) has been seriously challenged by those who support the concept of prenatal psychosexual differentiation (Money and Erhardt, 1972; Diamond and Sigmundson, 1997).

ABNORMAL SEXUAL DIFFERENTIATION

The classification of intersex disorders has undergone evolutionary change as understanding of the etiologic mechanisms of normal and abnormal sexual differentiation has improved. As a result, classification systems vary. We have borrowed from the system utilized by Grumbach and Conte (1998), which incorporates the historical emphasis on classification by gonadal morphology and introduced more descriptive contemporary terminology. The first category comprises disorders of gonadal differentiation, the second includes the masculinized female (female pseudohermaphroditism, i.e., ovaries present but external genitalia exhibiting evidence of masculinization), the third includes the undermasculinized

male (male pseudohermaphroditism, i.e., testes present but genital ducts and/or external genitalia incompletely masculinized), and the fourth category comprises unclassified forms. Within each category, remarkable advances in chromosomal and biochemical information have allowed subclassification of disorders based on etiologic mechanisms, contributing to a more rational classification system (Table 128–1).

Disorders of Gonadal Differentiation and Development

Seminiferous Tubule Dysgenesis (Klinefelter's Syndrome and Variants)

In 1942, Klinefelter, Reifenstein, and Albright described a syndrome characterized by eunuchoidism, gynecomastia, azoospermia, increased gonadotropin levels, and small, firm testes. By 1959, these patients were noted to have a 47,XXY karyotype (Jacobs and Strong, 1959).

Table 128–1. Abnormal Sexual Differentiation

Disorders of Gonadal Differentiation

Seminiferous tubule dysgenesis
Klinefelter's syndrome
46,XX male
Syndromes of gonadal dysgenesis
  Turner's syndrome
  Pure gonadal dysgenesis
  Mixed gonadal dysgenesis
  Partial gonadal dysgenesis (dysgenetic male
    pseudohermaphroditism)
  Bilateral vanishing testis/testicular regression syndromes
True hermaphroditism

Masculinized Female (Female Pseudohermaphroditism)

Congenital adrenal hyperplasia (21-hydroxylase, 11β-hydroxylase, 3β-
  hydroxysteroid dehydrogenase deficiencies)
Maternal androgens

Undermasculinized Male (Male Pseudohermaphroditism)

Leydig cell agenesis, unresponsiveness
Disorders of testosterone biosynthesis
Variants of congenital adrenal hyperplasia affecting corticosteroid and
    testosterone synthesis
  StAR deficiency (congenital lipoid adrenal hyperplasia)
  3β-Hydroxysteroid dehydrogenase deficiency
  17α-Hydroxylase deficiency
Disorders of testosterone biosynthesis
  17,20-Lyase deficiency
  17β-Hydroxysteroid oxidoreductase deficiency
Disorders of androgen-dependent target tissue
  Androgen receptor and postreceptor defects
  Syndrome of complete testicular feminization
  Syndrome of partial androgen resistance
  Androgen resistance in infertile men
Disorders of testosterone metabolism by peripheral tissues
  5α-Reductase deficiency
Disorders of synthesis, secretion, or response to müllerian-inhibiting
  substance
  Persistent müllerian duct syndrome

Unclassified Forms

In males
  Micropenis
In females
  Mayer-Rokitansky-Kuster-Hauser syndrome

Klinefelter's syndrome represents the most common major abnormality of sexual differentiation. **By definition, males with at least one Y chromosome and at least two X chromosomes have Klinefelter's syndrome.** The classic 47,XXY complement arises as a result of nondisjunction during meiosis; it occurs in 1 of 1000 liveborn males. But the phenotype is also associated with 48,XXYY and 49,XXXYY, and an exaggerated form of the phenotype is associated with 48,XXXY and 49,XXXXY. The mosaic form 46,XY/47,XXY is associated with a milder version of the phenotypic features of classic 47,XXY Klinefelter's syndrome. Perhaps as a result of phenotypic variability, Klinefelter's syndrome is believed to be underdiagnosed, with a 25% diagnostic rate in one Danish study (Bojesen et al, 2004).

In 47,XXY adults, seminiferous tubules degenerate and are replaced with hyaline. As a result, testes are small and firm, less than 3.5 cm in length. Histologically, Leydig cells appear to be present in large numbers, because they are seen in large clumps in certain areas of the testes, sometimes resembling Leydig cell tumors. However, the absolute volume of Leydig cells is not increased and is probably lower than normal. Serum levels of testosterone are low-normal and those of gonadotropins are elevated. Plasma estradiol levels tend to be high, with gynecomastia the result of an increased ratio of estradiol to testosterone. The vast majority of patients are azoospermic, and the presence of sperm suggests 46,XY/47,XXY mosaicism. Fertility, with the benefit of intracytoplasmic sperm injection, has been reported in patients with Klinefelter's syndrome (Kitamura et al, 2000). Some infertility experts advocate coupling intracytoplasmic sperm injection with pre-implantation diagnosis given the lower rate of normal embryos from Klinefelter's syndrome patients (54%) versus controls (77%) (Staessen et al, 2003).

The decreased androgen production prevents normal secondary sexual development. Muscle development is poor, and the fat distribution is more female than male. Normal amounts of pubic and axillary hair may be present, but facial hair is sparse. Patients tend to be taller than average, mainly because of the disproportionate length of their legs, which is present even in childhood. Otherwise, few if any distinguishing features are present in the prepubertal child.

Gynecomastia, which can be quite marked, is a common pubertal development in patients with Klinefelter's syndrome. As a result, these patients have eight times the risk for development of breast carcinoma compared with normal males (Harnden et al, 1971). In addition, they are predisposed to developing malignant neoplasms of extragonadal germ cell origin as well as Leydig and Sertoli cell tumors. Therefore, routine surveillance scrotal ultrasound has been advocated for postpubertal patients with Klinefelter's syndrome.

An intriguing area of research has been in the neuropsychiatric function of Klinefelter's syndrome patients. Studies have demonstrated depressed verbal ability and limitations in frontal executive functioning. Recent imaging studies have shown selective volume reduction in corresponding areas of Klinefelter's syndrome patients' brains versus normals (Shen et al, 2004). Other studies have demonstrated altered cerebral perfusion in Klinefelter's syndrome, corresponding to impaired verbal skills (Itti et al, 2003).

Management of Klinefelter's syndrome entails careful androgen supplementation in selected male patients to improve libido and reduction mammoplasty if necessary. Surveillance for testis tumor and breast carcinoma is also appropriate.

46,XX Males

The condition of 46,XX maleness, which occurs in 1 of every 20,000 males, may be closely related to that of Klinefelter's syndrome. Historically, the genetic analysis of subjects with sex reversal who had a phenotypic sex different from that anticipated based on karyotype was crucial for identification of the *SRY* gene.

XX maleness, first recognized by de la Chappelle and coworkers in 1964, is characterized by testicular development in subjects who have two X chromosomes and lack a normal Y chromosome. Most of these subjects have normal male external genitalia, but 10% have hypospadias and all are infertile. Among infertile adults, 2% have XX maleness (Van Dyke et al, 1991).

Two categories of patients with XX maleness have been identified: the 80% who are *SRY* positive and those who are *SRY* negative (Weil et al, 1994). The *SRY*-positive group rarely have genital abnormalities, but they have phenotypic features of Klinefelter's syndrome, including hypogonadism, gynecomastia, azoospermia, and hyalinization of seminiferous tubules with altered hormonal levels at puberty (low testosterone, increased follicle-stimulating hormone [FSH] and LH) (Fechner et al, 1993). Often, the diagnosis is made in a pubertal male who presents for evaluation of gynecomastia. **These patients differ from those with Klinefelter's syndrome in that they are shorter (mean height, 168 cm) and have normal skeletal proportions.**

Three mechanisms have been proposed to explain XX sex reversal. **The most common is translocation of Y chromosomal material, including *SRY*, to the X chromosome.** Clearly, this can be proven in the majority of patients. Alternatively, sex reversal could result either from the mutation of an autosomal or X chromosomal gene, permitting testicular differentiation downstream from *SRY*, or from undetected mosaicism with a Y-bearing cell line. Clinical studies have demonstrated XX sex reversal to be a genetically and phenotypically heterogeneous condition (Fechner et al, 1993). However, some series of XX sex reversal include genetically mosaic patients with ovotestes, who are by definition true hermaphrodites.

Treatment of XX maleness is similar to that for Klinefelter's syndrome. Androgen replacement benefits selected patients, and reduction mammoplasty may be beneficial. It is likely that these patients will also be at increased risk for breast carcinoma and testis tumor. Because of their lack of germ cell elements, those classic patients presenting with infertility would not benefit from testicular biopsy for potential intracytoplasmic sperm injection.

Syndromes of Gonadal Dysgenesis

Turner's Syndrome. In 1938, Henry Turner described the combination of sexual infantilism, webbed neck, and cubitus valgus (increased carrying angle at the elbows) as a distinct entity. Subsequently, gonadal dysgenesis was recognized as part of this syndrome (Hall and Gilchrist, 1990). It was not until 1959 that Ford recognized that one missing X chromosome was the etiologic basis for the syndrome. Subsequent chromosomal studies showed that **Turner's syndrome is characterized by the presence of only one normally functioning X chromosome.** The other sex chromosome may be absent or abnormal, or mosaicism may be present.

Turner's syndrome, with a 45,X karyotype, is associated with four classic features: female phenotype, short stature, lack of secondary sexual characteristics, and a variety of somatic abnormalities. But the clinical features of Turner's syndrome are quite variable, and almost any combination of physical features may be seen with any X chromosomal abnormality. The severity of phenotypic features does not necessarily correlate with karyotypic findings. The diagnosis of Turner's syndrome should be considered in any infant with lymphedema or any young woman with short stature or primary amenorrhea.

Turner's syndrome has an incidence of 1 in 2500 live births. Half of the patients have a 45,X karyotype in all cells; this is believed to be secondary to loss of an X chromosome through nondisjunction in gametogenesis or an error in mitosis. From 12% to 20% of patients with Turner's syndrome have an isochrome X (duplication of one arm of the X chromosome with loss of the other arm). Mosaicism—the presence of two or more chromosomally different cell lines—occurs in 30% to 40% of these patients, the majority (10% to 15%) being 45,X/46,XX and 2% to 5% being 45,X/46,XY (Zinn et al, 1993). **The presence of Y chromosomal material is of critical importance in patients with Turner's syndrome because it predisposes them to potential masculinization and gonadoblastoma.**

Turner's syndrome may be diagnosed prenatally on the basis of a variety of ultrasound findings (increased nuchal translucency, lymphedema, cystic hygroma, coarctation of the aorta, renal anomalies) or by abnormal results of fetal karyotyping. Affected fetuses often abort spontaneously. Whereas a 45,X fetus identified prenatally has a prognosis similar to that of a child with Turner's diagnosed postnatally, approximately 90% of fetuses in whom a 45,X/46,XX or 45,X/46,XY karyotype is incidentally diagnosed prenatally will have a normal female or male phenotype at birth. This so-called ascertainment bias in Turner's has profound implications for prenatal counseling.

It is postulated that in Turner's syndrome follicular cells that normally surround the germ cells and provide a protective mantle for the oocytes are inadequate (Stanhope et al, 1992). As a result, the rate of attrition of oocytes due to apoptosis is so rapid that by birth few or no oocytes remain in the **ovaries, which become streaks** (Epstein, 1990). Typically, these streaks are white, fibrous structures, 2 to 3 cm long and approximately 0.5 cm wide, located in the broad ligament. Histologically, the streak possesses interlacing waves of dense fibrous stroma that is devoid of oocytes but is otherwise indistinguishable from normal ovarian stroma. Both estrogen and androgen are decreased, and levels of FSH and LH are increased. Secondary sexual development does not occur in the majority of patients. Pubic and axillary hair fails to develop in normal abundance, and the well-differentiated external genitalia, vagina and müllerian derivatives, and breasts remain small (Saenger, 1996). Turner's syndrome is a common cause of primary amenorrhea, and the diagnosis is

frequently made because pubertal development never occurs. Spontaneous pubertal development may occur in up to 30% of Turner's patients, however.

The associated congenital anomalies that are thought typical in Turner's syndrome include short stature, broad chest, widespread nipples, webbing of the neck, peripheral edema at birth, short fourth metacarpal, hypoplastic nails, multiple pigmented nevi, coarctation of the aorta, bicuspid aortic valve, and renal anomalies (Fig. 128–13). The majority of the associated congenital anomalies can be explained by the presence of lymphedema at critical points in development, leading to an imbalance in growth forces. This may be secondary to failed opening of embryonic lymphatic channels (Zinn et al, 1993).

Of paramount importance in the assessment of the patient with Turner's syndrome is identification of Y chromosomal material or 45,X/46,XY mosaicism, whose detection has been enhanced by use of the polymerase chain reaction (PCR). **In patients with occult Y chromosomal material, the risk of gonadoblastoma, an in-situ germ cell cancer, is 7% to 30% and is being further defined** (Hall and Gilchrist, 1990; Gravholt et al, 2000). Gonadoblastoma is associated with dysgerminoma or other germ cell neoplasms in 50% to 60% of cases, sometimes associated with virilization. **Because the age of occurrence of gonadoblastoma is variable and has been reported as early as age 26 months** (Peters, 2005), **timely pro-**

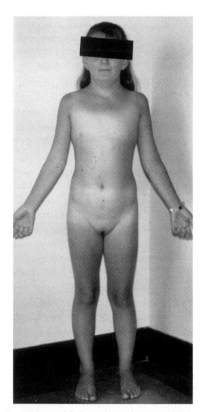

Figure 128–13. Patient with Turner's syndrome exhibiting short stature, low-set ears, webbed neck, shield chest, and widely spaced, hypoplastic nipples. (From Diamond D: Intersex Disorders: I and II. AUA Update Series, Vol IX, Lessons 9 and 10, Houston, TX, American Urological Association Office of Education, 1990.)

phylactic excision of the streak gonads in the Y mosaic Turner's patient is advised. This may be well performed laparoscopically. Streak gonads confirmed to be in 45,XO patients need not be removed.

KEY POINT: TURNER'S SYNDROME

In patients with Turner's syndrome and occult Y chromosomal material, the risk of gonadoblastoma, an in-situ germ cell cancer, is 7% to 30% and is being further defined (Hall and Gilchrist, 1990; Gravholt et al, 2000).

Between 33% and 60% of patients with Turner's syndrome have structural or positional abnormalities of the kidney; this occurs most frequently in the classic 45,XO karyotype (Hall and Gilchrist, 1990). Horseshoe kidney accounts for 10%, duplication or renal agenesis for 20%, and malrotation for 15% of these abnormalities. Multiple renal arteries have been noted in 90% of patients with Turner's syndrome as a result of their cardiovascular evaluation (Hall and Gilchrist, 1990).

The contemporary treatment of patients with Turner's syndrome has undergone considerable advances. In the neonate, it entails a concerted search for occult Y chromosomal material including fluorescent in-situ hybridization (FISH) or polymerase chain reaction (PCR) and, subsequently, prophylactic gonadectomy if necessary, as well as ultrasound screening for renal and cardiac abnormalities. In the child, human growth hormone has successfully been employed to achieve increased adult height (Saenger, 1993). At an appropriate age, typically between 12 and 15 years, exogenous hormonal therapy to induce puberty and then to maintain a normal female endocrine status is begun. An improved understanding of the long-term medical management of these patients, including cardiac surveillance and management of glucose intolerance and osteoporosis, has also resulted in considerable progress. Finally, with the remarkable advances in assisted reproductive technology, pregnancy is a realistic possibility for patients with Turner's syndrome, although spontaneous fertility is rare (Sybert and McCauley, 2004). A spectrum of potential gonadal function has been noted in large series of patients with Turner's syndrome (Kaneko et al, 1990). In one series, nonstreak gonads were reported in one third of such patients and were more commonly noted in girls with loss of only the short arm of the X chromosome. In 2% to 5% of Turner patients, spontaneous menses will occur with a potential to achieve pregnancy independently (Saenger et al, 2001). This appears most likely in women with mosaicism for a normal 46,XX cell line, a 47,XXX cell line, or distal Xp deletion. To date, more than 160 pregnancies have been reported among spontaneously menstruating Turner's syndrome patients. For the vast majority with true streak gonads, for whom egg donor implantation is used, 40% to 50% pregnancy rates have been reported by centers specializing in in-vitro fertilization (Saenger, 1993). However, among these rare pregnancies, the rates of miscarriage, stillbirth, and malformed infants is high (Abir et al, 2001). A recent area of interest has been the laparoscopic retrieval of follicles in girls with Turner's syndrome for cryopreservation (Hreinsson et al, 2002). The technique is regarded as experimental and not yet recommended for clinical use. One concern relates to confirmation of normalcy of the harvested oocytes.

It is of great interest that neuroanatomic imaging studies of 45,XO Turner's patients have demonstrated differences in parietal and temporal lobe anatomy and posterior fossa morphology that appear to correlate with certain established neurophysiologic and cognitive deficits (Brown et al, 2004; Rae et al, 2004).

46,XX "Pure" Gonadal Dysgenesis. Patients with 46,XX "pure" gonadal dysgenesis are closely related to those with Turner's syndrome. They are characterized by normal female external genitalia, normal müllerian ducts with absence of wolffian duct structures, a normal height, bilateral streak gonads, sexual infantilism, and a normal 46,XX karyotype. The streak gonads result in elevated serum gonadotropins. Because these subjects exhibit none of the somatic stigmata associated with Turner's syndrome and their condition entails gonadal dysgenesis only, it has been regarded by some authors as "pure."

A familial incidence of 46,XX gonadal dysgenesis has been reported as an autosomal recessive trait (Espiner et al, 1970). This suggests the possibility that autosomal genes in addition to genes on the X chromosome may be involved in ovarian maintenance.

Management of patients with 46,XX "pure" gonadal dysgenesis entails proper cyclic hormone replacement with estrogen and progesterone. In contrast to Turner's syndrome, growth is not abnormal with this condition, and therefore growth hormone should not be required. Because, by definition, these patients have no Y chromosomal material, gonadectomy is not required.

Mixed Gonadal Dysgenesis. The term *mixed gonadal dysgenesis* was coined by Sohval in 1963. In 1975, Zah and associates reported on their series of more than 100 patients with 45,X/46,XY karyotypes, 72 of whom had mixed gonadal dysgenesis with a streak gonad on one side and a testis on the other.

Mixed gonadal dysgenesis is characterized by a unilateral testis, which is often intra-abdominal, a contralateral streak gonad, and persistent müllerian structures associated with varying degrees of inadequate masculinization. Most patients with mixed gonadal dysgenesis have a 45,XO/46,XY karyotype, which is probably the result of anaphase lag during mitosis. The 45,X/46,XY mosaicism is the most common form of mosaicism involving the Y chromosome.

The phenotypic spectrum of patients with XO/XY mosaicism extends from phenotypic females with Turner's syndrome (25%), to those with ambiguous genitalia, to, rarely, those appearing as normal males (Berkovitz et al, 1991). In the newborn period, mixed gonadal dysgenesis is the second most common cause of ambiguous genitalia (after CAH) and must be in the differential diagnosis. The majority of these patients present with varying degrees of phallic enlargement, a urogenital sinus with labioscrotal fusion, and an undescended testis. In virtually all of these patients, a uterus, vagina, and fallopian tube are present. Short stature and associated somatic stigmata are variable features.

KEY POINT: MIXED GONADAL DYSGENESIS

In the newborn period, mixed gonadal dysgenesis is the second most common cause of ambiguous genitalia (after CAH) and must be in the differential diagnosis.

The phenotypic asymmetry of the internal ducts epitomizes the mechanism of local testosterone and MIS production on müllerian and wolffian duct regression and development. In the series of Mendez and colleagues (1993) comprising 16 patients, all had a fallopian tube accompanied by a streak gonad, consistent with absent MIS. **Therefore, although a dysgenetic or streak gonad is associated with ipsilateral müllerian derivatives (uterus, fallopian tube), a well-differentiated testis with functional Sertoli and Leydig cells will have ipsilateral wolffian but no müllerian ducts** (Davidoff and Federman, 1973). In addition, the presence of severe external genital ambiguity in many of these patients suggests that testosterone production in utero was inadequate to promote complete differentiation of the external genitalia. Paradoxically, the dysgenetic testis is capable of responding to gonadotropins and secreting testosterone in normal quantities at puberty. Yet, despite normal postpubertal endocrine function, it is postulated that fetal testicular endocrine function is either delayed or deficient. Histologically, the testes lack germinal elements, so infertility is the rule.

The risk of developing a gonadal tumor (gonadoblastoma, dysgerminoma) is increased in mixed gonadal dysgenesis, with an estimated incidence of 15% to 20% (Robboy et al, 1982; Wallace and Levin, 1990). Gonadoblastoma, a tumor of low malignant potential, is the most common. It was so named because it recapitulates gonadal development more completely than any other tumor (Scully, 1970). **Although germ cell tumors occur both in the dysgenetic testes and in the streak gonads of individuals with 46,X/46,XY mosaicism, the risk of tumor is higher in the former** (Verp and Simpson, 1987).

Patients with mixed gonadal dysgenesis are also at increased risk for Wilms' tumor. Rajfer (1981) reported that 50% of 10 patients with an intersex disorder and Wilms' tumor had mixed gonadal dysgenesis. He postulated that there was a genetic or teratogenetic defect involving the urogenital ridge, the common embryonic anlage of both kidney and gonad. This concept was borne out by improved understanding of the Denys-Drash syndrome, now clearly associated with mutations in the Wilms' tumor suppressor gene *(WT1)*. In 1967, Denys and colleagues described a child with XX/XY mosaicism, nephropathy, genital abnormalities, and Wilms' tumor. Drash and coworkers reported two further examples in 1970. **The full triad of the syndrome includes nephropathy, characterized by the early onset of proteinuria and hypertension, and progressive renal failure in most of the patients.** Renal histology demonstrates diffuse focal mesangial sclerosis. **Because incomplete forms of the syndrome may occur, the nephropathy has become regarded as the common denominator of the syndrome** (Habib et al, 1985). Wilms' tumor may be diagnosed before, after, or simultane-ously with presentation with nephropathy. The majority of the tumors are of favorable triphasic histology (Beckwith and Palmer, 1978). However, there is a high incidence of bilateral Wilms' tumor in this syndrome. The genital abnormalities include frank ambiguity, hypospadias, and cryptorchidism. **A large number of patients with Denys-Drash syndrome have been noted to have mixed gonadal dysgenesis.** A relatively new and consistent finding with Denys-Drash syndrome is that of caliceal blunting without obstruction (Jadresic et al, 1990). The high mortality rate associated with this syndrome has prompted an aggressive treatment approach with prophylactic bilateral nephrectomy in an attempt to improve the prognosis for these children (Jadresic et al, 1990).

Frasier syndrome, a related disorder due to mutations in the alternative splice donor site of exon 9 on *WT1*, presents in similar fashion to Denys-Drash syndrome but with certain important distinctions (Klamt et al, 1998). The nephropathy caused by focal segmental glomerulosclerosis occurs later in life with a more gradual progression to renal failure (Koziell and Grundy, 1999). There is no known predisposition to Wilms' tumor. Gonadoblastomas in 46,XY individuals are far more common in Frasier syndrome than in Denys-Drash syndrome. Because 46,XX individuals with Frasier syndrome have normal gonadal development, they would present with renal failure. But, it is presumed that many such 46,XX individuals go undiagnosed.

The management of mixed gonadal dysgenesis entails gender assignment, appropriate gonadectomy, and proper screening for Wilms' tumor. If the diagnosis is made in the neonatal period, the decision regarding sex of rearing should be based on the potential for normal function of the external genitalia and gonads. Historically, two thirds of patients with mixed gonadal dysgenesis have been raised as female. Potential fertility is not a significant issue in this disorder, and therefore the anatomy of the reproductive tract may direct the decision making. The likelihood of significant androgen imprinting is greater in association with a better-masculinized phenotype, and this may serve as the best clinical guide. For patients with Turner's stigmata and growth below the fifth percentile, growth hormone may be appropriate. If the male gender is elected and the testes can be brought to the scrotum, the decision between careful screening for gonadoblastoma (with physical examination and ultrasound) versus prophylactic gonadectomy and androgen replacement must be made.

The expanded use of prenatal diagnosis has changed the understanding of 45,X/46,XY mosaicism. Studies have shown that 90% to 95% of all infants with 45,X/46,XY mosaicism have normal-appearing male genitalia (Hsu, 1989). Approximately 25% have abnormal gonadal histology (Chang et al, 1990). Because only a small proportion of those with dysgenetic gonads actually have ambiguous genitalia, the possibility exists that some males with gonadal dysfunction have 45,X/46,XY mosaicism.

Partial Gonadal Dysgenesis (Dysgenetic Male Pseudohermaphroditism). In 1967, Federman coined the term *dysgenetic male pseudohermaphroditism,* which is a **condition closely related to mixed gonadal dysgenesis in that patients with abnormal sex differentiation have two dysgenetic testes rather than one dysgenetic testis and a streak gonad.** Others have applied the term *partial gonadal dysgenesis* to this condition, to distinguish it from mixed and complete forms of gonadal dysgenesis. As with mixed gonadal dysgenesis, these individuals typically have a 45,X/46,XY or 46,XY karyotype. They may present with a spectrum of external genital abnormalities, depending on the capability of the dysgenetic gonads to produce testosterone. Similarly, persistent müllerian structures are typically present, but to varying degrees depending on MIS secretion by the dysgenetic gonads.

On histology, the dysgenetic testis is found to be composed of immature hypoplastic seminiferous tubules and persistent stroma resembling that seen in the streak gonad.

Patients with partial gonadal dysgenesis (dysgenetic male pseudohermaphroditism) are at increased risk for gonadal malignancy. Manuel and colleagues (1976) reported that the incidence of gonadoblastoma or dysgerminoma was 46% by age 40 years. These patients are also at risk for Denys-Drash syndrome (Borer et al, 1995).

The management of partial gonadal dysgenesis (dysgenetic male pseudohermaphroditism), in terms of gender assignment and surveillance for malignancy, is similar to that for patients with mixed gonadal dysgenesis.

46,XY Complete (Pure) Gonadal Dysgenesis. Just as 46,XX males were of great importance in discovery of the TDF, so, too, have been the 46,XY females. **Patients with 46,XY complete gonadal dysgenesis are characterized by normal female genitalia, well-developed müllerian structures, bilateral streak gonads, and a nonmosaic karyotype.** Because there is complete absence of testicular determination in this condition, ambiguity of genitalia is not an issue but sexual infantilism is the primary clinical problem.

The etiology of 46,XY complete gonadal dysgenesis may well be an abnormality of the *SRY* gene that eliminates SRY function, or loss of another gene downstream from *SRY* that is necessary for SRY protein action. In either case, the absence of testicular determination would permit ovarian differentiation. To date, mutations in the *SRY* gene are the cause of 46,XX complete gonadal dysgenesis in 10% to 15% of cases. Recently, a mutation in the desert hedgehog *(DHH)* gene was noted in 3 of 6 patients with 46,XY complete gonadal dysgenesis, suggesting that the genetic origin of this entity is heterogeneous and the *DHH* is likely an important gene in gonadal differentiation (Canto et al, 2004). Investigation of a group of individuals with 46,XY complete gonadal dysgenesis has helped to narrow the chromosome interval containing the sex reversal gene to 9p24—a very small region (McDonald et al, 1997).

The majority of individuals with 46,XY complete gonadal dysgenesis present in their teens with delayed puberty. In addition to amenorrhea, breast development is usually absent. The serum concentration of gonadotropins is abnormally elevated, which leads the clinician to the determination of karyotype and the subsequent diagnosis (Grumbach and Conte, 1998). The high concentration of serum LH in these patients is thought to be responsible for the increased androgen levels that lead to clitoromegaly in some individuals (Fig. 128–14).

The histology of the streak gonad is similar to that of Turner's syndrome, with fibrous connective tissue resembling wavy ovarian stroma but without follicles. Some histologic variability has been noted, with more proliferative-appearing stroma in some and, rarely, preservation of intact primordial follicles. This variability in ovarian histology is thought to support the hypothesis that these gonads developed as ovaries

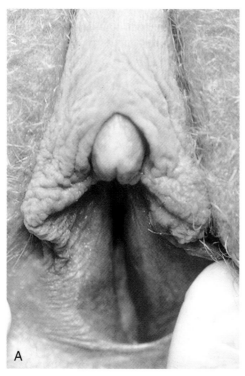 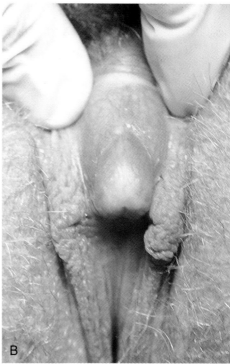

Figure 128–14. **A** and **B,** External genitalia of a 15-year-old female presenting with amenorrhea and hirsutism who was diagnosed with 46,XY gonadal dysgenesis, demonstrating clitoromegaly and urogenital sinus. (Courtesy of S. Bauer, MD.)

in utero (German et al, 1978). This would resemble the process that occurs in the streak gonad of Turner's syndrome.

Patients with 46,XY complete or pure gonadal dysgenesis are at significant risk for germ cell tumors. There appears to be a 30% risk of tumor development by age 30 years (Manuel et al, 1976). Gonadoblastoma is most common, and it is frequently bilateral (Fig. 128–15). Other tumors that may arise in this patient population include embryonal carcinoma, endodermal sinus tumor, choriocarcinoma, and immature teratoma. These more highly malignant tumors occur in fewer than 10% of patients with 46,XY complete gonadal dysgenesis (Scully, 1981).

Management of 46,XY complete gonadal dysgenesis entails removal of both streak gonads and proper cyclic hormone replacement with estrogen and progesterone.

Embryonic Testicular Regression and Bilateral Vanishing Testes Syndromes

The syndromes of embryonic testicular regression and bilateral vanishing testes are characterized by **patients with a 46,XY karyotype and absent testes in whom there is clear evidence of testicular function at some point during embryogenesis.** The syndrome entails the presence of testes that "vanish" during embryogenesis and is distinguished from pure gonadal dysgenesis, in which there is no evidence of testicular function in utero.

These syndromes have been regarded as synonymous by some authors. Other authors, including Migeon and colleagues (1994), have suggested a rational stratification

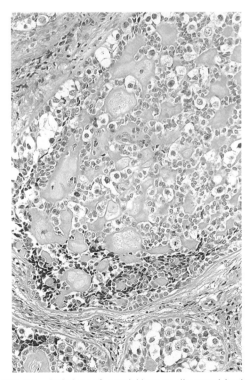

Figure 128–15. Pathology of gonadoblastoma discovered in the patient shown in Figure 128–14 with 46,XY gonadal dysgenesis. Encapsulated nests of gonadoblastoma comprise small sex cord–type cells arranged around rounded spaces of amorphous eosinophilic material and interspersed germ cells. (Courtesy of S. Bauer, MD.)

whereby "embryonic testicular regression" refers to loss of testicular tissue within the first trimester and is associated with ambiguity of external genitalia, whereas "bilateral vanishing testes syndrome" refers to individuals in whom male sexual differentiation of ducts and genitalia took place but loss of testicular tissue occurred subsequently in utero.

The etiology of these disorders remains unclear. **It is possible that regression of the testes in utero is caused by a genetic mutation, a teratogen, or bilateral torsion.** A genetic cause is supported by the finding of familial instances of XY agonadism that might be consistent with the rare recessive trait. Marcantonio and associates (1994) suggested the possibility that embryonic testicular regression represents a variant of 46,XY gonadal dysgenesis. They noted a group of patients with absent testes but evidence of incongruity between the extent of Leydig cell and Sertoli cell function, suggesting that gonadal tissue in these subjects was intrinsically abnormal before the testicular regression occurred. The occurrence of embryonic testicular regression in several subjects from one family in their series suggested a genetic basis for the condition, and the pattern of inheritance implicated the involvement of an X chromosome gene. In another group of patients, these authors noted multiple congenital anomalies, suggesting either a mutation in a single gene that functions in several developmental pathways or a defect of multiple genes that might be the result of a large chromosomal deletion.

Clinically, these two syndromes represent a spectrum of phenotypes ranging in severity from complete female, to varying degrees of genital ambiguity in the embryonic testicular regression syndrome, to a normal male phenotype with microphallus and empty scrotum in the bilateral vanishing testes syndrome (Edman et al, 1977). **The diagnosis can be made on the basis of a 46,XY karyotype and castrate levels of testosterone despite persistently elevated serum LH and FSH** (Jarow et al, 1986). In the most severe form of embryonic testicular regression syndrome, agonadism is discovered in a 46,XY phenotypic female with no internal genital structures. This picture is presumed to result when the testis has elaborated MIS but vanishes at approximately day 60 to 70 of gestation, before the elaboration of androgen. In this setting, a belated Jost model is created and the individual goes on to develop a sexually infantile female phenotype but lacks any internal ductal structures. At an intermediate point in the clinical spectrum is the 46,XY patient with absent gonads and internal ductal structures but with ambiguous genitalia owing to incomplete elaboration of androgen by the vanishing testes. Finally, in bilateral vanishing testes syndrome, patients may present as agonadal XY phenotypic males with fully developed wolffian structures, but an empty scrotum, absent prostate, and microphallus. This represents testicular loss after complete anatomic development of the male external genitalia within the first trimester.

On surgical exploration of patients with bilateral vanishing testes syndrome, rudimentary cord structures are usually identified and biopsy of their distal ends demonstrates no recognizable testicular tissue histologically (Bergada et al, 1962). Atrophic epididymal remnants are occasionally seen.

The management of patients with embryonic testicular regression syndrome or bilateral vanishing testes syndrome is dictated by their position in the clinical spectrum of either disorder. Sexually infantile phenotypic females require estrogen supplementation at the time of expected puberty for development of secondary sexual characteristics and may require vaginal dilation or vaginoplasty. Similarly, phenotypic males require long-term androgen replacement beginning at the time of expected puberty. A study of 21 males so treated demonstrated that replacement therapy started at the correct time caused a normal pubertal growth spurt with normal secondary sex characteristics including penile growth, together with normal bone maturation (Aynsley-Green et al, 1976). In addition, these patients may benefit from placement of testicular prostheses. Patients with embryonic testicular regression syndrome and ambiguous genitalia require individualized assessment to determine the optimal gender assignment.

True Hermaphroditism

True hermaphrodites are individuals who have both testicular tissue with well-developed seminiferous tubules and ovarian tissue with primordial follicles, which may take the form of one ovary and one testis or, more commonly, one or two ovotestes.

Both the external genitalia and internal duct structures of true hermaphrodites display gradations between male and female. **In most patients, the external genitalia are ambiguous but masculinized to variable degrees and 75% are raised as male.** Among those raised as male, hypospadias and chordee occur in approximately 80%. Among those patients raised as females, two thirds have clitoromegaly. Virtually all patients have a urogenital sinus, and in most cases a uterus is present (Figs. 128–16 and 128–17). The ovary is found in a normal location, more commonly on the left side. The testis or ovotestis may reside at any point along the path of testicular descent. Testes and ovotestes are more commonly located on the right side (Blyth and Duckett, 1991; Mittwoch, 2000). Sixty percent of gonads palpable in the inguinal canal or labioscrotal folds are ovotestes, which may be clinically suspected on the basis of a difference in firmness at either end of the gonad, consistent with polar segregation of ovarian and testicular tissue (Grumbach and Conte, 1998).

Approximately 60% of true hermaphrodites have a 46,XX karyotype; 33% are mosaics with a second cell line containing a Y chromosome (46,XX/46,XY; 46,XX/46,XXY), and 7% are 46,XY. Chimerism (mosaicism) has been thought to result from fertilization infusion of an ovum and its polar body, fusion of two nuclei, or double fertilization. It has also been suggested that true hermaphroditism may result from hidden mosaicism with a Y cell line. Ortenberg and colleagues (2002) demonstrated the *SRY* gene in ovotestes of all eight cases of true hermaphroditism studied, supporting somatic

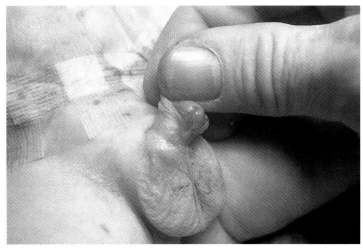

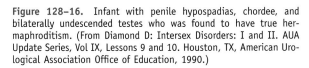

Figure 128–16. Infant with penile hypospadias, chordee, and bilaterally undescended testes who was found to have true hermaphroditism. (From Diamond D: Intersex Disorders: I and II. AUA Update Series, Vol IX, Lessons 9 and 10. Houston, TX, American Urological Association Office of Education, 1990.)

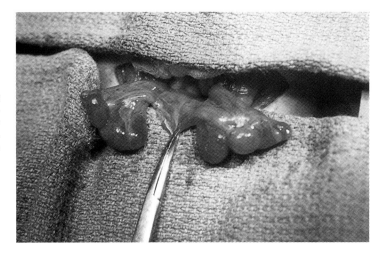

Figure 128–17. Laparotomy findings from true hermaphrodite noted in Figure 128–16; clamp is on uterus with bilateral, fimbriated fallopian tubes and bilateral ovotestes. (From Diamond D: Intersex Disorders: I and II. AUA Update Series, Vol IX, Lessons 9 and 10. Houston, TX, American Urological Association Office of Education, 1990.)

mosaicism. Other studies have demonstrated heterogeneity of Y-specific DNA regions detected in patients with true hermaphroditism (Hadjiathanasiou et al, 1994). This supports a non–Y chromosome–related mechanism responsible for 46,XX true hermaphroditism, such as mutation in an autosomal or X-linked gene involved in sex determination. Berkovitz and colleagues (1991) suggested that 46,XY true hermaphroditism may be a form of partial gonadal dysgenesis. According to this theory, a partial defect in testis determination results in both testicular and ovarian development. This is supported by the finding of ovarian stroma in some dysgenetic testes.

Just as the differentiation of external genitalia is variable in true hermaphroditism, differentiation of the internal ducts is also quite variable and is related to the function of the ipsilateral gonad. Fallopian tubes are consistently present on the side of the ovary, and a vas deferens is always present adjacent to a testis (Berkovitz et al, 1991). The ovotestis, which comprises two thirds of gonads in true hermaphroditism, is associated with a fallopian tube in two thirds of cases and with either a vas deferens only or both structures in one third of cases.

The ovarian portion of the ovotestis is frequently normal, whereas the testicular portion is typically dysgenetic. Therefore, although ovulation and pregnancy have been reported for female 46,XX true hermaphrodites, male fertility has not been clearly documented.

The incidence of gonadal tumors is approximately 10% in 46,XY true hermaphroditism and 4% in 46,XX true hermaphroditism. Both gonadoblastoma and dysgerminoma have been described (Verp and Simpson, 1987).

The most important aspect of management in true hermaphroditism is gender assignment. Sex assignment should be based on the functional potential of external genitalia, internal ducts, and gonads, according to the findings at laparoscopy or laparotomy. **Unlike patients with most other forms of gonadal dysgenesis, true hermaphrodites have the potential for fertility if raised as female with the appropriate ductal structures.** Pregnancies have been reported in patients with true hermaphroditism, the majority with the 46,XX karyotype (Starceski et al, 1988). If the patient is to be raised as female, all testicular and wolffian tissue should be removed. For those patients with an ovary, this is straightforward; if an ovotestis is present, surgical cleavage of the gonad with excision of the testicular portion has been performed successfully by Nihoul-Fekete and colleagues (1984). They recommend postoperative stimulation with human chorionic gonadotropin (hCG) to confirm that all testicular tissue has been removed. In some settings, the cleavage plane between testicular and ovarian tissues is unclear and gonadectomy is advisable. When ovarian tissue is preserved, normal ovarian function can occur at puberty, although hormonal replacement may be necessary. Careful surveillance for potential gonadal tumors in the patient raised as female is also advisable. If a male gender is assigned, as has been most common historically, all ovarian and müllerian tissue should be removed. Consideration should be given to gonadectomy at puberty with appropriate androgen replacement in this setting, given the high risk of malignancy and unlikelihood of male fertility. At the very least, long-term gonadal surveillance ultrasound for tumor development would seem appropriate.

Masculinized Female (Female Pseudohermaphroditism)

Masculinized female (female pseudohermaphroditism) is a disorder of phenotypic sexual development in which 46,XX individuals with ovaries have a partially masculinized phenotype and ambiguous genitalia. By far the most common cause of the masculinized female is CAH, which is the most common cause of ambiguous genitalia in the newborn. Two very rare causes of masculinized female (female pseudohermaphroditism) are maternal ingestion of androgens and virilizing tumors in the mother.

Congenital Adrenal Hyperplasia

The adrenogenital syndrome caused by CAH is a classic example of an inborn error of metabolism—in this case, an error involving cortisol synthesis. A defect in any one of the five enzymes involved in the cortisol biosynthetic pathway (cholesterol side chain cleavage enzyme, 3β-hydroxysteroid dehydrogenase, 17-hydroxylase, 21-hydroxylase, and 11-hydroxylase) may result in CAH. **The most commonly recognized syndromes result from a deficiency of one of the terminal two enzymes of glucocorticoid synthesis (21-hydroxylase or 11-hydroxylase)** (New and Levine, 1984) (Fig. 128–18). As a result of deficiency of either terminal enzyme, formation of hydrocortisone is impaired, causing a compensatory increase in the secretion of adrenocorticotrophic hormone (ACTH). This increase enhances formation of adrenal steroids proximal to the enzymatic defect and a secondary increase in the formation of testosterone, the active androgen in CAH.

> ## KEY POINT: CONGENITAL ADRENAL HYPERPLASIA
>
> The most commonly recognized syndromes of CAH result from a deficiency of one of the terminal two enzymes of glucocorticoid synthesis (21-hydroxylase or 11-hydroxylase) (New and Levine, 1984).

A deficiency of steroid 21-hydroxylase is responsible for 95% of cases of CAH; it occurs with an incidence ranging from 1 in 5,000 to 1 in 15,000 in the United States and Europe. The highest incidence, 1 in 490, is reported in the Yupik Alaskan Eskimo population (New et al, 1994). **Clinically, patients are divided into three categories: (1) salt wasters (patients with virilization and aldosterone deficiency), (2) simple virilizers (patients with virilization, but without salt wasting), and (3) nonclassic patients (those without evidence of virilization or salt wasting).** Dramatic progress has been made in understanding the molecular basis of CAH, and 95% of the mutations that account for CAH have been identified. The wide clinical spectrum of the disease appears to represent different degrees of enzymatic compromise conferred by specific, identifiable genetic defects.

The 21-hydroxylase gene *(CYP21)* is located on chromosome 6p21.3 within the major human leukocyte antigen (HLA) complex and is transmitted in an autosomal recessive

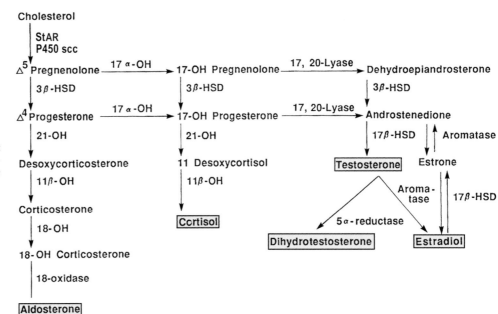

Figure 128–18. Steroid biosynthetic pathway for mineralocorticoid, glucocorticoid, and sex steroid hormone production.

pattern (Wilson et al, 1995). Adjacent to the *CYP21* gene, separated by 30 kb, and adjacent to and alternating with *C4B* and *C4A* genes encoding the fourth component of serum complement is the CYP21 pseudogene *(CYP21P)*, so called because it encodes no proteins and is therefore inactive (Tusie-Luna and White, 1995). The inactive *CYP21P* is 98% homologous to the active gene *CYP21*. During meiosis, a gene conversion may occur that transfers segments from the *CYP21P* gene to the *CYP21* gene, rendering it inactive. Thus far, all mutations causing 21-hydroxylase deficiency appear to result from either a complete deletion of the genes *C4B* and *CYP21B* (a product of misalignment and unequal crossing-over between chromatids during meiosis). To date approximately 15 mutations constitute 90% to 95% of alleles and are derived from intergenic recombination of DNA sequences between the *CYP21* gene and the highly homologous *CYP21P* while the remaining are spontaneous mutations (Forest, 2004). Approximately 100 different *CYP21* mutations have been reported.

The majority of patients with CAH secondary to 21-hydroxylase deficiency exhibit one of the two classic forms of the disease: **75% present with salt wasting and 25% with simple virilization** (Kohn et al, 1995). The higher proportion of patients with the salt-wasting form of the disease recognized in more recent series has been attributed to improved diagnostic capabilities and a high level of clinical suspicion as well as to increased survival owing to mineralocorticoid supplementation (Fife and Rappaport, 1983). Newborn screening programs for CAH have been credited with increasing the rate and shortening the time to diagnosis, particularly in males with the salt-wasting form of the disease. This has also proven to be an important means of diagnosing the simple virilizing (SV) form in the male and the nonclassic forms in some males and females (Brosnan et al, 1999).

In the female with the classic salt-wasting and simple virilizing form of the disorder, a masculinized female results. Because impaired steroidogenesis begins early in life—at the time of formation of the external genitalia (beginning at 10 weeks' gestation)—there is virtually always evidence of some degree of masculinization at birth. This is manifested by enlargement of the clitoris and varying degrees of labial fusion (Figs. 128–19 and 128–20). In addition, the vagina and urethra open into a common urogenital sinus. The enlargement of the clitoris may be so dramatic as to make it appear to be a hypospadiac penis with bilateral cryptorchidism, and cases of complete formation of a masculinized urethra to the tip of an enlarged clitoris have been reported. The severity of the virilization is usually greater in infants who experience salt wasting, but not uniformly so. Prader (1958) classified the degrees of virilization of external genitalia in females with CAH (Fig. 128–21). The müllerian structures in these patients are typically normal.

In both males and females with the salt-losing variant of CAH, symptoms begin within the first few weeks after birth, with failure to regain birth weight, progressive weight loss, and dehydration. In severely affected infants, adrenal crises occur within the first 10 to 21 days of life (Grumbach and Conte, 1998). **Vomiting is prominent and can be so extreme that a mistaken diagnosis of pyloric stenosis is made, particularly in the male.** Without therapy, death may rapidly ensue from hyperkalemia, dehydration, and shock. After birth, there is progression of masculinization of the untreated female; pubic and axillary hair develop prematurely, acne appears, and the voice deepens. There is rapid somatic maturation, resulting in premature epiphyseal closure and short adult stature. Although the internal genitalia are female, breast development and menstruation do not occur unless the excessive androgen production is suppressed by adequate steroid therapy.

In the male without salt wasting, the chief clinical manifestations are those of isosexual precocity. The infant appears normal at birth, but signs of sexual and somatic precocity appear within the first 2 to 3 years of life. Although the testes remain normal in size, enlargement of the penis, scrotum, and prostate occur, accompanied by the appearance of pubic hair, acne, and deepening of the voice. The musculature is well developed (prompting the descriptive term "little

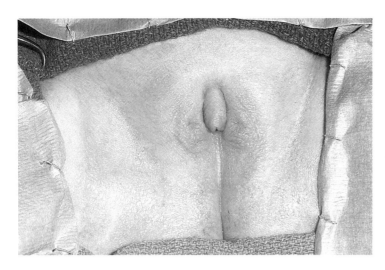

Figure 128–19. External genitalia of a patient with congenital adrenal hyperplasia secondary to 21-hydroxylase deficiency, showing labioscrotal fusion and clitoromegaly.

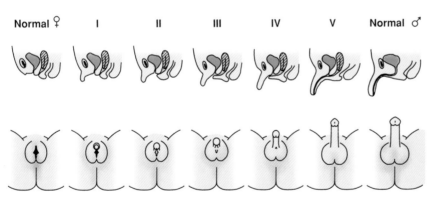

Figure 128–20. Patient with congenital adrenal hyperplasia secondary to 21-hydroxylase deficiency, demonstrating marked virilization of hypospadiac-appearing phallus.

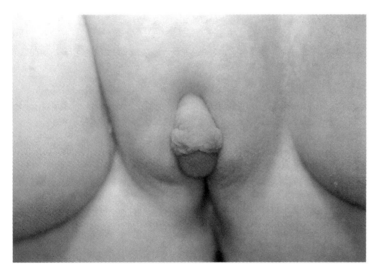

Figure 128–21. Classification by Prader of the various degrees of masculinization of the external genitalia in females with congenital adrenal hyperplasia, which has been applied by some authors to intersexual states in general. (From Prader A: Die Haufigkeit der kongenitalen androgenitalen Syndroms. Helv Pediatr Acta 1958;13:426.)

Hercules"), and bone age is more advanced than appropriate for the chronologic age. The syndrome often goes unrecognized in the non–salt-wasting male until signs of androgen excess, such as accelerated height and precocious sexual hair, appear later in childhood.

In the non–salt-wasting male, two major long-term implications are short stature and infertility. Premature epiphyseal closure will result unless early medical control is instituted. This emphasizes the value of newborn screening. Infertility has been noted in 30% of CAH males, often related to the finding of adrenal rest nodules on testicular examination or ultrasound. These nodules, present in 30% of males with CAH, represent hypertrophy of adrenal rests due to ACTH stimulation and when associated with impaired fertility warrant periodic scrotal ultrasound for these patients. In addition, poor control of the disease in boys with classic CAH has been associated with small testes and infertility with reduced sperm counts (New and Wilson, 1999). This is due to peripheral aromatization of excess androgen to estrogen that suppresses pituitary gonadotropins.

In classic 21-hydroxylase deficiency, plasma levels of progesterone and 17-hydroxyprogesterone are markedly elevated. Urinary levels of 17-ketosteroids and pregnanetriol are elevated. The diagnosis may be made biochemically with the use of radioimmunoassay of plasma 17-hydroxyprogesterone, which has replaced the more cumbersome 24-hour urine collection of metabolites (e.g., pregnanetriol). A pelvic ultrasound study demonstrating the presence of müllerian tissues is confirmatory. Some investigators have suggested that the finding of abnormally enlarged or "cerebriform"-appearing adrenal glands on neonatal ultrasonography, available before biochemical results, may represent the earliest diagnostic tool for CAH (Hernanz-Schulman et al, 2002).

More aggressive screening for 21-hydroxylase deficiency has provided considerable benefits. In one series, despite sexual ambiguity, one third to one half of the affected female newborns were not diagnosed as having 21-hydroxylase deficiency until they were identified by the screening test (Pang et al, 1985).

Nonclassic 21-hydroxylase deficiency represents an attenuated, late-onset form that is variable in its clinical severity and timing of onset. New and Wilson (1999) has found the nonclassic 21-hydroxylase deficiency to be the most common autosomal recessive disorder in humans, with an incidence of 1/100. The presenting symptoms in females are commonly hirsutism and oligomenorrhea, male pattern baldness, and polycystic ovaries. In men with the nonclassic form of 21-hydroxylase deficiency, oligospermia and subfertility have been presenting features and reversal of infertility with glucocorticoid therapy has been reported. Typically, lower doses of glucocorticoid are required for management of the nonclassic form of CAH.

A deficiency of 11β-hydroxylase accounts for roughly 5% of cases of CAH. Both classic and mild forms have been recognized. Unlike 21-hydroxylase, 11β-hydroxylase is not HLA linked. The defect results from mutations in the *CYP11B1* gene (Merke et al, 1998). To date, 11 mutations have been described that result in enzyme inactivation. Like 21-hydroxylase deficiency, the nonclassic variant of 11β-hydroxylase deficiency (late onset) is characterized by signs and symptoms of androgen excess in childhood or adolescence. Hypertension is a common finding in patients with this type of CAH, and it is believed to be secondary to increased serum levels of deoxycorticosterone (DOC). Although most of the patients are hypertensive, some are normotensive and others experience only intermittent hypertension. Marked virilization occurs in the severe form of the defect and may be as severe as in those patients with a 21-hydroxylase deficiency. In the late-onset form, mild virilization occurs in prepubertal and postpubertal patients.

The diagnosis of 11β-hydroxylase deficiency can be confirmed by finding increased plasma levels of 11-deoxycortisol and 11-DOC. Urinary levels of 17-ketosteroids and 17-hydroxycorticoids are increased. The treatment with glucocorticoids is identical to that of patients with 21-hydroxylase deficiency.

The least common enzyme deficiency responsible for a virilizing form of CAH is 3β-hydroxysteroid dehydrogenase. This deficiency affects the early steps in steroid biosynthesis in both adrenals and gonads, resulting in inability to convert 3β-hydroxysteroids to 3-ketosteroids. As a result, the severe form leads to impaired synthesis of aldosterone, cortisol, and sex steroids. Affected females exhibit mild clitoromegaly and labial fusion accompanied by symptoms of aldosterone and cortisol deficiency.

Two homologous genes have been identified for 3β-hydroxysteroid dehydrogenase, both of which contain four exons (Merke et al, 1998). A number of mutations giving rise to the syndrome have been described. This defect has an autosomal recessive inheritance pattern and is heterogeneous in its biochemical and clinical appearance. A non–salt-losing form and mild- and late-onset forms have been described, although the nonclassic form appears to be exceedingly rare.

The diagnosis of 3β-hydroxysteroid dehydrogenase is based on finding increased serum levels of 17-hydroxypregnenolone and dehydroepiandrosterone (DHEA). The pelvic ultrasound, confirming presence of müllerian tissue, would be supportive. Treatment is similar to that of patients with 21-hydroxylase deficiency.

Currently, one of the most exciting aspects of CAH is the capability of diagnosing and treating the disorder prenatally. Prenatal diagnosis of CAH in the at-risk fetus was initially made by a measurement of amniotic fluid for 17-hydroxyprogesterone at 16 to 17 weeks' gestation (Laue and Rennert, 1995). Currently, the diagnosis is made during the first trimester by HLA genotyping or by DNA analysis of genes within the HLA complex in cells obtained by chorionic villous sampling at 10 to 11 weeks' gestation (Hughes, 2002). Treatment of the mother with dexamethasone, which crosses the placenta, suppresses fetal secretion of ACTH, thereby preventing virilization of the genitalia. However, treatment should be instituted at 5 to 6 weeks of gestation, before initial development of the external genitalia. There are certain complexities to this form of management. The diagnosis of CAH in the fetus may be determined on chorionic villous cells or on cells from amniotic fluid for families in which a prior member was affected. Therefore, it is not possible to confirm the diagnosis before therapy is initiated. Because virilization is not a concern with the male fetus and three of four female fetuses at risk are unaffected, given the autosomal recessive pattern of inheritance, seven of eight fetuses may be treated unnecessarily. Therefore, one goal in therapy has been earlier diagnosis to avoid unnecessary treatment. A promising technique that may be applicable to the prenatal diagnosis of CAH is analysis of free fetal DNA, from circulating trophoblastic cells, in the maternal circulation.

A number of series have established the effectiveness of prenatal treatment for CAH with dexamethasone (Migeon, 1990; Pang et al, 1990; Speiser et al, 1990). In some neonates, there is no evidence of masculinization, suggesting totally successful therapy. In another group, there is milder masculinization than that noted in an affected sibling. Although compliance and timing of initiation of treatment have been variable from series to series, this heterogeneity of response to therapy raises intriguing questions about the mechanisms involved in virilization of the CAH fetus. In addition, prenatal treatment with dexamethasone has raised ethical concerns. Although there is no arguing its ability to prevent androgen effects on the genitalia and potentially the brain of affected females, the long-term effects of dexamethasone on unaffected fetuses undergoing treatment prenatally remain largely unknown. A recent study by Meyer-Bahlburg and colleagues demonstrated no cognitive or developmental motor impairment to have resulted from prenatal treatment of CAH fetuses. Miller (1999) and others have advocated the use of prenatal treatment for CAH only as an experimental therapy in large centers and under institutional review board scrutiny. The importance of long-term follow-up of these neonates has been emphasized (Speiser, 1999).

Hughes (2002) and others have emphasized the close correlation in CAH of genotype and phenotype, which has a number of practical implications. Molecular biologists can now predict not only the risk of a couple having an affected child, but also the likely clinical form of the disease. Therefore, genotypes of severe mutations would motivate prenatal treatment, whereas genotypes of less severe mutations would not. In addition, less severe genotypes in the newborn would allow for modification of steroid treatment to minimize side effects.

The treatment of affected children with hydrocortisone in childhood and adolescence achieves a number of goals, as noted by Bongiovanni and Root (1963): "to supply the deficient hormone; to suppress pituitary ACTH secretion and hence adrenal androgens and clinical virilization; to forestall abnormally rapid somatic growth and osseous advance; to permit normal gonadal development; and to correct salt-water loss or hypertension in the complicated forms." The required dose of glucocorticoid may be predicted by genotype, as noted by Hughes, but should be adjusted for the individual patient based on bone age, linear growth, 24-hour excretion of ketosteroids, and clinical evidence of glucocorticoid deficiency or excess (Grumbach and Conte, 1998; Hughes, 2002). The effectiveness of therapy may be assessed by measuring morning plasma 17-hydroxyprogesterone levels. Those children with the salt-losing form of the disease require increased salt intake and mineralocorticoid treatment in addition to hydrocortisone therapy. After control of electrolytes and blood pressure has been achieved in the acute setting, maintenance therapy with fludrocortisone (0.05 to 2.5 mg daily) should be instituted (Laue and Rennert, 1995; Grumbach and Conte, 1998). The administration of hydrocortisone and, when required, fludrocortisone is continued indefinitely in all patients. Typically, patients are instructed to triple their oral dose of hydrocortisone during stressful events such as surgery or infection.

In the majority of children (who will not have been diagnosed and treated prenatally), it is appropriate to perform feminizing genitoplasty at 3 to 6 months of age, when a well-established course of medical therapy has been instituted, the risks of anesthesia have become minimal, and the child has grown large enough to make the procedure technically feasible (Passerini-Glazel, 1990). **Long-term fertility in males and feminization, menstruation, and fertility in females can be anticipated in the well-treated patient.** Indeed, this potential in even the most masculinized female CAH patient has provided support for feminizing genitoplasty in virtually all 46,XX CAH patients.

An important area of recent research has been the potential imprinting of the brain by elevated prenatal androgen levels. A number of recent studies confirm that prenatal hyperandrogenization is associated with masculinization of gender-related behavior but not masculinization of gender identity. Hall and associates (2004) noted a close correlation between genotype and genital masculinization with behavioral masculinization. Furthermore, Berenbaum has noted that in females with CAH and virilized genitalia psychological development is not compromised in those who are reared as females and receive good medical care (Berenbaum and Bailey, 2003; Berenbaum et al, 2004). Therefore, the psychosexual evidence to date supports maintaining female gender in masculinized CAH patients diagnosed in infancy. Indeed, proper psychological support should be a component of long-term follow-up.

An intriguing area of surgical innovation in the management of CAH has been the experimental use of "prophylactic" adrenalectomy for selected patients. This approach is based on the premise that in certain patients it is more difficult to maintain adrenal suppression than to prevent adrenal crises. Clinically, these patients are the salt losers and extremely virilized females. For those with this most severe form of 21-hydroxylase deficiency, adequate suppression of adrenal production has required significant degrees of hypercortisolism, associated with poor growth, obesity, and infertility. For the 25% of CAH patients who completely lack 21-hydroxylase enzyme activity and therefore produce neither cortisol nor aldosterone, adrenalectomy may be a practical approach (VanWyk et al, 1996). In general, these patients may be identified genotypically as homozygotes or compound heterozygotes for "null alleles" of the *CYP21* gene (VanWyk et al, 1996). In a series of 18 patients with long-term follow-up, VanWyk and Ritzen (2003) noted bilateral adrenalectomy to be safe and effective in managing severe forms of CAH in which patients repeatedly escaped adrenal suppression. Most of these patients reported a better quality of life after bilateral adrenalectomy.

Although these patients are rendered addisonian by this surgery, those with the most severe form of CAH would have a poor intrinsic adrenal response to metabolic stress (Gunther et al, 1997). One theoretical disadvantage of this approach is that if gene therapy were to one day allow functional *CYP21* genes to be introduced into adrenal cortical tissue, adrenalectomized patients would not be candidates for such therapy (VanWyk et al, 1996).

Masculinized Female (Female Pseudohermaphroditism) Secondary to Maternal Androgens and Progestins and Maternal Tumors

The masculinization of a female fetus as a result of maternal administration of synthetic progestational agents or androgens is a rare occurrence; lessons have been learned from prior unfortunate experiences. Historically, progestational agents were used to prevent threatened abortion. In one large series, masculinization occurred in 2% of female infants whose mothers were treated with progestins during pregnancy (Ishizura et al, 1962). In addition, danazol, a testosterone derivative used to treat endometriosis, has been associated with virilization of the female fetus. **The degree to which any androgen or progestational agent affects female fetal development is a function of the strength of the agent, its maternal dosage, and timing and duration of administration** (Bongiovanni and McFadden, 1960).

Very rarely, a maternal ovarian or adrenal tumor has virilizing effects on a female fetus. More typically, such a tumor has virilizing effects on the mother but no apparent effect on the fetus. Ovarian tumors that have resulted in masculinization of the female fetus include arrhenoblastoma, hilar cell tumor, lipoid cell tumor, ovarian stromal cell tumor, luteoma of pregnancy, and Krukenberg's tumor (Calaf et al, 1994).

Rarer still are maternal adrenal tumors, which have masculinizing effects on the female fetus. Adrenocortical carcinoma and adenoma have been reported.

Aromatase deficiency represents an even rarer cause of transplacental transport of excess androgens to the fetus. The cytochrome P450 aromatase enzyme catalyzes the conversion of androgens to estrogens. Normally, weak androgens produced by the fetal adrenal gland are converted to estrogens by placental aromatase and pass to the maternal circulation. Mutations of the *CYP19* aromatase gene can result in profound virilization of the female fetus and mother during pregnancy. Although maternal virilization resolves postnatally, it recurs in subsequent pregnancies.

In any case of exogenous androgen effect on a female fetus, normal endocrine status is recognized postnatally and management is confined to external genital reconstruction, as required.

Undermasculinized Male (Male Pseudohermaphroditism)

The term *undermasculinized male (male pseudohermaphroditism)* refers to 46,XY individuals with differentiated testes who exhibit varying degrees of feminization phenotypically. Impaired male differentiation in these patients is secondary to inadequate secretion of testosterone by the testes at the necessary period in development, inability of target tissue to respond to androgen appropriately, or impaired production or action of MIS.

Leydig Cell Aplasia (Luteinizing Hormone Receptor Abnormality)

Leydig cell aplasia as a cause of undermasculinization of the male was first reported by Berthezene and colleagues in 1976. **In its pure form, this rare disorder is characterized by a normal 46,XY male karyotype associated with a normal-appearing female phenotype. Typically, testes are palpable in the inguinal canals or labia majora.** On investigation, there are no müllerian structures and the vagina is short. A low testosterone level is noted in conjunction with an elevated LH concentration. **The absence of a rise in serum testosterone level after hCG stimulation is characteristic of this disorder** (Brown et al, 1978). Physiologically, this disorder represents a spectrum between absent Leydig cells and Leydig cells with abnormal LH receptor (David et al, 1984). It is transmitted as an autosomal recessive trait expressed only in males. Incomplete forms of the syndrome occur, with the mildest form being expressed as primary hypogonadism with normal male external genitalia (Lee et al, 1982).

The clinical diagnosis of Leydig cell aplasia, or LH receptor abnormality, is typically made as a result of sexual infantilism and the absence of development of secondary sexual characteristics or the discovery of palpable gonads in the inguinal canal or labia on physical examination (Arnholt et al, 1985). The differential diagnosis includes androgen insensitivity syndrome or a terminal defect in androgen synthesis.

The histology of the abnormal testes demonstrates absence of Leydig cells in intratubular spaces with normal Sertoli cells.

Disorders of Testosterone Biosynthesis

A defect in any of the five enzymes required for the conversion of cholesterol to testosterone can cause incomplete (or absent) virilization of the male fetus during embryogenesis. The first three enzymes (cholesterol side chain cleavage, 3β-hydroxysteroid dehydrogenase, and 17β-hydroxylase) are present in both adrenals and testes. **Therefore, their deficiency results in impaired synthesis of glucocorticoids and mineralocorticoids in addition to testosterone.** For all five enzyme deficiencies, the pattern of inheritance is autosomal recessive.

StAR (Cholesterol Side Chain Cleavage Enzyme) *Deficiency.* The first step in gonadal and adrenal steroidogenesis is conversion of cholesterol to pregnenolone, which is mediated by a single cholesterol side chain cleavage enzyme known as 450SCC (previously known as 20-22 desmolase). A defect in this enzyme, first described by Prader and Gurtner in 1955, was believed to result in the rare condition congenital lipoid adrenal hyperplasia, so named because the adrenal glands became large and lipid laden. **However, more recent evidence suggests that a defect in cholesterol transport rather than a defective enzyme is etiologically responsible** (Saenger, 1997). The steroidogenic acute regulatory protein (StAR) stimulates cholesterol transport from the outer to the inner mitochondrial membrane (site of the cholesterol side chain cleavage complex). This appears to be the rate-limiting step in acute steroid synthesis.

Affected 46,XY individuals have female or ambiguous external genitalia with a blind-ending vaginal pouch; intra-abdominal, inguinal, or labial testes; and absence of müllerian structures, consistent with functioning Sertoli cells (Hauffa et al, 1985). Wolffian ducts are present but rudimentary. Infants often present in the first few weeks of life with severe adrenal insufficiency and salt wasting.

A diagnosis of StAR (cholesterol side chain cleavage enzyme) deficiency should be entertained in any newborn with nonvirilized female external genitalia and evidence of cortisol and aldosterone deficiency with hyponatremia, hyperkalemia, and metabolic acidosis. Abdominal computed tomography demonstrates large, lipid-laden adrenal glands.

Management is similar to that for 21-hydroxylase deficiency. To date, all surviving 46,XY patients with this disorder have been raised as females and have undergone gonadectomy (Laue and Rennert, 1995). Because testosterone production was never significant, brain imprinting is not a factor in gender assignment.

3β-Hydroxysteroid Dehydrogenase. 3β-Hydroxysteroid dehydrogenase catalyzes the 3β-hydroxysteroids (pregnenolone, 17-hydroxypregnenolone, and DHEA) to the three ketosteroids, progesterone, 17-hydroxyprogesterone, and androstenedione. A congenital deficiency of 3β-hydroxysteroid dehydrogenase was first described by Bongiovanni in 1962.

Affected individuals present with various degrees of incomplete masculinization resulting from a block in testosterone biosynthesis and with salt-wasting adrenal

insufficiency resulting from impaired synthesis of aldosterone and cortisol. The lack of salt-retaining hormone and cortisol results in a salt-losing crisis soon after birth. However, partial deficiencies associated with severe salt wasting occur, consistent with genetic heterogeneity. The gene has been cloned and localized to chromosome 1 at locus p11-p13 (Chang et al, 1993).

Males with this deficiency usually exhibit incomplete virilization of the external genitalia, with a small phallus, hypospadias with labioscrotal fusion, a urogenital sinus, and a blind-ending vaginal pouch. Testes are often scrotal, and wolffian ducts develop normally. As with other defects in testosterone biosynthesis, in which normal Sertoli cell function is preserved, müllerian structures are absent.

The diagnosis should be considered in 46,XY males with ambiguous genitalia and signs of adrenal insufficiency. Endocrine study demonstrating increased levels of 3β-hydroxysteroids confirms the diagnosis.

Management of 3β-hydroxysteroid dehydrogenase is similar to that for patients with 21-hydroxylase deficiency.

17α-Hydroxylase Deficiency. 17α-Hydroxylase catalyzes the conversion of pregnenolone and progesterone to 17α-hydroxypregnenolone and 17-hydroxyprogesterone, respectively, in adrenal and gonadal steroidogenesis. The first case of male pseudohermaphroditism due to this enzyme deficiency was reported by New in 1970. The gene for this enzyme has been localized to chromosome 10 (Laue and Rennert, 1995).

Affected 46,XY individuals usually have female external genitalia with absent to slight masculinization. **A deficiency in 17α-hydroxylase activity impairs cortisol production, causing ACTH hypersecretion and resulting in increased levels of DOC, corticosterone, and 18-hydroxycorticosterone in the adrenals. These compounds with mineralocorticoid activity produce excess salt and water retention, hypertension, and hypokalemia.**

The phenotype of affected individuals varies from female with external genitalia with a blind-ending vaginal pouch to male with perineal hypospadias and chordee. The diagnosis should be considered in a male pseudohermaphrodite with hypertension. Endocrine laboratory evaluation demonstrates elevated serum progesterone, DOC, corticosterone, 18-hydroxycorticosterone, and ACTH.

Therapy with glucocorticoid replacement brings blood pressure and hypokalemia back to normal by suppressing ACTH and hence adrenal cortical stimulation. Some patients have been raised as females with gonadectomy and estrogen replacement at puberty. In partial forms, typically with reasonable phallic size, patients may be raised as male with testosterone replacement at puberty. **Fertility has not been reported in patients with testosterone biosynthetic defects, and inadequate testosterone production makes androgen imprinting a less significant issue for these patients.** Therefore, the phenotype may dictate gender assignment.

17,20-Lyase Deficiency. The enzyme 17,20-lyase has been demonstrated to be related to 17α-hydroxylase in that the activities of both are linked to the same gene product on chromosome 10 (Laue and Rennert, 1995). However, in some patients with the genetic defect both biologic activities are absent, but with others only the 17,20-lyase function appears

deficient. Zachmann and colleagues first described this clinical entity in 1972.

In cases in which the deficiency primarily involves 17,20-lyase, cortisol and ACTH secretion are normal. Aldosterone is secreted normally, and hypertension does not result. **However, impaired biosynthesis of testosterone in the 46,XY individual results typically in ambiguous rather than totally female genitalia at birth.** The deficient masculinization of the external genitalia can range from severe, resulting in a female gender assignment in the neonate, to mild, resulting only in hypospadias. At puberty, the secretion of testicular androgen remains low. Zachmann and colleagues (1982) have postulated that there are two types of 17,20-lyase deficiency—one that is partial and another that is a complete defect.

The diagnosis may be suspected in male pseudohermaphrodites with absent müllerian derivatives and no defect in glucocorticoid or mineralocorticoid synthesis. At the time of expected pubertal development, the patients may present with failure to develop secondary sexual characteristics and elevated gonadotropin levels. The diagnosis may be made prepubertally using hCG and ACTH stimulation.

Management entails plastic reconstruction of the external genitalia and appropriate sex steroid replacement at puberty.

17β-Hydroxysteroid Oxidoreductase Deficiency. This last enzyme in the testosterone biosynthetic pathway catalyzes the conversion of androstenedione to testosterone, DHEA to androstenediol, and estrone to estradiol. Male pseudohermaphroditism resulting from a deficiency in 17β-hydroxysteroid oxidoreductase was first described by Saez and associates in 1971.

Clinically, this is the most interesting enzymatic defect in testosterone biosynthesis in its similarities to 5α-reductase deficiency. At birth, affected individuals appear to have a normal female phenotype, without significant evidence of virilization. Therefore, a female gender assignment is usually made. However, these individuals have well-differentiated testes located intra-abdominally, inguinally, or in the labia and no müllerian structures. Surprisingly, wolffian ducts are normally developed, which may be secondary to the action of androstenedione or minimal amounts of testosterone produced during embryogenesis (Boehmer et al, 2001). **At puberty, there is phallic growth and progressive development of male secondary sexual characteristics.** These include increased muscle mass and development of pubic, axillary, and facial and body hair with male distribution. Gynecomastia may occur, and the testes may become palpable (Saez et al, 1972). In some cases, gender reassignment to male has been reported (Imperato-McGinley et al, 1979; Rosler and Kohn, 1983).

The late onset of virilization is related to the pubertal increase in gonadotropin production, which may partially overcome the block in testosterone biosynthesis.

There is a characteristic hormonal profile in this disorder. In the prepubertal patient, plasma androstenedione and estrone levels may not be increased. At puberty, androstenedione, the immediate precursor of testosterone, is increased to 10 to 15 times the normal plasma concentration (Virdis and Saenger, 1984). Earlier precursors are within normal levels. Plasma testosterone is in the low-normal range. Serum LH and FSH are markedly elevated, typically four to six times normal.

As a result of biochemical characterization and molecular cloning, five different 17β-hydroxysteroid dehydrogenase isozymes have been identified to date. **The type III 17β-hydroxysteroid dehydrogenase isozyme, cloned by Andersson and colleagues (1997), catalyzes the biosynthesis of testosterone from androstenedione. A mutation involving this gene is responsible for male pseudohermaphroditism.** The type III isozyme is apparently expressed early in utero and is responsible for testosterone biosynthesis during the critical period of sexual differentiation, based on the observation that male adults homozygous for 17β-hydroxysteroid dehydrogenase type III gene defects have ambiguous genitalia (Zhu et al, 1998).

The diagnosis is rarely made in the newborn period. It may become apparent on discovery of a testis during a hernia repair in infancy or childhood. An hCG stimulation test resulting in an increased testosterone:androstenedione ratio would confirm the diagnosis and differentiate this condition from androgen insensitivity (Ahmed et al, 2000). **The primary management issue for patients with 17β-hydroxysteroid oxidoreductase deficiency has been gender assignment.** At this early stage, maintenance of the female sex of rearing with gonadectomy is usually elected. If the diagnosis is not made until puberty, when dramatic changes in virilization occur, certain families prefer a gender change to male. In an Arab cohort of 22 patients, Sobel and associates (2004) noted 7 to undergo spontaneous gender role reversal to male without parental consent or psychiatric intervention. Traditionally, this decision has been strongly culturally influenced.

If a female sex of rearing is elected, gonadectomy, plastic reconstruction of the genitalia as necessary, and estrogen replacement therapy at puberty are indicated. For the patient maintained in the male gender, orchidopexy and reconstruction of the external genitalia are required. This entails hypospadias repair and chordee correction, which can be quite successful. However, phallic size remains small and infertility is the rule. Some have suggested that childhood treatment with intramuscular testosterone may result in a larger phallus (Sobel et al, 2004). Usually endogenous androgen levels are adequate long term.

Two hypotheses have been proposed to explain the frequency of gender change from female to male with this enzyme deficiency, particularly among the cohort of Arab male pseudohermaphrodites with 17β-hydroxysteroid dehydrogenase type III deficiency. One entails the potential male imprinting of the brain in utero due to the conversion of androstenedione to estrone; this theory is supported by studies in rats and rabbits demonstrating that administration of estrogen or androstenedione is capable of inducing male sexual behavior (Reddy et al, 1974). The second is the possibility that 17β-hydroxysteroid dehydrogenase activity is not deficient in the brain, its effect being mediated by the conversion of androstenedione to testosterone or estrogen (Imperato-McGinley et al, 1979).

Androgen Receptor and Postreceptor Defects

Disorders of androgen receptor function represent the most common definable cause of the undervirilized male. These patients characteristically have a 46,XY karyotype and testes and present with a spectrum of phenotypic abnormalities that vary from complete external feminization (syndrome of complete androgen insensitivity), to ambiguous genitalia (partial androgen insensitivity), to the phenotypically infertile male.** Although the clinical presentations vary according to the severity of the disorder, the pathophysiology is similar (Wiener et al, 1997).

Syndrome of Complete (Severe) Androgen Insensitivity. The syndrome of complete androgen insensitivity (testicular feminization) is characterized clinically by a 46,XY karyotype, bilateral testes, female-appearing external genitalia, and absence of müllerian derivatives.** Wilkins first suggested in 1950 that the clinical features of this syndrome were the result of androgen resistance. This condition has an incidence of 1 in 20,000 to 1 in 60,000 males, and it is transmitted as an X-linked trait.

The androgen receptor regulates the transcription of other specific genes, once activated by testosterone or DHT. This results in new mRNA synthesis from the downstream genes and protein production. The androgen receptor has been mapped to the X chromosome at Xq11-12, spanning 90 kilobases and comprising 8 exons (Brown et al, 1989; Hiort, 2003). Males have only one copy of this gene. Point mutations of the gene account for more than 90% of cases of androgen insensitivity (Quigley et al, 1995). **The identifiable molecular alterations of the androgen receptor gene cannot predict the resulting phenotype of the affected individual unless there is total loss of the receptor, which occurs in only 1% of all patients** (Quigley et al, 1995).

Patients with complete androgen insensitivity have a normal female phenotype with the exception of diminished axillary and pubic hair. Their breast development and body habitus are feminine in character, and their external genitalia are unequivocally female, although the vagina is short and blind-ending. It had previously been believed that in-utero resistance to testosterone action prevented stabilization of the wolffian ducts. Hannema and associates (2004), however, have demonstrated wolffian duct derivatives in cases of complete androgen insensitivity. In 42% of patients, screening of the paratesticular area revealed well developed epididymis and/or vasa deferentia. The mutations found in these patients entailed a single amino acid substitution in the androgen receptor ligand binding domain, rather than frameshift mutations, premature stop codons, or mutations in the DNA-binding domain, all of which were associated with absence of well-developed wolffian duct structures. These investigators suggest that mutant receptors with residual activity in vivo stimulate wolffian duct development. As a result, they should be classified as having *severe* rather than complete androgen insensitivity. Because the fetal testes secrete MIS, müllerian structures are absent. The testes may be found in the labia, inguinal canal, or abdomen.

These patients are rarely diagnosed in the newborn period, unless a prenatal diagnosis is made on the basis of female phenotype and 46,XY karyotype on amniocentesis. With the increase in prenatal diagnostics, this is becoming a more common occurrence (Hughes and Patterson, 1994). More typically, however, the diagnosis is made as a result of primary amenorrhea or the finding of a testis at inguinal herniorrhaphy. Fifty percent of patients with complete (severe) androgen insensitivity syndrome have an inguinal hernia (Conte and Grumbach, 1989). Conversely, 1% to 2% of apparently female infants with inguinal hernia are found to have a 46,XY karyotype and complete androgen insensitivity syndrome (Wiener et al, 1997; Barthold et al, 2000). Therefore, routine vaginoscopy to confirm the presence of a cervix before inguinal herniorrhaphy in female patients is a prudent maneuver. Histologically, the testes exhibit incomplete or absent spermatogenesis, with normal or hyperplastic Leydig cells. They are comparable to immature, cryptorchid testes.

Endocrine evaluation in the newborn period demonstrates normal levels of testosterone, DHT, and gonadotropins. At puberty, gonadotropin levels rise, leading to increased levels of plasma estradiol, which results in feminization, including breast development.

Several types of receptor abnormality that would account for this syndrome have been described, including (1) a decreased amount of apparently normal receptor; (2) absence of receptor binding; (3) a qualitatively abnormal receptor (thermolabile, or unstable in the presence of molybdate); (4) other "receptor-positive" forms, including increased rate of dissociation of steroid receptor complex, defective upregulation of the androgen receptor, decreased affinity of ligand binding, and impaired nuclear retention of the ligand (Grumbach and Conte, 1998). In general, the severity of the defect in androgen receptor (quantity or quality) correlates with the phenotype. In addition, Hughes (2001) has noted the absence of co-regulator proteins, without the absence of the androgen receptor, in cases of complete androgen insensitivity, suggesting that for androgen effects to be optimal an integrated array of transcriptional factors, co-regulators, and ligands is required.

The diagnosis of complete (severe) androgen insensitivity may readily be made in the postpubertal patient on the basis of clinical and hormonal findings of amenorrhea, absence of pubic hair, or inguinal hernias containing testes. It is confirmed by a 46,XY karyotype and a normal male androgen and gonadotropin profile. Pelvic ultrasound examination confirms the absence of müllerian tissue, and a vaginal examination confirms a blind-ending vagina without a cervix.

In the prepubertal child, diagnosis is more difficult and requires an hCG stimulation test. Because of the time required for receptor binding quantification in genital skin, it is desirable to use PCR to characterize the androgen receptor gene in DNA obtained from a venous blood sample, to detect a genetic marker for androgen insensitivity syndrome.

Management of complete (severe) androgen insensitivity relates primarily to the optimal timing of gonadectomy. Because the testes produce estradiol, which results in the appropriate changes for the female phenotype, it is considered by many preferable to leave the testes in situ until puberty is complete. Potential exceptions to the policy of delayed gonadectomy are palpable testes or testes associated with an inguinal hernia. One important caveat in deciding to leave the testes in situ is the need to confirm with absolute certainty that complete rather than partial androgen insensitivity exists by PCR characterization of the androgen receptor gene in venous blood DNA. If an incomplete form should exist, virilization at puberty could result (Batch et al, 1993). Another important consideration is the anticipated need to discuss with a postpubertal female the presence of testes that require removal, rather than doing so when the

child is much younger and the psychosexual implications less charged.

A competing concern for retention of testicular tissue is the potential for malignant degeneration of the testes. In patients with complete androgen insensitivity who reach adulthood with a retained testis, the risk for development of a testis tumor—usually seminoma or gonadoblastoma—is thought to be 2% to 5%, only slightly higher than for a cryptorchid testis (Manuel et al, 1976; Muller and Skakkebaek, 1984). Before pubertal development the risk is extremely low; the youngest reported case of a germ cell tumor in an androgen insensitivity syndrome being in a 14-year old (Ahmed et al, 2000). Therefore, in general, delayed gonadectomy after puberty is believed to be safe.

After orchiectomy, cyclic estrogen/progestin therapy is begun. The majority of patients have successful treatment of their short vagina with progressive dilation. Some patients may benefit from vaginoplasty (Boehmer et al, 2001). **Currently, all studies of patients with complete androgen insensitivity support an unequivocal female gender identity, consistent with androgen resistance of brain tissue as well.** In one study, no statistical differences were found between the complete androgen insensitivity group and normal controls in any quality-of-life or gender-related behavior criterion (Hines et al, 2003). To date, there has been no report of a patient with complete androgen insensitivity raised as a female who needed gender reassignment to male (Meyer-Bahlberg, 1999).

Syndrome of Partial Androgen Resistance. The syndrome of partial androgen resistance includes syndromes that were once thought to represent separate entities: Reifenstein's, Gilbert-Dreyfus, Rosewater's, and Lubs' syndromes (Griffin, 1992). **These are X-linked disorders** of incomplete masculinization that represent a spectrum of phenotypic abnormalities. **The major finding is ambiguity of the external genitalia to varying degrees.** The partial form of androgen insensitivity may be expressed variably even within the same family. **The classic phenotype is that of a male with perineoscrotal hypospadias, cryptorchidism, rudimentary wolffian duct structures, gynecomastia, and infertility. However, the phenotypic spectrum can range from hypospadias and a pseudovagina to gynecomastia and azoospermia** (Wilson et al, 1974). The endocrine profile of partial androgen insensitivity syndrome is similar to that of the complete androgen insensitivity syndrome. At puberty, gynecomastia may develop. The phallus may enlarge slightly, but it remains small.

To date, over 300 mutations in the androgen receptor gene have been discovered. It has been well recognized in partial androgen insensitivity syndrome that these mutations produce a diversity of phenotypes between and within affected families, consistent with additional factors that modulate responsiveness to androgen. This seems consistent with prior studies in the 1980s on genital skin fibroblasts, demonstrating **two forms of receptor defect in the partial androgen insensitivity syndrome: (1) a reduced number of normally functioning androgen receptors and (2) a normal receptor number but decreased binding affinity** (Griffin and Durrant, 1982; Hughes, 2000).

The diagnosis of partial androgen insensitivity syndrome can be difficult. In the newborn period, it may be made in the setting of a 46,XY karyotype, ambiguous external genitalia, and absent müllerian structures on pelvic ultrasound.

Endocrine evaluation confirms normal testosterone and gonadotropin levels and a normal testosterone/DHT ratio. An hCG stimulation test and characterization of the androgen receptor gene in serum DNA by PCR should confirm the diagnosis. A family history consistent with X-linked inheritance of ambiguous genitalia is of great assistance.

Management must be individualized depending on the degree of genital ambiguity. In patients assigned a female gender, gonadectomy and surgical reconstruction of the external genitalia are indicated; at puberty, estrogen/progestin replacement is instituted. Those individuals raised as males would require treatment of their cryptorchidism, reduction of gynecomastia, and genitalia reconstruction. Phallic size remains small, however, and the effects of supraphysiologic doses of testosterone have been disappointing (Migeon et al, 1994). Of importance in considering gender assignment in patients with partial androgen insensitivity is the recognition that the receptor defect affecting the external genitalia appears to affect brain receptors for testosterone similarly. Unfortunately, because of the distinct phenotypic variability, even within families, gender assignment of patients with partial androgen insensitivity syndrome cannot be based on the specifically identified androgen receptor gene (Boehmer, 2001). The study by Melo and colleagues (2003) of 11 patients with partial androgen insensitivity syndrome (5 raised female, 6 raised male) demonstrated gender of rearing to be consistent with adult gender role. This suggests the possibility that in the setting of inadequate androgen imprinting of the fetal brain, sex of rearing may predominate in determination of gender identity. Unfortunately, this has not consistently proven to be the case.

The current recommendation with partial androgen insensitivity syndrome is to allow virilization of the external genitalia to serve as a guide in gender assignment, in that this may be the best means of assessing androgen imprinting of the brain, for lack of a more precise marker (Sobel and Imperato-McGinley, 2004).

The most recently discovered and mildest form of androgen receptor abnormality is that of the *infertile male syndrome* (Aiman et al, 1979). Recent studies have demonstrated a variety of mutations, usually quite discrete within the androgen receptor gene, to account for the infertility (Hiort et al, 2003). Men with this syndrome are normal phenotypically but are azoospermic or severely oligospermic. They have been found to have normal to elevated serum testosterone levels with normal to elevated LH levels. This suggests that infertility in otherwise normal males may be the clinical manifestation of partial androgen insensitivity—representing the far end of a variable phenotypic spectrum. To date, the pathophysiology of the abnormal spermatogenesis caused by androgen receptor mutations remains unknown (Hiort et al, 2003).

5α-Reductase Deficiency

The disorder of 5α-reductase deficiency is one of the most fascinating forms of male pseudohermaphroditism. The clinical presentation of this enzyme disorder was actually predicted in 1972, before the description of such patients in 1974 by Walsh and Imperato-McGinley and their colleagues (Wilson, 1972; Imperato-McGinley et al, 1974; Walsh et al, 1974). Extensive characterization of the disease has been achieved since that time.

5α-Reductase is a microsomal enzyme that catalyzes the conversion of testosterone to DHT. The condition is transmitted in an autosomal recessive pattern, and only homozygous males are affected. Two 5α-reductase genes have been cloned; they encode different isoenzymes. The type I isoenzyme, encoded on chromosome 5, is expressed in low levels in the prostate and external genitalia. The type II isoenzyme is encoded on chromosome 2 and is expressed in high levels in the prostate and external genitalia (Thigpen et al, 1992b). **Male pseudohermaphroditism due to 5α-reductase deficiency is secondary to mutations in the type II gene.** At least 40 mutations have been identified (Thigpen et al, 1992a; Imperato-McGinley, 2002). Identical mutations in individuals with widely different geographic and ethnic backgrounds support the concept of mutational "hot spots" on the gene.

Individuals with this disorder present as newborns with a 46,XY karyotype and a phenotype that may vary from penoscrotal hypospadias to, more commonly, markedly ambiguous genitalia. Typically, the phallus is quite small, appearing as a normal or enlarged clitoris (Fig. 128–22). A urogenital sinus is present, with separate vaginal and urethral openings and labioscrotal fusion (Fig. 128–23). The vaginal pouch is short and blind-ending. Testes and epididymides are located in the labia, inguinal canals, or abdomen; and the vasa terminate in the blind-ending vaginal pouch. At puberty, partial masculinization occurs with an increase in muscle mass, development of male body habitus, increase in phallic size, and onset of erections (Peterson et al, 1977). Sperm production and fertility in affected individuals have been reported

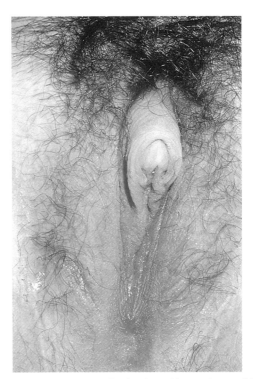

Figure 128–22. External genitalia of patient with 5α-reductase deficiency. Note clitoromegaly with marked labioscrotal fusion and small vaginal introitus. (From Diamond D: Intersex Disorders: I and II. AUA Update Series, Vol IX, Lessons 9 and 10. Houston, TX, American Urological Association Office of Education, 1990.)

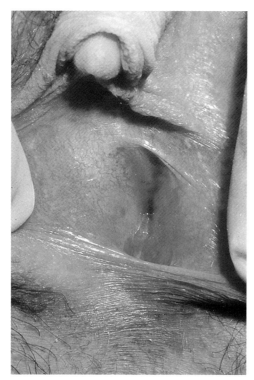

Figure 128–23. Intraoperative view of urogenital sinus in a patient with 5α-reductase deficiency; note enlarged clitoris, urogenital sinus with separate urethral and vaginal openings, and posterior labioscrotal fusion. (From Diamond D: Intersex Disorders: I and II. AUA Update Series, Vol IX, Lessons 9 and 10. Houston, TX, American Urological Association Office of Education, 1990.)

(Imperato-McGinley et al, 1982; Zhu et al, 1998). Other secondary sexual characteristics, including enlargement of the prostate and hairline recession do not develop.

On endocrine evaluation, these individuals have elevated mean plasma testosterone but low DHT levels. After hCG stimulation, the testosterone/DHT ratio increases from the range of 3 to 25 in normal subjects to a range of 75 to 160 (Kupfer et al, 1992). Genital skin fibroblast cultures demonstrate diminished to absent 5α-reductase activity (Migeon et al, 1994). At puberty, virilization is presumed to occur because the androgen receptor binds markedly higher levels of testosterone at low affinity or because of the normal increase at puberty in the activity of the 5α-reductase type I isoform resulting in sufficient DHT for virilization (MacLaughlin and Donahoe, 2004). Indeed, the enzyme abnormalities in this disorder have been shown to be biochemically heterogeneous, ranging from reduced affinity of the enzyme for testosterone and reduced affinity for reduced nicotinamide adenine dinucleotide phosphate (NADPH) to altered pH activity profiles (Kupfer et al, 1992).

The phenotypic characteristics of this disorder have helped to clarify the roles of testosterone and DHT in normal development. **Although DHT appears to be critical for the development of normal external genitalia in utero, testosterone alone appears sufficient for wolffian duct development.**

Individuals in the pedigree studied by Imperato-McGinley in the Dominican Republic underwent gender reversal at puberty and were known within the community as *guevedo-*

ces ("penis at 12") (Imperato-McGinley et al, 1979). This strong tendency toward reversal of gender identity in 5α-reductase deficiency has been one of the most intriguing aspects of the disorder. It has lent support to the concept that testosterone exerts the primary male imprinting effect on the brain. However, the discovery that there are two isoenzymes for 5α-reductase, only type II being deficient in this syndrome, allows for the possibility that 5α-reductase type I has some impact on the brain (Thigpen et al, 1992b). As a result, with early diagnosis of 5α-reductase deficiency, a male gender assignment is generally favored, bearing in mind that the studies strongly supporting male gender identity in this disorder were performed in sociologically unique environments (Zhu et al, 1998). The clinician must be open to familial cultural considerations regarding the value of male gender as well as the significance of penile size. In the setting of male gender assignment, cryptorchidism and hypospadias should be surgically corrected. Fertility is possible, particularly with the advent of intrauterine insemination (Katz et al, 1997). Exogenous DHT could be used at puberty in an attempt to promote phallic growth, but it would be likely to impair spermatogenesis. For some individuals, based primarily on extremely small phallic size, a female gender may be assigned. For these patients, gonadectomy should be performed as early as possible and certainly well before puberty to prevent virilization. Estrogen/progestin should be administered at the expected time of puberty. Vaginoplasty and clitoral reduction may be performed within the first year of life in those with a severe defect to provide for normal appearance of the external genitalia and to allay parental anxiety.

Persistent Müllerian Duct Syndrome

Persistent müllerian duct syndrome (PMDS), or *hernia uteri inguinale*, the term originally used by Nilson (1939), characteristically describes a group of **patients with a 46,XY karyotype and normal male external genitalia but internal müllerian duct structures. Typically, these phenotypic males have unilateral or bilateral undescended testes, bilateral fallopian tubes, a uterus, and an upper vagina draining into a prostatic utricle.** The condition is commonly diagnosed after müllerian tissue is encountered during inguinal herniorrhaphy or orchidopexy.

Clarnette and coworkers (1997) suggested three categories for patients with PMDS: (1) the majority (60% to 70%) with bilateral intra-abdominal testes in a position analogous to ovaries; (2) a smaller group (20% to 30%) in which one testis is found in a hernia sac or scrotum in association with a contralateral inguinal hernia (the classic presentation of hernia uteri inguinale); and (3) the smallest group (10%), in which both testes are located in the same hernia sac (as a result of transverse testicular ectopia) along with the fallopian tubes and uterus. Indeed, **PMDS is believed to be etiologically important in transverse testicular ectopia, occurring in 30% to 50% of cases** (Fujita, 1980).

The MIS gene was cloned in 1986 and localized on the short arm of chromosome 19 (Cates et al, 1986). It shows homology with the TGF-β super family of growth and differentiation factors (Imbeaud et al, 1995). **PMDS is thought to be a heterogeneous disorder genetically in which some subjects have a defect in the gene for MIS located on chromosome 19p13 and others have a defect in the gene for its type II** receptor located on chromosome 12q13 (MacLaughlin and Donahoe, 2004). The condition may occur sporadically or be inherited as an X-linked (or autosomal dominant, sex-limited) trait (Migeon et al, 1994).

The treatment of persistent müllerian duct syndrome is relatively straightforward, in that all patients are phenotypic males who require orchidopexy. The cases of adult patients with associated testis tumor (most commonly seminoma) probably reflect the increased risk of malignancy in intra-abdominal undescended testes. One treatment caveat relates to management of the rudimentary müllerian structures. **The vasa deferentia are in close proximity to the uterus and proximal vagina, and preservation of the necessary müllerian structures to avoid injury to the vasa is recommended to preserve fertility** (Sloan and Walsh, 1976). While fertility has been reported with this syndrome, only recently has a case of malignancy in retained müllerian structures been reported (Berkmen, 1997; Shinmura, 2002).

Unclassified Forms: Mayer-Rokitansky-Küster-Hauser Syndrome

The Mayer-Rokitansky-Küster-Hauser (MRKH) syndrome is a rare disorder entailing congenital absence of the uterus and vagina. It occurs in approximately 1 of every 4000 to 5000 female births. Patients with MRKH syndrome have a 46,XX karyotype and are normal-appearing females with normal secondary sex characteristics. The external genitalia appear normal, but only a shallow vaginal pouch is present. In the typical form of the syndrome, there is symmetrical anatomy with absence of both vagina and uterus. Normal ovaries and fallopian tubes are present, and ovarian function is normal, but only symmetrical uterine remnants are found (Griffin et al, 1976). The recent report of a *WNT4* mutation in a woman with a phenotype resembling MRKH suggests the importance of this gene in müllerian duct formation (Biason-Lauber et al, 2004).

The most common clinical presentation for MRKH syndrome is primary amenorrhea, but patients may present with infertility or dyspareunia. **Upper urinary tract anomalies occur in approximately one third of patients and include renal agenesis, pelvic kidney, and horseshoe kidney.**

Atypical forms of MRKH syndrome have been described in up to 10% of cases, in which asymmetrical uterine remnants and/or aplasia of one or both fallopian tubes is discovered. As a result, endometrial tissue or variable development of the uterus with hematometra may be present, resulting in a clinical presentation with cyclic abdominal pain. **Urinary tract anomalies occur more commonly in patients with the atypical form of MRKH.** In a study of 100 patients with MRKH syndrome, 38 of 56 patients (68%) with the atypical form of the condition had upper urinary tract abnormalities. Not one of 44 patients with the typical form of MRKH syndrome had an upper urinary tract anomaly (Strubbe et al, 1994).

A radiologic evaluation with ultrasound and MRI may define müllerian anatomy accurately in MRKH and distinguish between typical and atypical forms of the disorder (Nussbaum-Blask et al, 1991; Reinhold et al, 1997).

Treatment entails creation of a neovagina, surgically or by means of dilation, to allow for sexual function and drainage of menstrual fluid if necessary.

EVALUATION AND MANAGEMENT OF THE NEWBORN WITH AMBIGUOUS GENITALIA

The evaluation and initial management of the newborn with ambiguous genitalia must be regarded as a medical and psychosocial emergency and be handled with great sensitivity toward the family. Ideally, a medical team including a pediatric urologist, an endocrinologist, and a psychiatrist or psychologist experienced in managing intersex patients should work closely with the family. **The team's goal should be to make a precise diagnosis of the intersex disorder (which can be achieved in virtually every case) and, with the involvement of the parents, to assign a proper sex of rearing based on the diagnosis, the status of the child's anatomy, and the functional potential of the genitalia and reproductive tract.**

In obtaining the history, certain pieces of information may be particularly valuable. A history of infant death within the family might suggest the possibility of CAH, and infertility, amenorrhea, or hirsutism might also suggest possible familial patterns of intersex states. Certainly, maternal use of medications, in particular steroids or contraceptives, during the pregnancy is of great importance.

The critical finding on physical examination is the presence of one or two gonads. This finding effectively rules out overmasculinization of the female. Because ovaries do not descend, a distinctly palpable gonad along the pathway of descent is highly suggestive of a testis. Rarely, an ovotestis undergoes descent and may be suspected on the basis of asymmetry of tissue texture of the poles of the gonad. This suspicion may be further supported by ultrasound findings. **The patient with bilaterally impalpable testes or a unilaterally impalpable testis and hypospadias should be regarded as having an intersex disorder until proven otherwise, whether or not the genitalia appear ambiguous.** Kaefer and associates (1999) studied the incidence of intersex disorders in patients with cryptorchidism and hypospadias and without ambiguous genitalia. **With a unilateral cryptorchid testis, the incidence of intersex was 30% overall—15% if the undescended testis was palpable and 50% if it was impalpable. In the setting of bilateral undescended testes and hypospadias, the incidence of intersexuality was quite similar—32% overall but only 16% if both gonads were palpable. If one of two undescended testes was impalpable, the incidence of intersex tripled to 47%, comparable to the rate in those with a unilateral, impalpable, cryptorchid testis.** In addition, posterior urethral meatal position was noted to be a strong predictor of intersex in this group of patients—65%, versus 5% to 8% with a midshaft to anteriorly located hypospadiac meatus (Kaefer et al, 1999).

In addition to gonadal examination, penile size should be assessed and an accurate measure of stretched penile length recorded.

An additional important finding on physical examination is the presence of a uterus, which is noted as an anterior midline cord-like structure on rectal examination. **A more precise means of assessing müllerian anatomy is by pelvic ultrasound, which may be performed immediately in the newborn period.** In addition to defining müllerian anatomy and confirming the presence or absence of a uterus, the gonads and adrenals should be studied. Normal anatomy of an undescended gonad should be confirmed, and a cyst within the gonad, consistent with ovotestis, should be ruled out.

Within the immediate newborn period, a karyotype should be obtained. Typically this requires 2 to 3 days to perform. Therefore, an attractive approach to obtain chromosomal data quickly is FISH, which rapidly identifies X and Y chromosomes. It is typically used to confirm the presence of a second X chromosome. The technique is much more rapid than karyotyping, producing results in a few hours.

Serum studies should be immediately sent to rule out a salt-wasting form of CAH. In addition to serum electrolytes, testosterone and DHT should be measured early. Migeon and colleagues (1994) emphasized that the androgen levels may drop quickly, necessitating early study. In addition, they suggested that serum 17-hydroxyprogesterone should not be measured until day 3 or 4 to rule out 21-hydroxylase deficiency, because the stress of delivery may result in physiologic elevation of this steroid precursor in the first 1 or 2 days of life.

In the absence of palpable testes, the presence or absence of testicular tissue should be determined by documentation of a markedly elevated LH, consistent with anorchia, or by means of an hCG stimulation test, which can demonstrate normally functioning testicular tissue (Jarow et al, 1986). In addition to ruling out anorchia, the study can enable diagnosis of 5α-reductase deficiency (by virtue of an increased ratio of testosterone to DHT) and can help distinguish between impaired testosterone synthesis (deficient response to hCG) and androgen insensitivity (normal response to hCG). Serum MIS meas-

urement has been proposed as a reliable marker of the presence of testes, but the test is not yet universally available (Hughes, 2002).

Based on physical examination (largely, gonadal palpability) the presence or absence of müllerian structures on ultrasound, 17-hydroxyprogesterone concentration, and the karyotype, a reasonable differential diagnosis may be formulated (Fig. 128–24).

KEY POINTS: EVALUATION AND MANAGEMENT OF INTERSEX

The team's goal should be to make a precise diagnosis of the intersex disorder (which can be achieved in virtually every case) and, with the involvement of the parents, to assign a proper sex of rearing based on the diagnosis, the status of the child's anatomy, and the functional potential of the genitalia and reproductive tract.

The patient with bilaterally impalpable testes or a unilaterally impalpable testis and hypospadias should be regarded as having an intersex disorder until proven otherwise, whether or not the genitalia appear ambiguous.

Based on physical examination (largely, gonadal palpability) the presence or absence of müllerian structures on ultrasound, 17-hydroxyprogesterone concentration, and the karyotype, a reasonable differential diagnosis may be formulated.

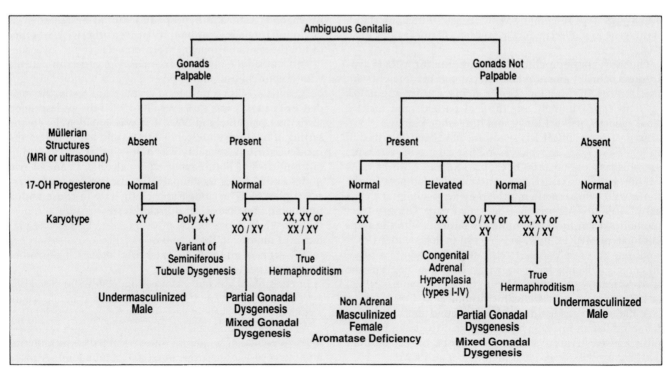

Figure 128–24. Diagnostic algorithm for a newborn with ambiguous genitalia based on gonadal palpability, presence or absence of müllerian structures, 17-hydroxyprogesterone concentration, and karyotype. (Modified from Grumbach MM, Conte FH: Disorders of sex differentiation. In Wilson JD, Foster DW [eds]: Williams Textbook of Endocrinology. Philadelphia, WB Saunders, 1998, p 1401.)

Laparotomy or laparoscopy and gonadal biopsy is usually the next definitive clinical step required when a firm diagnosis based on the aforementioned data is impossible. **Laparotomy or laparoscopy in this setting remains a diagnostic maneuver; removal of gonads or reproductive organs should be deferred until the final pathology report is available and a gender has been assigned.** PCR characterization of the androgen receptor in venous blood DNA may define the precise genetic abnormality responsible for a given intersex disorder, be it abnormal androgen receptor or an enzyme abnormality. These studies should be performed in specialized laboratories where normal values are well established.

Finally, anatomic definition of the urogenital sinus and ductal structures contributes to the correct diagnosis and is necessary before any surgical intervention. The urogenital sinus is well imaged by retrograde contrast injection, which also opacifies ductal structures, defines the entry of urethra and vagina into the sinus, and outlines the cervical impression within the vagina. Endoscopy can define these relationships further but is usually not necessary until surgical reconstruction becomes imminent.

Gender Assignment

After a definitive diagnosis has been reached, a thorough and candid discussion with the family regarding gender assignment should take place. **Issues related to the diagnosis-specific potential for normal sexual functioning and fertility and the risk of gonadal malignancy should be addressed.** Parents should understand that high-quality data regarding the long-term psychosocial outcomes of gender assignment for the majority of intersex conditions are lacking, although longitudinal studies are being pursued. Parental involvement in the decision-making process is essential. If the diagnosis of an intersex disorder is made prenatally, it is important to present a plan of management to the parents or risk termination of the pregnancy (Nihoul-Fekete, 2004).

In the setting of a 46,XX karyotype and masculinized female, gender assignment is usually appropriately female. In CAH, cortisol suppresses the undesired androgen, and if maternal androgen is responsible for virilization, its discontinued stimulation is corrective. In both cases there are normal ovaries and müllerian ducts and a normal reproductive potential exists. **If the karyotype is 46,XY, the issue is a more complex one and includes factors such as penile length and evidence of androgen insensitivity.** For example, 46,XY patients with complete (severe) androgen insensitivity are appropriately assigned a female gender, whereas those with 5α-reductase deficiency may be more appropriately assigned a male gender. The most frequent abnormal karyotype is 45,X/46,XY mosaicism, which presents a variable phenotypic spectrum. The degree of masculinization of the external genitalia appears to vary with the amount of testicular tissue present, and gender assignment depends on the functional potential of the gonadal tissue, reproductive tracts, and genitalia. Some investigators have suggested deferring the issue of gender assignment until patients reach an age at which they may declare their own gender identity. Such an approach, while rational, is difficult to implement given cultural norms.

As Elliott (1998) states, "we treat these children the way we do (as male or female) because this is the way we see the world…most importantly it is the way that the children, themselves, are taught to see the world."

Overall, it is well to remember in the management of ambiguous genitalia the parameters of optimal gender policy proposed by Meyer-Bahlburg (1998):

- **Reproductive potential (if attainable at all)**
- **Good sexual function**
- **Minimal medical procedures**
- **An overall gender-appropriate appearance**
- **A stable gender identity**
- **Psychosocial well-being**

Ultimately, management of patients with intersex disorders remains a challenging and humbling process. On the one hand, physicians have at their disposal sophisticated molecular biologic techniques that have enabled them to identify genetic disorders responsible for the majority of intersex conditions. On the other hand, the mysteries of brain dimorphism in the setting of sexual ambiguity remain to be solved to optimize the long-term psychosocial outcome of gender assignment for the individual patient.

KEY POINT: GENDER ASSIGNMENT

Overall, it is well to remember in the management of ambiguous genitalia the parameters of optimal gender policy proposed by Meyer-Bahlburg (1998):
- Reproductive potential (if attainable at all)
- Good sexual function
- Minimal medical procedures
- An overall gender-appropriate appearance
- A stable gender identity
- Psychosocial well-being

SUGGESTED READINGS

Hughes IA: Congenital adrenal hyperplasia: A continuum of disorders. Lancet 1998;352:752-754.

Hughes IA: Intersex. BJU Int 2002;90:769-776.

Jost A, Vigier B, Prepin J, Perchellet JP: Studies on sex differentiation in mammals: Recent progress in hormone research. Recent Prog Horm Res 1973;29:1-41.

Kaefer M, Diamond DA, Hendren WH, et al: The incidence of intersexuality in children with cryptorchidism and hypospadias: Stratification based on gonadal palpability and meatal position. J Urol 1999;162:1003-1007.

MacLaughlin DT, Donahoe PK: Sex determination and differentiation. N Engl J Med 2004;350:367-378.

Meyer-Bahlburg HF: Gender assignment and reassignment in 46,XY pseudohermaphroditism and related conditions. J Clin Endocrinol Metab 1999;84:3455-3458.

Pang S, Pollack MS, Marshall RN, Immken L: Prenatal treatment of congenital adrenal hyperplasia due to 21-hydroxylase deficiency. N Engl J Med 1990;322:111-115.

Sinclair AH, Berta P, Palmer MS, et al: A gene from the human sex determining region encodes a protein with homology to a conserved DHA-binding motif. Nature 1990;346:240-244.

Saenger P: Turner's syndrome. N Engl J Med 1996;335:1749-1754.

VanWyk JJ, Ritzen EM: The role of bilateral adrenalectomy in the treatment of congenital adrenal hyperplasia. J Clin Endocrinol Metab 2003;88:2993-2998.

Surgical Management of Intersexuality, Cloacal Malformation, and other Abnormalities of the Genitalia in Girls

RICHARD RINK, MD • MARTIN KAEFER, MD

As with all other organ systems, genital development in the female occurs in an orderly fashion through multiple complex steps that result in an anatomically and functionally normal child in the vast majority of cases. However, errors in development can occur, from minor, clinically insignificant disorders to severe abnormalities that are devastating to the child and parents. The abnormalities may affect the external genitalia alone or in combination with internal genital anomalies, and in some they may involve other organ systems. This chapter briefly describes normal urogenital and anorectal development and then discusses anomalies that arise when abnormal development occurs. Genital ambiguity is often the initial finding in these disorders. This chapter discusses only reconstruction along female lines; male reconstruction (i.e., hypospadias, chordee repair, and orchiopexy) is discussed in Chapter 125, "Hypospadias," and Chapter 127, "Abnormalities of the Testes and Scrotum and Their Surgical Management."

Genital reconstruction for intersex conditions at this time is very controversial. Although significant advances in surgical techniques have occurred since Young's early work (1937), well-controlled studies with regard to not just cosmetic results but also functional and psychological results are almost nonexistent. Historically, reconstruction of intersex conditions has been surrounded by secrecy, and decisions have been made without scientific studies and often without the patient's knowledge. Questions regarding genital sensitivity, orgasmic potential, gender identity, and psychological aspects in those undergoing early genital surgery currently exist. It is beyond the scope of this chapter to discuss all the pros and cons of this controversy, but it is clear that further studies are warranted.

The recently established multispecialty task force on intersex conditions may answer many of the questions surrounding treatment. It is strongly recommended that physicians honestly discuss with the parents of these children all aspects of care, including options, risks and benefits, and negative aspects of both observation and surgical therapy. A team of physicians, including a neonatologist, endocrinologist, geneticist, psychiatrist, psychologist, and pediatric urologist, should participate with the parents in decision-making. This writing addresses current surgical techniques that are available should surgical therapy be chosen for an intersex child. It also addresses other female genital anomalies not associated with genital ambiguity.

FEMALE REPRODUCTIVE AND CAUDAL EMBRYOLOGY

A comprehensive description of genitourinary embryology can be found in Chapter 106, "Normal Development of the Urogenital System," and Chapter 128, "Sexual Differentiation: Normal and Abnormal." To foster a deeper understanding of the complex combination of anomalies that can be found in patients with vaginal and cloacal anomalies, a brief review of relevant embryologic events is presented.

The cloaca is an endoderm-lined primordial organ that is first apparent at the beginning of the second week of gestation (Grosfeld, 1996). This structure, which represents a confluence of the primitive hindgut (dorsally) and the allantois (ventrally) just before the fourth week of gestation, receives the mesonephric ductal system. The urorectal septum, which first appears during the fourth week of development, serves to separate the urogenital sinus (ventrally) from the anal canal (dorsally) (Moore and Persaud, 1995). The urorectal septum actually consists of two components. The first is Tourneux's fold, which develops along the coronal plane in the angle between the allantois and the hindgut and grows in a caudal fashion toward the cloacal membrane. As this septum nears the cloacal membrane, infoldings of the lateral walls of the cloaca form Rathke's plicae, which coalesce in the coronal midline and form the urorectal septum caudally. By weeks 6 to 7 of development, the urorectal septum has fused with the cloacal membrane and divided it into a ventral urogenital membrane and a dorsal anal membrane. The fibromuscular node of tissue that results from contact of the septum with the cloacal membrane serves as a critical insertion site for the perineal muscles and as the dividing point of the primitive cloacal sphincter complex into anterior (urogenital diaphragm) and posterior (external anal sphincter) components. The common ontogeny of these two sphincter complexes explains why the pudendal nerve supplies all of these muscles.

While the urorectal anlage is undergoing division, the developing mesonephric ducts, which have contacted the cloaca, enter the urogenital sinus near the müllerian tubercle (Churchill and Hardy, 1978). An offshoot of the mesonephric duct, the ureteric bud, extends cranially to induce development of the metanephric blastema. The terminal branch point of the ureteral bud from the mesonephric duct is later absorbed into the wall of the urogenital sinus. Proper incorporation of this complex results in the ureters opening at the lateral aspect of the trigone.

During this critical phase of cloacal development, paired müllerian ducts, which form from the coelomic epithelium,

develop lateral to the mesonephric ducts and cross medially to fuse in the midline. The close proximity of these two ductal systems helps explain the common association of paramesonephric abnormalities and ipsilateral renal anomalies. The paired müllerian ducts then proceed caudally to join the urogenital sinus, where they produce an elevation called the müllerian tubercle. The caudal fusion of portions of these ducts normally leads to dissolution of the shared midline partition and the formation of a common uterovaginal canal, which as the name implies, gives rise to the uterus as well as the upper vagina.

As first delineated by Koff in 1933, contact of the uterovaginal primordium with the urogenital sinus forms the müllerian tubercle, which in turn induces the formation of paired caudal endodermal outgrowths called sinovaginal bulbs. Evidence suggests that these outpouchings may in fact represent the terminal segments of the wolffian ducts (Bok and Drews, 1983). Regardless of origin, the cells within these sinovaginal bulbs then proliferate to form a cord of tissue that develops into a distal vaginal plate, which is later canalized in a caudal-to-cranial direction to form the distal aspect of the vagina (Fig. 129–1). The portion of the urogenital sinus distal to the müllerian tubercle subsequently undergoes exstrophy and everts to become the vestibule. As a result of this process, the urethra and vagina acquire separate openings in the vulva. The lumen of the vagina is separated from the cavity of the urogenital sinus by the hymen, an invagination of the posterior wall of the urogenital sinus. Rupture of the hymen should occur during the perinatal period.

Various cystic structures may form along the luminal aspect of the vagina. Remnants of the prostatic ductal system and the wolffian duct give rise to the paraurethral glands of Skene and Gardner, respectively. Outgrowths from the urogenital sinus form the greater vestibular glands of Bartholin, which are homologues of the bulbourethral glands in the male.

Key events in skeletal formation occur concurrently with cloacal division and proper formation of the mesonephric and paramesonephric ductal systems (Churchill and Hardy, 1978). The vertebrae develop in a craniocaudal direction, with the lower extremity limb buds developing from condensation of somites 25 through 29. These somites undergo critical differ-

Figure 129–1. Formation of the vagina from the sinovaginal bulbs. (From Saler TW: Langman's Medical Embryology, 6th ed. Baltimore, Williams & Wilkins, 1990.)

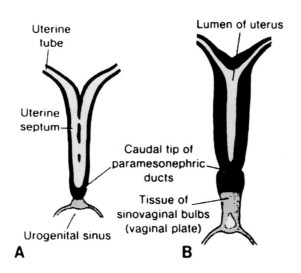
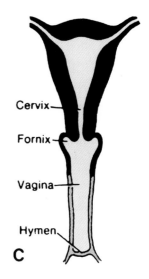

entiation from the fourth through the eighth weeks of development.

From the foregoing brief description of caudal embryology it should be evident that a disturbance in segmentation at the level of the caudal somites when the fetus is less than 10 mm in size (fourth to fifth weeks of human development) can affect many different organ systems. In 1960, Duhamel described the association of these "coincidentally" occurring congenital malformations and introduced the term *caudal regression syndrome* (Duhamel, 1961). Laboratory data with teratogens support the concept that a key event occurs between the fourth and fifth weeks of gestation that results in an error in the simultaneous development of the terminal bowel, kidney, bladder, paramesonephric ductal system, and lumbosacral spine (Mesrobian and Sessions, 1994). The actual inciting event remains unclear, although disordered mesodermal migration, reduced cellular proliferation, and premature apoptosis have all been proposed as potential mechanisms (Kallen and Winberg, 1974; Alles and Sulik 1993). Elements of the caudal regression syndrome are seen with increased frequency in infants of diabetic mothers, but the exact mechanism is still in question (Deuchar, 1978; Lynch et al, 1995). Specific gene deletions in the homeobox region of the mammalian genome (the region critical for proper mammalian spatial orientation and segmentation) have been shown to result in a constellation of anatomic findings, as predicted by Duhamel (Warot et al, 1997). Because differentiation of the somites progresses in a cranial-to-caudal direction, it would follow that the most complex anomalies (higher anorectal malformations) would occur as a result of aberrations at an earlier stage of development. This also helps explain the greater association of severe upper urinary tract malformations, internal genital duct abnormalities, and spinal anomalies in these patients than in those with less severe cases of imperforate anus.

Mesodermal disturbances are not limited to the caudal somites. As seen in the VATER (vertebral defects, anal atresia, tracheoesophageal fistula with esophageal atresia, and radial and renal dysplasia) and MURCS (müllerian duct aplasia, renal aplasia, and cervicothoracic somite dysplasia) associations, mesodermally derived organs as cranial as the C1 vertebra and tracheoesophageal anlagen can be affected in association with congenital abnormalities of the mesonephric and paramesonephric ductal systems (Quan and Smith, 1973; Duncan et al, 1979).

KEY POINTS: EMBRYOLOGY

- The close proximity of the mesonephric and paramesonephric ductal systems helps explain the common association of paramesonephric abnormalities and ipsilateral renal anomalies.

- The proximal part of the vagina forms from the paired müllerian ducts, whereas the distal portion forms from proliferating cells in the sinovaginal bulbs that later canalize.

STRUCTURAL ANOMALIES OF THE FEMALE INTERNAL GENITALIA

Anomalies of the female reproductive system can be grouped into three main categories: those resulting from either hypoplasia or agenesis, those caused by vertical fusion (canalization abnormalities resulting from abnormal contact of the müllerian structures with the urogenital sinus), and those resulting from lateral fusion (duplication). The clinical manifestations, physical findings, evaluation, and subsequent therapy vary considerably among these groups. Radiographic imaging is of central importance in determining the correct diagnosis. Ultrasound is helpful not only in identifying the genital anatomy but also in screening for associated upper urinary tract abnormalities (Rosenberg et al, 1986; Fernandez et al, 1996). Magnetic resonance imaging (MRI) is considered by many to be the "gold standard" for defining internal müllerian anatomy (Fedele et al, 1996; Russ et al, 1997; Lang et al, 1999). It is especially useful for determining the presence or absence of the cervix and the presence of functioning endometrium in complex anomalies. In complicated cases, additional information can be obtained by examination under anesthesia, vaginoscopy, hysteroscopy, and laparoscopy (Major et al, 1997). Obstructive anomalies typically require immediate intervention, but nonobstructive anomalies often do not require surgical intervention unless the patient has reached reproductive age and the condition affects intercourse or adversely affects fertility. Various systems have been proposed for the classification of these anomalies, with the system proposed by the American Society for Reproductive Medicine being the most inclusive (Anonymous, 1988).

Obstructive Genital Anomalies

Abnormalities of Vertical Fusion

Transverse Vaginal Septum. Transverse vaginal septa are believed to arise from a failure in fusion or canalization (or both) of the urogenital sinus and müllerian ducts. Many of the patients have amenorrhea and a distended upper vagina. A complete transverse vaginal septum may be located at various levels in the vagina, but there is a higher frequency in the second and upper third of the vagina. In one large series the distribution was 46% in the upper vagina, 40% in the middle vagina, and 14% in the lower vagina (Fig. 129–2) (Lodi, 1951). The septa are usually less than 1 cm thick and frequently have a small central or eccentric perforation (Suidan and Azoury, 1979). Even in cases in which a perforation is present, significant obstruction and ascending infection can occur.

Transperineal, transrectal, and abdominal ultrasonography and MRI may be beneficial in establishing the diagnosis and determining the location and thickness of a transverse vaginal septum (Ammann et al, 1983; Doyle, 1992; Meyer et al, 1995; Caloia et al, 1998; Fedele et al, 1999; Lang et al, 1999). MRI can help determine whether a cervix is present so that a high septum can be differentiated from congenital absence of the cervix. Failure to differentiate between these diagnoses can result in significant patient morbidity (Casey and Laufer, 1997).

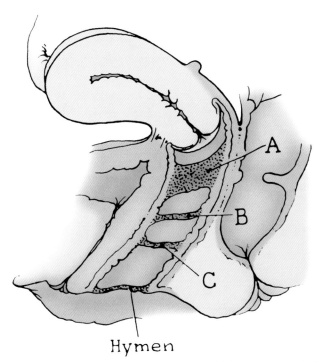

Figure 129–2. Transverse vaginal septum. A, high (upper vagina); B, middle; C, low. (From Yerkes EB, Rink RC: What urologists should know about pediatric gynecologic abnormalities. Contemp Urol 2002;14:12.)

Several surgical treatment modalities have been developed to treat congenital transverse vaginal septa. Techniques include simple incision (Brenner et al, 1965; Buttram, 1983), surgical excision of the septum followed by approximation of the corresponding portions of the transversely cut edges of the upper and lower mucosal membranes of the septum (Rock et al, 1982), the use of "Z"-plasties involving vaginal mucosa (Garcia, 1967), and the use of skin grafts to enlarge the vagina. The later technique has a higher rate of secondary tissue contracture, which often causes stenosis of the vagina (Garcia and Jones, 1977).

Vaginal Atresia (Distal Vagina). Vaginal atresia occurs when the urogenital sinus fails to contribute to formation of the lower (distal) portion of the vagina. This condition differs from vaginal agenesis and testicular feminization in that the müllerian structures are not affected. As a result, the uterus, cervix, and upper portion of the vagina are normal. A very shallow dimple caudal to the urethral opening may be appreciated on physical examination. Palpation of a distended vagina on rectal examination may help distinguish this condition from testicular feminization or vaginal agenesis. Radiographic evaluation in the form of ultrasound or MRI, or both, is mandatory to adequately define the müllerian anatomy before intervention.

Surgical correction consists of a transverse incision at the level of the hymenal ring. Dissection is carried out through the fibrous area of the absent lower vagina until the upper vagina is reached. As in treatment of a transverse vaginal septum, distention of the vagina with retained menstrual blood products can prove extremely beneficial in that it acts as a tissue expander. After the obstruction is drained and the vaginal mucosa is identified, a pull-through procedure can be performed to bring the distended vagina down to the introitus. The distance to bridge between the vagina and the perineal surface can almost always be successfully managed with perineal skin flaps or simple mobilization of the vagina (or both). Ramenofsky and Raffensperger (1971) described a combined abdominoperineal approach that can be of help in exposing and anastomosing the distal vagina to the perineal skin.

Vaginal Agenesis (Müllerian Aplasia)

General. Vaginal agenesis, which occurs at an incidence of approximately 1 in 5000 live female births, is congenital absence of the proximal portion of the vagina in an otherwise phenotypically (i.e., normal secondary sexual characteristics), chromosomally (i.e., 46,XX), and hormonally (i.e., normal levels of luteinizing hormone and follicle-stimulating hormone) intact female (Bryan and Nigro, 1949; Griffen et al, 1976). Although Realdus Columbus is credited by some authors as the first to describe a case of vaginal agenesis, Mayer was one of the first to report vaginal agenesis in stillborn children (Mayer, 1829; Lesavoy, 1985). In 1838, Rokitansky reported 19 adult autopsy cases of uterovaginal agenesis, including 3 with associated unilateral renal agenesis. In 1910, Kuster recognized urologic associations, such as renal ectopy and agenesis, along with skeletal deformities. Hauser and Schreiner (1961) brought further attention to the frequent association of renal and skeletal anomalies in these patients and stressed the differences between patients with these findings and those with testicular feminization.

The Mayer-Rokitansky-Kuster-Hauser (MRKH) syndrome, as the entity of müllerian aplasia has come to be known, results from failure of the sinovaginal bulbs to develop and form the vaginal plate (Fig. 129–3). This may be caused by improper induction of the sinovaginal bulbs from the neighboring uterovaginal primordium. Chronologically, the uterovaginal canal develops at a point in embryogenesis during which other critical mesodermally derived organ systems are also forming, which in part explains the many associated findings. Müllerian aplasia has also been associated with maternal deficiency of galactose 1-phosphate uridyltransferase (Cramer et al, 1996). In contrast to vaginal atresia, the hymenal fringe is usually present along with a small vaginal pouch because they are both derived embryologically from the urogenital sinus.

Most patients with MRKH syndrome are initially evaluated by the physician after the expected age of menarche because of primary amenorrhea. This syndrome is in fact second only to gonadal dysgenesis as a cause of primary amenorrhea. A minority of patients have cyclic abdominal pain caused by retention of menstrual blood in the uterus. Physical examination reveals absence of the vagina. Inguinal hernia is less common in this disorder than in the testicular feminization syndrome (Schmid-Tannwald and Hauser, 1973). The karyotype is that of a normal 46,XX woman. Radiographic evaluation is indicated to more fully delineate remnant müllerian structures and search for associated anomalies involving the renal and skeletal systems.

Associated Findings. MRKH syndrome is associated with variable absence or hypoplasia of the cervix, uterus, and fallopian tubes. In approximately 10% of patients, a normal but

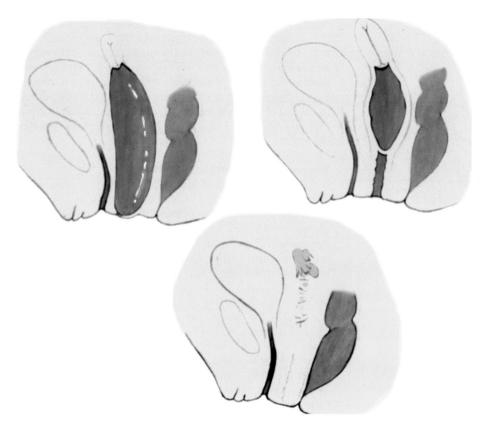

Figure 129–3. Forms of vaginal obstruction. *Upper left,* Imperforate hymen; *upper right,* transverse vaginal septum; *lower,* vaginal agenesis. (From Yerkes EB, Rink RC: What urologists should know about pediatric gynecologic abnormalities. Contemp Urol 2002;14:12.)

obstructed uterus or a rudimentary uterus with functional endometrium is present (Murray and Gambrell, 1979; Singh and Devi, 1983; Bates and Wiser, 1985). In one of the largest single series to date, Salvatore and Lodovicci (1978) reported that of 91 patients with vaginal agenesis, almost 25% lacked a uterus, 55% had a solid rudimentary uterus, and the remaining 30% had other abnormalities of this organ. In addition, they demonstrated that although the fallopian tubes were normal in 32% of cases, they were rudimentary in almost 50% and completely absent in 10%. Though occasionally cystic, the ovaries were almost always present and functional (Salvatore and Lodovicci, 1978). It was subsequently recognized, based on the morphology of the retained müllerian structures, that MRKH syndrome could be divided into typical and atypical forms (Schmid-Tannwald and Hauser, 1977).

In the typical form of MRKH syndrome (type A), the patient has symmetrical uterine remnants and normal fallopian tubes. The atypical form (type B) is characterized by asymmetric uterine buds or abnormally developed fallopian tubes. This distinction is important because the overwhelming majority of associated findings in other organ systems have been reported to be present with the atypical form whereas in the typical form, these findings are usually absent (Strubbe et al, 1992, 1993).

The association between vaginal agenesis and developmental abnormalities of the kidney was first recognized by Rokitansky (1838). Approximately a third of patients are found to have abnormal renal findings on intravenous pyelography or ultrasound examination (Strubbe et al, 1993). Renal anomalies are present almost exclusively in patients with the atypical subtype of vaginal agenesis (type B). In Strubbe's series, 34 of 51 patients with type B anatomy had renal anomalies, but none of the 40 patients with type A (symmetrical) anatomy demonstrated such a deformity (Strubbe et al, 1993). A meta-analysis published by Griffin and associates (1976) demonstrated that the renal anomaly consists of either unilateral renal agenesis or ectopia of one or both kidneys in 74% of those affected. The close proximity of the mesonephric and paramesonephric structures during the early phase of fetal development is thought to be the reason for this frequent association of renal anomalies. Not surprisingly, the converse is also true: the incidence of associated genital abnormalities in female patients with renal anomalies ranges between 25% and 89% (Thompson and Lynn, 1966).

Associated congenital abnormalities of the skeletal system have been described in 10% to 20% of cases (Turunen, 1967; Willemsen, 1982; Strubbe et al, 1987). Congenital fusion (failure of segmentation) of the cervical vertebrae is known as the Klippel-Feil syndrome and occurs approximately once in 30,000 to 40,000 live births (Gunderson et al, 1967). An association between this abnormality of cervical somite development and vaginal agenesis was first recognized by Duncan (1977). He proposed the term *MURCS association* to describe the combination of *mü*llerian duct aplasia, *r*enal aplasia, and *c*ervicothoracic *s*omite dysplasia, which many believe is caused by a generalized disordered development of mesodermal differentiation during the fourth week of fetal life (Duncan et al, 1979). Strubbe demonstrated that the Klippel-Feil abnormality was found only in patients with the atypical form of MRKH syndrome (type B). Additional, albeit less common skeletal abnormalities include scoliosis and abnormalities of the hands and face (Willemsen, 1982; Fisher et al, 2000).

Unlike müllerian anomalies that are associated with abnormal cloacal septation, vaginal agenesis is not associated with an increased incidence of lumbosacral spinal disorders or occult spinal dysraphism (Gunderson et al, 1967).

KEY POINTS: STRUCTURAL ANOMALIES OF THE FEMALE GENITALIA

- Anomalies of the female reproductive system can be grouped into three main categories: those resulting from (1) hypoplasia or agenesis, (2) vertical fusion, and (3) lateral fusion.

- Transverse vaginal septa are believed to arise from a failure in fusion or canalization (or both) of the urogenital sinus and müllerian ducts.

- Vaginal atresia occurs when the urogenital sinus fails to contribute to formation of the lower (distal) portion of the vagina.

- Vaginal agenesis is congenital absence of the proximal portion of the vagina in an otherwise phenotypically, chromosomally, and hormonally intact female.

- MRKH syndrome, as the entity of müllerian aplasia has come to be known, results from failure of the sinovaginal bulbs to develop and form the vaginal plate.

Creation of a Skin Neovagina. Both nonoperative and operative treatment options exist for this anomaly. Regardless of the method used, it can be very helpful to have the patient speak with someone who has previously undergone treatment before treatment is initiated (Ingram, 1981). **The nonoperative approach, initially popularized by Frank (1938), involves gentle pressure of graduated hard dilators against the perineal surface to create a progressive invagination of the vaginal dimple.** Ingram (1981) modified this technique by using a bicycle seat mounted on a stool. The nonoperative approach has greatest success when a vaginal dimple or pouch is already present (Williams et al, 1984, 1985). With proper patient compliance, this method can achieve a functional vagina in approximately 4 to 6 months.

Modifications of the Frank technique of perineal pressure have been developed that incorporate the surgical placement of tension sutures to aid in directing pressure from a Plexiglas dilator against the vaginal dimple (Vecchietti, 1979). The mold, often referred to as an "olive," has sutures attached to it that are guided in a cranial direction through the vesicorectal space into the perineal cavity and brought out through the abdominal wall (Vecchietti technique). Tension is progressively increased via the abdominal wall sutures until sufficient vaginal length has been achieved. To avoid a formal laparotomy, laparoscopic techniques have been described to assist in dissection of the tissue plane for the Vecchietti technique (Borruto, 1992; Gauwerky and Wallwiener, 1992; Fedele et al, 1996, 1999). In Fedele and colleagues' more recent series, all patients were found to have healthy vaginal mucosa, with the average vaginal length being almost 8 cm at 3 months. This technique has had limited use by urologists.

If the Frank method has been unsuccessful or is not accepted as a reasonable option by the patient or parents, creation of a functional vagina can be achieved by one of several techniques (Abbé, 1898; McIndoe and Banister, 1938; Hendren and Atala, 1994). The first landmark advance in vaginal reconstruction is attributed to Abbé in 1898. Abbé described dissecting a canal between the rectum and urethra and lining this area with split-thickness skin grafts. This method was later popularized by McIndoe, and the procedure that bears his name has gained wide acceptance in the United States (McIndoe and Banister, 1938). Preoperative preparation consists of full mechanical and antibiotic bowel preparation. A split-thickness skin graft is taken from the buttocks (0.018 to 0.022 inch) and tubularized over a stent (Fig. 129–4). A transverse incision is made at the level of the perineal dimple, and the potential space between the urethra and the rectum is carefully dissected up to the level of the peritoneal reflection. The graft and mold are then inserted into the potential space, and the labia minora are sutured around the stent to prevent extrusion during the initial healing phase (McIndoe, 1950). Many types of vaginal stents have been used for this purpose, including packed gauze, wood covered with a condom, silicone foam, acrylic, various metals, and an inflatable vaginal

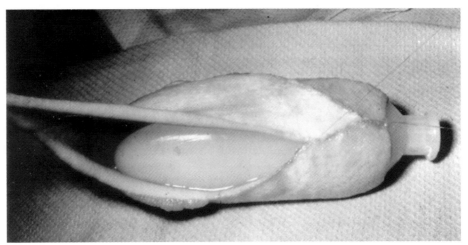

Figure 129–4. McIndoe skin vagina sewn over a vaginal stent.

stent (Concannon et al, 1993; Chen, 1994; Barutcu and Akguner, 1998). The Foley catheter is replaced by a suprapubic catheter, and postoperatively the patient is kept at strict bed rest for 1 full week. A high incidence of postoperative vaginal stenosis necessitates postoperative vaginal dilation (Ingram, 1981). Excellent patient satisfaction has been reported in most large series (Martinez-Mora, 1992; Strickland et al, 1993; Alessandrescu et al, 1996).

Other options for creation of a neovagina with local tissues include the use of full-thickness skin grafts from the buttocks or full-thickness skin flaps based on the labia majora. Those who champion the use of full-thickness skin grafts report a lower incidence of graft contracture than when split-thickness graft techniques are used (Sadove and Horton, 1988). The Williams vaginoplasty involves the creation of a vaginal pouch from the labia majora (Williams, 1964). The combination of this procedure and Frank-type dilation along the vaginal axis can provide a satisfactory result.

Many other surgical procedures have been developed for creation of a functional neovagina with various muscle flaps (e.g., pudendal thigh, rectus abdominis, buttock) (McCraw and Massey, 1976; Lilford et al, 1989; Dumanian and Donahoe, 1992; Wang and Hadley, 1993; Joseph, 1997). The pelvic peritoneum and human amnion are two other donor sites that have been used to create a neovagina (Davydov, 1977; Ashworth et al, 1986; Morton and Dewhurst, 1986; Tamaya and Imai, 1991).

Creation of an Intestinal Neovagina. Baldwin first described the use of bowel for creation of the vagina in 1907. The procedure involved anastomosis of a U-shaped segment of sigmoid colon to the perineum with subsequent division of the intervening septum (Hensle and Dean, 1992). Additional experience with this technique was reported by Fall in 1940, but it did not gain widespread acceptance until the 1970s because of high patient morbidity and mortality (Fall, 1940; Pratt, 1972). Subsequent improvements in technique and postoperative care resulted in renewed enthusiasm for these techniques (Turner-Warwick and Kirby, 1990; Hendren and Atala, 1994; Hensle and Reiley, 1998). Sigmoid, cecum, and small intestine have all been used successfully for the creation of a functional neovagina.

The day before surgery, the patient undergoes full mechanical and antibiotic cleansing of the alimentary tract. The procedure is performed with the patient supine, the legs spread, and the knees bent (frog-leg position). In an older child, Allen stirrups can be used. For a sigmoid vaginoplasty, the intraabdominal portion of the procedure commences by first identifying an appropriate length of distal sigmoid with a blood supply that will comfortably reach the perineum (Figs. 129–5 and 129–6). The distal end of the proposed segment is then divided and anastomosed to the perineum (Fig. 129–7). An intervening segment of sigmoid (approximately 3 cm) is then excised to create a space between the oversewn proximal edge of the bowel vagina and the end of the sigmoid, which is anastomosed to the rectum. This maneuver prevents an overlap of suture lines and thereby has the potential advantage of limiting the incidence of fistula formation. The bowel vagina is thereafter fixed to the posterior peritoneum to prevent prolapse.

Although we have had the most success with the sigmoid, a small-bowel segment may be chosen with a vascular pedicle

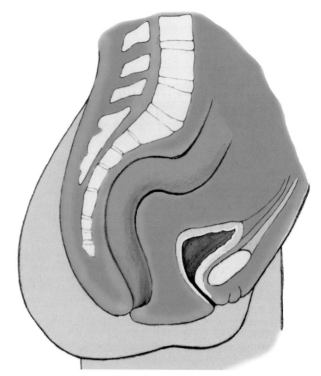

Figure 129–5. Vaginal agenesis.

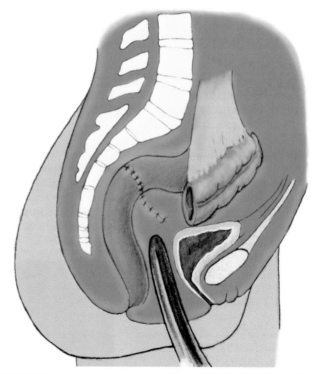

Figure 129–6. Bowel vagina: harvest of a colonic segment and creation of vaginal space.

that is of adequate length to reach the perineum. After isolating an appropriate length of ileum and reestablishing bowel continuity, the segment is detubularized and reconfigured in a conical arrangement to provide increased internal diameter (Figs. 129–8 and 129–9) (Hendren and Atala, 1994). The segment is then brought down to the perineum and sewn in place, as for a sigmoid neovagina. To avoid a formal laparotomy, laparoscopically assisted techniques have been described for harvest and delivery of the bowel segment to the perineal location (Ota et al, 2000).

If there is a perineal dimple (i.e., the segment of vagina contributed by the urogenital sinus is present), the bowel segment

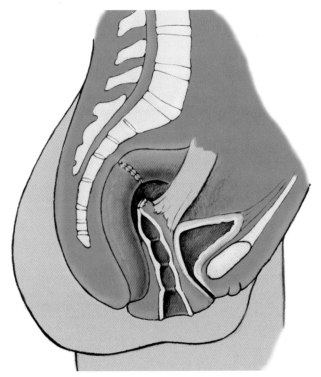

Figure 129–7. Bowel vagina: colonic segment sewn in place.

should be anastomosed directly to it. When a direct perineal anastomosis is required, it is of critical importance to create a large enough space between the rectum and bladder to avoid compromise of the intestinal blood supply. Creation of such a space can be facilitated by the use of progressively larger Hegar dilators.

Gentle passage of the intestinal segment into position is facilitated by placing the segment in a large lubricated Penrose drain before transfer to the perineum.

The functional results of bowel vaginoplasty have been excellent. Of the 65 patients reported by Hendren, 16 experienced mild eversion of the bowel segment, which in every case was amenable to simple trimming. Eight patients experienced mild stenosis that was later corrected by appropriate Z-plasties to increase the circumference of the mucocutaneous junction (Hendren and Atala, 1994). Patient satisfaction is high, and the majority of patients who are old enough to engage in sexual relations are able to achieve adequate coitus (Hensle and Reiley, 1998).

Stenosis has been reported more frequently after the use of ileum (Hensle and Dean, 1992). As a result, we and others believe that large intestine is the bowel segment of choice. Two specific indications for use of an ileal segment for bowel vaginoplasty are previous irradiation of the deep pelvis and the absence of large intestine (i.e., cloacal exstrophy). When ileum is used, various methods of reconfiguration can be used to increase the diameter (Hendren and Atala, 1994). Advantages of a bowel vagina over the McIndoe procedure include the lubricating properties of mucus (which may help facilitate intercourse) and the decreased incidence of postoperative contracture (and hence the reduced need for postoperative dilatation). Disadvantages include the frequent need to wear pads because of the chronic vaginal discharge. Daily douching may be necessary to evacuate the mucus. Finally, the

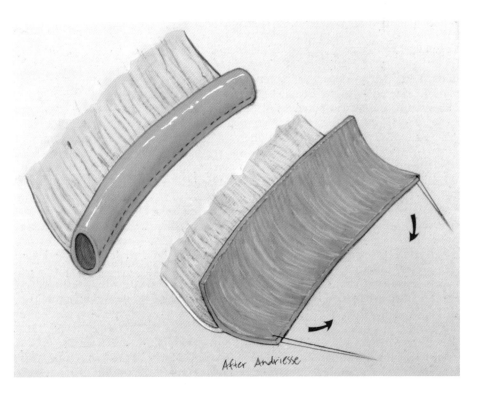

Figure 129–8. Bowel vagina: harvest of an ileal segment.

After Andriesse

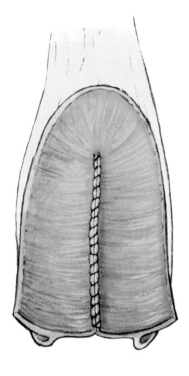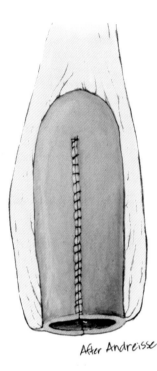

After Andreisse

Figure 129–9. Bowel vagina: reconfiguration of the ileal segment to create a larger luminal diameter.

potential transmission of blood-borne pathogens such as hepatitis and human immunodeficiency virus may be increased (in comparison to a squamous epithelium–lined vagina) because of the poor barrier effect of the gastrointestinal tract.

All patients undergoing creation of a functional vagina with perineal skin require annual examination because there have been reports of condylomata acuminata and squamous cell carcinoma involving grafts (Duckler, 1972; Rotmensch et al, 1983; Buscema et al, 1987). Annual examination of the bowel vagina is also indicated because adenocarcinoma has been identified after this procedure (Andryjowicz et al, 1985).

The optimal timing of surgery remains a source of debate. The majority of surgeons who favor the McIndoe procedure for construction of a neovagina believe that it is better to wait until adulthood to perform the procedure because a degree of maturity is required to consistently perform daily dilatations. Many surgeons who favor the use of bowel for neovaginal reconstruction do not believe that vaginoplasty should be deferred until the patient reaches adulthood. Hendren and Atala (1994) believe that delaying creation of a neovagina until adulthood may be psychologically traumatic to a young girl. We have based timing on the underlying diagnosis and need for a neovagina.

Special Considerations: Cervical Atresia. Cervical agenesis is an uncommon disorder that is associated with symptoms common to other obstructive entities of the female reproductive tract (i.e., primary amenorrhea, cyclic or chronic abdominal pain). Failure to establish the correct diagnosis and thereby choose the appropriate method of surgical intervention can be fraught with disaster and possible patient mortality. MRI is the most useful radiographic modality in establishing this diagnosis (Fig. 129–10). In many circumstances the patient is best served by hysterectomy with subsequent vaginal replacement by one of the previously described techniques (Rock et al, 1984; Cukier et al, 1986). Successful

KEY POINTS: VAGINAL REPLACEMENT SURGERY

■ The McIndoe procedure (skin neovagina) is associated with a higher incidence of postoperative vaginal stenosis than a bowel neovagina is.

■ Vaginal stenosis after creation of an intestinal neovagina is more common with ileum than with large bowel.

■ Vaginal reconstruction extending from the perineum to the uterus should be avoided in patients with cervical agenesis (because of the potential life-threatening complication of ascending bacterial infection).

direct anastomosis of the neovagina to the uterine remnant has been reported. Deffarges et al (2001), in describing their experience with uterovaginal anastomosis, reported a 40% pregnancy rate in patients attempting to conceive. Cerclage was performed in only one case. All pregnancies were delivered by cesarean section. Although this procedure appears to be successful in the majority of cases, absence of the normal endocervical barrier can leave the patient predisposed to the development of life-threatening ascending infection (Maciulla et al, 1978; Niver et al 1980; Casey and Laufer, 1997).

In cases in which it has not been possible to successfully achieve continuity between the uterus and vagina, in vitro fertilization plus transmyometrial embryo transfer has been performed, with subsequent delivery of a healthy fetus by cesarean section (Anttila et al, 1999; Lai et al, 2001). If this option is considered, hormonal blockade of the endometrium until the time at which the patient desires to initiate a

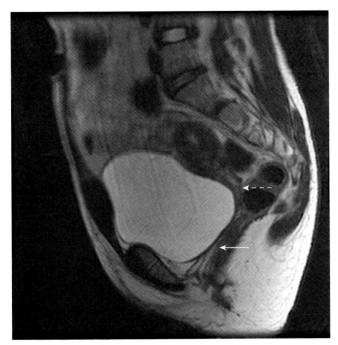

Figure 129–10. Magnetic resonance image of the pelvis in a 12-year old girl with Klippel-Feil syndrome and associated proximal vaginal and cervical atresia. The *solid arrow* points to the most cranial portion of the perineal vaginal pit. The *dashed arrow* points to the most inferior aspect of the uterus, where no cervical impression can be appreciated.

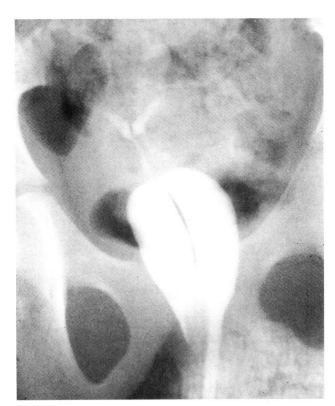

Figure 129–11. Genitogram of complete müllerian duplication (septated vagina and separate uteri).

pregnancy is indicated to minimize discomfort and reduce the incidence of endometriosis from retrograde menstrual flow in the fallopian tubes.

Abnormalities of Lateral Fusion

Most abnormalities of lateral fusion have no functional significance. With the exception of those with uterus didelphys and unilateral vaginal obstruction, most patients are asymptomatic. Although an exhaustive description of the defects of lateral fusion is beyond the scope of this chapter, some general comments can be made.

True duplication of the uterus is a rare event. This anomaly results from duplication of the müllerian ducts and subsequent doubling of the reproductive structures on one or both sides. The much more frequently encountered anomaly of uterine didelphys consists of two separate uterine cavities and cervices as a result of failed resorption of the common medial wall of the paired müllerian duct structures during development. Although up to 75% of patients also have a septate vagina, most have adequate reproductive outcomes and do not require surgical intervention. If later in life the patient experiences difficulty with intercourse, vaginal delivery, or the need to use two tampons, surgical excision of the vaginal septum should be undertaken. If only the most cranial portion of the septum remains, a bicornuate uterus will result. The vagina is typically normal, and surgical incision of the uterine septum is rarely indicated except in cases of recurrent pregnancy loss (DeCherney et al, 1986).

Duplication of the Uterus and Cervix with a Unilaterally Imperforate Vagina. Although the majority of obstructive

lesions are caused by abnormalities in vertical fusion, occasionally an obstructive process can be encountered in the context of an abnormality in lateral fusion (Figs. 129–11 and 129–12). More than 50 cases of uterus didelphys with a unilateral imperforate vagina have been reported in the world's literature (Allan and Cowan, 1963; Burbige and Hensle, 1984). As with other obstructive disorders, the patient may have cyclic or chronic abdominal pain. However, unlike other obstructive processes, duplication anomalies with unilateral obstruction do not result in primary amenorrhea. On physical examination, a unilateral abdominal-pelvic mass that terminates in a bluish bulge in the lateral vaginal wall is often appreciated (Eisenberg et al, 1982). Abdominal ultrasound and MRI are both excellent at defining the anatomy in a suspected case of unilateral noncommunicating uterine horn. Renal anomalies are frequently encountered on the side ipsilateral to the obstructed system, with renal agenesis being the most common (Eisenberg et al, 1982; Tridenti and Bruni, 1995). A prompt and accurate diagnosis is necessary to prevent injury to the genital organs as a result of chronic cryptomenorrhea and endometriosis. Treatment consists of wide incision of the vertical vaginal septum to release the entrapped menstrual blood.

Acquired Genital Obstructive Anomalies

Female Circumcision (Infibulation). Acquired vaginal obstruction may be secondary to a number of ritual female genital mutilation procedures that are widespread in many countries in Africa (stretching in a band from the Horn

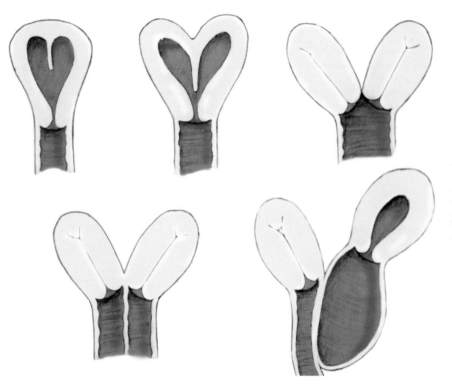

Figure 129–12.   Fusion anomalies of the müllerian system. *Upper left to lower right,* bicornuate uterus (partial), bicornuate uterus, uterine duplication, complete uterine and vaginal duplication, duplication of the uterus and cervix with a unilateral imperforate vagina. (From Yerkes EB, Rink RC: What urologists should know about pediatric gynecologic abnormalities. Contemp Urol 2002;14:12.)

of Africa through Central Africa to parts of Nigeria), the Middle East, and Muslim populations of Indonesia and Malaysia (Toubia, 1994; Dorkenoo, 1996). Although similar procedures were prescribed to U.S. and British women during the 19th century for the treatment of ailments ranging from epilepsy to lesbianism, all forms of genital mutilation are now illegal in these Western countries. Often referred to as "female circumcision," the procedure continues to affect an estimated 80 to 110 million women worldwide (Toubia, 1994).

The age at which this procedure is performed ranges from birth to just before marriage. However, it is typically performed on preadolescent children between the ages of 4 and 10 years, most commonly at age 7 (Anonymous, 1995). The procedure is usually performed without anesthesia in the context of a ceremony designating the rite of passage into adult society (Anonymous, 1995). The extent of the mutilation varies according to ritual, but the practice predates Islam and is therefore not part of a religion (McCaffrey et al, 1995). In many countries, the women have a deinfibulation procedure performed just before consummating the marriage.

The type of mutilation ranges from simple excision of the prepuce of the clitoris (termed "sunna") to complete excision of all elements of the vulvar region (McCaffrey et al, 1995).

Toubia (1994) classified the more extensive female genital mutilation procedures according to the amount of tissue destruction:

Type I: Complete or partial removal of the clitoris.

Type II: Excision of the clitoris and a portion of the labia minora.

Type III: Excision of the entire clitoris and labia minora with incision of the labia majora along its medial aspect

to create raw surfaces. The anterior two thirds of the labia majora are approximated to cover the urethra and introitus, with the lower third at the level of the posterior fourchette left for the passage of urine and menstrual fluid.

Type IV: Excision of the entire clitoris and labia minora with nearly complete approximation of the labia majora and only a pinhole opening left near the posterior fourchette for the passage of urine and menstrual fluid (Fig. 129–13).

Closing of the introitus, typically referred to as infibulation or pharaonic circumcision, is performed by a variety of means, including absorbable and nonabsorbable suture materials, thorns, and twigs. The child's legs are then bound for up to 40 days to ensure secondary healing in the ventral midline (McCaffrey et al, 1995).

The physical, psychological, and reproductive repercussions of these forms of genital mutilation are numerous and include immediate destruction and infection of local tissues (e.g., rectum, urethra). Long-term risks include chronic pain, recurrent urinary tract and vaginal infections, dysmenorrhea, dyspareunia, and apareunia. For individuals with the most narrowing, additional "surgeries" to revise the introital opening may be necessary for both intercourse and vaginal delivery (Aziz, 1980; Toubia, 1994).

Care of a patient who has undergone infibulation must be individualized, not only to provide functionality but also to respect the cultural and ritual desires of the woman. Educating the patient about the normal appearance of the external female genitalia is critical. Visual aids, including photographs or hand-drawn illustrations (or both) of the patient's anatomy and the planned revision, have been used as part of informed consent to avoid misunderstanding.

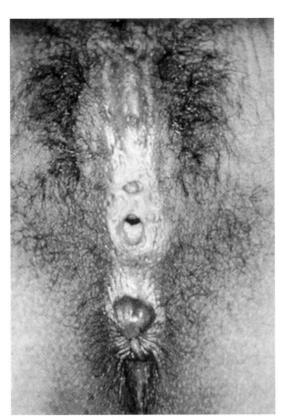

Figure 129–13. Female infibulation. Note the scarred labia majora with only a pinhole opening for the passage of menstrual fluid and urine. (From Gonzales ET, Bauer SB [eds]: Pediatric Urology Practice. Philadelphia, Lippincott Williams & Wilkins, 1999, p 599.)

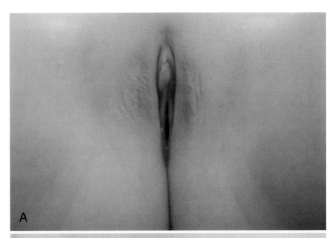

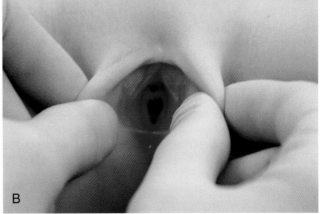

Figure 129–14. **A** and **B**, Photographs of the vaginal pull-down procedure. To aid in visualization of the female introitus, the labia majora are gently grasped and pulled caudally and laterally to enable funneling of the vagina.

Nonobstructive Genital Anomalies (Interlabial Mass)

The differential diagnosis of an interlabial mass in a neonate and young child is broad and requires a thorough understanding of the diagnostic possibilities and a systematic evaluation. The age and racial background of the patient can help narrow the differential diagnosis, but physical examination remains the most useful tool for determining the specific pathology.

The physician must be sure to specifically reassure the girl that the examination will not be painful. With the child in the frog-leg position, the physician should note the size of the clitoris, the configuration of the hymen, the location of the urethra, and the character of the interlabial mass (e.g., smooth, lobulated, hemorrhagic). To aid in visualization, the labia majora can be gently grasped and pulled caudally and laterally to enable funneling of the introitus and vagina (the so-called pull-down maneuver) (Fig. 129–14). Determining the nature of a specific mass can be facilitated by establishing the location of expected anatomic landmarks. In certain circumstances, the relationship of the mass to the vagina and urethra can be improved by gentle placement of a lubricated cotton applicator posteriorly or placement of a small feeding tube within the suspected urethral orifice, or both. Although an otoscope, nasal speculum, or pediatric vaginal speculum can be useful in evaluating the vagina while the patient is awake, complaints of vaginal origin (i.e., vaginal discharge or bleeding) are often best investigated with a carefully performed examination and vaginoscopy under anesthesia. Renal-pelvic sonography can be a useful adjunct in confirming or establishing the diagnosis in a few of these disorders.

Specific Lesions

Labial Adhesions. Labial adhesions are the most common interlabial abnormality identified in a pediatric urologic practice (Fig. 129–15). Fusion of the labia minora originates at the posterior fourchette and progresses for a variable distance toward the clitoris. It is important to differentiate this condition from the more serious entity of fusion of the labia majora, as is seen in certain intersex disorders. Hypoestrogenism is believed to play an important role in adhesion of the labia minora. This latter point appears to explain the fact that the overwhelming majority of cases occur in girls between the ages of 3 months and 7 years (Finlay, 1965). Labial adhesions have not been reported in newborn children, presumably because of the protective effect of maternal estrogen (Leung et al, 1993). Although hypoestrogenism appears to be important in the pathogenesis of this condition, other factors play a role (Papagianni and Stanhope, 2003). Local irritation and tissue trauma appear to be important inciting events in many cases of labial adhesions. Adhesions can rarely be associated with sexual abuse; in such cases, additional physical findings are often noted, including hematoma and lacerations (McCann et al, 1988). Although labial adhesions are usually asymptomatic, urine pooling within the vagina may lead to postvoid dribbling and perineal irritation and may make it difficult to obtain an accurate urinalysis.

Most children with labial adhesions do not require treatment unless they are symptomatic. When necessary, treatment ranges from the topical application of conjugated estrogens to surgical division. The 90% success rate that has been reported after the topical application of conjugated estrogens supports the concept that this disorder results from a relative hypoestrogenic state (Capraro and Greenberg, 1972). It is important to have the family place the cream directly on the labia minora. In addition, it is helpful to have the family perform the pull-down procedure a few times a day to put light stress on the midline adhesions and hence facilitate their separation. If separation is not noted after 2 weeks of treatment, manual separation in the outpatient setting may be indicated. After the application of EMLA cream to the introitus, gentle pressure is applied to the thin connecting membrane with the use of a lubricated probe. Rarely, in cases in which the adhesions are extremely dense, surgical division is required. Although one group has recently advocated oversewing the separated edges with 7-0 chromic (Nurzia et al, 2003), we have not found this to be necessary if the family is properly educated about keeping the labia separated (see Fig. 129–14) after the procedure.

KEY POINTS: NONOBSTRUCTIVE GENITAL ANOMALIES

■ Labial adhesions are thought to form as a result of low tissue levels of estrogen in a prepubertal girl.

■ Workup of a child with an introital (intralabial) mass that appears to be associated with the urethra should always include renal-pelvic ultrasonography.

■ Urethral prolapse occurs most often in prepubertal black girls and in postmenopausal white women.

Introital Cysts. Introital cysts in the newborn can represent one of three entities: paraurethral cysts (i.e., Skene's duct cyst), remnants of the mesonephric ductal system (Gartner's duct cyst), and a covered ectopic ureter. When the cyst is large and clearly emanating from the vaginal introitus, further investigation in the form of a renal-pelvic ultrasound is indicated to look for renal duplication.

Paraurethral cysts in a newborn represent a dilatation of the periurethral glands, which are located just inside the urethral meatus (Fig. 129–16). These glands are homologues of the male prostatic glands and number between 6 and 30, with the 2 largest termed the periurethral glands of Skene (Skene, 1880; Gottesman and Sparkuhl, 1979). In a newborn infant, the periurethral glands occasionally respond to maternal estrogen and secrete mucoid material, which can result in cyst

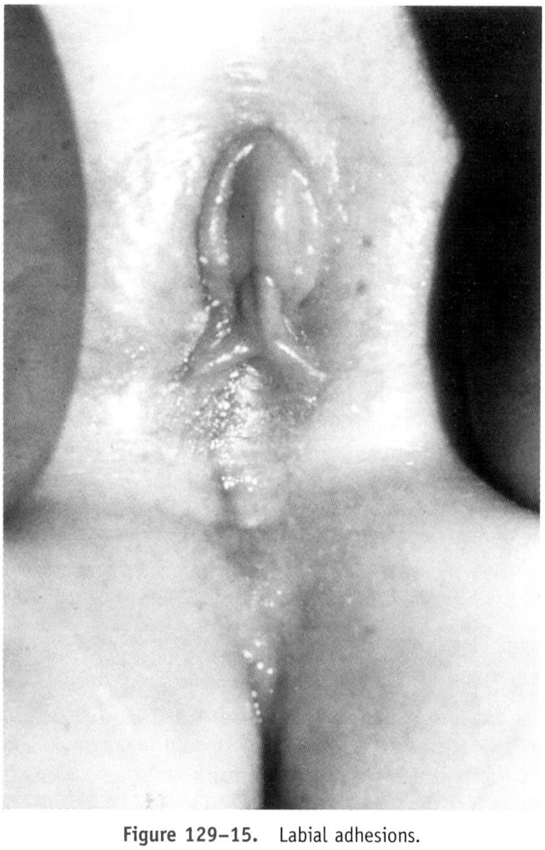

Figure 129–15. Labial adhesions.

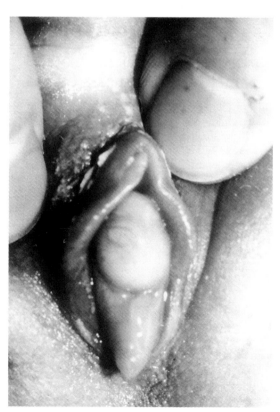

Figure 129–16. Paraurethral cyst. (From Yerkes EB, Rink RC: What urologists should know about pediatric gynecologic abnormalities. Contemp Urol 2002;14:12.)

formation. The main distinguishing feature of this condition is displacement of the urethral meatus by the mass and, consequently, an eccentric urinary stream. If the urethral meatus can be identified as being completely separate from the mass, radiographic evaluation is not needed to confirm the diagnosis (Nussbaum and Lebowitz, 1983). These cysts are frequently self-limited and often rupture spontaneously. If they are persistent, drainage by a small needle is easily achieved at the bedside.

Gartner's duct cysts represent cystic remnants of the wolffian duct system and can be found along the anteromedial wall of the vagina (Pradhan and Tobon, 1986). A cystic structure related to a Gartner's duct cyst is a *covered ectopic ureter* that enters into the vagina (Rosenfeld and Lis, 1993; Holmes et al, 1999). Embryologically, the ureter would not be expected to enter the vagina. However, an ectopically located ureter may end in a segment of the wolffian duct system, which in a female is represented by a Gartner's duct cyst. In most instances this cystic structure spontaneously ruptures before delivery, thereby resulting in direct communication between the ectopic ureter and the vagina. However, if the surface epithelium fails to rupture, a covered, urine-filled cyst will exist within the vagina. Intraoperative injection of the cystic structure with radiographic contrast material may be beneficial in outlining the anatomy (Fig. 129–17). Incision of the cystic structure relieves the obstruction. As a general rule, the more ectopic the insertion of the ureter, the more dysplastic the segment that it drains will be. However, renal moieties that ectopically insert into the vagina may produce urine. Subsequent upper pole heminephrectomy may be indicated if the child has significant urine production from the segment (resulting in incontinence) or an infection develops after decompression.

Hymenal Disorders. *Hymenal skin tags* are virtually a normal finding and are rarely symptomatic (Figs. 129–18 and 129–19). When symptomatic (i.e., bleeding), they should be excised to ensure that they do not represent a malignancy and to provide symptomatic relief. Congenital abnormalities of the hymen are not uncommon and range from an imperforate hymen to one with numerous small microperforations.

Imperforate hymen is probably the most common congenital obstructive anomaly of the female reproductive tract. The diagnosis is most frequently made at birth by noting the presence of a bulge along the posterior aspect of the introitus, which represents retained fluid within the vagina, or by palpation of a suprapubic mass from a distended vagina (Fig. 129–20). The buildup of retained vaginal secretions in the newborn period, which imparts a whitish appearance to the bulging hymenal membrane, is caused by maternal estradiol stimulation. If the diagnosis is made after the newborn period, the mucus will often have been reabsorbed and a bulge in the hymenal membrane may no longer be evident. On occasion, the diagnosis is not made until the adolescent period, when the patient experiences amenorrhea and possibly cyclic abdominal pain. In these circumstances, a bluish bulging hymen may be observed on genital inspection and a mass will be appreciated on rectoabdominal palpation.

In newborns, repair by incision of the hymenal tissue at the bedside is performed in the transverse direction to avoid inadvertent extension of the incision anteriorly or posteriorly

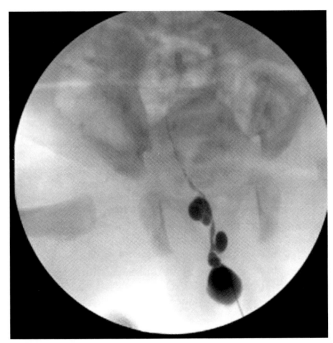

Figure 129–17. Retrograde injection of an ectopic ureter inserting into a Gartner's duct cyst. After injection of a vaginal cyst, contrast ascends cranially into an atretic, dysplastic ureter.

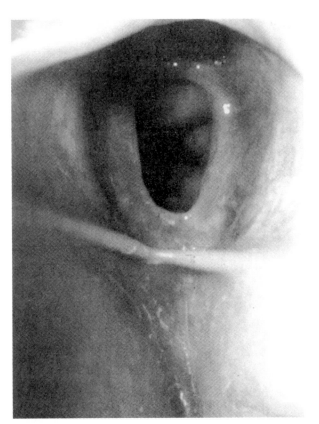

Figure 129–18. Normal hymenal ring. (From Emans SJ: Office evaluation of the child and adolescent. In Emans SJ, Laufer MR, Goldstein DP [eds]: Pediatric and Adolescent Gynecology, 4th ed. Philadelphia, Lippincott, Williams & Wilkins, 1998.)

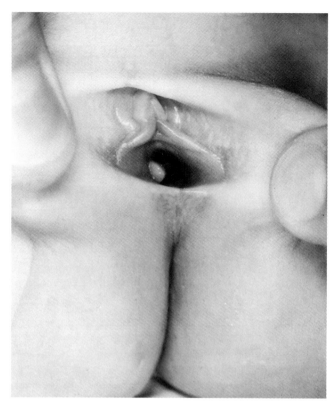

Figure 129–19. Hymenal skin tag.

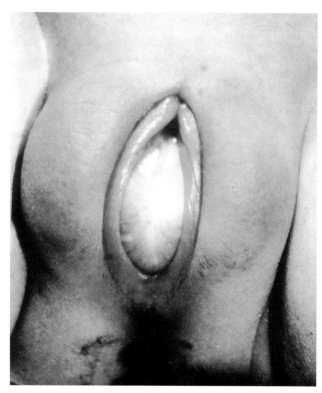

Figure 129–20. Imperforate hymen. Note the significant distention from vaginal secretions. (From Yerkes EB, Rink RC: What urologists should know about pediatric gynecologic abnormalities. Contemp Urol 2002;14:12.)

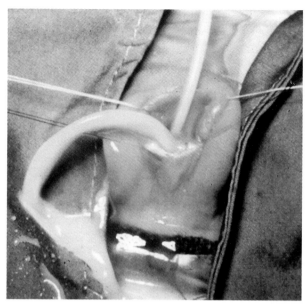

Figure 129–21. Intraoperative photograph showing incisional drainage of an imperforate hymen. (From Yerkes EB, Rink RC: What urologists should know about pediatric gynecologic abnormalities. Contemp Urol 2002;14:12.)

(which might injure the urethra or rectal structures). Simple aspiration of the vagina without a definite drainage procedure should be discouraged because incompletely evacuated material may be prone to ascending bacterial growth. In pubertal girls, general anesthesia with excision of excess hymenal tissue may be indicated (Fig. 129–21).

Acquired abnormalities of the hymenal ring usually result from sexual abuse. The associated finding of a hematoma, abrasion, or laceration in combination with hymenal transection should raise the possibility of this diagnosis. Proper examination under anesthesia and forensic swabbing of affected areas should be undertaken with the use of a standardized protocol.

Prolapsed Urethra. Urethral prolapse generally involves complete circumferential eversion of the urethral mucosa at the level of the external urethral meatus (Fig. 129–22) (Lowe et al, 1986). This entity, which was first described by Solinger in 1732, occurs most often in prepubertal black girls and in postmenopausal white women (Epstein and Strauss, 1937; Richardson et al, 1982). Various causes that have been proposed for urethral prolapse include hypoestrogenism (Desai and Cohen, 1997), abnormal connections between the inner longitudinal and outer circular muscle layers of the distal urethra (Lowe et al, 1986), and episodic increases in intraabdominal pressure (Lowe et al, 1986; Desai and Cohen, 1997; Valerie et al, 1999). The most common initial complaint is bleeding from the edematous and friable mucosa, which results in blood spotting on the underwear (Richardson et al, 1982; Chaouachi et al, 1989). Urethral prolapse is easily recognized as a doughnut-shaped mass with the urethral meatus at the center. If the diagnosis can be confirmed by passing a urethral catheter, radiographic evaluation is not indicated (Nussbaum and Lebowitz, 1983). Treatment options include observation, topical steroids, and surgical excision (Redman, 1982; Fernandes et al, 1993). Sitz baths may be helpful. Non-

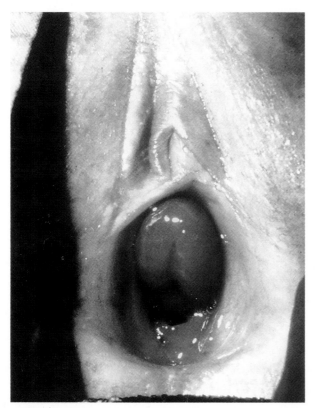

Figure 129–22. Urethral prolapse. (From Yerkes EB, Rink RC: What urologists should know about pediatric gynecologic abnormalities. Contemp Urol 2002;14:12.)

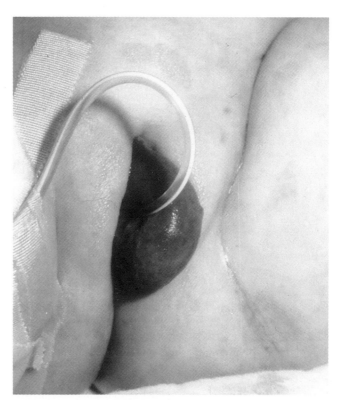

Figure 129–23. Prolapsed ureterocele. Note the catheter inserted in the urethra.

operative treatment may lead to spontaneous reduction of the prolapse, but a recurrence rate of up to 67% has been noted (Jerkins et al, 1984). Many methods of surgical repair have been described. Circumferential excision of the redundant mucosa with subsequent suturing of the normal urethra to the vestibule is the procedure of choice (Devine and Kessel, 1980). Other methods, including ligation over a transurethral catheter with subsequent sloughing and cryosurgery, should be discouraged (Owens and Morse, 1968; Klaus and Stein, 1973).

Prolapsed Ureterocele. An ectopic ureterocele is a cystic dilatation of the terminal portion of the ureter that occurs predominantly in white females (Mandell et al, 1980). Approximately 90% of ectopic ureteroceles are associated with the upper pole of a duplex collecting system. Although they normally remain positioned proximal to the bladder neck, some may prolapse through the urethra during micturition, almost always in infancy, and result in urinary retention and a relative urologic emergency (Gingell et al, 1971). Depending on the length of time that the ureterocele has been prolapsed, it may vary in color from pink to dusky purple (Fig. 129–23). If a prolapsed ureterocele is in the differential diagnosis, bladder-renal ultrasonography should be performed to look for upper pole hydronephrosis in a duplicated collecting system (Fig. 129–24).

Treatment of a prolapsed ureterocele consists of either needle decompression or incision and reduction and then placement of a urethral catheter. Although this can occasionally be achieved in the emergency room setting, abdominal

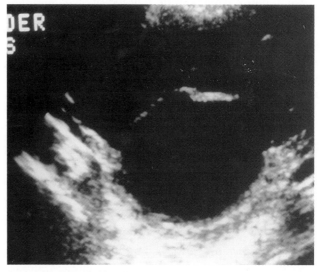

Figure 129–24. Bladder ultrasound demonstrating a ureterocele. (From Yerkes EB, Rink RC: What urologists should know about pediatric gynecologic abnormalities. Contemp Urol 2002;14:12.)

straining by the infant may make this procedure difficult, and treatment under general anesthesia is often preferable.

Injection of radiographic contrast material into the ureterocele can be helpful in identifying the relevant anatomy.

Urethral Polyp. The pediatric equivalent of a urethral caruncle, namely, a urethral polyp, is a rare lesion that can be manifested as an intralabial mass (Fig. 129–25). The etiology of true lesions has not been completely elucidated, but in a young

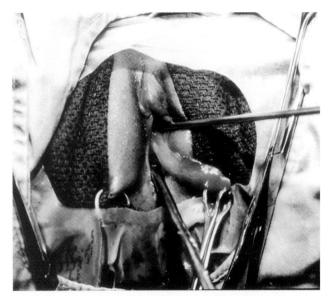

Figure 129-25. Urethral polyp: probe in urethra, Babcock clamp on urethral polyp (From Yerkes EB, Rink RC: What urologists should know about pediatric gynecologic abnormalities. Contemp Urol 2002;14:12.)

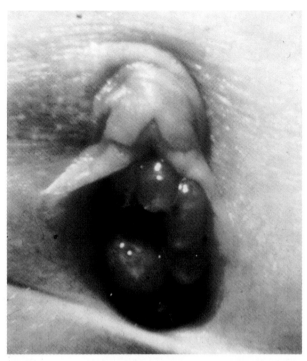

Figure 129-26. Vaginal rhabdomyosarcoma. (From Yerkes EB, Rink RC: What urologists should know about pediatric gynecologic abnormalities. Contemp Urol 2002;14:12.)

child they probably represent either hamartomatous growth or a response to inflammation.

We described two young girls with an interlabial mass. Histologic examination of each excised mass revealed a benign urethral polyp covered with transitional and squamous epithelium (Klee et al, 1993). Urethral polyps should be included in the differential diagnosis of an interlabial mass in young female patients.

Vaginal Rhabdomyosarcoma. Vaginal rhabdomyosarcoma is most often manifested as a grapelike cluster of tissue emanating from the posterior aspect of the vestibule (Fig. 129–26). The mean age of patients with primary vaginal tumors is younger than 2 years (Hays et al, 1988). Of all the female genital tract primary tumors, vaginal primaries appear to have the best prognosis. This excellent prognosis is thought to be a result of predominance of the embryonal cell type and relatively early detection because of symptoms of bleeding (Hays et al, 1988). Once a tissue diagnosis has been made by biopsy, proper staging with abdominal and pelvic computed tomography, chest radiography, and bone marrow biopsy is critical to optimal stratification of these patients into treatment protocols (Hays et al, 1985). Advances in chemotherapy have led to a reduction in the role of surgery for this disease with each subsequent Intergroup Rhabdomyosarcoma Study (IRS) trial: IRS-I, 100%; IRS-II, 70%; IRS-III, 30%; and IRS-IV, 13% (Andrassy et al, 1999). After chemotherapy, local resection may be required, but unlike other malignancies of the vagina, wide excision of the involved organ has no role except for persistent or recurrent disease (Hensley, 2000).

CLASSIFICATION OF UROGENITAL SINUS AND CLOACAL ANOMALIES

Persistent urogenital sinus anomalies are one of the more complex problems that a pediatric urologist will face, and they occur in a spectrum. Evaluation and management must be meticulous.

In urogenital sinus anomalies, there is a persistent communication of the vagina with the urinary tract. Communication of the vagina with the urinary tract may occur at any point from the urethral meatus to the bladder, but the majority occur within the mid to distal portion of the urethra. The two structures join and exit on the perineum as a single common urogenital sinus channel.

A persistent urogenital sinus is **seen in four entities.** Most commonly it occurs in **genital ambiguity states,** most frequently with congenital adrenal hyperplasia (CAH) (Fig. 129–27). It can also occur as a **pure urogenital sinus** with normal external genitalia (Fig. 129–28). In persistent **cloacal anomalies** there is the added complexity of rectal involvement, with all three systems—genital, urinary, and rectal—exiting as an isolated single perineal opening. More recently, **female exstrophy** has been thought to represent a form of persistent urogenital sinus (Adams, 2000).

Early descriptions of this confluence were based on previous medical training. Urologists described the vagina as entering the urethra, whereas gynecologists noted that the urethra entered the vaginal vestibule (Jones and Jones, 1954). Jaramillo and Lebowitz (1990) noted that on examination that the external cloacal orifice appears vaginal in nature in some but in others appears more like a normal urethral orifice (Figs. 129–29 and 129–30). **Regardless of how the confluence of the urinary and genital tracts is described, the confluence location in relation to the bladder neck is a more critical factor in surgical management than the length of the common channel** (Rink et al, 2005a).

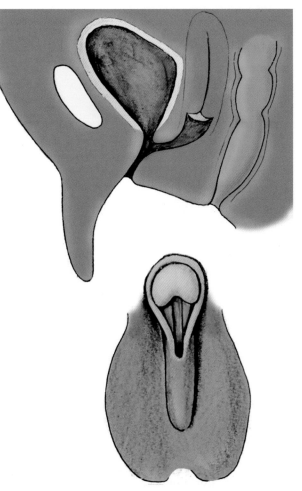

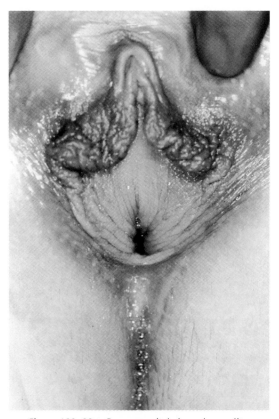

Figure 129–28. Pure urogenital sinus abnormality.

Figure 129–27. Urogenital sinus in a patient with intersex.

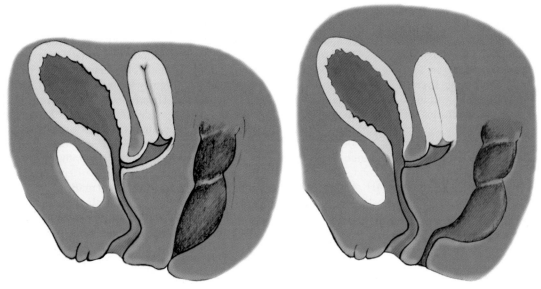

Figure 129–29. *Left,* Urethral-type urogenital sinus. *Right,* Urethral-type urogenital sinus with an anteriorly placed rectum.

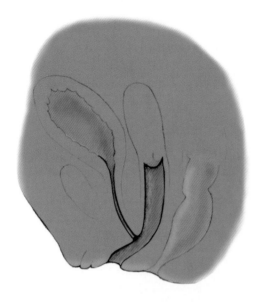
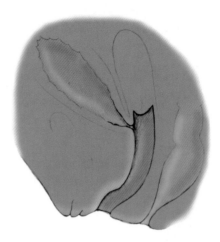

Figure 129–30. Vaginal-type urogenital sinus showing high (*right*) and low (*left*) confluence.

Evaluation

Urogenital sinus abnormalities are most often seen in intersex states, most commonly in association with CAH, which has been noted to have an incidence as high as 1 in 500 in the nonclassic, mild form (Hughes, 1988). The most common enzymatic defect in CAH resulting in genital ambiguity is 21-hydroxylase deficiency, which occurs in approximately 1 in 15,000 to 16,000 persons (Spieser and White, 2003; Merke and Bornstein, 2005). Therefore, initial management must focus on making an accurate diagnosis to allow proper gender identification. Every effort should be made to establish the genetic sex within 48 hours. Children with CAH require careful monitoring of fluid and electrolytes because 67% to 75% will have significant salt wasting (Spieser and White, 2003; Merke and Bornstein, 2005). Evaluation should include rapid karyotyping of cultured peripheral leukocytes, measurement of serum electrolyte levels, and determination of hormonal levels for CAH. All results are shared with the gender assignment team, which includes the parents, pediatric endocrinologist, pediatric urologist, neonatologist, child psychiatrist, and often clergy. The child should not be named until sex assignment is complete (Rink and Adams, 1998).

Cloacal anomalies are a much more complex problem involving multiple organ systems, but fortunately they occur in only 1 in every 40,000 to 50,000 patients (Karlin et al, 1989). They are the most challenging of the anorectal malformations and make up 13.6% of this group (Fleming et al,

1986). These children have a very broad spectrum of findings on examination of the external genitalia. Some may have a prominent phallic structure and also initially require evaluation for an intersex state.

History and Physical Examination

The history and physical examination are extremely helpful in cases of genital ambiguity and can often lead to the diagnosis itself. It is critical to determine whether the mother ingested any medications during pregnancy, especially androgenic substances. A family history of early infant death or fluid and electrolyte abnormalities suggests CAH. Have other children had genital ambiguity or gender dysphoria at puberty? Notation should be made of any family members with abnormal pubertal development.

The physical examination can at times be very useful in determining the appropriate gender and in helping to identify other organ systems involved. A general evaluation of the child's overall health should be completed before focusing on the genital examination. Abnormal facies suggesting a syndrome should be noted. **Hypertension can occur in children with genital ambiguity secondary to CAH with 11β-hydroxylase deficiency.** Therefore, blood pressure should be documented. Evidence of dehydration may also lead to a diagnosis of CAH. On abdominal examination, a mass, particularly a suprapubic mass, may be present because of a distended bladder or hydrometrocolpos, or both. **Hydrometrocolpos is frequently an initial sign and is often the only early finding in pure urogenital sinus abnormalities.**

In cloacal anomalies, abdominal distention may be severe secondary to hydrometrocolpos and bladder and intestinal distention. Hydrometrocolpos was noted commonly in early series (Chappell and Bleloch, 1973; Klugo et al, 1974); its incidence ranged from 29% of Pena's patients (1989) to 63% of those reported by Bartholomew and Gonzales (1978). It is caused most commonly by preferential flow of urine into the vagina (or vaginas) with voiding and associated poor vaginal drainage. Maternal estrogen stimulation of the cervical glands results in mucus production, thereby further adding to the distention. Urine flow can occur into the rectum also. This distention has resulted in edematous, cyanotic legs and respiratory distress, as well as acidosis (Raffensberger, 1988).

The lower part of the back should be examined to identify any evidence of spinal cord abnormalities, which can be associated with urogenital sinus abnormalities and are very common with cloacal anomalies. Such abnormalities may take the form of a sacral dimple, hair patch, or area of abnormal pigmentation, but more commonly there is evidence of a bone abnormality, such as an abnormal buttock crease or flattened buttocks as a result of sacral agenesis.

Genital examination should note the size of the phallus and the consistency of the erectile bodies. Any degree of curvature should be documented. Huffman multiplied the width of the glans times the length of the phallus to determine the "clitoral index," which he noted should be less than 3.5 mm to be normal and was of concern when greater than 10 mm (Huffman, 1976). The gonads should be sought, and when found, their number, location, and consistency should be noted. If both gonads are descended, it is extremely unlikely that a 46,XX chromosome makeup will be found. The labioscrotal folds should be examined for their relationship to the phallus and rectum, as well as for the degree of fusion. Increased pigmentation of the labioscrotal folds and areola may be seen in some cases of CAH as a result of increased levels of melanocyte-stimulating hormone.

In urogenital sinus anomalies, the location of the anus should be noted. Although it is usually in the normal location, anterior displacement is not uncommon, and this bridges the gap to cloacal anomalies (see Fig. 129–29). A gentle rectal examination is helpful in identifying a cervix.

Examination of a child with a persistent cloaca deserves special mention. There is a single perineal orifice because the rectum also enters this common channel. The appearance of the external genitalia assumes a much wider spectrum, from a nearly normal female appearance to much more bizarre appearances such as genital transposition or a blank-appearing perineum (doll-like) (Fig. 129–31) (Hendren, 1989). In some instances there is an enlarged phallic structure that gives the genitalia an ambiguous appearance. The single perineal opening may exit what appears to be a normal vaginal introitus, or it may extend to the tip of a phallic structure. We, as well as others, have encountered children with a secondary accessory channel that exits the tip of the phallus (Hendren, 1989; Karlin et al, 1989; Krstic et al, 2001; Rink et al, 2005b).

Cloacal anomalies are associated with a high incidence of related anomalies in other organ systems. The authors found 14 of 23 patients with renal anomalies, including 6 with solitary kidneys, 4 with renal dysplasia, 2 with ureteropelvic joint obstruction, 1 with duplication, and 1 with cross-fused ectopia. There were also two with bladder duplications (Rink et al, 2005b). Sixty percent have some degree of septation of the vagina and uterus (Warne et al, 2003). Kay and Tank (1977) reported that 13% of patients with cloacal anomalies have cardiovascular abnormalities, 10% have central nervous system problems, and respiratory abnormalities are noted in 5%; vertebral, particularly sacral anomalies are common. Many have the VACTERL association (vertebral abnormalities, anal atresia, cardiac abnormalities, tracheoesophageal fistula and/or esophageal atresia, renal agenesis and dysplasia,

and limb defects), so tracheoesophageal fistula is often present (Hendren, 1986, 1988). Other gastrointestinal anomalies have been noted, including doudenal atresia and rectal duplication in 2% (Karlin et al, 1989).

KEY POINTS: UROGENITAL SINUS ANOMALIES—EVALUATION

- Key points of the history and physical examination are findings of a family history of sudden infant death, fluid and electrolyte abnormalities, hypertension, lower extremity cyanosis, palpable gonads, and hyperpigmentation.

- The level of the urethrovaginal confluence and the location of the rectum must be identified radiographically and endoscopically, with note made of their relationship to the bladder neck. Ultrasonography is mandatory to look for the uterus, ovaries, and kidneys.

Radiographic and Endoscopic Evaluation

Urogenital Sinus Abnormalities

Certain critical details of the anatomy, including the length of the common urogenital sinus, the location of the vaginal confluence and its proximity to the bladder neck, the size of the vagina and the number of vaginas, the presence of a cervix, and bladder and urethral anatomy, must be defined by radiographic and endoscopic evaluation. The authors believe that the location of the vagina in relation to the bladder neck is the critical issue in determining the type of surgery, and this distance is more important than the length of the common channel. Vaginal confluence with the urinary tract occurs in a continuum from the bladder to a nearly normal location in the perineum. **It is not simply "high" (proximal/suprasphincteric) or "low" (distal/infrasphincteric)** (Powell et al, 1995; Hendren and Crawford, 1969; Rink and Kaefer, 2002) (Fig. 129–32).

A new urogenital sinus classification that measures the exact distance of the common channel and the distance of the bladder neck to the vagina has been devised to help delineate the exact level of the confluence, as well as clitoral size and appearance of the external genital (Rink et al, 2005a).

Ultrasonography of the urinary tract and pelvis is mandatory. The location and normalcy of the kidneys, ovaries, and uterus should be defined. Any bladder or vaginal distention should be noted. A cerebriform appearance with enlargement of the adrenal glands is indicative of CAH (Brock et al, 1998).

Filling the entire bladder, urethra, vagina, and sinus with contrast (i.e., **genitography**) **is critical in the anatomic evaluation of a child with a urogenital sinus** (Figs. 129–33 and 129–34). Genitography is performed by placing a Foley catheter with the balloon occluding the perineal meatus and injecting contrast. It is often helpful to pass a catheter into the bladder as for a voiding cystourethrogram. A cervical impression at the vaginal dome denotes normal female internal

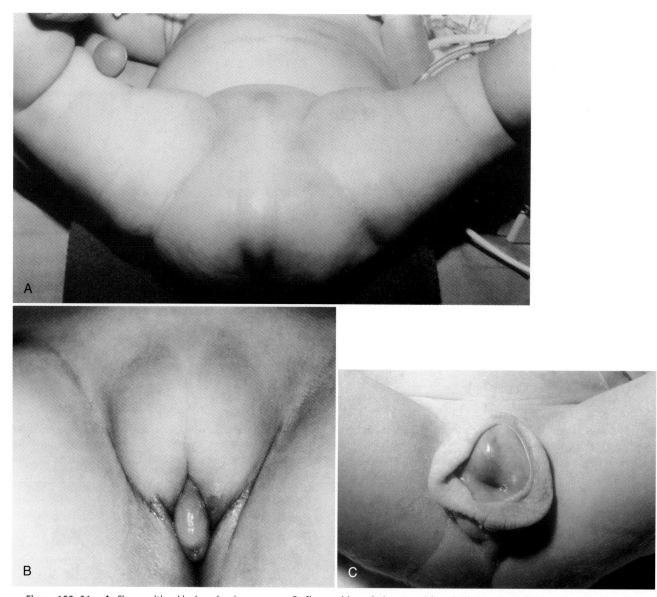

Figure 129–31. **A,** Cloaca with a blank perineal appearance. **B,** Cloaca with genital transposition. **C,** Cloaca, vaginal type, external appearance.

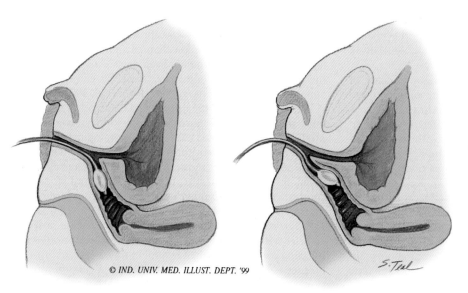

© IND. UNIV. MED. ILLUST. DEPT. '99

S. Teal

Figure 129–32. Fogarty catheter placed in the vagina in high confluence (*left*) and in low confluence (*right*). (Copyright 1999, Indiana University Medical Illustration Department.)

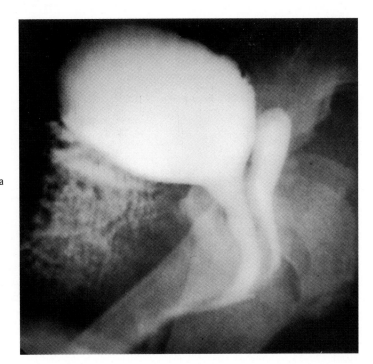

Figure 129–33. Genitography showing low confluence of the urethra and vagina.

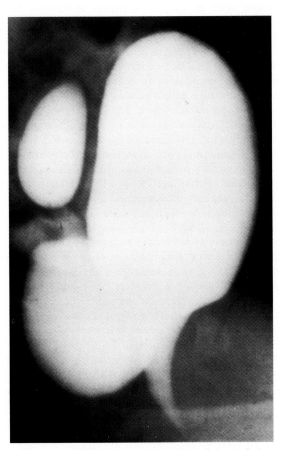

Figure 129–34. Genitography showing high confluence of the vagina entering near the bladder neck, with flow of contrast material into the uterus.

organs. MRI is of limited value in CAH but may be helpful to define the anatomy in pure urogenital sinus anomalies or intersex conditions.

The most helpful diagnostic study in defining the anatomy for surgical reconstruction is endoscopy. In patients with CAH, endoscopy is usually performed at the time of reconstruction but may be necessary as a separate early procedure to help with gender identity in intersex cases or in those with complex pure urogenital sinus anomalies or if the vagina is not identified on genitography (Rink and Kaefer, 2002). In the latter situation, multiple punctuate openings in the proximal portion of the urethra may be observed (Donahoe and Gustafson, 1994). We have found it helpful to pass a ureteral catheter into the opening and evaluate the vagina fluoroscopically in this situation (Rink and Kaefer, 2002). Again, the exact location, size, and number of the vaginas should be recorded (Fig. 129–35). Hendren has noted a malelike external sphincter in severely masculined children, with the vagina entering proximal to it in a verumontanum-like structure (Hendren and Crawford, 1969; Hendren and Atala, 1995). In our experience, only rarely have we seen such a well-defined sphincter (Adams and Rink, 1998).

Rarely, even with the evaluation described, some intersex children require gonadal biopsy or evaluation of the internal genitalia, which has historically been done by laparotomy but in most cases can now be easily performed laparoscopically. Regardless of the means, it should be carried out only when the findings would influence the gender of rearing (Rink and Adams, 1999). **If a biopsy is necessary, a deep incision should be made in the gonad because the ovarian component of ova-testes may completely surround the testicular component or be located at the poles** (Hensle and Kennedy, 1998; Schnitzer and Donahoe, 2001). Finally, scrotal skin biopsy may at times be helpful in males with incomplete androgen

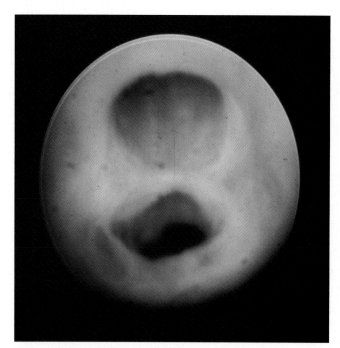

Figure 129–35. Endoscopic view of confluence. The urethra is superior; the vagina is inferior.

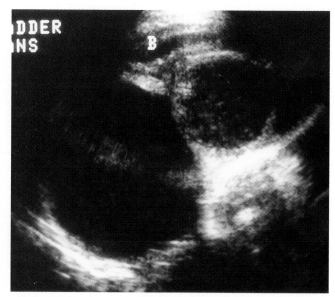

Figure 129–36. Pelvic ultrasound in a patient with a cloaca. Duplicate fluid-filled vaginas are seen posterior to the decompressed bladder (B).

insensitivity, decreased 5α-reductase activity, or decreased dihydrotestosterone binding (Griffin and Wilson, 1989).

Cloacal Anomalies

Evaluation for cloacal anomalies begins with antenatal ultrasound because there have now been several groups who have reported the prenatal diagnosis of persistent cloaca (Petrikovsky et al, 1986; Shalev et al, 1986; Cilento et al, 1994; Odibo et al, 1997; Adams and Rink, 1998; Cacciaguerra et al, 1998; Warne et al, 2002b). The diagnosis has been made as early as 19 weeks' gestation. **The finding of transient fetal ascites with bilobed or trilobed pelvic cystic structures, bilateral hydronephrosis, and decreased amniotic fluid is diagnostic** (Cacciaguerra et al, 1998; Warne et al, 2002a). The ascites is thought to develop via retrograde flow of urine into the uterus and out the fallopian tubes secondary to outlet obstruction from the distended vagina (Adams et al, 1998; Cacciaguerra et al, 1998).

Postnatal radiographic evaluation begins with a plain abdominal film (Jaramillo and Lebowitz, 1990). A pelvic mass may be obvious. Retrograde flow of urine and meconium, as described earlier, may result in the classic linear calcifications or calcified meconium. More granular calcifications may be noted along the course of the rectum as a result of urine flow into the rectum that yields calcified meconium (Jaramillo and Lebowitz, 1990).

Abdominal ultrasonography is very important to not only visualize the pelvic anatomy but also visualize the kidneys because hydronephrosis is common (Hendren, 1998). Hydronephrosis is usually related to hydrocolpos, with the distended vagina compressing the bladder neck and resulting in varying degrees of bladder outlet obstruction (Hendren, 1998). Ureteral compression may also occur; however, we have

seen hydronephrosis caused by primary obstructive megaureter in patients with cloacal anomaly.

Ultrasound may also detect other renal anomalies. **Renal anomalies such as dysplasia, fusion anomalies, ectopia, ureteropelvic junction obstruction, and duplication have been seen in 33% to 83% of children with a persistent cloaca** (Kay and Tank, 1977; Warne et al, 2002b; Rink et al, 2005b).

As with urogenital sinus abnormalities, genitography and endoscopy are mandatory to define the anatomy, which is even more complex with a cloacal anomaly. The technique and goals of genitography and endoscopy are the same but must now include identification of the rectal as well as the vaginal confluence. The length of the urethra and its communication with the cloaca are important for reconstructive purposes. In Hendren's patients, the urinary communication to the cloaca was urethral in 77%, but in 23% there was virtually no urethra, and the communication was noted at the bladder neck level (Jaramillo and Lebowitz, 1990). The vaginal anatomy is also much more complex and variable. In Hendren's report of 154 cloaca patients, 66 patients had one vagina, 68 had two vaginas, and the vagina was absent in 20 (Hendren, 1998). Vaginal duplication has been seen in nearly all of our own patient population (Rink and Yerkes, 2001) (Fig. 129–36). The duplication anatomy is also variable. Most authors have observed that the vaginas enter side by side with a single opening into the cloaca, but separate openings have been noted. The vaginas may be of different size, and one may enter the sidewall of the other. A cervix is usually seen at the top of each vagina. **The vaginal entrance into the cloaca again lies along a spectrum from the bladder to a location near the perineum.** Although the uterus is usually similar to the vagina (i.e., two vaginas with two uteri), the vagina may be absent with the uterus still present. Hall and associates (1985) found a bicornuate uterus, hypoplastic uterus, or uterus didelphys in 35% of their patients with persistent cloaca.

The rectal confluence is equally as complex, with the entrance in our experience most commonly located just at

the level of the vaginal confluence. This rectal opening may be broad, or it may have a long, narrow fistulous tract. It can even enter the vagina or bladder with no communication to the cloaca itself. The most common entrance in our experience is within the septum of a duplicated vagina, with all three joining the cloaca together (Rink and Kaefer, 2002). The various rectal entries are illustrated in Figure 129–37. The rectal communication has been found to be vaginal in 68% and cloacal in 11%, with the remainder in other locations (Jaramillo and Lebowitz, 1990). The length and configuration of the common cloaca should also be noted because it has important surgical as well as anatomic implications. At times, the common channel is narrow and appears very much like a urethra; in other instances, the channel is much larger and redundant and appears more like a vagina. The urethral appearance was found in 48% of patients and the vaginal appearance in 52% (Jaramillo and Lebowitz, 1990). **We and others have noted that the urethral types result in higher outlet resistance and are more likely to lead to hydrocolpos** (Warne et al, 2002a; Adams et al, 1998).

The frequent presence of associated organ system abnormalities necessitates further radiographic evaluation. Echocardiography should always be performed. MRI is necessary for evaluating the lumbosacral spine and assessing the pelvic anatomy and musculature. Historically, it has been well recognized that sacral anomalies are common. Pena (1989) noted a normal sacrum in only 35% of his 54 patients, and Jaramillo and Lebowitz (1990) reported sacral agenesis in 40% of Hendren's 65 patients. De Filippo and associates (1999) found 10 of 21 patients with imperforate anus or cloaca to have an abnormality of the sacrum and spine. **With the use of MRI, spinal cord abnormalities have been more commonly detected, with an incidence as high as 43%** (Jaramillo and Lebowitz, 1990). Hendren (1998) found that a third of his patients had a tethered spinal cord. Skin stigmata in the lumbosacral region were absent in 8 of 10 patients with spinal cord tethering in Morimoto and colleagues' report (2003). MRI has also been very helpful in defining the level of the rectal atresia and in identifying the degree of sphincteric muscle development (Sato et al, 1988).

Because of the complexity of the anatomy and the frequency of hydrometrocolpos, a child with a cloacal anomaly often needs endoscopy early as a separate procedure to decompress the vagina and bladder and to define the anatomy. As a general rule, visualization of the vagina (or vaginas) is easily accomplished, but entry into the bladder can be very difficult and even impossible at times in a newborn because it is compressed very anteriorly by the distended vagina. The vagina should always first be emptied. Identification of the rectal fistula can also be difficult at times. Once it is located, mucus and fecal material should be irrigated from the colon, which can be done by irrigation through the scope in combination with irrigation from the colostomy.

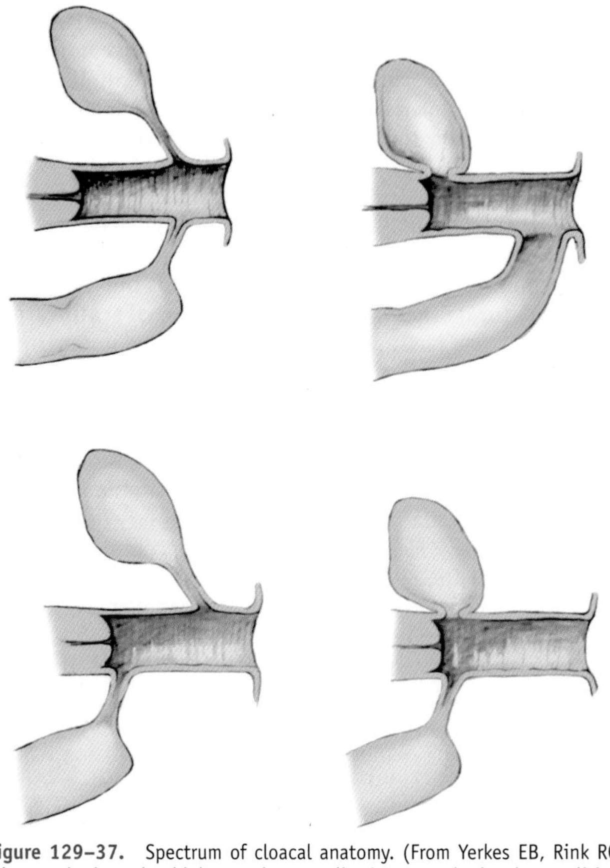

SURGICAL RECONSTRUCTION OF INTERSEX CONDITIONS AND UROGENITAL SINUS
Initial Management, Timing, and Principles

The majority of children born with a urogenital sinus have genital ambiguity, and this should be initially evaluated by the gender assignment team. It is extremely important that the family be made aware of all controversies surrounding genital surgery. Certainly, most families, physicians, and surgeons have historically made the decision to proceed with early feminizing procedures to "normalize" the child and allow a positive psychosocial adjustment (Schober, 1998). The thought has been that raising a child with genital ambiguity would be extremely difficult (Thomas, 2004). Recently, a number of advocacy groups and physicians have begun to question this wisdom. Informed consent is impossible with an infant, and many believe that the decision for genital surgery is a right of the patient, not the parents. The ethical issues involving parents' rights and responsibilities to make decisions for their child remain unresolved (Lee and Witchel, 2002). Unfortunately, there are no data on the impact of raising a child with genital ambiguity (Rangecroft, 2002).

At this time, excellent cosmetic results can be achieved by feminizing genitoplasty. However, it must be remembered that one's sexual identity is a result of many factors. It is known that the brain is the dominant organ in sexual orientation (Woodhouse, 2004). Schober (1999) has pointed out that little is known about how adults adjust to genitoplasty, nor are there any data in infants undergoing genitoplasty on what path they

Figure 129–37. Spectrum of cloacal anatomy. (From Yerkes EB, Rink RC: What urologists should know about pediatric gynecologic abnormalities. Contemp Urol 2002;14:12.)

might have chosen had the opportunity been given to them as adults. It is clear that genital surgery does not "cure" intersex.

Unfortunately, a dilemma remains for intersex surgery because there is no absolute correct answer at this time. Information should never be withheld from the parents, and counseling should be provided. Parents must be informed of all risks and options and be made aware of the current state of knowledge. They should also be given access to advocacy groups.

For the purposes of the remaining description of surgical techniques, it is assumed that all parties (parents and medical team) agree that surgery is warranted.

Children born with a urogenital sinus associated with genital ambiguity usually have clitoral hypertrophy, fusion of the labia with absence of the labia minor, and a common urogenital sinus (Fig. 129–38). **Therefore, genital reconstruction involves three steps: (1) clitoroplasty, (2) labioplasty, and (3) vaginoplasty.**

Most authors currently recommend that clitoroplasty be done early in life, but this has again been challenged by intersex advocacy groups. In the mid-1900s there was not thought to be an optimal timing for reconstruction (Jones and Jones, 1954; Lattimer, 1961), but more recently, clitoral reconstruction has been carried out progressively earlier. Gross and colleagues in 1966 and Spence and Allen in 1973 noted that clitoral surgery can ideally be performed when the child is 1 year old. By the 1980s, clitoral surgery was recommended as early as the first few months of life (Snyder et al, 1983). More

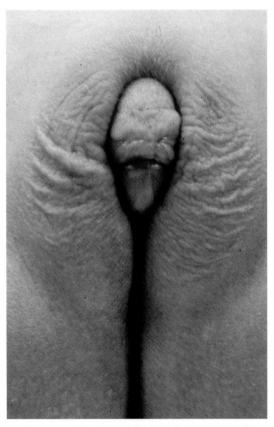

Figure 129–38. Moderately virilized external genitalia.

recently, de Jong and Boemers (1995) reported surgical correction at 1 to 3 weeks of age.

The optimal timing for vaginoplasty continues to be debated. Some have based the timing partly on the level of the vaginal confluence. A consensus statement on CAH from the Lawson-Wilkins Pediatric Endocrine Society and the European Society for Pediatric Endocrinology recommends surgery in the 2- to 6-month-old range for those with a high vaginal confluence, and surgery between 12 months and adolescence is not recommended (Consesus statement, 2002). **There is inadequate evidence at this time to give up our current practice of early vaginoplasty.**

Simultaneous performance of clitoroplasty, vaginoplasty, and labioplasty has been the standard practice for a child with a low (distal) vaginal confluence. Two separate schools of thought have been put forth for a high vaginal confluence. Some believe that the high rate of vaginal stenosis warrants delay of vaginal surgery until after puberty, which also avoids any need for vaginal dilatation (Sotiropoulos et al, 1976; Snyder et al, 1983; Alizai et al, 1999; Creighton et al, 2001; Rangecroft, 2002; Thomas, 2004). Others have found the incidence of vaginal stenosis to be higher in those who undergo surgery after puberty rather than during infancy (Eroglu et al, 2004). **We along with others believe that vaginoplasty, regardless of the vaginal location, is best combined with clitoroplasty and labioplasty in a single stage. This allows the surgeon flexibility in using redundant phallic skin for the reconstruction, which is compromised when the skin has previously been mobilized** (Mandell et al, 1988; Gonzalez and Fernandes, 1990; de Jong and Boemers, 1995; Hendren and Atala, 1995; Rink et al, 1997; Passerini-Glazel, 1998). **Furthermore, several authors have noted that maternal estrogen stimulation of the child's genitalia results in thicker vaginal tissue that is better vascularized, thus making it easier to perform early vaginal mobilization** (Passerini-Glazel, 1989; Donahoe and Gustafson, 1994; de Jong and Boemers, 1995; Rink and Adams, 1999; Farkas et al, 2001; Hensle and Bingham, 2002; Eroglu et al, 2004).

Today, when performing clitoroplasty, every effort is made to not only provide excellent cosmesis but also retain normal clitoral innervation for optimal sexual gratification. Clitoral surgery has undergone significant evolution. Initial efforts were primarily directed at not just amputating the clitoris but also completely excising all clitoral tissue to avoid any later painful erection (Jones and Jones, 1954; Gross and Randolf, 1966; Hendren and Crawford, 1969). Clitoral amputation was based on reports by both Hampson and Gulliver, who noted that the clitoris was not necessary for normal sexual response (Hampson, 1955). As recognition of the importance of the clitoris evolved, several ingenious clitoral recession techniques that preserved the innervation and all clitoral tissue were reported. Lattimer, in 1961, recessed the clitoris in subcutaneous fat and buried it beneath the skin. Kaplan (1967) reported an interesting technique of splitting the two corpora apart and closing in a transverse Henike-Mikulicz fashion. Randolph and Hung (1970) and also Pellerin (1965) buried the corpora beneath the pubis. Efforts to preserve the glans based on a flap were attempted as early as the 1930s by Young, but the glans sloughed (Young, 1937). In 1961, Schmid was the first to report excising corporal tissue yet preserving the neurovascular bundle with the glans intact.

Kumar et al (1974) later noted a similar technique proposed by Keifer the same year. Spence and Allen (1973) excised all of the clitoral shaft but left the glans intact to survive from the attached ventral urethral plate. **Virtually all techniques since have been based on Schmid's preservation of the neurovascular bundle** (Shaw, 1977; Barrett and Gonzales, 1980; Glassberg and Laungani, 1981; Mollard et al, 1981; Rajfer and Ehrlich, 1982). Although the glans often did well with these techniques, shrinkage and devascularization occurred at times. **Kogan and associates (1983) reported subtunical excision of the erectile tissue by incising laterally through Buck's fascia to resect the erectile corpus cavernosa tissue.** Clitoroplasty techniques exhibited only minor technical advances until the recent demonstration of the neurovascular anatomy of the clitoris by Baskin and coworkers (1999). This work suggests that a ventral incision would preserve not only the main dorsal neurovascular bundle but also the neural branches that fan out laterally (Fig. 129–39). Currently, much research is under way to further evaluate clitoral neuroanatomy, as well as techniques to evaluate sexual sensitivity.

Vaginoplasty techniques have similarly evolved, with all repairs based on a few landmark reports. **Almost every vaginal repair today uses a posteriorly based perineal flap proposed by Lattimer and originally described by Fortunoff and coworkers in 1964.** This wide-based Fortunoff flap has recently been modified to a more omega-shaped flap that has resulted in improved cosmesis (Jenak et al, 2001; Freitas-Filho et al, 2003). **In 1969, Hendren and Crawford reported a "pull-through" vaginoplasty for a high vaginal confluence.** Their efforts to establish the location of the vaginal confluence as the determining factor for the type of vaginoplasty remains the basis for all vaginoplasties today. Vaginal reconstruction techniques now generally take the form of one of four types. **(1) The cut-back vaginoplasty is rarely used and is appropriate for only simple labial fusion. (2) The flap vaginoplasty is applicable to a low (distal) vaginal confluence.** In this procedure, the posterior walls of the sinus and vagina are opened, but the anterior wall of the vagina is left intact. The posterior

perineal flap fits into the opened vagina. **This procedure does not change the level of confluence; it simply widely opens the introitus and urogenital sinus** (Rink and Adams, 1998). The authors and others believe that a flap vaginoplasty should never be used for patients with a very high vaginal confluence because it may result in a short hypospadiac urethra, vaginal voiding, many infections, and even incontinence (Hendren and Atala, 1995; Rink and Adams, 1999). **(3) The pull-through vaginoplasty is used for a very high confluence.** In this procedure, the vagina is separated from the urogenital sinus, and the sinus is used to create a urethra. The mobilized vagina may reach the perineum, but in most cases skin flaps have been required. **(4) Complete vaginal replacement can be achieved by several techniques, but it is used only for a rudimentary or absent vagina.**

Labioplasty techniques also continue to evolve. In CAH and other intersex states, the labia minora are absent and the labia majora are superior to the new vaginal introitus. Labia minora are created by using the split phallic skin as described by Marberger (1975). Both the labia majora and labia minor should be moved inferiorly by Y-V–plasty to create a normal cosmetic appearance of the vagina now located between the labia (Hendren and Donahoe, 1980; Rink and Adams, 1998) (Fig. 129–40).

Regardless of the surgeon's personal bias toward reconstruction or its timing, a balanced presentation of all pros and cons of surgery versus no surgery is imperative. All current data should be made available to the parents and the risks associated with each path clearly defined. The ultimate decision is the parents', but it should be made as a participant of a team. In the following sections, the techniques described are applicable to either infants or adolescents.

Current Operative Techniques for Intersex and Urogenital Sinus Repair

Preoperatively, it is important to ensure that the patient is metabolically stable, particularly a child with CAH. At a minimum, all children undergo an enema, and if there is any indication that a more significant vaginoplasty is required, complete bowel preparation with a polyethylene glycol–electrolyte solution (GoLYTELY) is warranted. All children receive preoperative broad-spectrum antibiotics. Children with CAH should undergo "stress dose" steroid replacement at the time of surgery. After general anesthesia, endoscopy is performed as described previously. **After passing a Fogarty catheter into the vagina, the balloon is inflated and the catheter is clamped and left indwelling. A Foley catheter is then anchored in the bladder.** Both are kept sterile, and the child is prepared with povidone-iodine (Betadine). Many surgeons prefer to place the child in lithotomy position, but we have found that this position limits vision to only the surgeon, hinders teaching, and does not allow manipulation of the child if a posterior or abdominal approach is unexpectedly needed. All children undergo a complete lower body preparation from nipples to feet. The child's legs are wrapped, and the lower part of the body is passed through the aperture in the drapes; this facilitates access to the entire perineum and abdomen and further allows the child to be rotated either supine or prone during the procedure (Fig. 129–41).

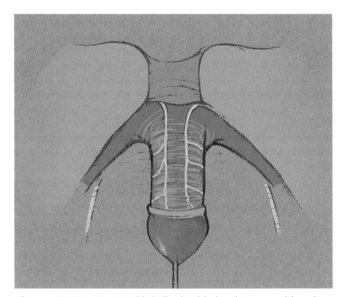

Figure 129–39. Hypertrophied clitoris with dorsal nerves and branches.

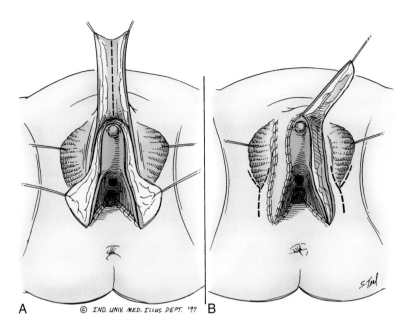

A   © IND. UNIV. MED. ILLUS. DEPT. '97   B

Figure 129–40. Labioplasty. **A,** Phallic skin unfurled. **B,** Preputial skin split and used to create the labia minora; proposed labia majora Y-V–plasty. (From Rink RC, Adams MC: Feminizing genitoplasty: State of the art. World J Urol 1998;16:212. Copyright 1997, Indiana University Medical Illustration Department.)

KEY POINTS: UROGENITAL SINUS ANOMALIES—RECONSTRUCTION

■ The three steps in surgical reconstruction are clitoroplasty, vaginoplasty and labioplasty.

■ Clitoroplasty is controversial. When performed, the glans and tunics with their neurovascular bundles must be preserved. Excision of erectile tissue, when performed, must be from the ventral aspect only.

■ Vaginoplasties consist of four types: cutback (no longer used), "flap" for a low to midlevel confluence, "pull-through" for a high confluence, and vaginal replacement for a rudimentary or absent vagina. The timing of vaginoplasties is controversial.

■ Labia minora are absent in urogenital sinus patients with genital ambiguity. They are reconstructed from phallic skin.

■ It is helpful to place a Fogarty catheter with the balloon inflated in the vagina. For a low confluence, an omega-shaped perineal flap provides better cosmesis. The flap is sewn into the posteriorly opened sinus, and this flap must reach to the more proximal normal-caliber vagina.

■ For a high confluence, the vagina is separated from the urinary tract at its confluence and "pulled through" toward the perineum. The sinus opening is closed to create a urethra.

Low Vaginal Confluence—Clitoral Hypertrophy

The vast majority of children who undergo surgery for intersex or urogenital sinus conditions have a low vaginal confluence amenable to flap vaginoplasty. They usually have clitoral hypertrophy. Clitoroplasty and classic flap vagino-

plasty are described. With the child in the supine position, a traction suture is placed through the glans, and the proposed incisions are outlined with a skin scribe. Along these lines, 0.5% lidocaine with 1:200,000 epinephrine is injected subcutaneously for hemostasis. Parallel longitudinal lines are drawn on either side of a ventral mucosal strip from around the meatus toward the glans and around the coronal margin. A perineal omega-shaped flap is outlined. A Y-incision line is drawn around the inferior aspect of each labia majora. The incision begins around the coronal margin with ample skin being left for a clitoral hood. This skin has been shown to be second only to the glans in sensitivity (Schober and Ransley, 2002). The clitoris is degloved while keeping the ventral strip intact. Dissection is carried out to the level of the bifurcation of the corporal bodies and the pubis dorsally, and care should be taken to not injure any neurovascular tissue (Fig. 129–42). It is important to recognize that the clitoral arterial supply branches from the internal pudendal artery from Alcock's canal near the ischial tuberosity. These arteries course ventrally and are on the medial aspect of the bifurcated corpora, where they then course dorsally along the phallic shaft (Schnitzer and Donahoe, 2001). The clitoral neural bundles ascend along the ischiopubic rami and meet as paired bundles that pass along the dorsal surface and then pass largely intact into the glans (O'Connell et al, 2005). A tourniquet is placed at the base of the clitoris. Longitudinal incisions are then made through Buck's fascia on the ventral-most aspect of each corporal body (Fig. 129–43); the incisions extend from the glans to the bifurcation to expose the corpora cavernosa tissue, which is dissected (often teased) from the tunics. The tunics are left undisturbed, except for the ventral incision. **No tunical tissue is excised. The dorsal neurovascular bundle should not be mobilized or disturbed in any way.** The proximal ends of the erectile tissue are suture-ligated. Efforts to decrease the size of the glans are controversial and, if attempted, should be done with great caution. Studies of Juskiewenski et al (1982) and Baskin et al (1999) would suggest that any glans excision should be performed ventrally near the midline (similar to

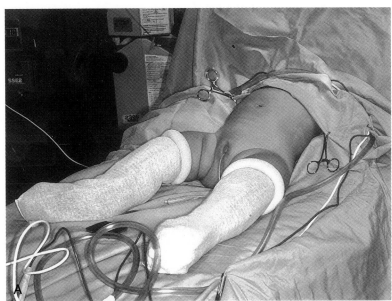

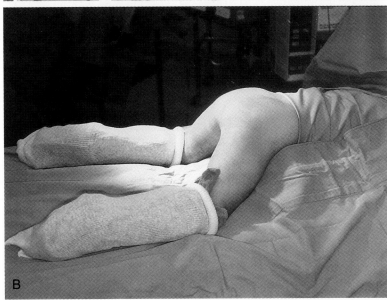

Figure 129–41. Total lower body preparation allows both supine (**A**) and prone (**B**) approaches. (From Rink RC, Adams MC: Feminizing genitoplasty: State of the art. World J Urol 1998;16:212.)

hypospadias glans wings). The glans is innervated by perforating branches entering at the dorsal junction of the glans and corpora (Baskin et al, 1999). Excision of glanular epithelium to conceal the glans is to be avoided because the sensory neuropeptides are located just beneath this layer. Furthermore, no data suggest that a large glans is detrimental to sexual function. The glans is now secured to the coronal stumps. In our experience, a glans sewn to the pubis results in an abnormally high prominent position (Rink and Yerkes, 2001).

With clitoroplasty completed, the flap vaginoplasty is started. The previously outlined omega flap is incised, and the underlying fat is mobilized with the flap to expose the urogenital sinus. The flap must be made long enough to provide a tension-free anastomosis to the vagina and wide enough to provide a normal-caliber introitus without compromising the blood supply of the perineal body. The posterior wall of the sinus and vagina is now dissected free from the underlying rectum. With stay sutures in the meatus, the posterior wall of the sinus is opened in the midline and extended proximally into the posterior wall of the vagina. **The distal third of the vagina is usually narrowed; therefore, the posterior wall incision must be carried proximally until normal-caliber vagina is encountered.** Sutures are placed individually through the perineal flap and then through the split posterior wall of the vagina and tied.

The phallic skin is unfurled and divided longitudinally in the midline while stopping short of the base to allow a clitoral hood. Labia minora are now created with this split preputial skin, which is moved inferiorly and anastomosed to the preserved ventral plate and the lateral vaginal wall. The proposed Y incisions are now made around the inferior aspect of each labia majora. The labia are mobilized and secured inferiorly alongside the vagina as a Y-V–plasty. The

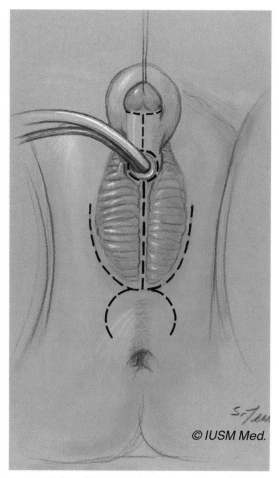

Figure 129–42. Proposed perineal flap, omega configuration.

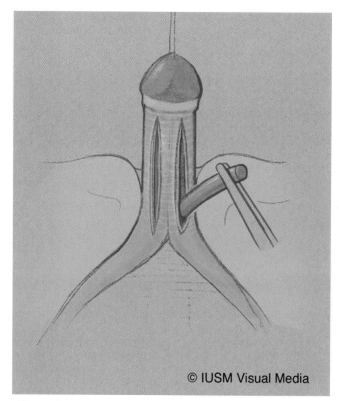

Figure 129–43. Proposed clitoral incisions. Note the ventral location.

vaginal introitus should now reside between the labia minora and majora.

High Vaginal Confluence—with or without Clitoral Hypertrophy

Most believe that complete separation of the vagina from the urogenital sinus with a "pull-through" vaginoplasty, as proposed by Hendren and Crawford (1969), is the best solution to a high vaginal confluence. Fortunately, this complex situation is found in only about 5% of patients with CAH (Dumanian and Donahoe, 1992). This high confluence can be seen in pure urogenital sinus abnormalities. Although the concept of vaginal separation and pull-through was a major advance, the operation as originally described frequently resulted in an isolated vaginal opening that appeared to be separate from the remainder of the genitalia, and a mucosal lining was lacking (Passerini-Glazel, 1989). It was also technically difficult because of poor vision at the critical points (Rink et al, 1997). Several authors have addressed these issues. Passerini-Glazel (1989) used the mobilized sinus by dividing it dorsally; when tabularized with the phallic skin and folded back toward the vagina, it would create a more normal cosmetic result and provide excellent coverage in the area of the vaginal separation while helping to prevent a urethrovaginal fistula. He later used this as a flap to form the anterior vaginal

wall rather than completely tubularizing it (Passerini-Glazel, 1994). Gonzalez and Fernandes (1990) used the preputial skin to construct the vaginal vestibule and anterior wall.

The critical and most technically demanding aspect of a pull-through vaginoplasty is separation of the anterior wall of the vagina from the urethra and bladder neck. There is no obvious plane of dissection, and great care must be taken to avoid injury to the urinary tract and its sphincteric mechanism. This area is also the most difficult to visualize, and poor exposure naturally leads to poor results, with the potential for a stricture, fistula, diverticulum, or retained distal vagina (Rink and Adams, 1998). Most surgeons have positioned the patient in the supine or lithotomy position. Several authors have reported means of improving exposure. Passerini-Glazel (1989, 1994) mobilized the vagina transtrigonally in difficult cases but has more recently reported that this approach is seldom necessary. Similarly, Di Benedetto (1997) and Rossi (1998) and their associates proposed an anterior sagittal transanorectal approach with a diverting colostomy. Hendren and Atala (1995) reported lateral mobilization of the rectum in 1995 but have since stopped because of the difficulty of this maneuver. Rink and colleagues reported a midline posterior prone approach with retraction but not division of the rectum that provides excellent exposure for critical aspects of the pull-through vaginoplasty and is described here (Rink et al, 1997). Endoscopy with Fogarty and Foley catheter placement and total-body preparation are as described for a flap vaginoplasty. If the child has associated clitoral hypertrophy, the clitoroplasty is performed with the child supine as described earlier for a low confluence. The child is then rotated to the prone position. In a patient with a pure urogenital sinus, the procedure is started with the patient in the prone position.

The perineal omega-shaped flap incision is made as previously described, and then the flap is retracted posteriorly, with dissection now carried out in the midline between the posterior wall of the sinus/vagina and rectum. As dissection proceeds proximally, the rectum is easily retracted with a small Deaver retractor (Fig. 129–44) to expose the entire urogenital sinus without the need to divide the rectum. The entire length of the sinus may be divided in the midline posteriorly to the normal caliber of the vagina. The Deaver retractor is now placed in the vagina and with upward retraction easily exposes the anterior wall of the vagina at its confluence with the sinus. This allows dissection of the vagina from the urethra under direct vision (Fig. 129–45). The tissues are quite thin in this area, and one should always err on the side of the vagina. More proximally, the dissection becomes easier. Excellent vision is also provided for tubularization of the sinus to create a urethra, which is closed in two or three layers over a Foley catheter. The anterior wall of the vagina is now mobilized inferiorly, closer to the perineum. "Pull-through" vaginoplasty is often a misnomer because frequently the separated vagina will not reach the perineum. In this situation, skin flaps have been used to reach up to the vagina (rather than the vagina "pulled through" to the perineum). Preputial skin may be sewn to the spatulated anterior vagina, as described by Gonzales and Fernandes (1990) (Fig. 129–46). When preputial skin is not available, a buttock flap or a laterally based skin flap can be used (Parrott and Woodard, 1991; Dumanian and Donahoe, 1992) (Fig. 129–47). The child is returned to the supine position, and the posterior perineal flap is anastomosed to the vagina as described for the flap vaginoplasty.

Labioplasty is now completed as described earlier. If a laterally based flap is required for the anterior wall, posterior relocation of the labia majora may be performed at a later stage.

In patients with a high confluence, particularly if multiple flaps have been used, the legs are bound together loosely postoperatively to prevent tension on the flaps.

Total and Partial Urogenital Mobilization

In 1997, Alberto Pena proposed a maneuver called ***total urogenital mobilization (TUM)*** as a means to repair the urogenital sinus component of a cloacal repair. **In this procedure, the entire sinus is dissected circumferentially and mobilized toward the perineum.** Pena noted a decrease in operative time by 70%, a superior cosmetic result, and less risk of fistula, vaginal stenosis, or acquired vaginal atresia with TUM because vaginal separation is not usually required. Since Pena's original description, TUM has been applied to several disorders, such as urogenital sinus, female exstrophy, and penile agenesis (Ludwikowski et al, 1999; Kropp and Cheng, 2000; Rink et al, 2000). Both Pena and Ludwikowski's group reported amputation of the mobilized sinus so that the vagina and urethra can be sewn flush to the perineum (Pena, 1997; Ludwikowski et al, 1999). **Rink and Adams (1999) reported using the mobilized sinus to provide a mucosa-lined vestibule or a Passerini flap to cover the anterior vaginal wall when a pull-through procedure is performed.** Jenak et al (2001) have since reported similar use of the mobilized sinus to create a mucosal vestibule, and Hamza et al (2001) have noted that the sinus may be used as a Passerini-like flap. There have been two recent descriptions of use of the mobilized sinus to replace the posterior perineal-based skin flap with a sinus flap. In one, the

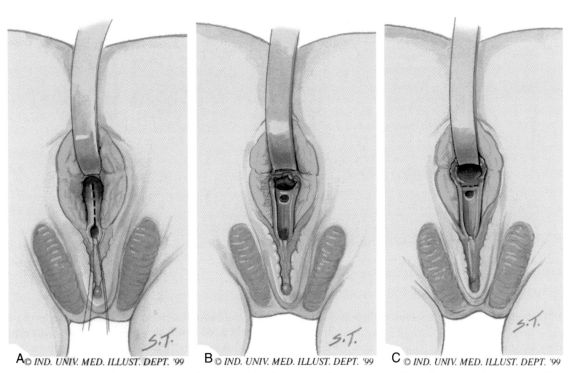

Figure 129–44. **A,** Posterior flap developed with the sinus exposed. **B,** Sinus opened in the posterior midline. **C,** Retractor in the vagina. (Copyright 1999, Indiana University Medical Illustration Department.)

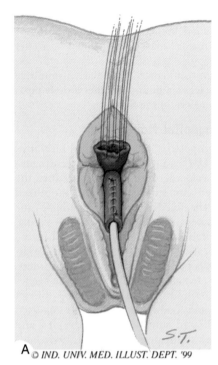
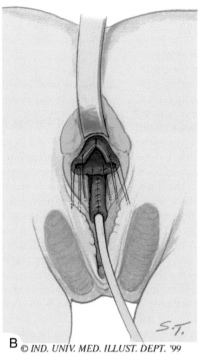

Figure 129–45. **A,** Vagina mobilized and the sinus tubularized to create a urethra. **B,** Posterior vagina spatulated. (Copyright 1999, Indiana University Medical Illustration Department.)

A © IND. UNIV. MED. ILLUST. DEPT. '99

B © IND. UNIV. MED. ILLUST. DEPT. '99

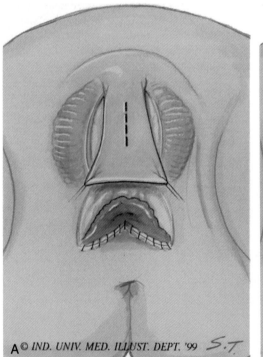
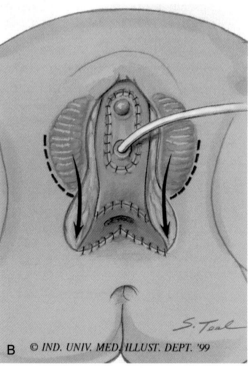

A © IND. UNIV. MED. ILLUST. DEPT. '99

B © IND. UNIV. MED. ILLUST. DEPT. '99

Figure 129–46. Modified Gonzalez preputial flap to create an anterior vaginal wall; the posterior flap has been anastomosed to the spatulated vagina. (Copyright 1999, Indiana University Medical Illustration Department.)

sinus is split laterally and rotated posteriorly (Rink and Cain, 2002). In the other, the sinus is split in half longitudinally and the two halves are rotated inferiorly (Gosalbez et al, 2005). At the Riley Hospital for Children, we have incorporated the TUM technique into many of our urogenital sinus repairs. **It allows a midlevel confluence to reach the perineum without requiring vaginal separation. The highest-level confluences may still need a pull-through procedure with separation of the vagina and urethra,** but it is much more easily performed after the urogenital sinus has been mobilized.

TUM is often thought of as its own type of vaginoplasty but is, in fact, a technique to allow vaginoplasty that may result in

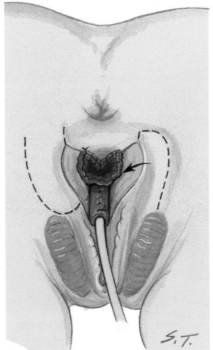 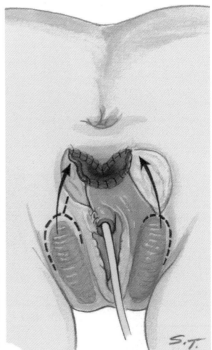

Figure 129–47. A buttocks- or labial-based flap may be used to create the anterior vaginal wall in a patient with a pure urogenital sinus. (Copyright 1999, Indiana University Medical Illustration Department.)

A © IND. UNIV. MED. ILLUST. DEPT. '99   B © IND. UNIV. MED. ILLUST. DEPT. '99

the vagina being sewn flush to the perineum; however, a flap or pull-through vaginoplasty may still be required. TUM is started, as in our previous descriptions, with endoscopy to evaluate the anatomy, to note the level of the confluence, and to place a Fogarty catheter in the vagina and a Foley catheter in the bladder. A sponge is placed in the rectum and the proposed incisions are outlined (see Fig. 129–42). Subcutaneous injection of 0.5% lidocaine with 1:200,000 epinephrine along the lines is carried out. Clitoroplasty is performed as previously described, except that the meatus of the urogenital sinus is circumscribed with stay sutures to allow mobilization of the sinus from the corporal bodies. The clitoroplasty is now completed as described earlier. The dissection is carried out in the midline posterior to the sinus until the peritoneal reflection is reached to allow access to the entire posterior wall of the vagina. The anterior wall of the sinus is now mobilized from the phallus (Figs. 129–48 and 129–49). This circumferential mobilization is done directly on the urogenital sinus and continues proximally beneath the pubis. As the avascular ligaments from the pubis to the sinus are divided in this area, the entire urogenital sinus is felt to "give" and move toward the perineum (Fig. 129–50).

The Fogarty balloon is now easily palpable in the vagina. The posterior wall of the vagina is opened between stay sutures. If the vagina is now near the perineum, it may be sewn flush to the perineum, or an omega-shaped perineal flap may be placed into the spatulated posterior wall to augment the vaginal caliber. We prefer the latter. Rather than discard the mobilized sinus, as previously reported, we have found it helpful to split the sinus ventrally and use it to provide a mucosa-lined vestibule (Fig. 129–51). If the vagina is still quite high, the anterior wall of the vagina should be separated from the urethra and bladder neck, as in the pull-through pro-

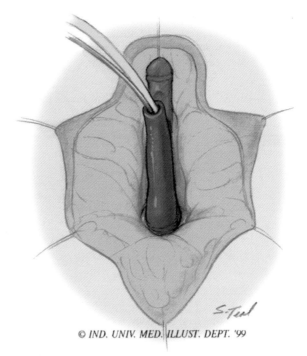

© IND. UNIV. MED. ILLUST. DEPT. '99

Figure 129–48. Skin mobilized with the sinus exposed. (Copyright 1999, Indiana University Medical Illustration Department.)

cedure (Pena, 1997; Rink and Kaefer, 2002). We believe that this is most easily performed with the child in the prone position to allow direct vision. The opening in the urethra is closed in two layers. The mobilized sinus in this situation is split anteriorly and then used as a Passerini-like flap to create the

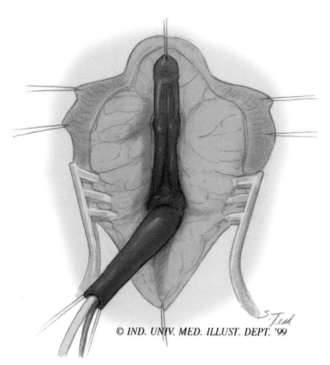

Figure 129–49. Total urogenital mobilization with the sinus mobilized. (Copyright 1999, Indiana University Medical Illustration Department.)

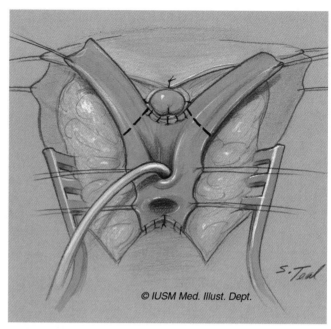

Figure 129–51. A ventral incision on the mobilized sinus allows the creation of a mucosa-lined vestibule.

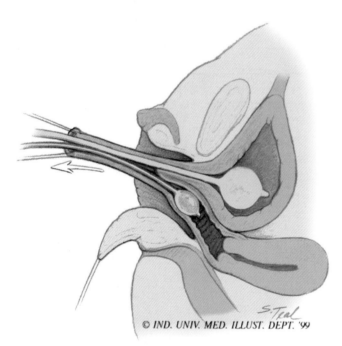

Figure 129–50. Total urogenital mobilization. The sinus is mobilized to a position beneath the pubis. (Copyright 1999, Indiana University Medical Illustration Department.)

anterior vagina wall (Rink and Adams, 1999) (Fig. 129–52). The posterior perineal flap is approximated to the spatulated posterior vaginal wall. Labioplasty is performed as previously described. TUM has achieved great popularity, and reports to date reveal excellent cosmesis and continence. No long-term

results are available. Some have expressed concern regarding the proximal circumferential dissection because of the potential risk for sphincteric musculature or nerve injury. There is concern for resultant stress incontinence or foreshortening of the vagina. **To address these concerns, Rink et al (2005c) proposed partial urogenital mobilization, which starts with the same circumferential dissection but stops at the level of the pubourethral ligament** (Fig. 129–53). This still allows use of the mobilized sinus as described earlier to improve cosmesis, yet it avoids the aggressive retropubic and suprapubic dissection and is applicable to the majority of patients. If more mobilization is necessary for a very high vagina, TUM is easily carried out.

KEY POINTS: UROGENITAL MOBILIZATION

- TUM is a technique applicable to both urogenital sinus and cloacal anomalies. The entire sinus is dissected circumferentially to above the pubis to allow the confluence to move inferiorly to the perineum.

- With the TUM technique, the mobilized sinus tissue can be used to create a mucosa-lined vestibule or an anterior or posterior vaginal wall. This sinus tissue should not be discarded.

- Partial urogenital mobilization circumferentially mobilizes the sinus to the level of the pubourethral ligament but does not extend above this level.

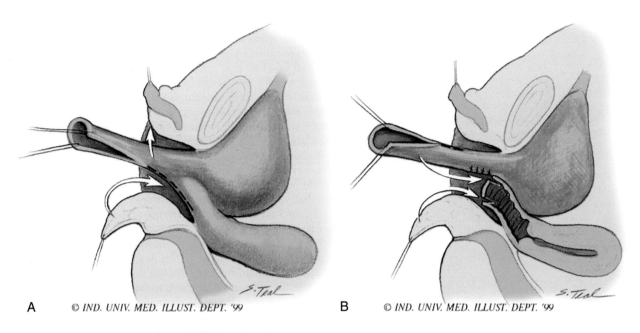

A   © IND. UNIV. MED. ILLUST. DEPT. '99   B   © IND. UNIV. MED. ILLUST. DEPT. '99

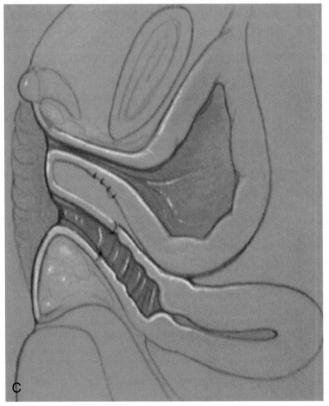

Figure 129–52. Total urogenital mobilization. **A,** The sinus is split ventrally to create a mucosa-lined vestibule in the flap vaginoplasty. **B,** The sinus is split dorsally to create an anterior vaginal wall for pull-through vaginoplasty. (From Rink RC: Journal of Pediatric Urology [in press] 2006.) **C,** The opened sinus now becomes the anterior vaginal wall.

Results of Urogenital Sinus and Intersex Surgery

Well-documented long-term outcomes of clitoroplasty and vaginoplasty are sorely lacking. Most articles look at success as an adequately open vagina with a feminized appearance. Success should include normal erotic sensation, lubrication, sexual satisfaction, and intercourse without discomfort. These latter factors are just beginning to be studied. **Cosmetic and early functional results have uniformly been reported to be good. Long-term outcomes are more concerning,** but in these studies it is often difficult to tell what procedures were done for what degree of severity of urogenital sinus, and none of the studies include data on the quality of endocrinologic control in these patients. Looking at what data are available, Jones and colleagues noted in 1976 that 25 of 84 patients undergoing vaginoplasty required a secondary procedure to provide a vaginal outlet satisfactory for intercourse; 5 of these

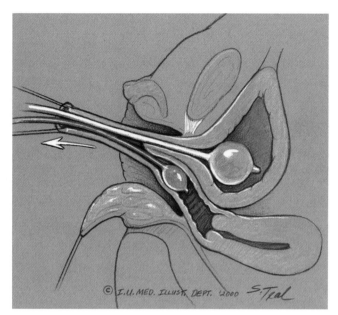

Figure 129–53. Partial urogenital mobilization. Dissection stops at the pubourethral ligament.

25 also required a third procedure. **The poor results were caused by failure to exteriorize the vagina initially or by scar formation.** Sotiropoulos and associates (1976) found that all patients undergoing prepubertal vaginoplasty required revision at puberty. Azziz and coworkers, in 1986, reported the results of attempted coitus in 42 women with CAH 23.6 years after vagina repair. Satisfactory coitus was noted in 62% (46% in salt wasters and 87% in those with the non–salt-losing form). There was a less favorable outcome when the initial procedure was performed before 1 year of age. Thirty secondary or tertiary procedures were needed to achieve the final results. These data are widely quoted, but almost all of these patients underwent a "cut-back" vaginoplasty initially ("incision of the urogenital sinus"), which is a procedure no longer used because it does not adequately open the vagina to the proximal normal caliber; specifically, the distal end of the vagina is narrowed and thus will be stenotic. Their revision involved the performance of a "flap" vaginoplasty, which currently would probably have been the initial procedure. In a series from Johns Hopkins, 28 patients (32% lost to follow-up) had adequate follow-up, 22 (78.6%) of whom needed further vaginal surgery (Bailez et al, 1992). The authors noted that if secondary surgery was needed for vaginal stenosis, success rates were high when the procedure was performed near puberty. This group also reported less favorable results in those younger than 1 year, with only 8 of 18 needing a secondary procedure requiring a flap. Nihoul-Fekete et al (1982) noted that 30% of 43 CAH patients required secondary surgery. Hendren and Atala (1995), reporting on 16 patients with high vaginal confluence, noted that 6 of 9 adults had satisfactory coitus and 2 had vaginal stenosis.

More recently, Alizai and colleagues (1999) assessed 14 girls with CAH under anesthesia, 11 to 15 years old, who had undergone genitoplasty at a mean age of 2.5 years and noted that 13 of 14 required additional vaginal surgery. Stenosis was seen in 43% and persistent urogenital sinus with or without fibrosis in 50%. Minto et al (2003) found that 39% of 28 patients required secondary surgery and a third procedure was required in 11%. It is tempting to assume that postpubertal vaginal surgery may result in better outcomes, but there are no data to support this assumption. Furthermore, Eroglu et al (2004) actually noted less vaginal stenosis in those who underwent early single-stage repair (3.4%) than in those who underwent late vaginoplasty (42.8%).

It seems clear that a "single-stage" early vaginoplasty will probably require a secondary repair after puberty, but this should be expected because the orifice is likely to remain the size that was created given that there is no flow through the orifice in childhood. In our experience, the secondary refinements are easily performed.

Surgical techniques to reduce clitoral size have dramatically improved and are now based on our current knowledge of clitoral neuroanatomy. Even though no long-term results are available for current techniques, some long-term results are now being reported for relatively modern techniques. Alizai et al (1999) found clitoroplasty results to be unsatisfactory in 46%. **Gearhart and coworkers (1995) looked at pudendal evoked potentials after clitoroplasty and noted that modern clitoroplasties preserve nerve conduction in the dorsal neurovascular bundle.** Barrett and Gonzales (1980) found intact sensation in all of their patients after clitoroplasty. Chase (1996) reported that even with normal evoked potentials there may be an absence of sensation and orgasm. We have not noted vascularization defects after modern clitoroplasty. It is clear that further long-term studies are necessary. Minto et al (2003) found the clitoris to be cosmetically normal in 59% who had undergone clitoral surgery, but it was excessive in 20%, large in 7%, small in 7%, and absent in 7%. This group also reported that hot, cold, and vibratory sensation was markedly altered as recorded by a genitosensory analyzer (Minto et al, 2003). Sensation alone may be a poor indication of clitoral normality after surgery. Further studies to analyze the newest techniques are warranted. The erotic sensitivity and potential for orgasm should be studied.

The results of TUM are very early. The procedure is technically easier and the cosmetic results are excellent, but the potential for stress incontinence or denervation of the sphincteric mechanisms is unknown. Most authors to date have not found continence to be altered by TUM (Rink and Adams, 1999; Hamza et al, 2001; Kryger and Gonzales, 2004). Until these results are available, this procedure should be used with caution.

Timing of vaginoplasty remains quite controversial. Although the few reported long-term studies suggest that delayed vaginoplasty may be preferable, most surgeons recommend early surgery. They argue that the available long-term studies are based on outdated techniques and that there are tremendous surgical advantages to a single-stage repair. Supporters of early vaginoplasty well recognize that secondary introitoplasty may be necessary, but this is usually accomplished easily. The argument, which will not be settled soon, contrasts two approaches: (1) a simple procedure in an infant (i.e., clitoroplasty) with a postpubertal extensive procedure (i.e., vaginoplasty) or (2) an extensive single-stage clitorovaginoplasty in an infant with a simple introitoplasty in the postpubertal period.

KEY POINTS: UROGENITAL SINUS ANOMALIES—OUTCOMES OF RECONSTRUCTION

■ It is clear that neonatal vaginoplasties will usually require a secondary procedure for stenosis after puberty (25% to 100%).

■ Successful coitus is often reported, but further studies should note sexual satisfaction, lubrication, and erotic sensitivity, as well as nonpainful coitus.

■ Current techniques of clitoroplasty seem unlikely to injure sensation, but newer studies question whether sensitivity is an adequate indication of clitoral function. Some studies note decreased sensation with newer techniques.

SURGICAL RECONSTRUCTION FOR CLOACAL MALFORMATIONS

Initial Management, Timing, and Principles

The initial management of cloacal anomaly involves stabilization because the child is often quite ill with abdominal distention that at times results in respiratory compromise. As with all other anomalies, its management has evolved. Historically, after decompression of the distended organs, it was common practice to perform a rectal pull-through procedure; genitourinary reconstruction followed at a later date, if at all (Okonkwo and Crocker, 1977). Hall and coauthors (1985) suggested that the vaginal surgery be done after puberty, when estrogen levels are higher. **Although it is tempting to perform a pull-through procedure only, it is now clear that this piecemeal repair of the cloaca is a disservice to the child and is absolutely contraindicated. It is optimal to repair all abnormalities (i.e., rectal, vaginal, and urethral) in a single stage** (Kay and Tank, 1977; Mollitt et al, 1981). **This allows the best exposure for the difficult rectal and vaginal separation.** Furthermore, the tissues have not been previously violated, and the rectum does not require remobilization. Hendren (1982, 1986) pointed out that rectal pull-through should never be done as a separate procedure. Of his 154 patients with cloacal anomaly, 60 were secondary cases, many of whom had undergone a previous pull-through procedure. Definitive repair in this situation often requires repeat rectal mobilization. Raffensberger (1988) proposed neonatal complete repair but later noted that this may not be appropriate. Levitt and Pena (2005) have recently stated that there are three pitfalls in the management of newborns with cloacas, including (1) failure to recognize and manage hydrocolpos, (2) colostomy or vesicostomy problems, and (3) clinical misdiagnosis.

Surgical management now involves four basic steps: decompression of the gastrointestinal tract, decompression of the genitourinary tract, correction of nephron-destructive or potentially lethal urinary anomalies, and definitive repair of the cloaca.

Decompression of the Gastrointestinal Tract

Decompression of the gastrointestinal tract is done by colostomy. Although all surgeons agree on the need for colostomy initially, the best anatomic location of the colostomy is debated. Hendren initially recommended a low-loop colostomy but more recently has performed a right transverse colon divided colostomy (Hendren, 1982, 1986, 1998). This change was prompted by difficulty in obtaining a bowel segment for vaginoplasty during the rectal pull-through procedure when a low colostomy has been performed. A divided transverse colostomy keeps the left colic blood supply intact (Hendren, 1992). Pena, as reported by Spitz and Coron, preferred a descending colostomy because there was less surface area for resorption of urine. A divided colostomy in the descending colon just after the colon takes off from its retroperitoneal attachment is recommended by Levitt and Pena (2005). This procedure maintains the availability of enough distal colon for future pull-through, and prolapse is less likely to occur. However, Pena did recommend leaving a long segment of sigmoid to prevent a difficult pull-through requiring abdominal exploration. We have favored a proximal colostomy but have at times found clinically challenging acidosis caused by urine absorption through the colonic mucosa.

At the time of colostomy, endoscopy may be performed to more clearly define the anatomy and to aid in decompression of the urinary tract. In our experience, as the cystoscope advances proximally through the cloacal channel, it tends to enter the vagina (or vaginas). In fact, entrance into the urethra/bladder can be extremely difficult in a neonate with a distended vagina because the vagina compressed the bladder to the anterior abdominal wall and obstructs the bladder neck. Drainage plus irrigation of the vagina (or vaginas) not only allows decompression and relief of abdominal distention but may allow visualization of the bladder as well. Often, the rectal fistula is also difficult to locate; as noted previously, it is more often found within the septum of the duplicated vaginas but can enter at almost any location. With a combination of irrigation through the fistula and through the distal limb of the colostomy, the inspissated mucus and meconium can easily be cleared. It is often helpful to leave small feeding tubes in all channels and then obtain radiographic studies to further delineate the anatomy. In our experience this is best done in the radiology suite with fluoroscopy.

Decompression of the Genitourinary Tract

Even after decompression of all structures draining into the cloaca, at times voiding continues into the vagina (or vaginas) or the rectum (or both) and results in rapid distention of these structures with subsequent poor urinary drainage, persistent hydronephrosis, abdominal distention, urinary infection, and hyperchloremic acidosis. This can generally be managed by intermittent catheterization. The catheter often enters the vagina rather than the bladder, but it still functions to drain and decompress the genitourinary tract (Hendren, 1992). If the desired decompression is not achieved, further maneuvers are required. We agree with

Hendren that in a long urethra-like cloaca, catheterization can at times be difficult and a cut-back procedure (opening the cloaca) may be helpful to aid catheterization (Fig. 129–54). If this approach fails, further decompression can be achieved by either vesicostomy or vaginostomy (Kay and Tank, 1977). Levitt and Pena (2005) have found vaginostomy helpful, but we believe that clean intermittent catheterization (CIC) or vesicostomy, or both, will usually keep the vagina adequately decompressed. Only when these maneuvers fail should vaginostomy be performed because it tethers the vagina to the abdominal wall and makes later pull-through or TUM difficult. It also necessitates an abdominal procedure. Levitt and Pena (2005) found that 25% of their cloaca patients had hydrocolpos but that in 59% of them, it was either not identified or mismanaged. This resulted in significant morbidity from ureteral obstruction, urinary tract infection, acidosis, and failure to thrive. Adequate vaginal drainage resulted in resolution of these problems.

Repair of Obstructive Urinary and Other Pathology

The third stage of care of a child with a cloacal anomaly is repair of any obstructive urinary tract pathology. Renal structural abnormalities have been identified in 60% to 83% of patients with persistent cloaca, some of which were obstructive in nature (Warne et al, 2003; Rink et al, 2005b). In those with a common channel longer than 3 cm, 91% had urologic defects (Pena et al, 2004). At times, these anomalies are

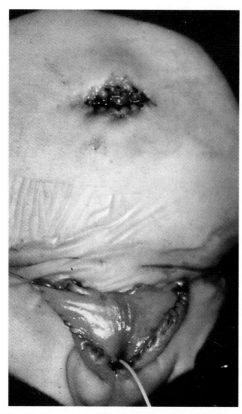

Figure 129–54. The urethra-like cloaca is opened, with a catheter in place; vesicostomy has also been performed.

ignored early on while awaiting definitive cloacal repair, but this practice should be avoided. Obstructive lesions should be treated promptly. However, vesicoureteral reflux, which is quite common, can generally be managed medically if urinary infection is prevented. Other organ system anomalies (e.g., cardiac, spinal cord) should be fully evaluated. Some may require repair during this phase.

Definitive Repair of Cloacal Malformations

Definitive repair of a cloaca is usually carried out at 6 to 12 months of age, but obviously, the child must be well nourished and thriving to proceed with repair. In healthy thriving children, Pena et al operate at 1 month of age. Definitive repair should never occur until the urinary tract has been evaluated and hydrocolpos has been ruled out (Pena et al, 2004). If endoscopy has not been performed previously, it may be helpful as a separate procedure before the definitive repair. Defining the anatomy can be tedious, and it is helpful to thoroughly cleanse the distal colonic segment, which usually requires irrigation from the mucous fistula, as well as the distal limb of the colostomy. A standard GoLYTELY bowel preparation should also be done.

Operative Technique—Cloaca

The definitive repair begins with endoscopy to reacquaint the surgeon with the anatomy. We have also found it is helpful to place a Foley catheter in the bladder and different-colored Fogarty catheters in the vagina (or vaginas) and rectum. The catheters are kept sterile during preparation. As described previously for urogenital sinus repair, a complete lower body Betadine preparation is done circumferentially from the level of the nipples to the toes, and the legs are wrapped sterilely. Such preparation allows prone and supine positioning for perineal and abdominal surgery.

The definitive posterior sagittal anorectovaginourethroplasty (PSARVUP) is begun with the child in the prone position and the pelvis elevated on rolls to achieve a jackknife position. An electrical stimulator is used to determine the area of maximal contraction, which is marked with a skin scribe and with stay sutures for later rectal placement. The proposed locations of the perineal body and vagina are also marked (Fig. 129–55). We agree with Hendren that it is at times helpful to have a sound in the common cloacal channel, but the Foley and Fogarty catheters usually suffice. The entire dissection is done in the midline until mobilization of the rectum and vagina is begun. The most important advances of Pena's PSARVUP procedure are that it allows identification of the external sphincter and muscle complex of the rectum and provides excellent exposure for separation of the rectum and vagina (or vaginas) from the cloaca.

The initial incision extends from the tip of the coccyx in the midline to the posterior aspect of the cloacal orifice. Sutures mark the sphincteric muscular structures on either side as they are encountered. We have found it helpful in the past to open the common cloaca in the midline posteriorly to the level of the confluences to allow easy identification of the rectal and vaginal insertions. With TUM, this is less appropriate because it may limit the options for use of the sinus in the recon-

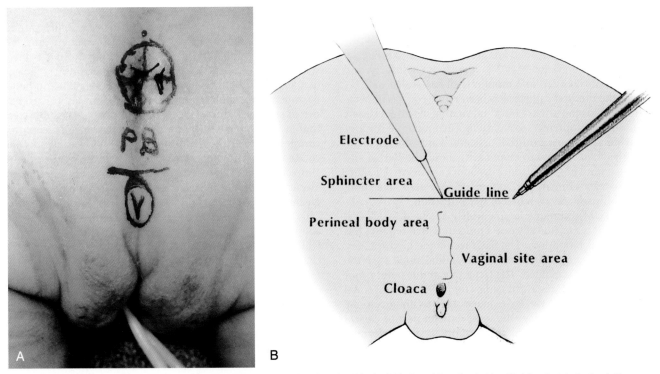

Figure 129–55. Cloaca—proposed location of the vagina (V) and perineal body (PB). Rectal location is identified by electrical stimulation.

struction as previously described for a urogenital sinus. When the rectal fistula is identified, it is opened posteriorly and multiple silk stay sutures are placed. These sutures are helpful in mobilizing the rectum away from the vagina (or vaginas). It is important to remember that the structures share a common wall initially and it is better to enter the vagina than either the rectum or urethra. Circumferential dissection of the rectum to well above the sacrum may be necessary. Separation of the peritoneum can be done from this position. Rarely, a child with a very high rectal confluence needs to be turned to the supine position for abdominal exploration to free the rectum more proximally. Once adequate rectal mobilization to allow a tension-free anastomosis to the perineal skin has been achieved, the rectal stay sutures are used to retract the rectum from the genitourinary structures.

In the classic PSARVUP procedure, the vagina is now separated from the sinus. This dissection is even more tedious and difficult than the rectal separation. With TUM (described later), which has now achieved widespread acceptance for cloacal repair, the vagina may not require separation. We now describe classic vaginal separation followed by the TUM technique. In classic vaginal separation as noted earlier, it is an error to enter the urinary tract during vaginal mobilization. In our experience, side-by-side vaginal duplication is most common, and the midline septum has been incised with electrocautery during the initial endoscopy. Hendren (1998) noted that 66 patients had a single vagina, 68 had two, and 20 had none. The Fogarty catheter (or catheters) within the vagina is easily palpable, and the posterior aspect of the vagina is opened at the level of the confluence. Again, circumferential stay sutures are very helpful in separating the vagina from the urethra and bladder. A malleable retractor inserted into the opened posterior vaginal wall exposes the anterior wall confluence for separation. Sharp dissection is less apt to injure the urinary tract than cautery is. Making dissection even more difficult is the realization that frequently the vagina almost encircles the urethra. Failure to recognize this situation can result in injury to these structures. Use of the stay suture for traction aids in further mobilization of the vagina (or vaginas). The outer wall of the vagina appears white, and identification of this color is helpful. Great care should be taken to avoid devascularization of the vagina during mobilization. Usually, vaginal mobilization allows the vagina to be "pulled through" to a position near the perineum. If after significant mobilization it still does not reach the perineum, skin flaps can be used to reach the spatulated vagina. With an extremely high vagina or the rare vaginal agenesis, it may be necessary to interpose a bowel segment to reach the perineum, which obviously requires abdominal surgery. With a very dilated vagina, a vaginal flap or vaginal "switch" can be created to reach the perineum, although care must be taken to avoid devascularization and stenosis (Hendren, 1986; Pena, 1989; Pena et al, 2004).

Before the vagina is brought to the perineum, the openings in the common cloacal channel should be closed in two to three layers with absorbable suture to create a urethra. If the cloaca is large and vagina-like, it needs to be opened in its entirety and tailored over the Foley catheter. The vagina is then secured to the perineum. If there is any concern about vaginal injury, the vagina should be rotated to avoid overlapping suture lines (Hendren, 1992). The Foley catheter is left indwelling for 2 weeks.

The perineal body is now reconstructed, and the rectum is pulled through to the perineum. Pena (1989) stressed the importance of tailoring the widened rectum. The amount of tailoring differs in each patient. The muscles must meet posterior to the rectum. The rectum is placed in the center of the sphincteric muscle mass and anastomosed to the skin. Rectal dilation is begun gradually at 2 to 3 weeks after surgery, and the colostomy is closed in 3 months if all has healed well.

Once the urethral catheter has been removed, it is imperative to monitor the urinary tract and voiding dynamics closely because poor emptying secondary to a neuropathic component is seen in almost a third of patients. If any concern arises about the child's ability to empty, CIC should be started and continued until normal bladder dynamics are ensured. Failure to do so can ultimately result in urinary tract infection, hydronephrosis, and even loss of renal function.

Pena's TUM technique is now widely accepted for cloacal anomalies. It is a technically easier procedure that requires less time with less blood loss. The basic technique involves 360-degree mobilization of the entire urogenital sinus after the rectum has been separated. The technique at this point is not different from that described earlier for TUM for urogenital sinus abnormalities. We have found this technique to be extremely helpful. It makes the most difficult part of cloacal surgery, vaginal separation, much more easily performed when necessary. If the confluence is only 2 to 3 cm from the perineum, separation may not be necessary. In those with a high vaginal confluence, separation may still be necessary, but it is much more easily accomplished (Rink et al, 1997). Concerns regarding continence have been raised, but to date the results have not been different than with standard repairs. Long-term results of the TUM procedure are needed.

KEY POINTS: CLOACAL RECONSTRUCTION

- Cloacal reconstruction involves four steps: decompression of the gastrointestinal tract (colostomy), decompression of the urinary tract (CIC, vesicostomy), correction of associated organ systems anomalies, and cloacal repair (PSARVUP).

- TUM is now commonly used for cloacal anomalies after the rectum is separated.

- The results of cloacal repairs are often based on the presence or absence of a normal spinal cord. CIC is frequently required, as is a bowel program, to achieve urinary and fecal continence.

Results of Cloacal Surgery

Cloacal anomalies are exceedingly challenging to repair. The anatomy is complex and differs from patient to patient. The surgeon must be prepared for a long, tedious procedure, must be imaginative, and must be willing to handle the tissues with great care. One might assume from this preface that the results would be dismal. On the contrary, most patients lead a productive life. We are indebted to Drs. W. Hardy Hendren and Alberto Pena for their pioneering work on children with cloacal anomalies, as well as their willingness to document their results.

Results have generally been reviewed in terms of urinary continence, fecal continence, and sexual capability; in the future, results should also focus on erotic sensitivity and fertility, as well as quality of life. Early results from a urinary standpoint were dismal: Chappel and Bleloch (1973) reported that all five of their patients had some degree of incontinence postoperatively, and Bartholomew and Gonzales (1978) had five of seven patients wet after reconstruction. **It is now clear that a high percentage of patients have a neuropathic component to their incontinence.** In 1999, De Filippo and colleagues reported urodynamic data on 26 patients with anorectal malformations (including 6 with cloacal anomalies). Twenty-one of the 26 had preoperative leak point pressures greater than 40 cm H_2O, and 15 had normal MRI of the spine. This means that even those not demonstrating a neurologic abnormality may have abnormally high outlet resistance, which adds to the risk for incontinence and upper tract changes. Of Hendren's 141 patients reported by De Filippo, 83 (59%) voided spontaneously with control, 40 (28%) required CIC, 4 (3%) had undergone urinary diversion, and 1 (0.7%) was continent with urinary diversion; only 5 (3.5%) were wet, and in 8 the results were too early to assess. Pena et al (2004) reported a review of 339 patients operated on for cloacal anomalies, 193 of whom were evaluated for urinary continence. They found that spontaneous voiding was related to length of the common channel. Overall continence with spontaneous voiding occurred in 54%. Another 46% were dry with CIC (24% with a native urethra, 22% with a Mitrofanoff channel). However, when the common channel was less than 3 cm, 28% required CIC; if greater than 3 cm, 78% required CIC. Warne et al (2002a) achieved 80% "social continence" but only 22% spontaneously voided, 12% performed CIC alone, and 46% required reconstructive urologic surgery to achieve continence (mean number of operations, 4.7). They likewise found that those with a common channel longer than 3 cm were less likely to void spontaneously (12% versus 31%). In our own series, 86% were dry but only a third were continent with spontaneous voiding. The remainder required CIC with or without lower urinary reconstruction (Rink et al, 2005b) (Table 129–1). Warne also noted that a good bladder neck, short common channel, normal sacrum, and two normal kidneys were all good prognostic signs for continence and spontaneous voiding. We are in agreement with Pena that voiding abnormalities are generally related to a noncontractile bladder and warrant CIC, but Warne et al (2002a) found hyperreflexia to be the predominant pattern in those with abnormal dynamics. It is important to note that 75% of their patients had an abnormal sacrum.

Fecal continence is directly related to neurologic status (Pena, 1989). **Hendren (1992) noted that certain factors bode well for continence: good perineal raphe, well-defined anal**

Table 129–1.	**Continence Rates after Cloacal Surgery**	
	Voiding Spontaneously	*Dry with CIC ± Continent Rec*
Hendren et al, 1998	0.62	0.34
Pena et al, 2004	0.54	0.46
Warne et al, 2002a	0.22	0.58
Rink et al, 2005b	0.33	0.53

dimple, normal spine, normal MRI, and brisk muscle reflex. In 105 patients, Hendren noted that 47 had normal bowel function, 27 required enemas, 7 had a colostomy, 7 had fecal soiling, and 4 with an anterior anus had normal control. Pena et al (2004) reported that 60% of 156 patients have voluntary bowel movements but only 28% of them never soil. The 40% who are fecally incontinent remain "clean" with a bowel management program.

Though not a direct result of reparative surgery, renal outcomes are worrisome. Renal insufficiency was found in 50% of the patients treated at Great Ormond Street Children's Hospital, and 17% of the patients progressed to end-stage renal failure (Warne et al, 2002b). In our own series, 18% had an abnormally elevated serum creatinine level and in another 26% it was borderline (Rink et al, 2005b). Lifelong yearly urologic evaluation is warranted, and prompt recognition plus treatment of any obstructive pathology or urinary tract infections is imperative. Bladder dynamics must be evaluated and abnormalities addressed. Of 24 reported adult patients, 17 had coitus and 6 had borne children (including 5 deliveries by cesarean section and 1 vaginal delivery (Hendren 1998).

SUMMARY

Management of urogenital sinus and cloacal anomalies can be exceedingly complex. In those with disorders of sex differentiation, prompt but very careful evaluation by an expert multidisciplinary team is mandatory. Family support and education with openness and respect for the child and family are required. Differing cultural practices must also be respected and accepted. Confidentially must be maintained. Surgical reconstruction requires great care of tissues, meticulous attention to detail, and a lifelong commitment by the surgeon. These complex anomalies require an entire team of physicians and nurses dedicated to the care of these problems. Urogenital sinus and cloacal anomalies are very challenging reconstructive problems. Those at the more severe end of the spectrum should be handled only in centers with great expertise and experience.

SUGGESTED READINGS

Consensus statement on 21-hydroxylase deficiency from the Lawson Wilkins Pediatric Endocrine Society and the European Society for Paediatric Endocrinology. J Clin Endocrinol Metab 2002;87:4048-4053.

Duhamel B: From the mermaid to anal imperforation: The syndrome of caudal regression. Arch Dis Child 1961;36:152.

Griffin J, Edwards C, Madden JD, et al: Congenital absence of the vagina: The Mayer-Rokitansky-Kuster-Hauser syndrome. Ann Intern Med 1976; 85:224-236.

Hendren W: Cloaca, the most severe degree of imperforate anus: Experience with 195 cases. Am Surg 1998;228:331-346.

Hendren W, Atala A: Use of bowel for vaginal reconstruction. J Urol 1994;152:752-755; discussion, 756-757.

Jaramillo D, Lebowitz R: The cloacal malformation: Radiologic findings and imaging recommendations. Radiology 1990;177:441-448.

McIndoe A, Banister J: An operation for the cure of congenital absence of the vagina. J Obstet Gynaecol Br Commonw 1938;45:490.

Pena A: Total urogenital mobilization: An easier way to repair cloacas. J Pediatr Surg 1997;32:267-268.

Pena A, Levitt MA, Hong A, Midulla P: Surgical management of cloacal malformations: A review of 339 patients. J Pediatr Surg 2004;39:470-479.

Quan L, Smith D: The VATER association: Vertebral defects, anal atresia, T-E fistula with esophageal atresia, radial and renal dysplasia: A spectrum of associated defects. J Pediatr 1973;82:104-107.

Rink RC, Herndon CD, Cain MP, et al: Upper and lower urinary tract outcomes after surgical repair of cloacal malformation: A three-decade experience. BJU Int 2005;96:131-134.

Schober JM: Feminizing genitoplasty for intersex. In Mouriquand PDE (ed): Pediatric Surgery and Urology: Long Term Outcomes. London, WB Saunders, 1998, pp 549-558.

Spieser P, White P: Congenital adrenal hyperplasia. N Engl J Med 2003;349:776-788.

130 Pediatric Urologic Oncology

MICHAEL L. RITCHEY, MD • ROBERT C. SHAMBERGER, MD

NEUROBLASTOMA

Neuroblastoma is the most common extracranial solid tumor of childhood. More than 95% of cases are diagnosed in children by 10 years of age, and regrettably, over half of these children have metastatic disease at diagnosis. Neuroblastoma is known to arise from cells of the neural crest that form the adrenal medulla and sympathetic ganglia. Tumors may occur anywhere along the sympathetic chain within the neck, thorax, retroperitoneum, pelvis, or adrenal gland. Seventy-five percent arise in the retroperitoneum, 50% in the adrenal, and 25% in the paravertebral ganglia. The variety of locations where these tumors arise and the spectrum of their differentiation result in a wide range of clinical manifestations and behavior (Brodeur, 1991). These tumors can undergo spontaneous regression (Brodeur, 1991), differentiate to benign neoplasms (Everson and Cole, 1966), or exhibit extremely malignant behavior.

Epidemiology and Genetics

Incidence

The most common extracranial solid tumor in children, neuroblastoma accounts for 8% to 10% of all childhood cancers. In the United States, the annual incidence is 10 cases per 1 million live births. It is the most common malignant tumor of infancy, with 50% of cases occurring in children younger than 2 years and 75% diagnosed by the fourth year of life (Fortner et al, 1968).

Genetics

A number of familial cases have been reported and are postulated to represent an autosomal dominant pattern of inheritance (Knudson and Strong, 1972; Robertson et al, 1991). The median age at diagnosis of neuroblastoma is 21 months, but in familial cases it is 9 months (Kushner et al, 1986). At least 20% of patients with familial neuroblastoma have bilateral adrenal or multifocal primary tumors, which is quite unusual in spontaneous cases. The risk for development of neuroblastoma in a sibling or offspring of a patient with neuroblastoma is less than 6% (Kushner et al, 1986).

Constitutional Chromosome Abnormalities

Numerous karyotypic abnormalities have been found in patients with neuroblastoma and are recognized to have prognostic significance. These changes occur in the form of chromosomal deletions, translocations, and cytogenetic evidence of gene amplification. Deletion of the short arm of chromosome 1 is found in 70% to 80% of patients with neuroblastoma and is an adverse prognostic marker (Brodeur et al, 1992; Caron et al, 1996). The deletions are of various lengths, but in a series of eight cases a consensus deletion included the segment 1p36.1-2, thus suggesting that genetic information related to neuroblastoma tumorigenesis is located in that segment (Weith et al, 1989). There have been two reports of constitutional abnormalities involving the short arm of chromosome 1 (Lampert et al, 1988; Laureys et al, 1990).

Aneuploidy of tumor DNA occurs in a significant number of cases and is a favorable prognostic indicator, whereas amplification of the N-*myc* oncogene is an adverse prognostic indicator (Look et al, 1991; Muraji et al, 1993). These findings have been so striking that neuroblastoma was the first tumor in which the intensity of chemotherapy for a patient was determined not only by the stage and histology of the tumor but by its "biologic markers," which were primarily chromosomal (Matthay et al, 1998).

Embryology and Spontaneous Regression

In 1963, Beckwith and Perrin coined the term *in situ neuroblastoma* for small nodules of neuroblasts found incidentally within the adrenal gland that are histologically indistinguishable from neuroblastoma. In situ neuroblastoma was found in 1 of 224 infants younger than 3 months during postmortem examination. This incidence is approximately 40 to 45 times greater than that of clinical tumors, which suggests that these small tumors regress spontaneously in most cases. Studies have subsequently shown that these neuroblastic nodules are found in all fetuses studied and generally regress (Ikeda et al,

1981). Neuroblastoma identified by prenatal ultrasound has also been shown to have a clinically favorable course (Ho et al, 1993).

The concept of in situ neuroblastoma has been used to support the argument that many neuroblastomas arise and regress spontaneously. This concept has been further supported by population-based studies in the province of Quebec and in Japan, where prospective screening of infants for neuroblastoma has been conducted on the basis of urinary catecholamine excretion. An increased number of children were identified with low-stage neuroblastoma, a higher frequency than found clinically, but there was no decrease in the incidence of advanced-stage tumors seen at an older age (Hayashi et al, 1995; Woods et al, 1996). Evaluation of adrenal tumors resected in the neonatal period, whether cystic or solid, showed that in most the "biologic markers" were favorable (Kozakewich et al, 1998). The highly favorable outcome of infants in whom neuroblastoma was diagnosed in the population screening studies first led to attempts at expectant observation. These trials demonstrated a high rate of spontaneous resolution (Yamamoto et al, 1998; Yoneda et al, 2001). Spontaneous regression of these perinatally identified lesions has also been demonstrated radiographically (Holgerson et al, 1996). A current prospective study by the Children's Oncology Group is evaluating infants with adrenal masses identified in the perinatal or neonatal period. Expectant observation for infants with small lesions and favorable catecholamine ratios is encouraged. These lesions are then monitored closely by serial ultrasound evaluation. The goal of this protocol is to document that expectant observation in these small stage I lesions in infants is safe and appropriate, as has been suggested by smaller retrospective studies.

Pathology

Neuroblastoma, ganglioneuroblastoma, and ganglioneuroma display a histologic spectrum of maturation and differentiation. A grading classification of neuroblastoma introduced in 1984 by Shimada and subsequently modified by him and others as the International Neuroblastoma Pathology Classification has helped define risk-based subtypes of ganglioneuroblastoma and neuroblastoma (Shimada et al, 1984, 1999a, 1999b). Ganglioneuroma is a histologically benign, fully differentiated counterpart of neuroblastoma. It is unclear whether ganglioneuroma arises de novo or by maturation of a preexisting neuroblastoma or ganglioneuroblastoma. Metastatic lesions from neuroblastoma have been observed to develop the histology of mature ganglioneuroma, thus supporting the latter theory (Hayes et al, 1989).

The Shimada classification is an age-linked histopathologic classification. One of its important aspects is determining whether the tumor is stroma poor or stroma rich. Patients with stroma-poor tumors and unfavorable histopathologic features have a very poor prognosis (less than 10% survival rate) (Shimada et al, 1984). **Stroma-rich tumors can be separated into three subgroups: nodular, intermixed, and well differentiated. Tumors in the latter two categories more closely resemble ganglioneuroblastoma or immature ganglioneuroma and carry a higher rate of survival.** Stroma-poor tumors can be divided into favorable and unfavorable subgroups based on the patient's age at diagnosis, the degree of histologic maturation, and the mitotic rate. When compared with other clinical features, these histologic patterns were independently predictive of outcome (Shimada et al, 1984).

In contrast to neuroblastomas, ganglioneuromas are most often diagnosed in older children and are usually located in the posterior mediastinum and retroperitoneum, with only a small number arising in the adrenal glands (Enzinger and Weiss, 1988). Ganglioneuromas often grow to very large size before they cause symptoms as a result of compression of adjacent structures or extension into the spinal canal (Benjamin et al, 1972) (Fig. 130–1).

Clinical Findings and Pattern of Spread

The clinical manifestations of neuroblastoma vary widely. Although most children have abdominal pain or a palpable mass, many have manifestations of their metastatic disease, including bone or joint pain and periorbital ecchymosis. Thoracic lesions may produce respiratory symptoms of cough or dyspnea. Direct extension of the tumor into the spinal canal may give rise to neurologic deficits as a result of cord compression.

Most primary tumors arise within the abdomen (65%); the frequency of adrenal tumors is slightly higher in children than in infants. Physical examination often reveals a fixed, hard abdominal mass. Pelvic neuroblastomas arising from the organ of Zuckerkandl account for only 4% of tumors (Haase et al, 1995). Extrinsic compression of the bowel and bladder can produce symptoms of urinary retention and constipation (Fig. 130–2).

Metastases are present in 70% of patients with neuroblastoma at diagnosis and can be responsible for a variety of the clinical signs and symptoms seen. A number of unique paraneoplastic syndromes have been associated with both localized and disseminated neuroblastoma. Symptoms produced by catecholamine release may mimic those seen in pheochromocytoma: paroxysmal hypertension, palpitations, flushing, and headache. Secretion of vasoactive intestinal polypeptide by the tumor can produce severe watery diarrhea

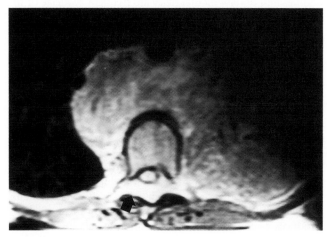

Figure 130–1. Magnetic resonance image of a child with thoracic ganglioneuroma extending into the spinal canal (*arrow*).

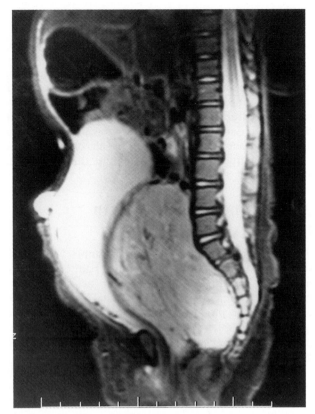

Figure 130–2. Magnetic resonance image demonstrating compression of the bowel and bladder by a pelvic neuroblastoma.

and hypokalemia (Cooney et al, 1982). Another unusual manifestation of neuroblastoma is acute myoclonic encephalopathy, in which myoclonus, rapid multidirectional eye movements (opsoclonus), and ataxia develop. It is thought to result from an interaction of antibodies produced against the neuroblastoma and normal neural tissue (Farrelly et al, 1984; Connolly et al, 1997). Although this syndrome is associated with a favorable outcome from an oncologic perspective (Altman and Baehner, 1976), prolonged neurologic impairment is the rule, and symptomatic therapy is often required (Koh et al, 1994; Russo et al, 1997). Learning disabilities and developmental delay are frequent sequelae of the syndrome. Adrenocorticotropic hormone (ACTH) is the most effective therapy, but other treatments include high-dose intravenous gamma globulin and cyclophosphamide. A current protocol of the Children's Oncology Group is evaluating the efficacy of intravenous gamma globulin and corticosteroids in the treatment of these children.

Diagnosis

Laboratory Evaluation

When sensitive techniques are used, increased levels of urinary metabolites of catecholamines, vanillylmandelic acid and homovanillic acid, are found in 90% to 95% of patients (Williams and Greer, 1963). Therapy with various modalities produces a reduction in catecholamine metabolite excretion in most patients (Gerson and Koop, 1974). These metabolites can be monitored to detect tumor relapse.

Anemia is noted in children with widespread bone marrow involvement. Studies suggest that marrow biopsies add substantially to the detection of marrow involvement by tumor as compared with marrow aspirates alone (Franklin and Pritchard, 1983). It is recommended that two marrow aspirates and two biopsies be performed. In the near future, it is likely that neuroblastoma-specific immunocytology of marrow aspirates will obviate the need for marrow biopsies in most patients (Moss et al, 1985; Hsiao et al, 1990).

Imaging

Imaging studies play an important role in the evaluation of a child with neuroblastoma. Plain radiographs may demonstrate a calcified abdominal or posterior mediastinal mass. Both bone scintigraphy and a skeletal survey should be performed to detect cortical bone metastases (Heisel et al, 1983). Metastatic lesions occur most commonly in the long bones and skull. If the skeletal films are negative, a radionuclide bone scan may detect metastases at an earlier stage. A newer method of imaging both the tumor and metastatic sites involves radiolabeled iodine I 131 metaiodobenzylguanidine (MIBG) (Geatti et al, 1985), which is taken up by the adrenergic secretory vesicles of the tumor cells in both primary and metastatic sites. MIBG scintigraphy can be used to determine the extent of disease and also to detect recurrence of tumor after the completion of therapy (Geatti et al, 1985). Others have reported that the findings of MIBG scans have little impact on patient treatment (Andrich et al, 1996). Ultrasound, computed tomography (CT), and magnetic resonance imaging (MRI) provide more information about the local extent of the primary tumors. Invasion of the renal parenchyma is not common, but it can be detected radiographically by CT (Albregts et al, 1994). MRI has advantages over CT in the evaluation of intraspinal tumor extension (see Fig. 130–1) and in demonstrating the relationship between the major vessels and the tumor (Azizhkan and Haase, 1993) (Fig. 130–3).

Screening

Mass population screening for neuroblastoma has been widely performed in Japan for more than 20 years (Nishi et al, 1987). The goal of screening programs is to detect disease at an earlier stage and decrease the number of older children with advanced-stage disease, thereby improving survival. In fact, children in whom neuroblastoma has been diagnosed as a result of screening studies have had almost uniformly favorable survival (>97%) (Suita, 2002). An increased number of infants younger than 1 year with neuroblastoma have been detected through the mass screening program (Ishimoto et al, 1990), and most of these patients have lower-stage tumors (Sawada, 1992). Before mass screening started, 20% of cases of neuroblastoma were diagnosed before 1 year of age as compared with 55% after its implementation. However, the number of children older than 1 year in whom advanced-stage disease is diagnosed has not decreased. These results suggest that the aggressive advanced-stage tumors in older children did not arise from the low-risk tumors seen in infants younger than 1 year.

There are biologic differences between tumors diagnosed by screening and those detected clinically (Hayashi et al, 1992). In one review of 48 cases discovered by screening, no tumors were observed to have amplified N-*myc* oncogene expression

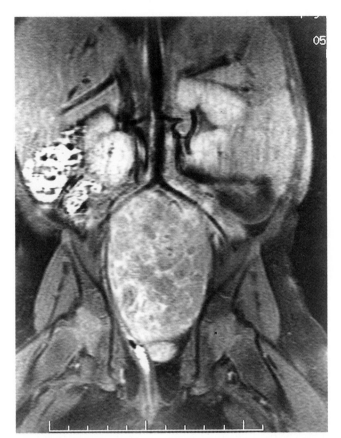

Figure 130–3. Magnetic resonance imaging of pelvic neuroblastoma. The bifurcation of the aorta and the iliac vessels are well delineated, as well as the relationship to the mass.

Table 130–1. **International Neuroblastoma Staging System**	
Stage	**Definition**
1	Localized tumor with complete gross excision, with or without microscopic residual disease; representative ipsilateral lymph nodes negative for tumor microscopically (nodes attached to and removed with the primary tumor may be positive)
2A	Localized tumor with incomplete gross excision; representative ipsilateral nonadherent lymph nodes negative for tumor microscopically
2B	Localized tumor with or without complete gross excision, with ipsilateral nonadherent lymph nodes positive for tumor. Enlarged contralateral lymph nodes must be negative microscopically
3	Unresectable unilateral tumor infiltrating across the midline,* with or without regional lymph node involvement; localized unilateral tumor with contralateral regional lymph node involvement; or midline tumor with bilateral extension by infiltration (unresectable) or by lymph node involvement
4	Any primary tumor with dissemination to distant lymph nodes, bone, bone marrow, liver, skin, and/or other organs
4S	Localized primary tumor (as defined for stage 1, 2A, or 2B), with dissemination limited to the skin, liver, and/or bone marrow (less than 10% tumor) in infants <1 year of age

*The midline is defined as the vertebral column. Tumors originating on one side and crossing the midline must infiltrate to or beyond the opposite side of the vertebral column.

(Ishimoto et al, 1991), and in a second review of 20 infants, only 1 who did poorly demonstrated amplification (Hase et al, 2002). Furthermore, 80% had a diploid chromosome pattern, which is also associated with a favorable prognosis. On follow-up, all 48 patients were still alive without tumor. In another series of 357 patients whose tumors were diagnosed by mass screening, the overall survival rate was 97% (Sawada, 1992). Given the favorable biologic characteristics of tumors discovered by screening, it is possible that many would spontaneously resolve without therapy, particularly given the increased incidence of neuroblastomas seen in the screened population.

Two large prospective population-based studies have now been completed in the province of Quebec and in Germany and have conclusively demonstrated that although urine screening at various ages was successful in identification of neuroblastoma, there was no decrease in the occurrence of neuroblastoma in older children and its subsequent mortality (Woods et al, 2002; Schilling et al, 2002).

Staging

Staging of neuroblastoma is an important aspect of management. The stage of the disease is a significant prognostic variable that determines adjuvant therapy. The International Neuroblastoma Staging System (INSS) is based on clinical, radiographic, and surgical evaluation of children with neu-

roblastoma (Brodeur et al, 1993) (Table 130–1). Earlier staging systems provided generally comparable results in terms of distinguishing low-stage, good-prognosis disease from high-stage, poor-prognosis disease. Use of a uniform international system, however, makes comparison of results from various studies much easier. The biggest differences arise when the various systems are applied to patients with intermediate-stage disease. It is in this cohort of children where use of the risk group classification, which combines pathologic findings, stage, and several of the biologic markers, best defines the child's risk for progressive disease (Katzenstein and Cohn, 1998). Although the classification appears complex (Table 130–2), it provides the most accurate assessment of how intense the chemotherapy and radiotherapy must be to cure the child.

Prognostic Factors

Many variables affect the prognosis of children with neuroblastoma. In addition to clinical features, many biologic studies can now be used to stratify patients for treatment.

Clinical Variables

Age still remains an important indicator of outcome, as originally reported by Breslow and McCann (1971). With current treatment, children 1 year or younger have better survival than older children do (Nitschke et al, 1988), which may be attributed to more favorable biologic parameters in tumors diagnosed at this age. Teenagers and adults with neuroblastoma have a particularly indolent and relentless form of the disease (Kushner et al, 2003; Gaspar et al, 2003). **The *site of origin* is of significance in that better survival is noted in children with nonadrenal primary tumors** (Haase et al,

Table 130–2. **Risk Group Classification**

Risk Group	INSS Stage	Age (Days)	N-myc Status	DNA Index	Shimada Histopathology
Low	1	Any	Any	Any	Any
	2A, 2B	<365	Any	Any	Any
	2A, 2B	≥365	Nonamplified	Any	Any
	2A, 2B	≥365	Amplified	Any	Favorable
	4S	<365	Nonamplified	>1.0	Favorable
Intermediate	3	<365	Nonamplified	Any	Any
	3	≥365	Nonamplified	Any	Favorable
	4	<365	Nonamplified	Any	Any
	4S	<365	Nonamplified	1.0	Favorable
	4S	<365	Nonamplified	Any	Unfavorable
High	2A, 2B	≥365	Amplified	Any	Unfavorable
	3	<365	Amplified	Any	Any
	3	≥365	Nonamplified	Any	Unfavorable
	3	≥365	Amplified	Any	Any
	4	<365	Amplified	Any	Any
	4	≥365	Any	Any	Any
	4S	<365	Amplified	Any	Any

INSS, International Neuroblastoma Staging System.

1995). Most children with thoracic neuroblastoma are initially seen at a younger age with localized disease and have improved survival even when corrected for age and stage (Adams et al, 1993). Tumors at this site are less likely to demonstrate N-*myc* amplification and more likely to have a DNA index greater than 1.0, both favorable prognostic indicators (Morris et al, 1995).

Stage of the disease is another powerful independent prognostic indicator. Virtually all stage I patients with complete resection of the primary tumor survive. Stage II patients also have a favorable survival prospect, even though there may be incomplete excision (Matthay et al, 1989). Children with advanced regional disease, stages III or IV, fare less well and require more intensive treatment. The proportion of patients initially seen with localized, regional, or metastatic disease is dependent on age (Nitschke et al, 1988). The overall survival rate of children with stages I, II, or IV-S is between 75% and 90%, whereas children with stage IV disease have a 2-year disease-free survival rate in the range of 19% to 30% despite intensive therapy, including bone marrow transplantation. The outcome for infants younger than 1 year is substantially better than that for older patients with the same stage of disease.

Stage IV-S (S = special) is a distinct category referring to infants with small primary tumors and liver, skin, and bone marrow metastases without radiographic evidence of bone metastases. It was first proposed by Evans and coworkers in 1971. This group of patients has a good prognosis with overall survival rates ranging from 80% to 88%. The INSS criteria later restricted this stage to children with less than 10% bone marrow involvement (Brodeur et al, 1993). This stage accounts for 7% to 10% of all cases of neuroblastoma. Many of these tumors undergo spontaneous regression (Evans et al, 1980, 1987; Haas et al, 1990). The tumors in children with stage IV-S neuroblastoma in general have favorable prognostic findings not typically seen in children with stage IV disease (Hachitanda et al, 1991; Nickerson et al, 2000). Poor outcome in stage IV-S patients is associated with elevated serum neuron-specific enolase (>100 nmol/mL), ferritin (>280 ng/mL), and urinary dopamine levels (>2500 nmol/mmol creatinine), as well as N-*myc* amplification and chromosome 1p deletion (Schleiermacher et al, 2003). Most deaths in this group occur in infants younger than 2 months with extensive abdominal involvement and respiratory compromise or disseminated intravascular coagulation (Nickerson et al, 2000).

Biologic Variables

The presence of homogeneously staining regions and double minute chromosomes was noted in approximately a third of neuroblastomas. These abnormalities are cytogenic manifestations of gene amplification, and it was subsequently found that the N-*myc* oncogene mapped to these regions. The association of N-*myc* amplification with the pathogenesis of neuroblastoma is unclear, but N-*myc* amplification is almost always present at the time of diagnosis (Brodeur, 1991). **Seeger and colleagues** (1985, 1988) **showed that N-*myc* amplification is associated with rapid tumor progression and a poor prognosis. Amplification is found in 5% to 10% of patients with low-stage or stage IV-S disease** (Hachitanda et al, 1991), **but in 30% to 40% of those with advanced-stage disease** (Brodeur and Fong, 1989; Brodeur, 1990). **The poor prognosis associated with N-*myc* amplification is independent of patient age or stage of disease at diagnosis.** However, not all patients with a poor outcome have N-*myc* amplification. Many advanced-stage tumors lack N-*myc* at diagnosis, and recurrence or progression of disease develops in most of these patients.

The DNA content of tumor cells and ploidy number have been reported to have prognostic value in patients with neuroblastoma (Cohn et al, 1990). Studies of DNA content measured by flow cytometry have shown that a "hyperdiploid" karyotype (or increased DNA content) was associated with a favorable outcome (Look et al, 1984; Kusafuka et al, 1994). DNA diploidy and tetraploidy were associated with decreased survival. Deletions of the short arm of chromosome 1 have been found in 70% to 80% of the near-diploid tumors that have been karyotyped (Brodeur and Fong, 1989; Brodeur, 1990). Preliminary studies suggest a correlation between 1p deletion and poor survival (Brodeur and Fong, 1989; Hayashi et al, 1989). Because there is an association between N-*myc* amplification and 1p deletion, it remains to be determined whether this finding has independent prognostic significance.

Children currently treated on protocols of the Children's Oncology Group are assigned to a risk group that is determined by age, stage of disease, N-*myc* status, histologic grade, and DNA ploidy (Katzenstein et al, 1998) (see Table 130–2). Other factors that have been demonstrated to have prognostic significance, although they are often associated with these genetic abnormalities, include expression of the gene encoding the high-affinity nerve growth factor receptor (termed the *TRKA* proto-oncogene) and the low-affinity nerve growth factor receptor (Tanaka et al, 1995). Both are favorable prognostic predictors and are inversely related to amplification of the N-*myc* oncogene (Nakagawara et al, 1993). Lack of expression of CD44 glycoprotein on the tumor cell surface and increased levels of serum ferritin, serum neuron-specific enolase, and serum lactate dehydrogenase are adverse prognostic factors (Chan et al, 1991; Silber et al, 1991). They have not, however, been shown by multivariate analysis to be independently predictive apart from age, stage, ploidy, and N-*myc* status.

KEY POINTS: NEUROBLASTOMA

- Neuroblastoma is the most common extracranial solid neoplasm in children.

- Metastatic disease occurs in 70% of patients. Children 1 year or younger have a better survival rate than older children do.

- Complete surgical resection is curative for low-stage disease.

- N-*myc* amplification, found in 30% to 40% of patients with advanced disease, is associated with tumor progression. This poor prognosis is independent of patient age and tumor stage.

Treatment

The treatment modalities primarily used for the management of neuroblastoma are surgery, chemotherapy, and radiation therapy. The role of each in individual patients varies depending on tumor stage, age, and biologic prognostic factors. These characteristics can be used to stratify patients into favorable and unfavorable categories by risk group (see Table 130–2).

Surgery

The goals of surgery are to establish the diagnosis, stage the tumor, excise the tumor (if localized), and provide tissue for biologic studies. Determination of resectability of the primary tumor should take into consideration tumor location, mobility, relationship to major vessels, and overall prognosis of the patient. With the efficacy of modern chemotherapy in reducing the size of primary tumors, sacrifice of vital structures to achieve resection at diagnosis should be avoided, particularly in young children in whom the prognosis is excellent.

Low-Risk Disease (Stages I, II, and IV-S). Children with stage I neuroblastoma have a disease-free survival rate of greater than 90% with surgical excision alone (O'Neill et al, 1985; Nitschke et al, 1988; DeBernardi et al, 1995). **Chemotherapy is indicated only in the event of recurrence, unless the child has N-*myc* amplification and unfavorable histology.** The Pediatric Oncology Group reviewed 101 children with localized neuroblastoma who underwent complete gross excision of the primary tumor (Nitschke et al, 1988). Nine patients experienced relapse, but six were salvaged with chemotherapy. Radiation therapy has no role in this subset of patients. With current use of risk factor grading, children with recurrence in the past may be identified now as the small number with adverse biologic markers. In a comparable study from the Children's Cancer Group, 374 stage I and II patients were treated primarily by resection (Perez et al, 2000). Event-free and overall survival for stage I patients was 93% ± 3% and 99% ± 1% versus 81% ± 4% and 98% ± 2% for stage II patients. Supplemental treatment was required in only 10% of stage I and 20% of stage II patients and achieved excellent overall survival in the stage II patients. N-*myc* amplification, unfavorable histology, age older than 2 years, and positive lymph nodes predicted lower overall survival.

Radical resection resulting in removal of normal organs, particularly the kidney, is not justified in this group of patients. Irradiation of the local tumor bed has been advocated for treatment of residual disease in stage II cases. However, a review of 156 patients with stage II neuroblastoma found a 90% 6-year progression-free survival rate regardless of whether radiation therapy was used (Matthay et al, 1989). Therefore, radiation therapy should be reserved for patients who fail to respond to either primary or secondary chemotherapy. In stage III disease, or in stage II with extensive tumor around the kidney and renal vessels, preoperative treatment with chemotherapy significantly decreases the risk for nephrectomy as a result of resection of the tumor (Shamberger et al, 1998) (Fig. 130–4).

The generally favorable behavior of stage IV-S disease has been explained with the understanding of biologic markers. The vast majority of these infants have tumors with entirely favorable markers, thus explaining their favorable behavior. However, a small percentage have adverse markers, and it is these children who have progressive disease that is often fatal. Resection of the primary is not mandatory (Nickerson et al, 1985; Evans et al, 1987). Although excellent survival has been reported after surgery (Martinez et al, 1992), information regarding histologic prognostic factors was not available for all of these patients. In a review of 110 infants with stage IV-S disease, the entire cohort had an estimated 3-year survival rate of 85% ± 4% (Katzenstein et al, 1998). This rate was significantly decreased to 68% ± 12% for infants whose tumors were diploid, to 44% ± 33% for those with N-*myc* amplification, and to 33% ± 19% for those with unfavorable histology. Of note, there was no statistical difference in survival rate for infants who underwent complete resection of their primary tumor versus those who had partial resection or only biopsy (Katzenstein et al, 1998; Nickerson et al, 2000; von Schweinitz et al, 2002). Patients with extensive

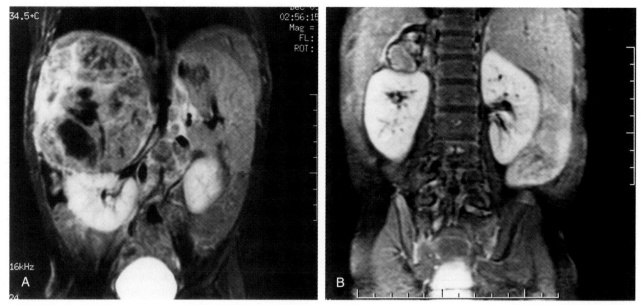

Figure 130–4. Magnetic resonance imaging before and after chemotherapy shows a marked reduction in size of a right suprarenal neuroblastoma. **A,** Before chemotherapy. **B,** After chemotherapy.

metastatic disease and N-*myc* amplification represent a high-risk group (Martinez et al, 1992). These patients should be considered for more aggressive treatment with multimodal therapy, according to the risk group classification (see Table 130–2) (Schleiermacher et al, 2003). Those with favorable biologic markers and no symptoms can be monitored and given supportive care, with limited chemotherapy and hepatic radiotherapy administered to infants with significant symptoms. Intensive chemotherapy is reserved for those with adverse markers, although these infants do poorly even with therapy.

High-Risk Disease (Stages III and IV). There is debate regarding the extent of surgical resection that is required for stage III lesions. A report of 58 patients with stage III disease from the Children's Cancer Group found that 8 of 12 patients with initial complete excision and 12 of 14 with subsequent resection of the primary tumor were long-term survivors (Haase et al, 1989). This outcome contrasts with only 9 of 32 survivors among patients in whom complete tumor excision could not be accomplished. Significant morbidity was reported in association with the surgical procedures, including 21 major complications. The Italian Cooperative Group for Neuroblastoma found that complete resection after chemotherapy for extensive unresectable neuroblastoma was associated with improved survival when compared with partial resection only (Garaventa et al, 1993). Similar results have been noted by others (LeTourneau et al, 1985; O'Neill et al, 1985; Powis et al, 1996). It has been suggested by some that even children with stage III disease do not need cytotoxic therapy if the biologic marker N-*myc* amplification is not present (Kushner et al, 1996). These results are not widely accepted, however, and confirmatory studies are required before this policy can be widely adopted.

Children with bulky pelvic tumors generally do quite well even with limited residual disease (Leclair et al, 2004). Extensive surgery at this site has been associated with long-term

neurologic sequelae, so the extent of resection must be balanced against this morbidity.

The evidence is conflicting in stage IV disease between studies that support (Cecchetto et al, 1983; LeTourneau et al, 1985; Haase et al, 1991; Tsuchida et al, 1992; LaQuaglia et al, 1994; Chamberlain et al, 1995; DeCou et al, 1995; Yokoyama et al, 1995; Adkins et al, 2004; Kuroda et al, 2003) and those that refute (Sitarz et al, 1983; Matsumura et al, 1988; Adams et al, 1993; Losty et al, 1993; Kiely, 1994; Kaneko et al, 1997; Castel et al, 2002; von Schweinitz et al, 2002) the role of extensive resection. In a retrospective review, Kiely (1994) compared the results of radical tumor resection with those of more conventional surgery in patients with stage III and IV disease. He found no difference in survival between 46 patients treated with radical surgical procedures and 34 patients treated with more conventional surgery. Shorter and colleagues (1995) also did not find any evidence that the extent of surgical resection had an impact on the survival of stage IV patients. In these nonrandomized studies, it has been difficult to determine whether the improved survival in those with complete resection has been due to more favorable intrinsic biology of the tumor allowing resection or truly due to the completeness of resection.

As the intensity of therapy increases, including the use of autologous bone marrow transplantation, and control of distant metastasis improves, the impact of maximal local control may become apparent. The combination of gross total resection and external beam irradiation has achieved local control in 84% to 90% of children (Wolden et al, 2000; Kushner et al, 2001). In another series of reports, intensive chemotherapy followed by double autologous bone marrow transplantation, aggressive surgical resection, and radiotherapy has achieved an overall survival rate of 56% and a local recurrence rate of only 2.6% (Marcus et al, 2003; von Allmen et al, 2005).

Usually, the safest approach for advanced tumors is to defer tumor resection until after initial chemotherapy

(Berthold et al, 1989; Shamberger et al, 1991; Shochat, 1992; LaQuaglia et al, 1994; Black et al, 1996). **After chemotherapy, the tumors are smaller and firmer, with less risk of rupture and hemorrhage, thereby resulting in a decreased rate of complications, particularly nephrectomy** (Shamberger et al, 1998) (see Fig. 130–4). One specific complication that is encountered after resection of extensive tumor surrounding the celiac axis and the superior mesenteric artery is diarrhea (Kiely, 1994). It is thought to result from resection of the autonomic nerves to the gut found anterior to the aorta at the base of the superior mesenteric artery and the celiac axis (Rees et al, 1998). Preoperative chemotherapy does appear to increase the proportion of children able to achieve complete resection (Adkins et al, 2004).

Surgery is usually performed 13 to 18 weeks after initiation of chemotherapy so that three to four courses of treatment can be completed (Azizkhan and Haase, 1993). Some tumors remain inoperable even after chemotherapy. Other attempts at local tumor control for unresectable disease have included the use of intraoperative radiation therapy. This technique has the advantage of delivering a higher dose of radiation to the operative field while sparing normal adjacent tissues (Leavey et al, 1997).

Infants younger than 1 year with extensive local or stage IV disease represent a special subset of patients. They have historically fared much better than children older than 1 year with comparable disease, but not as well as infants with stage IV-S disease. It is now recognized that biologic markers can be used to identify which infants have high-risk disease and require intensive therapy and which will have intermediate-risk disease requiring less intensive therapy.

In a large cohort (134 infants), N-*myc* amplification, serum ferritin, Shimada histopathologic classification, and bone marrow involvement by immunocytology were analyzed. Although each factor had prognostic significance by univariate analysis, only N-*myc* was significant by multivariate analysis; the event-free survival rate in infants without N-*myc* amplification was 93% ± 4% versus 10% ± 7% in those with amplification despite intensive therapy (Rubie et al, 2001; Schmidt et al, 2000).

Chemotherapy

A variety of multiagent treatment regimens have been developed to treat high-risk patients with neuroblastoma. The goal of such treatment intensification is better disease control. Although initial response rates are improving, with a prolonged time to progression of disease, relapse continues to be a major problem, and the 4-year overall survival rate in patients with stage IV disease is 20% (Ikeda et al, 1989; Haase et al, 1991). The dose intensification of chemotherapy needed for local tumor control results in significant myelosuppression, thus limiting the amount of therapy that can be given. This has prompted the use of autologous bone marrow transplantation after sublethal chemotherapy or total-body irradiation.

The use of marrow-ablative chemoradiotherapy followed by autologous marrow reinfusion has resulted in complete remission in up to 50% of patients with recurrent stage IV disease (Moss et al, 1987; Seeger et al, 1991; Dinndorf et al, 1992; Mugishima et al, 1994; Matthay et al, 1995; Grupp et al, 2000). However, a significant problem is the risk for late relapse. The presence of bulky disease results in increased failure. Tumor debulking via surgery or radiation therapy is warranted before autologous bone marrow transplantation. However, there are many questions yet to be resolved about this modality of treatment. The toxicity of bone marrow transplantation can be lethal, and the long-term complications in patients with successful transplantation are unknown. Nonetheless, these risks are acceptable given that long-term survival is difficult to achieve in these patients without such aggressive therapy.

New Innovative Biologic Therapies

Because increasing the intensity of chemotherapy appears to have reached its limit with the use of double autologous bone marrow transplantation, other routes of treatment must be identified. The use of biologic modifiers is being investigated (Villablanca et al, 1995). 13-*cis*-Retinoic acid produces differentiation of neuroblastoma in cell culture. It was given to children with advanced-stage disease for a 6-month period after cytotoxic therapy and significantly decreased the frequency of relapse (Matthay et al, 1999). Other avenues of treatment in current phase I and phase II trials include vaccine and antibody therapy against the G_{02} cell surface marker occurring in neuroblastoma. A new synthetic retinoid, fenretinide, which has produced apoptosis rather than differentiation in neuroblastoma cell lines, is also in early clinical trials.

Inhibition of angiogenesis is another appealing avenue of therapy for this very vascular tumor, particularly once there is minimal residual disease. Anti-angiogenic therapy has proved successful in animal models but has not yet been used clinically.

Another modality in the treatment of metastatic neuroblastoma is the use of ^{131}I-MIBG (Hutchinson et al, 1992). The finding that both the primary tumor and metastatic areas take up this radiotracer suggested the possibility that therapeutic doses can be delivered to the tumor. Preliminary analysis indicates that objective responses in terms of reduction of tumor volume do occur.

Radiotherapy

Radiotherapy is effective for local control of neuroblastoma, and risk for local relapse can be correlated with biologic markers. Although irradiation has not provided a benefit in low-stage tumors, it has increased local control in children with advanced stage IV or bulky stage III tumors (Matthay et al, 1989; Castleberry et al, 1991; Evans et al, 1996). A randomized controlled trial to evaluate the efficacy of local control with radiotherapy alone or surgery has not been performed. Doses of external beam radiation used have ranged between 15 and 30 Gy, depending on the patient's age and the location and extent of residual disease. Although the use of intraoperative radiotherapy has been promoted, it has not been convincingly demonstrated to be more favorable than external beam irradiation (Haase et al, 1991; Haas-Kogan et al, 2000).

Spinal Cord Compression

Extension of tumor into the spinal canal produces symptoms of spinal cord compression in up to 5% of patients with neuroblastoma (DeBernardi et al, 2001), and up to 13% of patients have evidence of extension into the spinal canal radiographically (Plantaz et al, 1998). These children have been treated by decompressive laminectomy, radiotherapy, or chemotherapy. Neurologic outcomes have been similar with all modalities, and regrettably, patients with severe motor deficits generally recover little function (DeBernardi et al, 2001; Katzenstein et al, 2001). Because of the delayed complication of scoliosis after laminectomy, current recommendations are to initiate treatment with chemotherapy and reserve laminectomy for children with progressive neurologic deterioration (Katzenstein et al, 2001). Radiotherapy is now generally avoided because of its adverse effect on growth of the spine.

Other Adrenal Lesions

Adrenocortical tumors are rare in children. The tumor types, adenomas or carcinomas, seen in children are similar to those in adults, and both can be hormonally active. They may produce cortisol, aldosterone, androgens, and estrogens. Adenomas are more likely to produce steroid hormones, but 50% of carcinomas in children older than 5 years secrete hormones (Driver et al, 1998). Hormonally active tumors will manifest stigmata of the associated hormone, such as hypertension, cushingoid features, and precocious puberty. Virilization and Cushing's syndrome are the most common manifestations.

Cushing's syndrome as a result of adrenal tumors is rare. However, children younger than 5 years are much more likely to have either an adrenal adenoma or an ectopic ACTH-secreting tumor (Bornstein et al, 1999).

Laboratory and imaging studies are invaluable in differentiating adrenal tumors from other causes of Cushing's syndrome. Pituitary ACTH production will be suppressed by the elevated cortisol produced by functioning adrenal adenomas or carcinomas. Imaging with CT or preferably MRI can detect most lesions (Ribeiro et al, 2000). T2-weighted imaging demonstrates enhancement of the lesion. Imaging can also distinguish these lesions from the micronodular form of adrenal hyperplasia, or Carney's disease.

Another rare adrenal tumor in children is pheochromocytoma arising from chromaffin cells in the medulla. It occurs primarily in children aged 6 to 15 years, with a slight male preponderance (Kaufman et al, 1983). The majority of children with pheochromocytoma have sustained hypertension. Approximately 10% of adrenal pheochromocytomas are malignant, and the diagnosis of malignancy is established by the presence of metastases. Tumors arising from the extra-adrenal sympathetic nervous system are called paragangliomas. Both tumors can synthesize catecholamines, which results in their clinical findings. These tumors are associated with several syndromes: multiple endocrine neoplasia (MEN IIA, MEN IIB), von Hippel-Landau (VHL) disease, and neurofibromatosis-1. Fortunately, genetic testing is available for patients with a family history because the genes responsible for pheochromocytoma in MEN, the *RET* proto-oncogene, and VHL, the *VHL* tumor suppressor gene, have been identified.

The diagnosis of pheochromocytoma also requires both laboratory and imaging evaluation. Plasma metanephrine levels are measured, but they may not be elevated if hypertension is paroxysmal. CT or MRI will detect most lesions, and T2-weighted images will demonstrate a bright lesion. MIBG scanning is very specific for pheochromocytoma and can

identify lesions, particularly in nonadrenal locations, that are missed on other imaging modalities (Sisson et al, 1981).

Treatment of adrenal tumors, as in adults, is primarily surgical. Laparoscopy has assumed a much greater role, particularly for small tumors and adenomas. Preoperative and postoperative medical management is important for functional tumors.

GENITOURINARY RHABDOMYOSARCOMA

Rhabdomyosarcoma (RMS) is the most common soft tissue sarcoma in infants and children, and it accounts for approximately half of all pediatric soft tissue sarcomas and 15% of all pediatric solid tumors. It is the third most common solid tumor in children after neuroblastoma and Wilms' tumor. **Fifteen percent to 20% of all cases of RMS arise from the genitourinary system** (Maurer et al, 1988; Crist et al, 2001). **The most common genitourinary sites are the prostate, bladder, and paratesticular region; involvement of the vagina and uterus is relatively unusual. Survival rates vary with the site, with certain sites such as the vagina and paratesticular region having a better prognosis than bladder/prostate primaries** (Rodary et al, 1988; Crist et al, 1990; Martelli et al, 1999; Arndt et al, 2001; Weiner et al, 2001; Ferrari et al, 2002). There is a bimodal age distribution, with a peak incidence in the first 2 years of life and again at adolescence, but two thirds of cases occur in children younger than 6 years (LaQuaglia et al, 1994). The botryoid variants arising from the bladder and vagina are seen almost exclusively in young children.

Etiology, Epidemiology, and Genetics

Subgroups of children with a genetic predisposition for the development of RMS have been identified. The Li-Fraumeni syndrome associates childhood sarcomas with mothers who have an excess of premenopausal breast cancer and with siblings who have an increased risk for cancer (Li and Fraumeni, 1969). **A mutation of the *p53* tumor suppressor gene was found in the tumors in all patients with this syndrome** (Malkin et al, 1990). An increased incidence of RMS has been found in association with neurofibromatosis (McKeen et al, 1978; Sung et al, 2004). In the fourth Intergroup Rhabdomyosarcoma Study (IRS-IV), 0.5% of children enrolled had neurofibromatosis.

The two major histologic subtypes of RMS, embryonal and alveolar, have been noted to have distinct cytogenetic abnormalities. Alveolar RMS is associated with a translocation between chromosomes 1 or 2 and 13, and it results in the formation of a chimeric protein (Parham, 1994). PAX3, a DNA binding protein on chromosome 2, or PAX7, a DNA binding protein on chromosome 1, is fused to the *FKHR* gene on chromosome 13 (Anderson et al, 2001). These genes may be involved in the pathogenesis of alveolar RMS and are prognostic factors as well. Expression of PAX3-FKHR is an adverse prognostic factor for children with metastatic alveolar RMS (Sorensen et al, 2002). In addition, patients with the t(1;13) translocation, *PAX7-FKHR* fusion, are often younger and have a better prognosis than do their counterparts with the t(2;13), *PAX3-FKHR* fusion abnormality (Barr, 1997; Kelly et al, 1997; Anderson et al, 2001; Sorensen et al, 2002).

Embryonal RMS demonstrates loss of heterozygosity (LOH) on chromosome 11p15, but at a different location than the *WT2* gene implicated in the development of some Wilms' tumors (Douglass et al, 1987; Scrable et al, 1990). This region is the location of the gene for insulin-like growth factor II (IGF-II). IGF-II overexpression has been documented in alveolar and embryonal RMS (Leiroth et al, 1995). IGF-II is a growth factor that can stimulate the growth of RMS tumor cells, and antibodies directed against IGF-II can inhibit tumor growth (El-Badry et al, 1990). Amplification of the transcription factor MYCN has been noted in neuroblastoma and recently in RMS (Williamson et al, 2005). Overexpression of MYCN was associated with an adverse outcome in patients with alveolar RMS.

Pathology and Patterns of Spread

The Intergroup Rhabdomyosarcoma Study Group (IRSG) has devised a pathology classification that recognizes three major histologic groups that have prognostic significance (Asmar et al, 1994). **Embryonal RMS is the most common subtype of RMS and accounts for most of the genitourinary tumors** (Maurer et al, 1977; Newton et al, 1988). **It may occur in solid form and arise in muscle groups such as the trunk and extremities or occur as the so-called sarcoma botryoides, a polypoid variety that develops in hollow organs or body cavities such as the bladder or vagina. A spindle cell, or leiomyomatous, variant is seen frequently in the paratesticular region. The botryoid and spindle cell variants of embryonal RMS are associated with excellent survival.** The second most common form is *alveolar*, which occurs more commonly in the trunk and extremity than in genitourinary sites and has a worse prognosis (Hays et al, 1983; Newton et al, 1988; Crist et al, 2001; Stevens et al, 2005). Alveolar RMS also has a higher rate of local recurrence and spread to regional lymph nodes, bone marrow, and distant sites. The third category consists of undifferentiated tumors, which also fare poorly. *Pleomorphic* RMS is now considered to be an anaplastic variant of the more common embryonal or alveolar RMS (Kodet et al, 1993).

RMS can occasionally be difficult to diagnosis with conventional histologic techniques. In such cases, histology may be complemented by other studies, including electron microscopy, cytogenetics, DNA flow cytometry, and immunochemistry (Shapiro et al, 1991). Alveolar RMS is associated with specific cytogenetic abnormalities, but this analysis can be technically difficult to perform. Immunohistochemical staining has been shown to be an effective adjunct for the diagnosis of alveolar RMS (Dias et al, 2000). Genes of the *MyoD* family are important in the differentiation of skeletal muscle (Parham, 1994). *MyoD* is important in the switch from proliferation to differentiation, and loss of this control and excess proliferation could lead to RMS (Sebire and Malone, 2003) Fetal myoblasts express MyoD and myogenin, another myogenic regulatory gene product, whereas adult myoblasts do not. MyoD and myogenin are expressed in patients with RMS and are believed to represent failure of differentiation. Myogenin has been proved to be a useful marker of alveolar RMS. Alveolar RMS demonstrates high levels of staining, whereas embryonal RMS is either negative or has a low level of staining (Dias et al, 2000). It is postulated that RMS may result from a block in the myogenic differentiation pathway. Embry-

onal RMS could be the result of an earlier block before the differentiation of myogenin (Dias et al, 2000).

Clinical Grouping and Staging

Tumor stage at diagnosis is most predictive of clinical outcome, and patients with localized disease have a better prognosis (Lawrence et al, 1987). Regional lymph node extension is fairly common and varies with site of the primary tumor. Metastatic spread of RMS is usually to the lungs. The clinical group staging system was developed by the IRSG in 1972 (Table 130–3). One of the difficulties inherent in this system is that the group is dependent to a large extent on the completeness of surgical excision. As treatment of RMS has evolved, more patients undergo biopsy only at the initial surgical procedure, with gross residual disease remaining. This results in shifting of more patients from group I to group III. Biologically equivalent tumors could end up in different categories, depending on the aggressiveness of the initial surgical resection.

A site-specific TMN staging system was devised by the IRSG for IRS-IV (Table 130–4) (Lawrence et al, 1997). The TMN

Table 130–3. Intergroup Rhabdomyosarcoma Study Group Clinical Grouping Classification

Group I	Localized disease completely resected Confined to the organ of origin Contiguous involvement
Group II	Total gross resection with evidence of regional spread Microscopic residual Positive nodes but no microscopic residual Positive nodes but microscopic residual in nodes or margins
Group III	Incomplete resection with gross residual disease After biopsy only After gross or major resection of the primary (>50%)
Group IV	Distant metastasis at diagnosis (lung, liver, bones, bone marrow, brain, and nonregional nodes) Positive cytology in cerebrospinal, pleural, or peritoneal fluid or implants on pleural or peritoneal surfaces are regarded as stage IV

Table 130–4. Intergroup Rhabdomyosarcoma Study Group Pretreatment TGNM Clinical Staging Based on Clinical, Radiographic, and Laboratory Examination and Histology of Biopsy Specimens

Stage 1: Favorable site, nonmetastatic
Stage 2: Unfavorable, small, negative nodes, nonmetastatic
Stage 3: Unfavorable, big or positive nodes, nonmetastatic
Stage 4: Any site, metastatic
Tumor:
  T1—Confined to the site of origin
  T2—Fixation to surrounding tissues
  ≤5 cm
  >5 cm
Histology:
  G1—Favorable histology (embryonal, botryoid, spindle cell)
  G2—Unfavorable histology (alveolar, undifferentiated)
Regional lymph nodes:
  N0—regional lymph nodes not clinically involved
  N1—regional lymph nodes clinically involved
Metastases:
  M0—No distant metastases
  M1—Metastases present

system was applied retrospectively to patients treated in IRS-III. The investigators found that distant metastases at diagnosis, involved regional lymph nodes, and large primary tumors (>5 cm) were relatively unfavorable prognostic signs. Patients with small tumors in unfavorable sites (e.g., genitourinary sites other than vulvovaginal and paratesticular) without tumor in the regional lymph nodes (i.e., stage 2 patients) fared as well as patients with stage 1 tumors that are located in favorable sites (Lawrence et al, 1997). A recent report found that age is also an independent prognostic factor in children with RMS (Joshi et al, 2004). Patients younger than 1 year and older than 10 years enrolled in IRS-III and IRS-IV had decreased survival. This poor prognosis persisted after adjustment for other known prognostic factors.

The staging classification relies on clinical findings from physical examination and laboratory and imaging studies. Proper assessment for determining the extent of disease includes chest radiography and CT, CT or MRI of the primary site and regional lymph nodes, a bone scan, and bone marrow aspiration or biopsy (or both).

Treatment

General Principles

The first effective treatment of RMS was radical surgical excision. The preferred treatment of pelvic genitourinary tumors consisted of total pelvic exenteration. RMS was later found to be radiosensitive, but local tumor control required high doses. In the 1960s, combination therapy was used, with chemotherapy and radiation therapy administered after attempts at complete surgical excision (Pinkel and Pickren, 1961). The first large study found that survival was significantly enhanced if chemotherapy was routinely administered after surgery (Heyn et al, 1974).

Because of the small numbers of patients encountered at any single institution, cooperative efforts were initiated to study the different therapeutic efforts for RMS (Maurer et al, 1977; Rodary et al, 1988). Once it was demonstrated that most patients would survive the disease, investigators explored the use of primary chemotherapy and radiation therapy to avoid the exenterative surgery used for genitourinary RMS (Ortega, 1979; Voute et al, 1981). A major aim of the protocols for patients with primary tumors in these sites in IRS-II (1978 to 1984) and the International Society of Paediatric Oncology (SIOP) RMS-75 study (1975 to 1984) was preservation of a functional lower urinary tract while maintaining the high survival rates achieved in IRS-I (Raney et al, 1990). Unfortunately, primary chemotherapy with vincristine (VCR), dactinomycin (AMD), and cyclophosphamide did not obviate the need for radical surgery or radiation therapy in patients with pelvic RMS. Three-year survival was the same for IRS-II as IRS-I (Maurer et al, 1993). In IRS-III (1984 to 1991), intensification of therapy using a risk-based study design significantly improved overall treatment outcomes. More intensive chemotherapy was required for stage III tumors, but selected patients were able to receive decreased therapy (Crist et al, 1995). In the SIOP MMT84 study, only 34% of patients received intensive local therapy, defined as wide-field radiotherapy or radical surgery, or both (Flamant et al, 1998). Treatment in MMT84 was based on response to initial chemotherapy and, despite an overall reduction in the use of local therapy, significantly improved survival for patients with nonmetastatic disease.

In IRS-IV (1991 to 1997), patients were stratified for treatment based on site, size, and stage. The role of hyperfractionated radiation therapy and the use of ifosfamide and etoposide were examined. Relapse-free survival for patients with embryonal RMS was improved in IRS-IV as compared with IRS-III (Crist et al, 2001). This improvement was predominantly for stage II/III, group 1/2 patients, 93% versus 76% (P < .001). There was no difference in the survival rates of patients treated with hyperfractionated or conventional radiation therapy.

A number of advances have been made by these cooperative group studies, including identification of prognostic factors, such as histology, site, biology, and extent of disease (Lawrence et al, 1987; Rodary et al, 1991); reduction or elimination of radiation therapy for special groups or sites (Flamant et al, 1998); reduced need for radical surgery, which led to a 25% to 60% increase in bladder salvage (Hays, 1993; Arndt et al, 2004; Stevens et al, 2005); and elimination of "routine" lymphadenectomy in some patients with localized paratesticular RMS (Crist et al, 2001; Ferrari et al, 2002). These advances are addressed in more detail later as they relate to specific genitourinary tumors. Options for managing new patients in IRS-V (1997 to present) are shown in Table 130–5.

Specific Sites

Bladder and Prostate Tumors. Urinary obstruction is a frequent clinical manifestation of RMS of the bladder or prostate (Meir et al, 2004) (Fig. 130–5). Signs and symptoms include urinary frequency, stranguria, acute urinary retention, and hematuria. On physical examination, an abdominal mass from either tumor or a distended bladder is often present. Tumors of the bladder usually occur as a botryoid form and grow intraluminally, generally at or near the trigone (Hays et al, 1982) (Fig. 130–6). Prostatic RMS tends to occur as a solid mass rather than the botryoid form seen in the bladder. Determining the actual site of origin can be difficult. Imaging studies show filling defects within the bladder or elevation of the bladder base in prostatic RMS. CT/MRI can delineate the extent of tumor, as well as evaluate the pelvic and retroperitoneal nodes. Cystoscopic evaluation establishes the diagnosis, and transurethral biopsy specimens can be obtained.

Treatment of bladder/prostate RMS has become focused on preserving an intact bladder. Most of these tumors arise from the trigonal area or prostate and are not amenable to local or partial resection. Only a small percentage of children with bladder RMS affecting the dome or sides of the bladder distant from the trigone are amenable to partial cystectomy as primary treatment. Anterior pelvic exenteration was once the initial therapy in most patients with pelvic RMS (Raney et al, 1993). However, even patients with bulky bladder/prostate RMS can be considered for bladder sparing after multimodal treatment. The IRSG approach is to use both chemotherapy and radiotherapy before surgical resection, with the exception of children amenable to partial cystectomy at diagnosis. **Although conservative surgical therapy for bladder/prostate tumors has not been as successful as for vaginal primaries, the bladder salvage rate has increased** (Hays et al, 1990; Hays, 1993). **With the intensification of treatment of pelvic RMS in IRS-III, 60% of patients retained a functional bladder at**

Table 130–5.	Intergroup Rhabdomyosarcoma Study Group V Risk Assignments								
Risk (Protocol)	**Stage**	**Group**	**Site***	**Size†**	**Age**	**Histology‡**	**Metastasis**	**Nodes§**	**Treatment¶**
Low, subgroup A	1	I	Favorable	a or b	<21	EMB	M0	N0	VA
(D9602)	1	II	Favorable	a or b	<21	EMB	M0	N0	VA + XRT
	1	III	Orbit only	a or b	<21	EMB	M0	N0	VA + XRT
	2	I	Unfavorable	a	<21	EMB	M0	N0 or NX	VA
Low, subgroup B	1	II	Favorable	a or b	<21	EMB	M0	N1	VAC + XRT
(D9602)	1	III	Orbit only	a or b	<21	EMB	M0	N1	VAC + XRT
	1	III	Favorable (excluding orbit)	a or b	<21	EMB	M0	N0 or N1 or NX	VAC + XRT
	2	II	Unfavorable	a	<21	EMB	M0	N0 or NX	VAC + XRT
	3	I or II	Unfavorable	a	<21	EMB	M0	N1	VAC (+ XRT, Gp II)
	3	I or II	Unfavorable	b	<21	EMB	M0	N0 or N1 or NX	VAC (+ XRT, Gp II)
Intermediate	2	III	Unfavorable	a	<21	EMB	M0	N0 or NX	VAC ± Topo + XRT
(D9803)	3	III	Unfavorable	a	<21	EMB	M0	N1	VAC ± Topo + XRT
	3	III	Unfavorable	a	<21	EMB	M0	N0 or N1 or NX	VAC ± Topo + XRT
	1, 2, or 3	I, II, or III	Favorable or unfavorable	a or b	<21	ALV/UDS	M0	N0 or N1 or NX	VAC ± Topo + XRT
	4	I, II, III, or IV	Favorable or unfavorable	a or b	<10	EMB	M1	N0 or N1	VAC ± Topo + XRT
High (D9802)	4	IV	Favorable or unfavorable	a or b	≥10	EMB	M1	N0 or N1	CPT-11, VAC + XRT
	4	IV	Favorable or unfavorable	a or b	<21	ALV/UDS	M1	N0 or N1	CPT-11, VAC + XRT

*Favorable = orbit/eyelid, head and neck (excluding parameningeal), genitourinary (not bladder or prostate); unfavorable = bladder, prostate, extremity, parameningeal, trunk, retroperitoneal, pelvis, other.

†a = tumor size 5 cm or less in diameter; b = tumor size greater than 5 cm in diameter.

‡ALV, alveolar rhabdomyosarcomas or ectomesenchymomas with alveolar rhabdomyosarcoma; EMB, embryonal, botryoid, or spindle cell rhabdomyosarcomas or ectomesenchymomas with embryonal rhabdomyosarcoma; UDS, undifferentiated sarcomas.

§N0, regional nodes clinically not involved; N1, regional nodes clinically involved; NX, node status unknown.

¶CPT-11, irinotecan; Gp, group; Topo, topotecan; VAC, vincristine, actinomycin D, cyclophosphamide; XRT, radiotherapy.

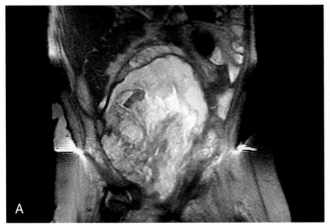 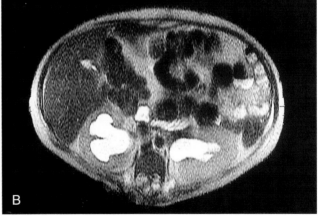

Figure 130–5. Magnetic resonance images of a large prostatic rhabdomyosarcoma extending into the upper part of the abdomen (**A**) with bilateral hydroureteronephrosis (**B**).

4 years from diagnosis, and overall survival exceeded 85% (Hays et al, 1995). One concern about a bladder-sparing approach is residual disease after partial cystectomy. Among 22 patients undergoing conservative surgery as primary treatment, local relapse occurred in 5 and distant relapse in 1 (Hays et al, 1990). All patients who relapsed died.

The results of bladder preservation in IRS-IV patients with bladder or prostate primaries were recently reported (Arndt et al, 2004). There were 88 patients with bladder/prostate primaries, including 17 patients undergoing partial cystectomy as the initial surgical procedure. Most patients underwent surgery after completion of x-ray therapy (XRT). The event-free survival rate at a mean of 6.1 years' follow-up was 77%. Overall, the bladder was retained in 55 patients. However, only 36 patients (41%) had no relapse and a normally functioning intact bladder at last follow-up. The reason for the less favorable results than those reported for IRS-III was attributed to longer follow-up and stricter definition of normal bladder function. Bladder function was determined by questionnaire, but it was completed by just 65% of patients with a retained bladder. Only one child had undergone urodynamic evaluation.

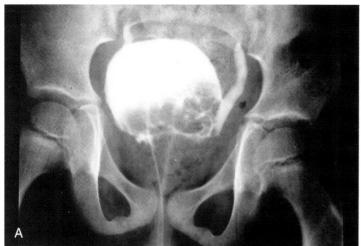

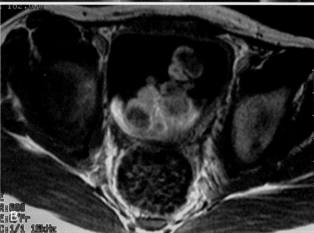

Figure 130–6. **A,** Excretory urogram demonstrating filling defects in the bladder from a botryoid rhabdomyosarcoma. (Courtesy of Dr. Stanford Goldman.) **B,** Magnetic resonance image of a botryoid-type sarcoma of the bladder.

More objective evaluation of bladder function with urodynamics after multimodal treatment of pelvic RMS has been reported (Yeung et al, 1994). Yeung and associates evaluated 11 children treated for pelvic RMS. After a mean follow-up of 6.6 years, the four unirradiated children had normal bladder function. All seven of the children who had undergone irradiation had a markedly reduced functional bladder capacity and abnormal voiding patterns.

Several reports have expressed concern regarding the routine use of radiation therapy before surgery for bladder/prostate RMS (Fisch et al, 1995; Meguerian et al, 1998; El-Sherbiny et al, 2000; Filipas et al, 2004). Although radiotherapy is important to prevent local treatment failure, it can affect bladder function in children with retained bladders and make subsequent reconstructive procedures more difficult. Merguerian and colleagues (1998) treated 10 patients with group III bladder/prostate RMS. Radiation therapy was reserved for patients with residual or metastatic disease. They reported a survival rate of 80% in their group III patients, and only four patients received XRT. El-Sherbiny and coauthors (2000) described a risk-based approach to the treatment of pelvic RMS. The response of the tumor to chemotherapy is used to stratify patients into low-risk patients with a complete or partial response and high-risk patients with a minimal response to chemotherapy. The latter group undergoes exenterative surgery without any attempt at bladder salvage. The low-risk group had an 85.7% 5-year disease-free survival rate. Low-risk patients were given radiation only for relapse. The group in Mainz also recommends assessment of the response of the primary tumor to chemotherapy after 7 to 9 weeks (Filipas et al, 2004). If there is less than a third reduction in tumor volume, radiation is given before surgery. Patients who have a good response and undergo complete resection do not receive XRT. They believe that this approach provides more complete tumor resection with excellent cure rates. Quality of life can be maintained in patients requiring exenterative surgery with the use of continent urinary diversion techniques.

The SIOP MMT89 protocol for treatment of RMS tried to limit the use of radiation therapy (Stevens et al, 2005). They also used tumor response to chemotherapy to stratify patients for therapy. Patients who did not receive XRT as part of the initial therapy had a lower 5-year event-free survival rate (64%), but overall survival was comparable to that of patients receiving XRT. IRS-IV also reported a greater incidence of local recurrence when XRT was omitted (Arndt et al, 2004).

A subset of patients with bladder RMS had a better prognosis. Leuschner et al (2001) found a 92% 10-year survival rate in patients with the botryoid subtype of RMS. Patients with diffuse endophytic intramural growth had a 68% 10-year survival rate. Prostatic RMS is associated with a poorer prognosis, and these tumors do not have the botryoid type of growth pattern (Crist et al, 2001; Stevens et al, 2005). Prostatectomy without cystectomy has been performed in selected patients with persistent disease or local relapse (Hays, 1993; Lobe et al, 1996; Meguerian et al, 1998). However, local relapse has occurred in 40% of these patients.

Assessing complete response to therapy after chemotherapy can present challenges. Completeness of surgical resection may be difficult to determine by frozen section. Some patients will have mature rhabdomyoblasts identified on post-treatment biopsy. Several reports of small numbers of patients have suggested that these patients can be safely observed with a low risk for recurrence (Atra et al, 1994, Heyn et al, 1997; Ortega et al, 2000; Smith et al, 2002). There is a report of two deaths occurring in patients with mature tumors after therapy (Leuschner et al, 2001). Also concerning is the finding by Godzinski and coworkers (1994) of a 51% relapse rate in RMS confirmed to have undergone complete remission by imaging and biopsy. Follow-up of patients with apparent complete remission should include serial imaging, endoscopy, and biopsy if indicated.

Patients undergoing cystectomy will require diversion. Most authors advocate an initial nonrefluxing colon conduit followed by later continent reconstruction after completion of therapy (Duel et al, 1996). Other authors have advocated performing continent reconstruction at the time of extirpative surgery (Lander et al, 1992; Meguerian et al, 1998). There are several concerns regarding early reconstruction. Frozen section may be unreliable in excluding residual disease (Meguerian et al, 1998), and treatment of a subsequent local recurrence could adversely affect reservoir function. Early reconstruction should be performed only if it is certain that no further local therapy will be required (Hensle and Chang, 2000). Enterocystoplasty may be necessary in some patients with contracted bladders as a result of radiation therapy (Hicks et al, 1993).

KEY POINTS: RHABDOMYOSARCOMA

- Embryonal RMS is the most common subtype of genitourinary RMS.

- Sixty to eighty percent of paratesticular RMS is stage I at diagnosis. Patients older than 10 years have a higher risk for retroperitoneal relapse and should undergo staging with ipsilateral retroperitoneal lymph node dissection (RPLND) before chemotherapy.

- An organ-sparing approach is preferred for bladder and genital RMS. Vaginal and uterine primaries are associated with a good prognosis.

Other Bladder Tumors. Transitional cell carcinoma of the bladder is rare in the first 2 decades of life (Javadpour and Mostofi, 1969; Hoenig et al, 1996). The etiology of transitional cell carcinoma in children is unknown for most patients. One specific cause is previous exposure to cyclophosphamide for both benign and malignant conditions (Travis et al, 1995; Kersun et al, 2004). The risk for bladder cancer after cyclophosphamide is dose dependent. Another recent report

described transitional cell carcinoma developing after enterocystoplasty at a mean interval of 19 years (Soergel et al, 2004). Gross hematuria is the most common manifestation of bladder tumors in children, but some tumors are detected incidentally on imaging evaluation for other problems. Most of these tumors are of low grade and stage and can be managed endoscopically. The risk for recurrence is low, presumably because of lack of exposure to carcinogens, except for carcinoma developing after cyclophosphamide therapy (Hoenig et al, 1996). For this reason, surveillance with urinalysis and ultrasound can avoid the need for repeat cystoscopy under anesthesia, although the real risk of recurrence in children is undefined.

Another bladder tumor occasionally found in children is nephrogenic adenoma (Ritchey et al, 1984; Heidenreich et al, 1999). These lesions appear to arise as a metaplastic response to chronic inflammation in the bladder. Transurethral excision is all that is needed in most patients, but periodic surveillance is recommended because of reports of recurrence.

Benign polyps of the prostatic urethra are the most common benign lesions of the prostate. Obstruction and hematuria are the most frequent manifestations (Gleason and Kramer, 1994). These fibroepithelial polyps arise from a stalk near the verumontanum. On histologic examination these lesions are covered by normal transitional epithelium. There have been no reports of recurrence when these lesions have been completely excised.

Paratesticular Rhabdomyosarcoma. Among primary genitourinary tumors, 7% to 10% are located in the paratesticular area (Bruce and Gough, 1991). The peak age at diagnosis is between 1 and 5 years (Wiener et al, 1994). Paratesticular RMS arises in the distal portion of the spermatic cord and may invade the testis or surrounding tissue. It is generally detected earlier than other genitourinary tumors. Paratesticular RMS is often manifested as a unilateral painless scrotal swelling or mass that is usually distinct from the testis. Ultrasound can confirm the solid nature of the lesion. **At diagnosis, 60% to 80% of paratesticular tumors are stage I, as compared with 13% of RMS overall** (Wiener et al, 1994, 2001; Ferrari et al, 2002). **More than 90% of paratesticular RMS are embryonal in histology and have a good prognosis. Patients with paratesticular RMS with alveolar histology do have a better prognosis than those with alveolar RMS found at other sites** (Ferrari et al, 2004).

Radical inguinal orchiectomy is recommended for initial treatment. If the tumor is removed through a prior transscrotal procedure, the risk for local recurrence and nonregional lymph node spread is increased. If cord elements remain after a trans-scrotal procedure, inguinal exploration with removal of the remaining spermatic cord and a partial hemiscrotectomy that includes the previous scrotal incision is performed (Dall'Igna et al, 2003).

Before effective chemotherapy, surgery alone produced a 50% 2-year relapse-free survival rate (Sutow et al, 1970). With current multimodal treatment, survival rates of 90% are expected (Wiener et al, 1994, 2001; Ferrari et al, 2002). An imaging evaluation is performed at diagnosis to detect or exclude metastasis. Extension to retroperitoneal lymph nodes occurs in up to 20% of patients. CT is most frequently used to evaluate the retroperitoneum for identification of nodal metastases (Raney et al, 1987). When enlarged nodes are found on CT, 65% to 94% are confirmed as positive by pathologic examination (Wiener et al, 1994; Ferrari et al, 2002). The converse is not always true. A review of 121 IRS-III patients with paratesticular RMS found a 14% false-negative rate of CT (Wiener et al, 1994). A more recent report of 198 patients treated by the Italian and German cooperative group noted better accuracy of CT in identifying node-negative patients (Ferrari et al, 2002). Of 72 patients undergoing routine surgical staging with negative imaging, only 1 patient had positive lymph nodes identified on pathologic evaluation.

The role of RPLND in paratesticular RMS is controversial (Olive et al, 1984; Goldfarb et al, 1994; Wiener et al, 1994, 2001; Ferrari et al, 2002). The first concern is the accuracy of imaging in detecting retroperitoneal nodal involvement, as outlined earlier. There can be significant morbidity associated with the surgery. Heyn and colleagues (1992) reported a 10% incidence of intestinal obstruction, 8% incidence of ejaculatory dysfunction, and edema of the lower extremities in 5% of patients who had undergone RPLND for paratesticular RMS. However, most of these patients underwent bilateral node dissection. A modified unilateral node dissection is appropriate for staging and, with the addition of nerve-sparing techniques, may avoid some of the reported morbidity associated with node dissection (LaQuaglia et al, 1989; Donohue et al, 1990). Others have suggested that multiple lymph node sampling is sufficient because they regard this as a staging and not a therapeutic procedure (Banowsky and Shultz, 1970; Ferrari et al, 2002).

Another major argument against routine RPLND is that microscopic nodal disease can be effectively treated by chemotherapy. An SIOP report of 46 children with completely excised tumors and negative CT or lymphangiography who were treated with intensive chemotherapy alone found that all children survived (Olive-Sommelet, 1989). However, it should be noted that most of the children did receive doxorubicin (DOX) or ifosfamide, which have potential for adverse late effects.

During IRS-III, 121 children who had paratesticular RMS and underwent RPLND were reported. The overall 5-year survival rate for the 98 patients with clinically negative nodes was 96%, and less than 10% of patients received DOX or alkylating agents. Patients found to have positive lymph nodes on pathologic evaluation were given radiotherapy to the retroperitoneum because of the increased risk for relapse (Wiener et al, 1994). **In IRS-IV, children with clinically negative nodes were treated primarily with chemotherapy, which resulted in a higher percentage of group I patients in comparison to IRS-III, 82% versus 68%** (Wiener et al, 2001). **However, adolescents were at higher risk for retroperitoneal relapse than were children younger than 10 years, and their relapse-free and overall survival was worse. Adolescents with group I tumors in IRS-IV had a 68% relapse-free survival rate. This compares with a 100% survival rate (overall or relapse-free) in adolescents with group II tumors who received radiotherapy and intensified chemotherapy. The IRSG subsequently recommended that children 10 years and older undergo ipsilateral RPLND as part of their routine staging before chemotherapy.** Patients with positive lymph nodes require intensified chemotherapy, as well as nodal irradiation (Wiener et al, 2001).

The Italian and German cooperative group treated 106 low-risk patients with chemotherapy only, avoiding RPLND (Ferrari et al, 2002). Low-risk patients were defined as having favorable histology and T1N0M0 disease and being in clinical group 1. Since 1988, these patients received only VCR and AMD. The 5-year survival rate was 99.1%. This study also reported a higher rate of retroperitoneal relapse in adolescents. SIOP treated low-risk patients with chemotherapy only in the MMT84 and MMT89 studies (Stewart et al, 2003). Of 156 clinical stage I patients, relapse developed in 14. Patient age older than 10 years and primary tumor size greater than 5 cm were identified as predictors of relapse. The larger tumors occur more often in adolescents, thus suggesting a delayed manifestation.

Vaginal and Vulvar Rhabdomyosarcoma. Vaginal and vulvar RMS are generally manifested in the first few years of life as vaginal bleeding, discharge, or a vaginal mass. The clinical findings can be quite striking if there is prolapse of the mass from the vaginal introitus (Fig. 130–7). The diagnosis is made by vaginoscopy and biopsy of the lesion. The vaginal lesions usually arise from the anterior vaginal wall in the area of the embryonic vesicovaginal septum (urogenital sinus). Vaginal tumors may invade the vesicovaginal septum or bladder wall because of their proximity. Cystoscopy is warranted during initial evaluation and at intervals during follow-up (Andrassy et al, 1994).

Vaginal lesions generally demonstrate embryonal or botryoid embryonal histology and have an excellent prog-

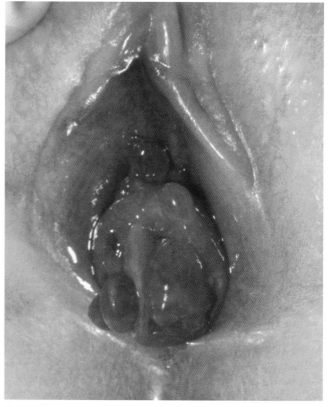

Figure 130–7. Mass protruding from the vaginal introitus in a young girl with vaginal rhabdomyosarcoma.

nosis (Andrassy et al, 1994; Martelli et al, 1999; Arndt et al, 2001). Vulvar lesions may display alveolar histology, but because most are localized, they also have a good prognosis. In addition to initial biopsy, clinical staging, imaging studies, and bone marrow examination are performed.

Anterior pelvic exenteration was frequently used to treat these patients in the past. With the development of effective chemotherapy, attempts to preserve the vagina have become a priority. Definitive surgery is delayed until after an initial course of therapy (Hays et al, 1988; Andrassy et al, 1994; Martelli et al, 1999; Arndt et al, 2001). Once an adequate response has been demonstrated, repeat biopsies are performed. If there is persistence of disease, delayed tumor resection is performed, which may consist of partial vaginectomy or vaginectomy with hysterectomy. In IRS-III, 24 patients with vaginal primaries were treated with a primary chemotherapy protocol. At subsequent surgery, seven patients underwent partial or complete vaginectomy. Six of these seven patients had no viable tumor in the resected specimen, and one had maturing rhabdomyoblasts. The presence of mature rhabdomyoblasts because of differentiation related to chemotherapy may not signify persistent active cancer (see earlier discussion) (Heyn et al, 1997; Ortega et al, 2000; Smith et al, 2002).

During IRS-IV (1988 to 1996), the rate of hysterectomy was only 26% as compared with 48% in IRS-I and IRS-II (Arndt et al, 2001). More than 50% of patients did receive XRT for local tumor control in IRS-IV, which probably reflects an attempt to achieve a complete response without surgery. Only 3 of 21 patients (14%) underwent surgical resection after primary chemotherapy. Age at diagnosis of 1 to 9 years, botryoid histology, and localized disease were predictive of a good prognosis (Andrassy et al, 1999; Arndt et al, 2001).

SIOP also uses initial chemotherapy for vaginal RMS. Only 12% of patients treated in MMT84 and MMT89 required hysterectomy. XRT was used in 11 girls, but 7 received intracavitary brachytherapy. Eleven girls did not require any local therapy, surgery, or XRT after chemotherapy (Martelli et al, 1999).

Uterine Rhabdomyosarcoma. Uterine RMS may be manifested in two ways, as a tumor originating from the cervix with vaginal bleeding or a mass or as a tumor originating in the uterine body with an abdominal mass. The diagnosis is made by incisional or excisional biopsy, usually by dilation and curettage and transvaginal biopsy. More than 90% of uterine tumors are of embryonal histology (Corpron et al, 1995; Martelli et al, 1999; Arndt et al, 2001). In addition to biopsy, staging requires a search for metastases, including pelvic examination and CT scans of the pelvis, abdomen, and chest; examination of bone marrow; cystoscopy; and vaginoscopy.

Older studies reported that uterine RMS occurs in a distinct group of patients who are older and have less response to treatment and thus a poorer prognosis than those with vaginal RMS (Hays et al, 1981, 1985). However, more recent reports suggest that patients with uterine RMS are of the same age group, a mean age of 5.5 years, as vaginal RMS patients (Arndt et al, 2001). As with vaginal RMS, patients with uterine RMS are treated by primary chemotherapy and delayed local therapy. With this approach it may be possible to salvage the uterus and vagina, as well as the bladder, in many of these patients (Martelli et al, 1999; Arndt et al, 2001).

WILMS' TUMOR

Wilms' tumor, or nephroblastoma, is the most common primary malignant renal tumor of childhood. This embryonal tumor develops from remnants of immature kidney. Although an excellent outcome is now expected in most children, there are subgroups of high-risk patients for whom more effective treatment is needed. Treatment of patients with nephroblastoma has been extensively investigated in a number of large randomized clinical trials in North America and Europe. Current management now emphasizes reducing the morbidity of treatment in low-risk patients while reserving more intensive treatment for high-risk patients for whom survival remains poor. This section outlines current recommendations for treatment and reviews the latest developments in the biology of Wilms' tumor.

Epidemiology

The annual incidence rate of Wilms' tumor in children younger than 15 years is about 7 to 10 cases per million, and it accounts for 6% to 7% of all childhood cancers (Breslow et al, 1993; Bernstein et al, 1999). Wilms' tumor typically affects young children (median age, 3.5 years), with more than 80% of cases occurring in those younger than 5 years. Nevertheless, older children and occasionally even adults can be affected (Arrigo et al, 1990; Kattan et al, 1994; Kalakapural et al, 2004a). The median age at diagnosis is highest for unilateral unicentric cases and lowest for bilateral cases (Breslow et al, 1993). Wilms' tumor occurs at an earlier age in males, with the mean age at diagnosis for those with unilateral tumors being 41.5 months versus 46.9 months in females. The mean age at diagnosis for those with bilateral tumors is 29.5 months for males and 32.6 months for females (Breslow et al, 1993).

Although Wilms' tumor is slightly more frequent in females than males in North America, the worldwide sex ratio is generally believed to be close to 1. With regard to ethnicity, the incidence of Wilms' tumor is lower in East Asian populations and higher in black populations than in the North American and European white populations (Breslow et al, 1994; Fukuzawa et al, 2004). However, the approximately 3- to 4-fold ratio in maximum to minimum rate worldwide is substantially less than the 10- to 20-fold ratios typically observed for adult epithelial tumors. The fact that such variations are more closely associated with race than geography suggests that environmental risk factors probably play a minor etiologic role, certainly in comparison to adult epithelial cancers (Breslow et al, 1993). Several epidemiologic studies have investigated occupational, environmental, and lifestyle issues as risk factors for Wilms' tumor. Several studies have suggested that a number of parental exposures might be associated with an increased risk for Wilms' tumor, but very few have been found to be conclusively associated (Breslow et al, 1993).

A number of recognizable syndromes are associated with an increased incidence of Wilms' tumor (Table 130–6) (Miller et al, 1964; Clericuzio, 1993). **These syndromes may be divided into those characterized by overgrowth and those lacking overgrowth. Genitourinary abnormalities (renal**

Table 130–6. Incidence of Congenital Anomalies in Patients with Wilms' Tumor Reported to the National Wilms' Tumor Study Group

Anomaly	Rate (per 1000)
Aniridia	7.6
Beckwith-Wiedemann syndrome	8.4
Hemihypertrophy	33.8
Genitourinary anomalies	
Hypospadias	13.4
Cryptorchidism	37.3
Hypospadias and cryptorchidism	12.0

fusion anomalies, cryptorchidism, hypospadias) are present in 4.5% of patients with Wilms' tumor (Breslow et al, 1993). These disorders are common in children, and prospective evaluation for the onset of Wilms' tumor is not necessary in most children with genital anomalies. However, one specific association of male pseudohermaphroditism, renal mesangial sclerosis, and nephroblastoma is the Denys-Drash syndrome (DDS) (Drash et al, 1970). The majority of these patients progress to end-stage renal disease. Nephropathy usually develops early in life, and renal biopsy demonstrates mesangial sclerosis (McTaggart et al, 2001). A specific mutation of the 11p13 Wilms' tumor gene has been identified in these children (Coppes et al, 1993). Although XY individuals have been reported most often, DDS has been found in genotypic/phenotypic females (McTaggart et al, 2001).

Aniridia is found in 1.1% of Wilms' tumor patients. Aniridia and Wilms' tumor are most commonly associated in patients with the WAGR syndrome (*Wilms' tumor, Aniridia, Genital anomalies, mental Retardation*) (Clericuzio, 1993). **Aniridia is caused by an abnormality of the *PAX6* gene located adjacent to the *WT1* gene** (see later). **Aniridia patients with deletions that include *WT1* are more prone to the development of Wilms' tumor** (Muto et al, 2002). **Wilms' tumor will develop in approximately 40% of aniridia patients with deletions of *WT1*. Conversely, Wilms' tumor does not develop in aniridia patients with normal *WT1*** (Grenskov et al, 2001). WAGR patients are more likely to have bilateral tumors, and the condition is diagnosed at a younger age (Breslow et al, 2003). **WAGR patients are more prone to the development of renal failure if they survive into puberty** (Breslow et al, 2000; Breslow et al, 2003).

An association between Wilms' tumor and horseshoe kidney has been noted. A review of National Wilms' Tumor Study Group (NWTSG) patients found a sevenfold increased risk for Wilms' tumor in patients with a horseshoe kidney (Mesrobian et al, 1985). The diagnosis of horseshoe kidney can be missed on preoperative imaging because of the location of the tumor (Neville et al, 2002). Wilms' tumor has been reported in patients with multicystic dysplastic kidney, but there is not sufficient evidence that it occurs at an incidence greater than that in children with two normal kidneys (Narchi, 2005). There is an increased risk for müllerian duct anomalies in girls with Wilms' tumor (Byrne and Nicholson, 2002). Approximately 10% of girls will have abnormalities such as duplication of the cervix or uterus or a bicornuate uterus.

Syndromes with overgrowth features that place patients at risk for the development of Wilms' tumor include hemihypertrophy, which may occur alone or as part of the Beckwith-

Wiedemann syndrome (BWS), and the Perlman, Soto, and Simpson-Golabi-Behmel syndromes (Perlman et al, 1975; Neri et al, 1998). **BWS is characterized by excess growth at the cellular, organ (macroglossia, nephromegaly, hepatomegaly), or body segment (hemihypertrophy) levels** (Beckwith, 1969; Wiedemann, 1983). Most cases of BWS are sporadic, but up to 15% exhibit heritable characteristics with apparent autosomal dominant inheritance. **The risk for nephroblastoma in children with BWS and hemihypertrophy is estimated to be 4% to 10%, with 21% of children having bilateral disease** (Beckwith, 1996; DeBaun and Tucker, 1998; Porteus et al, 2000). Adrenocortical neoplasms and hepatoblastoma also occur with increased frequency in BWS. Children with BWS found to have nephromegaly (kidneys in the 95th or greater percentile of age-adjusted renal length) are at greatest risk for the development of Wilms' tumor (DeBaun et al, 1998). More recently, investigators have been able to correlate genetic changes to identify which BWS patients are at risk for Wilms' tumor (DeBaun et al, 2002; Bliek et al, 2004). The mean age at diagnosis of Wilms' tumor in BWS and hemihypertrophy patients is similar to that of the general Wilms' tumor population (Breslow et al, 1993). Vaughan et al (1995) reported a 100% survival rate in BWS patients with Wilms' tumor and noted that all had favorable histology.

Screening with serial renal ultrasonography has been recommended in children with aniridia, hemihypertrophy, and BWS. Review of most studies suggests that 3 to 4 months is the appropriate screening interval. Tumors detected by screening will generally be of lower stage (Green et al, 1993a; Choyke et al, 1999). Retrospective reviews have been unable to determine whether early detection has an impact on patient survival. Nonmalignant renal lesions do occur at an increased rate in children with BWS, and recognition of these lesions is important to avoid unnecessary nephrectomy when new lesions are identified on screening ultrasound (Choyke et al, 1999). Medullary renal cysts have been noted in 13% of patients (Borer et al, 1999).

Biology

Children with Wilms' tumor have been the subject of intensive investigations to determine the role of genetic alterations in tumor development. Interest in Wilms' tumor was initially centered on patients with congenital anomalies and those with bilateral tumors. It was thought that these children had a germline mutation that predisposed to both the development of multiple tumors and an earlier age of onset than in the general population, as had been noted for children with retinoblastoma (Knudson and Strong, 1972; Strong, 2003). Knudson's model for tumor development predicts that two genetic events are rate limiting for tumor formation. Individuals with a genetic predisposition carry an initial lesion in their germline. Because all body cells have already been affected by the first event, only one new event in any one cell is required for tumor development. In the Knudson model, the two "genetic hits" constitute the inactivation of both alleles of a tumor suppressor gene (Cavanee et al, 1983). This second hit would result in a tumor occurring at a younger age than tumors that arise sporadically from somatic mutations.

However, it is now recognized that more than 90% of Wilms' tumors arise from somatic mutations restricted to tumor tissue. A much smaller percentage of Wilms' tumors are the result of germline mutations that can be inherited or occur de novo. Only 7% of children have bilateral Wilms' tumors (Blute et al, 1987) and 1% to 2% have a family history of Wilms' tumor (Green et al, 1982; Ruteshouser and Huff, 2004), both presumably the result of germline mutations. Unlike the genetic events leading to the development of retinoblastoma, the genetics of Wilms' tumor remains an enigma. It is likely that several genetic events are responsible for the development of Wilms' tumor (Dome and Coppes, 2002). The chromosomal abnormalities that have been most extensively studied in Wilms' tumor patients are discussed in the following sections.

WT1

Identification and subsequent cloning of *WT1* resulted from cytogenetic observations of gross chromosomal deletions in patients with the WAGR syndrome. These children were shown to have heterozygous germline deletions at 11p13 (Riccardi et al, 1978). Subsequent molecular analysis of DNA mapping of this specific region led to identification of *WT1* in 1990 (Bonetta et al, 1990; Call et al, 1990). *WT1* is present only in the kidneys, gonads, and heart. *WT1* encodes a zinc finger protein transcription factor important for gene regulation during normal renal and gonadal development (Pritchard-Jones et al, 1990; Dressler, 1995). *WT1* is necessary for ureteric bud outgrowth and is also important in nephrogenesis. Targeted mutation of the *WT1* gene in mice results in failure of kidney and gonadal development (Kreidberg et al, 1997). Loss of only one copy of *WT1*, as seen in WAGR and DDS, can result in significant genital abnormalities and renal disease. More than 90% of DDS patients harbor germline point mutations in only one *WT1* allele (Pelletier et al, 1991; Coppes et al, 1992). Therefore, the *WT1* mutation acts dominantly with respect to genitourinary abnormalities. The fact that the phenotype resulting from these heterozygous mutations is far more severe than that resulting from constitutional deletion of one *WT1* allele (i.e., WAGR patients) suggests that the Denys-Drash mutations do not result in inactivation of the WT1 protein, but rather in the production of a dysfunctional WT1 protein. It is postulated that this abnormally expressed protein alters regulation of transcription and urogenital development. Another implication of these *WT1* mutations is the late development of renal failure in WAGR patients and other Wilms' tumor patients with genitourinary abnormalities (Breslow et al, 2000).

WT1 was originally considered to be a classic tumor suppressor gene, and the loss of both copies or mutations of this gene would lead to the development of Wilms' tumor (Rauscher, 1993). Although this may be the case for some tumors, only a small percentage of patients with Wilms' tumor have a mutation in the germline or in tumor tissue (Diller et al, 1998; Huff, 1998; Varanasi et al, 1994). Patients with genitourinary anomalies have an increased risk for carrying a constitutional *WT1* mutation (Diller et al, 1998). The incidence of *WT1* mutations in patients with Wilms' tumor not associated with any genitourinary abnormality is approximately 2% (Little et al, 2004). Although there is no distinguishing phenotype for these patients, they do have an earlier age of onset and a stromal-predominant histology. *WT1* is involved in regulation of many other genes, including *EGFR*, *PDGF*, *IGF*, *N-MYC*, *PAX2*, *MDR1*, and *p-21*, all notable for their association with tumorigenesis (Lee and Haber, 2001).

WT2

A second Wilms' tumor gene, *WT2*, was identified at the 11p15 locus as a result of finding LOH at this site (Koufos et al, 1989; Mannens et al, 1990). **The *WT2* gene has been linked to BWS** (Koufos et al, 1989). The *WT2* locus has been extensively studied, and a number of genes have been identified, including *H19* and *IGF2* (Rainier et al, 1993; Ravenel et al, 2001; Feinberg, 2004). The latter genes are of importance in the epigenetic theory of cancer etiology. Epigenetic changes are modifications of the genome that do not involve a change in DNA sequence (Feinberg, 2004). Genomic imprinting is an epigenetic alteration in DNA. Imprinting of a specific parental allele of a gene in the zygote leads to silencing of that allele in somatic cells of the offspring. Loss of imprinting (LOI) is a common alteration in cancer that can lead to activation of a growth-promoting gene or silencing of a growth-silencing gene. *IGF2* encodes an embryonal growth factor that is normally expressed solely from the paternal allele. LOI of *IGF2* was first identified in Wilms' tumor, and it is overexpressed in a number of malignancies (Rainier et al, 1993; Feinberg, 2004). It is speculated that Wilms' tumors occurring at a later age are the result of these epigenetic changes, such as LOI for *IGF2* (Ravenel et al, 2001).

Ravenel and coworkers correlated LOI for *IGF2* and LOH of *WT1* with pathologic findings and age in patients with Wilms' tumor. They found LOI for *IGF2* in 9 of 10 (90%) Wilms' tumors classified as having a pathologic subtype associated with a later stage of renal development, from perilobar nephrogenic rests (PLNRs), and in only 1 of 15 (6.7%) Wilms' tumors with a pathologic subtype associated with an earlier stage of renal development, from intralobar nephrogenic rests (ILNRs). Remarkably, all nine (100%) of the tumors that showed LOH of 11p were ILNR-like. Furthermore, none of 12 PLNR-like tumors showed LOH of 11p. This finding is consistent with an earlier observation that tumors with ILNRs are associated with LOH (Grundy et al, 1996) (see later discussion on nephrogenic rests [NRs]). Children whose Wilms' tumors displayed LOI for *IGF2* were statistically significantly older at diagnosis (median of 65 months) than were children whose tumors displayed normal imprinting.

Familial Wilms' Tumor

As noted earlier, 1% to 2% of Wilms' tumor patients have a family history of Wilms' tumor (Green et al, 1982; Ruteshouser and Huff, 2004). Familial cases have an earlier age of onset and an increased frequency of bilateral disease. Two familial Wilms' tumor genes have been localized (Ruteshouser and Huff, 2004). *FWT1* is located at 17q12-q21 and *FWT2* at 19q13.4 (Rahman et al, 1996; McDonald et al, 1998). Penetrance of these genes appears to be moderate, and they do not follow the typical tumor suppressor gene pattern of LOH (Strong, 2003).

Other Chromosomal Abnormalities

Mutations of the tumor suppressor gene *p53* are frequently encountered genetic events in human cancer (Hollstein et al, 1991). Studies of *p53* mutations in Wilms' tumor have shown an increased frequency in patients with anaplastic histology

(Bardeesy et al, 1994, 1995). They have also been correlated with advanced-stage disease (Malkin et al, 1990; Sredni et al, 2001), but indexing of *p53* expression has not been shown to be an independent prognostic factor (Skotnicka-Klonowicz et al, 2001).

Loss of the long arm of chromosome 16 has been detected in approximately 20% of Wilms' tumors (Maw et al, 1992), **thus suggesting the presence of a gene at 16q involved in the biology of Wilms' tumor. Similarly, loss of the short arm of chromosome 1p has been found in approximately 10% of cases** (Grundy et al, 1994). **Grundy et al (1994) showed that these abnormalities were associated with an increased risk for tumor relapse and death.** However, the prognostic significance of these features has been questioned (Bown et al, 2002). A recent study found an association between LOI of the *IGF2* gene and 16q LOH (Mummert et al, 2005). This is the first association between a genetic (16q LOH) and an epigenetic (LOI of *IGF2*) alteration in Wilms' tumor. Confirming the utility of LOH of 16q and 1p to predict outcome was one of the major objectives of NWTS-5 (see discussion later).

KEY POINTS: RENAL TUMORS

- Deletions of *WT1*, located on chromosome 11p, are found in patients with aniridia and Wilms' tumor. Mutations of *WT1* occur in DDS. *WT1* is important for normal renal and gonadal development.

- A second Wilms' tumor gene, *WT2*, has been identified on chromosome 11p15 and is associated with BWS.

- LOH for chromosomes 1p and 16q is associated with an increased risk for relapse and death in Wilms' tumor patients.

- Local recurrence is increased in Wilms' tumor patients with local tumor spillage and those who do not undergo regional lymph node sampling. The 2-year survival rate after local recurrence is 43%.

- Congenital mesoblastic nephroma (CMN) is the most common renal tumor in infants. Recurrence has been reported in infants older than 3 months with a cellular variant of the tumor.

Pathology

Pathologists have made important contributions to the study of both the clinical behavior and the biology of Wilms' tumor (Farber, 1966; Beckwith and Palmer, 1978; Beckwith, 1983; Weeks and Beckwith, 1987; Zuppan et al, 1991; Schmidt and Beckwith, 1995; Ravenel et al, 2001). Wilms' tumor is characterized by tremendous histologic diversity, and classification of childhood tumors can be difficult. In fact, tumors thought to be variants of nephroblastoma, clear cell sarcoma of the kidney (CCSK) and rhabdoid tumor of the kidney (RTK), are now recognized to be distinctly separate entities (Beckwith and Palmer, 1978; Marsden et al, 1978). Recognition of these tumors, as well as Wilms' tumor with nuclear atypia or anaplasia, was an important milestone. These entities accounted for

almost half the tumor deaths in early NWTSG studies (Breslow et al, 1985). Separating patients with these tumors from those with more favorable histology (FH) has allowed for refinement of the staging system and better stratification of patients for treatment. As noted in the discussion earlier, correlation of the pathologic findings with genetic events is improving our understanding of the development of Wilms' tumor.

Favorable-Histology Wilms' Tumor

Wilms' tumor usually compresses the adjacent normal renal parenchyma to form a pseudocapsule composed of compressed, atrophic renal tissues. This intrarenal pseudocapsule can be helpful in distinguishing Wilms' tumor from NRs and other renal tumors. The tumors are generally soft and friable, with necrotic or hemorrhagic areas noted frequently. This consistency increases the risk for intraoperative tumor rupture. Most Wilms' tumors are unicentric, but 12% are multicentric unilateral tumors (Breslow et al, 1993). Extrarenal Wilms' tumor developing in the retroperitoneum and elsewhere is rare and thought to arise from displaced metanephric elements or mesonephric remnants. Derived from primitive metanephric blastema, Wilms' tumor is characterized by tremendous histologic diversity (Beckwith and Palmer, 1978). In addition to expressing a variety of cell types found in a normal developing kidney, Wilms' tumor often contains tissues such as skeletal muscle, cartilage, and squamous epithelium. These heterotopic cell types probably reflect the primitive developmental potential of metanephric blastema that is not expressed in normal nephrogenesis. **"Classic" Wilms' tumor is characterized by islands of compact, undifferentiated blastema and the presence of variable epithelial differentiation in the form of embryonic tubules, rosettes, and glomeruloid structures separated by a significant stromal component. The proportion of each of these components varies from infrequent to abundant within and among individual tumors. The coexistence of blastemal, epithelial, and stromal cells has led to use of the term "triphasic" to characterize the histologic composition of "classic" Wilms' tumor.** Some Wilms' tumors, however, are not triphasic but occur only in biphasic or even monomorphous patterns, so the diagnosis of Wilms' tumor need not be restricted to specimens in which all three cell lines are expressed (Schmidt and Beckwith, 1995). **Wilms' tumors with predominantly epithelial differentiation have a low degree of aggressiveness, and the majority are stage I tumors** (Beckwith et al, 1996). **However, these tumors may be more resistant to therapy if they are initially seen at an advanced stage. Blastemal-predominant tumors are highly aggressive, but very responsive to chemotherapy.**

Anaplastic Wilms' Tumor

As noted earlier, identification of tumors with unfavorable histologic features such as anaplasia was an important milestone (Beckwith and Palmer, 1978; Bonadio et al, 1985; Zuppan et al, 1991). Anaplasia is characterized by the presence of three abnormalities: nuclear enlargement to three or more times the diameter of the adjacent cells, hyperchromasia of enlarged nuclei, and abnormal mitotic figures. **Tumors with anaplastic features are rarely seen in patients younger than 2 years at diagnosis (incidence of about 2%), but their pres-**

ence increases to a relatively stable incidence of about 13% in those older than 5 years (Bonadio et al, 1985; Green et al, 1994). Anaplasia is associated with resistance to chemotherapy, as evidenced by the similar incidence of anaplasia (5%) in the NWTSG and SIOP studies (Vujanic et al, 1999). Although the presence of anaplasia has clearly been demonstrated to carry a poor prognosis, when the anaplastic component is completely removed, stage I, the outcome is generally excellent (Zuppan et al, 1988; Green et al, 1994). This confirms the observation that anaplasia is more a marker of chemoresistance than inherent aggressiveness of the tumor. Anaplasia has been further divided into focal and diffuse patterns to reflect the different prognosis of anaplasia that is present throughout the kidney or in an extrarenal location (Faria et al, 1996).

Nephrogenic Rests

More than a third of kidneys resected for Wilms' tumor contain precursor lesions, known as *nephrogenic rests* (Beckwith et al, 1990; Beckwith, 1993). NRs have also been detected in 1% of kidneys in infants on postmortem examination, most of which apparently undergo involution (Beckwith, 1998). NRs have a varied life, and most do not form Wilms' tumor. A rest can undergo maturation, sclerosis, involution, and complete disappearance.

NRs can be separated into two fundamentally distinct categories, *perilobar* (PLNRs) and *intralobar* (ILNRs) (Beckwith et al, 1990). These two types of NRs are distinguished by their position within the renal lobe (Fig. 130–8). Relative position within the lobe is a direct reflection of the chronology of the embryologic development of the kidney. PLNRs are found only in the lobar periphery, which is elaborated late in embryogenesis, whereas ILNRs are found anywhere within the lobe, as well as in the renal sinus and the wall of the pelvicalyceal system. Therefore, ILNRs are generally believed to be the result of earlier gestational aberrations. ILNRs are commonly stroma-rich and intermingle with the adjacent renal parenchyma. PLNRs are usually subcortical and sharply demarcated and contain predominantly blastema and tubules. Of particular interest is the observation that PLNRs are usually found in children with BWS, which is linked to the 11p15 Wilms' locus, whereas ILNRs are typically seen in children with aniridia, DDS, or other features associated with the 11p13 Wilms' tumor locus (Table 130–7). The age at diagnosis is lower for Wilms' tumor arising in association with ILNRs. These observations suggest that the different Wilms' tumor genes may be involved in distinct developmental pathways within the kidney and that their inactivation may interrupt normal kidney development at different time points. Both types of NRs are associated with bilateral Wilms' tumor, and the incidence of NRs is much higher than that seen in unilateral Wilms' tumor.

Multiple rests in one kidney usually implies that NRs are also present in the other kidney (Beckwith et al, 1990). Children younger than 12 months in whom Wilms' tumor is diagnosed and who also have NRs, in particular, PLNRs, have a markedly increased risk for the development of contralateral disease and require frequent and regular surveillance for several years (Table 130–8) (Coppes et al, 1999). Surveillance is likewise recommended for those in whom Wilms' tumor is diagnosed after 12 months of age and who

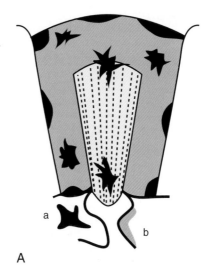

A

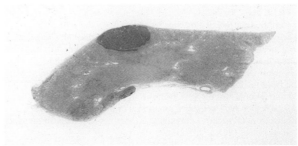

B

Figure 130–8. **A,** Illustration of the renal lobe showing characteristic locations of an intralobar nephrogenic rest (*dark gray*) and a perilobar nephrogenic rest (*black*). Label *a* indicates an intralobar nephrogenic rest in the renal sinus; *b* indicates an intralobar nephrogenic rest in the wall of the calyx. (From Beckwith JB: Precursor lesions of Wilms' tumor: Clinical and biological implications. Med Pediatr Oncol 1993;21:158-168.) **B,** Perilobar nephrogenic rest composed of blastemal cells just beneath the renal capsule (hematoxylin-eosin, magnification ×40.)

Table 130–7. **Approximate Prevalence of Nephrogenic Rests**		
Patient Population	*PLNR (%)*	*ILNR (%)*
Infant autopsies	1	0.01
Renal dysplasia	3.5	Unknown
Unilateral Wilms' tumor	25	15
Synchronous bilateral Wilms' tumor	74-79	34-41
Metachronous bilateral Wilms' tumor	42	63-75
Beckwith-Wiedemann syndrome, hemihypertrophy	70-77	47-56
Aniridia	12/20	84-100
Drash syndrome	11	78

ILNR, intralobar nephrogenic rest; PLNR, perilobar nephrogenic rest.
Adapted from Beckwith JB: Precursor lesions of Wilms' tumor: Clinical and biological implications. Med Pediatr Oncol 1993;21:158-168.

have NRs (D'Angio et al, 1993). The occurrence of metachronous Wilms' tumor in patients previously treated with conventional chemotherapeutic regimens suggests that NRs are not always eradicated.

NRs display a spectrum of appearances. Hyperplastic NRs can produce a renal mass that may be mistaken for a small

Table 130–8. **Recommended Follow-up Imaging Studies for Children with Renal Neoplasms of Proven Histology Who Are Free of Metastases at Diagnosis**

Tumor Type	Study	Schedule after Therapy
Favorable-histology Wilms' tumor		
Stage I anaplastic Wilms' tumor	Chest films	6 wk and 3 mo postop, then q3mo ×5, q6mo ×3, yearly ×2
Irradiated patients only	Irradiated bony structures*	Yearly to full growth, then q5yr indefinitely†
Without NRs, stages I and II	Abdominal ultrasound	Yearly ×3
Without NRs, stage III	Abdominal ultrasound	As for chest films
With NRs, any stage‡	Abdominal ultrasound	q3mo ×10, q6mo ×5, yearly ×5
Stage II and III anaplastic	Chest films	As for favorable histology
	Abdominal ultrasound	q3mo ×4, q6mo ×4
Renal cell carcinoma	Chest films	Like favorable histology
	Skeletal survey and bone scan	Like CCSK
CCSK	Brain MRI and/or opacified CT	When CCSK is established, then q6mo ×10
	Skeletal survey and bone scan	As for favorable histology
	Chest films	
Rhabdoid tumor	Brain MRI and/or opacified CT	As for CCSK
	Chest films	As for favorable histology
Mesoblastic nephroma§	Abdominal ultrasound	q3mo ×6

*To include any irradiated osseous structures.
†To detect second neoplasms, benign (osteochondromas) or malignant.
‡The panelists at the first International Conference on Molecular and Clinical Genetics of Childhood Renal Tumors, Albuquerque, New Mexico, May 1992, recommended a variation: every 3 months for 5 years or until age 7, whichever comes first.
CCSK, clear cell sarcoma of the kidney; CT, computed tomography; MRI, magnetic resonance imaging; NRs, nephrogenic rests.
§Data from the files of Dr. J.B. Beckwith reveal that 20 of 293 MN (7%) patients with mesoblastic nephroma relapsed or had metastases at diagnosis: 4 of the 20 in the lungs, 1 of the 4 at diagnosis. All but 1 of the 19 relapses occurred within 1 year. Chest films for patients with mesoblastic nephroma may be elected on a schedule such as every 3 months ×4 or every 6 months ×2.
Modified from D'Angio GJ, Rosenberg H, Sharples K, et al: Position paper: Imaging methods for primary renal tumors of childhood: Cost versus benefits. Med Pediatr Oncol 1993;21:205-212.

Wilms' tumor (Beckwith, 1998). Incisional biopsy of a hyperplastic rest is of little value in distinguishing this lesion from Wilms' tumor unless the interface between the rest and normal kidney is included. Wilms' tumor will have a pseudocapsule at the interface with normal parenchyma that compresses the normal elements. The appearance of the lesion can provide some help in distinguishing between NRs and Wilms' tumor. Wilms' tumor will have a spherical shape, whereas hyperplasic rests will retain the appearance of the original rest and be more elliptical or lenticular in shape. MRI may be of some value in distinguishing between the two lesions, but the utility of MRI needs to be confirmed prospectively in large numbers of patients (Gylys-Morin et al, 1993; Rorschneider et al, 1998).

The term *nephroblastomatosis* is used to refer to the presence of multiple NRs. Diffuse overgrowth of PLNRs may produce a thick rind that enlarges the kidney but preserves its original shape. These patients are prone to the development of FH Wilms' tumor, and bilateral lesions are common. Perlman and associates (2006) reviewed 52 cases of diffuse hyperplastic PLNRs reported to the NWTSG pathology center. Wilms' tumor developed in 23 patients at a median of 30 months. Of children receiving adjuvant therapy at diagnosis, Wilms' tumor developed in 17 of 33 (52%).

Preoperative Evaluation and Staging

A palpable smooth abdominal mass is present on physical examination in more than 90% of children. A family member or primary care provider often discovers the mass incidentally. Abdominal pain, gross hematuria, and fever are other frequent findings at diagnosis. Rupture of the tumor with hemorrhage

into the free peritoneal cavity can result in the occasional occurrence of an acute abdomen.

Compression or invasion of adjacent structures may result in an atypical manifestation. Extension of Wilms' tumor into the renal vein and inferior vena cava can cause varicocele, hepatomegaly as a result of hepatic vein obstruction, ascites, and congestive heart failure. Such symptoms are found in less than 10% of patients with intracaval or atrial tumor extension (Ritchey et al, 1988, 1990; Shamberger et al, 2001). Occasionally, children with Wilms' tumor have symptoms secondary to the production of bioactive substances by the tumor (Coppes, 1993). Hypertension is present in 25% of cases and has been attributed to elevated plasma renin levels (Voute et al, 1971). During the physical examination it is important to note signs of associated Wilms' tumor syndromes such as aniridia, hemihypertrophy, and genitourinary anomalies.

Emergency surgery is not necessary unless there is evidence of active bleeding or tumor rupture. Laboratory evaluation should include a complete peripheral blood count, renal and liver function tests, serum calcium, and urinalysis. Acquired von Willebrand's disease has been found in 8% of patients with newly diagnosed Wilms' tumor (Coppes, 1993). Elevated serum calcium levels can occur in children with CMN and RTK (Jayabose et al, 1988).

Imaging

A precise diagnosis cannot be obtained on the preoperative imaging studies. All of the solid renal tumors of childhood have some common radiographic features (Broecker, 1991; Glass et al, 1991; White and Grossman, 1991). **In the SIOP-9 study, 5.4% of patients in whom preoperative chemotherapy for Wilms' tumor was commenced before diagnostic biopsy**

were found to have renal malignancies other than Wilms' tumor (20 patients) or benign renal conditions (8 patients) on nephrectomy (Tournade et al, 2001). In the United Kingdom Children's Cancer Study Group (UKCCSG), 12% of renal tumors clinically and radiologically consistent with Wilms' tumor were found to have some other diagnosis on biopsy (Vujanic et al, 2003). Other clinical parameters can provide some clues to the diagnosis. The development of a renal tumor in a child known to have aniridia, hemihypertrophy, or other syndromes associated with an increased incidence of nephroblastoma is most likely to be Wilms' tumor. Bilateral or multicentric tumors are more typical of Wilms' tumor, but renal lymphoma can be manifested in this fashion. CMN is the most likely diagnosis in a neonate with a renal mass. However, FH Wilms' tumor and RTK can also occur in the first few months of life (Ritchey et al, 1995a). The renal origin of the mass is usually apparent on CT, but it can be mistaken for neuroblastoma.

The clinical findings (e.g., abdominal pain with tumor rupture) can create confusion regarding the preoperative diagnosis. In 2.5% of NWTS-3 patients, there was an erroneous diagnosis before surgical exploration, but the child had Wilms' tumor (Ritchey et al, 1992). Most of these children did not have any preoperative imaging studies performed, and this group of patients had an increased incidence of surgical complications. This emphasizes that defining the exact histology is not as important as establishing that the child has a solid renal tumor so that the surgeon can plan for a major cancer operation. Another important role of imaging is to confirm that the contralateral kidney is functioning before performing nephrectomy.

Ultrasound is the first study performed in most children with abdominal masses. It will demonstrate the solid nature of the lesion. Doppler ultrasound is particularly helpful to exclude intracaval tumor extension, which occurs in 4% of Wilms' tumor patients (Ritchey et al, 1988). MRI is the study of choice if extension of tumor into the inferior vena cava cannot be excluded by ultrasound (Fig. 130–9) (Weese et al, 1991). CT and MRI can further define the extent of the lesion

(Fig. 130–10) (Broecker, 1991; Glass et al, 1991; White and Grossman, 1991); however, the role of imaging studies in staging of the renal tumor continues to be defined (Cohen, 1993; D'Angio et al, 1993; Ditchfield et al, 1995). If preoperative imaging could accurately detect local extension of tumor beyond the renal capsule or into regional lymph nodes, it would obviate concerns regarding staging in patients treated with preoperative therapy. The local tumor burden (e.g., regional lymph node involvement) determines the intensity of the chemotherapy regimen and whether a child receives abdominal irradiation. Regional adenopathy can be identified on CT/MRI, but enlarged retroperitoneal benign lymph nodes are common in children, and correlation between pathologic findings and lymph node evaluation at surgical exploration in Wilms' tumor patients has found significant false-positive and false-negative error rates (Othersen et al, 1990). It should not be expected that CT/MRI would have greater accuracy than visual inspection of these enlarged nodes. Detection of extrarenal tumor extension into perirenal fat and adjacent structures is also problematic. Apparent extension of the tumor into adjacent structures is usually the result of compression and not frank invasion (Ng et al, 1991). Therefore, determination of inoperability must be made at surgical exploration.

Exploration of the contralateral kidney has been advised before proceeding with nephrectomy for presumed unilateral Wilms' tumor. This recommendation was made many years ago to identify lesions missed on preoperative imaging (Martin and Kloecker, 1961). If bilateral lesions are present, definitive surgical resection is deferred and chemotherapy is given (Blute et al, 1987). A review of NWTS-4 patients with bilateral Wilms' tumor found that 7% of lesions were missed on preoperative imaging studies (Ritchey et al, 1995b). The majority of these children underwent nephrectomy of the more involved kidney at diagnosis before exploration of the contralateral kidney. Failure to perform contralateral exploration before nephrectomy was also reported in a recent report of NWTS-5 patients (Ehrlich et al, 2005). Most of the missed contralateral lesions were managed with biopsy alone, yet extended follow-up of the children has not demonstrated any relapses (Ritchey et al, 2005). The conclusion was that

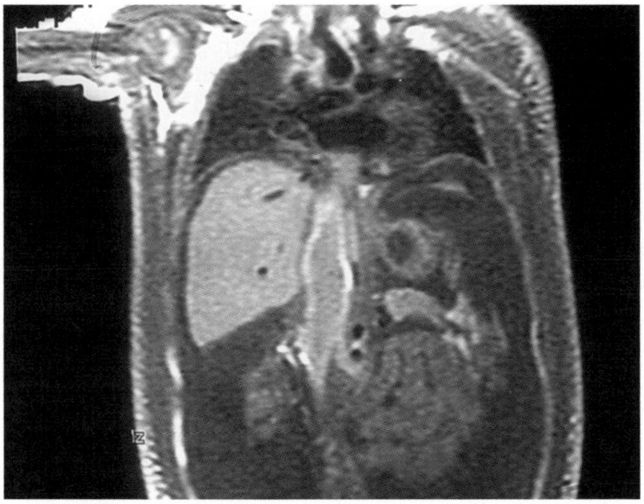

Figure 130–9. Magnetic resonance image depicting extension of Wilms' tumor into the inferior vena cava.

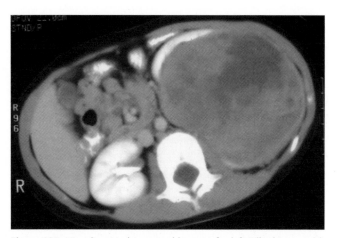

Figure 130–10. Computed tomographic scan of a left Wilms' tumor with a small rim of functioning renal parenchyma.

routine exploration is not necessary, provided that preoperative imaging with thin slices on multidetector helical CT scanners or MRI is performed.

The lung is the most common site of distant metastasis in children with Wilms' tumor, and CT of the chest, with or without plain chest radiographs, should be obtained before surgery. The clinical significance of lung nodules detected on CT scan alone is controversial (Wilimas et al, 1997; Meisel et al, 1999; Owens et al, 2002). Several reports have suggested that treatment of such patients with AMD and VCR is sufficient without the need for DOX or pulmonary irradiation. CT will clearly detect more lesions than a chest radiograph will, but not all of these lesions represent metastases (Ehrlich et al, 2005). Meisel and colleagues did note an increased number of deaths as a result of treatment toxicity in patients with CT-only lesions who received whole-lung irradiation (Meisel et al, 1999). CCSK and renal cell carcinoma have a propensity to metastasize to the skeleton (D'Angio et al, 1993; Indolfi et al, 2003). Skeletal surveys and bone scans are both recommended after the histologic diagnosis is confirmed (Feusner et al, 1990). Cranial CT or MRI is performed in all children with CCSK or RTK because both are associated with intracranial metastases (Weeks et al, 1989; Indolfi et al, 2003).

Staging

The most important determinants of outcome in children with Wilms' tumor are tumor histopathology and stage. Accurate staging of Wilms' tumor allows treatment results to be evaluated and enables universal comparison of outcomes. The staging system used by the Children's Oncology Group (Table 130–9) is based primarily on surgical and histopathologic findings. Examination for extension through the capsule, residual disease, vascular involvement, and lymph node involvement is essential to properly assess the extent of the tumor.

Stage I tumors are limited to the kidney and are completely resected. However, evidence of tumor extension can be subtle. Tumor invasion of blood and lymphatic vessels in the renal sinus is the first sign of spread outside the kidney in stage II tumors (Weeks et al, 1987). Penetration through the renal capsule is the next most common site of extrarenal spread. Clear demonstration of tumor cells in perirenal fat is required to document capsular penetration. In NWTS-5, the distribu-

tion by stage for patients with FH tumors was 24.9% with stage I, 29.9% with stage II, 30.6% with stage III, and 14.5% with stage IV. Patients with anaplastic tumors are twice as likely to have stage IV disease as those with FH tumors (Green et al, 1994).

Prognostic Factors

As treatment regimens for children with Wilms' tumor have become more effective, the ability of retrospectively determined prognostic factors to predict outcomes has diminished. The traditional staging factors relied on in the past to predict risk for tumor progression or relapse, such as tumor size, histology, and lymph node metastases, are now less able to stratify FH patients for treatment. The search is on for biologic factors that may predict tumor behavior. The NWTSG has established a central tumor bank that maintains biologic specimens from all patients in the NWTS-5 study. The clinical outcome is available for patients whose tumors are maintained in the bank, and this tremendous resource is available to potential investigators.

Chromosomal Abnormalities. LOH for a portion of chromosome 16q has been noted in 20% of Wilms' tumors (Maw et al, 1992). **A study of 232 patients registered in the NWTSG found LOH for 16q in 17% of the tumors** (Grundy et al, 1994). **Patients with tumor-specific LOH for chromosome 16q had a statistically significantly poorer 2-year relapse-free and overall survival than did those without LOH for chromosome 16q. This difference in outcome persisted after adjustment for histology and stage.** One of the primary goals of NWTS-5 was to verify these preliminary findings that LOH for chromosomes 16q and 1p is useful in identifying patients at increased risk for relapse and death. Among patients with stage I or II FH tumors, the relative risk for relapse and death was increased in patients with LOH of either 1p or 16q when compared with those lacking LOH at either locus (Grundy et al, 2005). The risk for relapse and death in patients with stage III or IV FH tumors was increased only with LOH for both regions. These results suggest that patients whose tumors demonstrate LOH for these chromosomal regions should have intensification of treatment.

Another potential marker is telomerase, a reverse transcriptase that maintains chromosome ends by compensating for the loss of DNA that occurs during replication. High telomerase activity has been found to be an unfavorable prognostic feature for several types of cancers. The enzyme, which plays a key role in cellular immortalization, is minimally composed of a catalytic subunit (TERT) and an RNA subunit (TERC/hTR) that provides the template for nucleotide repeat generation. In a case-cohort study of 78 patients with FH Wilms' tumor, TERT mRNA levels correlated with the risk for recurrence even after adjustment for tumor stage (Dome et al, 1999). A follow-up study involving 296 patients confirmed the correlation between TERT expression and recurrence but found that TERC expression was a more powerful prognostic indicator (Dome et al, 2004). Future studies will seek to evaluate how telomerase expression may be used in conjunction with other prognostic markers, such as LOH at 1p and 16q, to stratify patients into risk-appropriate treatment groups.

DNA Content. The proliferative rate of tumor cells can be estimated by measurement of the DNA content. Flow cytom-

Table 130–9. **Staging System of the Children's Oncology Group**
Stage
I   Tumor limited to the kidney and completely excised. The renal capsule is intact and the tumor was not ruptured prior to removal. There is no residual tumor.
II   Tumor beyond the kidney, but is completely resected. Extrarenal vessels may contain tumor thrombus or be infiltrated by tumor.
III   Residual nonhematogenous tumor confined to the abdomen: lymph node involvement, any tumor spillage, rupture or biopsy, peritoneal implants, tumor beyond surgical margin either grossly or microscopically, or tumor not completely removed.
IV   Hematogenous metastases to lung, liver, bone, brain, etc.
V   Bilateral renal involvement at diagnosis.

etry has been performed on Wilms' tumor specimens to predict which tumors are at risk for metastatic disease (Rainwater et al, 1987; Kumar et al, 1989). Aneuploidy occurs more frequently in tumors with anaplastic histology, but findings in FH tumors are inconclusive. The correlation between cellular DNA content and prognosis is being examined in the NWTS-5 cohort.

Cytokines. Growth of solid tumors is critically dependent on the induction of neovascularity by angiogenic cytokines. Vascular endothelial growth factor (VEGF) is an angiogenic cytokine detected with increased frequency and quantity in experimental and clinical specimens of Wilms' tumor (Kayton et al, 1999; Karth et al, 2000). In experimental animals, lung metastases were far more likely to occur in animals with VEGF-positive tumors. Anti-VEGF therapy has been shown to suppress tumor growth in mice and can prevent the development of metastases (Rowe et al, 2000; Frischer et al, 2004). Serum levels of VEGF have been found to decrease after nephrectomy, and rising levels portend a poor prognosis (Blann et al, 2001). Anti-angiogenesis therapy is a promising adjunctive future treatment for patients with Wilms' tumor.

Treatment

Surgical Considerations

The initial therapy for most children with Wilms' tumor is radical nephrectomy, which should be performed via a transperitoneal approach. The surgeon is responsible for determining tumor extent. Accurate staging is essential for subsequent determination of the need for radiation therapy and the appropriate chemotherapy regimen. Thorough exploration of the abdominal cavity is necessary to exclude local tumor extension, liver and nodal metastases, or peritoneal seeding. Exploration of the contralateral kidney is no longer mandated before nephrectomy if preoperative CT or MRI demonstrates a normal kidney (Ritchey et al, 2005). The renal vein and inferior vena cava are palpated to exclude intravascular tumor extension before vessel ligation. Wilms' tumor extends into the inferior vena cava in approximately 6% of cases and may be clinically asymptomatic in more than 50% (Ritchey et al, 1988). Selective sampling of suspicious nodes is an essential component of local tumor staging. Formal RPLND is not recommended (Othersen et al, 1990; Shamberger et al, 1999). Extensive lymph node dissection, particularly above the renal hilum, can result in chylous ascites (Weiser et al, 2003).

The other major responsibility when performing a nephrectomy for Wilms' tumor is complete removal of the tumor without contamination of the operative field. Gentle handling of the tumor throughout the procedure is mandatory to avoid tumor spillage because such patients have a sixfold increase in local abdominal relapse (Shamberger et al, 1999). **As risk factors for local tumor recurrence, Shamberger and colleagues identified tumor spillage, unfavorable histology, incomplete tumor removal, and absence of any lymph node sampling. The 2-year survival rate after abdominal recurrence was 43%, thus emphasizing the importance of the surgeon in performing careful and complete tumor resection.**

Removing a large renal tumor in a small child is associated with some morbidity. NWTS-4 patients undergoing primary nephrectomy had an 11% incidence of surgical complications (Ritchey et al, 1999). The most common complications encountered are hemorrhage and small bowel obstruction (Ritchey et al, 1992, 1993a, 1999). SIOP investigators have reported a lower rate of complications when nephrectomy is performed after preoperative chemotherapy (Godzinski et al, 1988).

Cooperative Group Trials

The finding in the 1960s that AMD and VCR were effective agents for treating Wilms' tumor radically altered the approach to management of children with this disease (Farber, 1966; Sutow, 1967). Since that time, multiple randomized clinical trials have been conducted by the NWTSG, SIOP, and UKCCSG to determine the appropriate role for each of the therapeutic modalities available. Patients are stratified into different treatment groups based on stage and pathology. The goals of these trials are to decrease the intensity of therapy for most patients in an effort to prevent late sequelae of treatment while maintaining overall survival.

National Wilms' Tumor Study Group. The NWTSG was formed in 1969 to study Wilms' tumor. The early NWTSG studies, NWTS-1 (1969 to 1973) and NWTS-2 (1974 to 1978), found that the combination of VCR and AMD was more effective than the use of either drug alone. The addition of DOX was found to improve survival for stage III and IV patients, and postoperative flank irradiation was unnecessary for group I patients (D'Angio et al, 1976, 1981). **A major accomplishment of the early trials was identification of prognostic factors that allowed stratification of patients into high-risk and low-risk treatment groups. Patients with positive lymph nodes and diffuse tumor spillage were found to be at increased risk for abdominal relapse and therefore considered stage III and given whole-abdomen irradiation. One of the most important findings was the identification of unfavorable histologic features that have a very adverse impact on survival.**

The findings of the first two NWTS-1 trials were incorporated into the design of NWTS-3 (1979 to 1986). Children with stage I FH Wilms' tumor were treated successfully with an 18-week regimen of AMD and VCR without irradiation (D'Angio et al, 1989). The 4-year relapse-free survival rate was 89%, with an overall survival rate of 95.6%. Stage II FH patients treated with the same therapy had an equivalent 4-year overall survival rate (91.1%) as children who also received DOX, with or without XRT. For stage III FH patients, 10.8 Gy of abdominal radiation was shown to be as effective as 20 Gy in preventing abdominal relapse if DOX was added to VCR and AMD. The 4-year relapse-free survival rate for stage III patients was 82% in NWTS-3, with a 90.9% 4-year overall survival rate. Children with stage IV FH tumors received abdominal (local) irradiation based on the local tumor stage and 12 Gy to both lungs. In combination with VCR, AMD, and DOX, the 4-year relapse-free survival rate was 79% with an 80.9% overall survival rate. There was no statistically significant improvement in survival when cyclophosphamide was added to the three-drug regimen.

NWTS-4 (1987 to 1994) compared a pulse-intensive single-dose schedule with divided-dose treatment regimens of AMD and DOX. The pulse-intensive regimens achieved equivalent survival while decreasing the cost of therapy through modification of the schedule of drug administration (Green et al, 1998a). Treatment durations of approximately 6 and 15 months were found to be equally effective in patients with stage II to IV/FH tumors (Green et al, 1998b). Overall, the 4-year survival rate for patients with all stages of FH Wilms' tumor now exceeds 90%.

Children with anaplastic Wilms' tumors were randomized in NWTS-3 and NWTS-4 to receive VCR, AMD, DOX, or these three drugs with the addition of cyclophosphamide. The results were analyzed after the tumors were reclassified with the criteria of Faria and Beckwith (Faria et al, 1996). There was no difference in outcome between the regimens for children with focal anaplasia, who had a prognosis similar to that for FH patients (Green et al, 1994). For stage II to IV diffuse anaplasia, the addition of cyclophosphamide to the three-drug regimen improved the 4-year relapse-free survival rate (27.2% versus 54.8%).

NWTS-5 (1995 to 2003) was a single-arm therapeutic trial. One of the major aims of the trial was to confirm the preliminary findings that LOH for chromosomes 16q and 1p is predictive of increased risk for tumor relapse and death (Grundy et al, 1994). These results were recently reported for the NWTS-5 cohort (Grundy et al, 2005). Among patients with stage I or II FH tumors, the relative risk (RR) of relapse and death was increased with LOH for 1p only (RR = 2.2 for relapse; RR = 4.0 for death), with LOH for 16q only (RR = 1.9 and 1.4), and with LOH for both regions (RR = 2.9 and 4.3) when compared with patients lacking LOH at either locus. The risk for relapse and death in patients with stage III or IV FH tumors was increased only with LOH for both regions (RR = 2.4 and 2.7). These results confirm that LOH for 16q and LOH for 1p are independent prognostic factors. When these findings are combined with the local tumor stage, further stratification of patients can be performed to increase the intensity of treatment in an attempt to decrease the risk for relapse. Another important result of NWTS-5 is that there is now a bank of tumor specimens available to evaluate new prognostic factors that may be identified in the future. The clinical outcomes of patients for whom there are banked specimens is available to determine whether newly defined biologic variables are predictive of outcome.

The treatment regimens used in NWTS-5 are summarized in Table 130–10. **Children with stage I or II FH and stage I anaplastic Wilms' tumor received an 18-week pulse-intensive regimen of VCR and AMD. Patients with stage III FH and stage II or III focal anaplastic Wilms' tumor were treated with AMD, VCR, DOX, and 10.8 Gy of abdominal irradiation. Patients with stage IV FH tumors received abdominal irradiation based on the local tumor stage, as well as 12 Gy to both lungs. The chemotherapy regimen used for patients with stage II to IV diffuse anaplasia did not result in improved survival for higher-stage patients** (Dome et al, 2005).

In NWTS-5, children younger than 2 years and weighing less than 550 g with stage I FH tumors did not receive chemotherapy after nephrectomy. This portion of the study was closed when the number of tumor relapses exceeded the limit allowed by design of the study (Green et al, 2001a). However, the 2-year overall survival rate of this cohort was 100% because of the high rate of retrieval of relapsed patients.

Table 130–10. Treatment Protocol Used in the National Wilms' Tumor Study-5

Stage/Histology	Radiotherapy	Chemotherapy
Stage I, II FH		
Stage I anaplasia	None	EE-4A—pulse-intensive AMD
Stage III, IV FH		plus VCR (18 wk)
Stage II-IV focal anaplasia	1080 cGy*	DD-4A—pulse-intensive AMD, VCR, and DOX (24 wk)
Stage II-IV diffuse anaplasia	Yes†	Regimen I: AMD, VCR, DOX, CPM, and etoposide
Stage I-IV CCSK		
Stage I-IV rhabdoid tumor of the kidney	Yes**	Regimen RTK: carboplatin, etoposide, and CPM

*Stage IV/FH patients are given radiotherapy according to the local tumor stage.
†Radiation therapy is given to all CCSK and RTK patients. Consult the protocol for specific treatment.
AMD, dactinomycin; CCSK, clear cell sarcoma of the kidney; CPM, cyclophosphamide; DOX, doxorubicin; FH, favorable histology, VCR, vincristine.

These results suggest that such an approach should continue to be evaluated in future trials.

Wilms' tumor is occasionally noted in adult patients. Earlier reports suggested that the outcome for adults with Wilms' tumor is poor and that they require more intensive therapy (Byrd et al, 1982, Arrigo et al, 1990). Recent reviews of adult patients with FH Wilms' tumor registered in NWTS-4, NWTS-5, and SIOP 93-01 found improved survival in comparison to previous reports (Kalakapurakal et al, 2004a; Reinhard et al, 2004). The recommendation is that adult patients receive stage-appropriate combined-modality therapy.

International Society Of Paediatric Oncology. In the randomized clinical trials conducted by SIOP, preoperative therapy is given before surgery. This approach usually results in tumor shrinkage (Fig. 130–11), thereby reducing the risk for intraoperative rupture or spillage (Lemerle et al, 1976). A greater number of patients have "postchemotherapy stage I" tumors because of treatment of micrometastases by the neoadjuvant therapy. This was thought to be a significant advantage in terms of decreasing the morbidity associated with treatment, particularly the late effects of radiotherapy.

Early SIOP studies evaluated prenephrectomy XRT (Lemerle et al, 1976). **SIOP-5 (1976 to 1980) showed that 4 weeks of AMD and VCR was as effective as prenephrectomy XRT in avoiding surgical tumor rupture and increasing the proportion of patients with low-stage disease** (Lemerle et al, 1983). **SIOP-6 (1980 to 1987) demonstrated that patients with "postchemotherapy stage I" disease can safely be treated with 18 weeks of AMD and VCR** (Tournade et al, 1993). **However, patients with "postchemotherapy stage II" tumors and negative lymph nodes were found to have a higher rate of abdominal relapse if postoperative irradiation was omitted** (Tournade et al, 1993). An anthracycline was subsequently added to the treatment of these children. SIOP-6 confirmed the need for a three-drug chemotherapy regimen after nephrectomy for patients with "postchemotherapy stage II" lymph node–positive and stage III tumors. SIOP-9 (1987 to 1993) evaluated the duration of prenephrectomy

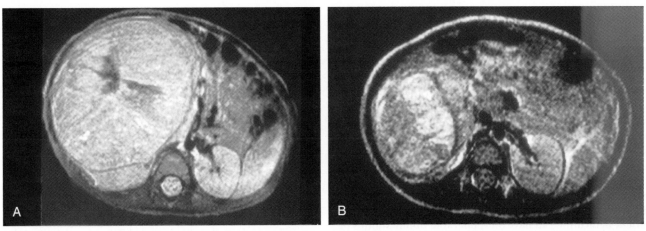

Figure 130–11.   A, Magnetic resonance image of a Wilms' tumor that was pretreated with chemotherapy. **B,** After 6 weeks of chemotherapy, the tumor is much smaller in size.

chemotherapy. They reported that the number of post-chemotherapy stage I patients was similar after either 4 or 8 weeks of preoperative AMD and VCR (64% versus 62%) and that 2-year relapse-free survival was equivalent (Tournade et al, 2001). The majority of tumor shrinkage was noted in the first 4 weeks of therapy. Patients with stage II and III FH tumors received three drugs (AMD, VCR, and epirubicin). Radiotherapy was limited to patients with stage II node-positive and stage III disease, with 18% of patients being irradiated (Graf et al, 2000). Abdominal relapses occurred in 6.6% of stage II N0 patients, and the 2-year relapse-free survival rate was 84%. The 2-year relapse-free survival rate for stage II N1 and stage III patients was 71%. There were 59 children with stage I to IV tumors who had complete tumor necrosis after chemotherapy, and 98% of these children had no evidence of disease at 5 years (Boccon-Gibod et al, 2000).

The latest SIOP study on Wilms' tumor, SIOP 93-01 (1993 to 2000), evaluated a reduction in postoperative therapy for patients with stage I intermediate-risk and anaplastic Wilms' tumor (deKraker et al, 2004). Patients were randomized to receive either 4 or 18 weeks of postoperative chemotherapy with AMD and VCR. The 2-year event-free survival rate was 91.4% after 4 weeks and 88.8% after 18 weeks of therapy, thus demonstrating that survival can be maintained while shortening the duration of postnephrectomy therapy. The current SIOP 2001 study is evaluating the ability to stratify patients for treatment based on postchemotherapy histologic findings (Weirich et al, 2001).

United Kingdom Children's Cancer Study Group. The UKCCSG trials use prenephrectomy chemotherapy, but unlike SIOP, they perform biopsy before treatment (Pritchard et al, 1995; Mitchell et al, 2000; Pritchard-Jones et al, 2003). Biopsy is performed to avoid giving chemotherapy for benign conditions, which account for 1% of lesions thought to be Wilms' tumor on imaging studies (Tournade et al, 2001). The other reason to perform biopsy is to avoid giving inappropriate chemotherapy to patients with non-Wilms' tumors. The UKW3 trial noted a 12% incidence of non-Wilms' tumors in patients with the typical features of Wilms' tumor on imaging study (Vujanic et al, 2003). The UKW1 and UKW2 studies evaluated the single agent vincristine for the treatment

of stage I FH tumors (Pritchard et al, 1995; Mitchell et al, 2000). The overall survival rate of 96% compares well with that of two-drug chemotherapy, but age older than 4 years was considered an adverse prognostic factor (Pritchard-Jones et al, 2003).

Preoperative Chemotherapy versus Immediate Nephrectomy

In summary, there is a different philosophic approach between the pediatric cancer cooperative groups. The common theme is identifying high-risk patients who require more intense therapy while minimizing treatment and thus morbidity for low-risk patients. Both groups want to reduce the number of patients receiving DOX and irradiation to avoid the late sequelae noted in extended follow-up of patients treated with these modalities (see later). Currently, approximately 50% of SIOP patients are treated with an anthracycline and 17% undergo irradiation, whereas approximately 35% of NWTSG patients have received both therapies (Pritchard-Jones, 2002; D'Angio, 2003). The NWTSG trials have relied on surgical and pathologic staging after immediate nephrectomy. Preoperative treatment can produce a dramatic reduction in the size of the primary tumor and thereby decrease the morbidity associated with surgery (Godzinski et al, 1998). However, the staging information obtained after prenephrectomy chemotherapy may inadequately define the risk for relapse (Tournade et al, 1993). The current SIOP approach is to use the histologic response of the tumor to preoperative therapy to determine postoperative treatment. The current strategy in North America will be to use biologic prognostic factors to stratify patients for therapy.

In some situations, preoperative chemotherapy is routinely recommended, including children with bilateral Wilms' tumors (Blute et al, 1987), tumors inoperable at surgical exploration (Ritchey et al, 1994), and tumor extension into inferior vena cava above the hepatic veins (Ritchey et al, 1993b; Shamberger et al, 2001; Szavay et al, 2004). The latter two conditions are associated with an increased risk for surgical complications if primary nephrectomy is undertaken (Ritchey et al, 1992). The rationale for preoperative chemotherapy in bilateral disease is to decrease the high rate of renal failure noted in these children (Ritchey et al, 1996; Breslow et al, 2000).

Inoperable Tumors. The surgeon must make the determination that a tumor is inoperable. **This decision should not be based on preoperative imaging studies, in which local tumor extension can be overestimated.** Also as noted earlier, not all renal masses in children represent Wilms' tumor (Vujanic et al, 2003). **If the tumor is found to be unresectable at surgical exploration, pretreatment with chemotherapy almost always reduces the bulk of the tumor and renders it resectable** (Ritchey et al, 1994; Grundy et al, 2004) (see Fig. 130–11). **Patients who are staged by imaging studies alone and receive preoperative chemotherapy before nephrectomy are also at risk for understaging** (Tournade et al, 1993). **A patient determined to have an inoperable tumor should be considered to have stage III and be treated accordingly** (Ritchey et al, 1994).

Repeat imaging is performed after 6 weeks of chemotherapy. Experience in SIOP has shown that the majority of the reduction in tumor volume occurs in the first 4 weeks (Tournade et al, 2001). After adequate shrinkage of the tumor has occurred, definitive resection can be completed. A clinically good response (by imaging) is usually associated with a pathologically good response in terms of regressive histologic changes (Zuppan et al, 1991; Weirich et al, 2001). The converse is not always true, however. The distribution of histologic subtypes is different after preoperative chemotherapy than after primary surgery because differentiation of the tumor occurs after chemotherapy. Stromal- and epithelial-predominant tumors are found more often after preoperative chemotherapy. These histologic subtypes may demonstrate a poor clinical response to therapy but have an excellent prognosis if the tumor is completely excised (Fig. 130–12). Patients with progressive disease have a very poor prognosis, and these patients will require treatment with a different chemotherapeutic regimen (Ritchey et al, 1994).

Bilateral Wilms' Tumors. Synchronous bilateral Wilms' **tumors occur in about 5% of children** (Blute et al, 1987; Coppes et al, 1989; Montgomery et al, 1991). **The preferred approach for patients with bilateral nephroblastoma is initial biopsy,** followed by preoperative chemotherapy (Blute et al, 1987; Coppes et al, 1989; Kumar et al, 1998). This strategy is recommended to decrease the incidence of renal failure, which occurs in 9.1% and 18.8%, respectively, of patients with synchronous and metachronous bilateral Wilms' tumor (Ritchey et al, 1996). The most common cause of renal failure was the need for bilateral nephrectomy for persistent or recurrent tumor in the remaining kidney after initial nephrectomy. Nephrectomy can be avoided entirely in almost 50% of patients who undergo initial biopsy followed by chemotherapy (Montgomery et al, 1991; Shaul et al, 1992).

After 6 weeks of chemotherapy, repeat imaging is performed to assess response. Experience in SIOP has shown that the majority of shrinkage occurs after 4 weeks of chemotherapy (Tournade et al, 2001). CT or MRI can assess the reduction in tumor volume and the feasibility of partial resection. Imaging cannot, however, predict the histology of the tumor based on changes in volume of the tumor after chemotherapy (Weirich et al, 2001; Olsen et al, 2004). Tumors not responding to therapy require open biopsy to determine their histology. Failure to achieve a reduction in volume is probably due to tumor differentiation (Weirich et al, 2001; Anderson et al, 2002). Differentiated tumors may show a poor clinical response to therapy, but they have an excellent prognosis if the tumor is completely excised. Tumors with complete necrosis and predominantly regressive changes can also increase in size during therapy.

At the time of the second-look procedure, partial nephrectomy or wedge excision of the tumors is performed. This should be done only if complete tumor resection with negative margins can be achieved and part of either or both of the kidneys can be salvaged. One area of controversy is the role of enucleation versus partial nephrectomy when renal salvage procedures are performed in these patients (Cozzi et al, 1996; Horwitz et al, 1996). The concern is that enucleation will be more likely to result in positive surgical margins (Horwitz et al, 1996). For FH tumors, adjuvant therapy may still provide a good outcome (Cozzi et al, 1996). However, if anaplasia is found in the resected specimen, a positive margin will adversely affect survival.

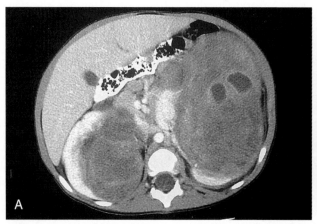
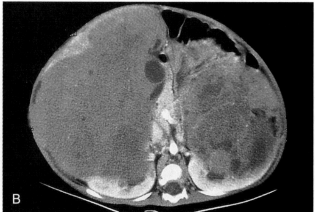

Figure 130–12. Patient with bilateral tumors who was treated by chemotherapy. **A,** Computed tomographic (CT) scan before treatment. **B,** CT scan after 6 months of chemotherapy showing an increase in size of the tumors. Bilateral partial nephrectomies were performed and revealed mature tumor elements with rhabdomyoblastic differentiation.

If extensive tumor involvement precludes partial resection, biopsy specimens are obtained. Patients with blastemal-predominant or anaplastic tumor should be changed to a different chemotherapeutic regimen. The patient should be reassessed after an additional 12 weeks of chemotherapy to determine the feasibility of resection. If it appears that either or both of the kidneys can be salvaged, partial nephrectomy or wedge excision of the tumors is performed. Radical nephrectomy is performed to remove the kidney with too extensive tumor involvement when only one of two can be preserved. Bilateral nephrectomy and dialysis may rarely be required when the tumors fail to respond to chemotherapy and radiation therapy. This is the most common cause of renal failure in patients with bilateral Wilms' tumor (Ritchey et al, 1996). The recommended interval between successful completion of treatment of Wilms' tumor and renal transplantation varies (Penn, 1979; Rudin et al, 1998). Some advocate a waiting period of 2 years to ensure that metastatic disease does not develop; others have found that a 1-year interval is sufficient. Patients in whom renal failure develops after renal-sparing surgery should have the remaining renal tissue removed before transplantation to prevent tumor recurrence after starting immunosuppression (Kubiak et al, 2004).

All patients treated for bilateral Wilms' tumor require close long-term follow-up. SIOP investigators have noted that late relapses have occurred in patients with bilateral Wilms' tumor more than 4 years after treatment and therefore recommend long-term follow-up (Coppes et al, 1989). These patients should also undergo frequent assessment of renal function, urine protein, and blood pressure.

Partial Nephrectomy for Unilateral Tumors. Several centers have explored the role of parenchymal-sparing procedures in children with unilateral Wilms' tumor (McLorie et al, 1991; Cozzi et al, 1996; Moorman-Voestermans et al, 1998; Haecker et al, 2003, Linni et al, 2003; Zani et al, 2005). The primary motivation for this approach is concern about the late occurrence of renal dysfunction after unilateral nephrectomy. Some studies have noted proteinuria and a decrease in creatinine clearance (Robitaille et al, 1985; Bertolone et al, 1987), but other investigators have failed to confirm these findings (Barrera et al, 1989; Bhisitkul et al, 1990). However, **the incidence of renal failure after treatment of unilateral Wilms' tumor is low. Median follow-up was 6 years from diagnosis (range 2 months to 22 years). In only 0.25% of NWTSG patients has renal failure developed after nephrectomy for unilateral tumors** (Ritchey et al, 1996). **Most of these patients were children with DDS who had intrinsic renal disease and often progressed to end-stage renal disease.** As noted earlier, this is due to mutation of WT1, which is necessary for normal renal development. **Patients with the WAGR syndrome also have an increased risk for renal failure, 38% at a median of 14 years from diagnosis** (Breslow et al, 2000). There is also an increased risk for renal failure in children with genitourinary anomalies and Wilms' tumor.

Most Wilms' tumors are too large at diagnosis to allow partial nephrectomy. After preoperative chemotherapy, partial nephrectomy can be performed in 10% to 15% of patients. Only an occasional child with Wilms' tumor will have a lesion small enough to allow partial nephrectomy at diagnosis, such as tumors detected as a result of screening studies for BWS

and aniridia. As noted before, there are concerns regarding staging after chemotherapy in that some patients need to receive added therapy to prevent local recurrence. Another concern is the increased risk for local recurrence after partial nephrectomy (Horwitz et al, 1996; Haecker et al, 2003). In NWTS-4, patients with bilateral Wilms' tumor who underwent partial nephrectomy had an 8% incidence of local recurrence (Horwitz et al, 1996). Patients in whom intra-abdominal relapse develops have markedly decreased survival. In past studies, only 42% of patients with local recurrence were retrieved by salvage chemotherapy protocols (Shamberger et al, 1999).

Cozzi and coauthors (2004) described a strict surgical protocol that should be followed when undertaking partial nephrectomy in children with unilateral Wilms' tumor. The lesion should be completely excised with a margin of normal renal parenchyma. These patients should not undergo partial nephrectomy if the tumor cannot be removed as stage I. They recommend frozen sections to confirm a negative margin and also to evaluate the histology. Patients with high-risk histologic patterns such as anaplasia or persistent blastemal-predominant tumor after chemotherapy should be treated by complete nephrectomy. Such patients have a greater risk for recurrence because these tumors have been demonstrated to be resistant to chemotherapy. The higher local recurrence rates noted in bilateral Wilms' tumor patients may reflect a more aggressive approach to sparing renal parenchyma, but they may also reflect a distinct tumor biology.

In summary, partial nephrectomy for patients with unilateral Wilms' tumor is controversial. It seems reasonable to consider partial nephrectomy for patients with bilateral Wilms' tumor, tumor in a solitary kidney, and renal insufficiency. For other children, this option should be approached with caution. Patients with aniridia and genitourinary anomalies, who have a known increased risk for late renal failure, might also be considered for such an intervention. As noted in the discussion earlier, the potential benefit of this approach must be weighed against the known risk for undertreatment and increased risk for local recurrence. Until there are more compelling data that the risk for renal failure or clinically relevant renal insufficiency in unilateral Wilms' tumor is significantly higher than what has been reported to date, a renal-sparing surgical approach should be considered investigational.

Late Effects of Treatment

Numerous organ systems are subject to the late sequelae of anticancer therapy. Clinicians must be aware of the spectrum of problems that these children face as they grow into adulthood. Musculoskeletal conditions such as scoliosis were a significant problem in children receiving XRT in the early NWTS trials (Evans et al, 1991). Hogeboom and colleagues (2001) studied the impact of treatment on stature in Wilms' tumor patients. They noted that reductions in stature directly correlated with the total radiation dose and age at treatment but concluded that currently recommended radiation doses should not result in clinically significant height deficits.

Gonadal irradiation can produce hypogonadism and temporary azoospermia in boys (Kinsella et al, 1989). The severity of damage is dependent on the radiation dose. Leydig cells are more radioresistant than germ cells, but higher doses can produce damage resulting in inadequate production of testosterone, which can lead to delayed sexual maturation. Chemotherapeutic agents can also adversely affect testicular function (Mustieles et al, 1995). A 12% incidence of ovarian failure was found in girls receiving abdominal XRT (Stillman et al, 1987). Abdominal XRT also increases the risk for adverse pregnancy outcomes (Li et al, 1983; Green et al, 2002). The offspring of irradiated female patients are at risk for low birth weight, premature birth, and congenital malformations. Radiation portals that include the pelvis and doses exceeding 20 Gy increase the risk for miscarriage (Kalapurakal et al, 2004b).

An increased incidence of second malignant neoplasms has been noted in children treated for Wilms' tumor. Two studies involving Wilms' tumor survivors have noted a 1% cumulative incidence 10 years after diagnosis and a rising incidence thereafter (Li et al, 1987; Breslow et al, 1988b). All but two occurred in irradiated patients, most often in the radiation field. All children in whom hepatocellular carcinoma developed had received flank irradiation (Kovalic et al, 1991). There is a greater risk for development of a second solid tumor over time. Secondary acute myelogenous leukemia occurred at a median of 3 years from initial diagnosis of the renal tumor (Shearer et al, 2001).

In recent years there has been increasing concern regarding the risk for congestive heart failure in children who receive treatment with anthracyclines such as DOX (Green et al, 2001b). In addition to the acute cardiotoxicity, cardiac failure can develop many years after treatment (Steinherz et al, 1991). In a preliminary review of patients entered in NWTS 1, 2, 3 and 4, the frequency of congestive heart failure was 4.4% in DOX-treated patients who received this drug as part of their initial chemotherapy regimen (Green et al, 2001b). The risk was increased if the patient received whole-lung or left flank irradiation.

OTHER RENAL TUMORS
Clear Cell Sarcoma of the Kidney

CCSK accounts for 3% of renal tumors reported to the NWTSG. Although CCSK can pose some serious challenges to the pathologist because it can mimic Wilms' tumor, RTK, and CMN, the classic pattern consists of a cellular lesion of polygonal cells with round oval nuclei having a delicate chromatin pattern and indistinct nucleoli (Schmidt and Beckwith, 1995). **Important predictors of improved survival are lower stage, younger age at diagnosis, treatment with DOX, and absence of tumor necrosis** (Argani et al, 2000). **The addition of DOX improved both overall and relapse-free survival** (D'Angio et al, 1989; Argani et al, 2000; Seibel et al, 2004). Patients with stage I tumors (using the current criteria of absence of renal sinus invasion) had a 98% survival rate. Unlike anaplastic Wilms' tumor, even stage I CCSK lesions are associated with increased rates of relapse and require postoperative irradiation. Long-term follow-up of CCSK patients is needed because 30% of relapses occurred more than 3 years after diagnosis and some as late as 10 years. Unlike Wilms' tumor, CCSK is associated with bone and brain metastases. Bilateral involvement has thus far not been reported, nor has the presence of Wilms' tumor–associated congenital anomalies such as aniridia or hemihypertrophy. Patients with CCSK were treated

in NWTS-5 with a regimen combining VCR, DOX, cyclophosphamide, and etoposide in an attempt to further improve the survival of this high-risk group, but the results of that trial are pending.

Rhabdoid Tumor of the Kidney

RTK is the most aggressive and lethal childhood renal tumor and accounts for 2% of renal tumors registered by the NWTSG. RTK is now considered a sarcoma of the kidney, yet the cell type of origin is unknown (D'Angio et al, 1989). RTK derives its name from the resemblance to rhabdomyoblasts, but the tumor is not derived from myogenic cells. It is characterized by large uniform cells with abundant acidophilic cytoplasm, frequently containing a discrete zone of pale eosinophilia and made up of fibrillary inclusion bodies, and large nuclei with very prominent nucleoli. RTK and CCSK both occur in renal and extrarenal locations, thus suggesting an origin from a non–organ-specific mesenchymal cell. Cytogenetic studies have shown that there may be a common genetic basis for renal and extrarenal rhabdoid tumors. Deletions and somatic mutations in the *INI1* gene on chromosome 22 in the region of 22q11 predispose to the development of this tumor (Biegel et al, 1999). Germline mutations of *INI1* have been identified in renal rhabdoid tumors. Staining for the products of the *INI1* gene can be useful because RTK is consistently negative (Hoot et al, 2004).

Typical clinical features include early age at diagnosis (median age <16 months), advanced stage, resistance to chemotherapy, and high mortality (Amar et al, 2001). **RTK is distinguished by its propensity to metastasize to the brain** (D'Angio et al, 1993). In addition, RTK is associated with second primary tumors in the brain, including cerebellar medulloblastomas, pineoblastomas, neuroblastomas, and subependymal giant cell astrocytomas (Bonnin et al, 1984).

Congenital Mesoblastic Nephroma

CMN is the most common renal tumor in infants, with a mean age at diagnosis of 3.5 months (Howell et al, 1982; Levin et al, 1982). CMN is a very firm tumor on gross examination, and the cut surface has the yellowish gray trabeculated appearance of a leiomyoma. There are three histologic subtypes: classic, cellular, and mixed (showing areas of both classic and cellular). The classic subtype, characterized by interlacing sheets of bland spindle cells, resembles infantile fibromatosis. The cellular variant, with a solid sheetlike growth pattern and frequent mitoses, is virtually histologically identical to congenital fibrosarcoma (Beckwith, 1986; Johsi et al, 1986; Gormley et al, 1989). Both tumors have a similar translocation that fuses the *ETV6* (*TEL*) gene from 12p13 with the 15q25 neurotrophin-3 receptor gene, *NTRK3* (Argani et al, 1998). In CMN, tumor induction is postulated to occur at a time when the multipotent blastema is predominately stromagenic (Snyder et al, 1981; Tomlinson et al, 1992). *WT1* is not expressed in CMN (Tomlinson et al, 1992).

The most important aspect of CMN is the usually excellent outcome with radical surgery only (Howell et al, 1982). The tumor can extend into the hilar or perirenal soft tissue; therefore, complete surgical resection is important (Beckwith, 1986). Local recurrence and metastasis can occur, particularly with the cellular variant of CMN (Johsi et al, 1986; Gormley et al, 1989; Fitchey et al, 2003). The risk for recurrence is thought to be less in children younger than 3 months at diagnosis, but metastases have been reported in a few infants (Heidelberger et al, 1993). Neither chemotherapy nor radiation therapy is routinely recommended (Howell et al, 1982), but adjuvant treatment should be considered in patients with cellular variants that are incompletely resected (Gormley et al, 1989). There are reports demonstrating response of both inoperable and recurrent tumors to chemotherapy (Loeb et al, 2002; McMahon et al, 2003).

Solitary Multilocular Cyst and Cystic, Partially Differentiated Nephroblastoma

Solitary multilocular cyst, or multilocular cystic nephroma, is an uncommon, benign renal tumor. Fifty percent of multilocular cysts are found in young children, usually boys. The second peak incidence occurs in young adult women (Johnson et al, 1973; Banner et al, 1981). Although the majority of cases of multilocular cystic renal disease have been unilateral, there are rare reports of bilateral cases (Ferrer and McKenna, 1994). The gross appearance of the tumor is its most distinguishing feature. The cut surfaces reveal a well-encapsulated multilocular tumor composed of various-sized cysts compressing the surrounding renal parenchyma. This tumor is distinguished by the finding of only mature cell types within the septa of the cyst wall. Multilocular cystic nephroma is cured by nephrectomy, but recurrence has occurred after incomplete excision by partial nephrectomy. If partial nephrectomy is considered, frozen section is indicated to exclude cystic, partially differentiated nephroblastoma.

Another entity reported in the literature with similar features is cystic, partially differentiated nephroblastoma. The majority of these lesions occur in the first 2 years of life (Joshi and Beckwith, 1989; Blakely et al, 2003). Eble and Bonsib (1998) recommend that multilocular cystic nephroma and cystic, partially differentiated nephroblastoma be considered the same entity. They are indistinguishable radiographically. Histologic examination reveals that blastemal cells or NRs may be found in the septa of both tumors. Surgery is curative in almost all patients, with recurrence being the result of incomplete resection (Eble and Bonsib, 1998; Blakely et al, 2003). In a review of 21 children with cystic, partially differentiated nephroblastoma reported to the NWTSG, there was a 100% survival rate. Eight were treated by surgery alone (Blakely et al, 2003). Thirteen patients received postoperative chemotherapy, including two patients with stage II disease.

Metanephric Adenofibroma

Another tumor with prominent stromal features that can resemble CMN is metanephric adenofibroma (Arroyo et al, 2000). The epithelial component of this tumor can range from inactive metanephric adenoma to Wilms' tumor. Other lesions contain areas morphologically identical to papillary renal cell carcinoma. This uncommon entity is thought to be derived from ILNRs (Arroyo et al, 2000). Metanephric adenofibromas with a composite Wilms' tumor component occur at a young age (mean of 12 months), similar to other ILNR-related Wilms' tumors that develop in patients with DDS and aniridia. None of these tumors have recurred after nephrectomy, but all have been treated with Wilms' tumor chemotherapy.

Renal Cell Carcinoma

Renal cell carcinoma is the most common renal malignancy in the second decade of life. Only 5% of renal cell carcinomas occur in children (Hartman et al, 1982; Broecker, 1991). An abdominal mass is the most frequent finding, but hematuria is more common than in Wilms' tumor (Broecker, 1991). Imaging studies cannot differentiate renal cell carcinoma from other solid renal tumors. **There is a higher incidence of papillary renal cell carcinoma in children** (Carcao et al, 1998; Renshaw et al, 1999). **These tumors, typically seen in adolescents or young adults, are genetically unique in that they have chromosome translocations involving a common breakpoint in the *TFE* gene located at Xp11.2** (Bruder et al, 2004). These tumors differ from adult renal cell carcinoma in that immunoreactivity for epithelial markers is reduced or absent.

Another type of renal cell carcinoma more commonly seen in children is renal medullary carcinoma, which is found in patients with sickle cell hemoglobinopathy (Swartz et al, 2002). The median age at diagnosis is 13 years, but it can be found in much younger children. It is a highly lethal tumor.

Complete tumor resection is the most important determinant of outcome in renal cell carcinoma. Raney and associates (1983) found that all children with stage I lesions survived, and others have reported 64% to 80% survival rates for stage I and II tumors (Dehner et al, 1970; Castellanos et al, 1974; Raney et al, 1983; Aronson et al, 1996). Younger age at diagnosis is a favorable prognostic factor (Raney et al, 1983). Regional lymph node involvement does not portend the same poor prognosis as adult renal cell carcinoma (Geller and Dome, 2004). Like renal cell carcinoma in adults, these tumors are not responsive to chemotherapy or radiation therapy.

Angiomyolipoma

Renal angiomyolipoma is a hamartomatous lesion that is only rarely seen in childhood. There is a clear association with the tuberous sclerosis complex (TSC), and it is more often bilateral in these patients (Blute et al, 1988; Ewalt et al, 1998). **Renal lesions of the TSC include angiomyolipoma, simple cysts, polycystic kidney disease, and renal cell carcinoma. Angiomyolipoma develops in up to 80% of patients with the TSC** (Ewalt et al, 1998). Two genes have been identified in the TSC, on chromosome 9 (*TSC1*) and chromosome 16 (*TSC2*) (Povey et al, 1994). It has been postulated that these genes act as tumor suppressor genes and that LOH of *TSC1* or *TSC2* may explain the progressive growth pattern of renal lesions seen in these patients (Henske, 2004).

The incidence of angiomyolipoma increases with age. Ewalt and colleagues (1998) reported on 60 patients with the TSC who were monitored with periodic ultrasound. The average age at which a normal ultrasound became abnormal was 7.2 years. Angiomyolipomas were found in 45 children. Growth of the lesion was observed in 28 children, with girls being

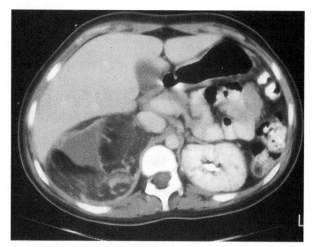

Figure 130–13. Angiomyolipoma of the right kidney in a patient with tuberous sclerosis.

Table 130–11. **Classification of Prepubertal Testicular Tumors**
Germ cell tumors
Yolk sac
Teratoma
Mixed germ cell
Seminoma
Gonadal stromal tumors
Leydig cell
Sertoli cell
Juvenile granulosa cell
Mixed
Gonadoblastoma
Tumors of supporting tissues
Fibroma
Leiomyoma
Hemangioma
Lymphomas and leukemias
Tumor-like lesions
Epidermoid cysts
Hyperplastic nodule secondary to congenital adrenal hyperplasia
Secondary tumors
Tumors of the adnexa

From Kay R: Prepubertal testicular tumor registry. J Urol 1993;150:671-674.

more likely to have an increase in size of the lesion. All patients with lesions larger than 4 cm in diameter were postpubertal. Annual ultrasound is recommended after puberty. **Children with growing lesions (Fig. 130–13) can be managed with embolization or partial nephrectomy before they become symptomatic with bleeding** (Lee et al, 1998). **The risk for serious bleeding appears to correlate with a diameter of greater than 4 cm** (Blute et al, 1988; Steiner et al, 1993; Dickenson et al, 1998). Nephron-sparing approaches are recommended in children with the TSC because of the presence of multiple, bilateral lesions and the risk for development of new lesions.

Miscellaneous Tumors

Tumors of the renal collecting system are also very uncommon in childhood. *Transitional cell carcinoma* of the renal pelvis has been reported, and these lesions are managed by nephroureterectomy (Hudson et al, 1981). Fortunately, most filling defects of the upper collecting system represent benign lesions. The most common lesion is a *fibroepithelial polyp* (Gleason and Kramer, 1994). These patients typically have symptoms secondary to obstruction. Management consists of segmental resection and reconstruction of the urinary tract.

TESTICULAR TUMORS

Testicular tumors are uncommon and account for 1% to 2% of all pediatric solid tumors. The annual incidence in boys younger than 15 years in the United States is 1 per 100,000 (Young et al, 1986). **Benign lesions represent a greater percentage of cases in children than in adults.** The American Academy of Pediatrics prepubertal testis tumor registry reported that benign tumors accounted for 38% of cases (Ross et al, 2002) (Table 130–11). Large series from single institutions report a higher percentage of benign lesions, thus suggesting that these entities were underreported to the tumor registry (Metcalfe et al, 2003; Shukla et al, 2004). **A recent multicenter report found that 74% of primary testis tumors in prepubertal children were benign** (Pohl et al, 2004). The incidence of childhood testicular tumors peaks at 2 years of age (Li and Fraumeni, 1972; Haas and Schmidt, 1995), tapers after 4 years of age, but then begins to rise again at puberty. Testis tumors are rare in black and Asiatic children.

Etiology and Genetics

A variety of chromosomal abnormalities have been identified in both adolescent and adult germ cell tumors (GCTs). Benign teratomas in children younger than 4 years usually demonstrate no abnormalities (Bussey et al, 1999). Yolk sac tumors (YSTs) in the same age group most commonly demonstrate gains of 1q and chromosome 3. The testicular GCTs of adolescents had abnormalities resembling those found in adult testicular GCT, including loss of chromosomes 11, 13, and 18 and gain of chromosomes 7 and 8 and the X chromosome (Bussey et al, 1999). The most frequent chromosomal abnormality is an isochromosome of 12p, or i(12p), which is characteristically composed of two copies of 12p. i(12p) is found in intratubular germ cell neoplasia, thus implying that this genetic event occurs early. Endodermal sinus tumors have been noted to have a deletion of the short arm of chromosome 1, specifically, 1p36, in 80% to 100% of cases (Perlman et al, 1996). DNA ploidy analysis reveals that most infantile testicular endodermal sinus tumors are diploid or tetraploid whereas adult GCTs are typically aneuploid (Silver et al, 1994).

Although the etiology of testicular cancer is unknown, a number of etiologic factors have been evaluated. The incidence of testicular cancer has been increasing in the past few decades (McKiernan et al, 1999). It is suggested that early or prolonged exposure to some carcinogenic stimuli might be implicated. **Patients with intersex disorders have an increased incidence of gonadal tumors. Such disorders include androgen insensitivity syndromes (e.g., complete testicular feminization) and gonadal dysgenesis. The risk for tumor formation in patients with gonadal dysgenesis is increased if there is a Y chromosome present, and the inci-**

dence of tumor development is approximately 10% by 20 years of age. The gonadoblastoma locus on the Y chromosome (GBY) predisposes the dysgenetic gonads to the development of in situ tumors (Page, 1987; Lau et al, 2000). It has been mapped to a critical interval on the short arm and adjacent centromeric region on the Y chromosome. GBY may have a physiologic function in normal testes, and in a dysgenetic gonad GBY might be oncogenic. **Intratubular germ cell neoplasia has been noted in 6% of children with intersex disorders, with a higher incidence after puberty** (Ramani et al, 1993).

The link between cryptorchidism and GCT of the testis is well known, but it is quite rare in childhood (Kay, 1993). Cortes and coworkers (2004) found testicular neoplasia in 7 of 182 (3.8%) children with abdominal undescended testes, abnormal external genitalia, or abnormal karyotype, but none in 1281 children without these characteristics. Neoplasia was found most often in children with bilateral cryptorchidism.

Pathology

Non–germ cell and germ cell neoplasms arise from the celomic epithelium and primordial germ cells, respectively. It is postulated that the totipotent germ cells can evolve into seminoma or embryonal carcinoma. Embryonal carcinoma is capable of differentiating into embryonic structures such as mature or immature teratomas and into extraembryonic structures such as endodermal sinus tumors and choriocarcinoma. Seminoma or dysgerminoma is a primitive germ cell neoplasm that lacks the capacity for further differentiation. These tumors are unusual in childhood except when related to gonadal dysgenesis.

YST is known by a number of other eponyms, including endodermal sinus tumor, embryonal adenocarcinoma, infantile adenocarcinoma of the testis, orchioblastoma, and Teilum's tumor. It is the most common malignant testis tumor in infants and young boys. Grossly, the tumor is firm and yellow-white on cross section, and hemorrhage is unusual. The microscopic appearance shows a mixture of epithelial and mesenchymal cells in a characteristic organoid pattern. The tumor cells produce the characteristic stages seen in the morphogenesis of extraembryonic membranes (yolk sac and allantoic mesoderm of the placenta). **The characteristic histologic finding in YSTs is Schiller-Duval bodies** (Wold et al, 1984). The latter are similar to the endodermal sinuses seen in the rat placenta. Eosinophilic cytoplasmic inclusions are common, and specialized staining techniques demonstrate the presence of α-fetoprotein (AFP).

Teratoma is a GCT composed of elements of more than one germ cell layer: endoderm, ectoderm, and mesoderm. Teratomas are classified as mature teratoma, immature teratoma, and malignant teratoma. Mature teratomas generally appear well encapsulated on gross examination. Multiple cysts are present, but consistency on cross section varies with the amount of solid tissue present between the cysts. The microscopic appearance varies with the relative amounts of tissue derived from the different germ layers and the degree of maturation (Mostofi and Price, 1973). Cartilage, bone, mucous glands, or muscle may be evident.

Epidermoid cysts occur within the testicular parenchyma and are filled with keratinous debris. Microscopically, well-differentiated stratified squamous epithelium lines the cysts. It is proposed that epidermoid cysts represent a monodermal teratoma (Ulbright, 2005). Intratubular germ cell neoplasia has not been found in the testis parenchyma adjacent to epidermoid cysts (Manivel et al, 1989).

Immature teratomas have a gross appearance similar to that of mature teratomas, but they contain various immature tissues. The latter is usually neuroepithelium; however, immature elements representative of other germ cell layers may be found (Heifetz et al, 1998). A grading system for teratomas has been developed (Gonzalez-Crussi, 1982). The incidence of foci of YST increases with the grade of the teratoma, and these patients frequently have elevated serum AFP levels preoperatively (Heifetz et al, 1998).

Leydig, Sertoli, and granulosa cells have a common embryologic origin from a mesenchymal stem cell. Pathologic diagnosis can be difficult because of incomplete differentiation (Goswitz et al, 1996). Leydig cell tumors appear well encapsulated with compression of the adjacent testicular tissue. They appear yellow to brown on cross section because of steroid production by the tumor. Their microscopic appearance is similar to that of adrenal rests. The pattern is that of closely packed eosinophilic cells with a granular cytoplasm. **The pathognomonic histologic feature of Leydig cell tumor, Reinke's crystals, is present in only about 40% of tumors** (Mostofi and Price, 1973). **Increased mitotic figures or other features suggestive of malignancy are absent in prepubertal Leydig cell tumors.** A review of 30 cases of Leydig cell tumors identified the following features associated with tumors that metastasized: increased mitotic activity, DNA aneuploidy, infiltrative margins, and angiolymphatic invasion (Cheville et al, 1998). Metastasizing tumors also had higher MIB-1 activity, a cell proliferation marker. In none of the prepubertal patients did metastatic disease develop.

Sertoli cell tumors are solid, usually without hemorrhage or necrosis. On cross section they are white to yellow and lobulated in appearance. On microscopic examination there are large polygonal cells with eosinophilic cytoplasm. Large cell Sertoli cell tumors can be confused with Leydig cell tumors because both are characterized by cells with abundant eosinophilic cytoplasm (Goswitz et al, 1996). The tumors of adrenogenital syndrome are also another confusing entity in the differential diagnosis (Srikath et al, 1992). Histology does not correlate with outcome in that Sertoli cell tumors often have high mitotic rates, nuclear pleomorphism, and increased cellularity.

Gonadoblastomas are small benign tumors found in patients with gonadal dysgenesis, including those who have at least a portion of the Y chromosome (Scully, 1970). They are bilateral in up to a third of cases. The tumors are composed of large germ cells similar to seminoma, sex cord derivatives resembling immature granulosa and Sertoli cells, and occasionally stromal elements.

Carcinoma In Situ

Carcinoma in situ (CIS), or intratubular germ cell neoplasia, is commonly found in adult patients with testicular cancer and is a precursor to the development of invasive GCT (Skakkebaek, 1975). CIS has been detected in adolescent cases of GCT (Jorgensen et al, 1995), but it has not been identified in children with YST of the testis. The seminiferous tubules adjacent to GCTs in prepubertal children frequently contain cells with enlarged nuclei and clear cytoplasm. However, staining for markers of CIS, placental alkaline phosphatase, and c-kit in seminiferous tubules adjacent to the GCT was negative in 28 prepubertal testes (Hawkins et al, 1997). CIS is also frequently detected in patients with androgen insensitivity disorders and dysgenetic gonads (Muller et al, 1985; Ramani et al, 1993). These differences suggest that the etiology of GCT in infants is different from that in adults.

There is an association between cryptorchidism and the development of CIS. The incidence of CIS is 1.7% in adults who have previously undergone orchidopexy (Giwercman et al, 1989). **Identification of CIS is more difficult in prepubertal patients.** Biopsies at the time of orchidopexy in prepubertal children have only rarely demonstrated CIS (Hadziselimovic et al, 1984). Giwercman and associates (1988) recommend repeat biopsy after puberty in prepubertal patients with CIS. An exception is a patient with androgen insensitivity or dysgenetic gonads.

Diagnosis and Staging

A painless testicular mass is the most common finding in a child with a testicular tumor. Disorders that must be excluded are epididymitis, hydrocele, hernia, and spermatic cord torsion. The latter can be manifested as a painless mass in a neonate with little scrotal wall inflammation if the event occurred prenatally. Acute abdominal pain can be the initial symptom with torsion of an abdominal undescended testicle containing a tumor. Some patients with hormonally active tumors may have small intratesticular lesions that are not palpable on physical examination.

Testicular ultrasound is routinely performed for the evaluation of testicular masses in children. Color Doppler ultrasound has been reported to be more effective than gray-scale ultrasound in detecting intratesticular neoplasms in the pediatric population (Luker and Siegel, 1994). **There are no sonographic features that can reliably distinguish benign and malignant tumors, but the finding of anechoic cystic lesions can suggest a benign lesion, such as a simple cyst, cystic dysplasia, teratoma, or cystic granulosa cell tumor. The ultrasound findings of epidermoid cyst are also unique** (Fig. 130–14). There is a heterogeneous intratesticular mass with concentric rings of alternating hypoechoic and hyperechoic layers that give rise to an "onion-skin" appearance. This corresponds to the multiple layers of keratin debris within the lesion. The mass is surrounded by a hypoechoic or echogenic rim and the absence of flow on color Doppler sonography (Langer et al, 1999). Ultrasound can also assess whether there is enough normal testis parenchyma remaining to warrant salvage. If a child is identified with a cystic lesion on ultrasound and the serum AFP level is normal, the surgeon can plan for a testis-sparing procedure (Rushton et al, 1990; Grunert et al, 1992; Valla, 2001; Metcalfe et al, 2003; Shukla et al, 2004). MRI may detect small functioning Leydig cell tumors not evident on ultrasound (Kaufman et al, 1990).

In addition to ultrasound, measurement of serum AFP can help identify tumors amenable to a testis-sparing procedure. AFP is an amino acid with a single polypeptide chain that is produced by the fetal yolk sac, liver, and gastrointestinal tract. YSTs invariably produce AFP, and all AFP-positive tumors are

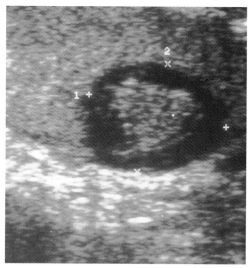

Figure 130–14. Testicular ultrasound demonstrating a cystic lesion that proved to be an epidermoid cyst of the testicle. The patient underwent a testis-sparing procedure.

considered to contain yolk sac elements (Huddart et al, 1990). Teratomas and other benign lesions are associated with normal AFP levels. AFP has a half-life of approximately 5 days, and degradation curves are followed after orchiectomy to assess for residual or recurrent disease. **It is important to note that AFP levels may be elevated in infant boys and do not always represent the presence of a malignant tumor or persistent disease after orchiectomy for YST. Normal adult reference laboratory values for AFP cannot be used in young children because AFP synthesis continues after birth** (Wu et al, 1981; Lahdenne et al, 1991; Brewer and Tank, 1993). **Normal adult levels (<10 mg/mL) are not reached until 8 months of age** (Wu et al, 1981). Human chorionic gonadotropin, β subunit (β-HCG), is a glycoprotein produced by embryonal carcinoma and mixed teratomas. The normal value of β-HCG is less than 5 IU/L. The half-life of β-HCG is approximately 24 hours. β-HCG is rarely elevated in preadolescent tumors.

The current staging system used by the Children's Oncology Group is listed in Table 130–12. Staging is based on both tumor markers and pathologic findings. AFP levels are determined at diagnosis and monitored after radical inguinal orchiectomy to determine whether an appropriate half-life decline has occurred. CT of the retroperitoneum and chest is obtained to exclude metastatic lesions. CT imaging of the retroperitoneum can identify most patients who have lymph node metastases, but there is a 15% to 20% false-negative rate (Pizzocara et al, 1987; Weiner et al, 1994).

Germ Cell Tumors

Mature Teratoma

Teratoma is the most common testis tumor in prepubertal children (Metcalfe et al, 2003; Pohl et al, 2004; Shukla et al, 2004). In a recent multicenter report, teratoma accounted for 48% of prepubertal tumors. **Prepubertal mature teratomas have a benign clinical course, in contrast to the clinical**

Table 130–12. Children's Oncology Group Staging System for Testicular Germ Cell Tumors

Stage	Extent of Disease
I	Tumor is limited to the testis and completely resected by high inguinal orchiectomy. No clinical, radiographic, or histologic evidence of disease beyond the testes. If scrotal orchiectomy has been performed, all margins are negative after resection of the proximal cord structures to the level of the internal inguinal ring. Tumor markers are negative after an appropriate half-life decline. Patients with normal or unknown tumor markers at diagnosis must have negative ipsilateral retroperitoneal node sampling to confirm stage I disease if radiographic studies demonstrate lymph nodes >2 cm
II	Microscopic residual disease is present in the scrotum or high in the spermatic cord (<5 cm from the proximal end). Tumor markers remain elevated after an appropriate half-life interval. Tumor rupture or scrotal biopsy before complete orchiectomy
III	Retroperitoneal lymph node involvement. Lymph nodes >4 cm by CT are considered metastases. Lymph nodes >2 cm and <4 cm need biopsy to document nodal metastases
IV	Distant metastatic deposits

behavior of teratomas in adults, which have the propensity to metastasize (Mostofi and Price, 1973; Grady et al, 1997; Gobel et al, 1998). As noted earlier, the presumptive diagnosis of teratoma can often be made on ultrasound examination. Other cystic lesions of the testis must be considered in the differential diagnosis. Teratoma appears more as complex hypoechoic areas surrounded by highly echogenic signals (Krone and Carroll, 1985).

Testicular teratomas are currently managed with testis-sparing procedures rather than radical orchiectomy (Marshall et al, 1983; Altadonna et al, 1988; Rushton et al, 1990; Pearse et al, 1999; Valla, 2001; Metcalfe et al, 2003; Shukla et al, 2004). There have been no recurrences reported to date. Frozen sections should be obtained intraoperatively and can reliably distinguish benign from malignant lesions (Valla, 2001; Elert et al, 2002). A detailed review of 21 cases of prepubertal teratoma at the Armed Forces Institute of Pathology did not reveal evidence of multifocal disease or CIS of the adjacent testis (Rushton et al, 1990).

Testis-sparing surgery should be performed via an inguinal incision with vascular control of the cord. An incision is made in the tunica albuginea and the mass is enucleated. Teratomas generally shell out easily because of the pseudocapsule around the lesion. The tumor is sent for frozen section and the tunica closed. The patient is not awakened until the results of frozen section are available.

Epidermoid Cyst

Epidermoid cysts account for 3% of pediatric testicular tumors (Ross et al, 1993). This monodermal teratoma follows a benign clinical course. Because of the lack of associated intratubular germ cell neoplasia in the surrounding testis, testis-sparing surgery has been advocated in both children and adults (Manivel et al, 1989; Ross et al, 1993; Pohl et al, 2004). AFP levels are normal, and the diagnosis of epidermoid cyst can be suggested by ultrasound. Frozen section diagnosis has been shown to be reliable in distinguishing this lesion (Valla, 2001; Elert et al, 2002).

Immature Teratomas

A less common tumor of the testis is immature teratoma. The most frequent extracranial site is in the ovary, with only 10% occurring in the testes. Immature teratomas have often been considered to be malignant tumors, but in children they appear to be benign unless they have foci of malignant cells. Because most patients with recurrent tumor can be salvaged with platinum-based chemotherapy, observation alone is recommended for completely resected immature teratomas (Gobel et al, 1998; Marina et al, 1999; Mann et al, 2000). Unlike at other sites, immature testicular teratomas have a low risk for relapse (Gobel et al, 1998). Incomplete resection of the tumor is a risk factors for relapse, but testis tumors are more amenable to complete resection than those at other sites. Recurrence of immature teratomas after resection is seen almost exclusively in patients with elevated AFP or foci of YST in the initial resection specimens. Recurrent tumors are typically YSTs.

Yolk Sac Tumor

YST is the second most common prepubertal testicular tumor of germ cell origin (Metcalfe et al, 2003; Shukla et al, 2004). This tumor occurs primarily in children younger than 2 years. Despite histologic similarities, the clinical behavior of YST varies considerably from the embryonal carcinoma seen in adults. The most common site of distant metastasis is the lung, and metastasis to the retroperitoneal lymph nodes occurs in 4% to 6% of children with YST (Bracken et al, 1978; Brosman, 1979). **More than 90% of prepubertal children are initially seen with stage I disease** (Haas et al, 1999).

The initial treatment for YST is radical inguinal orchiectomy. This treatment is curative in most children. Routine RPLND or adjuvant chemotherapy (or both) is not indicated (Mann et al, 1989; Haas and Schmidt, 1995; Haas et al, 1999). Staging of a patient with tumor markers and imaging studies is performed as outlined earlier.

Clinical stage I patients do not receive additional adjuvant treatment after radical orchiectomy. Chest radiography, CT, or MRI of the retroperitoneum is recommended monthly for 3 months, every 3 months, and then every 6 months. This surveillance is continued until 36 months after treatment. Tumor markers and physical examination are performed at more frequent intervals. Approximately 90% of YSTs produce positive serum levels of AFP. Scrotal orchiectomy with negative margins can be treated as stage I, but the proximal cord structures should be resected to the level of the internal ring (Rogers et al, 2004).

Patients who have previously undergone scrotal biopsy are considered stage II (Rogers et al, 2004). A completion orchiectomy with removal of all cord structures is performed. This approach has proved to be of benefit in adult patients with gross contamination during removal of GCTs (Giguere et al, 1988; Capelouto et al, 1995) Hemiscrotectomy is not required. All patients undergo abdominal CT to examine for retroperitoneal lymphadenopathy. Patients with enlarged lymph nodes should undergo lymph node sampling or biopsy. Patients who have persistent elevation of AFP and retroperitoneal adenopathy are presumed to have metastatic disease. These patients can be treated as though they have stage III disease.

Combination chemotherapy using platinum-based therapy—cisplatin, etoposide, and bleomycin (PEB)—has been used in pediatric patients with advanced GCTs (Ablin et al, 1991). Two intergroup studies for the treatment of localized and advanced GCTs in children conducted by the Children's Cancer Group and the Pediatric Oncology Group were recently published (Cushing et al, 2004; Rogers et al, 2004). The 6-year event-free survival and overall survival rate of children with stage II testicular tumors was 100%. For stage III disease, age younger than 15 years was associated with a better 6-year event-free survival rate than was age older than 15 years, 100% versus 83.3%, but both groups had a 100% overall survival rate. Patients with stage IV disease who were younger than 15 years of age also had improved 6-year event-free and overall survival rates, 94.4% and 100% versus 84% and 84%, respectively. The histology of tumors in patients younger than 15 years was pure YST in 83% of patients, whereas 80% of older patients had mixed GCT.

A number of patients experience significant ototoxicity with cisplatin-based chemotherapy regimens, and nephrotoxicity is also common (Pinkerton et al, 1990; Cushing et al, 2004). The UKCCSG used carboplatin instead of cisplatin in their second germ cell study, GCII (Mann et al, 2000). This trial was restricted to patients younger than 16 years. The 5-year event-free survival rate for testicular GCTs was 100%, with decreased toxicity when compared with the PEB regimen.

Persistent retroperitoneal masses after chemotherapy are uncommon (Uehling and Phillips, 1994; Kuo et al, 1999). However, children with clinically evident retroperitoneal disease or elevation of tumor markers after chemotherapy undergo surgery at 12 weeks to establish a histologic diagnosis. Patients with persistent viable tumor are then switched to another treatment regimen. Patients in whom relapse develops after initial treatment of a stage I tumor should also undergo biopsy for histologic confirmation.

Gonadal Stromal Tumors

Gonadal sex cord stromal tumors are the most common nongerminal testicular tumors in children (Cortez and Kaplan, 1993; Goswitz et al, 1996; Valla, 2001; Pohl et al, 2004). These benign non-GCTs are more common in children than adults. They arise from a common mesenchymal stem cell that can differentiate toward Leydig cells, Sertoli cells, granulosa cells, or a combination of these cells. An interesting feature of these tumors is their ability to secrete hormones.

Leydig Cell Tumor

Leydig cell tumor is the most common of the sex cord tumors, with a peak incidence at the age of 4 to 5 years. Leydig cells produce testosterone, and production of the hormone by the tumor can result in precocious puberty (Urban et al, 1978). This can lead to accelerated skeletal and muscle development and penile growth that does not resolve after treatment (Mengel and Knorr, 1983). Other hormones produced by Leydig cell tumors include corticosteroids, progesterone, and estrogens.

The differential diagnosis of precocious puberty includes pituitary lesions, Leydig cell hyperplasia, large cell Sertoli cell tumors, and hyperplastic testicular nodules that develop in boys with poorly controlled congenital adrenal hyperplasia (CAH) (Wilson and Netzloff, 1983; Cunnah et al, 1989; Srikath et al, 1992; Walker et al, 1997). Pituitary lesions can be excluded by finding increased serum testosterone with prepubertal luteinizing hormone and follicle-stimulating hormone levels. Children with Leydig cell hyperplasia have normal levels of urinary 17-ketosteroids. Testicular nodules tend to occur bilaterally in CAH patients, but there have been reports of bilateral Leydig cell tumors (Bokemeyer et al, 1993). A family history of CAH is helpful in making the diagnosis. The hyperplastic nodules that develop in patients with CAH resemble Leydig cells histologically but behave biochemically like adrenal cortical cells. Urinary ketosteroids are elevated in patients with 21-hydroxylase deficiency, and serum levels of 17-hydroxyprogesterone are elevated. Regression of the hyperplastic nodules in the testis is usually seen after glucocorticoid replacement (Srikath et al, 1992; Walker et al, 1997). Persistent nodules may result from fibrosis or calcification.

Inguinal orchiectomy has been performed most often for Leydig cell tumors. Testis-sparing surgery with enucleation of the tumor has now been reported in a number of children (Konrad and Schoenle, 1999; Valla, 2001). There is a report of local recurrence developing in one patient (Wegner et al, 1997). Malignancy has not been reported in Leydig cell tumors in children (Brosman, 1979).

Sertoli Cell Tumor

Sertoli cell tumor is the next most common gonadal stromal tumor in children (Young et al, 1998). This tumor develops at an earlier age than Leydig cell tumors, with the usual manifestation being a painless testicular mass. These tumors are not as metabolically active as Leydig cell tumors, but gynecomastia has been reported (Gabrilove et al, 1980). There are limited series of patients with Sertoli cells tumors occurring in children (Gabrilove et al, 1980; Goswitz et al, 1996; Thomas et al, 2001). Most recommend observation in infants because metastases are rare (Kolon and Hochman, 1997). The vast majority of patients have been managed with orchiectomy, but testis-sparing procedures have been performed in prepubertal children (Sugita et al, 1999; Nonomura et al, 2001; Valla, 2001). Examination of the retroperitoneum is warranted to exclude retroperitoneal spread (Rosvoll and Woodard, 1968). Large cell Sertoli cell tumors have been noted with increased frequency in patients with Peutz-Jeghers syndrome and the Carney complex (Chang et al, 1998).

Gonadoblastoma

Gonadoblastomas are the most common tumors found in association with intersex disorders. They occur in dysgenetic gonads and are associated with the presence of a Y chromosome in the karyotype (Manuel et al, 1976). **Children with mixed gonadal dysgenesis have a 25% risk for tumor formation** (Schellas, 1974), **and the incidence increases with age** (Manuel et al, 1976). **The germ cell component of gonadoblastoma is prone to malignant degeneration into seminoma and nonseminomatous tumors. All streak gonads in patients with gonadal dysgenesis should be removed** (Aarskog, 1970). Patients with gonadal dysgenesis who are raised as females should have the gonads removed at diagnosis (Olsen et al, 1988; Gourlay et al, 1994). Early gonadectomy is advocated because tumors have been reported in children younger than 5 years (Olsen et al, 1988; Gourlay et al, 1994).

In mixed gonadal dysgenesis patients reared as males, all streak gonads and undescended testes should be removed. Scrotal testes can be preserved because they are less prone to tumor development. It has been suggested that gonadal biopsy and histologic examination for CIS in children with gonadal dysgenesis can identify those at risk for the development of malignant GCTs (Muller et al, 1985). However, recognition of CIS in prepubertal gonadal biopsies can be difficult, and a negative biopsy does not preclude the later development of a GCT.

KEY POINTS: TESTICULAR TUMORS

- The majority of prepubertal testis tumors are benign.

- YST is the second most common testicular tumor in children. More than 90% of patients have stage I disease and do not require adjuvant chemotherapy. Monitoring serum AFP levels can detect tumor relapse.

- Gonadoblastomas are the most common tumors found in association with intersex disorders. They occur in dysgenetic gonads and are associated with the presence of a Y chromosome in the karyotype.

- Prepubertal patients with testis teratoma can be managed with a testis-sparing approach. Recognition of these tumors is feasible with testicular ultrasound.

Other Lesions

Leukemia and lymphoma are the most common malignancies that spread to the testis in children. Children with acute lymphoblastic leukemia who have bulky disease at diagnosis have been reported to have up to a 20% incidence of testicular relapse (Askin et al, 1981). A recent report found no relapses after systemic chemotherapy and a 4% relapse rate after total-body irradiation with a testicular boost (Quaranta et al, 2004). Routine testicular biopsy after treatment is no longer recommended (Trigg et al, 2000). Positive testis biopsies early in remission identify patients at a slightly higher risk for adverse events, but they do not have an impact on survival. Follicular lymphoma may occur as a primary tumor of the testis (Finn et al, 1999). The prognosis is favorable if the tumor is localized. Testicular involvement occurs in 4% of boys with Burkitt's lymphoma and may be the initial clinical finding (Lamm and Kaplan, 1974).

Testicular cystic dysplasia is a rare benign lesion in boys that has been reported with increasing frequency (Noh et al, 1999; Toffolutti et al, 1999). It is distinguished by the presence of multiple small irregular cysts localized in the rete testis. Renal agenesis or multicystic renal dysplasia has been noted in more than half the reported cases. A proposed etiology is a defective connection between the efferent ductules originating from the metanephros and the rete testis tubules originating from the gonad. Management options include testis-sparing surgery and nonoperative treatment (Noh et al, 1999; Eberli et al, 2002). If the latter approach is used, follow-up with serial testicular ultrasound is advised.

Testicular microlithiasis has been reported in association with testicular tumors but is present in more than 5% of healthy young men. It has been noted less often in children, and recommendations have been made for noninvasive ultrasound follow-up until adult age (Furness et al, 1998; Dell'Acqua et al, 1999; Leenen and Riebel, 2002). Patients with an increased risk for cancer are infertile men with atrophic testes and microlithiasis and patients with known testis cancer and microlithiasis in the contralateral testis (Holm et al, 2003; Hoei-Hansen et al, 2005). Routine screening ultrasound studies are not warranted for asymptomatic patients without known risk factors for testicular cancer (Rashid et al, 2004). Rashid and colleagues recommend monthly testicular self-examination and annual examination by a physician for all other patients.

SUGGESTED READINGS

Adkins ES, Sawan R, Gerbing RB, et al: Efficacy of complete resection for high-risk neuroblastoma: A Children's Oncology Group Study. J Pediatr Surg 2004;39:931-936.

Arndt CAS, Donaldson SS, Anderson JR, et al: What constitutes optimal therapy for patients with rhabdomyosarcoma of the female genital tract? Cancer 2001;91:2454-2468.

Arndt C, Rodeberg D, Breitfeld PP, et al: Does bladder preservation (as a surgical principle) lead to retaining bladder function in bladder/prostate rhabdomyosarcoma? Results from the Intergroup Rhabdomyosarcoma Study Group IV. J Urol 2004;171:2396-2403.

Beckwith JB: Nephrogenic rests and the pathogenesis of Wilms' tumor: Developmental and clinical considerations. Am J Med Genet 1998;79:268-273.

Crist WM, Anderson JR, Meza JL, et al: Intergroup rhabdomyosarcoma study–IV: Results for patients with nonmetastatic disease. J Clin Oncol 2001;19:3091-3102.

D'Angio GJ, Breslow N, Beckwith JB, et al: Treatment of Wilms' tumor: Results of the Third National Wilms' Tumor Study. Cancer 1989;64:349-360.

deKraker J, Graf N, van Tinteren H, et al: Reduction of postoperative chemotherapy in children with stage I intermediate-risk and anaplastic Wilms' tumour (SIOP 93-01 trial): A randomised controlled trial. Lancet 2004;364:1229-1235.

Green DM, Breslow NE, Beckwith JB, et al: Treatment with nephrectomy only for small, stage I/favorable histology Wilms' tumor: A report from the National Wilms' Tumor Study Group. J Clin Oncol 2001;19:3719-3724.

Hays DM, Lawrence W, Crist W, et al: Partial cystectomy in the management of rhabdomyosarcoma of the bladder: A report from the Intergroup Rhabdomyosarcoma Study (IRS). J Pediatr Surg 1990;25:719-723.

Mann JR, Raafat K, Robinson J, et al: The United Kingdom Children's Cancer Study Group's second germ cell study: Carboplatin, etoposide, and bleomycin are effective treatment for children with malignant extracranial germ cell tumors, with acceptable toxicity. J Clin Oncol 2000;18:3809-3818.

Marina NM, Cushing B, Giller R, et al: Complete surgical excision is effective treatment for children with immature teratomas with or without malignant elements: A Pediatric Oncology Group/Children's Cancer Group Intergroup Study. Am J Surg Pathol 1999;22:1115-1124.

Nickerson HJ, Matthay KK, Seeger RC, et al: Favorable biology and outcome of stage IV-S neuroblastoma with supportive care or minimal therapy: A Children's Cancer Group Study. J Clin Oncol 2000;18:477-486.

Perez CA, Matthay KK, Atkinson JB, et al: Biologic variables in the outcome of stages I and II neuroblastoma treated with surgery as primary therapy: A Children's Cancer Group Study. J Clin Oncol 2000;18:18-26.

Pohl HG, Shukla AR, Metcalf PD, et al: Prepubertal testis tumors: Actual prevalence rate of histological types. J Urol 2004;172:2370-2372.

Rogers PC, Olson TA, Cullen JW, et al: Treatment of children and adolescents with stage II testicular and stages I and II ovarian malignant germ cell tumors: A Pediatric Intergroup Study–Pediatric Oncology Group 9048 and Children's Cancer Group 8891. J Clin Oncol 2004;22:3563-3569.

Rushton G, Belman AB, Sesterhenn I, et al: Testicular sparing surgery for prepubertal teratoma of the testis: A clinical and pathological study. J Urol 1990;144:726-730.

Seeger RC, Brodeur GM, Sather H, et al: Association of multiple copies of the N-myc oncogene with rapid progression of neuroblastomas. N Engl J Med 1985;313:1111-1116.

Shamberger RC, Guthrie KA, Ritchey ML, et al: Surgery-related factors and local recurrence of Wilms tumor in National Wilms' Tumor Study 4. Ann Surg 1999;229:292-297.

Tournade MF, Com-Nogoue, deKraker J, et al: Optimal duration of preoperative chemotherapy in unilateral and nonmetastatic Wilms' tumor in children over 6 months of age: Result of the 9th SIOP Wilms' tumor trial and study. J Clin Oncol 2001;19:488-500.

Valla JS: Testis sparing surgery for benign testicular tumors in children. J Urol 2001;165:2280-2283.

Wiener ES, Anderson JR, Ojimba JI, et al: Controversies in the management of paratesticular rhabdomyosarcoma: Is staging retroperitoneal lymph node dissection necessary for adolescents with resected paratesticular rhabdomyosarcoma? Semin Pediatr Surg 2001;10:146-152.

Weirich A, Leuschner I, Harms D, et al: Clinical impact of histologic subtypes in localized non-anaplastic nephroblastoma treated according to the trial and study SIOP-9/GPOH. Ann Oncol 2001;12:311-319.

131 Pediatric Endourology and Laparoscopy

STEVEN G. DOCIMO, MD • CRAIG A. PETERS, MD

PEDIATRIC ENDOUROLOGY

PEDIATRIC LAPAROSCOPY

SUMMARY

Pediatric endourology, previously considered a controversial area, is an accepted part of the pediatric urology armamentarium. Instruction in minimally invasive techniques has become a standard part of many pediatric urology training programs. This acceptance has offered pediatric patients the advantages of less invasive means by which various urologic conditions may be treated, including stones, strictures, and nonfunctioning kidneys. This chapter reviews the current applications, techniques, and controversies regarding endourologic practice in children. This topic is divided into a discussion of general endourology, including ureteroscopy and percutaneous renal surgery, and then a review of laparoscopic techniques and their pediatric applications.

PEDIATRIC ENDOUROLOGY
Ureteroscopy

Instruments

Current ureteroscopic instruments permit safe access to the ureter in children as young as 4 months. The importance of appropriate working tools is magnified in the smaller patient. Unfortunately, there is a natural tradeoff with smaller instruments in the associated reduction in working channel size that often restricts any manipulation, even when access has been successful. With an appropriate working device, such as a stone basket, there is little room left for irrigation in the working channel and visualization may become limited. These issues must be recognized before a procedure is started, and they must be factored into the clinical balance regarding choice of therapy. Common pediatric ureteroscopic instruments are shown in Table 131–1. Although a range of instruments would be ideal, this is often not practical because of the cost. This is another limitation with pediatric compared with adult endoscopy: one size is largely suitable for adults, whereas the pediatric patient may be a 5-kg infant or a 70-kg adoles-

cent. A practical compromise has been the rigid 6.9-Fr cystoureteroscope. This instrument permits safe access to the distal ureter, even in smaller children and without dilation. It has 2-Fr and 3.5-Fr working channels to permit instrumentation with irrigation, thereby making it useful for older children. It can also be used for minipercutaneous access renal procedures. The 15-cm version is probably the most versatile, whereas the longer version is a useful semirigid ureteroscope for the upper tracts in the older child.

Accessory instrumentation is similar to that used in adult ureteroscopic applications, although the need for diagnostic visualization and biopsy in children is rare. Wire sizes need to be smaller to accommodate the generally smaller ureteroscopes, and they must include 0.28-inch and 0.18-inch wires. The rigidity of these wires may not always be sufficient to permit manipulations of the ureteroscope and passage of stents. Stone baskets and grasping devices are available as small as 1.7 Fr, but they are much less sturdy and may be frustrating to use. Balloon dilation of the ureteral orifice is occasionally needed, but there are few dilation balloons that are sufficiently small for young children. Use of a smaller ureteroscope is preferable, or pre-stenting the ureter can allow for passive dilation.

Indications

The need for ureteroscopic intervention in children is less than in adults and is largely limited to stone management. There is little need for diagnostic ureteroscopy or for tumor resection. Retrograde direct-vision endopyelotomy has not been used in any significant way in children. **The choice of ureteroscopic stone removal in a child is a complex one that should balance the relative need for a single-intervention treatment (in contrast to the risk of needing multiple procedures, as with extracorporeal shock wave lithotripsy [ESWL]) with the location and size of the stone.** Stones less than 5 mm have an approximately 60% likelihood of spontaneous passage in children (Pietrow et al, 2002). A stone that would appear proportionately to require intervention may actually pass spontaneously in a child as compared with an adult. The same indications for urgent intervention are applicable to children, including infection, intractable pain or nausea, and renal impairment. The potential for an associated or causative congenital impairment to urine flow should also be considered in the choice of treatment. The anatomic conditions may affect the utility of ureteroscopy.

Table 131–1.	**Endoscopes for Pediatric Applications**			
Type	**Name**	**Size**	**Channel Diameter (Fr)**	**Length (cm)**
Flexible cystoureteroscope	ACMI CAN-1	14.6	6.4	
Flexible ureteropyeloscope	ACMI AUR-7	7.2	3.6	65
Flexible ureteropyeloscope	ACMI AUR-9	9.8	3.6	65
Flexible cystoscope	ACMI AUR-PC	8.5	2.5	20
Semirigid ureteroscope	ACMI MICRO-6	6.9	3.4/2.3	33
Semirigid ureteroscope	ACMI MR-9	9.4	5.4/2.1	33
Semirigid cystoureteroscope	ACMI MRPC	6.9	3.4/2.3	15.5
Semirigid cystoureteroscope	ACMI MR 915	9.4	5.4/2.1	15
Operative ureteroscope	ACMI MRO-6	6.9/8.3	3.4/2.3	33
Rigid ureterorenoscope	Wolf	6/7.5	4.2	43
Rigid ureterorenoscope	Wolf	7.5/9.5	4.2	42
Flexible ureterorenoscope	Wolf	7.5	3.6	70/45/20
Flexible ureterorenoscope	Wolf	9	4.5	70/45
Cystourethroscope	Wolf	11	4	—
Cystourethroscope	Wolf	7.5	—	—
Cystourethroscope	Wolf	8.5	3	—
Cystourethroscope	Wolf	6/7.5	4	14
Cystourethroscope	Wolf	4.5/6	2.4	11
Semirigid ureterorenoscope	Wolf	4.5/6	2.4	31
Cystoureteroscope integrated	Wolf	10.5	5	16
Rigid cystoscope	Storz	7	3	—
Rigid cystoscope	Storz	7.5	3.5	11
Flexible cystoureteroscope	Storz	7.5	3.6	40

Stone location is not an absolute indicator of the potential use of ureteroscopy in children. The ureteroscopic management of proximal ureteral or renal pelvic stones has been described in several series; this is possible even in small children (Wollin et al, 1999; Wu and Docimo, 2004; Tan et al, 2005). It may be necessary to pre-place an indwelling stent to facilitate access. Renal pelvic stones are much more difficult to remove ureteroscopically in children than in adults because of the progressively limited manipulation ability with smaller, flexible instruments. These are largely technical problems that will become less important with improved instruments. The holmium laser is one such advance to facilitate ureteroscopic management of upper tract stones in the small child. The lower pole stone is a well-recognized challenge to ureteroscopic management, particularly in children, in whom functional access to the lower pole may be limited owing to limited space for endoscope deflection.

Access

The means of access should be determined by the instruments available for the application and the location of the stone to be removed. Complex procedures that may require several passages of the ureteroscope and prolonged manipulation of the stone and its fragments may benefit from placement of a ureteroscopic sheath to facilitate repeated placements and removals of the ureteroscope. These must be used with care in small children, and the smallest available size is a 9-Fr sheath. Once again, pre-stenting increases the safety of sheath passage.

Stone Manipulation and Removal

An appropriate means of stone fragmentation is essential for any pediatric stone manipulation and should be integrated with the ureteroscopic instruments available. The electrohydraulic lithotriptor (EHL) is a useful, all-purpose lithotripter, although it must be used carefully to avoid injury to the ureteral wall. Some surgeons do not use the EHL because of concern about ureteral wall injury; with low power settings and careful application, this is a limited risk. **The holmium: yttrium-aluminum-garnet (YAG) laser offers the potential for retrograde upper tract stone management in younger children** (Wollin et al, 1999; Reddy 2004; Tan et al, 2005). The principal benefit with the holmium laser is that stone fragments do not need to be extracted because they are small enough to pass spontaneously. Furthermore, the laser fiber is only 200 μm in diameter, which does not restrict irrigant flow or flexibility in smaller endoscopes. An initial concern regarding release of cyanide gas during uric acid stone lithotripsy appears to have been disproven (Teichman et al, 1998).

Postprocedure Management

A temporary indwelling ureteral stent is almost always appropriate after ureteroscopic stone manipulation. The goal is to provide adequate renal drainage until ureteral edema has diminished. This may be as brief as 1 to 2 days or as long as 2 weeks, depending on the degree of stone impaction and the complexity of removal. In children, stent removal usually requires a secondary cystoscopic procedure, except for short stenting periods in which a string attached to the stent may be used for withdrawal. After removal, ultrasound is used to monitor upper tract dilation, which may occur with ureteral obstruction. The timing of follow-up should be based on the complexity of the case, but it should not be delayed longer than 6 weeks after the stent is removed. If significant dilation is present, or if the child develops symptoms of obstruction, computed tomography (CT) is used to define the functional anatomy of the ureter and to rule out residual stone. Vesicoureteral reflux is a theoretical complication of ureteral dilation and manipulation, but it has not been reported to be a significant clinical issue (Caione et al, 1990; Scarpa et al, 1995). Routine cystography is not recommended.

KEY POINTS: URETEROSCOPY

■ Current ureteroscopic instruments permit safe access to the ureter in children as young as 4 months.

■ **The choice of ureteroscopic stone removal in a child is a complex one that should balance the relative need for a single-intervention treatment (in contrast to the risk of needing multiple procedures, as with extracorporeal shock wave lithotripsy) with the location and size of the stone.**

■ Stone location is not an absolute indicator of the potential use of ureteroscopy in children. The ureteroscopic management of proximal ureteral or renal pelvic stones has been described in several series; this is possible even in small children.

■ **The holmium:yttrium-aluminum-garnet laser offers the potential for retrograde upper tract stone management in younger children.**

■ A temporary indwelling ureteral stent is almost always appropriate after ureteroscopic stone manipulation.

Table 131–2. Results of Ureteroscopy

Study	No. Patients (age range)	No. Stone Free
Caione et al, 1990	7 (3 to 8 yr)	7
Scarpa et al, 1995	7 (10 yr)	7
Shroff et al, 1995	13	10 (single procedure)
Smith et al, 1996	11	9 (single procedure)
Fraser et al, 1999	16 (18 mo to 15 yr)	14
Jayanthi et al, 1999	12	11
Wollin et al, 1999	15 (4 to 17 yr)	12 (single procedure)
Van Savage et al, 2000	17 (6 mo to 17 yr)	17
Tan et al, 2005	21 (<14 yr)	20
Thomas et al, 2005	29 (5 mo to 12 yr)	25
Minevich et al, 2005	65 (1 to 12 yr)	64
Total	213	196 (92%)

Results

There are increasing reports of ureteroscopic stone manipulation in children (Table 131–2), and all have demonstrated good efficacy and a minimal complication rate. Stone-free rates are about 89%, although this depends on the selection of patients for ureteroscopic intervention. If distal stones alone are approached, a very high stone-free rate may be expected, whereas proximal and renal stones are more challenging to treat.

Percutaneous Nephrolithotomy

Instruments

A large initial investment in equipment is required for percutaneous renal procedures in children. The proper tools must be available, and assistants in the room must be familiar with both the equipment and the techniques for a successful procedure.

The technology for pediatric-specific applications of percutaneous nephroscopy has improved dramatically. Modern sheaths and endoscopes allow adequate access through small tracts, minimizing trauma to the infant kidney. The equipment for obtaining initial percutaneous access will not be discussed here. Many pediatric practitioners have their radiology colleagues obtain initial access to the kidney before the day of the procedure. There is evidence that this decreases blood loss, and it clearly decreases operating time. Access to the smaller pediatric kidney is facilitated by the ultrasonic and three-dimensional fluoroscopic equipment that is not usually available in the operating room. Obtaining access separately does usually require an additional anesthetic, however.

Once access has been achieved, equipment can be divided into that needed for dilation and sheath placement, the endo-scopes themselves, and equipment for stone manipulation, stone fragmentation or incision, and coagulation.

Traditionally, 24-Fr to 30-Fr percutaneous access sheaths and standard adult nephroscopic devices have been used in children with good success. In brief, once the nephrostomy tract has been established, a balloon or set of coaxial dilators is used to create a large enough tract into the kidney for placement of a plastic nephroscopy sheath (LeRoy et al, 1984). The nephroscopes are then introduced through this sheath and can be withdrawn and introduced without losing access to the intrarenal collecting system. The presence of a working sheath dramatically decreases working pressures within the renal pelvis, as measured manometrically, and thereby enhances the safety of percutaneous procedures (Saltzman et al, 1987). Concerns have been raised with the use of these large working sheaths in children, however, including potential damage to the small kidney from tract dilation. Smaller forms of access, including peel-away vascular access introducers, have been used as substitute nephroscopy sheaths (Helal et al, 1997; Jackman et al, 1998b). A purpose-built pediatric renal access sheath (Cook Urological, Spencer, IN) has been used for several years with excellent results even in infants (Jackman et al, 1998b) (Fig. 131–1). In combination with smaller endoscopes, the majority of pediatric percutaneous procedures can be performed through these or similar minipercutaneous sheaths.

Irrigation solutions must be warmed to prevent hypothermia, which can occur quickly in small children. Saline should be used as an irrigant in all cases to avoid dilutional hyponatremia, which can also develop quickly in the small child if extravasation should occur. With smaller endoscopes, irrigant can be introduced under pressure. If this is done, adequate low-pressure efflux via the nephroscopy sheath must be ensured or significant and life-threatening complications from extravasation may occur (Pugach et al, 1999).

Traditional nephroscopes are available in either rigid or actively deflectable configurations. Rigid nephroscopes have an offset lens system that allows the passage of probes necessary for stone fragmentation and retrieval. The tips of these endoscopes are rounded to decrease the possibility of renal injury. The telescopes come in 0- and 30-degree configurations. The outer diameter of the nephroscopes ranges in size from 17 to 24 Fr. Flexible nephroscopes were developed to

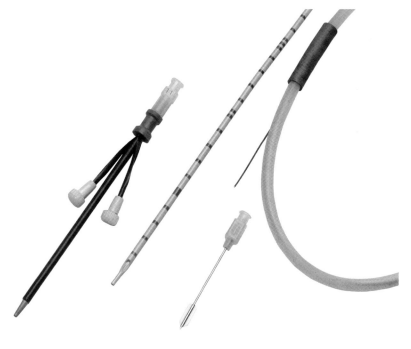

Figure 131–1. A commercially available set for minipercutaneous access to the kidney. The set includes floppy and stiff guide wires, a fascial incising needle, a dual-lumen dilating catheter, and the sheath/trocar combination. (Courtesy of Cook Urological, Inc.)

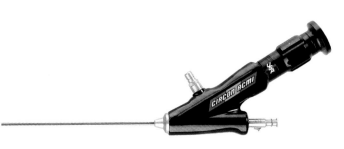

Figure 131–2. A very useful endoscope for pediatric percutaneous and transurethral procedures is this offset 7-Fr cystoscope with a 5-Fr working channel. (Courtesy of Circon, Inc.)

access all of the calyces of the intrarenal collecting system. These are 15-Fr actively deflectable endoscopes with a 6-Fr working channel. These instruments were specifically manufactured for use in the intrarenal collecting system and have a tip that has a very tight turning radius for working in a small space. In addition to the usual 15-Fr flexible nephroscope, smaller deflectable ureteroscopes can be used to obtain access through narrow infundibula. Also, if access to a calyx can be obtained by wire, a passive, flexible endoscope with a size as small as 5 Fr can be passed over the wire to visualize the difficult calyx.

Access to these adult nephroscopes is vital for an active percutaneous nephroscopy program, but the majority of pediatric procedures can now be done using one of a number of miniature endoscopes. The 7-Fr or 8-Fr offset cystoscopes with 5-Fr working ports allow almost any manipulation possible through larger telescopes (Fig. 131–2). The 7-Fr and 9-Fr flexible ureteroscopes double as nephroscopes, allowing access to all parts of the collecting system. All of these can be used through an 11-Fr access sheath with enough clearance to allow low-pressure irrigation.

The ideal instrument for intracorporeal lithotripsy at this time is the holmium laser (Reddy et al, 1999). Proper use of the laser often results in vaporization of the stones, leaving few fragments of significant size. The laser is an expensive instrument and therefore is not universally available for clinical use,

although it may be obtained on an as-needed basis from several companies.

Ultrasonic probes have a long track record for percutaneous lithotripsy, and they have the advantage that the larger probes aspirate stone fragments as they are created. Ultrasonic probes are used relatively infrequently in most series of pediatric stone procedures because of instrument size and length.

The EHL is perhaps the most universally available modality for stone fragmentation. Because EHL probes work equally well in normal saline and water, saline should always be used to decrease the risk of irrigant extravasation in the small child. EHL energy can perforate the renal pelvis or ureter very quickly, so it is imperative that it be used under direct vision at all times. Use of the EHL is by far the least expensive form of shockwave lithotripsy, and it is safe and effective under visual control (Denstedt and Clayman, 1990). The Swiss lithoclast, another energy source used mostly in adults, consists of a rigid probe that vibrates at a frequency of 12 cycles per second (Denstedt et al, 1992). This instrument acts as a percussive hammer to fragment stones. Probes as small as 3 Fr are available, and it appears that this device may fragment stones more rapidly and efficiently than ultrasonic lithotripsy.

Instruments for incision of ureteropelvic junction (UPJ) or ureteral strictures include cautery probes, laser fibers, small resectoscopes, and visual urethrotomes. A combination dilating balloon and cautery cutting wire (Accucise, Applied Medical, Laguna Hills, CA) has also been used for pediatric endopyelotomy, although its use is limited by the diameter of the uninflated device (Bolton et al, 1994).

Indications

Percutaneous access in children is used most commonly for stone removal (Docimo, 1996; Wu and Docimo, 2004). Because the ureter in the child is very distensible, allowing passage of relatively large stone fragments, ESWL is the first-line treatment for most renal calculi in children (Kroovand, 1997). There is no strict upper limit of stone burden that can be managed with ESWL in children, as there is in adults, although the larger the burden the less likely it is that success will be achieved with one procedure (Marberger and Hofbauer, 1996; Wu and Docimo, 2004). Percutaneous nephrolithotomy is most often used in the case of ESWL failure or in children whose anatomy would decrease the likelihood of ESWL success. This includes children with neurogenic bladder or bladder exstrophy who have had extensive reconstruction, including ureteral reimplantation or ureteroenterostomy (Cass et al, 1992). In these same children, percutaneous transrenal access may be the preferable route for removal of ureteral stones. Difficult access due to ureteral reimplantation, as well as the risk of causing recurrent vesicoureteral reflux after dilation of the reimplanted ureter (Garvin and Clayman, 1991), are relative contraindications to ureteroscopy, although access is relatively straightforward via a transvesical percutaneous approach (Santarosa et al, 1993).

Percutaneous access to the kidney is also used for ablation of calyceal diverticula, endopyelotomy, or ureterotomy for ureteral stricture. These techniques now can all be performed through miniaturized percutaneous access.

Access

Preoperative imaging of the urinary tract is essential to the planning and performance of endourologic procedures. Bowel preparation and/or simethicone may be used to optimize intraoperative fluoroscopic visualization of the urinary tract, especially in children with neurogenic bowel and bladder who have a tendency toward constipation. Infected urine should be sterilized before endourologic manipulation, and perioperative antibiotics should be used routinely. A ureteral access catheter may be introduced cystoscopically at the beginning of the procedure if it is believed necessary to visualize the collecting system for access. The pediatric ureter is small (Cussen, 1971), and the risk of ureteral injury or stricture, or both, is significant in this population. One should try to limit the number of catheters and wires traversing the ureter at any one time. Ureteral occlusion balloons or ureteral access catheters are not routinely required for percutaneous procedures in children. A Foley catheter is placed in the bladder. Free drainage of urinary stomas, if present, must be ensured when the patient is positioned; augmented bladders or intestinal neobladders should be catheterized with a tube large enough to allow easy passage of mucus to prevent potential rupture due to overdistention.

As mentioned earlier, initial access may be obtained preoperatively by an interventional radiologist. Alternatively, the urologist can obtain access in the operating room at the time of the procedure. Numerous techniques can be used to create a nephrostomy tract. Generally, access is achieved "blind" with the use of a C-arm fluoroscopic unit. The child is placed in the prone position on a fluoroscopic table. Appropriate padding is used for the chest, face, knees, and elbows to prevent injury during potentially prolonged procedures. The flank is prepared and draped with an occlusive drape with a water-collection system. A 22-gauge "finder" needle is introduced from a posterior position, lateral to the quadratus. When urine is aspirated, contrast material can be instilled through this needle to opacify the system. If the contrast agent extravasates, fluoroscopic visualization through the remainder of the case will be compromised; therefore, care should be used, and small amounts should be injected until intrarenal position has been confirmed. Alternatively, the contrast agent can be instilled via a previously placed ureteral catheter. Through either the finder needle or the ureteral catheter, air can be instilled instead of contrast material. The advantage of air is that it outlines first the posterior calyces, which are most advantageous for percutaneous procedures. Air should be instilled in small amounts to prevent the unlikely occurrence of air embolus.

An 18-gauge Chiba or diamond-tip needle is then introduced from a slightly more lateral position. The calyx is chosen for puncture, and the needle is lined up under the fluoroscopic image until it represents just a dot overlying the calyx. Without changing the direction of the needle, the C-arm is tilted to reveal a different view. When the needle tip reaches the calyx in this second dimension, its position is confirmed by aspiration. If urine is obtained, a 0.035- or 0.038-gauge Teflon-coated guide wire is introduced and the needle is withdrawn.

Alternatively, ultrasound guidance may be used to permit needle access to the collecting system. The appropriate calyx is selected and imaged with the use of an ultrasonic probe prepared in a sterile fashion on the operative field. The needle may be advanced under ultrasound guidance or with a biopsy guide placed on the probe to more precisely position the needle. The needle may be observed as it enters the collecting system.

At this point, the procedure is the same whether or not preoperative nephrostomy access has been obtained. Under fluoroscopic guidance, a 0.035-gauge Teflon-coated guide wire is situated in the kidney and the needle or nephrostomy tube is removed. The guide wire is manipulated down the ureter and into the bladder to obtain nephroureteral access if possible. An angle-tip catheter is sometimes required for this purpose (Kumpe, Cook Urological). For a minipercutaneous procedure, a 10-Fr dual-lumen catheter is passed over the wire after the fascia has been incised with a 4.5-mm fascial incising needle. A 0.035-gauge stiff guide wire is then placed alongside the original wire through the second lumen of the catheter, which is then removed. The Teflon-coated wire is sutured to the skin as a safety wire and put aside. Without further dilation, the 11-Fr pediatric access sheath is introduced over the guide wire and positioned appropriately in the kidney. The trocar is then removed, and access to the kidney is complete. If larger access is required, an appropriately sized fascial dilating balloon can be inserted over the stiff wire and inflated, with a standard percutaneous access sheath of 24 to 30 Fr introduced over the balloon. Visual confirmation of intrarenal position is always made with the endoscope.

KEY POINTS: PERCUTANEOUS NEPHROLITHOTOMY

- Percutaneous access in children is used most commonly for stone removal.

- Preoperative imaging of the urinary tract is essential to the planning and performance of endourologic procedures.

- As mentioned earlier, initial access may be obtained preoperatively by an interventional radiologist. Alternatively, the urologist can obtain access in the operating room at the time of the procedure.

- Irrigation solutions must be warmed to prevent hypothermia, which can occur quickly in small children. Saline should be used as an irrigant in all cases to avoid dilutional hyponatremia, which can also develop quickly in the small child if extravasation should occur.

- Access to these adult nephroscopes is vital for an active percutaneous nephroscopy program, but the majority of pediatric procedures can now be done using one of a number of miniature endoscopes.

- The ideal instrument for intracorporeal lithotripsy at this time is the holmium laser.

- As with any percutaneous nephrolithotomy, postoperative radiologic studies to ensure a stone-free status is imperative.

Stone Manipulation

Removal of calculi proceeds as indicated by the size, composition, and location of the stone. Small stones can be withdrawn with the use of baskets or three-prong graspers, or both. Tipless baskets improve access to stones in calyces and tight spaces (Honey, 1998). Lithotripsy may be performed by the techniques described earlier, depending once again on stone composition (which affects the ease of fragmentation) and available equipment. Smaller access sheaths have the disadvantage of requiring smaller stone fragments for removal. This is one of the reasons that the holmium laser, with its ability to vaporize stone, is ideal for use through the minipercutaneous sheath. Despite this, the first reported series of minipercutaneous procedures in children had a high rate of success with use of the EHL (Jackman et al, 1998b).

Postprocedure Management

At the end of the procedure, adequate drainage of the kidney and/or ureter must be achieved in most cases. After minipercutaneous nephrolithotomy, most patients are left with a 6-Fr nephroureteral stent with additional side holes created at the time of surgery to correspond to the location of the renal pelvis (Mitchell stent, Cook Urological) (Jackman et al, 1998b). This allows adequate drainage but can be capped and concealed under a bandage, thus preventing accidental dislodgment by the child. When a small stone has been removed intact, or after a brief procedure when there is no question of residual stone, one may elect to leave no drainage tube. If there

is any question, access via a nephrostomy or nephroureteral stent should be maintained until postoperative radiographs confirm the lack of obstruction and extravasation. A double-pigtail ureteral stent can be used as the primary form of postoperative drainage if percutaneous access is not needed subsequently.

After nephrolithotomy with a larger sheath, postoperative drainage may be achieved with a Foley catheter threaded over an angiographic catheter to provide both tamponade of the renal parenchyma and ureteral access (Docimo, 1996). Purpose-built nephroureteral catheters can also provide these functions.

As with any percutaneous nephrolithotomy, postoperative radiologic studies to ensure a stone-free status is imperative. A second-look procedure should be performed in any situation when there is concern about residual stone. The importance of removing all stone fragments may be greater in those children who have abnormal ureteral anatomy and are at higher risk for urinary stasis or poor passage of residual fragments.

Results

Modern series of percutaneous nephrolithotomy in children have demonstrated excellent results (Jackman et al, 1998b; Badawy et al, 1999; Jayanthi et al, 1999; Salah et al, 2004). Although any child who is going to undergo percutaneous renal procedures should have a blood sample that has been typed and screened in the blood bank, transfusion rates are quite low.

Endopyelotomy

Indications

Endopyelotomy is an option for the treatment of UPJ obstruction. The principle of the procedure borrows from the Davis intubated ureterotomy (Davis, 1943), in which the strictured ureter is incised longitudinally, stented, and allowed to regenerate over the stenting catheter. The difference in endopyelotomy is that the incision is made from inside the ureter, using endourologic access to achieve the same result.

The indications for endopyelotomy in children are still not clear (Docimo and Kavoussi, 1997). Despite an increasing number of reports, relatively few procedures have been documented in the literature, especially in young children. The success of open pyeloplasty in the infant and toddler (Hendren et al, 1980) far exceeds the expected success rate of endopyelotomy in the adult (Chow et al, 1999) or child (Schenkman and Tarry, 1998), and recommending primary endopyelotomy for this age group is premature. In addition, the adaptation of laparoscopic pyeloplasty to the young child gives a more satisfying minimally invasive alternative for managing the pediatric UPJ.

Endopyelotomy is generally acknowledged to be the procedure of choice after failed pyeloplasty in the adult, and it has a reasonable success rate (Jabbour et al, 1998). The same may be true in the pediatric population, although fewer cases have been reported (Capolicchio et al, 1997). Endopyelotomy should be attempted only when a lumen is recognizable and can be cannulated. Considering the difficulty and morbidity of reoperative pyeloplasty, an attempt at endopyelotomy in most cases is reasonable, although laparoscopic pyeloplasty may also be a useful option.

Although they are not specific contraindications to endopyelotomy, the presence of a large collecting system or poor renal function in the ipsilateral kidney, or both, portends a poorer likelihood of success (Danuser et al, 1998). It is controversial whether high insertion of the UPJ into the pelvis or anomalous crossing renal vessels (or both) is associated with failure (Tawfiek et al, 1998), but evidence suggests that these conditions should not necessarily preclude endopyelotomy (Chow et al, 1999; Nakada et al, 1998).

Access

Access for antegrade endopyelotomy is achieved essentially as described for percutaneous nephrolithotomy. The anatomy of the kidney must be carefully considered, with a posterolateral approach through a middle calyx usually the most effective choice (Bernardo and Smith, 2000). This maximizes the visibility of the UPJ and avoids the potential respiratory complications associated with upper pole access. Endopyelotomy may be effectively performed through a minipercutaneous access, using the holmium laser fiber or a small electrocautery probe to incise the strictured area. As mentioned earlier, access through the UPJ and into the bladder must be obtained before any attempt at incision is made.

Ureteroscopic endopyelotomy has been used with reasonable success in adults and older children (Tawfiek et al, 1998), but its use in younger children is limited by their small ureteral diameter. Very few cases of retrograde endopyelotomy have been reported in children (Gerber and Kim, 2000), so a recommendation cannot be made as to its use. Endopyelotomy by means of a balloon with an incorporated cutting wire has also been reported in children, but the large size of the catheter and the risk of vascular complications (Schwartz and Stoller, 1999) have dampened enthusiasm for this modality among pediatric urologists. For these reasons, only antegrade endopyelotomy is discussed here.

Incision

The incision of the UPJ must be through the full thickness of the ureteral wall to allow the strictured area to expand and reform around the indwelling ureteral stent. Consequently, renal parenchyma, surrounding structures, and large blood vessels may be encountered. To avoid these structures, a posterolateral incision usually is made in the UPJ. Endoluminal ultrasound has been used to identify vascular structures and modify the angle of incision accordingly, but this modality is not universally available (Tawfiek et al, 1998). The incision can be made with a hook blade, a straight cold knife, nephroscopic scissors, an electrocautery electrode, or a laser fiber (Clayman et al, 1990; Bernardo and Smith, 2000). Incision is made until the outside of the ureter can be seen and the ureteral lumen can be entered with the endoscope (Bernardo and Smith, 2000). Some recommend balloon calibration of the UPJ to ensure complete incision (Kavoussi et al, 1991).

After the incision is made, an appropriate stent is positioned across the UPJ. In adults, an endopyelotomy stent that is 14 Fr in its upper portion and 8.2 Fr in its lower portion is used (Bernardo and Smith, 2000), but this is clearly too large for pediatric use. A new pediatric endopyelotomy stent is now available but has had limited reports of use (Cook Urologi-

cal). There is evidence that the size of the stenting catheter may not correlate with success of the procedure (Moon et al, 1995; Anidjar et al, 1997), and in children a size appropriate to age may be used. The stent is conventionally left in situ for 6 weeks, although this might not be necessary, because 2- and 4-week periods have been reported with similar success rates (Kumar et al, 1999).

Postprocedure Management

If percutaneous endopyelotomy is performed, a nephroureteral stent is usually left in place to allow access to the kidney if needed. The stent can be capped and kept under a dressing once it has been demonstrated on a nephrostogram that there is no extravasation (Bernardo and Smith, 2000). It is easily removed after the requisite stenting period, and follow-up studies are obtained at 4 to 6 weeks to demonstrate patency. There is concern for late recurrence of obstruction, especially in the small child, so long-term follow-up with appropriate imaging studies is warranted (Capolicchio et al, 1997).

Results

As mentioned previously, the success rate for endopyelotomy in children is difficult to estimate because of the small numbers reported, but it seems to be approximately 85% at best (Motola et al, 1993; Tan et al, 1993; Bolton et al, 1994; Faerber et al, 1995; Capolicchio et al, 1997; Figenshau and Clayman, 1998; Schenkman and Tarry 1998; Gerber et al, 2000). The potential for serious complications exists, but they have been reported only rarely. One case of complete ureteral necrosis in an adolescent illustrates the care that must be taken in traversing the ureter, even in older children (Sutherland et al, 1992).

Percutaneous Management of Renal Calyceal Diverticula

Calyceal diverticula in children are uncommon but may manifest with infection, with pain due to stone, or, most often, incidentally on ultrasound examination for nonspecific symptoms (Kottasz and Hamvas, 1976; Siegel and McAlister, 1979). Their natural history is not well defined, but it is evident that they do persist and many increase in size. It is not determined that increasing size predicts the development of symptoms. Although the appearance on ultrasound may suggest compression of renal parenchyma, there is no evidence that this is associated with impaired renal function. The strict definition of a calyceal diverticulum includes evidence of accumulation of contrast material into the diverticulum, as seen on delayed intravenous pyelography or CT (Mosli et al, 1986). Otherwise, the diagnosis of a simple cyst is invoked. We have seen several confirmed calyceal diverticula with contrast agent accumulation that subsequently lost that property and were then considered to be simple cysts. This evolution raises the possibility that some simple cysts originated as calyceal diverticula. The clinical significance of this is unclear.

The indications for intervention in a calyceal diverticulum include infection, pain, and evidence of stone formation (Gauthier et al, 1983). Occasionally, evidence of stone formation is present as milk of calcium with layering of the echogenic debris (Yeh et al, 1992; Chen et al, 1997). Increasing stone size is a relative indication for intervention as well, although our practice is to continue to observe these stones, unless otherwise requested by parents.

Percutaneous intervention in children is based on obliteration and scarification of the epithelial lining of the diverticulum, rather than induced drainage through opening of the neck of the diverticulum, as is often performed in adults (Lang, 1991; Baldwin et al, 1998). Any procedure intending to establish free drainage requires temporary indwelling stents and runs the risk of reclosure of the neck. The impact of each of these elements in the child is greater than in the adult. We have therefore used a direct percutaneous access method to ablate the epithelial lining of the diverticulum (Shalhav et al, 1998; Monga et al, 2000).

Access is obtained percutaneously with ultrasound guidance directly into the cavity of the diverticulum, using methods similar to those for renal pelvic access. A flexible wire is coiled in the cavity, but it is unusual that a wire can be passed down the ureter. A working sheath is introduced, as with renal procedures, and the endoscope introduced. The neck of the diverticulum is sought, aided by retrograde instillation of methylene blue dye through a ureteral catheter if desired. The neck is then fulgurated with a Bugbee electrode, followed by cauterization of the epithelial lining. In larger patients, an adult resectoscope can be used to permit use of a roller-ball electrode to hasten the process. After fulguration, a Foley catheter is placed to allow collapse of the diverticulum. This is left in place for 2 to 3 days. The cavity may remain visible on ultrasound after the procedure and may shrink slowly.

Location of the diverticulum can present a technical challenge for access in that anteromedial diverticula require passage of the needle through the renal parenchyma. Laparoscopic resection of these diverticula may be a useful alternative (Gluckman et al, 1993; Ruckle and Segura, 1994; Harewood et al, 1996; Hoznek et al, 1998; Curran et al, 1999; Casale et al, 2004). There are few reports of percutaneous management of calyceal diverticula in children. Our experience with six cases suggests adequate outcome with minimal morbidity. In one case the diverticulum did not completely disappear, although its growth was halted. No significant complications were encountered. One patient required open resection owing to failure of percutaneous access and large size. Retrograde techniques have been described in adults but have not been employed in children. The comparative success rate of direct percutaneous ablation and the need for prolonged intubation and removal of stents in retrograde methods argue in favor of antegrade techniques for pediatric patients.

PEDIATRIC LAPAROSCOPY
Diagnostic Laparoscopy

Indications

Laparoscopic diagnosis has been employed in pediatric urology for 30 years, beginning with Cortesi and colleagues' report (1976) of using laparoscopic techniques to identify nonpalpable testes. Further uses in intersex conditions and hernia have been described as well.

Testis

Numerous reports have defined the anticipated outcomes and interpretation of laparoscopic findings associated with cryptorchidism (Garibyan, 1987; Castilho, 1990; Jones and Kern, 1993; Holcomb et al, 1994b; Moore et al, 1994; Tennenbaum et al, 1994; Brock et al, 1996). The true utility of diagnostic laparoscopy has not been completely determined, however, and debate continues (Ferro et al, 1996). **The primary aims of diagnostic laparoscopy are to identify the presence or absence, the location, and the anatomy of the nonpalpable testis.** Details of diagnostic laparoscopy for the nonpalpable testis are described in Chapter 127, "Abnormalities of Testis and Scrotum: Surgical Management."

Intersex

Diagnostic laparoscopy has been applied to intersex conditions (Yu et al, 1995) and has also been integrated with operative interventions (Martin et al, 1997; Lakshmanan and Peters, 2000). Diagnostic laparoscopy offers direct visualization of the internal genital structures in cases in which the anatomy may not be clear based on imaging studies. It also offers the ability to perform a diagnostic biopsy to establish a histologic diagnosis and the ability to remove aberrant gonadal or ductal structures if necessary.

The principal use of diagnostic laparoscopy for intersex is in conditions where gonadal development may be abnormal or discordant with the sex of rearing (Table 131–3). This includes various forms of gonadal dysgenesis and true hermaphroditism. The location and appearance of the gonad may help in making a diagnosis. In true hermaphroditism, the demonstration of testicular and ovarian tissue in one gonad is the diagnostic hallmark and may be established only with biopsy. In such cases, the biopsy should be longitudinal and deep enough to sample the entire gonad. In some situations, the gonad is inappropriate to the sex of rearing and should be removed (Droesch et al, 1990; Shalev et al, 1992; Gilliland et al, 1993; Long and Wingfield, 1993; McDougall et al, 1993). Similarly, gonadal removal may be needed in cases of tumor degeneration or risk of degeneration (Wilson et al, 1992). Laparoscopy may also be used when persistent müllerian

Table 131–3.	**Laparoscopic Evaluation of Intersex Conditions**	
Anatomic Findings	*Probable Diagnosis*	*Laparoscopic Role*
Palpable gonads, virilized, possible uterus	Deficiency of müllerian-inhibiting substance	Identify and excise müllerian structures
No palpable gonads, virilized	Gonadal dysgenesis, true hermaphroditism	Gonadal biopsy/ gonadectomy; define müllerian anatomy
Asymmetry/one palpable gonad, virilized	Gonadal dysgenesis (mixed)	Evaluate opposite gonad; gonadal biopsy/gonadectomy
Female	Male pseudohermaphrodite	
Testicular feminization	Gonadectomy	
5α-reductase deficiency	Orchiopexy	

ductal structures should be removed (McDougall et al, 1994; Ng and Koh, 1997; Wiener et al, 1997; Lima et al, 2004).

Occasionally the diagnosis of an unanticipated intersex case occurs intraoperatively, as in the finding of müllerian structures during herniorrhaphy in an apparent male. Laparoscopy permits immediate examination of the internal pelvic structures to facilitate clinical decision-making. Similarly, in the female child with a hernia, diagnostic laparoscopy can confirm the presence of normal müllerian structures.

KEY POINTS: DIAGNOSTIC LAPAROSCOPY

- The primary aims of diagnostic laparoscopy are to identify the presence or absence, the location, and the anatomy of the nonpalpable testis.

- The principal use of diagnostic laparoscopy for intersex is in conditions where gonadal development may be abnormal or discordant with the sex of rearing.

- Laparoscopic evaluation of the contralateral inguinal ring during hernia repair has emerged as a tool to determine specifically whether contralateral inguinal exploration is needed.

Hernia

Laparoscopic evaluation of the contralateral inguinal ring during hernia repair has emerged as a tool to determine specifically whether contralateral inguinal exploration is needed (Holcomb et al, 1994a; Wolf and Hopkins, 1994; Fuenfer et al, 1996; Miltenburg et al, 1998; Van Glabeke et al, 1999). Initially this technique was performed with the use of an umbilical laparoscope, but this incurred the small risk of umbilical access. Effective contralateral evaluation is readily accomplished by passing the endoscope through the ipsilateral hernia sac after it has been mobilized from the spermatic cord. A 70- to 90-degree endoscope is ideal and provides a direct view of the contralateral internal ring (Fig. 131–3). Flexible endoscopy has been used as well (Pavlovich et al, 1998). A patent processus vaginalis is evident by a gaping passage through the ring. It is usually readily seen, although there are ambiguous cases in which it may be necessary to pull on the contralateral testis to open a patent processus. Scrotal insufflation is an obvious but not universal indicator of a patent processus, as is inguinal crepitus.

Our technique is to isolate the ipsilateral hernia sac, pass the insufflating catheter (8 or 10 Fr) into the peritoneum, and instill carbon dioxide (CO_2) to a pressure of 8 to 10 mm Hg. The right-angle endoscope is passed alongside the catheter or through the sac after the catheter is removed. The spermatic vessels and vas permit rapid orientation and examination of the contralateral inguinal ring, and a diagnosis may be made. If there is any uncertainty, the inguinal canal is felt for crepitus and the testis is pulled to determine whether there is a subtle contralateral patent processus vaginalis. If the contralateral processus is patent, a conventional inguinal exploration is performed.

Published reports of diagnostic inguinal laparoscopy demonstrate the utility of laparoscopy in specifically identifying those patients in whom a contralateral inguinal exploration is needed (Kaufman et al, 1996). Although it is uncertain how many of these children would have developed a clinical hernia at some point in the future, it is clear that fewer unnecessary inguinal explorations will be performed with the use of this technique (Rowe et al, 1969). Concurrently, the number of delayed contralateral hernias requiring a subsequent operation will be reduced. Our experience has demonstrated an age-specific incidence of contralateral patent processus vaginalis that is contrary to what might be expected. The incidence of a patent processus in children younger than 2 years of age is less than in children older than 2 years until they reach 4 years. We have also observed 7 of 213 children (3.3%) in whom the processus was unambiguously closed yet developed a clinical hernia a mean of 35 months after surgery. This perhaps suggests that "congenital hernias" in children may actually be "acquired." It is also useful to note that we have

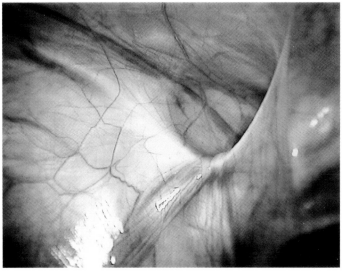

Figure 131–3. Patent processus vaginalis on the left seen laparoscopically during performance of a contralateral hernia repair. There was no clinical evidence of this patent processus.

identified a widely patent processus vaginalis in older patients (4 [15%] of 26 patients older than 8 years of age) with no clinical signs of a hernia, including a patient as old as 10 years. It is important to understand that laparoscopic exploration for contralateral patent processus is controversial because the number of children who will present with subsequent clinical hernia is much lower than the number with an identifiable patent processus. Parental preference may be an equally important indicator of its utility (Holcomb et al, 2004).

Operative Laparoscopy

Indications

The era of therapeutic laparoscopy in pediatric urology began with the introduction of spermatic vessel clipping for a first-stage Fowler-Stephens operation (Bloom, 1991) and then laparoscopic orchiopexy (Jordan and Winslow, 1994). Today, laparoscopic orchiopexy is a well-accepted part of the urologist's repertoire for dealing with the high testis (Jordan, 1997; Lindgren et al, 1998; Baker et al, 2001; Samadi et al, 2003). **Experience with laparoscopic techniques in adults led to the now common pediatric laparoscopic nephrectomy** (Clayman et al, 1991), **as well as laparoscopic partial nephrectomy** (Jordan and Winslow, 1993a). Attempts to manage vesicoureteral reflux in a minimally invasive fashion have included laparoscopic extravesical ureteral reimplantation (Atala et al, 1993; Lakshmanan and Fung, 2000) as well as the development and refinement of endoscopic techniques of ureteral manipulation within the bladder (Cartwright et al, 1996; Okamura et al, 1996; Lakshmanan et al, 1999; Gill et al, 2001; Peters and Wu, 2005; Yeung et al, 2005).

The reconstructive era of pediatric laparoscopic surgery is well underway. Upper tract operations, such as pyeloplasty, can be performed in this way but are technically demanding (Peters et al, 1995; Tan, 1999). Although the first laparoscopic bladder augmentation was performed in 1994 (Docimo et al, 1995), the technique is difficult enough that only a few have been performed since, and most of these were done in adults (Gill et al, 2000). Autoaugmentation of the bladder has also been applied laparoscopically (McDougall et al, 1995a; Braren and Bishop, 1998). Currently, the most feasible of these techniques is the laparoscopic-assisted bladder reconstruction, which combines the morbidity and cosmetic advantages of laparoscopy with the ability to perform complex tissue assembly through a low abdominal incision (Jordan and Winslow, 1993b; Cadeddu and Docimo, 1999; Hedican et al, 1999; Chung et al, 2004).

The field of therapeutic pediatric urologic laparoscopy will continue to expand as technology and experience improve. It is difficult to predict what the indications for minimally invasive abdominal surgery will be in the decades to come, but clearly this is a field that is changing almost daily. The introduction of a clinically useful robotic assistance system, the DaVinci Surgical System (Intuitive Surgical, Sunnyvale, CA), has presented the potential for wider application of complex reconstructive laparoscopy in pediatric urology (Peters 2003b, 2004b).

Instruments

Instruments used for therapeutic laparoscopy can be divided into those used for access and those that provide an extension of the surgeon's hands into the peritoneal cavity. Access can be obtained with the use of a Veress needle (Veress, 1938), followed by blind or visually aided trocar introduction; or, alternatively, an open access technique can be used. These techniques include the box stitch technique (Poppas et al, 1999), the Hasson cannula (Hasson, 1998), and the use of a radially dilating trocar system (Schulam et al, 1999; Cuellar et al, 2000). Each of these has its proponents and advantages and disadvantages. A more recently described technique, entering the peritoneum directly beneath the umbilicus at its attachment, has achieved popularity due to ease and safety (Franc-Guimond et al, 2003). This can be combined with a radially dilating trocar to achieve the benefits of both techniques (Docimo, 2004). **It is important that the surgeon be comfortable with at least one technique of access and preferably have some experience with both open and needle insufflation techniques.** Another option for diagnostic laparoscopy is the introduction of a 2-mm laparoscope through the Veress needle cannula (Molloy, 1995), obviating the need for secondary trocar placement.

Hand instruments for laparoscopy come in three basic sizes. The original laparoscopic hand instruments were almost all 10 mm in diameter. Five-millimeter hand instruments have been the standard for several years. Microlaparoscopic instruments may be either 2 or 3 mm in diameter, the former more conducive to needle trocar access, the latter somewhat sturdier and more varied in application.

Laparoscopic hand instruments mirror those used for open surgery. The difference, of course, is that the surgeon's actions need to be transmitted from outside of the body to the peritoneal cavity. For this reason, most hand instruments consist of a movable handle or grip, a long shaft, and a working end consisting of movable tips. These tips take the shape of scissors, graspers, or forceps of various types; right-angled instruments; or clamps. Most of the common hand instruments for open surgery have been duplicated in laparoscopic form. Many of these instruments can be connected to an electrocautery source for hemostatic maneuvers during laparoscopic surgery. For pediatric applications, shorter shaft lengths can be obtained for many of these instruments.

Suturing can be difficult laparoscopically. Laparoscopic needle drivers exist in 10-, 5-, and 3-mm sizes. Because of the constrained angle of approach, orienting the needle on the driver and the needle in relation to the tissue can be difficult. Automatic suturing devices have been developed that can increase speed and also make knot tying much easier (Adams et al, 1995). However, automatic suturing instruments remain rather large for pediatric applications. In addition, the most widely available of these incorporates a double-ended needle with a suture coming off at a right angle in the center of the shaft. This of necessity creates a large suture track, which is unacceptable for many pediatric reconstructive applications. For this reason, laparoscopic pyeloplasty continues to require hand suturing in pediatric patients, even though they are often accomplished with automatic suture devices in the adult (Chen et al, 1996). Self-righting needle drivers incorporate a curved face, forcing the similarly curved needle into an upright position as the jaws are closed. This removes at least one variable from the challenge of laparoscopic free-hand suturing, but these devices are not used widely.

Laparoscopic retraction can be difficult and has led to the creation of a number of devices, including fan retractors, instruments that form loops or rings after they are inserted into the body, and others. For most pediatric applications, patient positioning is adequate to allow exposure of the area of interest, but with more complex operations, laparoscopic retraction is a necessary part of the pediatric urologist's armamentarium.

More complex operations often require irrigation and/or suction to improve visualization. Suction devices come in 3-, 5- and 10-mm varieties. There are numerous interchangeable tips that allow effective suction under various circumstances. These irrigation-aspiration devices can be connected to reusable suction bottles and pressurized fluid bags, or disposable devices consisting of a battery powered pump directly plugged into a fluid bag can be used. These have the advantage of rapid setup should the unexpected need for suction and irrigation arise.

Hemostasis can be achieved laparoscopically with the use of electrocautery. Cautery can be delivered via hand instruments, such as scissors, or cautery wands. Both monopolar and bipolar cautery units are available with certain laparoscopic hand tools. Some surgeons prefer bipolar cautery because of theoretically lower risk of injury due to accidental touching of vital structures during cauterization. There are also suction devices that have a cautery tip to allow suction and hemostasis to be performed simultaneously. Larger vessels can be controlled using laparoscopic vascular clips (Nelson et al, 1992; Papaioannou et al, 1996). These can be introduced with reusable clip appliers or, more commonly, disposable clip appliers. They come in 5- and 10-mm sizes and should be considered standard equipment if procedures such as nephrectomy or two-stage orchiopexy are likely to be performed. Both titanium and plastic clips are available, including those with a locking mechanism (Hemaclips, Weck). Division of very large vessels, such as a renal vein in an adolescent or adult, might require a vascular gastrointestinal anastomosis stapler (Krasna and Nazem, 1991). These generally require a 12-mm laparoscopic port for introduction. Other methods of hemostasis have been applied, including the laser, the harmonic scalpel, and argon beam coagulation, all of which have been shown to be effective (Jackman et al, 1998a; Spivak et al, 1998; Gill and MacFadyen, 1999; Platt and Heniford, 2000). Newer hand-controlled harmonic forceps can be invaluable, especially in procedures requiring extensive dissection or division of small vessels or renal parenchyma. Specific needs will be dictated by the procedures being performed.

The myriad disposable laparoscopic products for specific indications cannot be covered here. Suffice it to say that the laparoscopic practitioner should remain aware of available devices but at the same time be aware of their potentially high cost.

Anesthetic Issues in Pediatric Laparoscopy

In general, laparoscopy is well tolerated by children, although concerns were raised initially. The principal issues in laparoscopy are the physiologic effects resulting from the creation of a surgical working space using a pneumoperitoneum or retroperitoneum. **Intra-abdominal pressure is increased significantly; and with the common use of CO_2 as the insufflating agent there is absorption of CO_2 across the peritoneum.** There are also risks of CO_2 embolus. In children, as compared with adults, the key difference from an anesthetic standpoint is the decreased pulmonary reserve in children, which results from a relatively low functional reserve capacity and lower oxygen reserve. **Their ability to withstand decreases in oxygen saturation is less than that of an adult, reducing the safety margin when any procedure reduces lung volume. Increased intra-abdominal pressure significantly reduces functional reserve capacity** (Tobias, 1998). It also increases airway pressures, which may impair ventilation and gas exchange. As a result, children may be more susceptible to oxygen desaturation during a laparoscopic procedure, and this susceptibility may be greater in younger children. Alterations in the mechanical characteristics of ventilation are induced during laparoscopy, reducing airway compliance and increasing resistance (Bergesio et al, 1999). It is important to recognize these issues and adjust intra-abdominal pressures accordingly. It is helpful that less pressure is required to produce abdominal distention in children because of their greater abdominal compliance.

Cardiovascular function is altered by pneumoperitoneum in children as a result of increased preload, afterload, and filling volumes. Systolic function is not markedly altered. The clinical effect in a child with normal cardiac function is insignificant, but it must be anticipated in the child with cardiac insufficiency (Gentili et al, 2000).

Hypercarbia caused by CO_2 absorption and decreased ventilatory clearance is well recognized to occur in laparoscopy and is well tolerated in healthy children. The principal effect of hypercarbia is on the myocardium, including inotropic, chronotropic, and arrhythmogenic effects. There is also catecholamine release, which may accentuate these effects and produce vasoconstriction. From a clinical standpoint, these effects are rarely significant in healthy children, but in the susceptible patient potential adverse effects should be anticipated and CO_2 levels adjusted. In general there is no strong indication to alter minute ventilation to control CO_2 levels as measured by the end-tidal CO_2 ($ETCO_2$), but this requires a clinical judgment by the anesthesiologist. CO_2 embolus may occur when a high volume of CO_2 enters the venous system as a result of vascular injury. Initially heralded by increasing $ETCO_2$ and decreasing oxygen saturation, cardiovascular collapse may soon follow. At that point, $ETCO_2$ falls to zero and rapid desaturation occurs. A CO_2 embolus should be suspected and acted on immediately. The classic "mill wheel" murmur gives evidence to the gas embolus that obstructs right-sided heart outflow and pulmonary circulation. Rapid placement of the patient into the right-side-up position with attempted aspiration of the embolus through a central venous line is appropriate.

Several studies have examined the use of laparoscopy and its impact on anesthetic management in children (Halachmi et al, 2003; Means et al, 2004). In studies of brief laparoscopic procedures used for diagnosis of contralateral hernia, 55 patients were monitored and were without anesthetic complications when endotracheal intubation was used (Tobias et al, 1995). A further study demonstrated that during this brief diagnostic laparoscopy an endotracheal tube was not necessary (Tobias et al, 1994, 1996). Our experience has included only one child who experienced oxygenation problems during laparoscopic orchiopexy. This child had multiple congenital anomalies and a small, kyphotic chest. He desaturated when the intra-abdominal pressure exceeded 10 mm Hg but then did well at 8 mm Hg, and the procedure was completed. **Neonates may be more prone to such desaturation because they have even less functional pulmonary reserve and higher oxygen consumption,** although experimental studies have not shown this to be a major risk (Rubin et al, 1996).

Temperature regulation is another concern in pediatric anesthesia, because children have a greater ratio of surface area to body mass and therefore lose heat more rapidly (Kaynan and Winfield, 2002). Attempts were initially made to warm the insufflating gas to reduce this risk. It has been our experience that heat loss is rare in children undergoing laparoscopic urologic procedures, and indeed it appears as if there are elevations in temperature during renal surgery in infants. The cause of this phenomenon is unknown but has been speculated to be activation of perirenal brown fat with release of catecholamines. We have not seen any adverse effects. For most laparoscopic cases, we do not routinely take extra measures to control temperature.

As with adults, increased intra-abdominal pressure in children reduces urine output, although this effect is transient and has not been observed to cause any permanent renal injury (Chang et al, 1994; Chiu et al, 1995, 1996; Razvi et al, 1996). As more procedures are performed in compromised patients, concern has arisen regarding the effect of pneumoperitoneum-induced oliguria on previously compromised renal function. Even in children with chronic renal insufficiency, significant alterations in function have not been observed. In an experimental study using a model of reduced renal function, pneumoperitoneum did not cause further permanent renal dysfunction (Cisek et al, 1998). That study also examined the physiologic basis for pneumoperitoneum-induced oliguria and suggested that the mechanisms for reduced renal blood flow may not be simple increases in pressure, as previously suggested (Kirsch et al, 1994; Razvi et al, 1996). Distinctly different patterns were seen between the renal circulation and the mesenteric or carotid circulation in response to changes in intra-abdominal pressure. Renal perfusion returned much more slowly than in the other vascular beds, suggesting regulation by factors other than pressure alone. Whether these are neural or humoral remains to be determined. It may be possible to pharmacologically control this response to provide the best possible protection to the kidney during laparoscopic surgery. There is no human evidence of renal injury related to pneumoperitoneum, even for prolonged procedures (Micali et al, 1999).

Complications of Pediatric Laparoscopy

The complications associated with pediatric laparoscopy are no different from those in adults, and similar precautions must be exercised. Several aspects of pediatric laparoscopy, however, increase the risk of certain problems that must be anticipated.

Complications Related to Access. Inadvertent injury to intra-abdominal structures may occur because of the different physical properties of the child's abdomen. The resistance to penetration is much less, and reduced force is needed for access, yet the peritoneum is more likely to separate from the abdominal wall. This may increase the risk of preperi-

---

KEY POINTS: PHYSIOLOGY OF LAPAROSCOPY

- Intra-abdominal pressure is increased significantly, and with the common use of CO_2 as the insufflating agent, there is absorption of CO_2 across the peritoneum.

- A child's ability to withstand decreases in oxygen saturation is less than that of an adult, reducing the safety margin when any procedure reduces lung volume.

- **Increased intra-abdominal pressure significantly reduces functional reserve capacity.**

- Hypercarbia caused by CO_2 absorption and decreased ventilatory clearance is well recognized to occur in laparoscopy and is well tolerated in healthy children.

- **Neonates may be more prone to such desaturation because they have even less functional pulmonary reserve and higher oxygen consumption.**

- Increased intra-abdominal pressure in children reduces urine output, although this effect is transient and has not been observed to cause any permanent renal injury.

---

toneal insufflation, and the temptation to push harder may be greater because the tip of the trocar is not yet visible in the field; puncture of abdominal viscera may be more likely. During retroperitoneal procedures, the peritoneum is more easily violated, because of its more posterior reflection and its lesser strength. This can occur even with excessive inflation of a balloon dissector. The relative size of any cannula is greater in a child than in an adult. Where a 5-mm port may not require closure in an adult, it does in a child; otherwise, postoperative hernia may occur (Bloom and Ehrlich, 1993; Waldhaussen, 1996). The lower limit of size requiring suture closure is not firmly established, but a 2-mm port does not require closure, whereas we would suture a 3.5-mm port site.

Open access technique is not without hazard, including inadvertent injury to a loop of bowel trapped during the opening (Sadeghi-Nejad et al, 1994). As with adult laparoscopy, there is greater risk with the use of Veress needle access (Peters, 1996), although it should be recognized that this is usually the result of injury from the subsequent blind placement of the first working cannula, rather than the Veress needle itself (Montero et al, 2001). With 2-mm instrumentation, diagnostic laparoscopy may be performed with the combination of a Veress needle and a 2-mm cannula. This requires only one puncture of the needle, whose sheath acts as the cannula for the telescope and insufflation. The radially dilating sheath system also obviates the need for a secondary blind trocar passage as the cannula is placed through the sheath inserted with the Veress needle. The abrupt stepoff of the sheath around the needle can cause hang-up on the fascia and cause the operator to push harder. Care should be taken to avoid excessive pressures that would permit abrupt past-pointing of the needle. When pushed against a nonyielding object such as the spine, the safety feature of the retractable needle is lost. We continue to use the saline test whereby a syringe with saline is attached to the needle and aspirated to assess for entry into a viscus or vessel; then a small amount of saline is instilled and the syringe is re-aspirated. The syringe is then removed and the abdominal wall lifted. If the needle is intraperitoneal, the drop of saline should fall quickly down the hub of the needle.

KEY POINTS: COMPLICATIONS

- Inadvertent injury to intra-abdominal structures may occur because of the different physical properties of the child's abdomen. The resistance to penetration is much less, and reduced force is needed for access; yet the peritoneum is more likely to separate from the abdominal wall.

- The principal cause of intraoperative complications in pediatric laparoscopy is likely to be the limited working space in most surgical procedures.

- The effect of pneumoperitoneum on ventriculoperitoneal shunt function has been an issue, yet there does not seem to be a significant risk.

Operative Complications. The principal cause of intraoperative complications in pediatric laparoscopy is likely to be the limited working space in most surgical procedures. Inadvertent injury with cautery or cutting instruments is the consequence of limited space. As a result, extra care is needed when operating in confined spaces. Attention to uninsulated parts of instruments used for cautery is essential. With smaller telescopes, visualization is more easily compromised by smoke, fluid spatter, and the light absorption of blood. All instrument changes must be done with greater care, because the safe range of movement is reduced. Smaller-diameter working instruments also increase the risk for the electrical effects of capacitance coupling, in which induced currents produce thermal injury, usually at port sites (Tucker et al, 1992; Grosskinsky et al, 1993). This is increased with smaller-diameter instruments because the current density is higher and with thinner abdominal walls because they disperse current less efficiently (Voyles and Tucker, 1992; Willson et al, 1997). Careful attention to the insulation on instruments is important, as is attempting to limit electrocautery use and power.

The effect of pneumoperitoneum on ventriculoperitoneal shunt function has been an issue, yet there does not seem to be a significant risk (Docimo, 1999). One early report suggested that increased intra-abdominal pressure would produce marked increases in intracranial pressure in a noncompliant, chronically drained ventricular system (Uzzo et al, 1997). The authors recommended exteriorization of these shunts during any laparoscopic procedure. However, clinical experience has not confirmed these concerns, and numerous procedures have been performed without ill effect. With a functioning valve in the shunt, there should be no risk of increasing pressure beyond what might be seen with temporary clamping of the shunt.

As a general practice, we have anticipated major complications by being prepared for emergency open access during laparoscopic procedures, particularly those involving the kidney. This means having blood available in the bank for major renal cases and having an abdominal instrument set with vascular instruments ready in the room. From a practical standpoint, it is essential to have backup laparoscopic instruments during all procedures, as well as two laparoscopic surgical clip appliers in the operating room at all times.

Renal Surgery
Access Techniques

Renal laparoendoscopic surgery may be performed transperitoneally or retroperitoneally. Initial procedures have been carried out transperitoneally with good success, yet retroperitoneal access has become equally used (Diamond et al, 1995; Valla et al, 1996; El-Ghoneimi et al, 1998; Kobashi et al, 1998; Borer et al, 1999; Lee et al, 2005). Concerns regarding creation of intra-abdominal adhesions with transperitoneal renal surgery have been raised, but in reality there have been no reported cases of postoperative complications from adhesions. Indeed, two reports suggest a very low incidence of postlaparoscopic adhesion formation, particularly in children (Moore et al, 1995b; Pattaras et al, 2002). Nevertheless, the usual open approach to the kidney is extraperitoneal, and the intuitive response is that perhaps this would be better for laparoendoscopic procedures as well. **As experience has grown with retroperitoneal laparoscopic renal surgery in children, its advantages have become evident: (1) it is the shortest distance to the kidney; (2) there is less risk of contamination of the peritoneum from any renal pathology (urinary leak, infection, or neoplasm); and (3) there are fewer exposure problems from liver, spleen, or bowel obscuring the operative field. On the other hand, transperitoneal anatomy may be more familiar with a wider working field and an anterior approach to renal pathology is sometimes advantageous.** There has been some examination of the physiologic effects of transperitoneal versus extraperitoneal laparoscopic surgery in adults (Chiu et al, 1995) but none in children. The current approach of one of the authors for almost all renal surgery is extraperitoneal, and for the other it is nearly always transperitoneal. As robotic renal surgery has emerged, transperitoneal access has been used more readily in children, but retroperitoneal access has been shown to be feasible in larger children (Olsen and Jorgensen, 2004).

Transperitoneal Access. Initial cannula placement is by open or closed technique in the umbilicus. Use of the superior aspect of the umbilicus avoids the three infraumbilical structures (urachus and obliterated umbilical arteries). A second cannula is placed in the ipsilateral lower quadrant, at the midclavicular line halfway between the umbilicus and pubis. The third cannula is placed above the umbilical port, near the midline, avoiding the falciform ligament. If this port is placed laterally, it is often too close to the upper pole of the kidney and liver edge to be as useful as needed. Three ports are usually adequate for all renal surgery, but a fourth may be placed in the anterior axillary line at the level of the kidney to facilitate exposure or for retraction of stay stitches (Fig. 131–4).

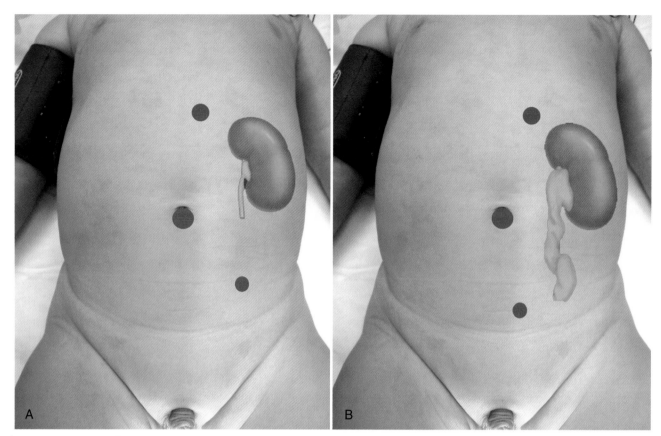

Figure 131–4. Diagram illustrating the port positions for a laparoscopic transperitoneal left renal surgery (**A**) and for nephroureterectomy (**B**). The midline position of the upper port site provides a more symmetrical approach to the kidney. The more medial position of the inferior port for the nephroureterectomy facilitates mobilization of the distal ureter.

Retroperitoneal Access—Prone. Retroperitoneal access may be gained by one of two methods, prone or flank. For the prone approach, initial access is gained with the patient in the full prone position using a subcostal incision at the edge of the paraspinous muscles that is developed with blunt dissection through the latissimus and oblique muscles (Borer and Peters, 2000; Urbanowicz et al, 2002). With a muscle-splitting technique, Gerota's fascia is eventually identified and entered. The yellow-brown perinephric fat is then evident, and a dissecting balloon is positioned into it. In children, the commercial balloons are too large; we use the finger of a surgical glove tied to a 12-Fr Mentor catheter. In an infant this is filled with 150 mL of saline; in older children up to 200 mL of saline is used. A box stitch of 3-0 absorbable suture is placed in the outer fascia to create a seal for the pneumoretroperitoneum and to ultimately close the site (Poppas et al, 1999). After a few minutes for hemostasis, the balloon is deflated, the camera port is placed into the retroperitoneum, and the suture is tightened but not tied. The retroperitoneal space is then insufflated to 15 or 20 mm Hg, and the space is inspected with the laparoscope. If the balloon has been positioned in Gerota's fascia, the kidney will be immediately visible. Blunt dissection with the camera develops the space to permit secondary port placement. Secondary ports are placed above the iliac crest just lateral to the paraspinous muscles and just medial to the peritoneal reflection, which should be specifically identified and swept medially. Dissection of the kidney may then begin (Fig. 131–5A).

Retroperitoneal Access—Lateral. In the flank approach, the patient is placed in the lateral decubitus position and flexed slightly (El-Ghoneimi et al, 1998). Retroperitoneal access is achieved through development of a small muscle-splitting incision off the tip of the 12th rib, with secondary ports placed either above the iliac crest or posteriorly and inferiorly (see Fig. 131–5B). Care must be taken to avoid injury to the peritoneal reflection, which would significantly hinder any retroperitoneal procedure because the peritoneum will be insufflated and the working space reduced. The lateral reflection of the peritoneum is the site most easily violated; this problem may be avoided by direct-vision blunt mobilization once the camera is placed within the retroperitoneal space.

Summary. Both approaches to the kidney appear to be safe and effective, and each has strengths and weaknesses (Borzi 2001; Borzi and Yeung, 2004). **The prone approach allows the kidney to fall anteriorly with gravity, exposing the hilar vessels without the need for further retraction** (Fig. 131–6). **The ureter and pelvis are directly posterior and easily accessed. There is less chance for peritoneal violation.** The working space is smaller, but in most cases this is not a significant hindrance. Theoretically, it would require more time to open from this position if emergency conversion were required. **The lateral approach provides a greater working space and slightly more access to the distal ureter.** The kidney must be retracted laterally to expose the hilum, and it is important not to mobilize the anterior aspect of the kidney until after the vessels have been controlled, or the kidney will fall onto the hilum. We have used both techniques and the prone approach is preferred for simple nephrectomy or partial nephrectomy, but when the ureter needs to be removed the lateral approach may be preferable.

KEY POINTS: RENAL LAPAROSCOPY

- Retroperitoneal laparoscopic renal surgery in children has several advantages: (1) it is the shortest distance to the kidney; (2) there is less risk of contamination of the peritoneum from any renal pathology (urinary leak, infection, or neoplasm); and (3) there are fewer exposure problems from liver, spleen, or bowel obscuring the operative field.

- Transperitoneal anatomy may be more familiar with a wider working field, and an anterior approach to renal pathology is sometimes advantageous.

- **Retroperitoneal access may be gained by one of two methods: prone or flank.**
  - The prone approach allows the kidney to fall anteriorly with gravity, exposing the hilar vessels without the need for further retraction. The ureter and pelvis are directly posterior and easily accessed. There is less chance for peritoneal violation.
  - The lateral approach provides a greater working space and slightly more access to the distal ureter.

- In transperitoneal nephrectomy, the colon is first reflected from the kidney by incision of the lateral line of Toldt. In most cases the ureter can be identified and used as a handle to lift the lower pole of the kidney. This facilitates access to the hilar vessels, which are then dissected free and independently ligated.

- In a cystic or massively hydronephrotic kidney, it is best to leave the cysts full until most of the dissection is complete to facilitate blunt dissection. Near completion, draining some of the fluid to permit grasping of the cyst walls for traction on the kidney is helpful.

- Removal of the ureter along with the kidney is readily accomplished laparoscopically, and may be best managed with a transperitoneal approach, although retroperitoneal approaches usually are adequate.

- In children, partial nephrectomy is usually performed for a nonfunctioning renal segment of a duplex system. The demarcation between the segments is usually very clear, and the affected unit is often hydronephrotic or cystic, with little blood flow. This facilitates separation of the two poles for removal. Careful attention is needed toward the renal vasculature of the **remnant** segment.

Nephrectomy

The surgical technique of laparoendoscopic nephrectomy is similar regardless of the approach used. **In transperitoneal nephrectomy, the colon is first reflected from the kidney by incision of the lateral line of Toldt. In most cases the ureter can be identified and used as a handle to lift the lower pole of the kidney. This facilitates access to the hilar vessels, which are then dissected free and independently ligated.** We have used surgical clips without problems, although some authors suggest using absorbable ties, harmonic energy, or bipolar cautery for smaller arteries. The security of clips is attractive, and they are efficiently placed. During hilar dissection there is a tendency in laparoendoscopic procedures to be very close to the kidney; this may lead to ligation of arterial branches, either anterior or posterior. One should always be alert for other branches still needing ligation before the kidney is removed. With dysplastic kidneys, aberrant arterial supply is common, and these small vessels should be sought. The renal vein can almost always be controlled with a medium or large clip in children and teenagers. It has not been our experience that a gastrointestinal anastomosis stapling device is needed as it can be in adults, although in a difficult nephrectomy staplers can be used in lieu of dissecting out individual vessels (Chan et al, 2001).

Further dissection of the perinephric tissues may be performed with a combination of rapid blunt and cautery-assisted dissection. **In a cystic or massively hydronephrotic kidney, it is best to leave the cysts full until most of the dissection is complete to facilitate blunt dissection. Near completion, it is helpful to drain some of the fluid to permit grasping of the cyst walls for traction on the kidney.** When the kidney is fully dissected, any remaining cysts should be drained to allow removal. In most cases, direct removal is possible through the umbilical port or through the initial port in retroperitoneal access. Larger kidneys may require bag extraction with morcellation.

Instrumentation used for nephrectomy is the same for either approach and includes scissors, delicate dissecting and grasping tools, and a heavy locking grasping device for specimen removal. In most children, 5-mm instruments are easily used and well tolerated. We have used 2-mm working instruments with a 5-mm endoscope, but these instruments are not sturdy enough for heavy use (Borer and Peters, 2000). As a compromise, 3.5-mm instrumentation has become available and seems to be effective without creating as large a defect as the 5-mm instruments. Stapling devices are limited to 5- and 10-mm instruments, so a 5-mm port will always be required. The radially expanding cannula system (Step, InnerDyne, Inc., Salt Lake City, UT) permits moving between 3.5-, 5- and 12-mm instruments with the same port, and the claim is made that these ports do not require suture closure, although we close all port sites over 2 mm. We have not experienced any complications with this system, but the valve mechanisms are fragile and may be damaged with multiple instrument changes.

Nephroureterectomy. Removal of the ureter along with the kidney is readily accomplished laparoscopically and may be best managed with a transperitoneal approach (see Fig. 131–4 B), **although retroperitoneal approaches usually are adequate.** The extent to which the ureter needs to be removed

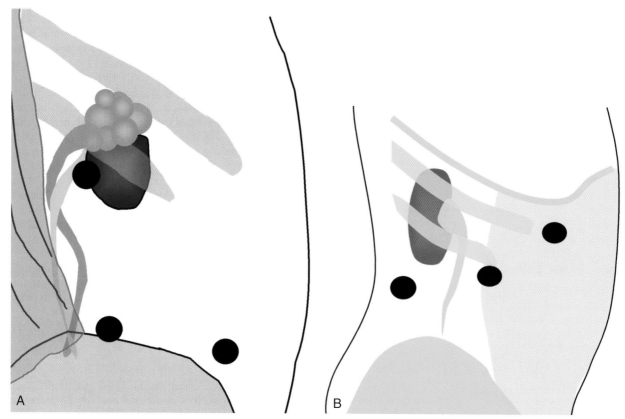

Figure 131–5. Diagram illustrating the port positions for prone retroperitoneal laparoendoscopic renal surgery (**A**) and for retroperitoneal laparoendoscopic nephrectomy from the flank position (**B**). The shaded area represents the approximate location of the lateral peritoneal reflection that needs to be mobilized.

depends on the pathology. In the setting of obstruction and reflux, the entire ureter must be removed, whereas free reflux with good drainage is unlikely to present any problems with a small, retained stump. In any case of reflux, the stump must be closed with suture. Reflux of urine into the peritoneum has occurred if this closure is not secure. Because clips can fall off readily, we recommend suture ligation or even double ligation. The ureter is usually transected just below the lower pole of the kidney and then removed separately, after the kidney has been fully dissected. If a concomitant bladder procedure is to be performed (e.g., contralateral ureteral reimplantation), the distal ureter is dissected from the bladder level, either intravesically or extravesically. Otherwise, the ureter is mobilized using the same three cannulas, with care being taken to pass the ureter under the gonadal vessels. In boys the vas is identified and avoided. The ureter is visualized to its insertion, at which point it is closed, with intracorporeal suturing for a large ureter or a ligature for a smaller one. A bladder catheter is left in place overnight.

Partial Nephrectomy. In children, partial nephrectomy is usually performed for a nonfunctioning renal segment of a duplex system. The demarcation between the segments is usually very clear (Fig. 131–7) and the affected unit is often hydronephrotic or cystic, with little blood flow. This facilitates separation of the two poles for removal. The critical feature in pediatric partial nephrectomy is the deli-

cacy of the renal vasculature of the remnant segment. Open partial nephrectomy is associated with a small but definite incidence of vascular compromise of the remnant pole due to vasospasm of the arterial supply. This may be induced by mobilization of the kidney or during dissection of the vessels to be ligated for removal of the affected pole. Any approach for laparoscopic partial nephrectomy must be done with extra care in protection of the remnant vessels. This is best accomplished by limiting the mobilization of the remnant pole and by isolating the affected vessels close to their renal unit and away from the remnant vessels. A potential advantage with laparoscopic approaches is that wide mobilization of the whole kidney is not necessary in most cases, and therefore the risk to the remnant pole is limited (Janetschek et al, 1997; Horowitz et al, 2001; Robinson et al, 2003; Lee et al, 2005).

After vascular control has been ensured, the affected pole is separated from the remnant pole with the use of either electrocautery or the harmonic scalpel. This instrument has been very effective in this procedure because it permits efficient cutting and vascular control of the junction between the affected and remnant renal units (Jackman et al, 1998a). The entire collecting system of the affected pole is removed, and this may be aided by development of the plane between the affected collecting system and the parenchyma of the remnant pole. The only residual tissue attaching the two poles is the thin rim of parenchyma, which may then be incised at its

Prone Retroperitoneal

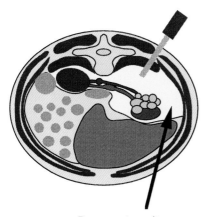

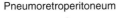

Pneumoretroperitoneum

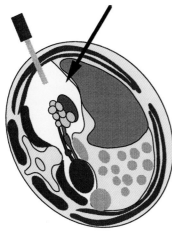

Flank Retroperitoneal

Figure 131–6. Diagram showing the relative positions of the kidney during retroperitoneal nephrectomy using the prone and flank positions. The kidney tends to fall forward and expose the hilum more readily in the prone position. (Reprinted from Peters CA: Laparoendoscopic renal surgery in children. J Endourol 2000;14:841-848.)

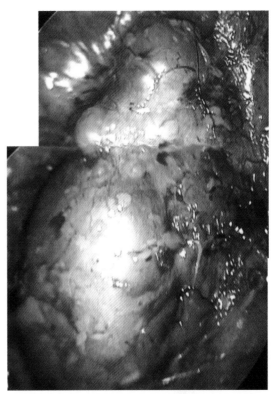

Figure 131–7. Prone retroperitoneal laparoendoscopic view of the upper pole of a duplex kidney in a child with an ectopic ureter. The healthy lower pole is visible at the bottom of the image.

margin with the harmonic scalpel. The edges of the remnant pole may be sutured together for further hemostasis. A retroperitoneal drain is optionally left in place.

Postoperative Management—Renal Laparoscopic Surgery

After a simple nephrectomy, some children may be discharged to home on the same day, depending on age. Younger children often return to their normal diet and exhibit adequate pain control within a few hours after the procedure. Others may need to stay overnight, in part based on parental anxiety. Older children continue to have some element of abdominal discomfort for up to 24 hours, perhaps as a result of the CO_2 distention for transperitoneal procedures. This seems less with retroperitoneal operations.

During the period of hospitalization, children need to be watched for signs of serious complications, which are made more dangerous by their infrequency and possible lack of early recognition. Hemorrhage is of most concern and is evidenced by alterations in the patient's vital signs. An appropri-

ate level of suspicion is the best means to permit early detection. Similarly, bowel injury may occur without intraoperative recognition during either transperitoneal or retroperitoneal procedures. Bowel injury may not become apparent until after discharge, when fever and evidence of intraperitoneal irritation develop, although usually with less severity than might be expected.

Miscellaneous Renal Surgery

Laparoscopic renal biopsy for nephrologic disease has been reported, although a comparison with ultrasound-guided needle biopsy has yet to be made. It is performed retroperitoneally, with few reported complications and rapid procedural time (Caione et al, 2000; Takeda et al, 2000; Mukhtar et al, 2005). Laparoscopic management of renal malignancy in children has been reported only in limited numbers of patients with Wilms' tumor after chemotherapy (Duarte et al, 2004) but may ultimately play a role in primary management of Wilms' tumor. Several cases of laparoscopic resection of neuroblastoma have been reported with good outcomes (Waldhausen et al, 2000).

Laparoscopic adrenal surgery in children has been reported in a few cases, primarily related to cortical adenoma and associated with congenital virilizing adrenal hyperplasia (Schier et al, 1999; Radmayr et al, 2000; Castilho et al, 2002; Gmyrek et al, 2002; Miller et al, 2002; Tobias-Machado et al, 2002). Resection of pediatric pheochromocytoma has been reported as well (Mirallie et al, 2001). The adrenal gland is readily visualized through both retroperitoneal and transperitoneal approaches (Steyaert et al, 2003). There is limited need for adrenalectomy in children, but laparoscopy appears to have a significant potential in this area, as it has in adult surgery.

Laparoscopic management of pediatric malignancies has been limited but is clearly emerging as a significant tool in the surgical armamentarium (Saenz et al, 1997; Waldhausen et al, 2000). The issue of port site seeding has been studied and found to be safe (Iwanaka et al, 2003). Recognizing the advance made in adult urologic laparoscopic oncologic surgery, it would seem appropriate to extend this to the pediatric realm as well.

Results

Overall results of laparoscopic renal surgery in children have been good as compared with open procedures (Hamilton et al, 2000; El-Ghoneimi et al, 2003; Lee et al, 2005). There remains uncertainty as to its advantages over conventional open surgery. From one perspective, children, and particularly infants, recover rapidly from most open renal surgery, and they are not saving any lost time at work. Subjectively, however, parents whose children have undergone laparoscopic renal surgery report recoveries that appear to be more rapid than seen in open surgery, and hospital stays are shorter (El-Ghoneimi et al, 2003; Lee et al, 2005). It is important to recognize that these parameters are subjective and depend on personal and institutional preferences. As laparoscopic renal surgery emerged, several reports of day surgical open nephrectomy in infants were published, indicating the rapidity of pediatric recovery, although these procedures were not without risk (Elder et al, 1995).

Operative times for laparoscopic renal surgery have declined with increasing experience and are now reported to be between 60 and 120 minutes in most series for simple nephrectomy. Partial nephrectomy requires somewhat longer but may be performed within 2 hours in many cases. There has been no formal comparison between transperitoneal and retroperitoneal nephrectomy in terms of operative duration, hospital stay, or complications. Age-matched comparison of laparoscopic and open partial nephrectomies showed initially longer operative times that came to match times for open surgery and clearly shorter hospital stays with less analgesic requirements (El-Ghoneimi et al, 2003; Lee et al, 2005). Similar success rates have been reported in small infants as well (Mulholland et al, 2005). Laparoscopic nephrectomy in high-risk patients, such as those with renal insufficiency, has been undertaken with good results (El-Ghoneimi et al, 2000) (Table 131–4).

The incidence of complications has been low in all published series (Ehrlich et al, 1994; Koyle et al, 1993; Diamond et al, 1995; Valla et al, 1996; El-Ghoneimi et al, 1998; Borer and Peters, 2000; Hamilton et al, 2000; Yao and Poppas, 2000; York et al, 2000). **The conversion rate is less than 5%.** No late morbidity has been reported. Pneumothorax has been reported in pediatric renal surgery, particularly involving the upper pole of the kidney, but also during a bladder procedure (Waterman et al, 2004).

Bladder Surgery

Laparoscopic surgery involving the bladder can be divided into procedures intended to remove or repair a portion of the bladder or urachus and reconstructive procedures such as bladder augmentation or continent urinary stoma formation. Intravesical surgery is covered in the section dealing with antireflux surgery. Operations to repair the bladder (e.g., diverticulectomy) have been rarely reported in children, so most of the cases in the literature involve adult patients (Jarrett et al, 1995; Zanetti et al, 1995; Iselin et al, 1996). This is also true of operations to excise urachal abnormalities (Trondsen et al, 1993; Redmond et al, 1994; Fahlenkamp et al, 1995; Hubens et al, 1995; Linos et al, 1997; Khurana and Borzi, 2002; Yohannes et al, 2003). The approach to the bladder may be extraperitoneal, working in the space of Retzius, but is more commonly transperitoneal, especially in children. The bladder is relatively easily accessible in children and therefore

Table 131–4. Results of Laparoscopic Nephrectomy

Study	Year	No.	Operating Time	Length of Stay	Conversion to Open Surgery	Comment
Koyle et al, 1993	1993	1				Case
Suzuki et al, 1993	1993	1				Case
Ehrlich et al, 1994	1994	14	2.25		1	
Nishiyama and Terunuma, 1996	1996	1				RP
Valla et al, 1996	1996	18	1.66		1	RP
Davies and Najmaldin, 1998	1998	36	1.4	2		RP
El-Ghoneimi et al, 1998	1998	31	1.75	2	0	RP
Ushiyama et al, 1998	1998	2	2.75			
Borer et al, 1999	1999	14	2.3	2	0	RP
Prabhakaran and Lingaraj, 1999	1999	6	3	2.3		
Hamilton et al, 2000	2000	10	3	1		Comparative
York et al, 2000	2000	11	2.75	2.4	0	
Borzi, 2001	2001	36	1			Compare post and lateral
Shanberg et al, 2001	2001	37	1.25	1.3	1	RP
Urbanowicz et al, 2004	2002	12	1.8		0	RP
Ku et al, 2004	2004			2.5	0	RP
Mulholland et al, 2005	2005	17	2.3	<1	0	Compared with open Infants <10 kg; one diaphragmatic injury

RP, retroperitoneal.

is well suited for laparoscopic approaches. For either urachal or bladder procedures, high abdominal access is necessary to allow exposure and room to manipulate instruments.

Bladder reconstructive procedures have taken three main forms to date: laparoscopic autoaugmentation techniques, laparoscopic enterocystoplasty, and laparoscopic-assisted reconstructive procedures. Augmentation of the bladder with tissue scaffolds (Calvano et al, 2000) or engineered bladder tissue may become important laparoscopic techniques, but they currently are experimental.

Laparoscopic Autoaugmentation. Autoaugmentation, or detrusorraphy, is a technique that involves dividing the bladder muscle and dissecting it free of the mucosa (Cartwright and Snow, 1989). This allows the development of a large bladder diverticulum, resulting in improved compliance and low-pressure storage. Because this is a form of bladder augmentation that does not involve the harvesting of gastrointestinal segments and requires very little suturing, it is adaptable to minimally invasive techniques. Laparoscopic autoaugmentation has been performed in animal models (Britanisky et al, 1995) and in children (Ehrlich and Gershman, 1993; Poppas et al, 1996; Braren and Bishop, 1998) and both transperitoneally and extraperitoneally (McDougall et al, 1995a). Bladder autoaugmentation requires a large incision of the detrusor with dissection of the underlying mucosa over a large surface area, often followed by fixation of the bladder muscle to the pelvic sidewall to prevent narrowing of the mouth of the newly formed bladder diverticulum. The process of separating bladder muscle from mucosa has been assisted with laser, with the theoretical advantage of a limited depth of tissue destruction (Poppas et al, 1996). This operation can be done with a very short hospital stay or on an outpatient basis, but it does require postoperative bladder drainage for some period of time because of the possibility of rupture and leakage. Autoaugmentation yields a bladder completely lined with uroepithelium, no mucus formation, no apparent increased risk of stones, and the ability to go on to other forms of augmentation should it become necessary. Autoaugmentation techniques have been combined with extravesical forms of ureteral reimplantation (Carr et al, 1999), and this could be readily performed laparoscopically (Lakshmanan and Fung, 2000).

Long-term results of open or laparoscopic autoaugmentation have not been consistent (Gonzalez, 1996), and autoaugmentation has not achieved wide acceptance as a reconstructive technique in children. This is, however, a minimally invasive technique of bladder enlargement, and it may be considered for patients with reasonable capacity but poor compliance and for those who do not require a large increase in bladder capacity. There is little disadvantage to an autoaugmentation if further reconstruction is necessary in the future, especially if it is performed laparoscopically.

Laparoscopic Enterocystoplasty. The first laparoscopic gastrointestinal bladder augmentation was performed using stomach (Docimo et al, 1995). The laparoscopic technique involved the use of endoscopic clips to dissect the gastroepiploic pedicle and endoscopic gastrointestinal anastomotic staplers to excise a wedge of stomach. The remaining stomach edge was oversewn with the previously described endoscopic suturing device, and the gastric patch was sewn to the bladder

in the same way. **Laparoscopic bladder augmentation has also been performed with the use of small or large intestine, usually with an extracorporeal bowel anastomosis** (Gill et al, 2000). These operations require a high degree of laparoscopic skill and involve difficult access for suturing. Development of innovative techniques for intestinal harvest (Elliott et al, 2002; Meng et al, 2002) or for bladder anastomosis including laser welding, tissue adhesives, newer suturing techniques, and robotic assistance may be required to bring laparoscopic bladder augmentation into the mainstream. It is not far-fetched to think that most bladder augmentations might be performed laparoscopically in the future.

Laparoscopic-Assisted Reconstructive Surgery. At the moment, the state of the art for minimally invasive reconstruction represents a compromise—the laparoscopic-assisted procedure. The concept is based on the premise that bladder reconstructive operations can be divided into two stages: in the first, the tissues for the augmentation and/or the continent stoma are freed and harvested; and in the second, the actual reconstruction is performed. The assembly of parts into a functional bladder unit takes place in the low pelvis and therefore can be accomplished through a small lower abdominal incision (Fig. 131–8). If no continent stoma is to be made and ileum or sigmoid is to be used for the augmentation, the entire operation can be done through this type of incision and laparoscopic assistance is not employed. If stomach, ureter, or appendix is to be used, an approach to the upper abdomen becomes necessary and laparoscopy obviates the need for a long midline incision or, in the case of ureter, two incisions. The principle of laparoscopic-assisted reconstructive surgery is simple: use laparoscopy to perform the parts of the operation that require upper abdominal access,

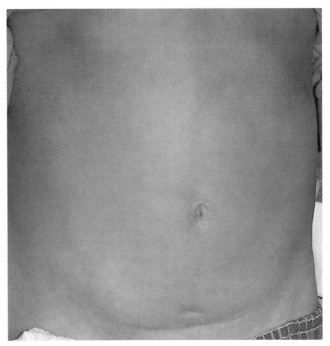

Figure 131–8. This 4-year-old boy with a history of ectopic ureter and poor bladder emptying has undergone laparoscopic nephroureterectomy and laparoscopic-assisted appendicovesicostomy.

and do the technically demanding reconstructive steps through an open lower abdominal incision (Hedican et al, 1999).

Laparoscopic-assisted surgery is widely applicable in patients who require bladder reconstruction and/or antegrade continence enema stoma. The majority of patients reported have had prior abdominal surgery, including ventriculoperitoneal shunt placement and bladder exstrophy closure (Cadeddu and Docimo, 1999; Hedican et al, 1999; Chung et al, 2004). The benefit of laparoscopic mobilization is not just cosmetic; in theory, less postoperative pain, more rapid recovery, and decreased intra-abdominal adhesions (Moore et al, 1995a, 1995b) can be expected. Therefore, even patients with a prior midline incision might benefit. The presence of a ventriculoperitoneal shunt is not a contraindication to laparoscopic surgery (Docimo, 1999; Jackman et al, 2000) and necessitates no special precautions or monitoring.

Laparoscopic-assisted surgery has been applied at only a few centers thus far (Jordan and Winslow, 1993b; Sanchez de Badajoz et al, 1995; Cadeddu and Docimo, 1999; Hedican et al, 1999; Chung et al, 2004). The results have generally been as good as those of open operations in terms of surgical outcome, and the cosmetic results are subjectively superior to a standard midline approach (Cadeddu and Docimo, 1999; Hedican et al, 1999). The only comparative series of laparoscopic-assisted versus open continent stoma procedures demonstrated a more rapid return to regular diet and a significant decrease in hospital stay with laparoscopy (Cadeddu and Docimo, 1999). In the largest series, 31 patients had 39 continent stomas created with a 7.7% revision rate at a mean of 32 months follow-up (Chung et al, 2004). Early experience with robotically assisted creation of continent stomas has been encouraging (Pedraza et al, 2004b; Peters, 2004b) (Fig. 131–9). Currently, all reconstructive operations that cannot be performed through a small lower abdominal incision can be done

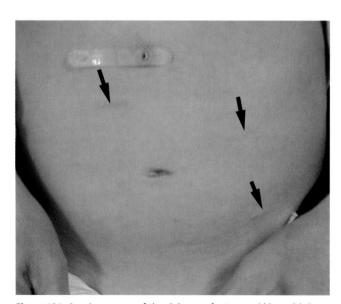

Figure 131–9. Appearance of the abdomen of a 5-year-old boy with Down syndrome and inadequate bladder emptying after robotically assisted laparoscopic appendicovesicostomy. Three port sites were used and were positioned to avoid his gastrostomy tube.

in this way, unless there has been extensive prior abdominal surgery.

Ureteral Surgery

Antireflux Surgery. Surgery for vesicoureteral reflux has long been a target for those interested in minimally invasive approaches. Most notable among these have been the injection methods (STING procedures) that have been employed for reflux, which are discussed in Chapter 117, "Vesicoureteral Reflux." This section deals specifically with the use of laparoscopic techniques in an attempt to correct reflux. These have taken two main forms: transvesical and extravesical techniques.

Strictly speaking, transvesical techniques are not "laparoscopic" or "peritoneoscopic" procedures but rather percutaneous bladder procedures that employ laparoscopic instruments and techniques. Smaller instrumentation has allowed experimentation and clinical experience in intravesical endoscopic surgery. One operation through this route has been the percutaneous endoscopic trigonoplasty, a modification of the Gil-Vernet procedure (Cartwright et al, 1996; Okamura et al, 1996). In this operation, a horizontal incision from ureteral orifice to ureteral orifice is closed vertically, incorporating detrusor, pulling the orifices toward the midline, and enhancing the fixation of the ureteral tunnel. Unfortunately, the initial promise of trigonoplasty has not been realized with long-term follow-up (Okamura et al, 1997; Gatti et al, 1999; Okamura et al, 1999). A modification of this approach has been described with sutured reinforcement of the back wall of the trigone after lifting the ureter. An 86% success rate with two ureteral injuries and prolonged catheterization was reported in the initial series (Tsuji et al, 2003). Taking this idea one step further, it has been shown both experimentally (Lakshmanan et al, 1999) and clinically that the ureters can be dissected free of the bladder muscle and reimplanted using endoscopic technique (Gill et al, 2001; Yeung et al, 2005). In a series of 16 patients with 23 refluxing ureters, Yeung and coworkers (2005) reported a 96% success rate with no significant complications. A limited number of other surgeons have undertaken this challenging procedure. Robotic assistance may show some promise in this area (Olsen et al, 2003; Peters and Woo, 2005).

The most widely applied laparoscopic approach to vesicoureteral reflux has been the laparoscopic extravesical reimplantation (Atala et al, 1993). This procedure has been used experimentally (Atala et al, 1993; McDougall et al, 1995b) and clinically at a number of centers (Janetschek et al, 1995; Lakshmanan and Fung, 2000). It is performed in the manner of the Lich-Gregoir operation (Gregoir, 1977). The ureterovesical junction is exposed transperitoneally by incision between the round ligament and the bladder (Lakshmanan and Fung, 2000). An incision is made in the bladder muscle adjacent to the ureter and is extended cephalad, staying outside the bladder mucosa. A trough is created with mucosa as its base. The bladder muscle is then closed over the ureter with interrupted laparoscopic suture and tying techniques to effectively create a submucosal tunnel. Results of the largest series to date suggest efficacy similar to that of open surgery (Lakshmanan and Fung, 2000). Robotically assisted extravesical antireflux ureteroplasty in a similar manner has shown high success rates with minimal invasive-

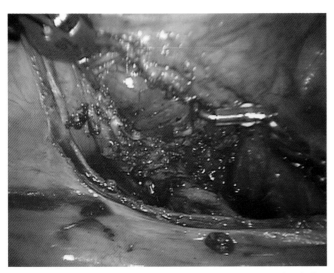

Figure 131–10. Laparoscopic appearance of robotically assisted antireflux procedure using the Lich-Gregoir approach. The detrusor has been incised and the mucosa exposed, and the trough is being developed before placement of the ureter within it.

ness (Fig. 131-10). Catheters and stents are not routinely used (Peters, 2004b; Peters et al, 2005).

It is not clear at this time whether any of these minimally invasive procedures will replace open surgery, which is performed through a small Pfannenstiel incision and requires a short hospital stay. The economics of reflux management are such that increased expense for minimally invasive approaches might further tip the balance away from surgical management if cost is the only factor considered (Mathews et al, 2000). Nevertheless, development of these techniques is vital if current reflux management is to be replaced by minimally invasive approaches. For those looking for minimally invasive reflux management, injection techniques have a lower success rate but are technically much easier. The more certain cure rates and known durability of conventional methods such as the transtrigonal or extravesical techniques, however, are appealing to some patients and families.

Perivesical Surgery

Seminal Vesicle Cyst/Retained Müllerian Remnants (Utricles). The potential for perivesical laparoscopic surgery is clear and there is an increasing number of reports to date. These procedures are mostly for persistent müllerian structures, seminal vesicle cysts, or prostatic utricles and are typically performed transperitoneally. The retrovesical peritoneum is incised to expose the structure retrovesically. The vas deferens may enter these structures or must be preserved. We have left a side wall of the cyst with the contralateral vas to attempt to protect the vas (Ikari et al, 1999; Yeung et al, 2001; Nanni et al, 2003; Valla et al, 2003; Willetts et al, 2003). Laparoscopy seems ideally suited to the management of these cases, which would otherwise require transtrigonal or posterior surgical approaches.

Vaginoplasty. There are numerous techniques for the creation of a neovagina in children with congenital absence of the vagina. Laparoscopic techniques have been used occasionally. Laparoscopy has been used as an adjunct to the

Vecchietti operation for creation of a neovagina in Mayer-Rokitansky-Küster-Hauser syndrome (Vecchietti, 1965). In this technique, an olive-shaped device is placed at the vaginal dimple and constant upward traction is applied transabdominally via sutures brought out through the anterior abdominal wall. This creates a neovaginal space in less than 2 weeks. Although this technique would rarely be applicable to pediatric urologic patients, it has been adapted laparoscopically, making it more widely applied for this specific adult population (Keckstein et al, 1995; Cooper et al, 1996; Fedele et al, 2000).

Much more commonly applied in children is the sigmoid (or ileal) vaginoplasty. These operations produce a mucosa-lined neovagina that can be expected to maintain a reasonable lumen without constant dilation. This operation is ideally suited to laparoscopic techniques, avoiding the often large abdominal incision used to harvest the segment of sigmoid (Urbanowicz et al, 2004). The sigmoid is ideally used and can be resected followed by circular stapler anastomosis via the rectum. Laparoscopic dissection of the retrovesical space can be combined with perineal dissection to facilitate creation of the neovaginal space (Ota et al, 2000). A similar dissection was used to facilitate skin graft vaginoplasty to an intact uterus in an adolescent girl (Lee et al, 1999). Laparoscopic access has been shown to permit combined repair of vaginal and anorectal malformations as well (Tei et al, 2003).

Robotic-Assisted Laparoscopic Surgery

The availability of a clinically useful surgical robotic system has permitted wider application of laparoscopy in pediatric urologic reconstruction. The limitation of inefficient suturing with free-hand laparoscopy can be readily overcome with the robotic system. The currently available system (DaVinci, Intuitive Surgical, Sunnyvale, CA) is a "master-slave" robotic manipulating device that permits the surgeon to have better control over the instruments by working through a mechanical device that translates the surgeon's movements into the laparoscopic instruments. Visual guidance with a three-dimensional binocular endoscope permits even more accurate control of movements. The system includes a stand that contains the three or four arms that hold the endoscope and working arms. The laparoscopic instruments are passed through cannulas that are attached to the working arms, and the instruments have an articulating end-effector under the surgeon's control (Fig. 131–11). The movements are controlled by the surgeon sitting at a console using two hand-held manipulator controls that permit movement throughout space while looking through the visual system. The positioning is very natural and movements are smooth with scaling and tremor filtering. The system is very expensive, and this current version is difficult to justify financially for only a few cases. When used regularly, the economics are more realistic. It is likely to be a rapidly advancing field however, as the potential is explored in these early cases.

To date, we have performed a wide variety of pediatric cases on the DaVinci system, including pyeloplasty (Lee et al, 2005), antireflux surgery, complex ureteral reconstructions, intravesical ureteral reimplantation, and both stone and adrenal cases. Although there is uncertainty about its ultimate place, the efficiency of laparoscopic manipulation and suturing in particular are very compelling arguments. The current system should

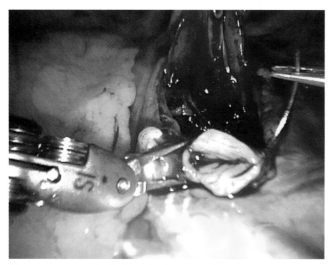

Figure 131–11. Robotically assisted laparoscopic pyeloplasty showing the accuracy of needle placement into the spatulated ureter in a child. The suture is 6-0 absorbable monofilament.

be viewed as demonstrating the "proof of principle" of robotic- or computer-assisted surgical technologies (Olsen and Jorgensen, 2004; Pedraza et al, 2004a, 2004b; Peters 2004a, 2004b; Peters and Woo, 2005).

SUMMARY

The continued expansion of applications of endourologic techniques in pediatric patients holds promise for enhancing care of these patients. Advances in technology will facilitate this expansion, but caution must be exercised so that enthusiasm for the novel does not cloud clinical judgment. It should be clearly evident or at least likely that the "minimally invasive" procedure offers a real advantage to the patient. There is

potential for significant harm in misguided applications of these technologies, particularly in inexperienced hands. Properly constructed clinical trials are difficult to accomplish in this setting (Mowatt et al, 1997; Peters, 2003a), but every effort should be made to evaluate in as objective a manner as possible the clinical outcomes of new surgical technologies. If this is not undertaken, new methods with real promise may never fulfill their potential.

SUGGESTED READINGS

Borer JG, Peters CA: Pediatric retroperitoneoscopic nephrectomy. J Endourol 2000;14:413-416; discussion 417.

Borzi PA, Yeung CK: Selective approach for transperitoneal and extraperitoneal endoscopic nephrectomy in children. J Urol 2004;171:814-816; discussion 816.

Chung SY, Meldrum K, Docimo SG: Laparoscopic assisted reconstructive surgery: A 7-year experience. J Urol 2004;171:372-375.

Cisek LJ, Gobet RM, Peters CA: Pneumoperitoneum produces reversible renal dysfunction in animals with normal and chronically reduced renal function. J Endourol 1998;12:95-100.

El-Ghoneimi A, Farhat W, Bolduc S, et al: Retroperitoneal laparoscopic vs open partial nephroureterectomy in children. BJU Int 2003;91:532-535.

Halachmi S, El-Ghoneimi A, Bissonnette B, et al: Hemodynamic and respiratory effect of pediatric urological laparoscopic surgery: A retrospective study. J Urol 2003;170:1651-1654; discussion 1654.

Holcomb GW, Brock JW, Morgan WM: Laparoscopic evaluation for a contralateral patent processus vaginalis. J Pediatr Surg 1994a;29:970-973; discussion 974.

Jackman SV, Hedican SP, Peters CA, et al: Infant and preschool age percutaneous nephrolithotomy: Experience with a new technique. Urology 1998b;52:697-701.

Lakshmanan Y, Peters CA: Laparoscopy in the management of intersex anomalies. Pediatr Endosurg Innov Tech 2000b;4:201-206.

Lee RS, Retik AB, Borer JG, et al: Pediatric retroperitoneal laparoscopic partial nephrectomy: Comparison with an age matched cohort of open surgery. J Urol 2005;174:708-711.

Minevich E, Defoor W, Reddy P, et al: Ureteroscopy is safe and effective in prepubertal children. J Urol 2005;174:276-279; discussion 279.

Peters CA: Robotically assisted surgery in pediatric urology. Urol Clin North Am 2004b;31:743-752.

Yeung CK, Sihoe JD, Borzi PA: Endoscopic cross-trigonal ureteral reimplantation under carbon dioxide bladder insufflation: A novel technique. J Endourol 2005;19:295-299.

132 Pediatric Genitourinary Trauma

DOUGLAS HUSMANN, MD

Traumatic injury, defined as the destruction of tissues or organs produced by external violence, is the primary cause of childhood death. In North America, blunt trauma is responsible for 90% of the genitourinary injuries in childhood, with approximately 90% of the patients with genitourinary injuries having coexisting injuries to the thorax, spine, pelvis/femur, or intra-abdominal organs (Buckley and McAninch, 2004; Heyns 2004; Santucci et al, 2004b). Traumatic injury to the kidney accounts for greater than 60% of the pediatric genitourinary injuries (Levy et al, 1993; Santucci et al, 2001, 2004a; Sahin et al, 2004).

SIMILARITIES AND DIFFERENCES IN EVALUATING PEDIATRIC VERSUS ADULT TRAUMATIC INJURIES

The Pediatric Kidney: Traumatic Renal Injuries and Congenital Renal Anomalies

The pediatric kidney is believed to be more susceptible to trauma because of a decrease in the physical renal protective mechanisms found in childhood. Specifically, the pediatric kidney is protected by an immature, more pliable thoracic cage and weaker abdominal musculature, has less perirenal fat, and sits in a lower position in the abdomen than its adult counterpart. Whether the incidence of renal injury after blunt abdominal trauma is truly increased in the pediatric compared with the adult patient population is controversial (Brown et al, 1998; Chopra et al, 2002; Heyns, 2004; McAleer et al, 2002). Statistical evaluations to confirm that children have an increased risk of renal damage after blunt trauma have revealed mixed results, and the question remains (Brown et al, 1998; Chopra et al, 2002; McAleer et al, 2002; Smith et al, 2003; Heyns, 2004).

What is known however is that preexisting renal abnormalities (i.e., ureteropelvic junction [UPJ] obstruction, hydroureteronephrosis, horseshoe kidney) are threefold to fivefold more common in pediatric patients undergoing screening computed tomography (CT) for trauma than in the adult population (Chopra et al, 2002; McAleer et al, 2002; Heyns, 2004; Santucci et al, 2004b). **Classically, patients with a preexisting congenital renal abnormality present with a history of hematuria disproportionate to the severity of trauma.** Although it has been hypothesized that a preexisting congenital genitourinary anomaly would be associated with a higher stage of renal injury, this has not been documented to be true, with the majority of the patients still sustaining only renal contusions or minor renal fractures (Chopra et al, 2002; McAleer et al, 2002).

Trauma-Induced Hematuria: Pediatric Compared with Adult Patients

After blunt abdominal trauma in the adult, up to 30% of the patients presenting with gross hematuria and up to 10% of patients with microscopic hematuria (>50 red blood cells per high-power field) with shock (systolic blood pressure <90 mm Hg) will be found to have a radiologically definable genitourinary injury. In fact, in the adult, either gross or microscopic hematuria with shock will be found in approximately 98% of patients with genitourinary injuries associated with blunt trauma and slightly greater than 90% of patients with genitourinary injuries associated with penetrating trauma (Mee and McAninch, 1989; Heyns, 2004; Santucci et al, 2004a). **In contrast, in children, hematuria is very unreliable in determining who to screen for renal injuries. Indeed, some studies have failed to find any evidence of either gross or microscopic hematuria in up to 70% of children sustaining grade 2 or higher renal injury. In essence, in the pediatric patient sustaining trauma, hematuria alone cannot be used to determine the need for radiographic screening studies** (Morey et al, 1996; Buckley and McAninch, 2004).

Indications for Imaging the Genitourinary Tract after Trauma: Pediatric Compared with Adult

At one time significant controversy existed regarding whether the screening criteria used to determine when to assess for renal injuries in adults could be applied to children (Mee et al, 1989; Quinlan and Gearhart, 1990; Levy et al, 1993; Stein et al, 1994; Morey et al, 1996; Brown et al, 2001; Santucci et al, 2004a). This controversy was based on three separate concerns; first, children will often have normal blood pressure in spite of significant blood loss. Indeed, in children a fall in serial hemoglobin or hematocrit values is a better determinant of blood loss than hypotension (Quinlan and Gearhart, 1990). Second, there is no consensus in the literature regarding the definition of an associated injury. For example, does an isolated closed-head injury indicate the need for a screening abdominal CT (Morey et al, 1996)? Third, there is no standard definition of a high-velocity or deceleration injury; for example, we use the combination of a rapid deceleration injury (from a motor vehicle accident or fall) or high-velocity impact (flank or back struck with high-velocity foreign object) to screen for a renal injury but some authors neglect the latter criterion.

To help end this controversy Santucci and associates (2004a) reviewed all of the published data regarding traumatic renal injuries in children. In this excellent review article, these authors found that the same screening criteria applied to adults are applicable to children. In view of this fact we recommend using the screening criteria outlined here be used in both children and adults.

Radiographic assessment of the genitourinary tract for a possible injury should occur after all penetrating abdominal trauma, as well as in blunt trauma victims who have one of four criteria (Mee and McAninch, 1989; Herschorn et al, 1991; Heyns, 2004; Santucci et al, 2004a):

1. **A significant deceleration or high-velocity injury such as one sustained in a high-speed motor vehicle** accident, a pedestrian/bicycle-motor vehicle accident, a fall from more than 15 feet, or a strike to the abdomen or flank with a foreign object (e.g., football helmet, baseball bat)
2. **Significant trauma that has resulted in fractures of thoracic rib cage, spine, pelvis, or femur, or bruising of the torso/perineum, or signs of peritonitis**
3. **Gross hematuria**
4. **Microscopic hematuria (>50 red blood cells per high-powered field) associated with shock (systolic blood pressure less than 90 mm Hg)**

RADIOGRAPHIC AND ENDOSCOPIC ASSESSMENT AND TREATMENT OF UPPER TRACT GENITOURINARY INJURIES

Use of Ultrasonography for Screening after Blunt Abdominal Trauma

In Europe, trauma physicians have touted Focused Assessment with Sonography for Trauma (FAST) combined with serial physical examinations as a screening modality after blunt abdominal trauma. Because of the easy access and availability of CT scanners within the major trauma centers in the United States, FAST evaluation to screen for the presence of intra-abdominal injuries after blunt abdominal trauma has been slow to be adopted within this country (Jang et al, 2004; Sirlin et al, 2004; Suthers et al, 2004; Nural et al, 2005). **The accuracy of FAST examinations is recognized to be operator and experience dependent** (Jang et al, 2004). **The sensitivity of this test ranges from 70% to 85%, and the specificity ranges from 93% to 100%** (Buchberger et al, 1993; Albrecht et al, 2004; Jang et al, 2004; Sirlin et al, 2004; Suthers et al, 2004; Nural et al 2005). **FAST examinations will, on average, miss somewhere between 5% to 10% of the clinically significant injuries involving the liver, spleen, kidney, adrenal gland, and small bowel** (Buchberger et al, 1993; Albrecht et al, 2004; Nural et al, 2005). **It is noteworthy, however, that a FAST scan that is negative for intra-abdominal injuries combined with normal serial physical examinations over a 24-hour period of observation will virtually rule out the presence of significant intra-abdominal injuries** (Sirlin et al, 2004). Therefore, the combination of FAST and 24-hour serial physical examinations may be of benefit, especially if radiologic resources are limited. At this time, some trauma centers use the combination of FAST and physical examination as screening tools to determine if the patient should be recommended for further radiologic workup with a CT evaluation or alternatively may be safely observed (Jang et al, 2004; Sirlin et al, 2004; Suthers et al, 2004; Nural et al, 2005).

Abdominal and Pelvic Computed Tomography and Single-Shot Intravenous Pyelography

The patient's hemodynamic stability determines whether, when, and occasionally what type of imaging studies should be done. In the clinically stable patient, triphasic abdominal

Grade of Renal Injury	Description
Table 132–1.	**Grading of Renal Injuries**
1	Renal contusion or subcapsular hematoma
2	Nonexpanding perirenal hematoma, less than 1 cm parenchymal laceration, no urinary extravasation; all renal fragments viable
3	Nonexpanding perirenal hematoma, more than 1 cm parenchymal laceration, no urinary extravasation; renal fragments may be viable or devitalized
4	Laceration extending into the collecting system with urinary extravasation; renal fragments may be viable or devitalized or Injury to the main renal vasculature with contained hemorrhage
5	Completely shattered kidney, by definition multiple major lacerations of more than 1 cm associated with multiple devitalized fragments or Injury to the main renal vasculature with uncontrolled hemorrhage, renal hilar avulsion

and pelvic CT (precontrast study, followed by a study immediately after injection of contrast agent, and then a 15- to 20-minute delayed study) is the most sensitive method for diagnosis and classification of genitourinary trauma. See Table 132–1 for classification of renal trauma (Mee and McAninch, 1989; Stein et al, 1994; Morey et al, 1996; Brown et al, 2001; Buckley and McAninch, 2004; Heyns, 2004; Santucci et al, 2004b). **In the clinically labile patient single-phase CT can be performed immediately after injection of a contrast agent. This test is beneficial in determining renal perfusion and the presence of major renal fractures but will be unable to accurately determine the presence of urinary extravasation and will miss the majority of the isolated ureteral injuries.** In the unstable patient requiring emergent laparotomy, once the patient is stabilized in the operating room, single-shot intravenous pyelography (IVP) (2 mL/kg intravenous bolus of contrast agent) with the radiograph taken 10 to 15 minutes after injection may be of benefit. We would caution the reader regarding the quality of the single-shot IVP, because this study frequently results in a suboptimal examination with poor excretion/visualization of contrast agent owing to the patient's clinical status. Single-shot IVP's chief benefit may be to detect a normally functioning contralateral kidney if unilateral nephrectomy is a consideration. As an alternative to single-shot IVP, the patient can be stabilized and a delayed CT evaluation obtained. Definitive surgical repair of any genitourinary injury is subsequently deferred for 12 to 24 hours (Azimuddin et al, 1997; Heyns, 2004).

Indications and Use of Arteriography

Approximately 25% of patients with grade 3 to grade 4 renal trauma, managed in a nonoperative fashion, will develop persistent or secondary (delayed) hemorrhage (Wessells et al, 1997a; Kansas et al, 2004). Classically, delayed hemorrhage develops 10 to 14 days after injury but may occur up to 1

month after the insult. Delayed hemorrhage usually arises from the development of arteriovenous fistulas or pseudoaneurysm malformations. Unlike the arteriovenous fistulas noted after renal biopsy, the vast majority of arteriovenous fistulas occurring after major renal trauma will not spontaneously resolve, with almost all cases of delayed hemorrhage secondary to trauma requiring active intervention (Heyns and Van Vollenhoven, 1992; Dinkel et al, 2002; Goffette and Laterre, 2002; Heyns, 2004). **Superselective angiographic embolization of isolated renal artery branches for persistent or secondary hemorrhage has a success rate approaching 80%. Although still controversial, it is believed that angiographic embolization results in a decreased risk of renal loss compared with open surgical exploration and is currently the preferred treatment method for this complication. Surgical exploration is reserved for embolization failure** (Heyns and Van Vollenhoven, 1992; Dinkel et al, 2002; Goffette and Laterre, 2002; Heyns, 2004).

Angiographic embolization will, on occasion, also be used to treat persistent urinary fistulas. In this scenario, a functional transected fragment of a grade 4 or 5 renal injury is completely separated from the renal collecting system, and a persistent urinary fistula has developed despite management by double-J stent and percutaneous nephrostomy tube placement. In these rare patients, selective angiographic embolization will resolve the urinary fistula by necrosing the isolated functional renal fragment (Pinto and Chimeno, 1998; Heyns, 2004).

Postembolization syndrome is a well recognized and self-limiting condition, manifested by pyrexia (up to 40° C [104° F]), flank pain, and an adynamic ileus. Symptoms will usually resolve within 96 hours after the embolization. Unlike angioinfarction for renal tumors in which up to 60% of the patients may develop postembolization syndrome, the syndrome may develop in approximately 10% of patients after angioinfarction after a traumatic injury. The decrease in the frequency of this syndrome after trauma is believed to be secondary to less pyrogens being released from the already partially necrotic tissue (Oesterling et al, 1986; Kehagias et al, 1998; Kalman and Varenhorst, 1999; Heyns, 2004; Mitra et al, 2004). **The problem when faced with persistent pyrexia after embolization is the need to rule out bacterial seeding of the necrotic tissue. It is therefore mandatory in the presence of a febrile response after embolization to obtain blood and urine cultures. Consideration for a repeat CT with possible aspiration, culture, and drainage of the hematoma/urinoma should be given if symptoms persist for more than 96 hours** (Heyns, 2004; Mitra et al, 2004).

Indications and Use of Retrograde Pyelography and Percutaneous Drainage

Two indications exist for the use of retrograde pyelography after renal trauma: (1) to rule out the presence of a partial/total ureteral disruption and (2) to aid in the management of a symptomatic urinoma (Boone et al, 1993; Heyns, 2004; Santucci et al, 2004b). In our experience, concern for a ureteral injury usually arises in a clinically labile patient who had undergone monophasic CT (no delayed films) or a patient who required emergent surgical exploration without antecedent radiographic evaluation. In this clinical scenario, the initial radiographic studies were either within normal limits or were suggestive of, but not conclusive for, a ureteral injury, and no further studies were performed at the time of the injury owing to the clinical status of the patient. Delayed CT 2 to 5 days after trauma reveal perirenal or upper ureteral extravasation of contrast agent, with no visualization of the ipsilateral distal ureter. In these situations, cystoscopy and retrograde pyelography are necessary to confirm or refute the diagnosis of a UPJ disruption versus laceration of the renal pelvis (Boone et al, 1993; Chopra et al, 2002; McAleer et al, 2002; Smith et al, 2003; Santucci et al, 2004b).

The second consideration for intervention with cystoscopy and retrograde pyelography occurs in the patient with a known renal injury associated with a urinoma. **Although most post-traumatic urinomas are asymptomatic and have a spontaneous resolution rate approaching 85%, they will occasionally persist and be associated with continued flank pain, adynamic ileus, and/or low-grade temperature.** Frequently we will manage these patients via endoscopic intervention, with cystoscopy, retrograde pyelography, and placement of a ureteral stent. Both percutaneous nephrostomy drainage and internal stenting are equally efficacious (Husmann and Morris, 1991; Husmann et al, 1993b; Philpott et al, 2003; Bozeman et al, 2004; Heyns, 2004; Keller et al, 2004). The advantage of an internal stent is that it prevents possible dislodgement of the draining tube and the need for external drainage devices. The two major disadvantages of internal drainage are that both stent placement and removal, in the pediatric patient population, require general anesthesia. In addition, the small size ureteral stents (4 to 5 Fr) placed in young children may become blocked with blood clots from the dissolving hematoma, resulting in persistence of the urinoma (Husmann and Morris, 1991; Husmann et al, 1993b).

Indications and Use of Dimercaptosuccinic Acid and Follow-up Radiographic Imaging after Renal Trauma

Follow-up renal imaging is not recommended for grade 1 and 2 renal injuries and for grade 3 lacerations in which all fragments are viable. In patients with grade 3 renal lacerations associated with devitalized fragments, grade 4 and salvaged grade 5 renal injuries, repeat CT with delayed images should be obtained 2 to 3 days after the traumatic insult. This study serves the purpose of assessing the extent of the hematoma/urinoma and will serve as a baseline evaluation in case secondary hemorrhage or infection should occur (Heyns, 2004; Santucci et al, 2004b). Irrespective of the grade of the injury, repeat imaging with triphasic CT is also recommended for patients with renal trauma who have a persistent and/or increased fever, worsening flank pain, or persistent gross hematuria more than 72 hours after the traumatic insult (Santucci et al, 2004b). We recommend a 3-month follow-up triphasic CT scan in all grade 3 renal lacerations associated with a devitalized fragment, grade 4, and salvaged grade 5

renal injuries. This latter study is obtained to verify resolution of any perinephric urinoma and to define the anatomic configuration of the residual functioning renal parenchyma (Buckley and McAninch, 2004).

Nuclear renal scanning using dimercaptosuccinic acid (DMSA) allows for the physician to quantify differential renal function. **Serial DMSA scans obtained after trauma have revealed that little if any renal parenchyma recovers function 1 week after injury; therefore, a DMSA scan obtained any time 1 week after trauma results in a valid prognosis of renal function** (Wessells et al, 1997b; Moog et al, 2003). **It is currently suggested that all patients with grade 3 injuries associated with devitalized fragments, all patients with grade 4 and 5 renal injuries, and all patients with persistent post-traumatic hypertension should be evaluated with a quantitative radionuclide scintigraphy, preferably DMSA, at 1 week after trauma** (Moog et al, 2003; Heyns, 2004). Provided the serum creatinine value is normal, a differential renal function greater than 29% typically demonstrates satisfactory function, which would prevent renal failure in the event that the uninjured kidney is lost (Wessells et al, 1997b; Heyns, 2004; Keller et al, 2004).

MANAGEMENT OF RENAL TRAUMA

Multiple studies have stated that the nephrectomy rate in patients with traumatic renal injuries was higher with surgical exploration than with nonoperative management (Cass and Ireland, 1973; Cass et al, 1987; Kristjanson and Pederson, 1993; Hammer and Santucci, 2003; Keller et al, 2004). **These papers suggested that hemorrhage from the severely injured kidney was held in check by a tamponade maintained by an intact Gerota fascia. Surgical exploration with disruption of the fascia resulted in uncontrollable renal bleeding and the need for emergent nephrectomy. Whether this is true is controversial. Specifically, with the enhanced ability of CT to accurately stage renal injuries and with the development and application of trauma-related severity scores, it is currently argued that the need for emergent nephrectomy during renal exploration is not due to intractable hemorrhage incited by the renal exploration; rather, emergent nephrectomy is usually due to either the severity of the initial renal injury and/or was performed in patients who had severe intraoperative hemodynamic instability due to multiple coexisting injuries. Nephrectomy in this latter situation was performed for expediency to save the hypothermic, coagulopathic, and clinically unstable patient** (Gonzalez et al, 1999; Husmann et al, 1993b; Santucci et al, 2001; Santucci and McAninch, 2001; Wessells and McAninch, 1996; Heyns, 2004; Santucci et al, 2004b).

Due to the controversy regarding whether renal exploration leads to an increased incidence of nephrectomy, three schools of thought arose regarding the management of coexisting intra-abdominal trauma and grade 3 or higher renal injuries:

1. Irrespective of the mechanism of injury, and provided no absolute indications for renal exploration are present, all renal trauma can be observed (Altiman et al, 2000; Hammer and Santucci, 2003; Keller et al, 2004).

2. Renal exploration and renorrhaphy of a grade 3 or higher renal injury should be carried out if a laparotomy

KEY POINTS: RADIOGRAPHIC AND ENDOSCOPIC ASSESSMENT AND TREATMENT OF PEDIATRIC UPPER TRACT GENITOURINARY INJURIES

■ After a traumatic insult, the same screening criteria can be used in both adults and children to determine if evaluation for a genitourinary injury is necessary.

■ Radiographic assessment of the genitourinary tract for a possible injury should occur after all penetrating abdominal trauma as well as in blunt trauma victims who have one of four criteria: (1) a history of a significant deceleration or high-velocity injury; (2) significant trauma that has resulted in fractures of thoracic rib cage, spine, pelvis, or femur or bruising of the torso/perineum or signs of peritonitis; (3) gross hematuria; and (4) microscopic hematuria (>50 red blood cells per high-power field) associated with shock (systolic blood pressure < 90 mm Hg).

■ Triphasic abdominal and pelvic CT is the most sensitive method for the diagnosis and classification of pediatric genitourinary trauma.

■ The two most likely genitourinary injuries to be missed by single-phase CT or single-shot IVP are urinomas and/or isolated ureteral injuries.

■ Approximately 25% of patients with grade 3 or 4 renal trauma, managed in a nonoperative fashion, will develop persistent or secondary (delayed) hemorrhage. Superselective angioinfarction of the bleeding vessel is the preferred method to manage this complication.

■ Most post-traumatic urinomas are asymptomatic and will spontaneously resolve. Approximately 15% will be associated with continued flank pain, adynamic ileus, and/or low-grade temperature and require endoscopic or percutaneous management.

■ Follow-up renal imaging is not recommended for grade 1 to 2 renal injuries and for grade 3 lacerations in which all fragments are viable. Grade 3 renal lacerations associated with devitalized fragments and grade 4 and grade 5 renal injuries should have a repeat CT scan, with delayed images obtained 2 to 3 days after the traumatic insult and again at 3 months.

■ A DMSA scan obtained any time 1 week after trauma results in a valid prognosis of renal function in the injured kidney.

was to be performed for a coexisting intra-abdominal injury (especially if the stomach, duodenum, pancreas, or colon were injured). If renal exploration and renorrhaphy were to be performed it was recommended that control of the renal vessels medial to Gerota's fascia be

obtained before surgical exploration for renal trauma (Corriere et al, 1991; Husmann et al, 1993b; Heyns, 2004; Santucci et al, 2004b). In this situation, it was believed that control of the renal vessels before opening Gerota's fascia would prevent life-threatening hemorrhage. **With the passage of time even the need to obtain vascular control before renal exploration has become controversial, with some studies revealing the incidence of nephrectomy being equivalent whether or not vascular control was used** (Corriere et al, 1991; Gonzalez et al, 1999; Heyns, 2004; Santucci et al, 2004b).

3. The third option is that renal exploration can be excluded in patients with concurrent intra-abdominal injuries, provided the trauma surgeon separates the enteric injury from the urinary tract by omentum or other alternative tissue and places perioperative drains. It is hypothesized that the separation of the two sites of injury and the placement of drains will prevent breakdown of enteric repairs by leaking urine and/or help prevent the development of urinary tract complications by removal of excess contaminating bacteria or pancreatic enzymes away from the site of genitourinary injury (Husmann et al, 1993b; Wessells and McAninch, 1996; Matthews et al, 1997; El-Khader et al, 1998; Santucci et al, 2004b).

As noted by the aforementioned controversies, the major problem facing the urologist in the patient with traumatic renal injury is in determining when to surgically intervene. The current recommendations on when to pursue operative intervention are based on three findings: (1) the hemodynamic stability of the patient, (2) an accurate radiographic staging of the renal trauma, and (3) the presence of associated organ injury (Table 132–2) (Husmann and Morris, 1991; Hussman et al, 1993b; Wessells et al, 1997a; Heyns, 2004; Santucci et al, 2004b).

Nonoperative Therapy for Renal Trauma

The ideal candidate for nonoperative management is the hemodynamically stable patient sustaining either blunt or penetrating trauma, with or without associated intra-abdominal injuries, who has a grade 1 or 2 renal injury. Genitourinary complications in this subset of patients are minimal (Wessells et al, 1997a; Santucci et al, 2004b; Heyns, 2004). **Patients with isolated grade 3, 4, and 5 renal injuries are also candidates for nonoperative treatment. Even identification of a large perinephric hematoma or urinoma is not an absolute contraindication for nonoperative management, provided the distal ureter is documented to be intact.** In patients with isolated grade 3 to 4 renal injuries, angiographic, endoscopic, or percutaneous intervention will be required in up to 55% of the patients. Intervention will be necessary for persistent or delayed bleeding in approximately 25% and for symptomatic urinomas in approximately 25%, and surgical exploration to control complications not amenable to nonoperative techniques will be required in approximately 5%. In essence, conservative management of isolated grade 3 or 4 renal injuries will save approximately 95% of the patients from open surgical intervention (Husmann and Morris, 1991; Hussman et al, 1993b; Wessells et al, 1997a; El-Khader et al,

Table 132–2.   Consensus Recommendations for Management of Renal Trauma

Clinical Findings and/or Grade of Renal Injury	Recommended Treatment
Grade 1 or 2 renal injury irrespective of traumatic etiology	Nonoperative
Isolated grade 3, 4, and hemodynamically stable grade 5 renal injuries	Nonoperative
Uncontrollable renal hemorrhage/vascular instability (usually grade 4 vascular or grade 5 injuries)	Absolute requirement for surgical intervention
Persistent or delayed hemorrhage not responding to angiographic embolization	Absolute requirement for surgical intervention
Expanding pulsatile retroperitoneal mass found on surgical exploration for coexisting intra-abdominal injuries	Absolute requirement for surgical intervention (verify contralateral renal function before exploration)
Penetrating trauma, inadequate preoperative radiographic staging due to vascular instability of patient, retroperitoneal hemorrhage found on exploration	Retroperitoneal (renal) exploration recommended (verify contralateral renal function)
Blunt trauma, inadequate preoperative radiographic staging due to vascular instability of patient, retroperitoneal hemorrhage found on exploration	Retroperitoneal (renal) exploration recommended (verify contralateral renal function)
Blunt/penetrating trauma, radiographic screening studies reveal grade 3 with devitalized renal fragments, grade 4 or 5 renal injury, coexisting intra-abdominal injuries, especially, duodenum, pancreas, and colon	Retroperitoneal (renal) exploration with renorrhaphy and repair recommended

1998; Buckley and McAninch, 2004; El-Sherbiny et al, 2004; Heyns, 2004; Santucci et al, 2004b).

Nonoperative therapy consists of bed rest, close monitoring of vital signs and urine output, serial abdominal examinations, serial hemoglobin/hematocrit determinations, and transfusion as indicated (Heyns, 2004; Santucci et al, 2004b). In patients with a renal injury secondary to penetrating trauma on a nonoperative protocol, intravenous broad-spectrum antibiotics are recommended owing to the risk of wound contamination. In renal injuries after blunt trauma, antibiotics may be considered if a large retroperitoneal hematoma or urinary extravasation is present. In this latter situation, the presence of a indwelling urethral catheter and/or multiple intravascular catheters may cause bacteremic colonization of the urine or blood and hypothetically result in an infected hematoma or urinoma (Wessells et al, 1997a; Buckley and McAninch, 2004; Heyns, 2004; Kansas et al, 2004; Santucci et al, 2004b).

Repeat CT of the kidney 2 to 3 days after trauma is recommended in patients with a grade 3 renal fracture with a devitalized fragment and in all grade 4 and salvaged grade 5 renal injuries. CT should be pursued earlier if prompted by clinical indications (see earlier). If the child becomes hemodynamically unstable or continues to have a falling hemoglobin/hematocrit despite transfusions, renal angiography with selective angioinfarction of the bleeding site is recommended. If the patient has a urinoma and complains of chronic or increasing flank pain and has a persistent low-grade fever and/or a persistent ileus, consideration for endoscopic or percutaneous management of the urinoma will need to be given. Ambulation is allowed as soon as gross hematuria has resolved; resumption of strenuous physical activity should be avoided for 6 weeks (Wessells et al, 1997a; Buckley and McAninch, 2004; Heyns, 2004; Kansas et al, 2004; Santucci et al, 2004b).

Operative Intervention for Renal Trauma

Absolute indications for renal exploration are hemodynamic instability due to a renal source, an expanding or pulsatile retroperitoneal hematoma, and inability to stop

persistent or delayed hemorrhage via selective vascular embolization. Relative indications are patients with a history of vascular instability resulting in inability to obtain adequate preoperative radiographic evaluations, where surgical exploration for intra-abdominal injuries reveals a retroperitoneal hematoma. Single-shot IVP to verify contralateral renal function is required before renal exploration. Another relative indication for surgical exploration is the presence of coexisting intra-abdominal injuries associated with grade 3 or higher renal injury (see Table 132–2) (Heyns, 2004; Santucci et al, 2004b). **In this latter situation it is the consensus that patients with a known grade 3 or higher renal injury undergoing exploratory laparotomy for multiple organ injury should undergo either renal exploration with renorrhaphy and the placement of retroperitoneal drains or separation of the urinary tract injury from adjacent enteric injuries by interposing omentum or other tissue with concurrent placement of adjacent drainage tubes. Although the surgeon can choose between these two options, he or she should be aware that it is the consensus that renal exploration and renorrhaphy are preferred** (Husmann et al, 1993b; Wessells and McAninch, 1996; Santucci and McAninch, 2001b; Noor and Ather, 2003; Buckley and McAninch, 2004; Heyns, 2004; Santucci et al, 2004b). (See Table 132–2.)

Renal salvage by renorrhaphy or partial nephrectomy requires complete exposure of the injured kidney, débridement of nonviable tissue, suture ligation of bleeding arterial vessels, and repair of collecting system injury. Defects in the renal parenchyma may be closed primarily with renal capsule. For larger defects we prefer the placement of Gelfoam and Surgicel pack into the parenchymal defect with coverage or closure of the renal capsule defect using woven polyglycolic acid mesh. Alternatively, perinephric fat, omentum, or thrombin-soaked Gelfoam may be used to pack the parenchymal defect. Watertight closure of the collecting system is not always possible and may be inadvisable. If the renal pelvis or ureter is closed with excessive stretch, further devascularization, tissue sloughing, and delayed urinary leakage may occur. If a major violation of the urinary drainage system is present, placement of intraoperative ureteral stents or a nephrostomy tube should be considered. Adequate drainage of the perinephric area after repair is vital. In the presence of concurrent duodenal, pancreatic, and colonic injuries, interposition of omentum or peritoneum between the site of the major renal injury and the site of the coexisting intra-abdominal injury is strongly advised. Nephrectomy should be considered in irreparable grade 4 and/or 5 renal injuries and in the hemodynamically unstable patient with multiple organ trauma. A nephrectomy in this latter situation may need to be performed to reduce operative time and help control bleeding in the hypothermic and coagulopathic patient (Heyns, 2004; Santucci et al, 2004b).

KEY POINTS: MANAGEMENT OF RENAL TRAUMA

- The ability of CT to accurately stage renal injuries combined with the application of trauma-related severity scores suggests that emergent nephrectomy at the time of surgical exploration is usually due to either surgical expediency in the unstable patient or preexisting vascular damage, not the consequence of intractable hemorrhage incited by the renal exploration.

- The need to obtain vascular control before renal exploration for a traumatically injured kidney is controversial.

- Nonoperative management is preferred in the hemodynamically stable patient with a grade 1 or 2 renal injury owing to either blunt or penetrating trauma, with or without associated intra-abdominal injuries. It is also the preferred treatment modality in isolated grade 3 and 4 renal injuries.

- Identification of a urinoma is not a contraindication for nonoperative management, provided the distal ureter is documented to be intact.

- Absolute indications for renal exploration after trauma are (1) hemodynamic instability due to renal bleeding, (2) an expanding or pulsatile retroperitoneal hematoma, and (3) inability to stop persistent or delayed hemorrhage via selective vascular embolization.

- Relative indications for renal exploration are (1) retroperitoneal hematoma found at the time of surgical exploration for intra-abdominal injuries in a patient with inadequate preoperative radiographic staging (a single-shot IVP to verify contralateral renal function is required before renal exploration) and (2) CT-documented presence of a grade 3 or higher renal injury coexisting with intra-abdominal injuries that require abdominal exploration.

RENAL VASCULAR INJURIES

In terms of arterial renal blood flow, the kidney is an end organ; only rarely is collateral blood flow outside of the main renal arterial supply sufficient to maintain renal function. **In a patient sustaining renal arterial trauma, the clinical triad**

of hemodynamic instability, inadequate collateral blood flow, and warm ischemic time almost invariably results in the inability to salvage renal function (Heyns, 2004; Santucci et al, 2004b). Because of these facts, no attempt to repair injuries to segmental renal vessels should be considered, and repair of the traumatically injured main renal artery is seldom indicated when a normal contralateral kidney is present. In essence, reconstruction of the main renal artery after trauma is only a primary consideration in patients who are hemodynamically stable with an injury to a solitary kidney or in patients with bilateral renal arterial injuries (Heyns, 2004; Santucci et al, 2004b). The infrequent exception to this rule is the presence of an incomplete arterial injury where perfusion to the kidney has been maintained by flow of blood through either the partially occluded main renal artery or via collateral vessels.

TRAUMA-INDUCED RENAL VASCULAR HYPERTENSION

The most common causes of post-traumatic renal hypertension are renal ischemia from segmental arterial occlusion, main renal artery occlusion with intact peripheral blood flow to the kidney, a traumatically induced arteriovenous malformation, or, on rare occasion, compression of the renal parenchyma by hematoma/fibrosis (the Page kidney model). **The presence of hypertension immediately after the traumatic insult may be secondary to pain, but persistent hypertension 30 days after injury could be due to a renal source and the diagnosis should be considered.** The incidence of traumatically induced hypertension after a grade 3 or higher renal injury is approximately 5% (Heyns, 2004; Santucci et al, 2004b).

Hypertension secondary to renovascular trauma will usually develop within 36 months after the injury (Heyns, 2004; Santucci et al, 2004b). **If sustained hypertension does develop, evaluation with a DMSA scan to determine differential renal function and radiographic studies (magnetic resonance imaging [MRI] or CT angiography) to rule out an arteriovenous fistula as the source of the hypertension should be performed. Hypertension found to be related to an arteriovenous malformation may be treated with angiographic embolization.** If consideration for surgical intervention is entertained, renal vein renin sampling for split renin ratios should be considered. The latter is especially helpful in the presence of segmental renal scarring when partial nephrectomy is a consideration for surgical management. In this situation, hypertension proven to be related to segmental renal ischemia can be treated by partial nephrectomy. **The most common clinical finding in post-traumatic hypertension is a small poorly functioning kidney (<20% function) associated with pan-nephric scarring; nephrectomy is the best surgical alternative** (Wessells et al, 1997a; Moog et al, 2003; Heyns, 2004; Keller et al, 2004; Santucci et al, 2004b). Treatment of hypertension due to a subcapsular hematoma or fibrosis by decortication of the kidney has been published, but the long-term results of this surgical treatment modality are extremely controversial (Heyns, 2004; Santucci et al, 2004b).

- In renal arterial trauma, the clinical triad of hemodynamic instability, inadequate collateral blood flow, and warm ischemic time almost invariably results in inability to salvage renal function. Therefore, repair of the traumatically injured main renal artery is seldom indicated when a normal contralateral kidney is present.

- Hypertension secondary to renovascular trauma will usually develop with 36 months after the injury. If sustained hypertension does develop, evaluation with a DMSA scan to determine differential renal function and radiographic studies (MRI or CT angiography) to rule out development of a arteriovenous fistula as the source of the hypertension should be performed. Hypertension found to be related to an arteriovenous malformation may be treated with angiographic embolization.

- The most common clinical finding in post-traumatic hypertension is a small poorly functioning kidney (<20% function) associated with pan-nephric scarring; nephrectomy is the best treatment alternative.

URETEROPELVIC JUNCTION DISRUPTION

Disruption of the UPJ is most commonly caused by acceleration-deceleration injuries (e.g., fall from >15 ft) or by a sudden extreme hyperextension of the trunk (e.g., pedestrian—motor vehicle accident, ejection injury associated with a motor vehicle accident). The mechanism of injury is hypothesized to be a sudden displacement of the more mobile kidney associated with a relatively fixed ureter, with force vectors from the traumatic impact interacting at the ureteropelvic junction (Boone et al, 1993; Chopra et al, 2002; McAleer et al, 2002).

Although it has been reported that preexisting hydronephrosis or a congenital UPJ obstruction renders the patient more susceptible to a UPJ disruption, this is controversial. The vast majority of patients with a history of trauma and preexisting UPJ or hydronephrosis will be found to have a renal contusion or grade 1 renal injury on evaluation. When urinary extravasation is seen, rupture of the renal pelvis or a major laceration extending through a thinned renal cortex into the collecting system (grade 3 renal injury) is the most common finding, not a UPJ disruption (Boone et al, 1993; Chopra et al, 2002; McAleer et al, 2002; Smith et al, 2003). The majority of patients sustaining a UPJ disruption will present with vascular instability, requiring emergent laparotomy with the patient unable to undergo preoperative imaging. Urinalysis on presentation will have

some degree of hematuria in 70% of patients; however, 30% of patients with UPJ disruption will have a completely normal urinalysis. Emergent exploratory laparotomy for coexisting intra-abdominal injury is usually necessary and exploration fails to reveal the presence of a retroperitoneal hematoma (Boone et al, 1993; Kattan, 2001; Chopra et al, 2002; McAleer et al, 2002). Because of the frequent association of this injury with life-threatening trauma the diagnosis of a UPJ disruption is delayed for more than 36 hours in more than 50% of patients (Boone et al, 1993; Kattan, 2001). Patients will eventually come to attention due to CT abnormalities found during the workup of persistent postoperative fever, chronic flank pain, continued ileus, or sepsis (Boone et al, 1993; Kattan, 2001; Chopra et al, 2002; McAleer et al, 2002). **Three classic findings on triphasic CT are associated with UPJ disruption: (1) good renal contrast agent excretion with medial extravasation of contrast agent in the perirenal and upper ureteral area; (2) absence of parenchymal lacerations; and (3) no visualization of the ipsilateral distal ureter** (Boone et al, 1993; Kattan, 2001; Chopra et al, 2002; McAleer et al, 2002; Heyns, 2004; Santucci et al, 2004b).

Children with preexisting hydronephrosis secondary to congenital hydronephrosis or a UPJ obstruction almost invariably have the site of the injury be a major laceration through the thinned renal cortex (grade 3 renal injury) or laceration of the renal pelvis; rarely is disruption of the UPJ present. These patients should undergo a retrograde pyelogram to confirm continuity of the ureteropelvic junction and then can be safely managed with either a percutaneous nephrostomy or double-J stent placement with delayed pyeloplasty performed after stabilization of the patient (Husmann and Morris, 1991; Matthews et al, 1997; McAleer et al, 2002; Smith et al, 2003).

In patients with a disruption of the UPJ, a delayed diagnosis can be reached up to 12 weeks after injury and will significantly increase the risk of nephrectomy (Boone et al, 1993; Kattan, 2001; Smith et al, 2003). In the clinically stable patient in whom the diagnosis is made within 5 days after the traumatic insult we prefer to proceed to immediate surgical repair with débridement of any devitalized tissue, spatulation and reanastomosis of the ureter over a stent, and placement of an intraoperative nephrostomy tube and retroperitoneal drain. Because the area of ureteral necrosis may extend for 2 to 3 cm, mobilization and downward displacement of the kidney may be necessary to obtain a tension-free anastomosis (Boone et al, 1993; Kattan, 2001). In patients with a delayed diagnosis of 6 or more days we prefer to place a nephrostomy tube and allow the patient and injury to stabilize for 12 weeks. Differential renal function is then obtained via a DMSA renal scan, and the length of the ureteral injury is ascertained by a combined antegrade and retrograde pyelogram. The combination of remaining renal function and the length of the surgical defect allow the surgeon to make the proper surgical planning. Surgical alternatives in this situation include primary uretero-ureterostomy, ileal ureter, autotransplantation, and nephrectomy. It should be noted that if at the time of delayed repair there is significant technical difficulty in mobilization of the kidney, renal pelvis, and blood vessels, nephrectomy as an option should always be discussed and may become necessary (Boone et al, 1993; Kattan, 2001; Heyns, 2004; Santucci et al, 2004b).

URETERAL TRAUMA
External Trauma Resulting in Ureteral Injury

In children, external trauma causing ureteral injuries is rare, occurring in less than 4% of penetrating injuries, and is reportable after blunt trauma (Kotkin and Brock, 1996; Velmahos et al, 1996; Velmahos and Degiannis, 1997; Hudolin and Hudolin, 2003). Ureteral injuries will be found to coexist with renal or bladder injuries in 10% and with other intraperitoneal organ injuries in 90% of the patients. Because of the frequent presence of multiple organ injury the mortality rate of a patient sustaining a ureteral injury from external trauma is in excess of 30% (Velmahos et al, 1996; Wessells et al, 1997a; Hudolin and Hudolin, 2003; Kansas et al, 2004).

Ureteral injuries associated with external trauma will lack the presence of hematuria in up to two thirds of the patients. The diagnosis is usually made via triphasic CT obtained to evaluate penetrating trauma and/or to rule out a genitourinary injury after high-velocity deceleration or impact trauma (Campbell et al, 1992; Kotkin and Brock, 1996; Velmahos and Degiannis, 1997; Medina et al, 1998; Palmer et al, 1999; Hudolin and Hudolin, 2003; Carver et al, 2004). **Gunshot wounds caused by a high-velocity missile (>350 m/s) deserve special mention. The kinetic energy of a high-velocity bullet creates a surrounding energy wave 30 to 40 times the missile diameter** (Al-Ali and Al-Hajaj, 2001; Perez-Brayfield et al, 2001; Hudolin and Hudolin, 2003; Santucci et al, 2004b). **In addition, the missile will frequently yaw or tumble during penetration. The combination of blast injury and missile tumbling results in extensive damage to the surrounding tissues at a significant distance from its path. Of concern regarding high-velocity gunshot wounds to the torso is that radiographic and/or surgical evaluation at the time of the assault may not reveal the presence of a genitourinary injury** (Al-Ali and Al-Hajaj, 2001; Medina et al, 1998; Perez-Brayfield et al, 2001; Hudolin and Hudolin, 2003; Carver et al, 2004; Santucci et al, 2004b). **In some patients with a high-velocity injury, the renal pelvis and/or ureter will appear intact or perhaps only slightly contused at the time of the radiographic examination and/or surgical exploration. As the high-velocity blast injury matures, necrosis of the ureter or portions of the renal pelvis may develop. The extent of the genitourinary injury finally comes to attention as urinary extravasation develops due to delayed necrosis. Classically, blast injuries to the urinary drainage system present as an increase in urine output from surgical placed drains 3 to 5 days after the injury** (Al-Ali and Al-Hajaj, 2001; Medina et al, 1998; Perez-Brayfield et al, 2001; Hudolin and Hudolin, 2003; Santucci et al, 2004b).

Iatrogenic Ureteral Injuries after Open, Laparoscopic, and Endoscopic Procedures

Iatrogenic traumatic ureteral injuries after laparoscopy or open surgical procedures are relatively common in adults after gynecologic and vascular surgery; however, literature reports of iatrogenic ureteral injuries after open procedures in pediatric patients are almost nonexistent. Our personal experience is limited to eight cases: four occurred secondary to resection of large retroperitoneal or osteogenic sarcomas, one was after a partial nephrectomy for a ruptured angiomyolipoma that could not be controlled by angiographic methods, two followed a laparoscopic appendectomy, and one occurred after laparoscopic orchiopexy. The four cases that occurred during resection of retroperitoneal or osteogenic sarcomas were immediately recognized, with 2 to 5 cm of ureter found to be present in the pathology specimen. All cases were treated with either a ureteral reimplantation or ureteral reimplantation with a psoas hitch. The remaining four cases had a delayed diagnosis of more than 6 days (range: 7 to 30 days). The complication was managed by placement of a temporary percutaneous nephrostomy tube and delayed definitive repair.

Because of the refinements in the techniques of ureteroscopy and ureteroscopic equipment, iatrogenic ureteral injuries such as ureteral perforation or avulsion are rare complications, occurring in less than 2% of all prepubertal ureteroscopic procedures (Schuster et al, 2002; Wu and Docimo, 2004; Minevich et al, 2005).

Operative Management of Ureteral Injuries

Ureteral perforation after ureteroscopy can almost invariably be managed with endoscopic intervention with ureteral stenting plus or minus nephrostomy tube placement if clinically indicated. Long-term results are excellent. In the very rare instances when ureteral avulsion has occurred the injury is managed depending on the site of the avulsion and the extent of ureteral devascularization. Treatment protocols are outlined here (Schuster et al, 2002; Wu and Docimo, 2004; Minevich et al, 2005).

If recognized at the time of surgery, ureteral contusions secondary to a high-velocity gunshot wound or inadvertent ligation of the ureter should be treated by removal of any offending clip or ligature and placement of a ureteral stent for 6 to 8 weeks. Long-term radiologic follow-up after removal of the stent is necessary because ureteral contusions may stricture or form fistulas over time.

Similar to the management of a traumatic UPJ disruption, if the diagnosis of a traumatic ureteral injury is made within the first 5 days after the insult, we prefer to proceed with immediate surgical repair. Primarily this consists of débridement of any devitalized tissue, ureteral spatulation, and reestablishment of urinary continuity with either an end-to-end ureteral anastomosis, anastomosis of the ureter to the renal pelvis, or a ureteral reimplantation. The type of procedure employed depends on the site and extent of the ureteral injury. The surgeon should be aware that the area of ureteral necrosis may extend for 2 to 3 cm, and mobilization of the kidney or creation of a bladder flap may be necessary to perform a tension-free anastomosis (Boone et al, 1993; Kattan, 2001). If the patient is hemodynamically unstable and unable to tolerate the additional operative time required for ureteral repair or if the ureteral injury is too extensive to allow for a direct anastomosis, we will tie off the damaged ureter and place a large clip at the proximal end. This maneuver aids in the dissection of the ureteral stump during the delayed repair.

The kidney may then be drained with either placement of an intraoperative or percutaneously placed nephrostomy tube. If a diagnosis of a ureteral injury is made 6 days or longer after the traumatic insult, we would place a percutaneous nephrostomy tube and, if possible, a ureteral stent. **Some authors have recommended management of all traumatic ureteral injuries be via percutaneous nephrostomy tube and stent placement** (Al-Ali and Hajaj, 2001; Ghali et al, 1999). **Other authors have challenged this recommendation, noting that management of traumatic ureteral injuries with endoscopic methods alone has a complication rate of approximately 40%, usually with obliterative ureteral strictures and fistula, whereas open repair has a complication rate of 10%** (Selzman and Spirnak, 1996; Campbell et al, 1992). Our own personal experience mirrors the latter data, and we firmly believe in early open repair as the best solution for this difficult problem.

Assessment of the extent of the ureteral injury and decision on the type of delayed repair that is necessary occurs approximately 12 weeks after the traumatic injury. Radiographic assessment at this time may employ a variety of modalities: antegrade and retrograde pyelography, nuclear renography for differential renal function, CT urography, and cystography. If we have used endoscopic or percutaneous intervention techniques and bridged the area of injury with a ureteral stent, we remove the stent 6 to 8 weeks after the traumatic insult and reassess the upper tract for developing hydronephrosis via ultrasound 6 weeks later. If progressive hydronephrosis is noted, temporary drainage of the upper tract with a nephrostomy tube is performed. Diagnostic radiographic studies to assess renal function and drainage are subsequently performed for 12 weeks after stent removal.

The type of delayed ureteral repair to be used is based on the location and the extent of ureteral damage. Options include ureteral anastomosis to the renal pelvis, primary ureteroureterostomy, transureteroureterostomy, ureteral reimplantation with or without a psoas hitch, ileal ureter, autotransplantation, and, on occasion, nephrectomy. We would caution that the use of transureteroureterostomy places the contralateral uninjured kidney and ureter at risk. This could convert a unilateral traumatic ureteral injury into a bilateral ureteral injury with an iatrogenic component, subsequently placing the surgeon at significant litigious risk. Based on this concern, we personally dislike this surgical alternative in managing these difficult problems.

BLADDER INJURIES

The urinary bladder is well protected from external trauma by the bony confines of the pelvis. Because of the extensive pelvic protective mechanisms, when bladder injuries do occur they are frequently associated with multiple organ trauma, with an average of three coexisting organ injuries and a mortality rate of 20% (Carroll and McAninch, 1984). Although it was once recommended that all patients with a history of blunt abdominal trauma presenting with either microscopic or gross hematuria should undergo bladder imaging, studies have revealed that this recommendation is associated with an extremely low yield for injury and is cost ineffective (Mokoena and Naidu, 1995; Cunningham et al, 1998; Iverson and Morey, 2001). **Absolute indications for bladder imaging after blunt**

abdominal trauma are currently limited to two indications: (1) the presence of gross hematuria coexisting with a pelvic fracture and (2) inability to void. Neither gross hematuria alone nor pelvic fracture alone is an absolute indication for screening. Relative indications for bladder imaging after blunt abdominal trauma are urinary clot retention, perineal hematoma, and a history of prior bladder augmentation (Mokoena and Naidu, 1995; Cunningham et al, 1998; Iverson and Morey, 2001). **Bladder imaging after penetrating trauma should be performed any time concern exists that the missile could have injured the bladder and/or if free abdominal fluid is found on the initial CT scan** (Cunningham et al, 1998).

Differences between Adults and Children in Traumatic Bladder Injuries: Lacerations through the Anterior Bladder Neck

Traumatic bladder lacerations in children are approximately two times more likely to extend through the bladder neck compared with the adult (Husmann et al, 1990; Boone et al, 1992; Koraitim, 1997, 1999; Chapple, 2000). The clinical importance of this fact is significant. Specifically, management

---

KEY POINTS: URETEROPELVIC JUNCTION DISRUPTION AND URETERAL INJURIES

- In patients sustaining a UPJ disruption, 30% will have a completely normal urinalysis.

- Owing to the frequent association of traumatic UPJ disruption with life-threatening trauma, the diagnosis of this injury is delayed for more than 36 hours in more than 50% of patients. Patients will eventually come to attention due to CT abnormalities found during the workup of persistent postoperative fever, chronic flank pain, continued ileus, or sepsis.

- Three classic findings on triphasic CT are associated with UPJ disruption: (1) medial extravasation of contrast agent in the perirenal and upper ureteral area; (2) contrast agent extravasation in the absence of parenchymal lacerations; and (3) no visualization of the ipsilateral distal ureter.

- In the clinically stable patient in whom the diagnosis of UPJ or ureteral disruption is made within 5 days after the traumatic insult, immediate surgical repair is the preferred treatment.

- In patients with a delayed diagnosis of UPJ or ureteral disruption made 6 or more days after the traumatic insult, placement of a nephrostomy tube with delayed repair at 12 weeks is preferred.

- The type of ureteral repair used is based on the location and extent of the ureteral injury.

of a bladder neck laceration with either a suprapubic tube alone and/or urethral catheter alone without coexisting repair of the bladder neck may result in the persistent extravasation of urine, with the possible development of a pelvic urinoma/abscess or pelvic osteomyelitis, and in the long term may result in a increased risk of urinary incontinence (Husmann et al, 1990; Boone et al, 1992; Koraitim, 1997; Chapple, 2000). The diagnosis of a bladder neck injury should be suspected any time extravasation of contrast agent is noted, and a competent bladder neck cannot be documented via radiographic studies. If concern for a bladder neck injury is present, the patient should undergo surgical exploration with opening of the bladder at the dome. Repair of the bladder neck should be via an intravesical approach with a multilayered closure. Great care should be given not to dislodge the pelvic hematoma to help prevent blood loss. The surgeon should be aware that anterior bladder neck lacerations are frequently associated with urethral injuries, and retrograde urethrography or cystoscopy to rule out this possibility should be considered. If a bladder neck laceration is repaired, a voiding cystourethrogram is necessary at the time of catheter removal to adequately visualize the bladder neck and confirm healing (Husmann et al, 1990; Boone et al, 1992; Kotin and Koch, 1995; Husmann, 1996).

Diagnosis of Bladder Injuries

The diagnosis of a traumatic bladder injury should be assessed by either standard or CT cystography. Either modality is accurate provided adequate bladder distention occurs. **In a child, the amount instilled within the bladder should, at a minimum, be equal to one half of the estimated bladder capacity for age (60 mL at birth and 30 mL for each year thereafter); instillation of contrast agent can stop at the maximum of bladder capacity for age, at a total of 300 mL, or if a bladder contraction occurs.** We would discourage performing a CT cystogram by plugging the catheter and evaluating the bladder at the time of the initial CT scan. Frequently the injured patient has oliguria secondary to hypovolemia, resulting in diminished urine output, with inadequate filling of the bladder. In our experience, performance of a CT cystogram by plugging the catheter alone has led to missing the diagnosis of a traumatic bladder injury on multiple occasions (Husmann, 1996; Haas et al, 1999; Peng et al, 1999; Deck et al, 2001; Iverson and Morey, 2001).

Classification and Treatment of Traumatic Bladder Injuries

All patients with traumatic bladder lacerations, either extraperitoneal or intraperitoneal, should initially be treated with intravenous antibiotics with oral antibiotic therapy continued for 48 hours after removal of bladder catheters. Extraperitoneal injuries are twice as common as intraperitoneal injuries and are almost invariably associated with a pelvic fracture. Classically, extraperitoneal bladder ruptures will have a starburst appearance on radiographic studies. **In the presence of an extraperitoneal bladder injury, consideration for open surgical intervention should be given if a bony spicule is found to protrude into the bladder on CT**

evaluation or if concern for a bladder neck laceration is present (Kotin and Koch, 1995; Husmann, 1996). **If these two complications are not present, management by an indwelling urethral catheter can be considered.** The age and size of the patient plays a major role in determining if the individual can be managed by an indwelling urethral catheter. In our experience a small-caliber urinary catheter placed in young children will frequently be occluded by blood clots. Placement of a large-bore urethral catheter to allow better drainage is a concern in young boys because of the possibility of producing a urethral stricture; therefore, a large-caliber suprapubic tube should be placed (Kotin and Koch, 1995). Urinary drainage via the bladder catheter is maintained for 7 to 10 days, and a cystogram should be obtained to verify healing of the injury before catheter removal.

Intraperitoneal bladder injuries will initially appear as free fluid in the abdomen on CT. Instillation of contrast agent in the bladder will result in extravasation of the contrast into the peritoneal cavity. Almost all intraperitoneal bladder ruptures occur at the dome of the bladder, the site of least support by the perivesical surrounding structures. Because these lacerations are usually large, the bladder neck's integrity frequently cannot be assessed by radiographic means (Husmann, 1996). **In intraperitoneal bladder injuries, open surgical repair of the laceration is the recommended treatment modality. This allows the surgeon to reduce any herniating omentum or small bowel from the confines of the bladder and allows careful intravesical inspection of the bladder neck at the time of surgical exploration.** In all patients, a perivesical drain is placed and a large-bore urinary catheter is used to provide urinary drainage. In younger females and/or boys, persistent gross hematuria with clots may occlude small-caliber urethral catheters and placement of a larger-bore suprapubic tube is usually merited. Urinary drainage for 7 to 10 days after injury should be provided and a cystogram obtained before catheter removal.

URETHRAL INJURIES
Differences between Pediatric and Adult Patients in Urethral Injuries

Owing to the immature pelvis and the relative intra-abdominal position of the child's bladder, children with a posterior urethral injury will differ from adults with this injury in four ways. **First, a pelvic fracture is more likely to be unstable and associated with a severely and permanently displaced prostatic urethra. Second, the severe displacement of the prostate off the pelvic floor makes a complete posterior urethral disruption more common in boys than men. Third, in children, concurrent bladder and urethral injuries may occur in up to 20% of the patients, with coexisting anterior longitudinal tears though the bladder neck and sphincteric complex being twofold more common in children compared with adults. Fourth, in prepubertal girls, pelvic fractures are four times more likely to be associated with a urethral injury than in adult women** (Husmann et al, 1990; Boone et al, 1992; Perry and Husmann, 1992; Koraitim, 1997, 1999; Chapple, 2000; Hemal et al, 2000).

The clinical impact of these differences is noteworthy. Permanent displacement of the prostate off the pelvic floor results

KEY POINTS: BLADDER INJURIES

- Absolute indications for bladder imaging after blunt abdominal trauma are currently limited to two indications: (1) the presence of gross hematuria coexisting with a pelvic fracture and (2) complaints of inability to void.

- Bladder imaging after penetrating trauma should be performed any time concern exists that the missile could have injured the bladder and/or if free abdominal fluid is found on the initial CT scan.

- Traumatic bladder lacerations in children are approximately two times more likely to extend through the bladder neck compared with the adult.

- Failure to repair a bladder neck injury may result in the persistent extravasation of urine with the possible development of a pelvic urinoma/abscess and osteomyelitis and increases the risk of permanent urinary incontinence.

- Traumatic bladder injuries can be accurately diagnosed by either standard or CT cystography, provided adequate bladder distention occurs. In a child, the amount instilled within the bladder should at a minimum be equal to one half of the estimated bladder capacity for age.

- In the presence of an extraperitoneal bladder injury, consideration for open surgical intervention should be given if a bony spicule is found to protrude into the bladder on CT evaluation or if concern for a bladder neck laceration is present. If these two complications are not present, management by an indwelling urethral catheter can be considered.

- In intraperitoneal bladder injuries, open surgical repair of the laceration is the recommended treatment modality. This allows the surgeon to reduce any herniating omentum or small bowel from the confines of the bladder and allows careful intravesical inspection of the bladder neck at the time of surgical exploration.

in an increased need for a transpubic, trans-symphyseal, or combined transpubic and perineal dissection for urethral reconstruction compared with the adult patient population. Hypothetically, the severe displacement of the prostate off of the pelvic floor raises concern that erectile dysfunction will be more common in children sustaining a urethral injury than adults (Husmann et al, 1990; Boone et al, 1992; Perry and Husmann, 1992; Koraitim, 1997; Chapple, 2000; Basiri et al, 2002). There is also apprehension that permanent urinary incontinence may be more likely in children after this injury owing to the increased risk of combined injuries to the posterior urethra, bladder neck, and sphincteric complex (Husmann et al, 1990; Boone et al, 1992; Perry and Husmann, 1992; Hemal et al, 2000).

Initial Presentation of Urethral Injury

Consideration for a urethral injury should arise any time a patient presents with a history of direct trauma to the penis, vagina, perineum, or pelvis. Radiographic or cystoscopic evaluations to rule out this injury are mandatory in the following circumstances: **(1) when the patient presents with the classic triad of findings of a perineal/penile hematoma, blood at the meatus/vaginal introitus, and inability to void; 2) when one or more pubic rami are fractured or symphyseal diastases are present; and (3) when radiographic findings suggest a bladder neck injury** (Chapple, 2000).

Association of Pelvic Fractures to Posterior Urethral Distraction Injuries

The risk of a urethral injury after pelvic fracture is directly related to the number of broken pubic rami, if there has been separation of the pubic symphysis, and whether there is displacement of the posterior pelvic arch (Colapinto, 1980; Kricum, 1990; Koraitim et al, 1996; Koraitim, 1999). The likelihood of a urethral injury after isolated fractures of the acetabulum, ilium, and sacrum that do not involving a fracture of a ramus or the separation of the pubic symphysis is essentially zero.

Diagnosis of Urethral Injuries

In males, retrograde urethrography (RGUG) is the diagnostic modality of choice to rule out the presence of a urethral injury (Fig. 132–1). In the prepubertal and postpubertal female, findings suggestive of a urethral injury are frequently noted on a CT evaluation, but we prefer to confirm the diagnosis by cystoscopy and vaginoscopy performed under general anesthesia (Husmann et al, 1990; Boone et al, 1992; Perry and Husmann, 1992).

When a urethral injury is found to coexist with a pelvic fracture a digital rectal examination is mandatory. The finding of blood in the stool signifies that an occult rectal injury may be present. In our experience, coexisting rectal and urethral injuries have been found in approximately 15% (11/73) of boys younger than age 16 years with traumatic posterior urethral injuries associated with pelvic fractures. Treatment of the rectal injury with a temporary diverting colostomy in this patient population is mandatory to prevent the disastrous consequences of pelvic abscess, pelvic osteomyelitis, and necrotizing fasciitis that can accompany an unrecognized rectal injury.

General Comments Regarding Repair of Urethral Injuries: Immediate, Delayed, and Late Urethroplasty

In the early phase of the injury the most important potential urologic complication is infection induced by bacterial contamination of the pelvic/perineal hematoma and extravasated urine. **Immediate treatment of urethral injuries should include the administration of broad-spectrum antibiotics, assessment of competence of the bladder neck, and establishment of urinary drainage.** Repair of the urethral injury

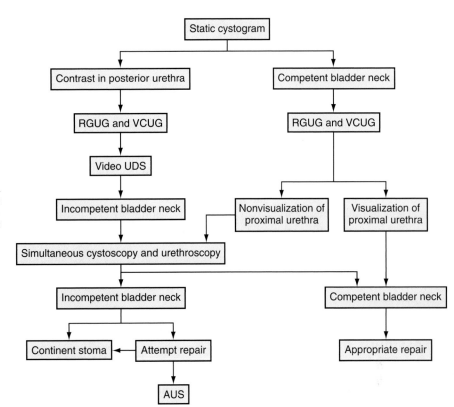

Figure 132–1. Algorithm for posterior urethral distraction injuries before delayed operative repair. RGUG, retrograde urethography; VCUG, voiding cystourethrography; AUS, anastomotic urethroplasty.

may be immediate (primary realignment or sutured primary end-to-end anastomosis, <2 days post injury), delayed (primary realignment or sutured end-to-end anastomosis) occurring 2 to 14 days after injury, or late (any type of repair occurring 3 months or more after injury) (Boone et al, 1992; Perry and Husmann, 1992).

Anterior Urethral Injuries

Anterior urethral injuries in children are usually iatrogenic, due to urethral instrumentation, circumcision, or injury occurring during the repair of a congenital anorectal malformation. If the anterior urethra was injured due to urethral instrumentation, acute management should be with antibiotic therapy, followed by establishment of urethral continuity with catheter drainage. Preferably, a urethral catheter is placed by either radiologic or endoscopic techniques and maintained for 5 to 21 days depending on the extent of the injury. If urethral continuity cannot be established, alternative treatments include temporary suprapubic tube placement or vesicostomy. If a urethral or suprapubic catheter is placed, a voiding cystourethrogram is obtained at the time of anticipated catheter removal. If no persistent urethral injury is noted, we obtain a follow-up RGUG in 3 months in infants; alternatively, in a child who is potty trained, a flow rate with ultrasound residual urine is adequate for follow-up. If a permanent urethral stricture develops we will usually defer definitive surgical repair until the child is either older than 1 year of age or, if the child is older than 1 year of age, wait at least 3 months since the time of the injury (i.e., a late urethroplasty). The delay in the repair allows the stricture to clearly delineate the extent of

the injury, allowing the physician to plan for the urethral reconstruction.

Three types of urethral injuries can result after a circumcision: meatal injury, loss of the distal urethra secondary to partial or complete glanular amputation, and the development of a urethrocutaneous fistula due to ischemic necrosis of the urethra. The latter injury usually occurs when the urethra was either crushed by a circumcision clamp or when a cautery or a suture ligature was used to stop bleeding from a vessel that was overlying the urethra (Baskin and Canning, 1997). Immediate repair of the acutely traumatized anterior urethra can be technically difficult. When the meatus is injured, a formal meatoplasty should be performed to prevent meatal stenosis from developing. When the glans with distal urethra has been amputated it may be reattached successfully using a direct spatulated suture anastomosis of the urethra and glans with urethral stenting, perioperative antibiotics, and compressive dressing for immobilization of the glans. When a partial distal urethral injury has occurred without substantial glans loss, suture reapproximation of the meatus (i.e., a meatoplasty) can be performed. After healing, a delayed repair using hypospadias techniques may be utilized if it is necessary. Urethrocutaneous fistulas are repaired using techniques similar to those used to close fistulas after a hypospadias repair; this surgery is usually delayed until the child is 6 to 9 months of age for technical reasons (Gluckman et al, 1995; Baskin and Canning, 1997).

We have had a number of children referred to us for repair of urethral injuries that occurred at the time of surgical correction of their congenital anorectal malformation. **In our experience this injury is usually due to one of two causes: no**

urethral catheter was in situ at the time of the rectal repair or the urethral catheter had been placed into the rectum via the urethrorectal fistula. In these circumstances, the proximal penile or bulbar urethra is usually excised or partially avulsed at the time of rectal dissection. The injury is frequently identified when the child is unable to void after surgery or voids through the perineal wound. The importance of an appropriately placed urethral catheter at the time of anorectal repair cannot be understated. Initial placement of the catheter before repair of the anorectal malformation may be difficult owing to the catheter hanging up at the site of the rectourethral fistula or inadvertently passing into the rectum. Placement of the catheter over a cystoscopically placed glide wire before the surgical repair of this congenital anomaly is frequently helpful. This allows for easy identification of the urethra; and if the urethral catheter becomes exposed during the case, the problem is recognized immediately and can usually be primarily repaired with rare long-term consequences (Spence, 1954; Williams and Grant, 1969; McLorie et al, 1998; Hong et al, 2002).

Assessment of Urethral Stricture before Delayed Repair

At the time surgical reconstruction is considered, usually 3 months after injury, RGUG followed by a simultaneous RGUG and VCUG are the first studies performed (if a suprapubic catheter or vesicostomy has been performed a static cystogram is also performed). Correctly performed RGUG will allow the physician to identify the location of the urethral stricture but may not allow the appropriate determination of the stricture's length, especially if an extremely tight bulbar or posterior urethral distraction injury is present. Proper interpretation of these three radiographic studies is essential for true estimation of the defect between the disrupted urethral ends. Without correct interpretation of the studies the urethral defect may be underestimated (contrast agent filling of a urinoma cavity associated with an incompetent bladder neck) or overestimated (nonfilling of the normal urethra due to failure of the bladder neck to open with voiding). When contrast agent from the static cystogram is found in the posterior urethra it arouses suspicion for a bladder neck injury and mandates further evaluation, as discussed below (see Fig. 132–1). If the bladder neck is competent, we obtain simultaneous RGUG and VCUG. Great care should be taken in interpreting these films. More often than not the pediatric patient will be unable to void and will fail to open the bladder neck. This results in nonvisualization of the proximal urethral segment and may cause a spurious estimation of a long distraction defect. If the posterior urethra fills with contrast agent on the static cystogram, this could be due to either a poorly felt or described detrusor contraction or an incompetent bladder neck. Because of the significant impact the latter has on the surgical prognosis, if contrast agent is seen in the posterior urethra, a video-urodynamic study is necessary. If the video-urodynamic study documents an incompetent bladder neck, or if the patient was unable to open up the bladder neck to see the posterior urethra during the VCUG, we perform a simultaneous flexible cystoscopy and urethroscopy. (On occasion, the physician may need to use flex-

ible ureteroscopes for this procedure in small children.) This examination allows the physician to confirm the anatomic detail of the bladder neck and allows determination of the extent of the urethral stricture. Specifically, we obtain anteroposterior and oblique pelvic films with the flexible scopes placed at the distraction margins; this allows the physician to see the extent and orientation of the distraction injury. Alternatively, a pelvic MR image with three-dimensional reconstruction can be obtained to evaluate the prostatic urethral dislocation and distal bulbar urethral position. The latter radiographic study lacks the ability to evaluate bladder neck competence. If cystoscopy and video-urodynamics demonstrate an incompetent bladder neck, we discuss with the patient and the family the options of urethral reconstruction, with the possible result of chronic incontinence or, alternatively, the performance of a continent abdominal stoma, appendicovesicostomy, as first-line therapy. See the later section, "Mitrofanoff Principle for Bladder Neck Incompetence after Posterior Urethral Injuries."

Endoscopic Repair of the Urethral Injury: Immediate Endoscopic Realignment, Delayed Urethroplasty with Direct Internal Visual Urethrotomy, and Delayed Urethroplasty with "Cut to Light Procedure"

Immediate endoscopic realignment using guide wires and urethral catheters for either partial or complete anterior or posterior urethral disruptions has been recommended by some authors (Husmann et al, 1990, 1993a; Koch, 1995; Elliott and Barrett, 1997). **We believe this technique is extremely reasonable for partial urethral injuries secondary to iatrogenic catheter or endoscopically induced urethral injuries, but in our hands endoscopic realignment for non-iatrogenic urethral trauma has resulted in abysmal long-term results. Indeed, in our patient population with non-iatrogenic urethral trauma managed by this technique the need for intermittent catheterization or repeated serial visual internal urethrotomies to maintain urethral patency was necessary in more than 90% of children during long-term follow-up. Owing to our personal poor experience with urethral realignment in children with non-iatrogenic traumatic urethral injuries, we have elected not to pursue this treatment modality in patients younger than 16 years of age** (Husmann et al, 1990; 1993a; Boone et al, 1992; Elliott and Barrett, 1997; Freitas Filho et al, 2003).

The "cut to light procedure," or antegrade and retrograde urethroscopy with either endoscopic incision or laser ablation of the obliterative urethral stricture, received publicity as a less-invasive form for treating obliterative posterior urethral distraction injuries in the late 1980s. Long-term follow-up has led most authorities in the field to abandon this treatment method. In our personal experience with cut-to-light urethroplasties for less than 1-cm obliterative urethral strictures, our long-term success in 22 patients younger than 16 years of age was 0%, with all individuals requiring either daily intermittent catheterization or a formal urethral reconstruction to maintain patency. At this point we would strongly recommend against treating obliterative urethral strictures by a cut-to-light procedure in children (Husmann et al, 1990; Boone et al, 1992; Kohrmann et al, 1994; Niesel et al, 1995; Levine and Wessells, 2001; Koraitim, 2004).

Endoscopic urethrotomy for short, less than 1-cm nonobliterative bulbar and penile urethral strictures is commonly performed for pediatric urethral stricture disease. Unfortunately, follow-up on these patients in adulthood is limited. Short-term follow-up of 1 year will frequently reveal success rates as high as 75% to 100%, but follow-up intervals of more than 5 years reveal success decreasing into the 20% to 35% range, with some studies suggesting that you can double your long-term success by repeating the urethrotomy on at least one occasion. **Repeating the urethrotomy more than one time does not appear to enhance its success and may in fact decrease the successful result of the eventual open urethral reconstruction** (Roehrborn and McConnell, 1994; Duel et al, 1998; Hsiao et al, 2003; Hafez, 2005).

Anastomotic Urethroplasty

The principles of anastomotic urethral reconstruction include complete excision of the scar tissue and a widely spatulated anastomosis with a tension-free epithelial-to-epithelial approximation associated with viable urethral margins. **An anastomotic urethroplasty through either the perineal, transpubic, trans-symphyseal, or combined approach has a reported success of more than 90% in the pediatric patient population.** The excellent outcome of this procedure verifies that the end-to-end anastomotic urethroplasty is the procedure of choice for distraction urethral injuries in both children and adults (Boone et al, 1992; Koraitim, 1997, 2004; Chapple, 2000; Holland et al, 2001; Levine and Wessells, 2001; Basiri et al, 2002). A direct end-to-end anastomosis of up to 2 cm may be performed in most children. Gaps of 3 cm or more usually require partial or complete pubectomy or symphysiotomy with or without splitting the penile crura to accomplish the anastomosis (Boone et al, 1992; Koraitim, 1997, 2004; Chapple, 2000; Holland et al, 2001; Levine and Wessells, 2001; Basiri et al, 2002). As noted previously, because of the propensity of the child's prostatic urethra to be permanently displaced off the pelvic floor after a posterior urethral distraction injury there will be a tendency for children to require either a partial pubectomy, symphysiotomy, or combined perineal and transpubic urethroplasty to complete the urethral reconstruction more often than in adults (Koraitim, 1997; Basiri et al, 2002; Park and McAninch, 2004).

Patch Urethroplasties: Flap versus Graft (One-, Two-, or Multiple-Stage Procedures)

Repair of traumatic urethral strictures of the bulbar, proximal, and penile urethra of more than 3 to 4 cm in length in children is usually pursued using a one-stage flap procedure from the prepuce or penile shaft skin (Orlandi procedure) or, if local skin is unavailable, a dorsal graft urethroplasty using a free skin graft or buccal mucosa (Schreiter and Noll, 1989; Barbagli et al, 2004; Park and McAninch, 2004; Schulte-Baukloh et al, 2004; Dubey et al, 2005). We prefer to do a single-stage repair, by approximating at least one side of the urethra and using the flap or graft on the opposing wall. If the defect is great enough that the flap or graft must be used in a circumferential manner (tube) we will opt for a two or multiple-stage approach. The use of a staged reconstruction is based on the realization that recurrent strictures are more likely to occur when any flap or graft is used in a circumferential manner (tube) as a single-stage procedure (Al-Ali and Al-Hajaj, 2001; Andrich and Mundy, 2001; El-Sherbiny et al, 2002; Dubey et al, 2003; Kessler et al, 2003; Manzoni et al, 2004). Staging the operation by performing a classic two-stage Johannson urethroplasty or preferentially a multiple-staged preputial flap or buccal graft urethroplasty allows the surgeon to verify flap/graft survival and provide time for neovascularity and the assessment of the urethral plate for possible hair-bearing skin before urethral closure. In general, the length of the urethral stricture, the availability of well-vascularized excess adjacent skin, and the health of the donor bed determine if we use a one-, two-, or multiple-stage approach (Schreiter and Noll, 1989; Roehrborn and McConnell, 1994; Koraitim, 1997; Kessler et al, 2003; Barbagli et al, 2004; Park and McAninch, 2004; Schulte-Baukloh et al, 2004; Dubey et al, 2005).

Female Urethral Injuries

Urethral injuries in females are invariably associated with an unstable pelvic fracture and are usually caused by a disruption of the pubic symphysis with a longitudinal laceration extending through the bladder neck and into the urethra or by dislocation of a bony fragment that lacerates the urethra, resulting in distraction of the two severed margins. Female urethral injuries may be quite insidious and are associated with concurrent vaginal laceration in 75% and concurrent rectal injuries in 30% (Venn et al, 1999; Chapple, 2000). **Blood at the vaginal introitus or the presence of a rectal injury in combination with a pelvic fracture should prompt the physician to consider a diagnosis of a female urethral injury.** Urethroscopy and vaginoscopy should be considered mandatory in these individuals. If the patient is clinically stable, immediate end-to-end urethroplasty for avulsion distraction injuries and primary bladder neck repair and repair of the longitudinal lacerated urethra over a urethral catheter should be performed. Concurrent repair of vaginal and rectal injuries (with a diverting colostomy) should be performed when indicated. Preliminary diversion with a suprapubic cystostomy without any treatment of the urethra will invariably result in either a urethral stricture, urinary fistula, or both. Delayed repairs of these injuries using a two-stage approach involving preliminary suprapubic cystostomy followed by a definitive reconstruction is less successful. Delayed urethral repair and establishment of urinary continence via bladder neck reconstruction, sling, or artificial urinary sphincter placement, frequently results in incontinence, urethral erosion with fistula formation, or proximal urethral obliteration. Indeed, the need for urinary diversion or a continent abdominal stoma to manage complications of the female bladder neck and urethral injuries occurs in up to 30% of

Mitrofanoff Principle for Bladder Neck Incompetence after Posterior Urethral Injuries

In patients with bladder neck incompetence and concurrent urethral stricture disease, we have pursued two different treatment options. Initially, reconstruction of the bladder neck with reestablishment of urethral continuity is performed. If subsequent urinary incontinence persists, as it almost inevitably does, we proceed with placement of an artificial sphincter or bladder neck sling. Alternatively, we may initially proceed with a continent catheterizable stoma using the Mitrofanoff principle with no attempt to reestablish urethral continuity (Cendron and Gearhart, 1991; Castera et al, 2001; Freitas Filho et al, 2003). Indeed, personal experience with these two techniques has resulted in our preference for a continent stoma. Unfortunately, placement of an artificial urinary sphincter or sling around the bladder neck or urethra after bladder neck reconstruction and end-to-end urethroplasty is technically difficult and fraught with the risk of delayed urethral erosion.

Erectile Dysfunction and Urinary Incontinence after Urethral Injuries

For decades it was argued that immediate repair of posterior urethral disruption injuries by primary urethral anastomosis and/or primary urethral realignment was directly associated with an increased incidence of erectile dysfunction and urinary incontinence. **Current studies have failed to reveal an association between the type of repair (immediate vs. late) and the incidence of erectile dysfunction and urinary incontinence. At this time it is believed that the severity of the primary injury and not the initial treatment modality chosen is the cause of these complications** (Husmann et al, 1990; Boone et al, 1992; Shenfeld et al, 2003).

The incidence of erectile dysfunction is increased when total disruption of the urethra occurs and/or when the prostate is grossly dislocated, both of which are more common in children than in adults (Boone et al, 1992; Husmann et al, 1990; Koraitim, 1997, 1999; Chapple, 2000; Hemal et al, 2000). Indeed, **long-term follow-up of children sustaining a posterior urethral disruption revealed erectile dysfunction may occur in up to 70% of children when severe dislocation and injury to the apical prostatic urethra occurred, compared with a 30% incidence of erectile dysfunction when significant prostatic dislocation did not occur** (Boone et al, 1992). As in erectile dysfunction, the etiology of urinary incontinence after urethral injuries is almost invariably related to the presence of a concurrent bladder neck/urethral injury or is found to be a consequence of pelvic or pudendal nerve damage resulting in denervation of the sphincteric complex (Husmann et al, 1990; Koraitim, 1997, 1999; Chapple, 2000; Hemal et al, 2000).

KEY POINTS: URETHRAL INJURIES

- A urethral injury should be ruled out in the following three circumstances: (1) if the classic triad of a perineal/penile hematoma, blood at the meatus/vaginal introitus, and inability to void is present; (2) if a pelvic fracture is associated with one or more fractured pubic rami and/or symphysis diastases; and (3) if radiographic findings are suggestive of a bladder neck injury.

- When a pelvic fracture and a urethral injury are present a digital rectal examination is mandatory. Blood in the stool signifies the possibility of a concurrent occult rectal injury and is found in approximately 15% of male and 30% of female pediatric patients with simultaneous pelvic fractures and a urethral injury.

- In a young girl with a pelvic fracture, if blood is noted at the vaginal introitus or if a concurrent rectal injury is present, urethral injury must be ruled out.

- Immediate treatment of urethral injuries should include the administration of broad-spectrum antibiotics, assessment of competence of the bladder neck, and the establishment of urinary drainage.

- Short, less than 1-cm nonobliterative bulbar and penile urethral strictures may be treated by a urethrotomy, with a success rate approaching 20% to 35%. Repeating the urethrotomy more than one time does not appear to enhance its success and may, in fact, decrease the success of an open urethral reconstruction.

- After a posterior urethral injury, the incidence of erectile dysfunction and urinary incontinence is directly related to the severity of the primary injury, that is, the severity of the prostatic dislocation, the concurrent presence of a bladder neck injury, or the presence of trauma-induced pelvic or pudendal nerve damage; it is not the result of the initial treatment modality chosen.

PENILE INJURIES

Penile trauma in the pediatric patient population is most commonly iatrogenic and caused by circumcision. **If excess penile skin is excised during circumcision, the majority of patients can be treated by wet-to-dry dressings and antibiotic ointment. Healing by secondary intention usually results in an excellent cosmetic appearance. If the penis is totally degloved, the penile shaft skin, if salvaged, can be defatted and replaced on the penis as a full-thickness skin graft** (Gluckman et al, 1995; Baskin and Canning, 1997).

Penile strangulation caused by a hair or thread is occasionally seen. In most cases it is hard to believe that this insult is purely accidental and consideration for social service investigation for possible child abuse should be given. The human hair-tie will result in the gradual onset of ischemia with little or no discomfort of the child. If seen early, the glans or distal penis will be edematous, erythematous, and ulcerated. The constricting hair or thread may not be noticeable without careful inspection. Removal of the constricting agent at this stage usually results in no long-term complications. Unfortunately, if the child presents in a delayed fashion or if the original diagnosis is missed, the hair may continue to cut through the penis, causing damage to the neurovascular bundle, corporeal bodies, and urethra. Injuries range from loss of glanular sensation to the development of a urethrocutaneous fistula and, in the extreme form, partial or complete penile amputation (El-Bahnasawy and El-Sherbiny, 2002; Radhakrishnan et al, 2002).

Domestic animal attack is the most severe form of penile trauma usually seen in childhood. These penile injuries are usually associated with significant tissue destruction and fraught with complications due to bacterial contamination. Treatment requires verification of a current tetanus vaccination and absence of rabies in the offending animal. The patient is treated with the liberal use of antibiotics, wound cleansing, and débridement and repair or reattachment of the penis as the injury would direct (El-Bahnasawy and El-Sherbiny, 2002; Radhakrishnan et al, 2002).

KEY POINTS: PENILE INJURIES

- During a circumcision excision of excess penile skin in the vast majority of patients can be treated by wet-to-dry dressings and antibiotic ointment with healing by secondary intension resulting in excellent cosmetic appearance.

- If during the circumcision the penis is totally degloved, the penile shaft skin, if salvaged, can be defatted and replaced back onto the penis as a full-thickness skin graft.

- Penile strangulation caused by a hair is occasionally seen, and consideration for social service investigation for possible child abuse should be given.

- Domestic animal attack is the most severe form of penile trauma seen in childhood. Treatment requires verification of a current tetanus vaccination and absence of rabies in the offending pet. The patient is treated with the liberal use of antibiotics, wound cleansing, débridement, and repair or reattachment of the penis as the injury would direct.

SCROTAL/VULVAR AND TESTICULAR TRAUMA

In the pediatric patient trauma to the scrotum/vulva is usually the result of athletic activities, an assault, or a fall. It is classi-

cally broken down into the two categories of penetrating or blunt trauma. If the patient has sustained penetrating scrotal or vulvar trauma, concern for associated injuries to the urethra and rectum exists (Husmann et al, 1993b). Evaluation should include a rectal examination with stool tested for occult blood and urinalysis. The presence of occult blood in the stool or hematuria should prompt further evaluations for coexisting urethral and rectal injuries. If sedation in the emergency department is inadequate in allowing the physician to perform a thorough physical examination of the genitalia, it may be necessary to bring the patient to the operative suite for general anesthesia. In all cases of penetrating trauma a meticulous examination to determine the depth of penetration, cleansing and débridement of the wound, administration of broad-spectrum antibiotics, and verification of an up-to-date tetanus immunization are employed.

Scrotal bruising and/or significant testicular discomfort should prompt concern for testicular injury and the use of either scrotal ultrasonography or MRI evaluation (Martinez-Pinero et al, 1992; Corrales et al, 1993; Mulhall et al, 1995; Srinivas et al, 2002). Radiologic evidence of a hematocele, rupture of the tunica albuginea, or intratesticular hematoma mandates surgical exploration (Martinez-Pinero et al, 1992; Corrales et al, 1993; Mulhall et al, 1995; Srinivas et al, 2002). We would stress that the presence of a hematocele alone even if no tunical lacerations can be visualized via radiographic evaluation should result in surgical exploration. Small tunical tears not seen via radiographic methods can result in extrusion of seminiferous tubules, the development of antisperm antibodies (clinical significance unknown), and testicular loss (Mulhall et al, 1995; Kukadia et al, 1996). Successful repair of a testicular injury is related to the extent of the testicular rupture and the time to repair. A delay in the diagnosis or treatment of testicular injury of more than 72 hours can result in a threefold to fourfold increased risk of testicular loss compared with immediate repair. Surgical treatment consists of removal and drainage of the scrotal hematoma, excision of necrotic tissue, and suture reapproximation of the tunica albuginea (Mulhall et al, 1995; Kukadia et al, 1996).

SUGGESTED READINGS

Buckley J, McAninch J: Pediatric renal injuries: Management guidelines from a 25-year experience. J Urol 2004;172:687-690.

Hemal A, Dorairajan L, Gupta N: Posttraumatic complete and partial loss of urethra with pelvic fracture in girls: An appraisal of management. J Urol 2000;163:282-287.

Koraitim M: Posttraumatic posterior urethral strictures in children: A 20-year experience. J Urol 1997;157:641-645.

Santucci R, Langenburg S, Zachareas M: Traumatic hematuria in children can be evaluated as in adults. J Urol 2004a;171:822-825.

Santucci R, Wessells H, Bartsch G, et al: Evaluation and management of renal injuries: Consensus statement of the renal trauma subcommittee. BJU Int 2004b;93:937-954.

INDEX

Note: Page numbers followed by the letter f refer to figures; those followed by t refer to tables.

Adrenal tumor(s) *(Continued)*
  oncocytoma as, 1843
  pheochromocytoma as. *See*
    Pheochromocytoma.
  testicular, 929-930
  testosterone-secreting, 1841-1842
Adrenal vein, 11f, 14, 23f, 24
  bleeding from, in radical nephrectomy, 1711
Adrenal vein sampling, in primary
  hyperaldosteronism, 1853-1854
Adrenalectomy
  clinical indications for, 1869, 1870t
  complications of
    postoperative, 1886, 1886t
    surgical, 1885-1886, 1885t
  contraindications to, 1869-1870
  for adrenal carcinoma, 1870t, 1871
  for Cushing's syndrome, 1870t, 1871
  for pheochromocytoma, 1870t, 1871
  history of, 1868
  laparoscopic. *See* Laparoscopic adrenalectomy.
  nonsurgical alternatives to, 1887
  obesity and, 1870
  open, 1871-1876
    complications of, 1886-1887
    flank retroperitoneal approach to, 1871-
      1873, 1872f, 1873f
    for specific tumors, 1870t
    indications for, 1870
    lumbodorsal posterior approach to, 1873-
      1874, 1874f
    subcostal anterior approach to, 1874-1875,
      1876f
    thoracoabdominal approach to, 1875-1876,
      1876f, 1877f
  outcomes of, 1885
  partial, 1887
  past surgical history and, 1870
  postoperative management of, 1884
  preoperative management of, 1871
    errors in, 1871t
  prophylactic, for congenital adrenal
    hyperplasia, 3820
  surgical options for, 1870, 1870t
  tumor size and, 1870
Adrenaline, 1821
Adrenergic agonists, effect of, on ureteral
  function, 1905-1906
α-Adrenergic agonists
  causing geriatric incontinence, 2308, 2308t
  for stress incontinence, 2075
  uropharmacology of, 1952
β-Adrenergic agonists
  for urethral sphincter dysfunction, in
    children, 3620
  uropharmacology of, 1952
Adrenergic antagonists, effect of, on ureteral
  function, 1906
α-Adrenergic antagonists
  causing geriatric incontinence, 2308-2309,
    2308t
  for benign prostatic hyperplasia, 2777-2787
    adverse events associated with, 2786
    classification of, 2777-2777, 2778t
    coexisting hypertension and, 2786
    comparison of, 2786-2787
    dose response of, 2778
    effects of
      in elderly, 2786
      on acute urinary retention, 2785-2786
      on bladder outlet obstruction, 2785
    future of, 2787
    literature review of, 2779-2785
    rationale for, 2777

α-Adrenergic antagonists *(Continued)*
    recommended dosage of, 2778t
    study designs for, 2778
  for bladder outlet obstruction, 2318-2319
  for pheochromocytoma, preoperative, 1866,
    1871
  for prostatitis, 321, 325t
  for smooth sphincter dysfunction, 2118-2119
  for urethral sphincter dysfunction, in
    children, 3620
  prophylactic, for postoperative urinary
    retention, 2040-2041
  uropharmacology of, 1952-1953, 1953f
β-Adrenergic antagonists
  erectile dysfunction caused by, 743, 744t
  preoperative, for pheochromocytoma, 1866
  uropharmacology of, 1952
Adrenergic receptors
  α-, 1952
  β-, 1952
α-Adrenoceptor agonists
  combination, 2111
  for stress incontinence, 2109-2111
  nonselective, 2109-2111
  selective, 2111
β-Adrenoceptor agonists
  for overactive bladder/detrusor overactivity,
    2093t, 2103-2104
  for stress incontinence, 2112
Adrenoceptor antagonists, for erectile
  dysfunction, 778-779
α-Adrenoceptor antagonists
  erectile dysfunction caused by, 743, 744t
  for overactive bladder/detrusor overactivity,
    2093t, 2103
β-Adrenoceptor antagonists, for stress
  incontinence, 2111
Adrenocortical tumors, in children, 3878
Adrenocorticotropic hormone (ACTH)
  ectopic, in Cushing's syndrome, 1831t
  production of, 1825-1826
  secretion of, 578, 637
Adrenocorticotropic hormone (ACTH)
  syndrome, Cushing's disease and, 1836-
    1837, 1837f
Adrenoreceptors, action of, on spinal cord,
  1962-1963
Advancement techniques, of hypospadias repair,
  3722, 3723f
Advancement test, in laparoscopic surgery, 180,
  180f
Afferent pathways, in lower urinary tract, 1938-
  1939, 1938f, 1939t
AG-013736, for renal cell carcinoma, 1630, 1630t
Age. *See also* Geriatric patients.
  altered bladder sensation with, 1970
  androgen deficiency and, 850-862. *See also*
    Hypogonadism, late-onset.
  at time of hypospadias repair, 3718
  bladder cancer and, 2409
  bladder contractility and, 1969-1970
  detrusor overactivity and, 1969-1970
  effect of, on ureteral function, 1916-1917,
    1917f
  erectile dysfunction and, 746
  germ cell tumor incidence and, 899-900
  gestational
    fractional excretion of sodium and, 3150
    glomerular filtration rate and, 3151
    maximal renal caliceal diameter according
      to, 1220t
  hormones affected by, 856-857, 856t
    historical perspective on, 850-851
  incontinence and, 2189, 2305-2306, 2306f

Age *(Continued)*
  of hypothalamic-pituitary axis, in males, 580
  onset of hypertension and, 1167
  pediatric urinary tract infections and, 3236
  pelvic organ prolapse and, 2189
  physiologic vs. chronologic, in orthotopic
    urinary diversion, 2616
  postpyelonephritic scarring and, 4338
  prostate cancer diagnosis and, 2856
  prostate cancer screening and
    discontinuation of, 2925-2926
    start of, 2924-2925
  renal calculi and, 1364
  vesicoureteral reflux and, 4324, 4325t
  voiding dysfunction and, 2043
Agenesis
  bladder, antenatal detection of, 3575
  of seminal vesicles, 1113-1114, 1114f
  of vas deferens, 3797-3798
  penile, 3756-3757, 3757f
    in bilateral renal agenesis, 3271
  renal, 3269-3276. *See also* Renal agenesis.
  sacral, 3644-3645, 3645f-3647f, 3647
  vaginal, 3833-3839. *See also* Vaginal agenesis.
Aging Male Survey (AMS), of late-onset
  hypogonadism, 853, 854f
AGTR2 gene, in vesicoureteral reflux, 4326
AIDS. *See* Acquired immunodeficiency
  syndrome (AIDS).
Albendazole
  for filariasis, 457
  for hydatid disease, 459
Alcock's canal, 71
Alcohol
  consumption of
    benign prostatic hyperplasia and, 2745
    erectile dysfunction caused by, 746
    male infertility and, 645
    patient history of, 88-89
    priapism associated with, 841
    prostate cancer associated with, 2863
  intraspinal injections of, for painful bladder
    syndrome/interstitial cystitis, 366
Aldosterone
  metabolism of, 1828
  secretion of
    in adrenal carcinoma, 1847-1848
    physiologic control of, 1826-1827, 1827f
Aldosterone:cortisol ratio, in primary
  hyperaldosteronism, 1854
Aldosterone-producing adenoma, treatment of,
  1856-1857
Aldosterone:renin ratio, in primary
  hyperaldosteronism, 1851-1852, 1854
Aldosterone-secreting adrenal tumor, 1842
Aldosteronism, glucocorticoid-remediable, 1848-
  1849
  diagnostic tests for, 1849
Alfuzosin
  for benign prostatic hyperplasia, 2784-2785
    dosage of, 2778t, 2785
    efficacy of, 2785t
  for prostatitis, 321, 327t
  uropharmacology of, 2119
  vs. other α-adrenergic blockers, 2787
Alginate, for tissue engineering, 555
Alkalemia, 1152
Alkalosis, 1152
  after augmentation cystoplasty, 3682
    in children, 3682
  metabolic, 1153, 1153t, 1154, 1154t
  renal tubular, 1153-1154
  respiratory, 1154
Allantois, embryology of, 3573

Cancer therapy. *See also specific type, e.g.,*
Chemotherapy.
spermatogenesis and, 611
targets for
death receptors as, 530
ligands as, 530
Cancer vaccines, 499-500
Candida
in intertrigo, 424, 424f
in prostatitis, 307
infection with. *See* Candidiasis.
Candida albicans
in pediatric urinary tract infections, 3265
in urinary sediment, 106f, 109
in vaginitis, 385
Candidemia
in children, 3265
kidney associated with, 462
predisposing factors for, 460
Candidiasis, 459-464
clinical manifestations of, 460, 460f, 462
cutaneous, 460
diagnosis of, 462-463
disseminated, treatment of, 461t, 464
epidemiology of, 459-460
in children, 462
of bladder, 460, 469f
of female genitalia, 460
of kidney, 462
management of, 300
of male genitalia, 460
of prostate, 460, 468f
of ureters, 462
predisposing factors in, 460
radiography of, 463, 463f
systemic, 462
treatment of, 463-464
treatment of, 463-464
antifungals in, 461t, 464t
vulvovaginal, 385, 460
Candiduria, 460
treatment of, 463
Cannula site, bleeding at, in laparoscopy, 209,
209f, 216
Cannulation, tubal, in evaluation of fertility, 612
Cantwell-Ransley repair, modified, of bladder
exstrophy, 3520, 3520f-3523f, 3523-3524
results of, 3531-3532
Capacitation, of sperm, 605
Capillary hemangioma, of male genitalia, 433
Capsaicin
efficacy of, vs. resiniferatoxin, 2107
for incontinence, 2072
for painful bladder syndrome/interstitial
cystitis, 362t, 364
intravesical therapy with, 2106-2107
uropharmacology of, 1958
Capsular artery, 63, 63f
Captopril, for cystinuria, 1425
Captopril test, for renovascular hypertension,
1169
Captopril-enhanced renography, of renovascular
hypertension, 1170
Caput epididymis, 597, 598. *See also* Epididymis.
Carbohydrate(s), intake of, in acute renal failure,
1338
Carbon dioxide, for pneumoperitoneum, in
laparoscopic surgery, 199
Carbon dioxide embolus, pediatric laparoscopy
and, 3917
Carbon dioxide lasers
for penile cancer, 973, 993
in lithotripsy, 1514
Carbon monoxide, in renal hemodynamics, 1135

Carbonated beverages, for nephrolithiasis, 1411-
1412
Carboplatin, for hormone-refractory prostate
cancer, 3105t
Carcinoembryonic antigen (CEA), T cell
recognition of, 496
Carcinogen(s), in bladder cancer, 2413, 2414
screening for exposure to, 2436-2437
Carcinogenesis
mutation and, 513, 513f
prostate, genes implicated in, 2861
Carcinoid(s)
of kidney, 1635-1636
of seminal vesicles, 1116
of testis, 930
Carcinoma. *See specific type, e.g.,* Transitional
cell carcinoma.
Carcinoma in situ
of bladder, 2418-2419, 2418f
BCG therapy for, 2455
of testes, 896-897, 899t
cryptorchidism associated with, 3773, 3902
in adolescents, 3901-3902
management of, 897, 899, 899t
of upper urinary tract, 1643, 1655
Carcinosarcoma
of bladder, 2444-2445
of prostate, 2881
Cardiac anomalies, in prune-belly syndrome,
3485t, 3486
Cardiac arrest, in laparoscopy, 211
Cardinal ligaments, 2197, 2198f
Cardiomyopathy, catecholamine-induced,
pheochromocytoma associated with, 1859
Cardiovascular disease
erectile dysfunction with, 777-778, 778f
in primary hyperaldosteronism, 1851
Cardiovascular system, effects of testosterone
therapy on, 859
Cardiovascular toxicity, of contrast media, 113
Cartilage cells, injections of, for bladder neck
reconstruction, in children, 3666
Caruncle, urethral, vs. urethral diverticula, 2384-
2385, 2384f
CASA (computer-assisted semen analysis), 617.
See also Semen analysis.
Casale continent catheterizable stoma, in
continent vesicostomy, 3698, 3699f
Cascade phenomena, of complement activation,
474
Case mix, in health care costs, 146-147
Caspases, in regulation of apoptosis, 531, 1205
Caspofungin, 469
cost of, 464t
dosage of, 461t
Cast(s), in urinary sediment, 107, 107f, 108f
Castration, for prostate cancer
medical, 3083, 3087-3088, 3087t
surgical, 3082-3083, 3085, 3085t
Catecholamine(s)
action of, 1829-1830, 1829t
metabolism of, 1829, 1830f
synthesis of, 1828-1829, 1829f
urinary, effects of drugs on, 1863t
Catecholamine receptors, action of, 1829t
Catheter(s). *See also specific catheter, e.g.,* Foley
catheter.
bacteriuria associated with, 296-297
condom, for geriatric incontinence, 2317-2318
dilating
in percutaneous nephrostomy, 1541, 1558-
1560, 1558f, 1559f
postoperative removal of, in renal
transplant recipient, 1313-1314

Catheter(s) (*Continued*)
in urodynamic studies, 1988-1989
indwelling, urinary tract infection associated
with, 238
intraurethral, stenting with, 2806
removal of, after orthotopic urinary diversion,
2633
single/dual, in postoperative vesicovaginal
fistula drainage, 2333
ureteral
commonly used, 170f
for ureteroscopy, 1511t, 1512, 1512f
urethral. *See* Urethral catheter.
Catheterization
bladder calculi related to, 2665-2666
clean intermittent
for bladder filling/storage disorders, 2294-
2295
for cloacal disorders, 3865-3866, 3866f
for urethral sphincter dysfunction, in
children, 3620
in renal transplant recipients, 1300
continuous, for bladder filling/storage
disorders, 2295-2297
ureteral, in localizing site of bacteriuria, 241,
241t
urethral. *See* Urethral catheterization.
Catheterizing pouches, continent, for continent
urinary diversion, 2586-2591
care of, 2588-2589
methodology of, 2587-2588
patient's questions regarding, 2588
surgical principles in, 2586-2587, 2587f
Cation(s), transport of, effect of ureteral
obstruction on, 1202-1203
Cauda equina syndrome, 2031
Caudal embryology, 3830-3832, 3831f
Caudal regression syndrome, 3832
Cautery wire balloon endopyelotomy, for
ureteropelvic junction obstruction
complications of, 1238-1239
indications for and contraindications to, 1237,
1237f
postoperative care following, 1237
results of, 1237-1238
technique of, 1237, 1238f
Cautery wire balloon incision
in endopyelotomy, 1237
in ureteral stricture repair, 1257-1258
Caveolae, ureteral, 1891
Caveolin, 540
Cavernosal fibrosis, penile prosthesis for, 798-
800, 799f, 800f
Cavernosography, pharmacologic, 762, 762f
Cavernosometry, pharmacologic, 761-762
Cavernous artery, 721, 721f, 1035, 1035f
occlusive pressure of, evaluation of, 760,
761f
pharmacologic arteriography of, 760-761, 761f
Cavernous (subcutaneous) hemangioma, of
male genitalia, 3760
Cavernous nerve, 724, 725f
stimulation of, 724-725
Cavernous vein, 723f, 1034, 1034f
Cavitation mechanism, of stone fragmentation,
1476
CD (cluster of differentiation) markers, 475-477,
476t
CD4+ T cell(s)
activation and expansion of, 485, 485f
dendritic cell activation of, 485f
in HIV infection, 389, 391, 392
in painful bladder syndrome/interstitial
cystitis, 341

Genitourinary tract *(Continued)*
 parasitic, 448-459
 pediatric, 3232-3268
 tuberculous, 436-447. *See also* Tuberculosis.
 injury to, in children, 3929-3945. *See also specific anatomic site; specific injury.*
  assessment and treatment of, 3930-3932
  grading of, 3931t
  imaging of, indications for, 3930
  vs. adult injury, 3929-3930
 pediatric urinary tract infections and, 3240-3241. *See also* Urinary tract infection, in children.
  recurrent, 3261-3262
  radiation-induced, 3016t
Gentamicin
 for pediatric urinary tract infections, 3248t
 intravenous, 3249
 prophylactic, prior to pediatric genitourinary procedures, 3242t
Geriatric patient
 bacteriuria in, 293-296, 295f, 1138f
 benign prostatic hyperplasia in, α-adrenergic blockers for, 2786
 detrusor hyperactivity with impaired contractility in, 2310
 frequency in, 2311
 incontinence in, 2306-2309
  cause(s) of
   detrusor overactivity as, 2309-2310
   detrusor underactivity as, 2310
   DIAPERS mnemonic for, 2306, 2307t
   established, 2309-2311
   functional, 2310-2311
   lower urinary tract, 2309-2310
   outlet obstruction as, 2310
   pathologic, 2306-2308, 2307t
   pharmaceutical, 2308-2309, 2308t
  diagnostic categorization of, empirical, 2313-2314
  diagnostic evaluation of, 2059-2070, 2311-2313
  functional, 2310-2311
  history-taking in, 2311-2312, 2312t
  laboratory investigation of, 2313
  physical examination for, 2312-2313
  stress, 2310
  stress testing in, 2313
  transient, causes of, 2059t, 2306-2309, 2307t, 2308t
  treatment of, 2314-2320, 2314f
   adjunctive measures in, 2317-2318
   behavioral therapy in, 2314-2316
   stepwise approach to, 2315t
   urodynamic testing in, 2314
   voiding diary in, 2312, 2312f
 nocturia in, 2311-2312, 2312t
 tension-free vaginal tape procedure in, 2254
Germ cell(s)
 aplasia of, infertility and, 634
 primordial, migration of, 579, 3803, 3803f
 Sertoli cells associated with, 588, 589f, 591-592, 591f
 transformation of, 3803-3804
Germ cell tumor(s), testicular, 893-925. *See also specific type.*
 acquired causes of, 901
 clinical manifestations of, 902-903
 clinical staging of, 903-904, 904t, 905t, 938
 congenital causes of, 900-901
 diagnosis of, delay in
 differential diagnosis of, 903
 epidemiology of, 899-900
 etiology of, 900-901

Germ cell tumor(s), testicular *(Continued)*
 high-stage
  fertility in, 957
  post-chemotherapy pathologic findings in, 951t
  surgery for
   complications of, 955-956
   high-risk post-chemotherapy patients and, 953-954
   histologic findings and controversies in, 950-951
   late-relapse and, 953
   lung resection as, 955
   mediastinal resection as, 955
   neck resection as, 955
   nonseminomatous tumors and, 950-956
   post-chemotherapy RPLND as, 954-955
   predicting necrosis in, 952-953
   preoperative preparation for, 950
   reoperative retroperitoneal, 954-955
   teratomas and, 951-952
   timing of, 950
 histologic classification of, 893-895, 894t
 imaging of, 905
 in children, 3902-3904, 3903t
 incidence of, 899
 intratubular, 896-897, 899, 899t
 low-stage
  fertility in, 949
  treatment options for, 948-949
 natural history of, 901, 938
 nongonadal, 924-925
 nonseminomatous, 895-896. *See also* Nonseminomatous germ cell tumor(s).
 pathogenesis of, 901
 patterns of spread of, 901-902, 939
 scrotal ultrasonography of, 903
 seminomatous, 894-895. *See also* Seminoma(s).
 signs and symptoms of, 903
 treatment of, 936-950. *See also* Orchiectomy; Retroperitoneal lymph node dissection (RPLND).
  anatomic considerations in, 939, 939f
  for nonseminomatous tumors, 913-924, 950-956
   options in, 948-949
  for seminomas, 909-913, 956-957
  organ-preserving surgery in, 908-909
  principles of, 908-924
 tumor markers for, 893, 906-908
Gerota's fascia, 26, 27f, 28
Gestational age
 fractional excretion of sodium and, 3150
 glomerular filtration rate and, 3151
 maximal renal calyceal diameter according to, 1220t
GH (growth hormone), affected by aging, 856t, 857
Gibson incision, in renal transplantation, 1310
Giggle incontinence, in children, 3612
Gil-Vernet procedure, in antireflux surgery, 4366
Ginkgo biloba, for erectile dysfunction, 770t
Ginseng, for erectile dysfunction, 770t
Girlie disease, 1160. *See also* Perimedial fibrodysplasia.
Gishiri cutting, vesicovaginal fistula following, 2325
Gitelman's syndrome, in children, 3229
Gittes bladder neck suspension, for stress incontinence, 2212-2213
Glands of Littre. *See* Periurethral glands.

Glans penis. *See also* Penis.
 anatomy of, functional, 721
 cutaneous lesions of, 960
 in erection, hemodynamics of, 724
 lymphatic drainage of, 1035
 partial removal of, with Mogen clamp, 3748
 poor support of, in penile prosthesis implantation, 797, 798f
 squamous cell carcinoma of, 1012, 1012f
Glansectomy, partial, for squamous cell carcinoma, 1012-1013, 1013f
Glanuloplasty. *See also* Meatoplasty and glanuloplasty (MAGPI) technique.
 in hypospadias repair, 3718
Gleason grading
 of adenocarcinoma of prostate, 2876, 2877f
 of prostate cancer, 2926, 2928t-2929t
Glenn-Anderson technique, of antireflux surgery, 4356, 4356f
Glial cell line–derived neurotrophic factor
 in ureteral development, 1891
 in ureteric bud outgrowth, 3129, 3129f
Global Response Assessment, of painful bladder syndrome/interstitial cystitis, 355, 356t
Globulin, sex hormone–binding, 767
 assessment of, in females, 872
Glomerular circulation, effect of angiotensin II on, 1163
Glomerular filtration rate
 autoregulation of, 1132
 clinical assessment of, 1132-1133
 determinants of, 1131-1132, 1326
 estimation of
  by creatinine clearance, 3230t
  mathematical formulas in, 1133
 factors influencing, 1195
 in acute renal failure, 1325-1326
 in chronic renal failure, 1341-1342, 1342t
 in fetus, 3149-3150
 in infant and child, 3153
 in neonate, 3151-3152, 3152f, 3153f
  regulation of, 3158, 3158f
 oncotic pressure in, 1132
 permeability in, 1132
 plasma markers in, 1133, 1133f
 regulation of, 1132
 renal clearance in, 1132-1133
 renal plasma flow and, 1132
 transglomerular (hydraulic) pressure in, 1131-1132
 tubuloglomerular feedback in, 1132
 urinary tract obstruction and, 1195-1196
Glomerulations, in painful bladder syndrome/interstitial cystitis, 352-353, 352f
Glomerulocystic kidney disease
 familial hypoplastic, 3329
  characteristics of, 3314t
 sporadic, 3350-3351
  characteristics of, 3314t
  conditions associated with, 3350t
Glomerulonephritis
 acute, 1327-1328, 1328t
 focal. *See* IgA nephropathy (Berger's disease).
 membranoproliferative, in chronic renal failure, 1345-1346
 membranous, retroperitoneal fibrosis associated with, 1270-1271
 postinfectious, in children, 3226
 rapidly progressive, differential diagnosis of, 1328t
Glomerulosclerosis
 focal segmental, in children, 3225-3226
 in renal transplant recipient, 1297-1298

Glomerulotubular balance, 1138
Glomerulus(i)
    disorders of, hematuria associated with, 98-
        99, 99f, 99t
    foam cells of, 1344
    injury to, in children, management of, 3597-
        3598
    microscopic anatomy of, 31, 32f
Glucocorticoids
    actions of, 1827-1828, 1828t
    excess of, male infertility and, 638
    for cutaneous diseases, of external genitalia,
        406
    hypercalcemia associated with, 1376-1377
Glucose
    in urine, 103-104
    metabolism of, 852-853
    renal reabsorption of, in proximal convoluted
        tubules, 1140, 1141f
    tubular reabsorption of, in neonate, 3156
Glue, fibrin-based, in laparoscopy, 193
Glutamate
    in spinal cord, 1964
    uropharmacology of, 1962-1963
γ-Glutamyl transpeptidase, in testicular tumors,
    907
Glutaraldehyde cross-linked bovine collagen
    (GAX-collagen) injections, for
    incontinence, 2274
    adverse effects of, 2284t
    efficacy of, 2282-2283
    safety of, 2285
Glutathione S-transferase, in prostate cancer,
    2866
Gluteal artery, inferior, 50f, 51
Glycosaminoglycan(s), in painful bladder
    syndrome/interstitial cystitis, 343-345, 363
Glycosaminoglycan layer, of urothelium, 1932-
    1933
Glycosides, effect of, on ureteral function,
    1920
GMP. See Guanosine monophosphate (GMP).
GnRH. See Gonadotropin-releasing hormone
    (GnRH).
Gomco clamp, 1045, 3215
Gonad(s). See also Ovary(ies); Testis(es).
    descent of
        in females, 3144f, 3145
        in males, 3143-3145, 3144f
    in sexual differentiation, 3803-3804, 3803f
        disorders in, 3808-3816. See also specific
            disorder.
    function of, 3804-3805, 3805f
    renin-angiotensin-aldosterone system and,
        1163
Gonadal artery, 11f, 13, 13t
Gonadal dysgenesis syndrome(s), 3809-3814
    mixed, 3811-3812
    partial, 3812-3813
    "pure," 3811
    Turner's syndrome as, 3809-3811, 3810f
    46,XY complete, 3813-3814, 3813f, 3814f
Gonadal stromal tumor(s), testicular, 927-928
Gonadal vein, 11f, 13
    excision of, in left-sided laparoscopic RPLND,
        946-947
Gonadal vessels, dissection of, in right-sided
    laparoscopic RPLND, 946
Gonadoblastoma(s), 926t, 928-929
    in children, 3901, 3904-3905
    in complete androgen insensitivity syndrome,
        risk of, 3824
    in 46,XY complete gonadal dysgenesis, 3814,
        3814f

Gonadoblastoma(s) (Continued)
    in mixed gonadal dysgenesis, 3812
    in Turner's syndrome, 3810-3811
Gonadotropin(s). See also specific hormone.
    therapy with, for male infertility, 636, 646
Gonadotropin-releasing hormone (GnRH)
    for cryptorchidism, 3776
    in male reproductive axis, 577, 578f
    in males, 618
    therapy with, for male infertility, 636, 646
Gonadotropin-releasing hormone (GnRH)
    stimulation test, in males, 619
Gonorrhea, 379
    rates of, 372
Goodwin technique, transcolonic, of
    ureterointestinal anastomosis, 2556,
    2556f
Gouty diathesis, 1405, 1405f
    treatment of, 1424
Gouverneur's syndrome, 2351
Graft(s). See also Allograft(s); Xenograft(s).
    for vesicovaginal fistula repair, 2332, 2340
    free, in hypospadias repair, 3716
        neourethral formation and, 3734, 3736-
            3738, 3738f
        reoperative, 3741
    full-thickness, 1025
    imbibition of, 1023
    in penile curvature repair, 3714, 3715f
    in penile reconstruction
        saphenous interposition, 1095
        split-thickness, 994, 996, 996f
    in reconstructive surgery, 1023, 1024f-1025f,
        1025-1026
    in urethral stricture repair, 1062, 1064-1066f,
        1067
    in vaginal prolapse surgery
        biologic, 2216
        synthetic, 2216, 2216t
    in vaginal repair surgery, 2220t, 2222, 2223f
    inosculation of, 1023, 1025
    interposition nerve, in radical retropubic
        prostatectomy, 2976-2977
    kidney. See Kidney graft.
    mesh, 1025
    saphenous interposition, in penile
        reconstruction, 1095
    split-thickness, 1025
        in penile reconstruction, 994, 996, 996f
        in reoperative hypospadias repair, 3741
    vascular, placement of, ureteral obstruction
        due to, 1223
Granular cell myoblastoma, of bladder, 2445
Granulocyte(s), 477
Granulocyte-macrophage colony-stimulating
    factor, source and activity of, 486t
Granuloma
    after vasovasostomy, 678
    sperm, 1102, 1108
Granulomatous disease, hypercalcemia
    associated with, 1376
Graspers, laparoscopic, 190, 191f
Gravimetric flowmeter, 1989
Grayhack shunt, for priapism, 848, 848f
Great vessels, anatomy of, 6f, 9, 11f, 13-14, 13t,
    14f
    anatomy of. See also specific vessel, e.g.,
        Aorta.
Greater omentum, in vesicovaginal fistula repair,
    2339-2340
Green tea
    for prostate cancer, chemopreventive, 2871
    in prevention of bladder cancer, 2443
GRHPR gene, in hyperoxaluria, 1378

Growth
    and development, detrimental effect of
        conduit urinary diversion on, 2574
    delayed, after augmentation cystoplasty, in
        children, 3682
    of prostate. See also Prostate, growth of.
        endocrine control of, 2684-2689
        regulation of
            balance of cell replication and death in,
                2711-2715
            steroid receptors in, 2696-2705
            steroids and protein growth factors in,
                2689-2696
Growth factor(s). See also specific growth factor.
    in benign prostatic hyperplasia, 2731-2732,
        2731f
    in bladder cancer, 2428-2429
    in prostate, 2705-2711
    in renal cell carcinoma, 1590
    mechanism of action of, 2706, 2707f
    properties of, 2706t
Growth factor receptors, 2706, 2708-2711
Growth hormone (GH), affected by aging, 856t,
    857
Growth pathways, in hormone-refractory
    prostate cancer, 3115-3116
Guaifenesin calculi, 1389
Guanosine monophosphate (GMP), cyclic
    in penile smooth muscle relaxation, 732
    in smooth muscle relaxation, 1954
    in ureteral smooth muscle contraction,
        1901
Guanylyl cyclase, in male sexual function, 735
Guarding reflex, 1975
    in continence, 2049
Gubernaculum
    development of, 3762
    female, 3145
    in testicular descent, 3768-3769
    innervation of, 3145
    male, 3143-3145
Guide wires
    for ureteroscopy, 1509, 1510f, 1511t, 1512,
        1512f
        safety, 1515-1516
            cystoscopic placement of, 1515
    in percutaneous nephrostomy, 1541
Guillain-Barré syndrome, voiding dysfunction
    in, 2035
Gunshot wounds
    to kidney, 1274
    to penis, 1050, 2650-2651
    to ureters, hematuria with, 1284-1285
Gynecomastia, 613
    androgen deprivation therapy causing, 3091
    germ cell tumors associated with, 903
    in Klinefelter's syndrome, 3809
    testosterone therapy causing, 859

H

H flap. See also Flap(s).
    in Peyronie's disease surgery, 833, 835f, 836,
        836f
HAART (highly active antiretroviral therapy)
    for HIV infection, 401
        immune-based strategies with, 403-404
    for HIVAN, 398
Haemophilis ducreyi, in chancroid, 374
Hailey-Hailey disease, 417, 417f
Hair, in penile strangulation injury, 2652
Hair growth, intraurethral, after hypospadias
    repair, 3740
Hald-Bradley classification, of voiding
    dysfunction, 1984, 1984t

Immunity (Continued)
    phagocytosis in, 474
    role of, 496
  passive, 502
  primary, 478
  secondary, 478
  T-cell receptor in, 479-480
  to infections, 500-502, 502t
  to uropathogens, 235-236
Immunobead test, for antisperm antibodies, 624t
Immunobiology, of renal cell carcinoma, 1588-1589
Immunoglobulin(s). See also Antibody(ies).
  classes of, 478
  in seminal plasma, 2724
Immunoglobulin A, secretion of, 475
Immunohistochemistry, in diagnosis of oncology, 547-548
Immunologic infertility, in males, 649-650
Immunology, molecular, 502-503, 504f
Immunosuppressants
  in renal transplantation, 1316-1317
    infection and peptic ulcer prophylaxis and, 1317, 1318t
    mechanism of action of, 1316t
    potential drug interactions among, 1317, 1317t
    protocol for, 1317, 1317f
    sites of action of, 1316f
    toxicity of, organ targets for, 1317, 1318t
  pregnancy safety and, 1323t
  secretion of, as mechanism of tumor escape, 497-498, 498f
Immunotherapy
  for bladder cancer, non–muscle-invasive, 2455-2458
    bacille Calmette-Guérin in, 2455-2457, 2457t, 2458t
      chemotherapy with, 2460
    interferon in, 2457
    investigational agents in, 2457-2458
  for painful bladder syndrome/interstitial cystitis, 360t, 361
  for prostate cancer, 3030
    hormone-refractory, 3116-3117
  for renal cell carcinoma, 1588-1589
    metastatic, 1629
  for retroperitoneal fibrosis, 1217, 1272
  for tumors, 499-500
  for urothelial tumors, 1651, 1651t
Imperforate anus, 3647, 3647t
  associated findings in, 3647-3648
  evaluation of, 3648, 3649f
  in neonate, 3195
  in unilateral renal agenesis, 3275, 3275f
Imperforate hymen, 3843-3844, 3844f
  with hydrocolpos, 3194
Imperforate vagina, cervix and uterine duplication with, 3839, 3839f, 3840f
Impetigo, in HIV patients, 396-397
Implant, penile. See Penile prosthesis.
Implantable microballoons
  for bladder filling/storage disorders, 2292
  for incontinence, 2286-2287
Impotence, 86. See also Erectile dysfunction; Penile detumescence; Priapism.
  after urethral distraction injuries, 2661
  arteriogenic, 740-742
  hormonal, 740
  in end-stage renal disease, 1301
  neurogenic, 739-740
  patient history of, 87

Impotence (Continued)
  psychogenic, 739
  venogenic, 742
In vitro fertilization. See also Assisted reproductive techniques (ARTs).
  with intracytoplasmic sperm injection, 650, 651, 652, 717-718, 718f
Incision(s). See also specific incision.
  electrosurgical, 191
  in adrenal surgery
    flank, 1871-1873, 1872f, 1873f
    lumbodorsal, 1873, 1874f
    subcostal, 1874, 1875f
    thoracoabdominal, 1875-1876, 1876f
  in antireflux surgery, 4351
  in radical nephrectomy, thoracoabdominal, 1709-1710, 1711f, 1712f
  in radical retropubic prostatectomy, 2959-2960
    endopelvic fascia, 2960-2961, 2961f
  in renal surgery
    abdominal, 1695-1698, 1697f-1701f
    dorsal lumbotomy, 1695, 1696f
    flank, 1691-1694, 1691f-1695f
    thoracoabdominal, 1698, 1701f-1702f, 1703
  in simple nephrectomy
    flank, 1703, 1703f-1705f
    transperitoneal, 1703, 1707, 1707f
  sites of, in varicocele repair, 659, 660f
Incisional hernia
  after laparoscopy, 217-218
  after radical nephrectomy, 1720
Inconspicuous penis, 3749f, 3751, 3751f
Incontinence, 2046-2077. See also Fecal incontinence; Voiding dysfunction.
  after cryotherapy, 3049-3050
  after robotic-assisted laparoscopic radical prostatectomy, 2999, 2999t
  after urethral injury, 3944
  age-related changes and, 2189, 2305-2306, 2306f
  assessment of, initial, 2059
  bladder abnormalities in, 2053-2056, 3658-3659
    conditions causing, 2054-2056, 2055t, 2056f-2058f, 2056t
    urodynamic observation of, 2053-2054, 2053f, 2054f
  causes of, 2049t
    established, 2309-2311
    functional, 2310-2311
    lower urinary tract, 2309-2310
  classification of, 2046-2047
  clinical evaluation of, 2202-2203, 2202t
    self-administered questionnaire in, 2203t
    self-administered short forms in, 2203t
  continuous, 86, 2047
  definition of, 2187
    International Continence Society, 2046, 2082
  detrusor overactivity causing. See also Overactive bladder.
    medical treatment of, 2071-2073
    surgical treatment of, 2073-2074
  diagnostic evaluation of, 2059-2070, 2311-2313
    empirical categorization in, 2313-2314
    history in, 2311-2312, 2312t
    laboratory examination in, 2313
    physical examination in, 2312-2313
    stress testing in, 2313
    urodynamic testing in, 2314
    voiding diary in, 2312, 2312f

Incontinence (Continued)
  during abdominal pressure increase, 1975-1976
  dye testing for, 2063
  effect of, on quality of life, 2062, 2062t
  endoscopy in, 2069-2070
  epidemiology of, 2047-2049, 2187-2190
  etiology of, 2053-2059
  extraurethral, 2047
  eyeball urodynamics in, 2064, 2064f
  female, 1936, 2047-2048, 2048f
    physical examination for, 2059-2060
    retropubic suspension surgery for, 2168-2185. See also Retropubic suspension surgery, for female incontinence.
    sphincter abnormalities and, 2058-2059
  geriatric. See Geriatric patient, incontinence in.
  history of, 2059-2060, 2060t
  impact of, 2124-2125, 2125t
    on sexual function, 2204-2205
  in children, 3612
    giggle, 3612
    injection therapy for, 2273
      intraurethral technique of, 2280
    urinary tract infection associated with, 3263
  in schizophrenia, 2041
  in stroke patients, 2014-2015
  in ureterovaginal fistula, 2341
  in urethrovaginal fistula, 2347-2348
  in valve patients, 3597
  incidence of, 2187, 2188, 2188t
  laboratory investigation in, 2313
  leak point pressures in
    abdominal, 2066, 2066f
    detrusor, 2067, 2067f
  low bladder compliance causing, treatment of, 2071-2074
  male, 2048-2049
    physical examination for, 2060
    prosthesis for, history and development of, 2392-2393
    sphincter abnormalities and, 2059
    surgical treatment of, 2391-2403. See also Artificial urinary sphincter; Perineal sling.
      contraindications to, 2392
      indications for, 2391-2392
  micturition diary in, 2062
  mixed, 2046, 2084, 2084f, 2202
    management of, 2145
    tension-free vaginal taping for, 2256-2257
  multichannel videourodynamic monitoring of, 2068-2069, 2069f
  myelodysplasia and, management of, 3636-3639, 3638f
  neurologic examination in, 2060
  overflow, 86, 2047
  pad testing for, 2063
  pathophysiology of, 2053-2059
  patient history of, 86
  pelvic examination in, 2060
  physical examination in, 2060-2061, 2312-2313
  postvoid residual volume in, 2060
  pressure-flow relation in, 2068
  prevalence of, 2187, 2188, 2188t
  radical retropubic prostatectomy causing, 2974
  recurrent
    artificial sphincter placement–induced, 2400-2401
    perineal sling procedure causing, 2396

Obesity (*Continued*)
  morbid
    affecting renal calculi surgery, 1447-1448
    as contraindication to laparoscopy, 174
    definition of, 1447, 1499
    percutaneous nephrolithotomy and, 1499
    ureteroscopy and, 1520
  nephrolithiasis and, 1413-1414
  open vs. laparoscopic adrenalectomy and,
    1870
  orthotopic urinary diversion and, 2616
  pelvic organ prolapse associated with, 2189
  prostate cancer associated with, 2863
  tension-free vaginal tape procedure and,
    2254-2255
Oblique muscle, 8-9, 9t, 10f
  external, 40, 42f
Observation, therapeutic, of renal cell
  carcinoma, 1618-1619, 1618t
Obstetrical implications, of exstrophy, in female
  patient, 3552-3553
Obstructive urinary symptoms, in patient
  history, 84-86, 85t
Obturator artery, 50f, 51
Obturator internus muscle, 43-44, 46f
Obturator lymph nodes, 52, 52f
Obturator nerve, 18f, 19, 53, 53t
Occlusive devices, for bladder filling/storage
  disorders, 2292
Occupation
  bladder cancer associated with, 2413
  HIV infection associated with
    epidemiology of, 400
    interventions to decrease, 400-401
    postexposure chemoprophylaxis for, 401
    specific exposures and, 400, 400t
  renal stones associated with, 1365
  urothelial tumors associated with, 1639
Occupational exposure(s), infertility due to, 644
Ochoa (urofacial) syndrome, in children, 3613
Office management, of premature ejaculation,
  786, 787t
Office surgical procedures, for pediatric urologic
  patient, 3215, 3215f
Office-based endoscopy, of bladder cancer,
  non–muscle-invasive, 2454
Ofloxacin
  for *Chlamydia trachomatis* infection, 378
  for gonorrhea, 379
  for mollicute infections, 384
  for prostatitis, 320t
Oligoasthenoteratospermia
  conditions associated with, 611
  evaluation of, 623
Oligohydramnios
  etiologies of, 3184-3185
  in bilateral renal agenesis, 3271
  in neonate, 3195
  second-trimester, 3181
  timing of onset of, 3186
Oligomeganephronia, 3310, 3311f
Oligospermia
  evaluation of, 622
  in XYY syndrome, 639
  vasography in, 627
  Y chromosome microdeletions in, 632, 717
Oliguria, with pneumoperitoneum, 201
Olmstead County Study, of benign prostatic
  hyperplasia, 2763
Omniport device, hand-assist, 186, 186f
Omphalocele
  closure of, in cloacal exstrophy, 3542
  in exstrophy-epispadias complex, 3503
Onchocerca volvulus, 455. See also Filariasis.

Onchocerciasis, 458
Oncocytoma
  adrenal, 1843
  renal, 1577-1578, 1577f
    vs. renal cell carcinoma, 1577-1578
Oncogene(s), 513-514. *See also specific oncogene.*
  definition of, 508t
  in bladder cancer, 2410
  in prostate cancer, 2865, 2866
  mutation of, 514
  tumorigenesis induced by, 546
Oncotic pressure, in glomerular filtration rate,
  1132
One-kidney, one-clip constriction, of renal
    artery, renovascular hypertension in, 1164-
    1165, 1165t
One-stage proximal procedure, in hypospadias
    repair, 3729-3734
  onlay techniques for, 3729-3731
  tubularization techniques for, 3731-3732,
    3732f-3733f, 3734
Onlay technique(s), of hypospadias repair,
    3725-3726, 3728, 3728f-3729f
  split prepuce in-situ technique of, 3725 40,
    3728, 3730f-3731f
Open biopsy
  of kidney, 1753, 1754f
  of testis, 655-657, 656f, 657f
Open donor nephrectomy, 1303
Open stone surgery, 1505-1506, 1505t
  for renal calculi, 1506
  for ureteral calculi, 1506
Open-ended vasectomy, 1102. *See also*
  Vasectomy.
Operating room setup, for laparoscopic surgery,
    176, 176t
Operative team placement, for laparoscopic
    surgery, 177-178, 177f
Opiate(s), erectile dysfunction caused by,
    746
Opiate antagonist, for painful bladder
    syndrome/interstitial cystitis, 360t, 361
Opioid(s)
  for painful bladder syndrome/interstitial
    cystitis, 362
  in male sexual function, 730
  uropharmacology of, 1964, 1965
Opioid receptor antagonists, to facilitate bladder
    emptying, 2117
Opsonin, for phagocytes, 474
Optical magnification, in repair of hypospadias,
    3719
Oral cavity, mucocutaneous lesions of, in
    Behçet's disease, 418, 418f
Oral thrush. *See* Candidiasis.
Orchialgia
  chronic, 1107-1108
    definition of, 1107
    of undetermined etiology, 1108, 1109f
    post-vasectomy, 1108
  in children, 3207
  patient history of, 83
  post-hernia repair, 1108
Orchidopexy (orchiopexy)
  complications of, 3787
  for high undescended testes, 3779, 3781
  for prune-belly syndrome, 3492-3493
    Fowler-Stephens, 3492-3493
    transabdominal, 3492, 3493f
  Fowler-Stephens, 3781
    laparoscopic, 3786
  in adults, 1106-1107
    for intermittent torsion, 1107
    for retractile testes, 1107

Orchidopexy (orchiopexy) (*Continued*)
  laparoscopic, 3785-3786
  reoperative, 3787
  standard, 3776-3777, 3776f-3780f, 3779
Orchiectomy
  delayed, for germ cell tumors, 938
  for complete androgen insensitivity, timing of,
    3824
  for germ cell tumors, 936-938, 937f
    findings at, 904-905
    prior scrotal violation and, 938
  for prostate cancer, 3082-3083, 3085, 3085t
  partial, for germ cell tumors, 938
  radical
    for germ cell tumors, 936-938, 937f
    for Leydig cell tumors, 926t, 927
    for yolk sac tumors, 3903
Orchitis
  classification of, 327, 327t
  definition of, 327
  diagnosis of, 328
  in HIV patients, 396
  infertility due to, 643
  pathogenesis and etiology of, 327-328
  pediatric urinary tract infections and, 3264-
    3265
  treatment of, 328
Orciprenaline, effect of, on ureteral function,
    1905
Organ entrapment
  in laparoscopic nephrectomy, 1769
    hand-assisted, 1798
    transperitoneal approach to, 1784, 1786-
      1787, 1786f, 1787f
  in laparoscopic surgery, 195, 196f
Organomegaly, as contraindication to
    laparoscopy, 175
Organophosphate, for hypercalciuria, 1419
Organ-preserving surgery
  for penile cancer, 972-973
  for testicular tumors, 908-909
Orgasm, absence of, 87
Orgasmic disorder, in females, 864
Orthopedic anomalies, in prune-belly syndrome,
    3485t, 3487
Orthopedic hardware, indwelling, antibiotic
    prophylaxis for, 254, 254t
Orthoplasty, in hypospadias repair, 3712-3714,
    3713f, 3715f
  two-stage, 3734, 3736f-3737f
Osmolality, of urine, 97
Osteogenic sarcoma, of kidney, 1634
Osteomalacia, conduit urinary diversion
    causing, 2574
Osteopontin, as calcium oxalate crystal inhibitor,
    1367, 1371
Osteoporosis, androgen deprivation therapy
    causing, 3089
Osteotomy
  in exstrophy patient, 3513, 3514f-3516f,
    3515
    complications of, 3515-3516
    urinary reconstruction and, 3543, 3543f
  with cloacal exstrophy, 3543, 3543f
Ostlin's folds, 3360, 3361f
Ototoxicity, cisplatin-induced, 924
Ouabain, effect of, on ureteral function, 1920
Outpatient procedures, in pediatric urologic
    patient, 3214-3215
Outpatient surgery, laparoscopic adrenalectomy
    as, 1884-1885
Outpatient therapy, for urinary tract infections,
    in children, 3247-3249, 3248t
Ovarian cyst, ureteral obstruction due to, 1221

Testicular appendage torsion, in acute scrotum, 3792

Testicular artery, 74, 75f, 581, 582-583, 583f
  injury to, varicocelectomy and, 665

Testicular cancer, 93, 893-934
  adenocarcinoma in, 929, 932t
  cryptorchidism associated with, 3772-3773
  germ cell tumors in, 893-925. See also Germ cell tumor(s), testicular.
  gonadoblastoma as, 926t, 928-929. See also Gonadoblastoma(s).
  in AIDS patients, 399-400
  leukemic infiltration in, 930-931
  lymphoma in, 930, 932t
  mesenchymal origin of, 929
  metastatic, 931
  sex cord–mesenchymal tumors in, 925-928, 926t
  surgery for, 936-957. See also specific procedure.
  teratoma as, 895. See also Teratoma(s).

Testicular cystic dysplasia, in children, 3905

Testicular dysfunction, pathology of, 3794-3795

Testicular failure, primary, micropenis due to, 3753

Testicular hormone replacement, 569, 569f

Testicular microlithiasis, in children, 3905

Testicular pain
  patient history of, 83
  post-hernia repair, 1108

Testicular regression, embryonic, 3814-3815

Testicular torsion, 93
  cryptorchidism and, 3773
  infertility with, 641
  intermittent, orchidopexy for, 1107

Testicular tumor(s)
  adenomatoid, 930
  adrenal rest tumors as, 929-930
  carcinoids as, 930
  epidermoid cysts as, 929
  in children, 3900-3905. See also specific tumor.
    classification of, 3900t
    diagnosis of, 3902
    etiology of, 3900-3901
    evaluation of, 3199
    genetics of, 3900
    pathology of, 3901-3902
    staging of, 3902, 3903t
  malignant. See Testicular cancer; specific neoplasm.
  surgery for, 936-957. See also specific procedure.

Testicular vein, 74, 75f, 583-584, 583f
  thrombophlebitis of, ureteral obstruction due to, 1223
  tortuosity and dilation of. See Varicocele.

Testis(es), 73-74, 74f, 75f, 77
  absent (vanishing), 3765
    laparoscopic assessment of, 3783-3784
  androgen production by, 2685-2686, 2686t, 2687f
  atrophy of, 621-622
    mumps-associated, germ cell tumors due to, 901
  biopsy of, 633-634, 633f
    complications of, 658
    indications for, 655
    open, 655-657, 656f, 657f
      sperm retrieval through, 701
    percutaneous, 657, 657f
  blood barrier of, 589-591, 590f, 591f
  blood supply to, 1099t
  cancer of. See Testicular cancer; specific neoplasm.

Testis(es) (Continued)
  cryoarchitecture of, 584-596
  delivery of, in varicocele repair, 662
  descent of, 3143-3145, 3144f
    calcitonin gene–related peptide in, 3769
    developmental defect in. See Cryptorchidism.
    endocrine factors in, 3766-3768
    epididymis related to, 3769-3770
    genitofemoral nerve in, 3769
    gubernaculum in, 3768-3769
    intra-abdominal pressure and, 3770
    normal, 3762-3763
      definition of, 3764
    theories of, 3766
  dimensions of, examination of, 613, 613t
  dysfunction of, tissue engineering for, 569, 569f
  ectopic, 3765
  embryology of, 3761-3763
  endocrinology of, 579-580
  end-stage, infertility and, 634
  fetal, endocrine function of, 3804, 3805f
  fine-needle aspiration of, sperm retrieval through, 701, 703, 705-706, 705f-707f
  function of, 584-596
  in prune-belly syndrome, 3485
  innervation of, 77, 581
  interstitium of, 581, 581f, 584-585, 585f-587f, 587
  intra-abdominal, 3765
    laparoscopic assessment of, 3784
    laparoscopic orchidopexy for, 3785-3786
  ipsilateral, varicocele associated with, 641
  lymphatic drainage of, 14, 583-584
  mumps-associated atrophy of, germ cell tumors due to, 901
  non-palpable, 3765
    diagnostic laparoscopy for, 3782
    laparoscopic assessment of, 3782-3784, 3783f
  normal, 633, 633f
  ovoid, 581
  prenatal development of, 592
  rete, 581, 582f
  retractile, 3765
    in adults, orchidopexy for, 1107
    in children, 3208
  seminiferous tubules of, 581, 587. See also Seminiferous tubules.
  structure of, 581-584, 581f-583f
  tissue extraction from, sperm retrieval through, 706, 707f
    microsurgical, 705-706, 706f
  torsion of. See Testicular torsion.
  tuberculosis of, 440
  tumors of. See Testicular tumor(s).
    malignant. See Testicular cancer.
  undescended, 3763-3787. See also Cryptorchidism.
    surgical management of. See Orchidopexy.
  vanishing (absent), 640, 3765, 3814-3815
    laparoscopic assessment of, 3783-3784
  vascularization of, 581-584, 583f

Testis cords, 3136
  in puberty, 3136-3137

Testis-determining factor, 3799-3800, 3800f, 3801f
  SRY gene in, 3801

Testis-sparing surgery, for teratomas, 3903

Testicular injury
  diagnosis of, 2652-2653, 2653f
  etiology of, 2652
  in children, 3945

Testicular injury (Continued)
  management of, 2653-2654, 2653f
  outcome and complications of, 2654

Testoderm gel, for erectile dysfunction, 772

Testoderm patch, for erectile dysfunction, 771-772

Testolactone, for male infertility, 646-647

Testosterone. See also Dihydrotestosterone.
  assays for, 855-856, 855t, 856f
  bioavailability of, measurement of, 767
  biosynthesis of
    disorders of, 3821-3823
    errors in, cryptorchidism associated with, 3767
  circulation of, 3084, 3085t
  commercial formulations of, 861
  fetal secretion of, 3761-3762, 3804
  for erectile dysfunction, 771-772, 771t
    injectable, 771
    oral, 772
    "rescue" therapy with, 776
    transdermal delivery of, 771-772
  for Kallmann syndrome, 635
  for late-onset hypogonadism, 857-858, 858t
    adverse effects of, 859-860
    body composition/strength changes with, 858-859
    bone mineral density changes with, 859
    buccal delivery of, 858, 858t
    cardiovascular changes with, 859
    intramuscular injections of, 857, 858t
    objective effects of, 858-859
    oral preparations of, 857-858, 858t
    sexual function changes with, 859
    transdermal delivery of, 858, 858t
  for micropenis, 3753
  for sexual dysfunction
    in perimenopausal and postmenopausal women, 880-881
    in premenopausal women, 876-878
  in regulation of spermatogenesis, 595-596
  in testicular descent, 3766-3767
  in utero deficiency of, 3767
  increased levels of, following varicocele repair, 664
  metabolism of, 851-852, 852-853, 852f
  plasma levels of, 2686, 2686t
  production of
    diurnal pattern in, 767
    luteinizing hormone in, 585, 586f
    regulation of, central mechanisms in, 851-852
  serum range of, 767-768
  synergism of, with PDE-5 inhibitors, 859
  synthesis and metabolism of, 2686, 2687f
  transport of, 851, 852f

Testosterone-secreting adrenal tumor, 1841-1842

Tetanus, for human and animal bite wounds, 2651

Tethered cord syndrome
  definition of, 2030
  voiding dysfunction with, 2030

Thalidomide
  as inhibitor of angiogenesis, 545
  for prostatitis, clinical trial data on, 322

Therapeutic cloning strategy, in tissue engineering, 570-572, 571f, 572f

Therapeutic observation, of renal cell carcinoma, 1618-1619, 1618t

Thermal ablative therapy, for localized renal cell carcinoma, 1616-1618, 1617t

Thermal mapping, in transurethral microwave therapy, 2814-2815

Transverse preputial island flap. *See also* Flap(s).
   in hypospadias repair, 3731-3732, 3732f-
      3733f, 3734
Transverse resection, in partial nephrectomy,
   1724-1725, 1727f
Transversus abdominis muscle, 8-9, 9t, 10f
Transvesical infiltration, of pelvic plexus, 2291
Trapped penis, 3750f, 3751
   resulting from circumcision, 3750f
Trauma. *See also at anatomic site; specific type of*
   injury.
   germ cell tumors due to, 901
   ulcerative, to genitalia, 418-419
Tray agglutination test, for antisperm antibodies,
   624t
Trazodone, for erectile dysfunction, 782
Tremor, in early graft dysfunction, 1318
Treponema pallidum, in syphilis, 375. *See also*
   Syphilis.
Trestle stent, 2806
Triage, of pediatric urologic patient, 3198-3204,
   3199t
   emergent evaluations in, 3198-3200, 3200t-
      3201t, 3202t, 3203, 3203t
   routine evaluations in, 3203-3204
   semi-urgent evaluations in, 3203
   urgent evaluations in, 3203
Triamterene calculi, 1389
Triazoles, 469
Trichlormethiazide
   for absorptive hypercalciuria, 1418
   for calcium oxalate stone prevention,
      1421t
   for calcium oxalate stones, 1421t
Trichloroacetic acid, for genital warts, 381
Trichloroethylene, exposure to, renal cell
   carcinoma associated with, 1584
Trichomonas, in prostatitis, 307
Trichomonas vaginalis, 380
   in urinary sediment, 109, 109f
Trichomoniasis, 380
Trichomycosis axillaris, of male genitalia, 423-
   424, 424f
Tricyclic antidepressants. *See also*
   Antidepressants; *specific agent.*
   erectile dysfunction caused by, 744
   for urethral sphincter dysfunction, in
      children, 3620
Trigone, 59f, 60, 60f
   formation of, 3132-3133, 3134f
Trigonosigmoidostomy, in exstrophy patient,
   3537-3538
Trimethoprim, for pediatric urinary tract
   infections, prophylactic, 3250t, 3252
Trimethoprim-sulfamethoxazole
   for cystitis, 256-257, 256t
   for urinary tract infections, 245, 245t, 246t,
      247t
      in children, 3248t
         prophylactic, 3250t, 3251, 3251t
      low-dose prophylactic, for recurrent urinary
         tract infections, 262t, 263
      prophylactic, for vesicoureteral reflux,
         4348
Trimetrexate, for bladder cancer, metastatic,
   2478
Trisphosphate, in ureteral smooth muscle
   contraction, 1901, 1902f
Trocar(s)
   blind insertion of, 180
   complications related to, 206-209, 207t,
      208f
   closure of, in hand-assisted laparoscopic
      nephrectomy, 1798

Trocar(s) *(Continued)*
   configuration of, in robotic-assisted
      laparoscopic radical prostatectomy,
      2986f, 2988-2989, 2989f
   placement of
      in laparoscopic antireflux surgery, 4366
      in laparoscopic nephrectomy, 1762, 1764f,
         1765f
         hand-assisted, 1791, 1792f-1796f
         retroperitoneal approach, 1788-1789,
            1789f, 1790f
         transperitoneal approach, 1781
      initial, 187
      secondary, 187-189, 188f, 189f
         complications related to, 209-210, 209f,
            210f
   recurrence of, after laparoscopic surgery, 1779,
      1779f, 1780t, 1781, 1781t
   technology of, 185-187, 186f
   types of, 185, 185f
Tropical pulmonary eosinophilia, in filariasis,
   457
Tropical spastic paraparesis, voiding dysfunction
   in, 2035-2036
Tropomyosin, of smooth muscle, 1898
Troponin, of smooth muscle, 1898
Trospium
   for incontinence, in elderly, 2316, 2317t
   for overactive bladder/detrusor overactivity,
      2093t, 2095-2096
TRUS. *See* Transrectal ultrasonography
   (TRUS).
TSC1 gene, in tuberous sclerosis, 3306, 3330,
   3331, 3899
TSC2 gene, in tuberous sclerosis, 1599, 3306,
   3330, 3331, 3899
TSH (thyroid-stimulating hormone), secretion
   of, 578
Tuberculin reaction, CDC definition of, 440,
   441t
Tuberculin test, for genitourinary tuberculosis,
   440, 441t
Tuberculosis, 436-447
   arteriography of, 443
   biopsy in, 443
   clinical features of, 437-438, 440
   computed tomography of, 442, 443f
   cystoscopy of, 443
   development of, 437
   diagnosis of, 440-441
   epidemiology of, 436-437
   history of, 436
   immunology of, 437
   incidence of, 436-437, 437t
   intravenous urography of, 441-442, 442f
   magnetic resonance imaging of, 443
   microbiology of, 440
   multidrug-resistant, 444
   of bladder, 438, 439f
   of epididymis, 438, 440
   of kidney, 438, 438f
      in AIDS patients, 396
   of penis, 440
   of prostate, 440
   of testis, 440
   of ureter, 438, 439f, 440f
   of urethra, 440
   pathogenesis of, 437
   pathology of, 437-438, 438f-440f, 440
   percutaneous antegrade pyelography of,
      443
   radiography of, 437f, 441
   retrograde pyelography of, 443
   transmission of, 437

Tuberculosis *(Continued)*
   treatment of
      antituberculous drugs in, 443-444, 445t
      excision of diseased tissue in, 444-446
      intravesical BCG therapy in, 447
      medical, regimens in, 444
      reconstructive surgery in, 446-447
      surgical, 444-447
      vaccine prospects in, 447
   tuberculin test for, 440, 441t
   ultrasonography of, 442-443
   urine examination in, 440-441
Tuberous sclerosis, 3329-3332, 3330t
   angiomyolipoma in, 1578, 1579f, 1580, 3331
   characteristics of, 3314t
   clinical features of, 3331-3332
   evaluation of, 3331
   genes responsible for, 3306
   genetics of, 3330-3331
   histopathology of, 3331
   pheochromocytoma associated with, 1861
   renal angiomyolipoma with, 3899-3900, 3900f
   renal cell carcinoma associated with, 3332
      screening for, 1599
   renal cysts in, 3329, 3329f, 3330t, 3331-3332,
      3331f
Tubo-ovarian abscess, ureteral obstruction due
   to, 1220
Tubular interstitial disease, in chronic renal
   failure, 1346-1347
Tubularization techniques, of hypospadias
   repair, 3722-3723, 3724f, 3725, 3729, 3731-
   3732, 3732f-3733f, 3734
Tubularized flap technique, dismembered, of
   laparoscopic pyeloplasty, 1253
Tubularized incised plate (TIP) urethroplasty, in
   hypospadias repair, 3722, 3724f, 3725
Tubulogenesis, cell-cell interactions in, 3130-
   3131, 3130f
Tubuloglomerular feedback, 3172
   in glomerular filtration rate, 1132
TUIP. *See* Transurethral incision of prostate
   (TUIP).
Tumor(s). *See also named tumor and at anatomic*
   site.
   formation of, after augmentation cystoplasty,
      3684
Tumor biology, of renal cell carcinoma, 1588-
   1591
Tumor DNA, somatic mutations in, 2865-2867
Tumor immunology, 495-500
   adoptive cell therapy in, 499
   allogeneic bone marrow transplantation in,
      500
   antigens in, 495-496, 496t
   cancer vaccines in, 499-500
   cytokines and interferons in, 499
   immunotherapy in, 499-500
   mechanism(s) of tumor escape in, 497-498,
      498f
      impaired antigen presentation as, 497
      induction of apoptosis of T cells as, 498-
         499
      secretion of immunosuppressive products
         as, 497-498, 498f
   mechanisms of tumor evasion in, 496-497
   monoclonal antibodies in, 500
   role of NK cells in, 496
   role of T cells in, 495
Tumor marker(s). *See also specific tumor marker.*
   clinical applications of, 907
   combination of, 2430
   histologic subtype prediction with, 907-908
   monitoring response of, 907